ASCO-SEP®

MEDICAL ONCOLOGY SELF-EVALUATION PROGRAM

FOURTH EDITION

EDITOR
Charles L. Loprinzi, MD

ASSOCIATE EDITORS
Frederick R. Appelbaum, MD
Martee L. Hensley, MD, MSc
Joseph T. Ruggiero, MD

AUTHORS
Amy P. Abernethy, MD
Frederick R. Appelbaum, MD
Jan Buckner, MD
Bruce E. Clurman, MD, PhD
Harvey J. Cohen, MD
David R. Gandara, MD
Matthew P. Goetz, MD
Axel Grothey, MD
Martee L. Hensley, MD, MSc
Joleen M. Hubbard, MD
Arif H. Kamal, MD
Sani Kizilbash, MBBS
Charles L. Loprinzi, MD
Bhoomi Mehrotra, MD
Matthew I. Milowsky, MD
Alfred I. Neugut, MD, PhD
Beth Overmoyer, MD
Oliver W. Press, MD, PhD
S. Vincent Rajkumar, MD
Arati V. Rao, MD
Jonathan W. Riess, MD
Lynn M. Schuchter, MD
Scott M. Schuetze, MD, PhD
Barry E. Storer, PhD
Pierre L. Triozzi, MD
Eric Winer, MD, FASCO

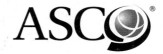

Cover photograph: Light micrograph of cancer cells of the human breast. Jonathan Ashton/Science Source.

LETTER FROM THE EDITOR

Dear Participant:

On behalf of ASCO, I am pleased to present the fourth edition of *ASCO-SEP®: Medical Oncology Self-Evaluation Program*. This self-assessment resource was designed to help you assess your level of knowledge in areas of oncology as preparation for your board exams, as you move through the maintenance of certification (MOC) process, for assistance in the care of individual patients with cancer, and as a means of staying current with oncology issues. This year, due to great demand, there will be a new ASCO University® eLearning course associated with *ASCO-SEP 4th Edition*, which will allow the user to receive MOC points after completion (university.asco.org/maintenance-certification).

ASCO-SEP is a comprehensive learning tool that includes 21 chapters focused on specific disease sites and oncology topics, as well as more than 180 multiple-choice questions that can be used for self-study. For this fourth edition, all of the self-assessment questions are new, so learners will have unique opportunities for review. Also available is the *ASCO-SEP 4th Edition* Online Question Bank, which can be accessed on ASCO University (university.asco.org/SEP). This convenient online study tool includes the questions contained in this book as well as 100 bonus questions, presented in an interactive format. Another valuable resource is the ASCO Flashcards app on your mobile device or tablet; the *ASCO-SEP 4th Edition* Flashcards Deck includes 200 digital flashcards and provides short, convenient opportunities for self-study based on content from the book.

A new feature in the fourth edition is a section at the onset of chapters that identifies key updates relevant to that topic area from the previous edition. The "Updates from 2012" section includes references to allow the reader to stay up-to-date on the latest information in our field.

This *ASCO-SEP 4th Edition* would not have been possible without the efforts of three outstanding Associate Editors, who dedicated substantial time and commitment to ensure the high quality of the content: Frederick R. Appelbaum, MD, Martee L. Hensley, MD, MSc, and Joseph T. Ruggiero, MD. The success of this publication has relied on the time and talents of many contributors, including chapter authors and peer reviewers who graciously shared their expertise. ASCO staff also contributed an enormous amount of time, effort, and expertise to the publication.

Thank you for participating in this worthwhile continuing medical education program. If you have comments or suggestions regarding *ASCO-SEP*, please email university@asco.org.

Sincerely,

Charles L. Loprinzi

Charles L. Loprinzi, MD
Editor, *ASCO-SEP 4th Edition*

EDITOR BIOGRAPHIES

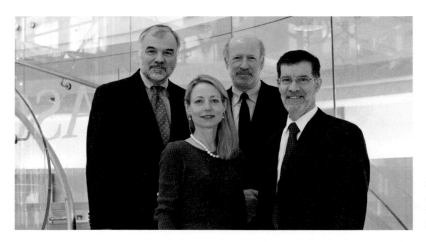

Back row: Joseph T. Ruggiero, MD, and Frederick R. Appelbaum, MD; *front row:* Martee L. Hensley, MD, MSc, and Charles L. Loprinzi, MD.

Charles L. Loprinzi, MD, is the endowed Regis Professor of Breast Cancer Research at the Mayo Clinic, where he has served as Chair of the Division of Medical Oncology and Vice-Chair of the Department of Oncology. He serves as the Chair of the Alliance for Clinical Trials in Oncology Symptom Intervention Program and Co-Director of the Mayo Cancer Center Prevention and Control Program. He was the founding editor of the "Art of Oncology" section in the *Journal of Clinical Oncology*.

Frederick R. Appelbaum, MD, is the Deputy Director of the Fred Hutchinson Cancer Research Center and Executive Director of the Seattle Cancer Care Alliance. He is the past Chair of the Board of Scientific Advisors of the National Cancer Institute and has served on the Board of Directors for ASCO, the American Society of Hematology, and the American Association for Cancer Research.

Martee L. Hensley, MD, MSc, is Professor of Medicine at Weill Cornell Medical College and Attending Physician in the Gynecologic Medical Oncology service at Memorial Sloan Kettering Cancer Center. She is Co-Chair of the Uterine Task Force of the National Cancer Institute's (NCI) Gynecologic Cancer Steering Committee, and Co-Chair of the NCI-European Organisation for Research and Treatment of Cancer-Cancer Research UK International Rare Cancer Initiative for Gynecologic Sarcomas.

Joseph T. Ruggiero, MD, is Associate Professor of Clinical Medicine in the Division of Hematology Oncology at New York-Presbyterian Hospital, Weill Medical College of Cornell University. He is the Clinical Director of the Solid Tumor Oncology Practice at Weill Cornell. He is a medical oncologist at the Jay Monahan Center for Gastrointestinal Health and the Center for Advanced Digestive Care at New York-Presbyterian Hospital. Dr. Ruggiero has been actively involved with issues of certification and recertification in both internal medicine and medical oncology. From 1998 until 2005, Dr. Ruggiero served on the American Board of Internal Medicine committee responsible for authoring the oncology portion of the exam.

CONTRIBUTORS

EDITOR

Charles L. Loprinzi, MD
Mayo Clinic
Rochester, MN

ASSOCIATE EDITORS

Frederick R. Appelbaum, MD
Fred Hutchinson Cancer Research
 Center
Seattle, WA

Martee L. Hensley, MD, MSc
Memorial Sloan Kettering Cancer
 Center
New York, NY

Joseph T. Ruggiero, MD
Weill Cornell Medical College
New York, NY

AUTHORS

Amy P. Abernethy, MD
Duke University Medical Center
Durham, NC

Frederick R. Appelbaum, MD
Fred Hutchinson Cancer Research
 Center
Seattle, WA

Jan Buckner, MD
Mayo Clinic
Rochester, MN

Bruce E. Clurman, MD, PhD
Fred Hutchinson Cancer Research
 Center
Seattle, WA

Harvey J. Cohen, MD
Duke University Medical Center
Durham, NC

David R. Gandara, MD
University of California Davis Cancer
 Center
Sacramento, CA

Matthew P. Goetz, MD
Mayo Clinic
Rochester, MN

Axel Grothey, MD
Mayo Clinic
Rochester, MN

Martee L. Hensley, MD, MSc
Memorial Sloan Kettering Cancer
 Center
New York, NY

Joleen M. Hubbard, MD
Mayo Clinic
Rochester, MN

Arif H. Kamal, MD
Duke University Medical Center
Durham, NC

Sani Kizilbash, MBBS
Mayo Clinic
Rochester, MN

Charles L. Loprinzi, MD
Mayo Clinic
Rochester, MN

Bhoomi Mehrotra, MD
St. Francis Hospital
Roslyn, NY

Matthew I. Milowsky, MD
University of North Carolina at Chapel Hill
Chapel Hill, NC

Alfred I. Neugut, MD, PhD
Columbia University
New York, NY

Beth Overmoyer, MD
Dana-Farber Cancer Institute
Boston, MA

Oliver W. Press, MD, PhD
Fred Hutchinson Cancer Research
 Center
Seattle, WA

S. Vincent Rajkumar, MD
Mayo Clinic
Rochester, MN

Arati V. Rao, MD
Duke University Medical Center
Durham, NC

Jonathan W. Riess, MD, MS
University of California Davis Cancer
 Center
Sacramento, CA

Lynn M. Schuchter, MD
University of Pennsylvania Cancer
 Center
Philadelphia, PA

Scott M. Schuetze, MD, PhD
University of Michigan Health System
Ann Arbor, MI

Barry E. Storer, PhD
Fred Hutchinson Cancer Research Center
Seattle, WA

Pierre L. Triozzi, MD
Cleveland Clinic Taussig Cancer Institute
Cleveland, OH

Eric Winer, MD, FASCO
Dana-Farber Cancer Institute
Boston, MA

PEER REVIEWERS

Alex A. Adjei, MD, PhD
Roswell Park Cancer Institute
Buffalo, NY

Edward P. Balaban, DO
University of Pittsburgh Medical Center
  Cancer Centers
Coraopolis, PA

Al B. Benson III, MD
Northwestern University
Chicago, IL

Jonathan S. Bleeker, MD
Mayo Clinic
Rochester, MN

Mary Bretscher, MD
Springfield Clinic
Springfield, IL

Renier J. Brentjens, MD, PhD
Memorial Sloan Kettering Cancer Center
New York, NY

Jonathan C. Britell, MD
Southlake Clinic
Renton, WA

Paul B. Chapman, MD
Memorial Sloan Kettering Cancer Center
New York, NY

Jennie Robertson Crews, MD
Beaufort County Hospital
Washington, NC

William L. Dahut, MD
National Cancer Institute
Gaithersburg, MD

Mary Daly, MD, PhD
Fox Chase Cancer Center
Philadelphia, PA

Patrick J. Donovan, MD, FACP
Scottsdale Medical Specialists
Scottsdale, AZ

Leon H. Dragon, MD
Kellogg Cancer Care Center
Highland Park, IL

Mario A. Eisenberger, MD
Johns Hopkins University
Baltimore, MD

Suzanne George, MD
Dana-Farber Cancer Institute
Boston, MA

Shawn D. Glisson, MD
Norton Cancer Institute
Louisville, KY

Wiliam J. Gradishar, MD
Northwestern University
Chicago, IL

Peter R. Graze, MD
Annapolis Oncology Center
Annapolis, MD

Robert I. Haddad, MD
Dana-Farber Cancer Institute
Boston, MA

Lee P. Hartner, MD
University of Pennsylvania Abramson
  Cancer Center
Philadelphia, PA

Richard M. Ingram, MD
Virginia Cancer Specialists
Winchester, VA

Jeffrey J. Kirshner, MD
Hematology/Oncology Associates of
  Central New York
East Syracuse, NY

Richard A. Larson, MD
University of Chicago
Chicago, IL

Hillard M. Lazarus, MD, FACP
University Hospital of Cleveland
Cleveland, OH

John P. Leonard, MD
Weill Cornell Medical College
New York, NY

Mark A. Lewis, MD
MD Anderson Cancer Center
Houston, TX

Stuart M. Lichtman, MD
Memorial Sloan Kettering Cancer Center
New York, NY

Thomas A. Marsland, MD
Orange Park Cancer Center
Orange Park, FL

Ann Mauer, MD
Creticos Cancer Center
Chicago, IL

Kenneth R. Meehan, MD
Dartmouth-Hitchcock Medical Center
Lebanon, NH

Joseph J. Muscato, MD
Missouri Cancer Association
Columbia, MO

Antonio M.P. Omuro, MD
Memorial Sloan Kettering Cancer Center
New York, NY

Paul G. Richardson, MD
Dana-Farber Cancer Institute
Boston, MA

Daniel J. Sargent, PhD
Mayo Clinic
Rochester, MN

Bryan J. Schneider, MD
Weill Cornell Medical College
New York, NY

Mikkael A. Sekeres, MD, MS
Cleveland Clinic
Cleveland, OH

David B. Solit, MD
Memorial Sloan Kettering Cancer Center
New York, NY

Scott T. Tagawa, MD, MS
Weill Cornell Medical College
New York, NY

Howard R. Terebelo, DO
Providence Hospital
Southfield, MI

Carrie A. Thompson, MD
Mayo Clinic
Rochester, MN

Linda Van Le, MD
University of North Carolina at Chapel
  Hill
Chapel Hill, NC

Charles F. Von Gunten, MD, PhD
San Diego Hospice
San Diego, CA

ASCO STAFF

Publisher
Lisa Johnson

Content Development Manager
Allison Burg

Managing Editor
Virginia Anderson

Art Director
Leigh Hubbard

Production Manager
Donna Dottellis

Permissions Coordinator
Stephanie Wamsley

DISCLOSURE INDEX

In compliance with standards established by the Accreditation Council for Continuing Medical Education (ACCME), it is ASCO's policy to ensure balance, independence, objectivity, and scientific rigor in all of its educational activities through the disclosure of financial relationships, among other measures. All *ASCO-SEP 4th Edition* editors, authors, and peer reviewers are required to disclose relationships with commercial interests that may have a direct bearing on relevant subject matter. The financial interests or relationships requiring disclosure are outlined in ASCO's Conflict of Interest Policy (asco.org/rwc).

The intent of this policy is to identify relationships openly, so readers can form their own judgments about the publication in light of these relationships. It remains for readers to determine whether the contributor's outside interests reflect a possible bias in the publication or the conclusions presented. The categories of relationships that contributors are required to disclose are detailed here as a guide to the disclosure statements that appear in the following Disclosure Index.

ITEMS REQUIRING DISCLOSURE

- **Employment or Leadership Positions (Commercial Firms):** Any full- or part-time employment or service as an officer or board member for an entity having an investment, licensing, or other commercial interest in the subject matter under consideration must be disclosed.
- **Consultant or Advisory Role:** Consultant or advisory arrangements with an entity having an investment, licensing, or other commercial interest in the subject matter under consideration must be disclosed.
- **Stock Ownership:** Any ownership interest (except when invested in a diversified fund not controlled by the covered individual) in a start-up company, the stock of which is not publicly traded, or in any publicly traded company must be disclosed if the company is an entity having an investment, licensing, or other commercial interest in the subject matter under consideration.
- **Honoraria:** Honoraria are reasonable payments for specific speeches, seminar presentations, or appearances. Disclosure of honoraria is required when paid directly to the covered individual by an entity having an investment, licensing, or other commercial interest in the subject matter under consideration and when provided within 2 years of the activity or subject matter in question.
- **Research Funding:** All payments associated with the conduct of the clinical research project in question must be disclosed if provided by the trial sponsor or agents employed by the sponsor.

- **Expert Testimony:** Provision of expert testimony must be disclosed when the testimony relates to the subject matter under consideration.
- **Other Remuneration:** The value of trips, travel, gifts, or other in-kind payments not directly related to research activities must be disclosed if received from an entity having an investment, licensing, or other commercial interest in the subject matter under consideration and when received within 2 years of the activity or subject matter in question. These payments exclude research-related costs and travel.

EDITORIAL BOARD DISCLOSURES

Financial relationships reported by members of the *ASCO-SEP* Editorial Board are provided below. During all phases of planning, areas of conflict were managed through a peer-review process and/or through individual recusal when appropriate.

All relationships are considered self-held and compensated unless otherwise noted. *(Legend: I, immediate family member; B, self and immediate family; U, uncompensated.)*

CHARLES L. LOPRINZI, MD
- *Consultant or Advisory Role: Helsinn Healthcare Data Monitoring Committee (B)*
- *Research Support: Pfizer and Competitive Technologies*

FREDERICK R. APPELBAUM, MD
- *No relevant relationships to disclose*

MARTEE L. HENSLEY, MD, MSC
- *Employment or Leadership Position: Sanofi (I)*
- *Consultant or Advisory Role: GlaxoSmithKline, Arnotherapeutics*

JOSEPH T. RUGGIERO, MD
- *No relevant relationships to disclose*

AUTHOR DISCLOSURES

The *ASCO-SEP* Editorial Board has reviewed all author disclosure reports, identified potential conflicts of interest, and implemented strategies to manage those areas of conflict, where they exist.

All relationships are considered self-held and compensated unless otherwise noted. *(Legend: I, immediate family member; B, self and immediate family; U, uncompensated.)*

AMY P. ABERNETHY, MD
- *Consultant or Advisory Role: Novartis, Pfizer; Corporate Board of Directors—Advoset, Orange Leaf Associates, LLC.*
- *Research Funding: DARA BioSciences Inc., MiCo; Pending Research—Genentech, Dendreon, BMS*

FREDERICK R. APPELBAUM, MD
- *No relevant relationships to disclose*

JAN BUCKNER, MD
- *Consultant or Advisory Role: Genentech (U), EMD Serano*

BRUCE E. CLURMAN, MD, PHD
- *No relevant relationships to disclose*

HARVEY J. COHEN, MD
- *No relevant relationships to disclose*

DAVID R. GANDARA, MD
- *Consultant or Advisory Role: Amgen, AstraZeneca, Boehringer-Ingelheim, BMS/ImClone, Celgene, GlaxoSmithKline, Genentech, Merck, Novartis, Pfizer, Sanofi-Aventis, Synta, Response Genetics, Inc.*
- *Research Funding: Abbott, BMS/ImClone, Genentech, Lilly, Merck, Novartis, Pfizer*

MATTHEW P. GOETZ, MD
- *Consultant or Advisory Role: DNA Direct, Pathwork Diagnostics, Roche, Pfizer (U), Eli Lilly (U)*

AXEL GROTHEY, MD
- *No relevant relationships to disclose*

MARTEE L. HENSLEY, MD, MSC
- *Employment or Leadership Position: Sanofi (I)*
- *Consultant or Advisory Role: GlaxoSmithKline, Arnotherapeutics*

JOLEEN M. HUBBARD, MD
- *Consultant or Advisory Role: Genomic Health*

ARIF H. KAMAL, MD
- *No relevant relationships to disclose*

SANI KIZILBASH, MBBS
- *No relevant relationships to disclose*

CHARLES L. LOPRINZI, MD
- *Consultant or Advisory Role: Helsinn Healthcare Data Monitoring Committee (B)*
- *Research Support: Pfizer and Competitive Technologies*

BHOOMI MEHROTRA, MD
- *No relevant relationships to disclose*

MATTHEW I. MILOWSKY, MD
- *Research Funding: Bind Biosciences, Johnson & Johnson, Merck, Astellas, Agenus, Dendreon, Exelixis*

ALFRED I. NEUGUT, MD, PHD
- *Consultant or Advisory Role: Executive Health Exam*

BETH OVERMOYER, MD
- *No relevant relationships to disclose*

OLIVER W. PRESS, MD, PHD
- *Consultant or Advisory Role: Roche, Algeta, BIND Biosciences*
- *Stock Ownership: PhaseRx, Emergent*
- *Research Funding: Genentech/Roche (paid to Fred Hutchinson Cancer Research Center)*

S. VINCENT RAJKUMAR, MD
- *No relevant relationships to disclose*

ARATI V. RAO, MD
- *No relevant relationships to disclose*

JONATHAN W. RIESS, MD, MS
- *Consultant or Advisory Role: Celgene*
- *Honorarium: Roche/Genentech*
- *Research Funding: Onconova Therapeutics and Millennium*
- *Travel/Expenses: Roche/Genentech*

LYNN M. SCHUCHTER, MD
- *No relevant relationships to disclose*

SCOTT M. SCHUETZE, MD, PHD
- *Research Funding: Amgen, ASCO Foundation, Ziopharm, SARC, AB Science, Janssen*
- *Honorarium: Novartis, Amgen, GlaxoSmithKline*

BARRY E. STORER, PHD
- *No relevant relationships to disclose*

PIERRE L. TRIOZZI, MD
- *No relevant relationships to disclose*

ERIC WINER, MD, FASCO
- *Research Funding: Genentech*

PEER REVIEWER DISCLOSURES

The *ASCO-SEP* Editorial Board has reviewed all peer reviewer disclosure reports, identified potential conflicts of interest, and implemented strategies to manage those areas of conflict, where they exist.

All relationships are considered self-held and compensated unless otherwise noted. *(Legend: I, immediate family member; B, self and immediate family; U, uncompensated.)*

ALEX A. ADJEI, MD, PHD
- *No relevant relationships to disclose*

EDWARD P. BALABAN, DO
- *Consultant or Advisory Role: Truven Health Analytics (Micromedex)*

AL B. BENSON III, MD
- *Consultant or Advisory Role: Genentech, Genomic Health, Gilead Sciences, Lilly/ImClone, Bristol Myers Squibb, Sanofi*
- *Honoraria: Amgen*
- *Research Funding: Advanced Accelerator Applications, Amgen, Astellas Pharma, Bayer, Genentech, Gilead Sciences, MDS Nordion*

JONATHAN S. BLEEKER, MD
- *No relevant relationships to disclose*

MARY BRETSCHER, MD
- *No relevant relationships to disclose*

RENIER J. BRENTJENS, MD, PHD
- *Research Funding: Amgen*

JONATHAN C. BRITELL, MD
- *No relevant relationships to disclose*

PAUL B. CHAPMAN, MD
- *Consultant/Advisory Role: GlaxoSmithKline, Roche/Genentech, Bristol Myers*
- *Research Funding: Genentech, GlaxoSmithKline*

JENNIE ROBERTSON CREWS, MD
- *No relevant relationships to disclose*

WILLIAM L. DAHUT, MD
- *No relevant relationships to disclose*

MARY DALY, MD, PHD
- *No relevant relationships to disclose*

PATRICK J. DONOVAN, MD, FACP
- *No relevant relationships to disclose*

LEON H. DRAGON, MD
- *No relevant relationships to disclose*

MARIO A. EISENBERGER, MD
- *Consultant or Advisory Role: Astellas, Medivation*
- *Research Funding: Sanofi, Genentech, Tokai*

SUZANNE GEORGE, MD
- *Consultant or Advisory Role: Novartis, Bayer, ARIAD, Pfizer*
- *Research Funding: Bayer, Novartis; Pfizer, ARIAD*

SHAWN D. GLISSON, MD
- *No relevant relationships to disclose*

WILIAM J. GRADISHAR, MD
- *Consultant or Advisory Role: Abraxis BioScience, Celgene, Eisai, Genomic, Novartis, Onyx, sanofi-aventis*
- *Honoraria: Abraxis BioScience, Amgen, Genentech, GlaxoSmithKline, Novartis, Roche*
- *Research Funding: Bayer/Onyx, Breast Cancer Research Foundation, ImClone Systems*

PETER R. GRAZE, MD
- *Honoraria: Amgen*

ROBERT I. HADDAD, MD
- *Consultant or Advisory Role: Boehringer-Ingelheim*

LEE P. HARTNER, MD
- *No relevant relationships to disclose*

RICHARD M. INGRAM, MD
- *No relevant relationships to disclose*

JEFFREY J. KIRSHNER, MD
- *Consultant or Advisory Role: Amgen*

RICHARD A. LARSON, MD
- *Consultant or Advisory Role: Bristol-Myers Squibb, Caremark, Celgene, Novartis, Pfizer, Sanofi-aventis*
- *Research Funding: Amgen, ARIAD, Novartis, Erytech*

HILLARD M. LAZARUS, MD, FACP
- *Consultant or Advisory Role: Actinium, Pluristem*
- *Speakers' Bureau: Celgene*

JOHN P. LEONARD, MD
- *Employment or Leadership Position: Weill Cornell Medical College*
- *Consultant or Advisory Role: PharmaCyclics, MedImmune, Celgene, BioTest, Genentech, Gilead, Hospira*

MARK A. LEWIS, MD
- *No relevant relationships to disclose*

STUART M. LICHTMAN, MD
- *No relevant relationships to disclose*

THOMAS A. MARSLAND, MD
- *Consultant or Advisory Role: Celgene, Lilly, Spectrum Pharmaceuticals*
- *Stock Ownership: Johnson & Johnson (I), Novartis (I), Pfizer (I), Raintree Oncology Services, Seattle Genetics (B)*
- *Honoraria: Oncology Business Review*

ANN MAUER, MD
- *No relevant relationships to disclose*

KENNETH R. MEEHAN, MD
- *No relevant relationships to disclose*

JOSEPH J. MUSCATO, MD
- *No relevant relationships to disclose*

ANTONIO M.P. OMURO, MD
- *Consultant or Advisory Role: Novocure, Roche*

PAUL G. RICHARDSON, MD
- *Consultant or Advisory Role: Celgene, Johnson & Johnson, Millennium, BMS, Novartis*

DANIEL J. SARGENT, PHD
- *No relevant relationships to disclose*

BRYAN J. SCHNEIDER, MD
- *Honoraria: Genentech, Pfizer*
- *Research Funding: Celgene, Boehringer-Ingelheim*
- *Consultant or Advisory Role: Genentech*

MIKKAEL A. SEKERES, MD, MS
- *Consultant or Advisory Role: Celgene, Amgen*

DAVID B. SOLIT, MD
- *No relevant relationships to disclose*

SCOTT T. TAGAWA, MD, MS
- *Consultant or Advisory Role: Medivation/Astrellas, Janssen, Dendreon, Amgen*
- *Research Funding: Sanofi-Aventis, Janssen, Medivation/ Astellas, Amgen*

HOWARD R. TEREBELO, DO
- *Honoraria: Amgen, Celgene, Millennium*

CARRIE THOMPSON, MD
- *No relevant relationships to disclose*

LINDA VAN LE, MD
- *Consultant or Advisory Role: Biologics Inc.*
- *Honoraria: Merck*

CHARLES F. VON GUNTEN, MD, PHD
- *Consultant or Advisory Role: Salix*
- *Honoraria: Salix*

CONTINUING EDUCATION INFORMATION

PROGRAM OVERVIEW

The *ASCO Self-Evaluation Program®* (*ASCO-SEP®*) is a comprehensive resource designed to help physicians assess their level of knowledge in the various areas of oncology and provide a current understanding of cancer, its treatment, and the supportive care needed to optimize the quality of life for people with cancer. This program includes 21 chapters and a companion self-assessment tool with rationales covering the full range of topics in oncology, including major cancer types, epidemiology and cancer prevention, management strategies for geriatric cancers, clinical trial design and statistics, molecular biology, and an overview of biologic therapy.

TARGET AUDIENCE

ASCO-SEP® is targeted to Fellows certifying for the subspecialty exam as well as practicing oncologists who are enrolled in a Maintenance of Certification program. *ASCO-SEP®* is also appropriate for use as a self-assessment tool for individual professional development, or as a teaching tool for training and continuing education purposes.

NEEDS STATEMENT

The number of Americans with a history of cancer, estimated to be 13.7 million in 2012, will grow to approximately 19 million by 2024, according to a report by the American Cancer Society in collaboration with the National Cancer Institute (NCI). The report, *Cancer Treatment & Survivorship Facts & Figures, 2014-2015*,[1] and accompanying journal article published in *CA: A Cancer Journal for Clinicians*, used data from the NCI-funded Surveillance, Epidemiology, and End Results (SEER) Program[2] to generate new estimates of cancer survivor prevalence in the United States. The reports find that even though cancer incidence rates are decreasing, the number of cancer survivors is growing due to the aging and growth of the population and improvements in early detection and treatment, as well as improving cancer survival rates.

ASCO-SEP® reflects within its chapters the state of oncology today. It is not meant to be used as a textbook and does not typically include future directions for research. Rather, this publication serves as a comprehensive overview of the subspecialty of oncology for use in review, self-assessment, and teaching activities; to validate current knowledge; and to improve overall competency in oncology.

LEARNING OBJECTIVES

Upon completion of this educational activity, participants will be able to:
- Apply the basic principles of epidemiology, molecular biology, clinical pharmacology, and clinical trial design to the practice of oncology;
- Incorporate appropriate imaging and diagnostic techniques to accurately identify and stage neoplastic disease;
- Discuss current treatment options with patients diagnosed with cancer and recommend approaches based on current evidence; and
- Assess and mitigate potential symptoms affecting quality of life and relating to treatment toxicity, comorbidities, or late effects.

CME ACCREDITATION STATEMENT

The American Society of Clinical Oncology is accredited by the Accreditation Council for Continuing Medical Education to provide continuing medical education for physicians.

The American Society of Clinical Oncology designates this enduring material for a maximum of *51 AMA PRA Category 1 Credits™*. Physicians should claim only the credit commensurate with the extent of their participation in the activity.

DATE OF ORIGINAL RELEASE

The original release date for this material is October 15, 2014. The Continuing Medical Education credit availability expires April 30, 2016.

MEDIUM USED AND METHOD OF PARTICIPATION

The *ASCO-SEP®* program consists of text, images, written self-assessment items, and an online self-assessment component. After completing the book, the participant is encouraged to respond to questions about the content of the activity and complete an evaluation of the activity. This evaluation can be filled out online by visiting ASCO University® at university.asco.org/SEP.

ESTIMATED TIME TO COMPLETE THE ACTIVITY

It is estimated that the time to complete this activity ranges from 1 to 3.5 hours for each chapter. It is estimated that the time required to complete the entire self-evaluation program is 51 hours.

OBTAINING CONTINUING MEDICAL EDUCATION CREDIT

In order to receive a Continuing Medical Education (CME) certificate or Participation certificate, please complete the evaluation and credit request. These forms can be completed online by visiting ASCO University® at university.asco.org/SEP and logging in using the access code provided in the front cover of the book.

Questions can be directed to the ASCO CME staff at 571-483-1403 or cme@asco.org

UNLABELED USAGE STATEMENT

The information presented is that of the contributing authors and does not necessarily represent the views of the American Society of Clinical Oncology. Specific therapies discussed may not be approved and/or specified for use as indicated. Therefore, before prescribing any medication, please review the complete prescribing information including indications, contraindications, warnings, precautions, and adverse effects.

COMMERCIAL SUPPORT STATEMENT

No commercial support was received for this activity.

References
1. American Cancer Society. *Cancer Facts & Figures 2014.* Atlanta, GA; American Cancer Society: 2014
2. DeSantis CE, Lin CC, Mariotto AB, et al. Cancer treatment and survivorship statistics, 2014. *CA Cancer J Clin.* 2014;64:252-271. PMID: 24890451.

CONTENTS

21

PALLIATIVE AND END-OF-LIFE CARE   **529**
Arif H. Kamal, MD, and Amy P. Abernethy, MD, PhD

————————

SELF-EVALUATION

INDEX

COMMONLY USED ABBREVIATIONS

EPIDEMIOLOGY AND PREVENTION

Alfred I. Neugut, MD, PhD

Updates from 2012

▶ The use of low-dose computed tomography scans for screening reduces mortality from lung cancer among smokers and has been recommended for use by the U.S. Preventive Services Task Force (Moyer VA, *Ann Int Med* 2014).

▶ Daily multivitamin use was associated with a small reduction in total cancer risk (Gaziano JM, *JAMA* 2012).

▶ A randomized trial has shown that, for patients with Barrett esophagus and low-grade dysplasia, radiofrequency ablation reduces the risk of progression to esophageal adenocarcinoma as compared with endoscopic surveillance (Phoa KN, *JAMA* 2014).

Epidemiology is the study of disease in populations, including its distribution, determinants, natural history, and survival. Rather than the individual patient, its perspective is that of public health. The traditional focus and goal of epidemiology has been the determination of the incidence and mortality rates of cancer in different populations and subgroups, as well as the identification of risk factors for the purpose of disease prevention and control through primary prevention and screening interventions; more recently, the methods of epidemiology have been applied to clinical questions, including the assessment of treatment outcomes, such as survival, and the long-term sequelae of cancer and its treatment.

Because of its emphasis on populations, epidemiology typically uses rates (with denominator populations—rates standardized to a population—and time frames) or relative measures rather than absolute figures to measure relevant statistics. Descriptive epidemiology, the usual starting point for epidemiologists, encompasses incidence and mortality rates, survival rates, and time trends. Incidence and mortality rates are commonly expressed as the number of newly diagnosed patients or deaths per 100,000 in the group at risk.

These rates are usually age- and gender-adjusted, meaning they are mathematically adjusted to a standard population to remove the effects of a population's age and gender distribution, which may change over time. Cancer is primarily a disease of older people. With the extensive increase during the past 30 years in the number of people in the United States who are age 70 and older, the number of cancer cases occurring annually also has increased or only slightly diminished because cancer is an age-dependent disease. Furthermore, because women have a life expectancy 7 years longer than men, there are substantially more older women than men, so a difference in gender distribution would magnify or diminish with age as well. Thus, adjusting cancer rates for age and gender removes the effects of gender and age. As a result, a true change in cancer rates because of prevention, treatment, or new etiologic factors must be assessed by

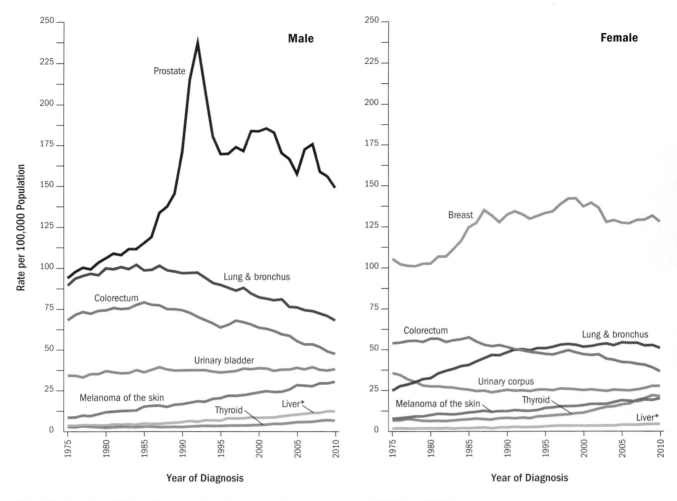

Fig. 1-1 Trends in U.S. incidence rates for selected cancers by sex (1975 to 2009).

Rates are age-adjusted to the 2000 U.S. standard population and adjusted for delays in reporting.

*Liver includes intrahepatic bile duct.

Reproduced from John Wiley & Sons, Inc., copyright 2014: Siegel R, Ma J, Zou Z, et al. Cancer Statistics, 2014; 64(1):9-29.

increases or decreases in age- and gender-adjusted incidence and mortality rates (Figs. 1-1, 1-2, and 1-3).[1,2]

Survival is defined as the time from diagnosis to death. A commonly used measure is the proportion of people alive at 5 years after diagnosis (Table 1-1). For some cancers, such as breast or prostate cancer, this time frame may be too short, as recurrences and deaths may continue to occur long after 5 years, and for these, 10-year survival may occasionally be a useful measure

The American Cancer Society (ACS) publishes an annual estimate of the absolute number of new cancer cases and deaths.[2] These numbers are widely quoted, especially by the lay press. As noted above, these figures are not rates and are subject to fluctuations in the age and gender distribution of the population. ACS also publishes time trends of incidence and mortality rates for major cancers during the past 75 years; these figures can give interesting insight on the inroads made by primary prevention, screening, and treatment, as well as the changes brought about by increases or decreases in risk factors (Figs. 1-1, 1-2, and 1-3).[1,2]

Table 1-1 **Definition of Terms Related to Survival**	
Survival time	Time from the initial diagnosis of cancer to death
Disease-free survival	Time from complete remission to relapse of disease
5-year survival rate	Proportion of patients who are alive 5 years after the time of diagnosis
Disease-specific survival rate	Proportion of patients who have not died of the specific disease (does not take into account deaths unrelated to the disease)
Overall survival rate	Proportion of patients who are alive at a specific time after the diagnosis (takes into account all causes of death)

Figures 1-2 and 1-3 show the changes in mortality for selected cancers since 1930. They illustrate the dramatic rise in mortality for lung cancer that accompanied the rise in tobacco use in the 20th century, peaking in men around 1985 and then

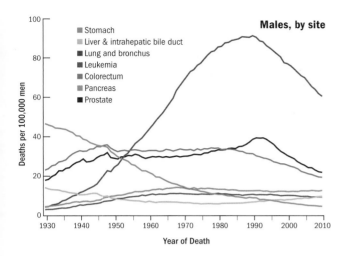

Fig. 1-2 Trends in death rates among U.S. males for selected cancers (1930 to 2009).

Rates are age-adjusted to the 2000 U.S. standard population. Due to changes in International Classification of Diseases (ICD) coding, numerator information has changed over time. Rates for cancers of the lung and bronchus, colorectum, and liver are affected by these changes.

Reproduced from John Wiley & Sons, Inc., copyright 2014: Siegel R, Ma J, Zou Z, et al. Cancer Statistics, 2014; 64(1):9-29.

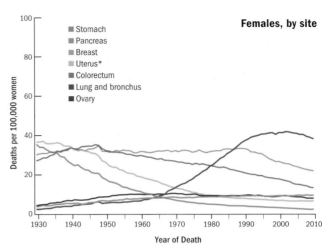

Fig. 1-3 Trends in death rates among U.S. females for selected cancers (1930 to 2009).

Rates are age-adjusted to the 2000 U.S. standard population. Due to changes in International Classification of Diseases (ICD) coding, numerator information has changed over time. Rates for cancers of the uterus, ovary, lung and bronchus, and colorectum are affected by these changes.

*Uterus includes uterine cervix and uterine corpus.

Reproduced from John Wiley & Sons, Inc., copyright 2014: Siegel R, Ma J, Zou Z, et al. Cancer Statistics, 2014; 64(1):9-29.

falling 20 years after the Surgeon General's reports of 1964 and 1968, which publicized the hazards of cigarette smoking and its link to lung cancer. As tobacco use has fallen to around 20% in males, the lung cancer incidence and mortality rates have fallen and will continue to fall for the foreseeable future. Another dramatic change has been the fall in gastric cancer, which was the leading cause of cancer mortality in the United States prior to World War II. Most experts attribute this decline to the increased availability of the electric refrigerator and the concomitant increased consumption of fresh meat, fruits, and vegetables, as opposed to smoked and cured foods, which contain nitrites and other potentially carcinogenic agents.[3] One can also see among women a dramatic fall in uterine cancer, primarily reflecting the uterine cervix, and attributable to the widespread use of the Pap smear for screening after World War II. A decline in breast cancer mortality after the mid-1980s has been attributed to a combination of mammographic screening and advances in treatment, such as the use of adjuvant therapy.[4,5]

KEY POINTS

- Epidemiology is the study of the distribution, etiology, and natural history of disease in populations.
- Epidemiology can include assessment of treatment outcomes, disease prevention, and disease screening.
- Epidemiology addresses these issues with a public health and public policy perspective as opposed to the perspective of the individual patient.

On the incidence figures (Fig. 1-1), the rise in prostate cancer incidence after 1985 is the most salient curve and reflects the introduction of prostate-specific antigen (PSA) testing to the clinical laboratory and its widespread use for screening. A rise in the incidence of cutaneous melanoma in men and women has been attributed to both a change in sun exposure patterns in the population and increased skin screening.[6,7]

RISK

Much of epidemiology involves the assessment of cancer risk. A person can be at increased risk of cancer because of either extrinsic or intrinsic factors, or a mix thereof.

- Extrinsic influences are factors outside of the individual's own body, such as environmental pollutants, cultural/lifestyle habits, medication use, infectious factors, and diet.
- Intrinsic influences are factors unique to each person, such as genetics.
- To assess etiology, risk is usually reported relative to another population. For example, in 2005, the breast cancer mortality rate for black women was 35.6 per 100,000, and the rate for non-Hispanic white women was 25.8 per 100,000. During that period, the relative risk of death for black women was 1.38 times that of white women (35.6 divided by 25.8).[8]

From an epidemiologic perspective, an etiologic agent or risk factor is anything that increases the probability that an individual will develop the disease. These risk factors can include demographic characteristics (e.g., increasing age or race/ethnicity) or lifestyle and behavioral factors, such as smoking.

They also include endogenous factors, such as genetic mutations that have been identified as predisposing a person for a disease, such as *BRCA1* and *BRCA2*. Most cancers undoubtedly arise from a combination of genetic and exogenous factors that interact to define certain demographic patterns. These patterns are recognized as the populations in which a specific cancer is most likely to occur.

Certain genetic mutations occur with relatively high frequency but convey only a slight increase in probability of the cancer occurring. These are referred to as genetic polymorphisms and are usually thought to provide increased susceptibility to an environmental carcinogen or to modify risk in some other way. For example, genetic polymorphisms for the cytochrome P450 enzyme system that metabolizes carcinogens in cigarette smoke can cause variability in susceptibility to the effects of cigarette smoke. Better known are the uncommon genetic mutations that convey high risk for the development of malignancy, such as the mutations of the *BRCA* or familial adenomatous polyposis (FAP) genes. *BRCA1* and *BRCA2* are genes with well-defined DNA sequences. Some *BRCA1* and *BRCA2* mutations increase the risk of breast and ovarian cancers and of certain other malignant diseases compared with risk for individuals without the mutations.[9] Advances in our knowledge regarding DNA methylation, histone modification, and other epigenetic phenomena may provide new insights on the effect of environmental factors on carcinogenesis and may suggest new targets for interventions.[10-12]

Knowledge regarding genetic risk factors for a particular cancer and the ability to predict the development of a particular cancer can help oncologists develop and select intervention options and to target high-risk populations for interventions. Table 1-2 lists selected low-prevalence, high-penetrance genetic syndromes with their associated cancers. Discussions of specific genetic syndromes related to cancers of different organ sites are to be found in the disease-specific chapters.

Knowledge of the risk factor also may present ethical dilemmas. Examples include whether to convey knowledge of risk to third parties in a patient's family, how to handle selection of embryos for implantation during in vitro fertilization on the basis of genetic testing, or the use of amniocentesis for testing of known genes, the results of which could be followed by termination of the pregnancy. However, knowledge of the risk factor may allow for early interventions that could prevent disease or limit its severity.

To address risk from genetic factors, it is critical to take a good family history from patients with cancer. This is particularly important for younger patients, who are more likely to harbor a mutation. Such a history should include a census of all first-degree relatives at a minimum (i.e., parents, siblings, and children), with their genders, current age or age at death, any cancers diagnosed, and age at diagnosis. Family histories with cancers among the relatives that fit the pattern of a known genetic mutation or early age at diagnosis for certain cancers should lead to referral to a genetic specialist for further evaluation and testing. The results of these evaluations have implications for the patient regarding risk of further

Table 1-2 Selected Hereditary Neoplastic Syndromes (Clinical Tests Available)

Syndromes	Site(s) of Most Common Cancer(s)	Associated Gene(s)
Hereditary breast-ovarian cancer	Breast, ovary	*BRCA1*, *BRCA2*
Cowden	Breast, thyroid	*PTEN*
Li-Fraumeni	Brain, breast, adrenal cortex, leukemia, sarcoma	*TP53*
Familial adenomatous polyposis	Large bowel, small bowel, brain (Turcot), skin, bone (Gardner)	*APC*
Hereditary nonpolyposis colorectal cancer	Colorectal and endometrium, also ovary, pancreas, stomach, small bowel	*MSH2, MLH1, PMS1, PMS2, MSH6*
Multiple endocrine neoplasia (MEN1)	Pancreatic islet cell, pituitary adenoma, parathyroid adenoma	*MEN1*
MEN2	Medullary thyroid, pheochromocytoma	*RET*
Neurofibromatosis-1	Neurofibrosarcoma, pheochromocytoma	*NF1*
Von Hippel-Lindau	Hemangioblastoma, nervous system, renal cell	*VHL*
Retinoblastoma	Eye, bone	*RB1*
Melanoma, hereditary	Skin	*CDKN2/p16, CDK4*
Basal cell	Skin	*PTCH*

cancers, as well as implications for other blood relatives in the patient's family.

Just as with genetic information, the clinician should make an effort to collect other relevant risk-factor information for patients with cancer or for healthy patients who are undergoing wellness exams. Risk information should include, at a minimum, tobacco and alcohol use, height and weight, family history, and occupational history. Other factors should be included as relevant to a specific symptom or diagnosis (e.g., exposure to organic solvents, such as benzene, in those diagnosed with leukemia; exposure to exogenous estrogens in women with postmenopausal bleeding; sexual history in those with human papillomavirus [HPV]-related disease). This information can be used to provide advice and guidance to the patient (e.g., regarding tobacco cessation), to identify patients at high risk for certain cancers, to guide early detection and prevention strategies, and to assist with diagnosis of certain cancers.

Chemoprevention and screening are options for certain high-risk populations, as is the modification of high-risk behavior. People at high risk for cancer may engage in intensive screening for the cancer in question. Although such screening may be clinically prudent, it may be less effective for patients at very high risk. In theory, a screening test might benefit those at risk for sporadic cancers and may not benefit patients at genetically high risk for a cancer. Alternatively, a screening test proven effective for average-risk individuals is likely to be of greater value in those at higher risk. Certain screening tests may be of value in those at higher risk, but would not be useful in average- or lower-risk individuals because of cost or other problems, such as high rates of false-positive results.

Population categorization is important in epidemiology. Populations can be delineated by gender, nationality, culture, race and ethnicity, socioeconomic status, age, and other characteristics. This is the basis of descriptive epidemiology—along with time trends—and is used to provide clues as to etiology. For example, a cancer that has a strong predominance in men may have a specific occupational component to it. Differences in incidence rates for various cancers found in both Japan and the United States have suggested hypotheses regarding diet and the consumption of green tea.[13]

Race and ethnicity are common ways of dividing populations in the United States. It should be remembered that race is a sociopolitical categorization.[14] The definitions used by U.S. investigators when generating population statistics are not formulated scientifically on the basis of characteristics such as genes, but rather reflect self-report by the individual and a mix of anatomical traits that often encompasses varying degrees of racial admixture. Much concern has arisen in the past 10 to 15 years regarding outcome disparities, in particular for a wide range of cancers and for black patients compared with white patients. In some instances, these disparities also reflect differences in incidence, but, in others, they may reflect differences in stage at diagnosis, access to treatment, or tumor biology. Race and ethnicity can correlate with other methods of categorization, such as poverty or prosperity, both of which are capable of changing the incidence of cancer and its related mortality.

Socioeconomic status and education also can be related to the risk of disease and death. Higher rates of breast cancer among white women in the San Francisco Bay area in California and on Long Island in New York were linked to a higher prevalence of professional women in those areas who, as a cohort, are less likely to have a full-term pregnancy by age 30, a known risk factor for breast cancer.[15] Socioeconomic status also has been related to type of treatment received and subsequent outcomes for various cancers, although this variable is heavily confounded with race/ethnicity and education.[16] In a classic study, Ayanian et al[17] found that women with breast cancer who were uninsured or on Medicaid had a 49% (95% CI 20, 84) and 40% (95% CI 4, 89) higher risk of death, respectively, than women with private insurance. A similar effect for socioeconomic status was found for survival of patients with colorectal cancer[18] and for quality of life for prostate cancer survivors.[19]

In analytic epidemiology, observational studies are carried out to ascertain whether associations exist between an exposure and an outcome. Although a statistical association may exist between the two, there is always concern that this may reflect bias in the way the study was conducted or the presence of confounding factors. Confounding factors are those associated with both the exposure and the outcome and can lead to an observed association, which is not truly a relationship between the two. For example, a study may show that asbestos workers have an elevated risk of lung cancer compared with the general population. However, one must be concerned that asbestos workers may be heavier smokers than other individuals in the general population and cigarette smoking is associated with lung cancer risk; thus, smoking may confound the observed association. Therefore, it is mandatory in a study that looks at this exposure and outcome to collect smoking information so that it can be statistically controlled and the individual effect of asbestos exposure can be appropriately measured.

Epidemiologic observational studies fall into two broad categories: cohort studies and case-control studies. Participants in cohort studies are categorized on the basis of their exposure and then followed to determine whether the outcome develops differently in the exposed and unexposed groups. Case-control studies enroll participants who have the outcome or disease under study, in addition to a control group of healthy participants. Both groups are then assessed for exposure. Both types of studies have their advantages and disadvantages. In both types, one must try to avoid bias or directional error. For example, in a case-control study, a patient with cancer may be inclined to give a positive answer more frequently than a control participant to a question regarding smoking history—this is referred to as recall bias.

As a general rule, cohort studies are preferred when the exposure is uncommon and the outcome is common, while case-control studies are preferable with uncommon outcomes. Since the incidence of most cancers—even the most common ones—is relatively low, case-control studies commonly are used in cancer research. Their disadvantage is that they are often ambiguous on the temporal relationship between the exposure and the cancer. If you compare 100 patients with colon cancer to 100 patients without colon cancer for their intake of saturated fat, it can be unclear whether a decreased intake in the cases is related to the disease or preceded the disease. In a cohort study, where the exposure is ascertained before the subjects have developed the cancer, one can be more confident that any observed association preceded the development of disease. On the other hand, because of the low incidence of most cancers, a cohort study requires tens of thousands of subjects to be followed for years. One of the best-known cohort studies, the Nurses' Health Study, followed almost 90,000 nurses for 4 years to generate enough endpoints to determine the risk associated with dietary fat and breast cancer, the most common cancer.[20]

Molecular epidemiology—the use of sophisticated molecular and genetic markers in conjunction with the traditional tools of analytic epidemiology to investigate etiologic or other questions in cancer epidemiology—is a major field within cancer epidemiology. Biomarkers can be used to measure exposures or endpoints in place of the more traditional answers to questionnaires, and, in some instances, biomarkers can give a more objective unbiased assessment.

Many contemporary studies in clinical oncology use epidemiologic methodology to address clinical questions in oncology. When randomized trials may be difficult to conduct, observational studies, such as cohort or case-control studies, may be used to answer typical questions regarding the efficacy of a drug or the incidence of an adverse event from a drug and also to ascertain the cost-effectiveness of a particular intervention. Therefore, an understanding of these analytic tools is imperative for the modern oncologist.

PATTERNS OF CARE, DISPARITIES, AND OUTCOMES RESEARCH

Although descriptive epidemiology and the determination of etiologic risk factors have been the traditional domains of epidemiology, the assessment of treatment outcomes in populations has become an important aspect of epidemiology. Clinical trials demonstrate "efficacy" of a treatment. How well the intervention works in the population as a whole in routine practice is referred to as "effectiveness." A phase II clinical trial can demonstrate the efficacy of a treatment intervention (e.g., tumor shrinkage), and a phase III study compares two interventions to determine which is superior. Prevention trials usually require phase III studies to show efficacy.

The study of patterns of care or treatments used is an aspect of outcomes research. Numerous studies often demonstrate geographic and regional differences in the preferred treatment of cancers. For example, for women with localized breast cancer, the decision to treat with lumpectomy and radiation therapy or with mastectomy may vary depending on the patient's geographic location.[21] Similar regional differences have been noted for prostate cancer screening and for the types of treatment used for localized prostate cancer.[22]

Health disparities generally can be defined as differences in outcomes related to a disease among a segment of the population compared with the general population. In current usage, the term is often used for subpopulations that are thought to be disadvantaged in some way, such as by race/ethnicity, increasing age, socioeconomic status, sexual orientation, rural residence, etc., and the public policy interest in disparities stems from an interest in finding avoidable and correctable causes for the disparities. For cancer-related disparities, such causes may reflect differences in risk-factor exposure, screening utilization, access to care, quality of care, or tumor biology. Most notably in this area, black patients are at increased risk of mortality from a wide variety of cancers.[23,24] Differences in tobacco usage have been responsible for disparities in mortality from squamous cell carcinoma of the esophagus between black and white patients.[25] A study from the Southwest Oncology Group found persistent racial disparities for women with breast and ovarian cancers entered on phase III trials despite similar stage, treatment, and follow-up, suggesting that biologic differences may also play a role.[26]

Many of the disparities in outcomes among groups defined by race and socioeconomic status have been linked to differences in patterns of care. For example, treatment is less than optimal for a substantial proportion of patients with cancer who are poor or of certain ethnic backgrounds.[27] The reasons for these variations in care are complex. Some are the result of sociocultural differences in attitudes toward therapy. Patient–physician communication also can play a major role.[28] In other cases, poverty, lack of insurance, or underinsurance can make access to care difficult.[17,29] Logistical difficulties, such as a lack of adequate transportation to a treatment center, may play a role. Patients with severe comorbid disease or poor performance status may justifiably not be offered aggressive cancer treatments because they are at higher risk of a treatment-related morbidity.

CANCER PREVENTION

Prevention is intended to reduce cancer incidence and mortality. Primary cancer prevention is best defined as the use of interventions to reduce cancer incidence. Important to prevention is the fact that carcinogenesis is not a distinct event but rather a process that occurs over time. It is a cumulative continuum of discrete cellular changes resulting in uncontrolled growth. Primary prevention involves interventions or manipulations of the genetic, biologic, and environmental factors in the causal pathway of carcinogenesis. Smoking cessation, sun avoidance, diet modification, weight loss and increased physical activity, cancer virus vaccination, and chemoprevention (e.g., tamoxifen for breast cancer prevention) are primary prevention activities. Screening for asymptomatic cancers, which is intended to detect cancers earlier so that treatment can be introduced more promptly and effectively to reduce mortality, is considered secondary prevention. For some cancers, such as cervix cancer and colorectal cancer, intraepithelial neoplasia is an intermediate step in carcinogenesis, and treatment of this condition is a form of cancer prevention.[30]

SMOKING CESSATION

Tobacco use is the most avoidable risk factor for cardiovascular disease, pulmonary disorders, and cancer. Smoking cessation and avoidance have the potential to save and extend more lives than any other public health activity. A smoker has a one-in-three lifetime risk of dying prematurely of a smoking-related disease. More human lives are lost because of cardiovascular disease caused by smoking than from smoking-related cancer. In addition to lung cancer, cigarette smoking has been linked to cancer of the larynx, oropharynx, esophagus, kidney, bladder, pancreas, and colon.[31]

The risk from tobacco smoke is not necessarily limited to the smoker. Epidemiologic studies suggest that environmental tobacco smoke, often called secondhand or passive smoke, may cause lung cancer and other pulmonary diseases in nonsmokers. The amount of smoke exposure, as well as the degree of inhalation of cigarette smoke, is correlated with the risk of mortality associated with lung cancer. Light and low-tar cigarettes are not safer because smokers tend to inhale them more frequently and more deeply. Compared with their nonfiltered counterparts, filtered cigarettes allow smaller particles to get into the peripheral parts of the lung and cause different histologic subtypes of cancer,[32-34] specifically adenocarcinomas. Those who stop smoking almost immediately stop increasing their risk of cancer, although it takes some time before their risk of cancer declines. Some carcinogen-induced gene mutations, however, may persist for years.

The vast majority of adult U.S. smokers begin smoking before age 18; two-thirds are nicotine-dependent in their high school years.[35] Therefore, communicating health messages to the pediatric and adolescent population is a major public health challenge. Studies show that a physician's simple advice to avoid or quit smoking can improve the quit rate by two-thirds.[36] Despite this, a recent survey found that although more than 80% of oncologists assess smoking behavior in their patients, fewer than 20% feel confident enough to intervene in this important area.[37]

Among the most effective smoking cessation interventions are governmental actions. Tax increases on cigarettes and restrictions on venues where smoking is permitted have been very effective in reducing smoking prevalence rates.[38] Current smoker rates are down to 20% or less in the United States, and most tobacco-related cancers in this country now occur in former smokers. However, smoking remains a major factor globally, especially in Asia, and lung cancer is the leading cause of cancer mortality worldwide. Much concern has been raised in particular about smoking rates in India and China, and global efforts to reduce smoking rates are being initiated.[39,40]

Smoking is an addiction. It is easier for light smokers—the less addicted—to quit. Experts believe that heavy smokers typically need an intensive, broad-based cessation program that includes counseling, behavioral strategies, and drug therapy; if drug therapy is needed, the recommended first-line therapies are nicotine-replacement therapy, bupropion, and varenicline, with clonidine and nortriptyline as possible second-line therapies.[36] Most U.S. smokers who successfully quit smoking do so on their own, without participation in an organized cessation program, but this process can be strongly enhanced by even a small amount of encouragement from a health care provider. Smokers who stop completely are more likely to be successful than smokers who gradually reduce the number of cigarettes smoked or change to cigarettes containing lower amounts of tar or nicotine. The smoker who is quitting goes through a process with identifiable stages that include contemplation of quitting, an action phase during which the smoker quits, and a maintenance phase. As noted above, there now exist numerous effective strategies beyond counseling for advising and assisting the cooperative patient with his or her goals.[41,42] Use of the electronic or e-cigarette has recently been growing as another tool to enhance tobacco cessation. This device, which provides nicotine for the user who is addicted but without the harmful carcinogenic exposures, is controversial in that some see it as an improvement over regular smoking, while others oppose its use because they feel that it provides a more acceptable alternative to total tobacco cessation.[43]

Much of the literature focuses on the risks of cigarette smoking. Cigar smokers do not inhale, but the health risks associated with cigars are similar to those of cigarettes, especially the risks of oropharyngeal cancers.[44] Smokeless tobacco, or chewing tobacco, is the fastest-growing segment of the tobacco industry and represents a serious health risk. Chewing tobacco has been linked to dental caries, gingivitis, oral leukoplakia, and oral cancer. In addition, the nitrosamines found in this product have been shown to cause lung cancer in animal studies. Esophageal cancer is linked to the carcinogens in tobacco that dissolve in saliva, are swallowed, and then come into contact with the esophagus. Smoking opium in certain parts of the world, presumably from the polycyclic aromatic hydrocarbons in the smoke, has also been associated with esophageal cancer etiology.[45]

ALCOHOL

It is worth recognizing that alcohol ingestion plays a substantial role in cancer etiology.[46] A major carcinogenic role for alcohol has been as a cofactor with tobacco in cancers of the upper aerodigestive tract, where the joint utilization of tobacco and alcohol can lead to synergistic risks. It is a significant carcinogen in its own right for hepatocellular carcinoma (HCC) by the induction of cirrhosis or as a risk factor for breast cancer.[47]

Recent data have accumulated particularly with regard to moderate alcohol use and breast cancer risk. As a consequence, it appears to have an attributable risk for breast cancer that approaches 5% in Europe and overall to be responsible for 10% or more of overall cancer.[48]

SUN AVOIDANCE

Results of epidemiologic studies show a correlation between the risk of nonmelanoma skin cancers (basal and squamous cell) and cumulative exposure to ultraviolet radiation. Possible risk factors for melanoma include a propensity to sunburn, a large number of benign melanocytic nevi, and atypical nevi. A history of severe sunburns, especially in childhood and adolescence, is associated with increased risk of melanoma in adulthood. Recently, concern has been raised about the increasing use of indoor tanning and tanning beds, and measures calling for their regulation have been sounded.[49,50] Reduction of sun exposure through the use of protective clothing and a change in one's pattern of outdoor activities to avoid the most intense and direct sunlight have been advocated as ways to reduce the risk of skin cancer. Although past studies have been inconclusive, a recent randomized trial confirmed that sunscreen use can reduce the risk of melanoma.[51]

DIET MODIFICATION

Rates of cancers of the breast, colon, endometrium, and prostate are higher in North America and western Europe than in Asia. Immigrants from Asia and their offspring acquire a higher risk for these cancers after they have been in the United States for some time. These observations, as well as data from animal studies, are the basis for the belief that dietary modification can significantly lower cancer risk for individuals in the United States.[52] Diet is a highly complex exposure to many nutrients and chemicals. Low-fat diets, which are usually low in red meat and high in fruits and vegetables, may render some protection through anticarcinogens found in vegetables, fruits, legumes, nuts, and grains. Potentially protective substances found in foods include phenols, sulfur-containing compounds, and flavones.[53] Although the cancer-prevention benefits are theoretical and not fully demonstrated, such a diet does lower the risk of cardiac disease. However, vitamins, minerals, or nutritional supplements in amounts greater than those provided by a good diet have not been demonstrated to be of value. Most randomized trials of vitamin supplements have not shown benefit in terms of prevention and in some instances have even shown harm (discussed in the Chemoprevention section below).

Despite correlative data, the dietary fat–cancer hypothesis has not been definitively demonstrated. Case-control and cohort epidemiologic studies yield conflicting results. No prospective clinical trial has demonstrated that cancer can be prevented through lowering dietary fat or increasing fiber intake. Studies, including randomized trials, have consistently shown no effect of dietary fiber intake on colon cancer risk.[54,55] The Women's Health Initiative, which included a randomized trial with a low-fat diet intervention, also did not indicate an effect on breast cancer or colon cancer risk.[56,57] Nonetheless, a randomized trial of more than 2,400 women with early-stage breast cancer showed that patients randomly assigned to a low-fat diet, in addition to standard adjuvant therapy, had a significantly improved survival compared with women on a regular diet (hazard ratio [HR] 0.76, 95% CI 0.60, 0.98).[58]

WEIGHT REDUCTION AND PHYSICAL ACTIVITY

A major public health concern has centered on the obesity epidemic in the United States. Obesity represents the effects of an individual's net caloric intake, which is the amount consumed versus the amount expended through physical activity. Changes in either of these variables will impinge on the measure of obesity, thereby affecting cancer risk. Obesity affects cancer risk through a number of mechanisms, including hormone metabolism, thereby affecting breast, endometrial, and prostate cancer risk, or by increasing esophageal reflux, which affects the occurrence of Barrett metaplasia and esophageal adenocarcinoma.[59,60] Many consider obesity the second most important risk factor for cancer in the United States, after tobacco.[61]

Although obesity does appear to be related to the incidence and prognosis of a number of cancers, there is very little data on whether weight loss can ameliorate the risk.[62] Recent studies in this area have focused more on weight loss in cancer survivors than on the use of weight loss to prevent cancer incidence.

Physical activity has been studied for 2 decades and has been shown to be protective for breast cancer, colorectal cancer, lung cancer, and prostate cancer. For those who develop these cancers, increases in physical activity appear to be helpful to survivors, although large elegant phase III trials remain lacking. Its strongest associations appear to be for cancers of the alimentary tract.[63]

OCCUPATIONAL CARCINOGENS

Since Percival Pott recognized an increased risk of scrotal cancer among chimney sweeps in 18th-century London, it has been understood that occupational exposures can increase the risk of certain cancers. The most important of the occupational carcinogens has been asbestos—exposure to which is prominent among construction workers, pipefitters, and shipyard workers. It has been closely linked to the incidence of mesothelioma, lung cancer, and probably gastrointestinal tract malignancies. Another classic exposure has been radon inhalation, which occurs in uranium miners and potentially from home radon exposure and increases the risk of lung cancer. Various other organic and aromatic chemicals are linked to the risks of leukemia and cancers of the urinary collecting system.

IONIZING RADIATION

As noted above, inhaled radon exposure can be carcinogenic to the lungs. The effects of other sources of radiation exposure and radiation carcinogenesis have been well recognized since their discovery at the turn of the 19th to 20th centuries, particularly on hematologic malignancies. The most prominent source of such exposure stemmed from the atomic bomb explosions in August 1945 in Japan, and much of what we know about radiation dosimetry, latency, and carcinogenic effects comes from the careful and meticulous studies undertaken in the wake of those events. The other major source of radiation exposure is therapeutic radiation, mainly in treatment of malignancies—hence the observation of second malignancies as a consequence. Exposure to ionizing radiation is associated with increased risk of breast, lung, esophageal, and bladder cancers, leukemia, sarcoma, and brain tumors. It has also been linked to thyroid cancer when there is exposure to radioactive iodine, as in the aftermath of the Chernobyl nuclear accident, which released radioactive iodine into the atmosphere.[64] Efforts to reduce the use of radiation therapy, to minimize the fields, and to avoid the joint use of an alkylating agent in combination with radiation therapy are well known to reduce the risk of these second malignancies. Recent concern has also arisen about the increased use of diagnostic scans in medical care and the carcinogenic risks arising from this cumulative exposure. On a population scale, sophisticated modeling has suggested that a significant increase in cancers can be anticipated from this widespread phenomenon.[65]

CANCER VIRUS VACCINATION

Virally induced cancer has been recognized since the early part of the 20th century, with the discovery of Rous sarcoma virus in chickens. In humans, several viruses, including hepatitis B (HCC), hepatitis C (HCC), Epstein-Barr (Burkitt lymphoma), and HPV (cervix cancer, other anogenital squamous cell malignancies, and head and neck carcinoma) have been clearly established as carcinogenic. An understanding of retroviruses has broadened our appreciation of other viral agents, such as human herpesvirus-8 and Kaposi sarcoma.[66,67] In addition, the bacterium *Helicobacter pylori (H. pylori)* was found to be associated with gastric cancer. These are particularly exciting findings because these agents provide targets for vaccination as a means of primary prevention. This has been achieved for hepatitis B[68] and for HPV.[69] In Taiwan, where hepatoma is the leading cancer, hepatitis B vaccine was introduced in 1984 and the risk of hepatoma has so far been reduced by over 70% among those vaccinated.[70]

Another success has been the introduction of a vaccine for several subtypes of HPV. Vaccination for HPV is now recommended for young girls prior to becoming sexually active, which should reduce the incidence of cervix cancer by 70% or more. The U.S. Centers for Disease Control and Prevention recently recommended the vaccine for boys as well. More recent studies have suggested that one or two vaccinations may suffice to give an adequate immune response versus the recommended three vaccinations, so compliance should increase.[71] Because these same viruses are involved in other cancers, the incidence of anal, vaginal, penile, and oropharyngeal cancers may also decline, particularly if vaccination of boys becomes common.[72,73]

KEY POINTS
■ Avoidance of carcinogens is the most efficient way to prevent cancer.
■ Smoking is the cause of nearly one-third of all cancers in the United States.
■ Other environmental influences, such as sun overexposure, certain chemicals, and certain infectious agents, are associated with cancer causation.

CHEMOPREVENTION

Cancer chemoprevention is the use of natural or synthetic chemical agents to reverse, suppress, or prevent carcinogenesis before the development of an invasive malignant process.[74] Cancers are prevented through chemoprevention or, in certain cases, through surgical removal of the organ at risk. Although the concept that pharmacologic agents can prevent a cancer is relatively new, the idea that a compound can prevent chronic disease is not. Antihypertensive agents are used to prevent heart disease, kidney disease, and stroke. Lipid-lowering drugs are prescribed to prevent coronary artery disease.

The initial genetic changes of carcinogenesis are termed "initiation." This alteration can be inherited or acquired. Acquired genetic damage is the result of physical, infectious, or chemical carcinogens (Table 1-3). The influences that cause the initiated cell to change phenotypically are called promoters. Known promoters include androgens linked to prostate cancer and estrogen linked to breast and endometrial cancers. The distinction between the initiator and promoter can sometimes blur; some components of cigarette smoke are referred to as "complete carcinogens" and serve as both initiators and promoters. Cancer can be prevented or controlled through interference with the factors causing disease initiation, promotion, or progression.

Compounds of interest in chemoprevention include anti-inflammatory agents, antioxidants, differentiating agents, or hormone antagonists. A long-term, randomized, placebo-controlled clinical trial is usually necessary to establish the efficacy of a chemopreventive agent, and several large clinical trials have been completed.[75-77] As discussed in the following sections, tamoxifen,[75] raloxifene,[77] and aromatase inhibitors[78] have been shown to reduce the incidence of breast cancer. In addition, nonsteroidal anti-inflammatory drugs, particularly aspirin, can reduce the occurrence of colorectal adenomas in various circumstances and have also been shown to reduce the

Table 1-3 Examples of Initiators and Promoters of Cancer

Carcinogen	Associated Cancer or Neoplasm
Alkylating agents	Acute myelocytic leukemia, bladder
Androgens	Prostate
Aromatic amines (dyes)	Bladder
Arsenic	Lung, skin
Asbestos	Lung, pleura, peritoneum
Benzene	Acute myelocytic leukemia
Chromium	Lung
Diethylstilbestrol (prenatal)	Vaginal (clear cell)
Epstein-Barr virus	Burkitt lymphoma, nasopharynx
Estrogens	Endometrium
Estrogen plus progesterone	Breast
Ethyl alcohol	Liver, esophagus, head and neck
Helicobacter pylori	Gastric
Hepatitis B virus	Liver
Hepatitis C virus	Liver
Human T-cell leukemia (HTLV)-1 virus	Adult T-cell leukemia, lymphoma
Human herpesvirus-8 (HHV-8)	Kaposi sarcoma
Human immunodeficiency virus (HIV)	Non-Hodgkin lymphoma, Kaposi sarcoma, squamous cell carcinoma of cervix
Human papillomavirus (HPV)	Squamous cell carcinoma of cervix, anogenital area, oropharynx
Immunosuppressive agents (azathioprine, cyclosporine, corticosteroids)	Non-Hodgkin lymphoma
Nitrogen mustard gas	Lung, head and neck, nasal sinuses
Nickel dust	Lung, nasal sinuses
Phenacetin	Renal pelvis, bladder
Polycyclic aromatic hydrocarbons	Lung, skin (especially squamous cell)
Schistosomiasis	Bladder (squamous cell)
Sunlight (ultraviolet)	Skin (squamous cell and melanoma)
Tobacco (including smokeless)	Upper aerodigestive tract, bladder, pancreas
Vinyl chloride	Liver (angiosarcoma)

These agents are thought to act as cancer initiators or promoters for the cancers with which they have been associated.

incidence of colon cancer, breast cancer, and a variety of other cancers.[79,80] Finasteride and dutasteride reduce the incidence of prostate cancer.[76,81] Retinoids may inhibit head and neck cancers.[82] Selenium and vitamin E were shown not to reduce prostate cancer risk.[83] Recent agents of interest for

chemoprevention of breast, colon, and other cancers include calcium and vitamin D.[84,85] Most observational studies have not shown a benefit to the use of multivitamin uptake. However, in a prospective randomized trial of a daily multivitamin compared with placebo for U.S. male physicians, there was a small but statistically significant reduction in the incidence of cancer among the men assigned to multivitamin treatment.[86] Table 1-4 contains a list of selected large, randomized chemoprevention trials that have been conducted.[75-78,81-83,87-108]

CANCERS OF THE LUNG, HEAD AND NECK, AND ESOPHAGUS

Tobacco smoking is the major cause of squamous cell cancers of the lung, head, neck, and esophagus. The risk of a second cancer of the lung, head, or neck is high—as great as 5% per year of smoking—for patients cured of these diseases. This is because of "field cancerization," meaning the carcinogens in tobacco smoke affect all tissues exposed to them. Even after smoking cessation, the tissues that have come in contact with smoke have residual molecular damage. For the esophagus, head, and neck, alcohol ingestion has an interactive effect with smoking. Other cancers of the lung (e.g., small cell and adenocarcinoma) also are associated with tobacco use. Very high rates of oral cancer are found in India in association with betel nut chewing. HPV infection, particularly the HPV-16 subtype, has been linked to oropharyngeal cancer[109]; a significant increase in incidence is anticipated in the coming years as a consequence, though the introduction of HPV vaccination may reduce this incidence.

In the United States, incidence rates for esophageal adenocarcinoma are among the most rapidly increasing since the late 1970s. This cancer occurs as a sequelae of Barrett esophagus and is thought to be the result of gastroesophageal reflux disease.[110] Esophagogastroduodenoscopy often is used as regular surveillance to detect Barrett esophagus in patients with gastroesophageal reflux disease; however, there is no convincing evidence that demonstrates a reduction in the subsequent incidence or mortality of esophageal adenocarcinoma.

Rates of squamous cell carcinoma of the esophagus have been declining concomitant with the rise of adenocarcinoma, reflecting the decline of smoking prevalence. Very high rates of squamous cell carcinoma have been identified in a belt spanning central Asia from northern Iran to China,[111] with evidence implicating local risk factors, such as very hot tea ingestion and the smoking of opium.[45,112]

Several large-scale studies have been launched to assess potential chemopreventive agents for patients at high risk for lung cancer. The Alpha-Tocopherol, Beta-Carotene Cancer Prevention Trial (ATBC)[88] and the Beta-Carotene and Retinol Efficacy Trial (CARET)[89] were prevention trials that showed the importance of testing even seemingly harmless chemoprevention agents, such as vitamins, before widespread use. The results of both trials are in contrast to numerous observational studies. The ATBC trial enrolled Finnish male smokers between ages 50 and 69. Participants received alpha-tocopherol, beta-carotene, both, or placebo in a randomized, 2×2 factorial design. After

Table 1-4 Randomized Chemoprevention Trials

Author (Year, Trial Name)	Study Setting/ Endpoint	Number of Patients	Intervention	Primary Outcome
Head and Neck				
Hong et al (1990)[82]	Prior SCC	103	Isotretinoin (100 mg/m^2/d)	Positive (SPT)
Bolla et al (1994)[87]	Prior SCC	316	Etretinate (50, 25 mg/d)	Negative
Lung				
Virtamo et al (2003; ATBC Cancer Prevention Study)[88]	Lung cancer	29,133	Carotene (20 mg/d); vit E (50 mg/d)	Negative
Omenn et al (1996; CARET)[89]	Lung cancer	18,314	Carotene (30 mg/d); vit A (25,000 IU/d)	Negative
Pastorino et al (1993)[90]	Prior NSCLC	307	Vit A (300,000 IU/d)	Positive (SPT)
van Zandwijk et al (2000)[91]	Prior HNC, NSCLC	2,592	Vit A (300,000/150,000 IU/d); NAC (600 mg/d)	Negative
Lippman et al (2001)[92]	Prior NSCLC	1,166	Isotretinoin (30 mg/d)	Negative
Karp et al (2013)[93]	Prior NSCLC	1,561	Selenium (200 µg/d)	Negative
Skin				
Levine et al (1997)[94]	Prior BCC/SCC	524	Isotretinoin (5-10 mg/d); vit A (25,000 IU/d)	Negative
Greenberg et al (1990)[95]	Prior BCC/SCC	1,805	Carotene (50 mg/d)	Negative
Tangrea et al (1992)[96]	Prior BCC	981	Isotretinoin (10 mg/d)	Negative
Moon et al (1997)[97]	AK	2,298	Vit A (25,000 IU/d)	Positive
Bavinck et al (1995)[98]	Renal transplant	38	Acitretin (30 mg/d)	Positive
Clark et al (1996)[99]	Prior BCC/SCC	1,312	Selenium (200 µg/d)	Negative
Breast				
Fisher et al (1998; BCPT)[75]	High risk/BC	13,388	Tamoxifen (20 mg/d)	Positive
Veronesi et al (1998)[100]	BC	5,408	Tamoxifen (20 mg/d)	Negative
Powles et al (1998)[101]	High risk/BC	2,471	Tamoxifen (20 mg/d)	Negative
Fisher et al (1999)[102]	DCIS/BC	1,804	Tamoxifen (20 mg/d)	Positive
Veronesi et al (1999)[103]	CBC	2,972	Fenretinide (200 mg/d)	Negative
Vogel et al (2006; STAR)[77]	High risk/BC	19,747	Raloxifene (60 mg/d) vs. tamoxifen (20 mg/d)	Equal
Goss et al (2011)[78]	High risk/BC	4,560	Exemestane (25 mg/d)	Positive
Colorectal				
Wactawski-Wende et al (2006)[104]	Colorectal cancer	36,282	Calcium (500 mg bid); vit D3 (200 IU bid)	Negative
Prostate				
Thompson et al (2003; PCPT)[76]	Prostate cancer	18,882	Finasteride (5 mg/d)	Positive
Andriole et al (2010)[81]	Prostate cancer	6,729	Dutasteride (0.5 mg/d)	Positive
Lippman et al (2009; SELECT)[83]	Prostate cancer	35,533	Selenium (200 mcg/d); vit E (400 IU/d)	Negative
Esophagus/Stomach				
Blot et al (1993; Linxian)[105]	Geographic risk	29,584	Multiple vitamins/minerals	Negative
Li et al (1993)[106]	Geographic risk	3,318	Multiple vitamins/minerals	Negative
All Cancer				
Hennekens et al (1996; PHS)[107]	Healthy men	22,071	Carotene (50 mg qod)	Negative
Lee et al (1999)[108]	Healthy women	39,876	Carotene (50 mg qod)	Negative

Abbreviations: AK, actinic keratosis; BC, breast cancer; BCC, basal cell carcinoma; bid, twice daily; CBC, contralateral breast cancer; d, day; DCIS, ductal carcinoma in situ; HNC, head and neck cancer; NAC, N-acetylcysteine; NSCLC, non-small cell lung cancer; SCC, squamous cell carcinoma; SPT, second primary tumor; qod, every other day; vit, vitamin.

Adapted from: Kufe DW, Bast RC Jr, Hait W, et al (eds). Holland-Frei Cancer Medicine, 7th Edition. *Hamilton, ON, and Lewiston, NY: BC Decker; 2006.*

a median follow-up of 6 years, there was a significant increase in lung cancer incidence and mortality for the participants who received beta-carotene. Alpha-tocopherol had no effect on lung cancer mortality. CARET enrolled 17,000 smokers and workers exposed to asbestos. Participants were randomly assigned to four arms and received beta-carotene, retinol, both, or placebo in a 2×2 factorial design. The results of the trial demonstrated a 28% increase in lung cancer and a 17% increase in deaths for the participants receiving beta-carotene. The reason for this outcome is uncertain; it occurred despite beta-carotene's role as both an antioxidant and as a precursor to retinol.

Retinoids have proven to be effective as chemopreventive agents for squamous cell malignancies of the head and neck, possibly by promoting terminal differentiation.[82] A study randomly assigned 102 patients with a first primary squamous cell carcinoma of the head and neck to 13-*cis*-retinoic acid, a retinoid analogue, or to placebo. At 3 years, there were two second primary head and neck cancers in the intervention group versus 12 in the placebo group (p = 0.005). Despite this study and later supportive trials, the retinoids have not become standard of care, mainly because of toxicities.

GASTRIC CANCERS

Heavy intake of smoked and cured meats and foods, limited consumption of fresh fruits and vegetables, and infection with *H. pylori* are associated with an increased risk of gastric cancer.[110] Gastric cancer was the most common cancer in the United States prior to World War II, but it is now much less common. This decline is thought to be caused by increased consumption of fresh meats, fruits, and vegetables and decreased consumption of cured/smoked foods. Experimental evidence of causality is scarce. Gastric cancer remains a very common malignancy in Japan, Latin America, China, and in other parts of the developing world. A randomized trial in China of eradication of *H. pylori* infection with a combination of omeprazole, amoxicillin, clavulanate, and metronidazole did not show a reduction in subsequent gastric cancer incidence. Nonetheless, patients who had no gastric pathology at study entry did show a significant reduction in gastric cancer incidence in subgroup analysis.[113] There are no randomized trial data to support screening for groups at high risk for *H. pylori* (e.g., Asian individuals), which would lead to the institution of eradication procedures to reduce the subsequent risk of gastric cancer. Studies are underway to further elucidate this question. Furthermore, the rates of cancer of the gastric cardia and esophageal adenocarcinoma are rising, and there is evidence to suggest that this may be a consequence of recent declines in the prevalence of *H. pylori*.[114] The reasons the cancers of the proximal stomach and distal stomach may have inverse associations with the presence of *H. pylori* are unclear. Nonetheless, it may be one reason why the incidence of distal gastric cancer in the United States has been declining while the incidence of proximal and gastroesophageal junction cancer incidence has been rising.[115]

COLON CANCER

Findings from epidemiologic studies suggest that nonsteroidal anti-inflammatory agents, such as piroxicam, sulindac, and aspirin, have protective effects against adenomatous polyps and invasive cancer.[79,80,116] The results of prospective intervention trials have demonstrated positive effects on the prevention of polyps; meta-analyses of randomized trials of aspirin designed to assess other endpoints have demonstrated that these agents prevent colon cancer.[79,80] In a placebo-controlled trial, high-dose celecoxib, a cyclooxygenase-2 (COX-2) inhibitor, was found to reduce the occurrence of colorectal polyps for patients with familial adenomatous polyposis.[117] A prospective randomized trial of patients with a history of colorectal adenomas demonstrated a 20% reduction in recurrence of polyps for patients who received celecoxib.[118] Trials to assess COX-2 inhibitors and other nonsteroidal anti-inflammatory agents for the prevention of colorectal adenomas have shown preventive benefits; however, these agents are associated with increased cardiovascular risk. A recent study suggested that the risk of colon cancer can be reduced even by doses of aspirin as low as 80 mg daily.[119] One observational study suggested that COX-2 inhibitors could improve mortality when used in patients with node-positive colon cancer[120]; a randomized trial is in progress to confirm this finding. This may be partly because of a beneficial effect on cancer metastasis.[121]

The Women's Health Initiative was a prospective, randomized study involving postmenopausal women randomly assigned to either combination estrogen plus progestin or to placebo. The rate of colorectal cancer was lower for women taking the study drug compared with women taking placebo.[122] However, the effect is offset by the life-threatening cardiovascular and breast cancer risks associated with treatment with estrogen plus progestin.[123]

The results of epidemiologic studies indicate that diets high in calcium are associated with a lower risk of colon cancer. However, in the Women's Health Initiative study, calcium and vitamin D supplementation did not lower the incidence of colorectal cancer.[104] Evidence from prospective randomized studies shows that calcium supplementation decreases the risk of recurrence of adenomatous polyps by approximately 20%.[124] Calcium binds bile and fatty acids, reducing intraluminal exposure to compounds that cause hyperproliferation of the colonic epithelium.

Obesity is associated with an increased risk of colorectal cancer. However, in another Women's Health Initiative randomized controlled trial, there was no difference in the incidence of colorectal cancer among women assigned to a low-fat diet as compared with control participants.[57]

Colectomy is used as a preventive measure for individuals at extremely high risk of colon cancer as a result of a history of ulcerative colitis or of a genetic predisposition to the disease, such as familial adenomatous polyposis.[125]

No chemopreventive agent is currently recommended for prevention of colorectal cancer for individuals at average risk. The use of nonsteroidal anti-inflammatory agents for patients with familial adenomatous polyposis following colectomy may be reasonable in conjunction with endoscopic screening.

LIVER CANCER

Hepatitis B–induced HCC is one of the most commonly diagnosed cancers in Asia. The hepatitis B vaccine has been advocated for its ability to prevent the disease. Reductions in the incidence of HCC in Taiwan and elsewhere suggest some success.[68] Although HCC is much less common in the United States, there has been a rise in incidence rates because of an epidemic of hepatitis C, which also leads to HCC, but for which no vaccine is available.

BREAST CANCER

Tamoxifen has mixed estrogenic and anti-estrogenic activities. It acts as an estrogen agonist in the endometrium and bone and as an estrogen antagonist in breast tissue. It also up-regulates transforming growth factor-beta, which decreases breast cell proliferation. In randomized, placebo-controlled trials to assess tamoxifen as adjuvant therapy for patients with early-stage breast cancer, this drug was found to prevent new cancers in the contralateral breast. The Breast Cancer Prevention Trial was a randomized, placebo-controlled study of more than 13,000 women at high risk of breast cancer. After a median treatment of 69 months, tamoxifen was found to decrease the period risk of breast cancer by 49%. It also was associated with a reduction in bone fractures and with a small increase in risk of endometrial cancer, stroke, pulmonary emboli, and deep vein thrombosis.[75,126] A trial to compare tamoxifen with another selective estrogen-receptor modulator, raloxifene, for postmenopausal women, was completed (the Study of Tamoxifen and Raloxifene [STAR] Trial). Raloxifene decreased the risk of invasive breast cancer by amounts similar to tamoxifen but did not decrease the risk of noninvasive breast cancer. Compared with tamoxifen, raloxifene was associated with less risk of endometrial cancer, as well as with lower risk of thromboembolic events and cataracts.[77] Another randomized trial showed that an aromatase inhibitor, exemestane, could also prevent breast cancer.[78] In a trial with 4,560 postmenopausal women randomly assigned to exemestane or placebo, exemestane reduced the risk of breast cancer compared to placebo by 65% (95% CI 0.18, 0.70). Despite these trials, uptake of these drugs for breast cancer prevention has been relatively low.[127]

The Women's Health Initiative was discontinued early partially because of the increased risk of breast cancer (odds ratio 1.26) among women who were postmenopausal and who were taking active hormone-replacement estrogens with progestins.[122] A parallel trial of estrogen alone compared with placebo for women with a prior hysterectomy did not show an increased risk of breast cancer among women taking estrogen.[128] A recent analysis of the Women's Health Initiative concluded that there was no overall benefit of postmenopausal estrogens for women except perhaps for reduction of hot flashes.[129]

Obesity also is associated with an increased risk of breast cancer, related to aromatase activity in fat tissue and increased estrogenic production.

Prophylactic bilateral mastectomy to prevent breast cancer has not been assessed by randomized trials. In a prospective series of 139 women with BRCA1 and BRCA2 mutations, 76 chose prophylactic bilateral mastectomy, and 63 chose close surveillance. At 3 years, there was no breast cancer diagnosed in those who chose surgery; eight women in the surveillance group had been diagnosed with breast cancer. This study is small, of short duration, and, by design, prone to selection biases. However, it is fair to say that the short-term risk of breast cancer appears to be lower for women with certain BRCA1 and BRCA2 mutations who choose prophylactic mastectomy. Because this surgery leaves some breast tissue behind, a patient's risk is not reduced to zero. When coupled with prophylactic bilateral salpingo-oophorectomy, ovarian cancer risk is markedly decreased, and there is an added benefit for breast cancer prevention. Retrospective analysis of mastectomies for 214 women at high risk of breast cancer because of family history suggests that prophylactic mastectomy can lead to a 90% reduction in risk.[130] One large study of patients from 11 centers investigated 1,079 women with deleterious BRCA mutations and compared those who self-selected salpingo-oophorectomy to those who did not. With 3 years of follow-up, the prophylactic surgery was associated with an 85% reduction in risk of gynecologic cancer and a 72% reduction in risk of breast cancer in the BRCA1 group, but there was no clear benefit for BRCA2 carriers.[131]

A recent Cochrane review concluded that bilateral prophylactic mastectomy for those at very high risk of breast cancer (e.g., those with deleterious BRCA mutations) was effective in reducing the incidence and subsequent mortality from breast cancer.[132]

PROSTATE CANCER

Androgens stimulate prostate cell proliferation and, in laboratory animals, cause prostate carcinogenesis. Finasteride decreases androgenic stimulation of the prostate by inhibiting the production of 5-alpha-reductase. This enzyme, which is found in high amounts in the prostate, converts testosterone to the more potent dihydrotestosterone. Finasteride was tested as a preventive agent for prostate cancer in the Prostate Cancer Prevention Trial, a 10-year, randomized, placebo-controlled study involving 18,000 men age 55 and older. Results of the study showed that this drug was associated with a 24.8% reduction in the risk of prostate cancer during the treatment period. There were some initial concerns regarding an observed increased incidence of high-grade tumors that developed while patients were treated with finasteride.[76] Later re-analyses showed that these observations were a result of statistical methods, and that there are no true increases in high-grade tumors.[133,134] A recent study of another 5-alpha-reductase inhibitor, dutasteride, also found a protective effect against prostate cancer.[81] Long-term follow-up of the finasteride study showed that, despite the reduction in incidence of prostate cancer, there was not an improvement in overall survival.[135] It raises the interesting question of whether the use of a chemopreventive agent is worthwhile solely for prevention of incidence if mortality benefit does not accompany it.[136]

Findings from epidemiologic studies indicate a correlation between high intake of antioxidants, such as selenium and vitamin E, and lower risk of prostate cancer. The results of a small, randomized skin cancer prevention trial of selenium compared with placebo showed a significant decrease in the number of prostate cancers in men treated with selenium compared with men receiving placebo.[137] Eight years into the ATBC Prevention Trial, which enrolled 29,000 men, there were 99 cases of prostate cancer reported among men receiving vitamin E and 151 cases reported among men taking placebo. The cancers diagnosed were almost all detected as a result of the work-up of symptoms because there is no routine prostate cancer screening in Finland.[138]

The prostate cancer findings in both of these trials were incidental results of a secondary analysis. A prospective, randomized, placebo-controlled trial—the Selenium and Vitamin E Cancer Prevention Trial (SELECT)—assessed these drugs in 32,400 participants and reported no reduction in prostate cancer incidence.[83]

GYNECOLOGIC CANCER

Laser ablation, conization, or hysterectomy is used to treat cervix dysplasia or intraepithelial neoplasia, both of which are precursors to invasive cervix cancer. Vaccines for HPV have been approved for young girls and will undoubtedly lower the incidence of cervix cancer.[69]

Studies have shown a strong protective effect against ovarian cancer for oral contraceptive hormone preparations.[139] However, there is no current recommendation for their use on a routine basis for prevention. For women at very high risk of ovarian cancer because of a *BRCA* genetic mutation, bilateral salpingo-oophorectomy after completion of child-bearing remains the treatment of choice (including fallopian tube removal).[140] Women with Lynch syndrome, associated with large and small bowel polyps and cancers, are also at elevated risk for endometrial cancer. For these women, prophylactic hysterectomy and bilateral salpingo-oophorectomy may also be recommended.

KEY POINTS

- Most randomized trials of vitamins or nutritional supplements as chemopreventive agents have proven negative.
- Hormone inhibitors for hormone-dependent cancers have proven efficacious as preventive agents and may have a role in clinical practice, though the benefits must be weighed against potential side effects.
- Drugs and vitamins to be used for prevention need to undergo the same rigorous assessment of efficacy and toxicity as do therapeutic agents prior to recommendation. Indeed, because they are typically administered to a healthy population, their toxicity profile must be safer than those of drugs used in the therapeutic setting.

CANCER SCREENING

Cancer screening is an attempt to detect cancer or its precursors early in asymptomatic individuals, with the goal of intervening and decreasing morbidity and mortality. A screening test is not typically diagnostic for cancer; rather, it determines whether cancer might be present and if additional testing, including a biopsy and staging, is necessary. To be of true benefit, screening must lead to earlier treatment that offers a better outcome, usually reduced mortality, compared with treatment that would occur at the onset of symptoms. Because of various biases (discussed in the Potential Biases section below), the ideal evaluation of a screening technology is through the assessment of disease-specific and overall mortality in a randomized clinical trial.

Early detection of an apparently localized cancer does not automatically confer benefit. There are screening tests for some diseases that have been found to be of no benefit, such as chest x-ray screening for lung cancer[141,142] or urine screening for vanillylmandelic acid to detect neuroblastoma.[143] A number of common screening tests used in the United States offer undetermined benefit.

POTENTIAL BIASES

The evaluation of the benefits of a screening test is subject to several biases, including lead-time, length, and selection biases, the influences of which are reduced in a randomized trial.[144] These biases can lead one to believe that there is a benefit to a screening test when, in truth, there is none; there may even be a net harm. Screening, regardless of benefit, will usually increase the number of specific cancers diagnosed. It also can produce a shift in stage toward lower stages that will appear to improve survival statistics without reducing mortality (i.e., the number of deaths of a given cancer per number of people at risk of the disease). In such a case, the apparent duration of survival, measured from the date of diagnosis, would increase without lives truly being saved or life expectancy being changed.

When pure lead-time bias occurs, survival—the time from diagnosis to death—is increased, but treatment does not prolong life. Patients do not live longer; they are merely diagnosed at an earlier date. The screening test only prolongs the time the individual is aware of the disease and the time the individual is treated as a patient.

Length bias occurs when slow-growing, less-aggressive cancers are detected during screening. Cancers diagnosed as the result of the onset of symptoms between scheduled screenings are, on average, more aggressive, and treatment outcomes are not as favorable. An extreme form of length bias is termed overdiagnosis bias, or detection of pseudodisease. Some undetected slow-growing tumors fulfill the histologic criteria for cancer but would never be clinically significant or cause death. This phenomenon is compounded by the fact that the most common cancers are most frequent among older people. Other competing causes of death, such as heart disease, become more relevant. This is particularly common in prostate cancer.

Selection bias must be considered when assessing the results of any clinical trial. The group most likely to seek entry in the study may differ from the general population to which the study results might be applied. In an assessment of a group of individuals undergoing screening, individuals may have volunteered because of a particular risk factor not found in the larger population, such as a strong family history. In general, volunteers are more health-conscious and are likely to have better prognoses or lower mortality rates regardless of actually being screened; this trend is referred to as the "healthy volunteer effect."

ASSESSMENT OF SCREENING TESTS

As a result of the biases above, a screening intervention is best evaluated in a population-based, randomized, controlled screening trial with cause-specific mortality as the endpoint.[144] Because gold-standard randomized screening trials for cancer are perforce large (often involving thousands of people) and last for years, less-definitive study designs often are used to estimate the efficacy and effectiveness of screening practices. In order of strength of evidence, efficacy can by assessed using the following:

- Findings of internally controlled trials in which intervention-allocation methods other than randomization are used, such as allocation determined by birth date or by date of clinic visit;
- Results of cohort or case-control analytic observational studies;
- Findings of multiple time series studies, with or without the intervention; and
- Opinions of respected authorities based on clinical experience, descriptive studies, or consensus reports of experts.

The last form of evidence is the weakest, because even experts can easily be misled by the biases described above.

POTENTIAL HARMFUL EFFECTS

Subjects can be harmed as a result of screening. A harmful effect can be associated with the test itself, the work-up of positive results of screening tests (both true-positive and false-positive results), and injuries from the treatment of true-positive results. Screening can detect some cancers that would never have caused medical problems; the unnecessary treatment of these cancers can be harmful. Aside from the adverse effects of screening and the subsequent work-up and extra treatment, there are the financial costs associated with screening and all of the above extra tests and treatments.

ACCURACY

The accuracy of any medical test is usually described using four indices: sensitivity, specificity, positive predictive value, and negative predictive value. The results of screening tests can be classified into four categories (Tables 1-5 and 1-6). Sensitivity and specificity are relatively independent of the underlying prevalence or risk of the population being screened, but the positive and negative predictive values are highly dependent on prevalence (Table 1-7). In other words, screening is most beneficial, efficient, and economical when targeting a cancer

Table 1-5 Indices for Describing the Accuracy of Screening Tests

Term	Definition	Ability of Test	Equation
Sensitivity	Proportion of people with the disease who have a positive result on a screening test	To detect disease when it is present	A / (A+C)
Specificity	Proportion of people who do not have the disease who have a negative result on a screening test	To correctly identify the absence of disease	D / (B+D)
Positive predictive value	Proportion of people with a positive result on a screening test who actually have the disease	To accurately predict the presence of disease	A / (A+B)
Negative predictive value	Proportion of people who have a negative result on a screening test who truly do not have the disease	To accurately predict the absence of disease	D / (C+D)

Abbreviations: A, true-positive result; B, false-positive result; C, false-negative result; D, true-negative result.

Table 1-6 Types of Results of Screening Tests

	Condition Present	Condition Absent
Positive Results	True positive (A)	False positive (B)
Negative Results	False negative (C)	True negative (D)

Table 1-7 Influence of Prevalence on Predictive Value

Positive Predictive Value for a Disease with Prevalence of 5 Affected Individuals per 1,000 Population			Positive Predictive Value for a Disease with Prevalence of 1 Affected Individual per 10,000 Population		
	Sensitivity			Sensitivity	
	0.8	0.95		0.8	0.95
Specificity			Specificity		
0.95	7%	9%	0.95	0.2%	0.2%
0.999	80%	83%	0.999	7%	9%

common to the general population or groups with a high prevalence (or high risk) of the specific disease being screened. Sensitivity need not be extremely high (Table 1-7). However, it is worth reiterating that the key criterion for the public health recommendation of a screening test is that it is able to reduce cancer mortality.[145]

A screening test that is not efficacious in reducing mortality in an average-risk population does not become efficacious if used in a high-risk population. It is certainly preferred to utilize screening tests in higher-risk populations (e.g., those with family history, or a lung cancer screening test in smokers), but this is because the yield will be higher, and thus the cost-effectiveness and, more importantly, the positive predictive value will be better (i.e., there will be fewer false positives). But if the screening test is not effective (i.e., does not reduce mortality), it will also not reduce mortality in higher-risk populations and should not be utilized. A good example is chest x-ray screening, which has been shown to not reduce lung cancer mortality. Its use in heavy smokers or asbestos workers would not make it "work" any better in those populations and it should not be used in these patients. The Prostate, Lung, Colorectal, and Ovarian (PLCO) Cancer Screening Trial recently demonstrated that CA-125 and transvaginal ultrasound screening are not effective in reducing the mortality from ovarian cancer (discussed below). Thus, the use of such screening in *BRCA* carriers would not be indicated despite their high risk.

KEY POINTS

- Evaluation of the benefits and efficacy of a cancer screening test is far more complicated than simply the performance of the test and the yield of localized cancers.
- The biases of screening are volunteer selection, lead-time, length, and overdiagnosis. These biases can make a screening test appear beneficial when there is actually no benefit, or even harm.
- To offset these biases, a randomized trial is the best way to assess a screening test with the endpoint of reduction in cancer-related mortality.

SCREENING FOR SPECIFIC CANCERS

Results from well-executed studies are convincing that screening for cervix, colorectal, and breast cancers is beneficial at certain ages for people at average risk. Although special surveillance of individuals at high risk for some specific cancers because of family history or genetic risk may be prudent, few studies have been carried out to assess its true worth.

A number of organizations have evaluated certain screening tests and considered whether to endorse routine use of such measures. The U.S. Preventive Services Task Force (USPSTF)[146] and the Canadian Task Force on Preventive Health Care[147] published screening recommendations after a rigorous review process. Each recommendation is made with a thorough, structured evaluation of the literature by screening experts. ACS publishes the most commonly quoted screening guidelines (Table 1-8).[148]

BREAST CANCER

Studies of breast self-examination have not shown that this practice decreases mortality.[149] The results of the largest randomized, controlled study of breast self-examination reported to date showed both an increased rate of biopsy and enhanced detection of benign lesions but little or no stage shift and no reduction in breast cancer mortality.[150]

Findings from several randomized trials indicate that screening women older than 50 with normal risk using mammography alone or mammography and clinical breast examination every 1 to 2 years decreases mortality by 20% to 30%. Each trial has been criticized for a certain aspect of its design, but there is power in the consistency of the observations.[151]

Experts disagree on whether women of average risk between ages 40 and 49 benefit from screening (Table 1-8). A meta-analysis of seven large randomized trials showed no benefit from mammography screening for women in this age group when assessed 5 to 7 years after trial entry.[152] There was a small benefit for women at 10 to 14 years after entry, which may have been the result of screening these women after they turned 50.[153] Nonetheless, current U.S. guidelines recommend initiating screening at age 40. There is no consensus on the age at which to cease screening. A recent re-analysis sponsored by the USPSTF suggested that screening before age 50 was not necessarily beneficial.[154] Although there was a potential 18% reduction in mortality, the number needed to screen to achieve this and the concomitant number of false positives that needed to be evaluated were so high that the USPSTF argued that the risk-benefit ratio for screening before age 50 was not worthwhile. The resulting disagreement from women's groups, political agencies, radiologists, and others has caused these guidelines not to be implemented as policy.

The results from outcomes studies show that there is substantial variation among U.S. radiologists regarding recommendations for additional testing or biopsy. This disparity is especially notable among younger women. In large cohorts, nearly one-half of all women between ages 40 and 49 screened annually for 10 years will have false-positive mammograms necessitating repeat mammography, ultrasound examination, magnetic resonance imaging (MRI), or biopsy. In addition, the diagnosis of ductal carcinoma in situ has risen dramatically since the widespread introduction of mammographic screening for women younger than 50.

Mammography may not be as sensitive for detecting breast cancers among women with *BRCA1* or *BRCA2* mutations, possibly because these women tend to develop cancers at a younger age, when mammography is less sensitive. Studies have suggested that MRI has greater sensitivity than mammography or ultrasound. Its high cost and unproven survival benefit make it undesirable for general use, but it can increase yield in a cost-effective fashion for young *BRCA* mutation carriers[155,156] and for

Table 1-8 Screening Recommendations for Asymptomatic Patients with Normal Risk*

Test or Procedure	U.S. Preventive Services Task Force	Canadian Task Force on Preventive Health Care	American Cancer Society
Fecal occult blood testing (FOBT) for colorectal cancer	Annual FOBT for individual age 50 or older	FOBT every 1 to 2 years for individual age 50 or older	Annually, FOBT or fecal immunochemical test (FIT) starting at age 50 (FIT preferred)
Flexible sigmoidoscopy for colorectal cancer	Flexible sigmoidoscopy every 5 years for individual age 50 or older	Flexible sigmoidoscopy every 5 years for individual age 50 or older	Flexible sigmoidoscopy every 5 years, starting at age 50
Double contrast barium enema (DCBE) for colorectal cancer	Every 5 years for individual age 50 or older	No recommendation	Every 5 years, starting at age 50
Colonoscopy for colorectal cancer	Every 10 years for individual age 50 or older	Insufficient evidence	Every 10 years, starting at age 50
CT colonography for colorectal cancer	Insufficient evidence	Insufficient evidence	Every 5 years, starting at age 50
Digital rectal examination (DRE)	No recommendation	Poor evidence to include or exclude for men older than age 50	No recommendation
Prostate-specific antigen (PSA) and DRE for prostate cancer	Insufficient evidence to recommend	Insufficient evidence to include PSA in periodic health exam (PHE). Poor evidence to include or exclude DRE from PHE	Shared decision between physician and patient. Annually, starting at age 50 in men with a life expectancy of 10 or more years
Pap test for cervix cancer	Begin 3 years after the onset of sexual activity or age 21, whichever first. Pap smear every 3 years from age 21 to age 65, or alternatively Pap smear combined with HPV testing every 5 years starting at age 30	Annual screening to begin following initiation of sexual activity or at age 18. After two normal smears, screen every 3 years to age 69	Begin at age 21. Screen every 3 years with conventional Pap tests or liquid-based Pap tests. At or after age 30, women with three normal tests in a row may screen every 3 years with cervix cytology alone, or every 5 years with HPV DNA test plus cervix cytology. Women age 65 and older who have had three or more normal Pap tests and no abnormal tests in the last 10 years and women who have had a total hysterectomy may choose to stop cervix cancer screening
Breast self-examination (BSE) for breast cancer	Recommends against clinicians teaching women how to perform BSE	Insufficient evidence to make recommendation	Beginning in their early 20s, women should be advised about the limitations and benefits of BSE. Women may choose not to do BSE or to do BSE irregularly or regularly
Clinical breast examination (CBE) for breast cancer	Insufficient evidence to recommend adding over and above mammography	Recommended with mammogram	Every 3 years for women in their 20s and 30s, annually for women age 40 and older
Mammography for breast cancer	Every 2 years for women age 50 to 74. Screening before age 50 should take into account patient context and patient values regarding specific benefits and harms	Mammogram and CBE every year for women age 50 to 69	Annually, starting at age 40
Low-dose CT scan for lung cancer	No recommendation	No recommendation	For those age 55 to 75 with a 30-pack-year smoking history, a discussion should be held regarding potential benefits and harms of screening. Smoking cessation should be emphasized.
Cancer-related check-up	No recommendation	No recommendation	On the occasion of a PHE, cancer-related check-up should include exam for cancers of the thyroid, testicles, ovaries, lymph nodes, oral cavity, and skin. Counseling about tobacco cessation, sun exposure, diet and nutrition, risk factors, sexual practices, and environmental and occupational exposures should occur at the time of the health exam

*These recommendations were made for the general population—asymptomatic people who have no risk factors, other than age or gender, for the targeted condition.

Abbreviation: CT, computed tomography; HPV, human papillomavirus.

other women at increased risk for breast cancer.[157] ACS has developed guidelines[158] for the use of MRI for women who have a lifetime risk of breast cancer that is 20% to 25% or greater as determined by the BRCAPRO statistical model[159] or in some other way.

CERVIX CANCER

No randomized clinical trial has been conducted to determine whether cervix cancer screening with a Pap test reduces mortality, but findings from several cohort and case-control studies have shown the utility of this test in reducing mortality. Indeed, the introduction of this test in the late 1940s was accompanied by a dramatic decline in the incidence of cervix cancer in the United States (Fig. 1-1). Routine Pap testing is recommended for women who are sexually active and 21 or older. The recommended interval for Pap testing has recently been increased to 2 to 3 years by several organizations (Table 1-8). An upper age limit at which screening ceases to be effective is not known. In the United States, Pap testing has resulted in a decrease in cervix cancer incidence because screening usually finds and eliminates the precursor lesion, cervix intraepithelial neoplasia.

Current guidelines recommend that screening for cervix cancer with cytology (Pap testing) should start at age 21, regardless of the age of first intercourse.[160,161] In March 2012, the ACS, USPSTF, and the American College of Obstetrics and Gynecology jointly released updated guidelines that endorsed screening every 5 years for women over age 30 with combined cytologic testing and HPV DNA testing. If normal by age 65, women could stop further screening. Women with certain risk factors, such as infection with HIV, might be screened more frequently.

The association of cervix cancer with HPV has led to the use of HPV DNA testing as the sole means of screening for cervix neoplasia. This has been recommended for use in resource-poor environments where Pap tests are difficult to conduct properly. In addition, HPV testing can be used to identify women at higher risk for development of cervical intraepithelial neoplasia when the Pap test cytologic diagnosis is atypical squamous cells of undetermined significance.[162]

COLORECTAL CANCER

Several methods are recommended for colorectal cancer screening:

- Fecal occult blood testing
- Sigmoidoscopy
- Colonoscopy
- Radiographic barium contrast studies
- Computed tomography (CT) colonography

The results of randomized studies indicate that annual fecal occult blood testing can reduce colorectal cancer mortality by one-third.[163] The rate of false-positive results for fecal occult blood testing is 1% to 5%. Fewer than 10% of patients with occult blood found in stool analysis have cancer, and approximately one-fifth to one-third have adenomas.

Findings from two case-control studies found that screening sigmoidoscopy is associated with a decrease in mortality among participants 50 and older.[164] The results from other studies show that approximately one-half of all polyps are found with the 35-cm flexible scope and two-thirds to three-quarters are found with a 60-cm scope. Diagnosis of polyps by sigmoidoscopy should lead to evaluation of the entire colon with colonoscopy.

Three randomized trials of sigmoidoscopy have published their findings. One from Great Britain[165] showed a clear-cut mortality benefit for sigmoidoscopy that was quite dramatic, and may justify the use of sigmoidoscopy as a routine screening test, perhaps even as an alternative to colonoscopy. A second trial from Italy showed an 18% statistically significant reduction in colorectal cancer incidence and a 22% reduction in overall mortality that was not statistically significant.[166] The PLCO trial in the United States has also reported the results of its randomized trial of sigmoidoscopy, the largest of the three studies with over 150,000 participants.[167] This study showed significant 21% and 26% reductions in overall colorectal cancer incidence and mortality. All three randomized trials showed dramatic and significant reductions in distal colon cancer incidence and mortality, but there was no benefit for cancers in the proximal colon.

Several recent reports, all well-conducted observational studies, explored the benefits of colonoscopy in reducing mortality. At least four such reports found that although colonoscopy did reduce incidence and mortality in the left colon, it did not have the expected benefits on the right side of the colon that are the reasons for its use. The reasons for this finding are unclear and may represent differences in the biology of right-sided versus left-sided lesions or differences in the expertise of endoscopists in examining the right side of the colon.[168] One recent study from Germany[169] did suggest a reduced incidence of right-sided neoplasia with the use of colonoscopy, so perhaps it is a population-specific phenomenon. A case-control study by Baxter et al[170] demonstrated an overall reduction in colorectal cancer mortality of about 60% with the use of screening colonoscopy and showed a benefit of screening for the right colon; presumably this was because the vast majority of colonoscopies in the United States are done by gastroenterologists who have greater expertise. A recent study from the Harvard cohort studies has confirmed the overall benefit of colonoscopy as well as its benefit on the right side of the colon.[171]

Although no study results have clearly demonstrated benefit, it is prudent to use colonoscopy as a screening tool for individuals at average risk for colorectal cancer. This rationale is an extension of the available data for sigmoidoscopy, which show a mortality benefit almost exclusively for left-sided cancers and no benefit for the right side of the colon where the sigmoidoscope does not reach.[172] Colonoscopy should be used for those at high risk, such as those with a genetic predisposition to colorectal cancer and those with inflammatory bowel disease. Little information is available on the utility of the barium enema as a screening tool. Recent interest has centered on

CT (virtual) colonography as well. The evidence suggests that, in certain instances, it may substitute for colonoscopy.

Guidelines for colorectal cancer screening continue to evolve. Although ACS currently recommends the full range of screening tests listed above as options for screening, new guidelines were published in November 2008 by a working group composed of members from ACS and the American College of Radiology and experts in gastroenterology.[173] These guidelines put increased emphasis on structural tests that could "detect adenomatous polyps and cancer" as opposed to "tests that primarily detect cancer," essentially suggesting that the fecal tests, guaiac-based occult blood testing and fecal immunochemical testing, were less desirable than endoscopy or CT colonography. It is notable that CT colonography was recommended along with endoscopy. Almost simultaneously, the USPSTF released its newest recommendations,[174] which include fecal occult blood testing, sigmoidoscopy, and colonoscopy, and conclude that the evidence is currently insufficient to recommend CT colonography. An excellent discussion of the relative merits and approaches of these two sets of recommendations can be found in an editorial accompanying the USPSTF report.[175]

LUNG CANCER

Screening for lung cancer with chest x-ray and sputum cytologic testing was evaluated in four randomized lung cancer screening trials in the 1960s and 1970s. No reduction in lung cancer mortality was seen in those studies.[176,177] A randomized trial of chest x-ray screening was recently conducted as part of the PLCO study to re-evaluate its value. The results of this study reaffirmed the absence of benefit for chest x-ray screening.[141]

Studies have shown that spiral CT can diagnose lung cancers at early stages, but it is unclear whether it will save lives.[178-180] This technology was evaluated in a large, randomized clinical trial of heavy smokers which compared CT screening to chest x-ray screening. These results were reported from the NLST trial[181] and showed a 20% reduction in mortality for the arm screened with CT. Spiral CT also can detect many benign processes that cause noncalcified lung radiodensities; these are false-positive findings. Spiral CT does increase the number of lesions diagnosed and, thus, will increase the number of diagnostic and therapeutic procedures performed (see Fig. 7-3 in Chapter 7: Lung Cancer). Recently, overall policy reviews have been conducted for spiral CT screening, and they conclude that the benefits for certain subgroups of heavy smokers outweigh the negatives of overdetection and false positives. The USPSTF recommends CT screening for current or former heavy smokers of more than 30-packs per year.[182,183]

OVARIAN CANCER

Adnexal palpation, transvaginal ultrasound, and measurement of serum CA-125 have been considered for ovarian cancer screening. No randomized prospective trial of screening for ovarian cancer has shown an improvement in ovarian cancer mortality. The results of such studies could lead to futile invasive diagnostic testing that might include laparotomy. A recent clinical trial (PLCO) randomly assigned more than 78,000 women to screening with CA-125 and transvaginal ultrasound for 4 years or usual care, and it found no difference in ovarian cancer mortality.[184]

PROSTATE CANCER

The digital rectal examination (DRE) and measurement of serum PSA are commonly used in the United States, although most professional organizations advise caution in the use of such screening tools (Table 1-8). No well-designed, -conducted, and -analyzed study has been completed to test the true benefits of screening and treatment of prostate cancer.[185] Prostate cancer is prone to lead-time bias, length bias, and overdiagnosis. Whereas screening using PSA levels and DRE clearly detects many asymptomatic cancers, its ability to reliably distinguish tumors that could be lethal but are still curable from those that pose little or no threat to health is limited. It has been estimated that more than 30% of localized prostate cancers diagnosed during screening are indolent and clinically insignificant. Treatment of screen-detected cancers may cause morbidity, such as impotence and urinary incontinence, and carries a small risk of death.[186]

Most expert organizations do not recommend screening for prostate cancer. The USPSTF examined the evidence in support of screening and found there was insufficient evidence to recommend it.[186,187] ACS and the American Urological Association recommend that men older than 50 at normal risk be offered screening and be allowed to make a choice after being informed of its potential risks and benefits (Table 1-8).

The interim results of two large randomized trials of prostate screening have been reported. The PLCO trial randomly assigned 76,693 men to 6 years of annual screening with PSA or regular management according to community standards. In essence, 85% of the men in the intervention group were screened, and more than 40% of the men in the control arm were screened. After 7 to 10 years, there was no mortality benefit (HR 1.13, 95% CI 0.75, 1.70).[188] The European Randomised Study of Screening for Prostate Cancer (ERSPC) randomly selected 182,000 men in seven countries; each country had slight differences in study design. The intervention group was offered PSA screening every 4 years (every 2 years in Sweden), and 82% participated; a cut-off of 3 was used for the PSA rather than the usual 4. With a median follow-up of 9 years, the HR for mortality was 0.80 (95% CI 0.65, 0.98). It is notable that 1,410 men needed to be screened (16% of patients being screened had an abnormal PSA and required biopsy and further evaluation) to prevent one death, and 48 cases of prostate cancer were detected among those 1,410 men to save that one life.[189]

SKIN CANCER

No randomized study has been conducted to assess whether screening for skin cancer decreases mortality. Screening programs in Scotland and Australia may have caused the stage shift in diagnosed melanomas.[190] These programs also may reinforce sun avoidance and other prevention behaviors.

OTHER CANCERS

The dramatic rise in the incidence of esophageal adenocarcinoma during the past 2 decades has raised concerns about prevention. These tumors are known to arise from Barrett esophagus, a metaplastic change in the esophageal mucosa that later progresses to dysplasia and malignancy. The main risk factor for Barrett esophagus is gastroesophageal reflux disease, a condition that has increased dramatically, perhaps partially because of the epidemic of obesity. Thus, there has been a major effort to conduct esophagogastroduodenoscopy on patients with persistent gastroesophageal reflux disease to detect early-stage Barrett esophagus and to intervene in this pathway with the use of proton pump inhibitors and close surveillance with endoscopy. This has become a recommendation of the American Gastroenterological Association, despite the absence of any randomized trial or other high-quality evidence demonstrating a significant benefit from the point of view of cancer prevention or survival benefit.[191]

Although this chapter has focused on cancer screening in the United States, it is worth noting that screening for some cancers may be worthwhile in other countries where these cancers are more common. One example is oral cancer, which is the most common cancer among men in India, largely because of the chewing of betel nuts. A randomized trial has shown that in this region the use of visual screening of the oral cavity reduced mortality significantly.[192] HCC is a common cancer in large portions of East Asia and Africa, related to chronic hepatitis B infection. A trial was conducted in Shanghai of over 18,000 carriers of hepatitis B, who were randomly assigned to a serum alpha-fetoprotein (AFP) test plus ultrasonography every 6 months or no screening. At 5 years, the HCC mortality was reduced by 37% in the screened group (HR 0.63, 95% CI 0.41, 0.98).[193]

Another common screening test is the use of photofluorography in Japan to screen for gastric cancer. No randomized trial has been conducted to confirm the efficacy of this test in reducing mortality.[194]

SURVIVORSHIP

It is estimated that there are currently 12 million cancer survivors in the United States, and this number is likely to grow in the coming years. This is a good thing, of course, to the degree that it reflects the increasing success of treatment in curing (or at least prolonging life for) those diagnosed with cancer. The number of cancer survivors is also increasing because of the aging of the population with a concomitant increase in cancer cases and because of the increased use of screening and diagnostic tests, and thus the increased diagnosis of subclinical disease.

Cancer survivors share a substantial number of issues and problems that are currently the subjects of intensive research efforts, including their psychologic needs, employment issues, appropriate surveillance, and management of long-term toxicities of treatment. It is also critical to bear in mind that they are at increased risk for second malignancies as an overall group. Some may be at increased risk for certain specific cancers.[195] They require, at the least, special attention to make sure that they obtain the screening studies that are recommended for the general population. For those who have special risks, they may require that special screening protocols be utilized. For example, MRI screening may be recommended for young breast cancer survivors who are at very high risk for a contralateral breast cancer.

It is mandatory that a good working relationship be established between the oncologist and the primary care physician.[191] Some studies have shown that regular wellness care may be neglected for cancer survivors under the stress and pressure of a cancer diagnosis and its treatment.[192-194] The standard protocols of good medical care, including hypertension, lipid, and other screening and vaccination protocols, should be followed for cancer survivors as they would be for any other adult. In addition, there is increasing evidence that improved lifestyle and other prevention activities, such as weight loss, tobacco cessation, increased physical activity, and a moderate diet, may improve the incidence of second malignancies and may reduce the recurrence of the initial primary cancer. In coming years, the medical oncologist is likely to play an increasing role as a

KEY POINTS

- The PLCO study yielded new data on screening for four cancers. It has confirmed that chest x-ray screening is ineffective for lung cancer, confirmed that sigmoidoscopy is efficacious in reducing mortality for colorectal cancer, provided definitive evidence that CA-125 and transvaginal ultrasound screening for ovarian cancer are not effective, and provided negative data on prostate-specific antigen (PSA) screening for prostate cancer.

- Although mammography screening for breast cancer in women older than 50 has significant evidence in its support, screening in women younger than 50 and PSA screening in men for prostate cancer both remain controversial. In both circumstances, the absolute mortality reduction is small and the number needed to screen is large, making the risk-benefit ratio a major concern from a policy standpoint.

- New data from a randomized trial suggest that low-dose spiral computed tomography screening may be a future approach to reducing lung cancer mortality among heavy smokers.

- The use of human papillomavirus DNA testing in conjunction with Pap smear testing for women 30 and older can allow the prolongation of the interval between screening for cervix cancer to extend to 5 years.

- Randomized trial data is now substantial enough to support the use of both fecal occult blood testing and sigmoidoscopy as screening modalities for colorectal cancer.

- Despite its widespread use, the evidence supporting the use of colonoscopy for colorectal cancer screening is modest but growing.

primary and secondary prevention expert, similar to the ways in which cardiologists counsel their patients on tobacco cessation, weight loss, physical activity, and lipid management.[196]

References

1. Howlader N, Noone AM, Krapcho M, et al. SEER Cancer Statistics Review, 1975-2009. Bethesda, MD: National Cancer Institute. seer.cancer.gov/csr/1975_2009. Accessed November 5, 2012.

2. Siegel R, Maj J, Zou Z, et al. Cancer statistics, 2014. *CA Cancer J Clin.* 2014;64:9-29. PMID: 24399786.

3. Crew KD, Neugut AI. Epidemiology of gastric cancer. *World J Gastroenterol.* 2006;12:354-362. PMID: 16489633.

4. Cronin KA, Feuer EJ, Clarke LD, et al. Impact of adjuvant therapy and mammography on U.S. mortality from 1975 to 2000: comparison of mortality results from the cisnet breast cancer base case analysis. *J Natl Cancer Inst Monogr.* 2006;36:112-121. PMID: 17032901.

5. Berry DA, Cronin KA, Plevritis SK, et al. Effect of screening and adjuvant therapy on mortality from breast cancer. *N Engl J Med.* 2005;353:1784-1792. PMID: 16251534.

6. Jemal A, Devesa SS, Hartge P, et al. Recent trends in cutaneous melanoma incidence among whites in the United States. *J Natl Cancer Inst.* 2001;93:678-683. PMID: 11333289.

7. Simard EP, Ward EM, Siegel R, et al. Cancers with increasing incidence trends in the United States: 1999 through 2008. *CA Cancer J Clin.* Epub 2012 Jan 4. PMID: 22281605.

8. Whitman S, Ansell D, Orsi J, et al. The racial disparity in breast cancer mortality. *J Community Health.* 2011;36:588-596. PMID: 21190070.

9. Lux MP, Fasching PA, Beckmann MW. Hereditary breast and ovarian cancer: review and future perspectives. *J Mol Med (Berl).* 2006;84:16-28. PMID: 16283147.

10. Feinberg AP. An epigenetic approach to cancer etiology. *Cancer J.* 2007;13:70-74. PMID: 17464249.

11. Risch A, Plass C. Lung cancer epigenetics and genetics. *Int J Cancer.* 2008;123:1-7. PMID: 18425819.

12. Ahmed FE. Colorectal cancer epigenetics: the role of environmental factors and the search for molecular biomarkers. *J Environ Sci Health C Environ Carcinog Ecotoxicol Rev.* 2007;25:101-154. PMID: 17558783.

13. Weisburger JH. Worldwide prevention of cancer and other chronic diseases based on knowledge of mechanisms. *Mutat Res.* 1998;402:331-337. PMID: 9675332.

14. Brawley OW. Population categorization and cancer statistics. *Cancer Metastasis Rev.* 2003;22:11-19. PMID: 12716032.

15. Kulldorff M, Feuer EJ, Miller BA, et al. Breast cancer clusters in the northeast United States: a geographic analysis. *Am J Epidemiol.* 1997;146:161-170. PMID: 9230778.

16. Link BG, Northridge ME, Phelan JC, et al. Social epidemiology and the fundamental cause concept: on the structuring of effective cancer screens by socioeconomic status. *Milbank Q.* 1998;76:375-402, 304-305. PMID: 9738168.

17. Ayanian, JZ, Kohler BA, Abe T, et al. The relation between health insurance coverage and clinical outcomes among women with breast cancer. *N Engl J Med.* 1993;329:326-331. PMID: 8321261.

18. Hodgson DC, Fuchs CS, Ayanian JZ. Impact of patient and provider characteristics on the treatment and outcomes of colorectal cancer. *J Natl Cancer Inst.* 2001;93:501-515. PMID: 11287444.

19. Penson DF, Stoddard ML, Pasta DJ, et al. The association between socioeconomic status, health insurance coverage, and quality of life in men with prostate cancer. *J Clin Epidemiol.* 2001;54:350-358. PMID: 11297885.

20. Willett WC, Stampfer MJ, Colditz GA, et al. Dietary fat and the risk of breast cancer. *N Engl J Med.* 1987;316:22-28. PMID: 3785347.

21. Gilligan MA, Kneusel RT, Hoffmann RG, et al. Persistent differences in sociodemographic determinants of breast conserving treatment despite overall increased adoption. *Med Care.* 2002;40:181-189. PMID: 11880791.

22. Lu-Yao G, Albertsen PC, Stanford JL, et al. Natural experiment examining impact of aggressive screening and treatment on prostate cancer mortality in two fixed cohorts from Seattle area and Connecticut. *BMJ.* 2002;325:740. PMID: 12364300.

23. Albano JD, Ward E, Jemal A, et al. Cancer mortality in the United States by education level and race. *J Natl Cancer Inst.* 2007;99:1384-1394. PMID: 17848670.

24. DeLancey JO, Thun MJ, Jemal A, et al. Recent trends in Black-White disparities in cancer mortality. *Cancer Epidemiol Biomarkers Prev.* 2008;17:2908-2912. PMID: 18990730.

25. Brown LM, Devesa SS. Epidemiologic trends in esophageal and gastric cancer in the United States. *Surg Oncol Clin N Am.* 2002;11:235-256. PMID: 12424848.

26. Albain KS, Unger JM, Crowley JJ, et al. Racial disparities in cancer survival among randomized clinical trials patients of the Southwest Oncology Group. *J Natl Cancer Inst.* 2009;101:984-992. PMID: 19584328.

27. Shavers VL, Brown ML. Racial and ethnic disparities in the receipt of cancer treatment. *J Natl Cancer Inst.* 2002;94:334-357. PMID: 11880473.

28. Liang W, Burnett CB, Rowland JH, et al. Communication between physicians and older women with localized breast cancer: implications for treatment and patient satisfaction. *J Clin Oncol.* 2002;20:1008-1016. PMID: 11844824.

29. Gornick ME, Eggers PW, Reilly TW, et al. Effects of race and income on mortality and use of services among Medicare beneficiaries. *N Engl J Med.* 1996;335:791-799. PMID: 8703185.

30. Greenwald P. Lifestyle and medical approaches to cancer prevention. *Recent Results Cancer Res.* 2005;166:1-15. PMID: 15648179.

31. Thun MJ, Apicella LF, Henley SJ. Smoking vs other risk factors as the cause of smoking-attributable deaths: confounding in the courtroom. *JAMA.* 2000;284:706-712. PMID: 10927778.

32. Shields PG. Tobacco smoking, harm reduction, and biomarkers. *J Natl Cancer Inst.* 2002;94:1435-1444. PMID: 12359853.

33. Wynder EL, Muscat JE. The changing epidemiology of smoking and lung cancer histology. *Environ Health Perspect.* 1995;103 Suppl 8:143-148. PMID: 8741774.

34. Carpenter CL, Jarvik ME, Morgenstern H, et al. Mentholated cigarette smoking and lung-cancer risk. *Ann Epidemiol.* 1999;9:114-120. PMID: 10037555.

35. Hu MC, Davies M, Kandel DB. Epidemiology and correlates of daily smoking and nicotine dependence among young adults in the United States. *Am J Publ Health.* 2006;96:299-308. PMID: 16380569.

36. Mahvan T, Namdar R, Voorhees K, et al. Clinical Inquiry: which smoking cessation interventions work best? *J Fam Pract.* 2011;60:430-431. PMID: 21731922.

37. Weaver KE, Danhauer SC, Tooze JA, et al. Smoking cessation counseling beliefs and behaviors of outpatient oncology providers. *Oncologist.* 2012;17:455-462. PMID: 22334454.

38. Stoner WI, Foley BX. Current tobacco control policy trends in the United States. *Clin Occup Environ Med.* 2006;5:85-99, ix. PMID: 16446256.

39. Jha P, Chaloupka FJ, Corrao M, et al. Reducing the burden of smoking worldwide: effectiveness of interventions and their coverage. *Drug Alcohol Rev.* 2006;25:597-609. PMID: 17132576.

40. Jha P, Jacob B, Gajalakshmi V, et al. A nationally representative case-control study of smoking and death in India. *N Engl J Med.* 2008;358:1137-1147. PMID: 18272886.

41. Law M, Tang JL. An analysis of the effectiveness of interventions intended to help people stop smoking. *Arch Int Med.* 1995;155:1933-1941. PMID: 7575046.

42. A clinical practice guideline for treating tobacco use and dependence: A US Public Health Service report. The Tobacco Use and Dependence Clinical Practice Guideline Panel, Staff and Consortium Representatives. *JAMA.* 2000;283:3244-3254. PMID: 10866874.

43. Fairchild AL, Bayer R, Colgrove J. The renormalization of smoking? E-cigarettes and the tobacco "endgame". *N Engl J Med.* 2014;370:293-295. PMID: 24350902.

44. Baker F, Ainsworth SR, Dye JT, et al. Health risks associated with cigar smoking. *JAMA.* 2000;284:735-740. PMID: 10927783.

45. Nasrollahzadeh D, Kamangar F, Aghcheli K, et al. Opium, tobacco, and alcohol use in relation to oesophageal squamous cell carcinoma in a high-risk area of Iran. *Br J Cancer.* 2008;98:1857-1863. PMID: 18475303.

46. Schütze M, Boeing H, Pischon T, et al. Alcohol attributable burden of incidence of cancer in eight European countries based on results from prospective cohort study. *BMJ.* 2011;342:d1584. PMID: 21474525.

47. Allen NE, Beral V, Casabonne D, et al. Moderate alcohol intake and cancer incidence in women. *J Natl Cancer Inst.* 2009;101:296-305. PMID: 19244173.

48. Schutze M, Boeing H, Pischon T, et al. Alcohol attributable burden of incidence of cancer in eight European countries based on results from prospective cohort study. *BMJ.* 2011;342:1584. PMID: 21474525.

49. Lazovich D, Vogel RI, Berwick M, et al. Indoor tanning and risk of melanoma: a case-control study in a highly exposed population. *Cancer Epidemiol Biomarkers Prev.* 2010;19:1557-1568. PMID: 20507845.

50. Lim HW, James WD, Rigel DS, et al. Adverse effects of ultraviolet radiation from the use of indoor tanning equipment: time to ban the tan. *J Am Acad Dermatol.* 2011;64:e51-e60. PMID: 21295374.

51. Green AC, Williams GM, Logan V, et al. Reduced melanoma after regular sunscreen use: randomized trial follow-up. *J Clin Oncol.* 2011;29:257-263. PMID: 21135266.

52. Greenwald P, Clifford CK, Milner JA. Diet and cancer prevention. *Eur J Cancer.* 2001;37:948-965. PMID: 11334719.

53. Key TJ, Schatzkin A, Willett WC, et al. Diet, nutrition and the prevention of cancer. *Public Health Nutr.* 2004;7:187-200. PMID: 14972060.

54. Schatzkin A, Lanza E, Polyp Prevention Trial Study Group. Polyps and vegetables (and fat, fibre): the polyp prevention trial. *IARC Sci Publ.* 2002;156:463-466. PMID: 12484235.

55. Park Y, Hunter DJ, Spiegelman D, et al. Dietary fiber intake and risk of colorectal cancer: a pooled analysis of prospective cohort studies. *JAMA.* 2005;294:2849-2857. PMID: 16352792.

56. Prentice RL, Caan B, Chlebowski RT, et al. Low-fat dietary pattern and risk of invasive breast cancer: the Women's Health Initiative Randomized Controlled Dietary Modification Trial. *JAMA.* 2006;295:629-642. PMID: 16467232.

57. Beresford SA, Johnson KC, Ritenbaugh C, et al. Low-fat dietary pattern and risk of colorectal cancer: the Women's Health Initiative Randomized Controlled Dietary Modification Trial. *JAMA.* 2006;295:643-654. PMID: 16467233.

58. Chlebowski RT, Blackburn GL, Thomson CA, et al. Dietary fat reduction and breast cancer outcome: interim efficacy results from the Women's Intervention Nutrition Study. *J Natl Cancer Inst.* 2006;98:1767-1776. PMID: 17179478.

59. Bianchini F, Kaaks R, Vainio H. Weight control and physical activity in cancer prevention. *Obes Rev.* 2002;3:5-8. PMID: 12119660.

60. Polednak AP. Estimating the number of U.S. incident cancers attributable to obesity and the impact on temporal trends in incidence rates for obesity-related cancers. *Cancer Detect Prev.* 2008;32:190-199. PMID: 18790577.

61. Schottenfeld D, Beebe-Dimmer JL, Buffler PA, et al. Current perspective on the global and United States cancer burden attributable to lifestyle and environmental risk factors. *Annu Rev Public Health.* 2013;34:97-117. PMID: 23514316.

62. Birks S, Peeters A, Backholer K, et al. A systematic review of the impact of weight loss on cancer incidence and mortality. *Obes Rev.* 2012;13:868-891. PMID: 22672203.

63. Wei EK, Wolin KY, Colditz GA. Time course of risk factors in cancer etiology and progression. *J Clin Oncol.* 2010;28:4052-4057. PMID: 20644083.

64. Brenner AV, Tronko MD, Hatch M, et al. I-131 dose response for incident thyroid cancers in Ukraine related to the Chornobyl accident. *Environ Health Perspect.* 2011;119:933-939. PMID: 21406336.

65. Brenner DJ. Minimising medically unwarranted computed tomography scans. *Ann ICRP.* 2012;41:161-169. PMID: 23089015.

66. Serraino D, Piselli P, Scognamiglio P. Viral infections and cancer: epidemiological aspects. *J Biol Regul Homeost Agents.* 2001;15:224-228. PMID: 11693428.

67. Parkin DM. The global health burden of infection-associated cancers in the year 2002. *Int J Cancer.* 2006;118:3030-3044. PMID: 16404738.

68. Chien YC, Jan CF, Kuo HS, et al. Nationwide hepatitis B vaccination program in Taiwan: effectiveness in the 20 years after it was launched. *Epidemiol Rev.* 2006;28:126-135. PMID: 16782778.

69. Roden R, Wu TC. How will HPV vaccines affect cervical cancer? *Nat Rev Cancer.* 2006;6:753-763. PMID: 16990853.

70. Chang MH, You SL, Chen CJ, et al. Decreased incidence of hepatocellular carcinoma in hepatitis B vaccines: a 20-year follow-up study. *J Natl Cancer Inst.* 2009;101:1348-1355. PMID: 19759364.

71. Kreimer AR, Rodriguez AC, Hildesheim A, et al. Proof-of-principle evaluation of the efficacy of fewer than three doses of a bivalent HPV16/18 vaccine. *J Natl Cancer Inst.* 2011;103:1444-1451. PMID: 21908768.

72. Garland SM, Hernandez-Avila M, Wheeler CM, et al. Quadrivalent vaccine against human papillomavirus to prevent anogenital diseases. *N Engl J Med.* 2007;356:1928-1943. PMID: 17494926.

73. FUTURE II Study Group. Quadrivalent vaccine against human papillomavirus to prevent high-grade cervical lesions. *N Engl J Med.* 2007;356:1915-1927. PMID: 17494925.

74. Greenwald P. Cancer chemoprevention. *BMJ.* 2002;324:714-718. PMID: 11909790.

75. Fisher B, Costantino JP, Wickerham DL, et al. Tamoxifen for prevention of breast cancer: report of the National Surgical Adjuvant Breast and Bowel Project P-1 Study. *J Natl Cancer Inst.* 1998;90:1371-1388. PMID: 9747868.

76. Thompson IM, Goodman PJ, Tangen CM, et al. The influence of finasteride on the development of prostate cancer. *N Engl J Med.* 2003;349:215-224. PMID: 12824459.

77. Vogel VG, Costantino JP, Wickerham DL, et al. Effects of tamoxifen vs raloxifene on the risk of developing invasive breast cancer and other disease outcomes: the NSABP Study of Tamoxifen and Raloxifene (STAR) P-2 trial. *JAMA.* 2006;295:2727-2741. PMID: 16754727.

78. Goss PE, Ingle JN, Alés-Martínez JE, et al. Exemestane for breast-cancer prevention in postmenopausal women. *N Engl J Med.* 2011;364:2381-2391. PMID: 21639806.

79. Rothwell PM, Price JF, Fowkes FG, et al. Short-term effects of daily aspirin on cancer incidence, mortality, and non-vascular death: analysis of the time course of risks and benefits in 51 randomised controlled trials. *Lancet.* 2012;379:1602-1612. PMID: 22440946.

80. Algra AM, Rothwell PM. Effects of regular aspirin on long-term cancer incidence and metastasis: a systematic comparison of evidence from observational studies versus randomised trials. *Lancet Oncol.* 2012;13:518-527. PMID: 22440112.

81. Andriole GL, Bostwick DG, Brawley OW, et al. Effect of dutasteride on the risk of prostate cancer. *N Engl J Med.* 2010;362:1192-1202. PMID: 20357281.

82. Hong WK, Lippman SM, Itri LM, et al. Prevention of second primary tumors with isotretinoin in squamous-cell carcinoma of the head and neck. *N Engl J Med.* 1990;323:795-801. PMID: 2202902.

83. Lippman SM, Klein EA, Goodman PJ, et al. Effect of selenium and vitamin E on risk of prostate cancer and other cancers: the Selenium and Vitamin E Cancer Prevention Trial (SELECT). *JAMA.* 2009;301:39-51. PMID: 19066370.

84. Speers C, Brown P. Breast cancer prevention using calcium and vitamin D: a bright future? *J Natl Cancer Inst.* 2008;100:1562-1564. PMID: 19001596.

85. Grant WB, Garland CF, Gorham ED. An estimate of cancer mortality rate reductions in Europe and the US with 1,000 IU of oral vitamin D per day. *Recent Results Cancer Res.* 2007;174:225-234. PMID: 17302200.

86. Gaziano JM, Sesso HD, Christen WG, et al. Multivitamins in the prevention of cancer in men: the Phyisicians' Health Study II randomized controlled trial. *JAMA.* 2012;308:1871-1880. PMID: 23162860.

87. Bolla M, Lefur R, Ton Van J, et al. Prevention of second primary tumours with etretinate in squamous cell carcinoma of the oral cavity and oropharynx. Results of a multicentric double-blind randomised study. *Eur J Cancer.* 1994;30A:767-772. PMID: 7917535.

88. Virtamo J, Pietinen P, Huttunen JK, et al. Incidence of cancer and mortality following alpha-tocopherol and beta-carotene supplementation: a postintervention follow-up. *JAMA.* 2003;290:476-485. PMID: 12876090.

89. Omenn GS, Goodman GE, Thornquist MD, et al. Risk factors for lung cancer and for intervention effects in CARET, the Beta-Carotene and Retinol Efficacy Trial. *J Natl Cancer Inst.* 1996;88:1550-1559. PMID: 8901853.

90. Pastorino U, Infante M, Maioli M, et al. Adjuvant treatment of stage I lung cancer with high-dose vitamin A. *J Clin Oncol.* 1993;11:1216-1222. PMID: 8391063.

91. van Zandwijk N, Dalesio O, Pastorino U, et al. EUROSCAN, a randomized trial of vitamin A and N-acetylcysteine in patients with head and neck cancer or lung cancer. For the EUropean Organization for Research and Treatment of Cancer Head and Neck and Lung Cancer Cooperative Groups. *J Natl Cancer Inst.* 2000;92:977-986. PMID: 10861309.

92. Lippman SM, Lee JJ, Karp DD, et al. Randomized phase III intergroup trial of isotretinoin to prevent second primary tumors in stage I non-small-cell lung cancer. *J Natl Cancer Inst.* 2001;93:605-618. PMID: 11309437.

93. Karp DD, Lee SJ, Keller SM, et al. Randomized, double-blind, placebo-controlled, phase III chemoprevention trial of selenium supplementation in patients with resected stage I non-small cell lung cancer: ECOG 5597. *J Clin Oncol.* 2013;31:4179-4187. PMID: 24002495.

94. Levine N, Moon TE, Cartmel B, et al. Trial of retinol and isotretinoin in skin cancer prevention: a randomized, double-blind, controlled trial. Southwest Skin Cancer Prevention Study Group. *Cancer Epidemiol Biomarkers Prev.* 1997;6:957-961. PMID: 9367070.

95. Greenberg ER, Baron JA, Stukel TA, et al. A clinical trial of beta carotene to prevent basal-cell and squamous-cell cancers of the skin. The Skin Cancer Prevention Study Group. *N Engl J Med.* 1990;323:789-795. PMID: 2202901.

96. Tangrea JA, Edwards BK, Taylor PR, et al. Long-term therapy with low-dose isotretinoin for prevention of basal cell carcinoma: a multicenter clinical trial. Isotretinoin-Basal Cell Carcinoma Study Group. *J Natl Cancer Inst.* 1992;84:328-332. PMID: 1738183.

97. Moon TE, Levine N, Cartmel B, et al. Effect of retinol in preventing squamous cell skin cancer in moderate-risk subjects: a randomized, double-blind,

controlled trial. Southwest Skin Cancer Prevention Study Group. *Cancer Epidemiol Biomarkers Prev.* 1997;6:949-956. PMID: 9367069.

98. Bavinck JN, Tieben LM, Van der Woude FJ, et al. Prevention of skin cancer and reduction of keratotic skin lesions during acitretin therapy in renal transplant recipients: a double-blind, placebo-controlled study. *J Clin Oncol.* 1995;13:1933-1938. PMID: 7636533.

99. Clark LC, Combs GF Jr, Turnbull BW, et al. Effects of selenium supplementation for cancer prevention in patients with carcinoma of the skin. A randomized controlled trial. Nutritional Prevention of Cancer Study Group. *JAMA.* 1996;276:1957-1963. PMID: 8971064.

100. Veronesi U, Maisonneuve P, Costa A, et al. Prevention of breast cancer with tamoxifen: preliminary findings from the Italian randomised trial among hysterectomised women. Italian Tamoxifen Prevention Study. *Lancet.* 1998;352:93-97. PMID: 9672273.

101. Powles T, Eeles R, Ashley S, et al. Interim analysis of the incidence of breast cancer in the Royal Marsden Hospital tamoxifen randomised chemoprevention trial. *Lancet.* 1998;352:98-101. PMID: 9672274.

102. Fisher B, Dignam J, Wolmark N, et al. Tamoxifen in treatment of intraductal breast cancer: National Surgical Adjuvant Breast and Bowel Project B-24 randomised controlled trial. *Lancet.* 1999;353:1993-2000. PMID: 10376613.

103. Veronesi U, De Palo G, Marubini E, et al. Randomized trial of fenretinide to prevent second breast malignancy in women with early breast cancer. *J Natl Cancer Inst.* 1999;91:1847-1856. PMID: 10547391.

104. Wactawski-Wende J, Kotchen JM, Anderson GL, et al. Calcium plus vitamin D supplementation and the risk of colorectal cancer. *N Engl J Med.* 2006;354:684-696. PMID: 16481636.

105. Blot WJ, Li JY, Taylor PR, et al. Nutrition intervention trials in Linxian, China: supplementation with specific vitamin/mineral combinations, cancer incidence, and disease-specific mortality in the general population. *J Natl Cancer Inst.* 1993;85:1483-1492. PMID: 8360931.

106. Li JY, Taylor PR, Li B, et al. Nutrition intervention trials in Linxian, China: multiple vitamin/mineral supplementation, cancer incidence, and disease-specific mortality among adults with esophageal dysplasia. *J Natl Cancer Inst.* 1993;85:1492-1498. PMID: 8360932.

107. Hennekens CH, Buring JE, Manson JE, et al. Lack of effect of long-term supplementation with beta carotene on the incidence of malignant neoplasms and cardiovascular disease. *N Engl J Med.* 1996;334:1145-1149. PMID: 8602179.

108. Lee IM, Cook NR, Manson JE, et al. Beta-carotene supplementation and incidence of cancer and cardiovascular disease: the Women's Health Study. *J Natl Cancer Inst.* 1999;91:2102-2106. PMID: 10601381.

109. D'Souza G, Kreimer AR, Viscidi R, et al. Case-control study of human papillomavirus and oropharyngeal cancer. *N Engl J Med.* 2007;356:1944-1956. PMID: 17494927.

110. Crew KD, Neugut AI. Epidemiology of upper gastrointestinal malignancies. *Semin Oncol.* 2004;31:450-464. PMID: 15297938.

111. Kamangar F, Malekzadeh R, Dawsey SM, et al. Esophageal cancer in Northeastern Iran: a review. *Arch Iran Med.* 2007;10:70-82. PMID: 17198458.

112. Islami F, Pourshams A, Nasrollahzadeh D, et al. Tea drinking habits and oesophageal cancer in a high risk area in northern Iran: a population based case-control study. *BMJ.* 2009;338:b929. PMID: 19325180.

113. Wong BC, Lam SK, Wong WM, et al. Helicobacter pylori eradication to prevent gastric cancer in a high-risk region of China: a randomized controlled trial. *JAMA.* 2004;291:187-194. PMID: 14722144.

114. Abrams JA, Sharaiha RZ, Gonsalves L, et al. Dating the rise of esophageal adenocarcinoma: analysis of Connecticut Tumor Registry data, 1940-2007. *Cancer Epidemiol Biomarkers Prev.* 2011;20:183-186. PMID: 21127287.

115. Abrams JA, Gonsalves L, Neugut AI. Diverging trends in the incidence of reflux-related and Helicobacter pylori-related gastric cardia cancer. *J Clin Gastroenterol.* 2013;47:322-327. PMID: 22914345.

116. Chan AT, Arber N, Burn J, et al. Aspirin in the chemoprevention of colorectal neoplasia: an overview. *Cancer Prev Res (Phila).* 2012;5:164-178. PMID: 22084361.

117. Steinbach G, Lynch PM, Phillips RK, et al. The effect of celecoxib, a cyclooxygenase-2 inhibitor, in familial adenomatous polyposis. *N Engl J Med.* 2000;342:1946-1952. PMID: 10874062.

118. Bertagnolli MM, Eagle CJ, Zauber AG, et al. Celecoxib for the prevention of sporadic colorectal adenomas. *N Engl J Med.* 2006;355:873-884. PMID: 16943400.

119. Rothwell PM, Wilson M, Elwin CE, et al. Long-term effect of aspirin on colorectal cancer incidence and mortality: 20-year follow-up of five randomised trials. *Lancet.* 2010;376:1741-1750. PMID: 20970847.

120. Chan AT, Ogino S, Fuchs CS. Aspirin use and survival after diagnosis of colorectal cancer. *JAMA.* 2009;302:649-658. PMID: 19671906.

121. Rothwell PM, Wilson M, Price JF, et al. Effect of daily aspirin on risk of cancer metastasis: a study of incident cancers during randomised controlled trials. *Lancet.* 2012;379:1591-1601. PMID: 22440947.

122. Chlebowski RT, Wactawski-Wende J, Ritenbaugh C, et al. Estrogen plus progestin and colorectal cancer in postmenopausal women. *N Engl J Med.* 2004;350:991-1004. PMID: 14999111.

123. Nelson HD, Humphrey LL, Nygren P, et al. Postmenopausal hormone replacement therapy: scientific review. *JAMA.* 2002;288:872-881. PMID: 12186605.

124. Grau MV, Baron JA, Sandler RS, et al. Vitamin D, calcium supplementation, and colorectal adenomas: results of a randomized trial. *J Natl Cancer Inst.* 2003;95:1765-1771. PMID: 14652238.

125. Lynch HT, Lynch JF. Hereditary cancer: family history, diagnosis, molecular genetics, ecogenetics, and management strategies. *Biochimie.* 2002;84:3-17. PMID: 11900873.

126. Fisher B, Costantino JP, Wickerham DL, et al. Tamoxifen for the prevention of breast cancer: current status of the National Surgical Adjuvant Breast and Bowel Project P-1 study. *J Natl Cancer Inst.* 2005;97:1652-1662. PMID: 16288118.

127. Hortobagyi GN, Brown PH. Two good choices to prevent breast cancer: great taste, less filling. *Cancer Prev Res.* 2010;3:681-685. PMID: 20522797.

128. Stefanick ML, Anderson GL, Margolis KL, et al. Effects of conjugated equine estrogens on breast cancer and mammography screening in postmenopausal women with hysterectomy. *JAMA.* 2006;295:1647-1657. PMID: 16609086.

129. Manson JE, Chlebowski RT, Stefanick ML, et al. Menopausal hormone therapy and health outcomes during the intervention and extended post-stopping phases of the Women's Health Initiative randomized trials. *JAMA.* 2013;310:1353-1368. PMID: 24084921.

130. Hartmann LC, Schaid DJ, Woods JE, et al. Efficacy of bilateral prophylactic mastectomy in women with a family history of breast cancer. *N Engl J Med.* 1999;340:77-84. PMID: 9887158.

131. Kauff ND, Domchek SM, Friebel TM, et al. Risk-reducing salpingo-oophorectomy for the prevention of BRCA1- and BRCA2-associated breast and gynecologic cancer: a multicenter, prospective study. *J Clin Oncol.* 2008;26:1331-1337. PMID: 18268356.

132. Lostumbo L, Carbine NE, Wallace J. Prophylactic mastectomy for the prevention of breast cancer. *Cochrane Database Syst Rev.* 2010;(11):CD002748. PMID: 21069671.

133. Lucia MS, Epstein JI, Goodman PJ, et al. Finasteride and high-grade prostate cancer in the Prostate Cancer Prevention Trial. *J Natl Cancer Inst.* 2007;99:1375-1383. PMID: 17848673.

134. Sarvis JA, Thompson IM. Prostate cancer chemoprevention: update of the prostate cancer prevention trial findings and implications for clinical practice. *Curr Oncol Rep.* 2008;10:529-532. PMID: 18928669.

135. Thompson IM Jr., Goodman PJ, Tangen CM, et al. Long-term survival of participants in the prostate cancer prevention trial. *N Engl J Med.* 2013;369:603-610. PMID: 23944298.

136. LeFevre M. A role for finasteride in the prevention of prostate cancer? *N Engl J Med.* 2013;369:670-671. PMID: 23944306.

137. Clark LC, Dalkin B, Krongrad A, et al. Decreased incidence of prostate cancer with selenium supplementation: results of a double-blind cancer prevention trial. *Br J Urol.* 1998;81:730-734. PMID: 9634050.

138. The effect of vitamin E and beta carotene on the incidence of lung cancer and other cancers in male smokers. The Alpha-Tocopherol, Beta Carotene Cancer Prevention Study Group. *N Engl J Med.* 1994;330:1029-1035. PMID: 8127329.

139. Bernstein L. The risk of breast, endometrial and ovarian cancer in users of hormonal preparations. *Basic Clin Pharmacol Toxicol.* 2006;98:288-296. PMID: 16611204.

140. Søgaard M, Kjaer SK, Gayther S. Ovarian cancer and genetic susceptibility in relation to the BRCA1 and BRCA2 genes. Occurrence, clinical importance and intervention. *Acta Obstet Gynecol Scand.* 2006;85:93-105. PMID: 16521688.

141. Oken MM, Hocking WG, Kvale PA, et al. Screening by chest radiograph and lung cancer mortality: the Prostate, Lung, Colorectal, and Ovarian (PLCO) randomized trial. *JAMA.* 2011;306:1865-1873. PMID: 22031728.

142. Marcus PM, Bergstralh EJ, Fagerstrom RM, et al. Lung cancer mortality in the Mayo Lung Project: impact of extended follow-up. *J Natl Cancer Inst.* 2000;92:1308-1316. PMID: 10944552.

143. Woods WG, Gao RN, Shuster JJ, et al. Screening of infants and mortality due to neuroblastoma. *N Engl J Med.* 2002;346:1041-1046. PMID: 11932470.

144. Prorok PC. Epidemiologic approach for cancer screening. Problems in design and analysis of trials. *Am J Pediatr Hematol Oncol.* 1992;14:117-128. PMID: 1530116.

145. Kramer BS, Brawley OW. Cancer screening. *Hematol Oncol Clin North Am.* 2000;14:831-848. PMID: 10949776.

146. U.S. Preventive Services Task Force. Recommendations for adults. www.uspreventiveservicestaskforce.org/adultrec.htm. Accessed July 25, 2012.

147. Canadian Task Force on Preventive Health Care. www.canadiantaskforce.ca/recommendations_current_eng.html. Accessed July 25, 2012.

148. Smith RA, Brooks D, Cokkinides V, et al. Cancer screening in the United States, 2013: a review of current American Cancer Society guidelines, current issues in cancer screening, and new guidance on cervical cancer screening and lung cancer screening. *CA Cancer J Clin.* 2013;63:88-105. PMID: 23378235.

149. Barry H. Breast self-examination does not reduce mortality. *Am Fam Physician.* 2003;67:1784.

150. Thomas DB, Gao DL, Ray RM, et al. Randomized trial of breast self-examination in Shanghai: final results. *J Natl Cancer Inst.* 2002;94:1445-1457. PMID: 12359854.

151. Green BB, Taplin SH. Breast cancer screening controversies. *J Am Board Fam Pract.* 2003;16:233-241. PMID: 12755251.

152. Fletcher SW, Black W, Harris R, et al. Report of the International Workshop on Screening for Breast Cancer. *J Natl Cancer Inst.* 1993;85:1644-1656. PMID: 8105098.

153. Humphrey LL, Helfand M, Chan BK, et al. Breast cancer screening: a summary of the evidence for the U.S. Preventive Services Task Force. *Ann Intern Med.* 2002;137:347-360. PMID: 12204020.

154. US Preventive Services Task Force. Screening for breast cancer: U.S. Preventive Services Task Force recommendation statement. *Ann Intern Med.* 2009;151:716-726, W-236. PMID: 19920272.

155. Le-Petross HT. Breast MRI as a screening tool: the appropriate role. *J Natl Comp Cancer Netw.* 2006;4:523-526. PMID: 16687098.

156. Plevritis SK, Kurian AW, Sigal BM, et al. Cost-effectiveness of screening BRCA1/2 mutation carriers with breast magnetic resonance imaging. *JAMA.* 2006;295:2374-2384. PMID: 16720823.

157. Granader EJ, Dwamena B, Carlos RC. MRI and mammography surveillance of women at increased risk for breast cancer: recommendations using an evidence-based approach. *Acad Radiol.* 2008;15:1590-1595. PMID: 19000876.

158. Saslow D, Boetes C, Burke W, et al. American Cancer Society guidelines for breast screening with MRI as an adjunct to mammography. *CA Cancer J Clin.* 2007;57:75-89. PMID: 17392385.

159. Parmigiani G, Berry D, Aguilar O. Determining carrier probabilities for breast cancer-susceptibility genes BRCA1 and BRCA2. *Am J Hum Genet.* 1998;62:145-158. PMID: 9443863.

160. Saslow D, Solomon D. Lawson HW, et al. American Cancer Society, American Society for Colonoscopy and Cervical Pathology, and the American Society for Clinical Pathology screening guidelines for the prevention and early detection of cervical cancer. *CA Cancer J Clin.* 2012; 62:147-172. PMID: 22422631.

161. Saslow D, Runowicz CD, Solomon D, et al. American Cancer Society guideline for the early detection of cervical neoplasia and cancer. *CA Cancer J Clin.* 2002;52:342-362. PMID: 12469763.

162. Wright TC Jr, Schiffman M, Solomon D, et al. Interim guidance for the use of human papillomavirus DNA testing as an adjunct to cervical cytology for screening. *Obstet Gynecol.* 2004;103:304-309. PMID: 14754700.

163. Mandel JS, Church TR, Bond JH, et al. The effect of fecal occult-blood screening on the incidence of colorectal cancer. *N Engl J Med.* 2000;343:1603-1607. PMID: 11096167.

164. Ault MJ, Mandel SA. Screening for colorectal cancer. *N Engl J Med.* 2000;343:1652; author reply 1652-1654. PMID: 11184983.

165. Atkin WS, Edwards R, Kralj-Hans I, et al. Once-only flexible sigmoidoscopy screening in prevention of colorectal cancer: a multicentre randomised controlled trial. *Lancet.* 2010;375:1624-1633. PMID: 20430429.

166. Segnan N, Armaroli P, Bonelli L, et al. Once-only sigmoidoscopy in colorectal cancer screening: follow-up findings of the Italian Randomized Controlled Trial--SCORE. *J Natl Cancer Inst.* 2011;103:1310-1322. PMID: 21852264.

167. Schoen RE, Pinsky PF, Weissfeld JL, et al. Colorectal-cancer incidence and mortality with screening flexible sigmoidoscopy. *N Engl J Med.* 2012;366:2345-2357. PMID: 22612596.

168. Neugut AI, Lebwohl B. Colonoscopy vs sigmoidoscopy screening: getting it right. *JAMA.* 2010;304:461-462. PMID: 20664047.

169. Brenner H, Chang-Claude J, Seiler CM, et al. Protection from colorectal cancer after colonoscopy: a population-based, case-control study. *Ann Intern Med.* 2011;154:22-30. PMID: 21200035.

170. Baxter NN, Warren JL, Barrett MJ, et al. Association between colonoscopy and colorectal cancer mortality in a US cohort according to site of cancer and colonoscopist specialty. *J Clin Oncol.* 2012;30:2664-2669. PMID: 22689809.

171. Nishihara R, Wu K, Lochhead P, et al. Long-term colorectal-cancer incidence and mortality after lower endoscopy. *N Engl J Med.* 2013;369:1095-1105. PMID: 24047059.

172. Neugut AI, Forde KA. Screening colonoscopy: has the time come? *Am J Gastroenterol.* 1988;83:295-297. PMID: 3278596.

173. Levin B, Lieberman DA, McFarland B, et al. Screening and surveillance for the early detection of colorectal cancer and adenomatous polyps, 2008: a joint guideline from the American Cancer Society, the US Multi-Society Task Force on Colorectal Cancer, and the American College of Radiology. *CA Cancer J Clin.* 2008;58:130-160. PMID: 18322143.

174. U.S. Preventive Services Task Force. Screening for colorectal cancer: U.S. Preventive Services Task Force recommendation statement. *Ann Intern Med.* 2008;149:627-637. PMID: 18838716.

175. Pignone M, Sox HC. Screening guidelines for colorectal cancer: a twice-told tale. *Ann Intern Med.* 2008;149:680-682. PMID: 18840787.

176. Humphrey LL, Deffebach M, Pappas M, et al. Screening for lung cancer with low-dose computed tomography: A systematic review to update the U.S. Preventive Services Task From Recommendation. *Ann Intern Med.* 2013;159: 411-420. PMID: 23897166.

177. Marcus PM, Bergstralh EJ, Zweig MH, et al. Extended lung cancer incidence follow-up in the Mayo Lung Project and overdiagnosis. *J Natl Cancer Inst.* 2006;98:748-756. PMID: 16757699.

178. Manser RL, Irving LB, Byrnes G, et al. Screening for lung cancer: a systematic review and meta-analysis of controlled trials. *Thorax.* 2003;58:784-789. PMID: 12947138.

179. International Early Lung Cancer Action Program Investigators, Henschke CI, Yankelevitz DF, et al. Survival of patients with stage I lung cancer detected on CT screening. *N Engl J Med.* 2006;355:1763-1771. PMID: 17065637.

180. Bach PB, Jett JR, Pastorino U, et al. Computed tomography screening and lung cancer outcomes. *JAMA.* 2007;297:953-961. PMID: 17341709.

181. National Lung Screening Trial Research Team, Aberle DR, Adams AM, et al. Reduced lung-cancer mortality with low-dose computed tomographic screening. *N Engl J Med.* 2011;365:395-409. PMID: 21714641.

182. Bach PB, Mirkin JN, Oliver TK, et al. Benefits and harms of CT screening for lung cancer: a systematic review. *JAMA.* 2012;307:2418-2429. PMID: 22610500.

183. Aberle DR, Abtin F, Brown K. Computed tomography screening for lung cancer: has it finally arrived? Implications of the national lung screening trial. *J Clin Oncol.* 2013;31:1002-1008. PMID: 23401434.

184. Buys SS, Partridge E, Black A, et al. Effect of screening on ovarian cancer mortality: the Prostate, Lung, Colorectal and Ovarian (PLCO) Cancer Screening Randomized Controlled Trial. *JAMA.* 2011;305:2295-2303. PMID: 21642681.

185. Andriole GL, Reding D, Hayes RB, et al. The prostate, lung, colon, and ovarian (PLCO) cancer screening trial: Status and promise. *Urol Oncol.* 2004;22:358-361. PMID: 15283897.

186. Lin K, Lipsitz R, Miller T, et al. Benefits and harms of prostate-specific antigen screening for prostate cancer: an evidence update for the U.S. Preventive Services Task Force. *Ann Intern Med.* 2008;149:192-199. PMID: 18678846.

187. U.S. Preventive Services Task Force. Screening for prostate cancer: U.S. Preventive Services Task Force recommendation statement. *Ann Intern Med.* 2008;149:185-191. PMID: 18678845.

188. Andriole GL, Crawford ED, Grubb RL 3rd, et al. Mortality results from a randomized prostate-cancer screening trial. *N Engl J Med.* 2009;360:1310-1319. PMID: 19297565.

189. Schröder FH, Hugosson J, Roobol MJ, et al. Screening and prostate-cancer mortality in a randomized European study. *N Engl J Med.* 2009;360:1320-1328. PMID: 19297566.

190. MacKie RM, Hole D, Hunter JA, et al. Cutaneous malignant melanoma in Scotland: incidence, survival, and mortality, 1979-94. The Scottish Melanoma Group. *BMJ.* 1997;315:1117-1121. PMID: 9374883.

191. Wani S, Sharma P. The rationale for screening and surveillance of Barrett's metaplasia. *Best Pract Res Clin Gastroenterol.* 2006;20:829-842. PMID: 16997164.

192. Sankaranarayanan R, Ramadas K, Thomas G, et al. Effect of screening on oral cancer mortality in Kerala, India: a cluster-randomised controlled trial. *Lancet.* 2005;365:1927-1933. PMID: 15936419.

193. Zhang BH, Yang BH, Tang ZY. Randomized controlled trial of screening for hepatocellular carcinoma. *J Cancer Res Clin Oncol.* 2004;130:417-422. PMID: 15042359.

194. Hamashima C, Shibuya D, Yamazaki H, et al. The Japanese guidelines for gastric cancer screening. *Jpn J Clin Oncol.* 2008;38:259-267. PMID: 18344316.

195. Robinson E, Neugut AI. Clinical aspects of multiple primary neoplasms. *Cancer Detect Prev.* 1989;13:287-292. PMID: 2663155.

196. Neugut AI. Preventive oncology–lessons from preventive cardiology. *Lancet.* 2004;363:1004-1005. PMID: 15051278.

2

MOLECULAR BIOLOGY

Bruce E. Clurman, MD, PhD

Molecular oncology is rapidly evolving. Many of the genes that drive tumorigenesis, and the biologic pathways and processes affected by oncogenic mutations, have now been identified. Moreover, new molecular approaches have enabled the development of therapeutics that target specific oncogenic mutations, and advances in large-scale molecular biology are providing comprehensive descriptions of cancer genomes and allowing targeted therapies to be rationally applied to treat individual cancers. The goal of this chapter is to outline the current framework of the molecular basis of cancer, as well as the technologies being used to develop and guide therapy.

BASIC PRINCIPLES OF MOLECULAR BIOLOGY

Deoxyribonucleic acid (DNA) is a macromolecule composed of four nucleotides: adenine (A), guanine (G), cytosine (C), and thymine (T; Fig. 2-1).[1,2] Each nucleotide base is connected to a deoxyribose sugar, and phosphodiester bonds between the sugar moieties form the DNA strand. The nucleoside components of one DNA strand form hydrogen bonds with nucleosides on the complementary strand (C pairs with G, and A pairs with T) to create a double-stranded DNA molecule. When DNA is replicated, the strands separate and each provides a template for an exact complement to be synthesized.

From a molecular viewpoint, the term *gene* refers to a DNA sequence that encodes a protein or a functional ribonucleic acid (RNA). Most genes are discontinuous and arranged in segments called exons and introns. The first step in protein synthesis is transcription of the DNA template into a linear RNA copy, during which the introns are subsequently spliced out to generate a messenger RNA (mRNA) that contains a continuous coding sequence composed of exons (Fig. 2-2). The mRNA is a template for the attachment of ribosomes, and nucleotide triplets—termed codons—specify which amino acids will be incorporated into a nascent polypeptide chain. The 5' and 3' extremities of mRNA extend beyond the coding regions and have regulatory functions, such as determining mRNA stability and translational efficiency.

mRNA expression is controlled by numerous regulatory elements such as promoters (which direct the site of transcription initiation) and enhancers (which increase transcription), and these may be located large distances from the genes they control (Fig. 2-2).[3] Promoters and enhancers are composed of nucleotide sequences that are recognized by proteins called transcription factors, which establish the timing and tissue-specific characteristics of gene expression. Many transcription factors bind directly to these DNA elements and subsequently recruit regulatory proteins into the transcription complex. Proteins that mediate the assembly of active transcription complexes by recruiting factors or facilitating chromatin changes that favor transcription are termed coactivators,[4] whereas corepressors inhibit transcription.[5] Individual cell types express only a subset of

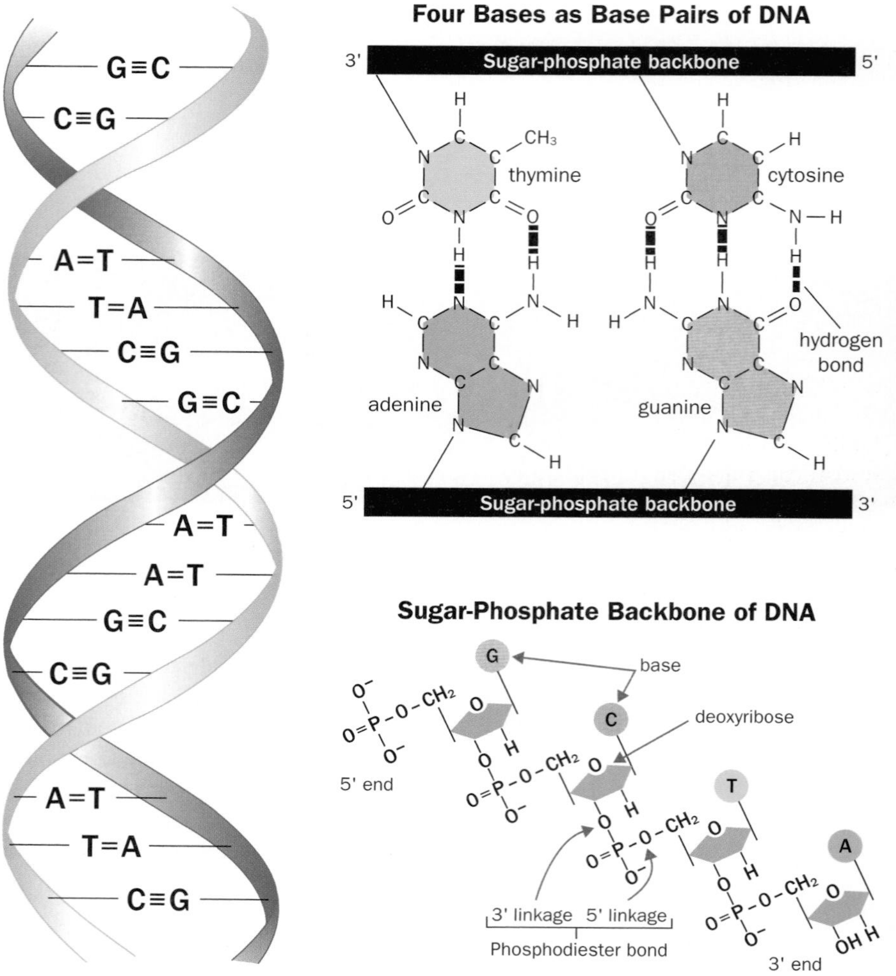

Four Bases as Base Pairs of DNA

Fig. 2-1 The double helix structure of DNA includes hydrogen bonding between adenine (A) and thymine (T) bases and between guanine (G) and cytosine (C) bases.

Right top: Close-up of hydrogen bonds between the two pairs of bases. Right bottom: A single strand of DNA showing the molecular structure of the backbone made of phosphodiester bonds between sugar molecules.

Reprinted with permission from Alberts B, Bray D, Lewis J, et al. Molecular Biology of the Cell, 1st edition. New York, NY: Garland Publishing, Inc.; 1983.

Sugar-Phosphate Backbone of DNA

the full complement of genes, and this restricted gene expression underlies cellular differentiation. The control of gene expression is critical during growth and development, during maintenance of tissue specificity, and during neoplastic transformation.

DNA is compacted into chromatin by winding around proteins called histones, which maintain the DNA in nucleosomal complexes (Fig. 2-3A). Chromatin is highly dynamic and undergoes modification and remodeling—known as epigenetic gene regulation—that profoundly influence gene expression.[6] Histones are modified covalently (i.e., acetylation, methylation, phosphorylation, and ubiquitylation), by changes in subunit composition (e.g., replacement of core histones by specialized histones), and by repositioning. Each of these modifications renders DNA more or less accessible to RNA polymerase (Fig. 2-3B).[7,8] Histone methylation occurs on lysine (K) residues and is highly regulated by opposing methylating and demethylating enzymes: methylation on some sites (e.g., H3K4) facilitates transcription, whereas others (e.g., H3K27) repress transcription.[9] Acetylation is another modification that is also regulated by groups of opposing enzymes. Histone acetylation is found in actively transcribed genes, whereas histone deacetylation correlates with repression. Epigenetic regulation also involves DNA modifications, most commonly cytosine

methylation within CG dinucleotides.[10] DNA regions that contain many CGs are termed CpG (cytosine-phosphate-guanine) islands, and CpG methylation is found in transcriptionally repressed loci. Importantly, promoter methylation is one way that cancer cells inactivate tumor suppressor genes (discussed further in the Detection of Tumor Suppressor Gene Inactivation and Cell Cycle Control sections). There is widespread crosstalk between epigenetic modifications of DNA and histones, and genome-wide analyses are revealing how these complex patterns of epigenetic "marks" establish differential gene expression.[11,12]

Because of their influence on gene expression, the enzymes that catalyze epigenetic modifications are important targets for cancer therapeutics.[13] For example, histone deacetylase inhibitors are being evaluated as therapeutic agents[14] and include vorinostat, which is approved for the treatment of cutaneous T-cell lymphoma.[15] DNA methylation is another important drug target: 5-azacytidine and 5-aza-2′deoxycytidine, which are approved for treatment of myelodysplastic syndrome, inhibit DNA methylation and re-establish expression of genes that were repressed by methylation.[16]

The human genome contains approximately 3 billion nucleotides partitioned among 23 chromosomes. Although the

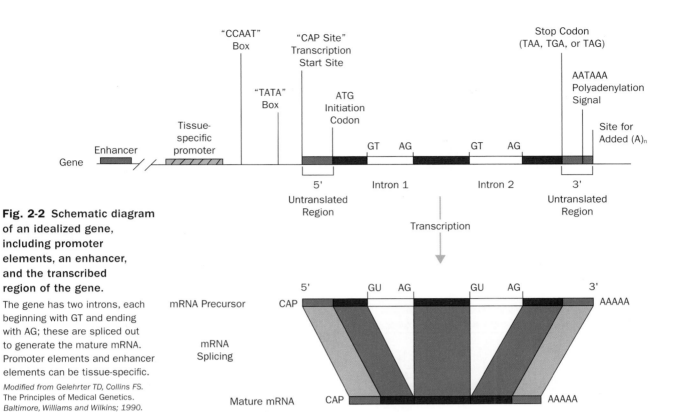

Fig. 2-2 Schematic diagram of an idealized gene, including promoter elements, an enhancer, and the transcribed region of the gene.

The gene has two introns, each beginning with GT and ending with AG; these are spliced out to generate the mature mRNA. Promoter elements and enhancer elements can be tissue-specific.

Modified from Gelehrter TD, Collins FS. The Principles of Medical Genetics. Baltimore, Williams and Wilkins; 1990.

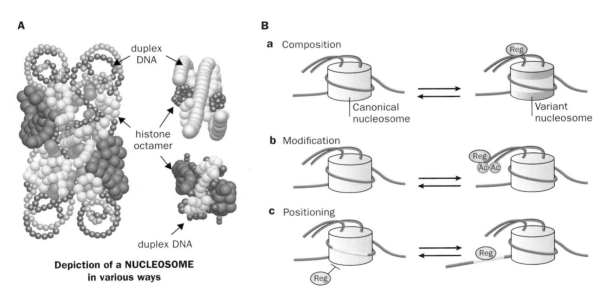

Depiction of a NUCLEOSOME in various ways

Fig. 2-3 Nucleosome structure and regulation.
(A) Nucleosome structure. View is down the molecular two-fold axis; DNA is represented by a tube that almost completely occludes the protein. **(B)** Nucleosome regulation. **(a)** Remodeling complexes can remove the canonical H2A–H2B dimers and replace them with variant histones (indicated in green), forming a variant nucleosome with unique tails that might bind unique regulatory proteins. **(b)** Nucleosome modification (only acetylation [Ac] is depicted for simplicity) allows the binding of regulatory factors, which have specialized domains that recognize acetylated histone tails. **(c)** Nucleosome repositioning allows the binding of a regulatory factor to its site on nucleosomal DNA (light-blue segment).

Reprinted by permission from Macmillan Publishers Ltd: Nat Rev Mol Cell Biol. Saha A, Wittmeyer J, Cairns BR. Chromatin remodeling: the industrial revolution of DNA around histones. 2006;7(6):437-447.

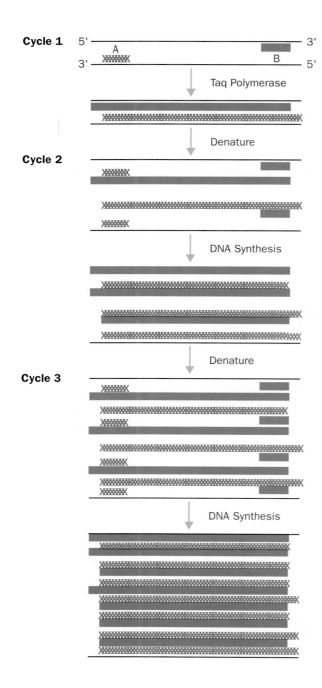

Fig. 2-4 Polymerase chain reaction (PCR).

The DNA (target) to be amplified is shown as a double-stranded DNA molecule with complementary segments (in blue). Cycle 1: The DNA is denatured and then allowed to reanneal to short oligonucleotide fragments complementary to the region surrounding the segment to be amplified. Taq DNA polymerase then extends from the primer, making perfect complementary copies of the segments of DNA (in blue), yielding two copies of the target DNA. Cycle 2: The DNA from cycle 1 is denatured and reannealed, and the steps in cycle 1 are repeated, yielding four copies of target DNA. Cycle 3: The DNA from cycle 2 is denatured, and the steps in cycle 2 are repeated, yielding eight copies of DNA. With n cycles, the amount of DNA increases exponentially as 2^n.

Reprinted with permission from Gelehrter TD, Collins FS. The Principles of Medical Genetics. Baltimore, MD: Lippincott Williams & Wilkins; 1990.

Human Genome Project was completed in 2003, the exact number of human genes remains unclear, and most estimates are in the range of 25,000. However, because many genes express alternatively processed mRNAs that encode different protein isoforms, the number of proteins in the human proteome greatly exceeds the number of genes. Most human cells contain a complete genomic copy of DNA, but there are exceptions. For example, erythrocytes contain no genomic DNA, mature lymphocytes delete fragments of DNA within either immunoglobulin (Ig) or T-cell receptor genes to generate antigen-recognition proteins, and megakaryocytes contain extra copies of the genome that results from the process of endoreduplication.

KEY POINTS

- Genes are functional units contained within DNA that specify the production of proteins and RNAs.
- Cells only express a subset of the genes contained within their genomes. Genes are transcribed into mRNA, and this is controlled by regulatory DNA elements (i.e., enhancers, promoters, and insulators).
- Gene expression is regulated by epigenetic modifications of DNA and histones. These types of chromatin modifications, which include methylations and acetylations, play a major role in determining the timing and amount of gene expression. The enzymes that catalyze epigenetic modifications are important targets for the development of cancer therapies.

ANALYZING NUCLEIC ACIDS AND DETECTING CANCER-ASSOCIATED MUTATIONS

DNA

Polymerase Chain Reaction

The polymerase chain reaction (PCR) is a powerful technique that can synthesize a large quantity of specific DNA fragments from minute amounts of template.[17,18] In its most basic form, PCR relies on (1) annealing synthetic DNA primers to DNA sequences that flank the target DNA to be amplified, and (2) DNA polymerase enzymes isolated from thermophilic bacteria that can survive high temperatures. Multiple cycles of DNA-strand synthesis, heat denaturation, and primer reannealing allow for the repeated replication of the target sequence, resulting in exponential amplification of the DNA fragment (Fig. 2-4). For example, 20 PCR cycles produce approximately 1 million double-stranded copies of the original DNA, whereas 30 cycles produce more than 1 billion copies. A wide variety of PCR-based techniques have revolutionized virtually all methods used to manipulate, detect, and analyze nucleic acids.

DNA Polymorphisms Facilitate Genetic Analyses of Complex Diseases

DNA sequences that exhibit a high degree of variability in a population are termed polymorphisms and are used to

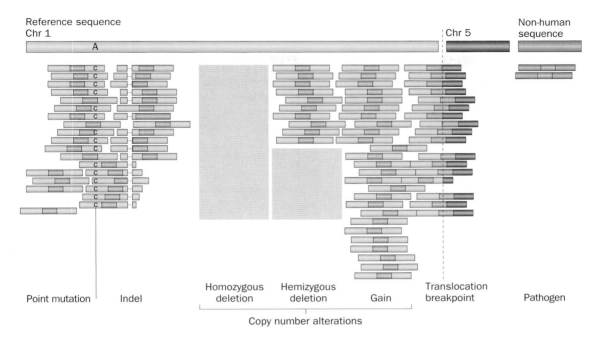

Fig. 2-5 Types of mutations discovered by genomic sequencing.
Sequenced fragments are depicted as bars with colored tips representing the sequenced ends and the unsequenced portion of the fragment in grey. Reads are aligned to the reference genome (mostly chromosome 1 in this example). The colors of the sequenced ends show where they align to. Different types of genomic alterations can be detected, from left to right: point mutations (in this example A to C) and small insertions and deletions (indels; in this example a deletion shown by a dashed line) are detected by identifying multiple reads that show nonreference sequence; changes in sequencing depth (relative to a normal control) are used to identify copy number changes (shaded boxes represent absent or decreased reads in the tumor sample); paired-ends that map to different genomic loci (in this case, chromosome 5) are evidence of rearrangements; and sequences that map to non-human sequences are evidence for the potential presence of genomic material from pathogens.

Reprinted by permission from Macmillan Publishers Ltd: Nat Rev Genet. Meyerson M, Gabriel S, Getz G. Advances in understanding cancer genomes through second-generation sequencing. 2010 Oct;11(10):685-96.

distinguish alleles in genetic analyses. Dense maps of polymorphic markers throughout the human genome facilitated the mapping of genetic traits, such as cancer predisposition, because large family cohorts could be analyzed for polymorphic markers that segregated with the trait of interest. This general approach—although labor–intensive—identified many of the genes responsible for hereditary cancer syndromes. Single nucleotide polymorphisms (SNPs) are the most common polymorphisms used in mapping genetic traits, and current approaches typically utilize microarray-based chips and/or DNA sequencing methods that analyze SNPs on a genome-wide scale (see below).[19-21] Cytosine–adenine (CA) dinucleotide repeats, called microsatellites, are another type of polymorphism. These regions are susceptible to imperfect duplication by DNA polymerase, leading to variability in the lengths of CA repeat regions. Mutations in DNA mismatch repair enzymes that normally suppress these replication errors are found in some cancers—such as hereditary nonpolyposis colon cancer (HNPCC)—and cause altered microsatellites that form the basis of diagnostic tests.

DNA Sequencing: Beyond the Human Genome Project
The completion of the Human Genome Project in 2003 heralded a new era in molecular medicine. Obtaining the human genome with 99.9% accuracy took 13 years and nearly $3 billion, and the completed sequence has enabled revolutionary insight on human biology and disease. The technology used to obtain the reference human genome sequence used the Sanger dideoxy DNA sequencing method and required large-scale automation and a large consortium of international sequencing centers. Although a remarkable achievement, these methods are not practical to apply toward goals such as sequencing cancer cell genomes or "personal genomes" because of the time and expense required. However, new technologies, termed next-generation sequencing, are transforming the landscape of genome-wide analyses and realizing the long-awaited goal of allowing chemotherapy to be based on the specific mutations present in an individual tumor.[22,23]

Although a detailed description of these methodologies is beyond the scope of this text, these methods apply massively parallel sequencing technologies to obtain millions of sequence reads in single instrument runs.[24] Several different technology platforms are in use for different applications and in different institutions. A common feature of these technologies is that the length of the sequence read for each DNA molecule is relatively short, and their power relies on the pre-existing reference human genome sequence for positioning and alignment

A

ChIP-Seq data

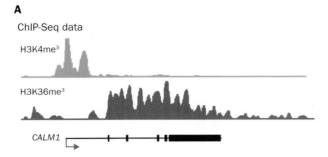
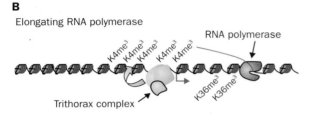

B

Elongating RNA polymerase

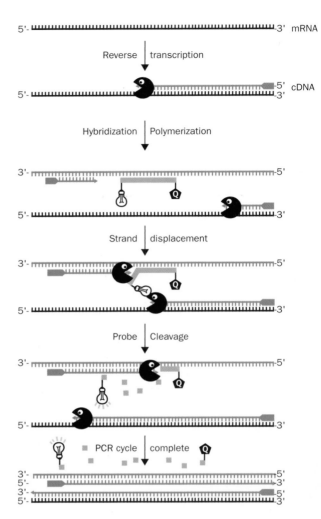

Fig. 2-6 Chromatin state maps reveal a stereotypical pattern at active genes.

(A) In mouse ES cells, the transcription start site for the *CALM1* gene (blue arrow) is marked by H3K4 trimethylation, a trithorax-associated mark, while the remainder of the transcribed region is marked by H3K36 trimethylation. (B) Evidence from model systems supports a central role for initiating and elongating RNA polymerase II in recruiting the relevant histone methyltransferase enzymes.

Reprinted from Current Opinion in Genetics & Development, *Volume 18(2). Mendenhall EM, Bernstein BE. Chromatin state maps: new technologies, new insights. Pages 109-15, copyright 2008. With permission from Elsevier.*

of millions of short reads, which also requires sophisticated bioinformatics tools. The cost and speed of next-generation sequencing are rapidly improving. For example, in 2008, two studies reported human genome sequences that were completed in a few months but cost approximately $1 million per genome.[25,26] As of late 2012, it seems likely that rapid human genome sequencing will soon be available with costs in the range of several thousand dollars and time frames measured in days to weeks, and this has enormous implications for cancer biology and treatment strategies. Indeed, these techniques have already been applied to cancer genomes with great success (discussed further in the Modern Oncogenomics section). Because these methods are quantitative, they can be used to detect structural changes, such as chromosomal gains and losses and translocations in cancer cells, in addition to point mutations (Fig. 2-5).

Next-generation sequencing platforms also allow epigenetic studies at a genome-wide scale. ChIP-Seq is a method that uses antibodies that recognize specific modifications (e.g., histone K4 methylation) to precipitate fragments of DNA associated with the modified histone, and then applies massively parallel sequencing to identify all DNA regions that contain the modification.[27] This strategy has revealed highly detailed maps of the epigenetic marks that regulate gene expression and fundamental new insight on cellular differentiation (Fig. 2-6). Massively

Fig. 2-7 The principle of the 5' nuclease (TaqMan) assay, a type of real-time PCR reaction.

The RT step synthesizes a cDNA copy of the RNA template. After denaturation, primers and probe anneal to their targets. The probe contains a reporter dye at the 5' end and a quencher (Q) at its 3' end. During the polymerization step, the 5' nuclease activity of the Taq polymerase displaces and cleaves the probe. This physically separates the reporter dye and quencher dyes, resulting in reporter fluorescence. The increase in signal is directly proportional to the number of molecules released during that cycle. Accumulation of PCR products is detected directly by monitoring the increase in fluorescence of the reporter dye.

Reproduced with permission from Bustin SA, Mueller R. 2005. Real-time reverse transcription PCR (qRT-PCR) and its potential use in clinical diagnosis. Clin Sci (Lond). 2005;109(4):365-79. Copyright © the Biochemical Society (http://clinsci.org).

parallel sequencing also has been used to map genome-wide DNA methylation patterns, and this revealed that CpG methylation is a highly dynamic process that changes dramatically during cellular differentiation.[28] Importantly, next-generation sequencing–based strategies are being used in the Encyclopedia of DNA Elements (ENCODE) project, which has made remarkable progress toward identifying all sites of transcription factor binding and chromatin and histone modifications in the human genome.[29] Overall, these technologies are providing an

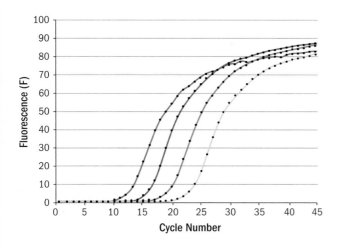

Fig. 2-8 Detection of amplified DNA in real-time PCR reactions.

Fluorescence is a function of cycle number. Fluorescence (arbitrary units) is measured in four different samples (serial dilutions) at the end of the elongation step of each cycle.

Reprinted from Methods in Enzymology, Volume 410. Lutfalla G, Uze G. Performing Quantitative Reverse-Transcribed Polymerase Chain Reaction Experiments. Pages 386-400, copyright 2006. With permission from Elsevier.

entirely new understanding of how gene expression is regulated in health and disease.

RNA
Real-Time Polymerase Chain Reaction

Many PCR-based methods for RNA analyses use reverse transcription, in which the reverse transcriptase enzyme and DNA primers are used to convert mRNA to a DNA copy, called cDNA. These cDNAs are used as templates for PCR techniques to quantitate specific RNAs or for other applications, such as sequencing. This general strategy is termed reverse transcription-PCR (RT-PCR) to reflect both the reverse transcription and PCR steps. RT-PCR methods are widely used to precisely measure RNA abundance in cells and tissues. Several different "real-time" PCR assays use fluorescent dyes to accurately measure the amount of PCR products synthesized in various amplification cycles (Figs. 2-7 and 2-8).[30,31] The amount of RNA in a sample is determined by measuring how many amplification rounds are needed for the fluorescent signal to exceed a standardized threshold. The advantages of real-time PCR include extreme sensitivity, technical ease, and the ability to accurately quantitate DNA and RNA over a range of at least five orders of magnitude. Real-time PCR is often the method of choice for analyzing the abundance of specific mRNAs in tumor samples, such as monitoring the expression of the *BCR-ABL* transcript in patients undergoing therapy for chronic myeloid leukemia, and for detecting minimal residual disease in leukemias and lymphomas. RT-PCR can also simultaneously determine the expression of multiple genes. For example, one approved diagnostic test uses RT-PCR to assess the expression of 21 genes to predict recurrence risk in women with early-stage estrogen receptor–positive breast cancer.[32]

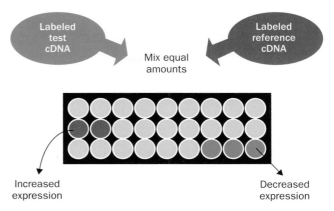

Fig. 2-9 Expression microarray.

Standard RNA and tumor RNA are converted to cDNA and labeled with different fluorescent probes. These are hybridized to arrays of microscopic dots containing DNA or oligonucleotide probes representing different genes. The resulting array of fluorescent signals is read electronically and the output suggests differential expression of a subset of genes in the two samples.

Microarrays, Next-Generation Sequencing, and Global Analyses of Transcription

Real-time PCR methods are used for studies involving relatively small numbers of genes or specific and/or abnormal mRNAs. However, other approaches are needed to study the expression of thousands of genes simultaneously, and these typically utilize either microarrays or next-generation sequencing. Microarrays use chips, which are small slides on which either oligonucleotides or cDNAs are spotted in defined arrays.[33] These arrays are interrogated by hybridizing cDNA made from tumor and control cells, each labeled with a different fluorescent dye. A computerized reader assesses the fluorescence intensity, which depends on the relative abundance of the mRNAs in two samples cells (Fig. 2-9). In some cases, small amounts of RNA from limited clinical specimens are first amplified by PCR prior to hybridization. Microarrays can simultaneously measure the abundance of nearly all genes that are expressed in a tissue or tumor sample, termed the transcriptome, and are essential tools in molecular oncology research. Microarray studies can also define prognostic groups in clinically challenging populations, such as using gene expression signatures to predict time to metastases in women with node-negative breast cancer.[34] Similarly, array-based mRNA signatures can separate morphologically indistinguishable large-cell lymphomas into high- and low-risk groups on the basis of their gene expression patterns, which reflect their cell of origin.[35] Genome-wide microarray analyses are expensive and complex, which makes this a difficult technique to bring to the clinic. However, gene subsets can be used to accurately report prognostic or diagnostic information, and these can be arrayed on smaller chips that are more easily adapted to clinical labs. For example, the expression profiles of 70 genes derived from the genome-wide profiling of breast cancers provide a tool for predicting metastasis and survival (Fig. 2-10).[36]

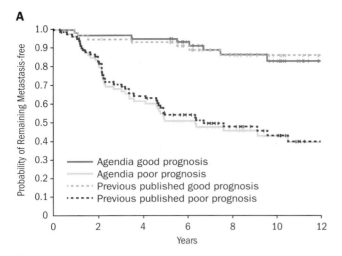

A

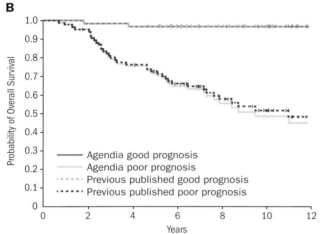

B

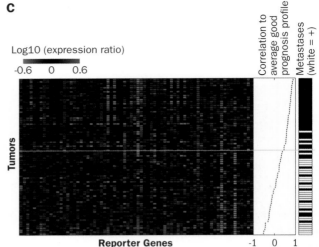

C

Fig. 2-10 Gene expression profiles as a predictive tool.

(A) Kaplan-Meier analysis of the probability that patients would remain free of distant metastases among 145 patients with lymph node–negative breast cancer. Light blue: current good prognosis profile group; green dashed: previous good prognosis profile group; yellow: current poor prognosis profile group; dark blue dashed: previous poor prognosis profile group. (B) Kaplan-Meier analysis of the probability of overall survival among 145 patients with lymph node–negative breast cancer. (C) Expression data matrix of 70 prognostic marker genes from tumors of 78 patients with breast cancer hybridized using the custom microarray. Each row represents a tumor and each column a gene. Genes are ordered according to their original ordering. Tumors are ordered by their correlation to the average profile of the good prognosis group. The metastases status for each patient is shown in the right panel. White indicates patients who developed metastases within 5 years after the initial diagnosis, black indicates patients who continued to be metastasis-free for at least 5 years.

Reprinted with permission from Glas AM, Floore A, Delahaye LJ, et al. Converting a breast cancer microarray signature into a high-throughput diagnostic test. BMC Genomics. 2006;7:278-288.

Because next-generation sequencing is quantitative, it provides new ways to assess mRNA abundance at genome scale that are not prone to many of the technical limitations of microarrays. Thus, as high-throughput sequencing becomes more widely available, sequencing-based approaches will replace microarrays as the method of choice for quantitating mRNAs in tumors.

MicroRNAs and Small Interfering RNAs

MicroRNAs (miRNAs) are RNAs with fundamental roles in regulating gene expression. miRNAs are small RNAs (18 to 24 nucleotides) that regulate the expression of other genes by base-pairing to their target mRNAs and inhibiting their expression. This inhibition is usually accomplished either by interfering with mRNA translation or by catalyzing mRNA destruction by cellular nuclease complexes (Fig. 2-11).[37] Most miRNAs are encoded within longer primary transcripts that are processed to form the final miRNAs. Humans have more than 400 miRNA genes that regulate most cellular processes.[38,39] Rapid progress in developing bioinformatic and experimental approaches to identify miRNA target genes have revealed that individual miRNAs can target many genes

(dozens to hundreds), and that as many as 30% of all genes are thought to be under miRNA control. The complexity of the miRNA regulatory network is thus immense. Studies of miRNA expression patterns indicate that specific cancers exhibit characteristic and abnormal patterns of miRNA expression. Indeed, aberrant miRNA expression is thought to play causal roles in human neoplasia,[40] and miRNA deregulation causes cancers in mouse models.[41] Global analyses of miRNA expression likely will become an important tool in cancer diagnosis and prognosis.

Small interfering RNAs (siRNAs) are synthetic double-stranded miRNAs that are vital tools for molecular oncology research. Because siRNAs efficiently catalyze the degradation of their cognate mRNAs, researchers can design siRNAs that inhibit the expression of any desired gene. These techniques are revolutionizing studies of gene function, and genome-wide siRNA screens are widely used to dissect biologic pathways to ascertain gene function and identify drug targets in cancer cells.[42,43]

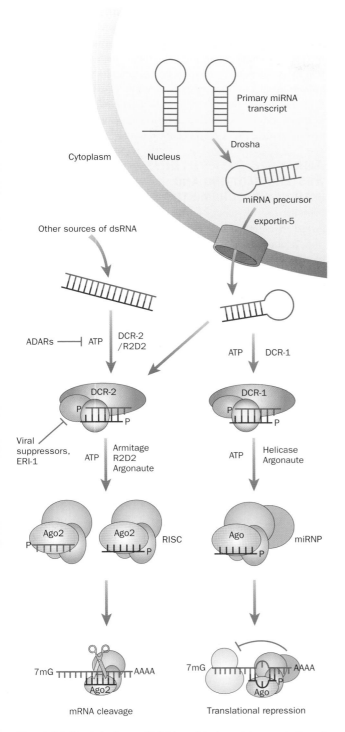

Cytoplasm   Nucleus

Primary miRNA transcript

Drosha

miRNA precursor

exportin-5

Other sources of dsRNA

ADARs ⊣ ATP   DCR-2 /R2D2

ATP   DCR-1

DCR-2

DCR-1

Viral suppressors, ERI-1

ATP   Armitage R2D2 Argonaute

ATP   Helicase Argonaute

Ago2   Ago2   RISC

Ago   miRNP

7mG ——AAAA
Ago2

mRNA cleavage

7mG ——AAAA
Ago

Translational repression

CHROMOSOME ANALYSIS
KARYOTYPING

Cancer cells often exhibit chromosome abnormalities that are pathognomonic for specific diseases. Karyotype analyses examine an individual's entire chromosome complement, and classical analyses identify chromosomes in metaphase spreads based on banding patterns and morphology. Although these techniques are still widely used, they are often augmented with newer techniques that are more sensitive and/or comprehensive. Several cytogenetic methods employ fluorescence in situ hybridization (FISH), in which fluorescently labeled nucleic acid probes are hybridized to their homologous sequences in either metaphase or interphase cells, allowing specific genes to be examined. For example, chromosome- and gene-specific probes are used to determine the copy number of specific oncogenes, such as the *HER2* gene in breast cancers. Another common FISH technique uses probes that detect gene fusions and chromosome translocations, such as the *BCR-ABL* fusion. The ability of FISH-based methods to identify rare cells with abnormal karyotypes makes them useful for detecting residual disease when malignant cells harbor a cytogenetic marker. Spectral karyotyping (SKY) is a FISH method for characterizing

Fig. 2-11 Model of small-RNA–guided post-transcriptional regulation of gene expression.

Primary miRNA transcripts are processed to miRNA precursors in the nucleus by the RNase-III–like enzyme Drosha. The miRNA precursor is subsequently exported to the cytoplasm by means of the export receptor exportin-5. The miRNA precursor is further processed by Dicer to siRNA-duplex–like intermediates. The duplex is unwound while assembling into miRNP/RISC. Mature miRNAs bind to Ago proteins, which mediate translational repression or cleavage of target mRNAs. Other sources of long dsRNA in the cytoplasm of a cell are viral RNAs, artificially introduced dsRNA, dsRNAs generated by RdRPs, and genomic sense and antisense transcripts. Like miRNA precursors, long dsRNA is processed by the RNase-III enzyme Dicer into 21–23 nucleotide dsRNA intermediates. Assisted by the RNA helicase Armitage and R2D2, the single-stranded siRNA-containing RISC is formed. The stability of the dsRNA and its recognition by Dicer can be regulated by specific ADARs and the exonuclease ERI-1.

Adapted by permission from Macmillan Publishers Ltd: Meister G, Tuschl T. Mechanisms of gene silencing by double-stranded RNA. Nature. 2004;431(7006):343-349.

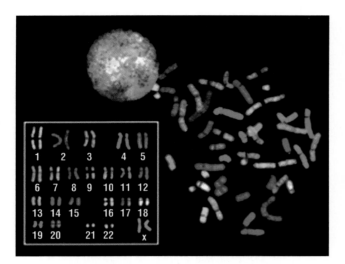

Fig. 2-12 Spectral karyotype showing different dyes characteristic for each chromosome.

This technique allows for rapid analysis of metaphase spreads for subtle chromosomal losses, gains, and translocations.

Reprinted with permission from the National Human Genome Research Institute; http://www.genome.gov/pages/hyperion/dir/vip/glossary/illustration/pdf/sky.pdf. Accessed May 27, 2014.

chromosome aberrations that cannot be appreciated by classic techniques. SKY uses a panel of chromosome-specific probes that are labeled with different fluorochromes and hybridized to metaphase chromosomes. Each chromosome is thus visualized by color, which allows the identification of chromosomes affected by subtle and/or complex rearrangements (Fig. 2-12).

COPY NUMBER VARIATIONS

Comparative genomic hybridization (CGH) is a technique that identifies DNA gains and losses in a tumor by using DNA hybridization to compare it with a normal sample. To perform CGH, differentially labeled tumor and normal DNA are hybridized to a reference sample, and amplifications or deletions of tumor DNA are identified by deviations in the ratio of signal provided by

KEY POINTS

- Karyotyping reveals gross DNA structural anomalies in tumor cells, such as translocations and chromosomal deletions.
- Methods that incorporate hybridization techniques, such as spectral karyotyping and comparative genomic hybridization, greatly increase the sensitivity of cytogenetic analyses.
- FISH techniques detect structural abnormalities in tumor DNA, such as translocations, deletions, and copy number variations. These sensitive methods are also used to detect residual disease in hematologic cancers.

the normal and tumor probes. In array CGH, labeled tumor and normal DNA are hybridized to chips containing arrays of DNA fragments representing entire genomes.[44] Because array CGH detects copy number changes in DNA fragments too small for detection by cytogenetic techniques and at genome scale, it provides unique insight on the complex genomic gains and losses that drive neoplastic transformation. However, as discussed above, next-generation sequencing approaches may soon become the preferred means of detecting copy number changes in cancers.

ANALYSIS OF PROTEINS
WESTERN BLOTTING AND IMMUNOHISTOCHEMISTRY

Proteins can be separated by gel electrophoresis and transferred to membranes, which can then be exposed to detection probes, most commonly antibodies (termed Western blotting).[45] These probes can detect changes in protein size, post-translational modifications (e.g., phosphorylation), and abundance. Pathology departments routinely employ antibody-based immunohistochemical methods to detect the expression of specific proteins in tumor cells. Examples include antibodies to intermediate filament proteins that are used to define the origins of poorly differentiated cancers, immunodetection of neuron-specific enolase and synaptophysin used to distinguish neuroendocrine cancers, and studies of steroid-hormone receptor expression in breast cancer. Another important immunohistochemical diagnostic technique, particularly for hematologic cancers, is flow cytometry, which simultaneously detects multiple cell surface markers in complex cell populations, such as bone marrow. These features make flow cytometry especially useful for applications such as the immunophenotyping used to classify leukemias and lymphomas based on their cell surface proteins. Because flow cytometry has extremely high sensitivity and can analyze large numbers of cells, it is often used to detect small numbers of tumor cells, such as residual leukemia in normal bone marrow. Immunohistochemistry is also used as a surrogate to detect certain oncogene mutations, such as *HER2* amplifications in breast cancer and mutations of the *p53* tumor suppressor that cause increased p53 abundance.

MASS SPECTROMETRY AND PROTEOMICS

The methods described previously are used to study the expression of individual proteins in biologic samples. However, analogous to the large-scale genomic analyses of DNA sequence or RNA expression, proteomics involves global studies of protein abundance and modifications. Mass spectrometry forms the core of modern proteomics and is used in combination with bioinformatics to quantitate and identify the large numbers of proteins present in complex biologic samples.[46] These methods are informed by genome-wide sequencing that allowed construction of the comprehensive databases used to identify the peptides analyzed by mass spectrometry. Mass spectrometry can also interrogate signaling processes such as protein phosphorylation on a very large scale. One intense area of proteomics research involves early cancer detection based

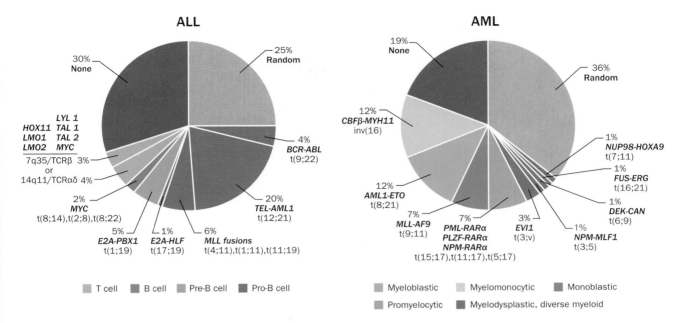

Fig. 2-13 Distribution of translocation-generated oncogenes among the acute leukemias of children and young adults.
The products of these aberrant genes are most often nuclear proteins active in transcription, with the notable exception of BCR-ABL, which encodes a cytoplasmic protein containing the activated ABL tyrosine kinase domain. In acute lymphocytic leukemia (ALL), gene fusions tend to be specifically associated with one of the commonly recognized immunologic subtypes of the disease, as indicated by the color coding on the chart. The T-cell leukemias (light green) are characterized by translocations that dysregulate the expression of proto-oncogenes. The *MYC* gene is also dysregulated through translocation into the vicinity of one of the immunoglobin (Ig) loci in B-cell leukemia (dark green) and Burkitt lymphoma. In the pre-B (light teal) and pro-B (dark teal) immunologic subtypes of ALL, fusion genes encoding chimeric oncoproteins are produced. The *BCR-ABL* and *MLL* gene fusions have also been identified in the chronic (CML) and acute myeloid leukemias (AML), respectively, suggesting that they arise in primitive stem cells with multilineage potential. "Random" refers to sporadic translocations that have been observed only in leukemic cells from single cases. "None" refers to leukemias that lack identifiable gene abnormalities. In AML, the genes show specific associations with disease subtypes corresponding to the morphologic stages of normal myeloid cell development. Although both the *AML1-ETO* and *CBFbeta-MYH11* fusion genes lead to alterations in the CBF transcription complex, they appear to disrupt hematopoiesis through distinct mechanisms, because they are associated with different morphologic subtypes of AML. Other rearrangements affect the *RARalpha* gene on chromosome 17 in promyelocytic progenitors, resulting in fusions with *PML* or, rarely, *PLZF* or *NPM*. Less frequent translocations give rise to fusion genes associated with myelodysplastic syndrome progressing to AML (*NPM-MLF1, DEK-CAN, and NUP98-HOXA9*).

From Look AT. Oncologic transcription factors in the human acute leukemia. Science. *1997;278(5340):1059-1064. Reprinted with permission from AAAS.*

on defining protein signatures indicative of early-stage cancers in tissues, such as peripheral blood.[47] Proteomic methods likely will be an important tool in cancer detection, diagnosis, and prognosis in the near future.

KEY POINTS

- Protein analyses reveal protein abundance, functional modifications such as phosphorylation and acetylation, and information such as subcellular localization.
- Immunohistochemical techniques that detect protein expression are used for a wide variety of diagnostic tests, including immunophenotyping for diagnosis and classification, and detection of minimal residual disease.
- Mass spectrometry–based proteomics allow for large-scale analyses of protein expression and modifications in tumor tissues.

ONCOGENES: THE ENGINES OF CANCER

Transforming a normal cell into a malignant cell requires a series of mutations in genes, termed oncogenes, which contribute to neoplasia when their functions are altered.[48,49] To date, perhaps several hundred human genes have been implicated as proto-oncogenes, which are genes that have the potential to be converted into oncogenes. Oncogenes are either dominant or recessive, and they normally function in cellular processes such as cell division, apoptosis, and differentiation. Dominant oncogenes sustain gain-of-function mutations in cancers, whereas recessive oncogenes—also called tumor suppressor genes—sustain loss-of-function mutations in cancers.

ACTIVATION AND IDENTIFICATION OF DOMINANT ONCOGENES

Dominant oncogenes are activated by numerous mechanisms. Many of the first known oncogenes were discovered in experimental cancer models, and many of the same genes first identified in model systems were subsequently found to be activated in human cancers by mechanisms such as translocation,

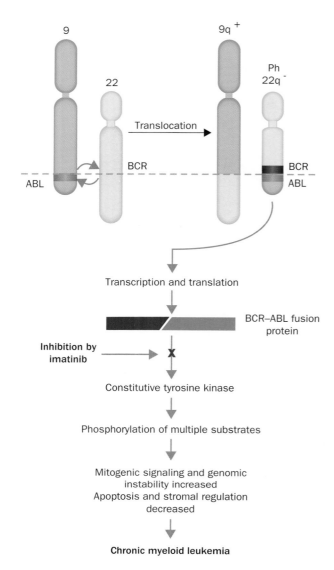

Fig. 2-14 Translocation leading to the Philadelphia (Ph) chromosome and the role of *BCR-ABL* in the pathogenesis of chronic myeloid leukemia.

The Ph chromosome is a foreshortened chromosome 22 resulting from an exchange between the long arms of chromosomes 9 and 22.

From New Engl J Med, Savage DG and Antman KH. Imatinib Mesylate—A New Oral Targeted Therapy, 346;9:683-693. Copyright © (2002) Massachusetts Medical Society. Reprinted with permission from Massachusetts Medical Society.

amplification, and point mutations. These different types of mutations lead to distinct functional outcomes and often provide important diagnostic and prognostic information.

Experimental Cancer Models: Retroviruses and Transfections

Many dominant oncogenes were first discovered through studies of animal cancers induced by retroviruses, called RNA tumor viruses. One class of RNA tumor viruses carries viral oncogenes within their viral genomes, and several dozen viral oncogenes were identified in the 1970s and 1980s. The major breakthrough with respect to human cancer came with the realization that viral oncogenes represent mutated versions of host proto-oncogenes that were captured by the viral genomes during their life cycle. Many viral oncogenes are the counterparts of extremely important human oncogenes, and the identification of their cellular homologues established the framework within which we understand the role of dominant oncogenes in tumorigenesis.

The second class of RNA tumor viruses causes animal cancers by a mechanism termed insertional mutagenesis, in which the integration of a viral genome into a host chromosome activates a cellular proto-oncogene. Insertional mutagenesis is a powerful genetic tool for oncogene discovery, and a host of new approaches have been developed in the post-human and mouse genome era that are identifying many previously unknown proto-oncogenes.

Another experimental strategy initially used to identify oncogenes is called DNA transfection. In this approach, DNA is extracted from tumor cells and introduced into recipient cells by a technique called transfection. The recipient cells used in these experiments, such as murine NIH3T3 cells, undergo morphologic and growth alterations when they are transfected with an oncogene and are said to become transformed. The transfected tumor cell DNA is subsequently isolated and sequenced from the transformed cells, allowing the identification of the transferred oncogene. Many critical human oncogenes, including *RAS*, were originally isolated from transfection experiments.

Chromosome Translocations

Cancers often contain recurrent chromosome translocations; this is particularly true for hematologic malignancies, which are characterized by chromosome translocations that often involve Ig and T-cell receptor genes (Fig. 2-13).[50] Specific translocations have important diagnostic and prognostic implications, and they serve as molecular markers for the detection of residual disease and relapse. The regions of DNA commonly involved with translocations are termed breakpoints and often contain proto-oncogenes that are activated by the DNA rearrangement.

Chromosome translocations activate proto-oncogenes in two general ways.[51] The most common mechanism involves the creation of fusion genes when the translocation joins two genes normally found on separate chromosomes in the same translational reading frame and results in a novel protein encoded by the two fused genes. Fusion proteins often involve transcription factors or tyrosine kinases and have biologic activities that differ from the parental proto-oncogene. An example of this type of translocation is the *BCR-ABL* fusion that results from the reciprocal exchange of DNA between chromosomes 9 and 22, t(9;22), known as the Philadelphia chromosome (Fig. 2-14). The translocation juxtaposes the 5' end of the *BCR* gene on chromosome 22 and the 3' end of the *c-ABL* oncogene on chromosome 9. The resultant novel gene produces a hybrid mRNA that codes for the BCR-ABL oncoprotein, which deregulates the tyrosine kinase activity normally associated with the c-ABL protein.

Translocations also activate proto-oncogenes by deregulating their expression without altering their protein structure. An example of this type of translocation is found in Burkitt

Table 2-1 The Immunoglobulin and T-Cell Receptor Gene-Associated Translocations

Translocation	Genes	Major Structures	Disease
t(8;14)(q24;q32)	MYC	BHLH	Acute lymphoid leukemia
t(2;8)(p12;q24)	IGH; IGK	BHLH	Acute lymphoid leukemia
t(8;22)(q24;q11)	MYC; MYC	BHLH	Acute lymphoid leukemia
t(14;19)(q32;q13)	IGH; IGL	IkB homology	Chronic lymphoid leukemia (B-cell)
t(5;14)(q31;q32)	BCL-3; IL-3	Cytokine	Chronic lymphoid leukemia (pre B-cell)
t(7;14)(q21;q32)	IGH; THE (CDK6)	Cyclin-dependent kinase	Chronic lymphoid leukemia (B-cell)
t(9;14)(p21;q11)	IGH; p16/p19^{ARF}	TS activity	Acute lymphoid leukemia (B-cell)
t(7;19)(q35;p13)	TCRd; TCRb	BHLH	Acute lymphoid leukemia (T-cell)
t(1;14)(p32;q11)	LYL1; TAL1/SCL	BHLH	Acute lymphoid leukemia (T-cell)
t(7;9)(q35;q34)	TCRa; TCRb	BHLH	Acute lymphoid leukemia (T-cell)
t(11;14)(p15;q11)	TAL2; LMO1/rbtn1/Tgt1	Lim domain	Acute lymphoid leukemia (T-cell)
t(11;14)(p13;q11)	TCR; LMO2/rbnt2/Tgt2	Lim domain	Acute lymphoid leukemia (T-cell)
t(7;11)(q35;p13)	TCR; TCRb; LMO2/rbnt2/Tgt2	Lim domain	Acute lymphoid leukemia (T-cell)
t(7;10)(q35;q24)	TCRb	Homeodomain	Acute lymphoid leukemia (T-cell)
t(14;21)(q11;q22)	HOX11; TCRa	BHLH	Acute lymphoid leukemia (T-cell)
t(10;14)(q24;q11)	BHLHB1; HOX11	Homeodomain	Acute lymphoid leukemia (T-cell)
t(14;18)	TCRd; IGH	BCL2 protein	B-cell lymphoma
(q32;q21)	BCL2; CCDN1	Cyclin D1	Mantle cell lymphoma
t(11;14)(q13;q32)	IGH	Cyclin D1	Mantle cell lymphoma

Abbreviations: BHLH, basic helix-loop-helix; TS, thymidylate synthase.

lymphoma, which is characterized by translocations that cause the *c-MYC* oncogene—located on chromosome 8—to be juxtaposed to Ig genes that are located on chromosomes 14, 2, and 22. In each case, the translocation deregulates *c-MYC* expression by placing it under the control of transcriptional elements contained within the Ig locus. Other examples of proto-oncogenes that are activated by translocations involving Ig genes include cyclin D1 (found in mantle cell lymphoma) and *BCL-2* (in follicular lymphoma). Table 2-1 lists representative proto-oncogenes involved in translocations with Ig and T-cell receptor loci.

Recurrent chromosome translocations also occur in solid tumors. In Ewing sarcoma (EWS), translocations fuse the *EWS* gene on chromosome 22 to the *FLI-1* gene on chromosome 11, creating a transcription factor containing a DNA-binding domain derived from *FLI-1* and transcriptional activation domain from *EWS*.[52] Alveolar rhabdomyosarcomas also contain a pathognomonic translocation, which fuses the *PAX3* and *FHK4* transcription factors. Translocations that join the androgen-responsive *TMPRSS2* gene with two *ETS* transcription factors—*ETV1*

and *ERG*—occur frequently in prostate cancer and result in abnormal *ETS* expression driven by the androgen-responsive regulatory elements in the *TMPRSS2* gene.[53]

DNA Amplification

DNA amplification results in the increased copy number of a gene and is another mechanism by which cancer cells increase the expression of a gene product, and many solid tumors exhibit amplification of known proto-oncogenes (Table 2-2).[54] Gene amplification can be detected by many methods, including CGH, FISH, and genomic sequencing. In some cases, the detection of amplified genes provides important prognostic and treatment-related information, as in the case of *HER2* amplification in breast cancer and *N-Myc* gene amplification in neuroblastoma.

Point Mutations

Dominant oncogenes are frequently activated by point mutations that increase or alter (neomorphic) their activity. For example, recurrent mutations of amino acids that alter *KRAS* function are found in a large number of human cancers. Because

Table 2-2 Oncogenes Amplified in Human Cancers

Gene Amplified	Locus	Tumors
AKT2	19q13.2	Ovarian cancer
CCND1 (Cyclin D1)	11q13.3	HNSCC, esophageal, breast, HCC
CCNE (Cyclin E)	19q12	Gastric cancer
CDK4	12q14	Sarcoma, glioblastoma
ERBB1 (EGFR)	7p12	Glioblastoma, HNSCC
ERBB2 (EGFR2)	17q11.2-q12	Breast, ovarian, cervix cancer
FGFR1	8p11.1-p11.2	Breast cancer
FGFR2	10q25.3-q26	Breast cancer
HRAS	11p15.5	Colorectal cancer
KRAS	12p13	Colorectal, gastric cancer
MDM2	12q14	Soft tissue sarcomas, osteosarcoma, esophageal cancer
MET	7q31	Gastric cancer
MYB	6q23.3-q24	Colorectal cancer
MYC	8q24.12-q24.13	Ovarian, breast, SCLC, HNSCC, esophageal, cervix cancer
N-MYC	2p24.3	Neuroblastoma

Abbreviations: HNSCC, head and neck squamous cell carcinoma; HCC, hepatocellular carcinoma; SCLC, small cell lung cancer.

Reproduced with the permission of the McGraw-Hill Companies: Scriver CR, Sly W (eds.), et al. Metabolic and Molecular Basis of Inherited Disease, 8th Edition. 2001.

some common oncogenes, such as *RAS*, are activated by only a few specific point mutations, these genes were some of the first that were routinely screened for in cancer specimens, because they can be identified with relatively simple techniques. However, genome-scale sequencing has now made it possible to identify nearly all potentially oncogenic point mutations in primary tumor samples.

Detection of Tumor Suppressor Gene Inactivation

Loss of tumor suppressor gene alleles occurs commonly in cancers.[55] Delineating a locus involved by allelic loss in a tumor type often is the first step toward identifying a tumor suppressor gene. Sites of allelic loss have traditionally been determined by analyzing polymorphic markers or using CGH to analyze tumor and normal DNA from an individual. These analyses define the smallest region of allelic loss that is common to a number of patients, thereby localizing the disease

gene (among other candidate genes within a deleted region). However, this is another area of cancer genetics that is being affected by next-generation sequencing, which is rapidly becoming the method of choice for detecting allelic losses in tumors. Sequence-based approaches can be targeted toward known tumor suppressor genes, all expressed genes (exomes), or genome-wide (see Modern Oncogenomics section).

Many tumor suppressor genes were first identified by virtue of their association with hereditary cancer syndromes. Importantly, the effect of these studies extends far beyond hereditary cancer syndromes because the genes responsible for familial cancers often are the same tumor suppressor genes that are inactivated in sporadic cancers. In most familial cancer syndromes, a mutant copy of a recessive oncogene is inherited, followed by mutation of the remaining normal allele in cancers that develop in these individuals. Thus, the molecular signature of a classic tumor suppressor is loss of heterozygosity and inactivating mutations within the remaining allele in tumors. This is known as a Knudson two-step tumor suppressor, named after classic studies of the *Rb* tumor suppressor in retinoblastoma. In fact, the failure to find biallelic loss in tumors often was used as evidence against the assignment of a putative locus as a tumor suppressor.

However, there are important exceptions to the Knudson model that expand our understanding of how tumor suppressor genes are mutated in cancers. In some cases, loss of a single allele of a tumor suppressor is sufficient to confer cancer susceptibility or contribute to neoplastic progression, even when a normal allele persists. In the case of these haploinsufficient tumor suppressor genes, intragenic mutations in the remaining allele will not be found, and this initially can confuse the identification of important human tumor suppressors, such as the *p27Kip1* cell cycle inhibitor. Another situation when a tumor suppressor will not conform to the Knudson model is when tumor suppressors are inactivated by epigenetic mechanisms, such as when the *p16INK4A* cell cycle inhibitor is silenced by DNA methylation in cancers.

FUNCTIONS OF ONCOGENES

Genes that can become oncogenes through mutations normally function in a wide array of biologic processes, such as

KEY POINTS

- Proto-oncogenes are normal cellular genes that can be converted into oncogenes by mutation or by epigenetic mechanisms, which alter their normal functions or expression.
- Dominant oncogenes encode proteins that are activated in tumors by mechanisms such as amplification, point mutations, and translocations.
- Tumor suppressor genes are recessive oncogenes that are inactivated in tumors by diverse mechanisms including deletions, point mutations, and silencing.

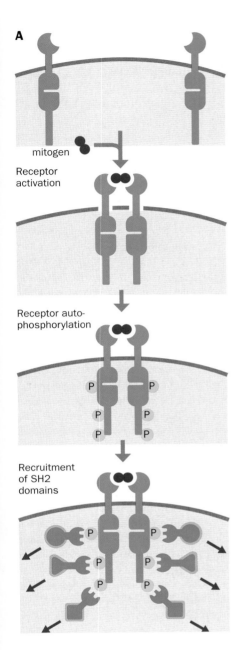

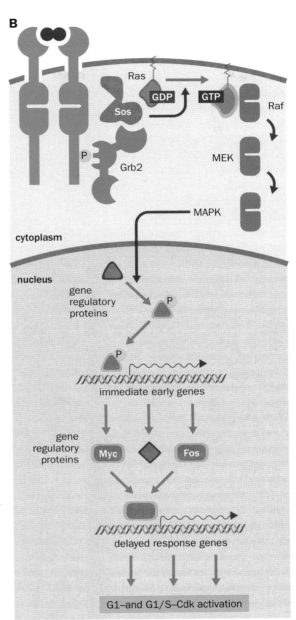

Fig. 2-15 Mitogenic signaling.

(A) Origin of the mitogenic signal at the cell membrane. The binding of growth factors to receptor tyrosine kinases causes receptor dimerization and autophosphorylation. The receptor tyrosine phosphorylation then recruits binding proteins that contain SH2 domains, and these transmit the mitogenic signal (see text). **(B)** Mitogenic signaling by the RAS pathway. RAS activation stimulates the MAP kinase pathway, which leads to the activation of downstream transcription factors such as JUN and MYC (see text).

Reproduced by permission of the New Science Press. From Figures 10-11 and 10-12 from Morgan, David O. The Cell Cycle: Principles of Control (New Science Press, 2007).

transduction, cell division, DNA repair, and apoptosis. Many of the major cellular pathways that contain dominant oncogenes and tumor suppressor genes are summarized in the following subsections.

MITOGENIC SIGNAL TRANSDUCTION PATHWAYS

Cell division is triggered by signal transduction pathways that are stimulated when protein growth factors bind to specific cell-surface receptors, and these pathways contain proto-oncogenes throughout the signaling chain (Table 2-3).[56] Most growth factor receptors are anchored in the cell membrane such that an extracellular domain is available for growth factor (ligand) binding and an intracellular domain interacts with downstream signaling molecules. The intracellular portions

of a class of growth factor receptors, called receptor tyrosine kinases (RTKs), contain a kinase domain that catalyzes the addition of phosphate to tyrosine residues. Ligand binding causes RTKs to dimerize and leads to autophosphorylation (Fig. 2-15A). RTK tyrosine phosphorylation recruits proteins that contain SH2 domains, which recognize the phospho-tyrosine motifs and then transmit the mitogenic signal down several parallel pathways, including the phosphatidylinositol 3-kinase (PI3K) and mitogen-activated kinase (MAP kinase) pathways. Constituents of these signaling pathways were some of the earliest identified oncogenes, and dominant mutations in these proto-oncogenes lead to unrestrained mitogenic signaling that subverts the normal growth factor signals needed to stimulate these pathways.

Table 2-3 **Oncogenes**

Oncogene	Lesion	Neoplasm	Proto-Oncogene
Growth Factors			
v-sis		Glioma/fibrosarcoma	B-chain *PDGF*
int 2	Proviral insertion	Mammary carcinoma	Member of *FGF* family
KS3	DNA transfection	Kaposi sarcoma	Member of *FGF* family
HST	DNA transfection	Stomach carcinoma	Member of *FGF* family
int-1	Proviral insertion	Mammary carcinoma	Possible growth factor
Receptors Lacking Protein Kinase Activity			
mas	DNA transfection	Mammary carcinoma	Angiotensin receptor
Tyrosine Kinases: Integral Membrane Proteins, Growth Factor Receptors			
EGFR	Amplification	Squamous cell carcinoma	Protein kinase (tyr) *EGFR*
v-fms		Sarcoma	Protein kinase (tyr) *CSF-1R**
v-kit		Sarcoma	Protein kinase (tyr) stem cell factor R
v-ros		Sarcoma	Protein kinase (tyr)
MET	Rearrangement	MNNG-treated human osteocarcinoma cell line	Protein kinase (tyr) *HGF/SFR*
TRK	Rearrangement	Colon carcinoma	Protein kinase (tyr) *NGFR*
NEU	Point mutation; amplification	Neuroblastoma, carcinoma of breast	Protein kinase (tyr)
RET	Rearrangement	Carcinoma of thyroid Men 2A, Men 2B	Protein kinase (tyr) *GDNFR*
Tyrosine Kinases: Membrane-Associated			
SRC		Colon carcinoma	Protein kinase (tyr)
v-yes		Sarcoma	Protein kinase (tyr)
v-fgr		Sarcoma	Protein kinase (tyr)
v-fps		Sarcoma	Protein kinase (tyr)
v-fes		Sarcoma	Protein kinase (tyr)
BCR/ABL	Chromosome translocation	Chronic myeloid leukemia	Protein kinase (tyr)
Membrane-Associated G Proteins			
HRAS	Point mutation	Colon, lung, pancreas carcinoma	*GTPase*
KRAS	Point mutation	Acute myeloid leukemia, thyroid carcinoma, melanoma	*GTPase*
NRAS	Point mutation	Carcinoma, melanoma	*GTPase*
gsp	Point mutation	Carcinoma of thyroid	*Gsalpha*
gip	Point mutation	Ovary, adrenal carcinoma	*G1alpha*
GEF Family of Proteins			
Dbl	Rearrangement	Diffuse B-cell lymphoma	GEF for *Rho* and *Cdc42Hs*
Ost		Osteosarcomas	GEF for *RhoA* and *Cdc42Hs*
Tiam-1	Metastatic and oncogenic	T-cell lymphoma	GEF for *Rac* and *Cdc42Hs*
Vav	Rearrangement	Hematopoietic cells	GEF for *RAS*?
Lbc	Oncogenic	Myeloid leukemias	GEF for *Rho*

Table 2-3 **continued**

Oncogene	Lesion	Neoplasm	Proto-Oncogene
Serine/Threonine Kinases: Cytoplasmic			
v-mos		Sarcoma	Protein kinase (ser/thr)
v-raf		Sarcoma	Protein kinase (ser/thr)
pim-1	Proviral insertion	T-cell lymphoma	Protein kinase (ser/thr)
Cytoplasmic Regulators			
v-crk			SH-2/SH-3 adaptor
Nuclear Protein Family			
v-myc		Carcinoma myelocytomatosis	Transcription factor
N-MYC	Gene amplification	Neuroblastoma, lung carcinoma	Transcription factor
L-MYC	Gene amplification	Carcinoma of lung	Transcription factor
v-myb		Myeloblastosis	Transcription factor
v-fos		Osteosarcoma	Transcription factor API
v-jun		Sarcoma	Transcription factor API
v-ski		Carcinoma	Transcription factor
v-rel		Lymphatic leukemia	Mutant NFgammaB
v-ets		Myeloblastosis	Transcription factor
v-srbA		Erythroblastosis	Mutant thioredoxine receptor

Abbreviations: CSF-1R, macrophage colony-stimulating factor-1 receptor; EGFR, epidermal growth factor receptor; FGF, fibroblast growth factor; GEF, guanine nucleotide exchange factor; GDNF, glial-derived neurotropic factor; HGF/SF, hepatic growth factor/scatter factor; NGF, nerve growth factor; PDGF, platelet-derived growth factor.

Reproduced with the permission of the McGraw-Hill Companies: Vogelstein B, Kinzler K. The Genetic Basis of Human Cancer, 2nd Edition. *2002.*

Kinases are attractive therapeutic targets in cancers, and several therapeutic strategies that target aberrant RTKs are in clinical use. One approach utilizes antibodies that bind to and inhibit RTKs. Examples include trastuzumab, which antagonizes HER2 activity and is used in the treatment of breast cancers with *HER2* amplification,[57] and cetuximab, an inhibitory antibody that binds to the epidermal growth factor receptor (EGFR) and is approved for use in metastatic colon cancer and head and neck cancers.[58,59] Another strategy to target RTKs in cancers utilizes small molecule inhibitors, such as imatinib (see below), gefitinib, and erlotinib, which bind to RTKs and inhibit their catalytic activity. Small molecule RTK inhibitors that have been designed against a specific target have the greatest efficacy in tumors that contain mutations with the target kinase. For example, gefitinib efficacy is closely associated with mutations in *EGFR* that are found in a small fraction of patients with lung cancers.[60]

RAS proteins transduce mitogenic signals downstream of RTKs.[61] One key SH2 protein that binds to phosphorylated RTKs is the Grb2 adaptor protein (Fig. 2-15B). The GRB2/RTK complex is bound by Son of Sevenless (SOS), a guanine nucleotide-exchange factor (GEF) that activates RAS by exchanging guanosine triphosphate (GTP) with guanosine diphosphate (GDP). RAS activity also is regulated by interaction with guanosine triphosphatase-activating proteins (GAPs) that mediate

hydrolysis of RAS-bound GTP to GDP. GDP-bound RAS is inactive until a GTP molecule replaces GDP in an exchange reaction mediated by a guanine exchange factor such as SOS. The amount of RAS activity is thus determined by the balance between GEF and GAP activity (Fig. 2-15). Oncogenic *RAS* mutations affect amino acids 12, 13, and 61, which are all critical for interaction with GAPs. Because reduced GAP function prolongs RAS signaling, GAPs may function as recessive oncogenes. For example, the *NF-1* gene is a GAP that acquires a loss-of-function mutation in neurofibromatosis. Because *RAS* pathway mutations are so frequent in cancers (e.g., 80% of pancreatic cancers, 40% of lung cancers, 50% of colon cancers), anti-RAS therapy has been pursued aggressively. Most efforts to block RAS activity have focused on agents that inhibit an essential post-translational modification of RAS proteins by a fatty acid moiety that is required to localize RAS to its site of action at the inner plasma membrane.[62]

RAS activity drives three parallel pathways: the MAP kinase pathway (which activates transcription factors), the RAL/CDC42 pathway (which regulates membrane and cytoskeletal changes), and the PI3K pathway (which affects many cellular functions, including protein synthesis and apoptosis; Fig. 2-16). The MAP kinase pathway is stimulated by the RAF serine/threonine kinase and signals to additional downstream cytoplasmic serine-threonine kinases that ultimately activate MAP

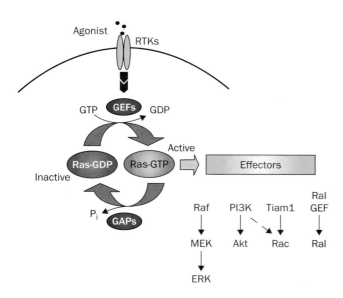

Fig. 2-16 RAS upstream and downstream signaling.
Extracellular stimuli signal through cell surface plasma membrane receptors, for example, RTKs. Through a variety of adaptor proteins, these signals cause guanine nucleotide exchange factors to replace the GDP-bound to inactive RAS with GTP. GAPs trigger the hydrolysis of GTP back to the inactive GDP-bound form. GTP-bound RAS binds to a plethora of downstream effector molecules to stimulate intracellular signaling of several pathways. Those with established roles in *RAS* oncogenesis include the RAF serine/threonine kinases, the PI3K lipid kinases, RAL GEFs, and Tiam1. Activation of these pathways and others has been shown to cause changes in many mechanisms leading to transformation, invasion, and metastasis.

Reprinted with permission from Campbell PM, Der CJ. Oncogenic Ras and its role in tumor cell invasion and metastasis. Semin Cancer Biol. 2004;14(2):105-114, Elsevier.

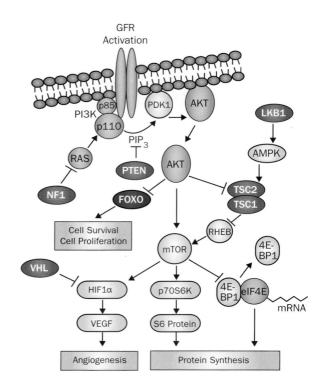

Fig. 2-17 Alterations of the AKT pathway in human cancer.

Activation of growth factor receptors (GFRs) such as the epidermal growth factor receptor, either by ligand stimulation or receptor overexpression/mutation, is one of the major mechanisms responsible for upregulation of AKT signaling. Other common mechanisms include activation of oncoproteins and inactivation of tumor suppressors intersecting the AKT signal transduction pathway. Proteins shown in green indicate oncoproteins for which overexpression and/or activating mutations have been implicated in many sporadic human cancers. Proteins in red are tumor suppressors whose loss and/or inactivation have been found to contribute to deregulation of the AKT pathway and tumor formation. FOXO transcription factors (shown in dark blue) have also been implicated as tumor suppressors (see text), although mutations have not been observed in any hereditary cancer syndrome to date.

Adapted by permission from Macmillan Publishers Ltd: Altomare DA, Testa JR. Pertubations of the AKT signaling pathway in human cancer. Oncogene. 2005;24(50):7455-7464.

kinases and other effectors. Mutations of the *BRAF* gene are found in approximately 50% of melanomas, and studies have found remarkable responses when BRAF inhibitors are used to treat patients with melanomas that harbor *BRAF* mutations.[63] MAP kinase signaling ultimately activates nuclear proto-oncogenes that are transcription factors, such as *FOS*, *JUN*, and *MYC*. Each of these oncogenic transcription factors stimulates a transcriptional program by binding to target genes that contain sequence-specific DNA elements, and their oncogenic activation has far-reaching effects on gene expression.

The PI3K-AKT pathway is also mutated in cancer cells and stimulates transcriptional and translation responses that promote cell growth and division (Fig. 2-17).[64,65] AKT is a protein kinase that is downstream of PI3K and is often amplified and/or overexpressed in cancers. Moreover, many cancers exhibit elevated AKT activity caused by mutations in genes that regulate AKT. For example, the PTEN tumor suppressor opposes PI3 kinase and prevents AKT activation, and PTEN is deleted in many cancers.[66] AKT phosphorylates many substrates that regulate cell division, apoptosis, and protein synthesis. The PI3K-AKT pathway is widely viewed as an important therapeutic target, and AKT and PI3K inhibitors are being studied in clinical trials.

The nonreceptor tyrosine kinases are cytoplasmic tyrosine kinases that include several proto-oncogenes, including *SRC*, *FES*, *YES*, and *LCK* (Table 2-3). The c-ABL protein is a cytoplasmic tyrosine kinase that is fused with the *BCR* gene in chronic myeloid leukemia. The BCR-ABL kinase domain is the target for drugs such as imatinib that inhibit its activity by preventing ATP from binding to the active site.[67] Because of homologies among kinases, "specific" kinase inhibitors often affect kinases other than their original target, and this can result in undesired consequences, such as toxicity, or unanticipated clinical benefits. For example, imatinib inhibits *c-KIT* and platelet-derived growth factor receptor in addition to *ABL*, and *c-KIT* inhibition by imatinib underlies its use in the treatment of gastrointestinal stromal tumors.

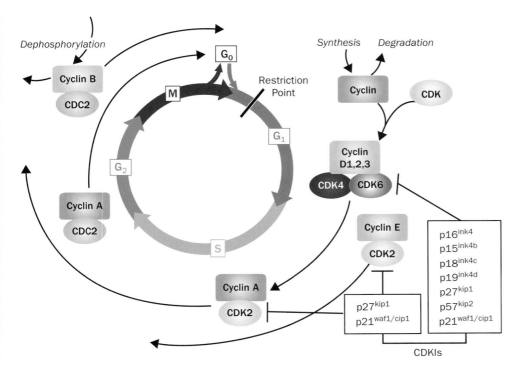

Fig. 2-18 The cell cycle.

The cell cycle is divided into four phases (G1, S, G2, and M). Progression through the cell cycle is promoted by cyclin-dependent kinases (CDKs), which are regulated positively by cyclins and negatively by CDK inhibitors (CDKIs). The restriction point is the point at which cells progress through the cell cycle independent of external stimuli.

Reproduced with permission from Schwartz G, Shah M. Targeting the cell cycle: A new approach to cancer therapy. J Clin Oncol. 2005;23(36): 9408-9421.

CELL CYCLE CONTROL

Cell cycles are divided into four phases that coordinate cell growth, DNA replication, and cell division (Fig. 2-18). G1 phase is a period of growth between mitosis and the onset of DNA synthesis during which cells integrate mitogenic signals and commit to the onset of DNA replication. S-phase is the period of DNA synthesis during which a cell replicates its genomic complement. G2 phase follows S-phase and is a second period of cell growth. In mitosis, chromosomes are segregated to daughter cells and cell division occurs. It is critically important that cells execute the cell division cycle faithfully, and mutations in the genes that regulate the cell cycle are among the most common genetic changes in cancer cells.[68-70]

The cyclin-dependent kinases (CDKs) orchestrate cell cycle transitions by phosphorylating large numbers of proteins involved in various cell cycle functions, and each cell cycle phase contains a unique profile of cyclin-CDK activities. CDKs are holoenzymes composed of two subunits: a catalytic subunit (the CDK) and a regulatory subunit (the cyclin) that activates the CDK. The best-known CDK substrate is the retinoblastoma protein (pRb), which governs G1 progression, and the Rb pathway is mutated in most cancer cells (Fig. 2-19). CDK inhibitor proteins oppose cyclins and prevent CDK activity (Fig. 2-18). The INK4 proteins inhibit only CDK4 and CDK6, whereas the Cip/Kip proteins (p21, p27, p57) bind to most cyclin-CDKs.

Cyclins and CDKs can act as dominant oncogenes. The cyclin D1 gene (*CCND1*) is rearranged by chromosome inversion in parathyroid adenomas, translocated to the IgG heavy chain locus in mantle cell lymphomas and amplified in 10% to 15% of solid tumors. Similarly, the cyclin E gene (*CCNE1*) was found to be the second most commonly amplified gene in ovarian

cancers,[71] and cyclin E is deregulated in cancers by increased transcription or prolonged protein stability.[72] CDKs themselves also can undergo oncogenic mutation, such as a *CDK4* mutation found in familial melanomas that prevents its inhibition by INK4 proteins.

Genes encoding proteins that inhibit CDKs are recessive oncogenes, including CKIs and *pRb* itself. The INK4 proteins frequently exhibit allelic loss in cancers; *p15* and *p16* are linked and are often codeleted in many tumor types. Another potent tumor suppressor, termed ARF, also is contained within the

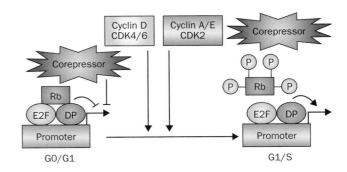

Fig. 2-19 Rb and E2F function.

Rb binds the transcription factor E2F and its associated subunit DP. Rb represses E2F-mediated transcription by recruiting chromatin remodeling complexes to the promoter in resting cells. At the G1–S-phase transition, Rb is thought to be phosphorylated by CDK2, CDK4, and CDK6. Hyperphosphorylated Rb releases E2F, allowing it to activate transcription of its target genes.

Adapted by permission from Macmillan Publishers Ltd: Classon M, Harlow E. The retinoblastoma tumour suppressor in development and cancer. Nat Rev Cancer. 2002;2(12):910-917.

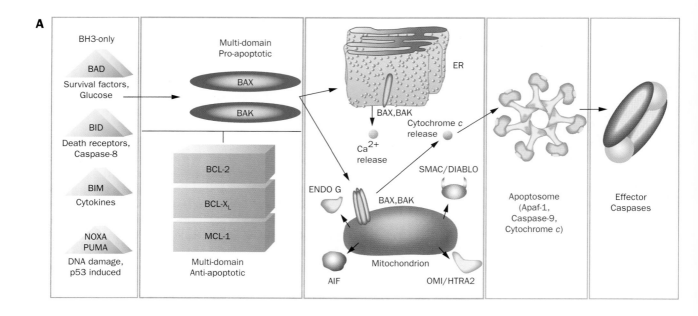

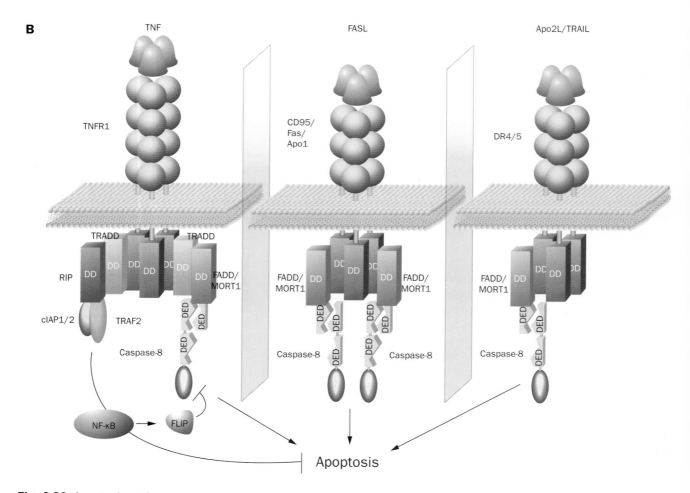

Fig. 2-20 Apoptosis pathways.

(**A**) The intrinsic apoptosis pathway (see text for details). (**B**) Extrinsic death receptor pathways. The distinct composition of the Death-Inducing-Signaling Complex (DISC) downstream of the various death receptors TNFR1, CD95, and DR4/5 is illustrated.

Reprinted from Cell, *Volume 116(2). Danial NN, Korsmeyer SJ. Cell death: critical control points. Pages 205-219, copyright 2004. With permission from Elsevier.*

p16 locus and contributes to the biologic selection for its allelic loss.[73] In addition to deletions and point mutations, the *p16* gene also is epigenetically inactivated in tumors by promoter methylation, most notably in colon and lung cancers.

The p27Kip1 CDK inhibitor is a tumor suppressor whose abundance has prognostic significance in many tumor types.[74] *p27* is an example of a tumor suppressor that is rarely mutated itself, but instead is inactivated by mutations in the pathways that regulate its degradation and/or subcellular localization. *pRb* is the prototype tumor suppressor, and its role in hereditary retinoblastoma provided the basis for the Knudson two-step model. Importantly, *pRb* often is mutated in many sporadic cancers, such as lung cancer. The realization that virtually all cancer cells contain mutations in the genes that regulate the cell cycle led to the widespread belief that drugs targeting cell cycle proteins would rapidly become important chemotherapeutic agents.[75] Although numerous clinical trials are currently testing CDK inhibitors, this promise has not yet been fulfilled.

APOPTOSIS

Tumor growth is a consequence of both unrestrained cell division and decreased cell death, and the pathways that mediate cell death contain proto-oncogenes that are mutated in cancers. Apoptosis is a physiologic process whereby complex biochemical pathways mediate cell death, and it is triggered by two distinct pathways (Fig. 2-20).[76] Cell death through the extrinsic pathway is signaled when ligands, such as tumor necrosis factor (TNF)-alpha and FAS-ligand, bind to cell-surface death receptors, such as TNF-R1 and FAS. Ligand binding to death receptors initiates a sequence of events leading to activation of proteases, termed caspases, which execute the apoptotic response. In contrast, the intrinsic or mitochondrial pathway results from a number of stimuli, such as radiation therapy or chemotherapy, and involves changes in the mitochondrial membrane that affect the release of cytochrome C into the cytoplasm. The intrinsic pathway also activates a caspase cascade that ultimately leads to DNA fragmentation and cell death.

The BCL-2 family is composed of proteins that regulate apoptosis and are either pro-apoptotic (promote cell death) or anti-apoptotic (promote cell survival).[77] BCL-2 itself is anti-apoptotic and first identified as the gene activated by the 14:18 translocation found in follicular lymphomas. The precise mechanisms by which BCL-2 prevents cell death are not fully elucidated, but they involve interactions with pro-apoptotic family members and mitochondrial functions. One important consequence of BCL-2 overexpression in tumorigenesis is that it prevents the apoptosis normally triggered by dominant oncogenes, such as *c-MYC*, and this likely underlies the aggressive behavior of "double-hit" lymphomas, which contain activating translocations of both the *MYC* and *BCL-2* genes. The realization that BCL-2 prevents apoptosis was pivotal in the evolution of understanding of the relationship between apoptosis and cancer. Because of their potential to induce apoptosis in tumor cells, drugs that target the BCL-2 family are being widely studied in clinical trials.[78]

Many oncogenes interact with the core apoptotic pathways. The most common mutations that impair apoptosis in tumors involve the *p53* tumor suppressor gene. Apoptosis is one outcome of *p53* activation by cellular stresses, and impaired cell death is an extremely important consequence of *p53* loss in cancer. Another frequently mutated pathway that negatively regulates apoptosis is the PI3-kinase-AKT pathway. AKT's interaction with apoptotic signaling is complex and includes direct effects on the mitochondrial membrane, as well as functional interactions with BCL-2 family members, FOXO transcription factors, nuclear factor-kappa B, and *p53*.

UBIQUITIN-MEDIATED PROTEOLYSIS

Many short-lived proteins are degraded in a proteolytic structure called the proteasome. Conjugation of a protein to ubiquitin is the signal for its delivery to the proteasome, and this is catalyzed by a multistep reaction in which ubiquitin is transferred to lysine side chains of the target protein (Fig. 2-21).[79,80] Ubiquitin, a 76-amino acid protein, is first attached to the ubiquitin-activating enzyme, called E1, and then transferred to approximately one dozen carrier proteins called E2s, or ubiquitin-conjugating enzymes. Each of the E2 enzymes recognizes and transfers ubiquitin only to particular proteins, thereby imposing some degree of selectivity on the process of ubiquitin-dependent proteolysis. Further selectivity arises from the fact that the ubiquitylation of many proteins requires an additional enzyme called an E3, or ubiquitin ligase. Cells contain hundreds of E3s that often recognize their targets after they have been modified by specific signals (e.g., phosphorylation). This system provides an enormous amount of specificity over which proteins are degraded in specific contexts.

E3s are classed into several groups, including the RING- and HECT-type ubiquitin ligases. Perhaps the most commonly mutated E3 ligase pathway in cancers involves MDM2, a HECT-type ubiquitin ligase that degrades p53. RING-finger–type E3 complexes also are tumor suppressors. The von Hippel-Lindau (VHL) syndrome is an autosomal-dominant hereditary cancer syndrome in which affected individuals develop renal cell carcinoma, central nervous system hemangioblastomas, pheochromocytoma, pancreas tumors, and other neoplasms. VHL syndrome is diagnosed by the presence of germ-line inactivating *VHL* mutations, and the remaining allele is inactivated in tumors

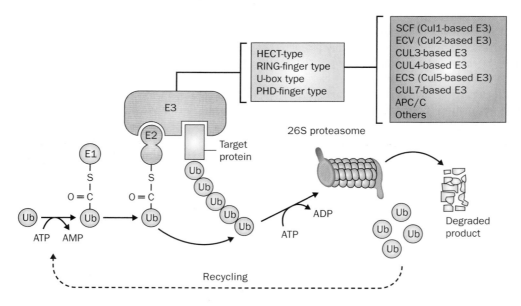

Fig. 2-21 Overview of the ubiquitin-proteasome pathway.

Ubiquitin (Ub) is a small protein, which is first transferred to the ubiquitin-activating enzyme, E1, in an ATP-dependent manner. This activated ubiquitin is then transferred to the ubiquitin-conjugating enzyme, E2. Finally, the ubiquitin is covalently attached to the target protein by an E3 ubiquitin ligase, leading to formation of a polyubiquitin chain. The polyubiquitinated protein is recognized by the 26S proteasome, and is destroyed in an ATP-dependent manner. There are many E3 ubiquitin ligases, which are categorized into four major classes: HECT-type, RING-finger type, U-box type, and PHD-finger type. RING-finger ligases are further divided into subfamilies, including cullin-based E3s. There are seven cullin-based E3s, including the SCF-type ligases and the anaphase-promoting complex/cyclosome (APC/C).

Adapted by permission from Macmillian Publishers Ltd: Nakayama KI, Nakayama K. Ubiquitin ligases: Cell-cycle control and cancer. Nat Rev Cancer. 2006;6(5):369-381.

by mutation. Importantly, *VHL* is also implicated in most spontaneous renal cell carcinomas, which have VHL allelic loss and mutations. VHL functions as the substrate recognition component of a RING-finger E3 that is inactivated by mutations in renal cancers.[81] One critical VHL target is hypoxia-inducible factor-1 alpha (HIF-1-alpha). Oxygen causes HIF-1-alpha to be hydroxylated on proline, which generates the VHL binding site and facilitates HIF-1-alpha degradation. HIF-1-alpha is a transcription factor that regulates genes in response to hypoxia—many of which promote angiogenesis. The angiogenic transcription program of HIF-1-alpha contributes to the highly vascular tumors associated with VHL loss and provides a rationale for trials of antiangiogenic agents for patients with renal cell carcinoma.

FBW7/hCDC4 is another RING-finger ubiquitin ligase that is a tumor suppressor, and it functions as the substrate recognition component of an E3 that targets several proto-oncogenes for degradation, including cyclin E, *c-MYC*, *Notch*, and *c-JUN*.[82] *Fbw7* mutations are found in approximately 6% of all human cancers and include both allelic loss and point mutations. Some cancers exhibit a higher rate of *Fbw7* mutation: *Fbw7* is the fourth most common mutation in colorectal cancer,[83] and *Fbw7* is mutated in approximately 35% of T-cell acute lymphoblastic leukemias.

Proteasome inhibitors are emerging as important antineoplastic agents. Bortezomib was the first pharmacologic proteasome inhibitor in clinical use and is approved for the treatment of patients with multiple myeloma and mantle cell lymphoma.

Carfilzomib is a second-generation proteasome inhibitor recently approved for the treatment of multiple myeloma, and other inhibitors of the proteasome itself or more specific proteasomal pathways are in clinical trials. However, the mechanism(s) that account for the therapeutic index associated with proteasome inhibitors remain unclear because these compounds affect a very large number of proteins normally degraded by the proteasome.

WNT/BETA-CATENIN SIGNALING

The Wnt/beta-catenin pathway is a signaling pathway with vital roles in development and cellular self-renewal.[84] Consistent with these functions, abnormal Wnt signaling contributes to the pathogenesis of many diseases, including cancers. In its simplest form, the canonical Wnt pathway refers to a signal transduction pathway in which soluble Wnt proteins bind to membrane-bound receptors, and this prevents the degradation of beta-catenin by the proteasome. Beta-catenin then translocates to the nucleus, where it stimulates a transcriptional program in concert with the TCF transcription factor. In reality, this pathway is quite complex, and many proteins function to augment or restrain Wnt pathway activation. The best-characterized role of Wnt pathway activation in human cancer is in familiar adenomatous polyposis (FAP), a hereditary colon cancer syndrome caused by deletion of the *APC* tumor suppressor. *APC* functions within the complex that instigates beta-catenin degradation, and its loss in cancers upregulates Wnt signaling by increasing beta-catenin

Fig. 2-22 A model for the interactions of APL fusion proteins with the N-CoR–mSin3–histone deacetylase (HD) complex.

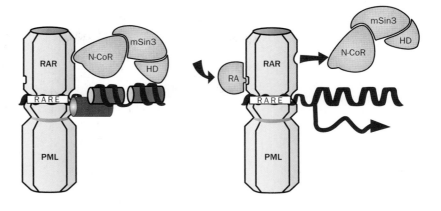

DNA-bound PML–RARalpha interacts with N-CoR (or SMRT) and recruits the mSin3–HD complex, decreasing histone acetylation and producing repressive chromatin organization and transcriptional repression. RA induces dissociation of the N-CoR–mSin3-HD complex, recruitment of coactivators with histone acetyl-transferase activity (not shown), increased levels of histone acetylation, chromatin remodeling, and transcriptional activation.

Adapted by permission from Macmillian Publishers Ltd: Grignani F, De Matteis S, Nervi C, et al. Fusion proteins of the retinoic acid receptor-alpha recruit histone deacetylase in promyelocytic leukemia. Nature. 1998;391(6669):815-818.

abundance. Although first described in FAP, *APC* mutations are found in most sporadic colon cancers, where they are thought to function early during colorectal cancer progression. Many other human cancers also have aberrant Wnt signaling, including brain cancers and leukemias. Because many of the cellular regulators of Wnt signaling are enzymes, the small molecule inhibitors of the Wnt pathway are being heavily studied for cancer therapy.

DIFFERENTIATION

Most somatic cells are in a terminally differentiated, postmitotic state, and this is regulated by complex transcriptional pathways. Many proto-oncogenes affect the pathways that regulate differentiation, and these often are transcription factors and/or coactivators involved in leukemias and lymphomas.[85] For example, the retinoic acid receptor (RAR)-alpha is rearranged in several translocations found in acute promyelocytic leukemia (APL), most commonly t(15;17), which produces a PML-RAR-alpha fusion protein (Fig. 2-22). This fusion protein acts as a "dominant negative" mutant that inhibits RAR-alpha target genes by recruiting corepressors. This dominant negative RAR-alpha fusion is targeted by all-trans retinoic acid (ATRA), which is used in conjunction with combination chemotherapy to induce remission in patients with APL. ATRA binds to the fusion protein and prevents it from bringing corepressors to RAR-alpha target genes. ATRA treatment thus reverses the differentiation block caused by the translocation product and allows promyelocytes to proceed down their differentiation pathway. Core-binding factor (CBF) is another transcription factor that regulates hematopoietic differentiation and is commonly mutated by translocations in leukemias. Both components of CBF (RUNX1/AML1 and CBF-beta) are involved in translocations found in acute leukemia. Like RAR-alpha, these translocations produce dominant negative proteins that inhibit CBF target gene expression, which is thought to impair hematopoietic cell differentiation.

The *Notch* genes are proto-oncogenes involved in cell-fate and differentiation pathways. *Notch* genes encode transmembrane receptors that stimulate transcriptional programs after they bind to ligands.[86] Ligand binding causes Notch proteins to be cleaved, forming intracellular domains that translocate to the nucleus. Notch proteins play important roles in lymphoid differentiation and are implicated in hematologic cancers. *Notch1* was first described as an oncogene by virtue of its involvement in the t(7;9) translocation found in a subset of patients with T-cell acute lymphoblastic leukemia. However, *Notch1* mutations occur in up to 50% of patients with this disease.[87] The precise mechanisms through which *Notch* promotes leukemia are unknown, but they are thought to involve impaired differentiation and enhanced self-renewal, and data suggest that *c-MYC* is a critical mediator of *Notch* activity.[88]

DNA REPAIR PATHWAYS

Mammalian cells use three major DNA-repair pathways to maintain genomic integrity (Fig. 2-23). Mutations that disrupt these pathways cause genetic instability and are associated with diseases characterized by sensitivity to DNA-damaging agents and predisposition to cancer. Ultraviolet light–induced nucleotide dimers and other DNA adducts are recognized and repaired by the nucleotide excision repair (NER) pathway. DNA-recombination repair is involved in the restoration of double-stranded breaks induced by ionizing radiation and radiomimetic agents. Finally, the DNA mismatch repair pathways correct errors during DNA replication by the removal of the mismatched strand and subsequent repair of the DNA.

Nucleotide Excision Repair Pathway

NER pathways correct nucleotide lesions induced by ultraviolet light and adducts induced by chemical carcinogens.[89] There are two NER pathways: a global repair pathway and a transcription-coupled repair pathway that repairs DNA damage that occurs during transcription. Mutations affecting these pathways give rise to sun-sensitive and developmental disorders, including xeroderma pigmentosum, Cockayne syndrome, and trichothiodystrophy. Xeroderma pigmentosum is an autosomal-recessive disorder with an estimated incidence rate of one in 70,000. Affected individuals have progressive neurodegeneration, sensitivity to ultraviolet light, abnormalities in skin

Fig. 2-23 DNA lesions and repair mechanisms.

(Top) Common DNA damaging agents. (Middle) Examples of lesions that can be introduced by these agents into the DNA double helix. (Bottom) The most frequently used repair mechanisms for such lesions. Distinct damaging sources can induce similar types of DNA lesions, and any one agent often induces more than one type of damage. The lesion spectrum of different repair pathways may overlap.

Abbreviations: BER, base excision repair; NER, nucleotide excision repair.

Reproduced with permission from Oxford University Press: de Boer J, Hoeijmakers JH. Nucleotide excision repair and human syndromes. Carcinogensis. 2000;21(3):453-460.

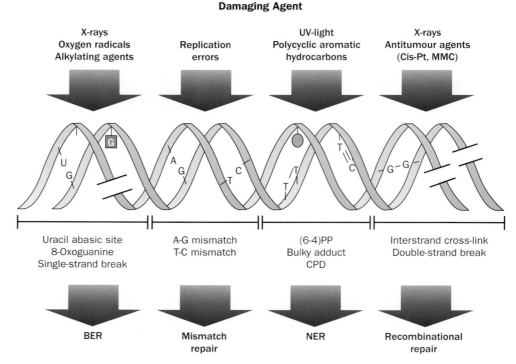

pigmentation, and a predisposition to skin cancer. Approximately one-half of affected individuals have clinical symptoms by 18 months, and the average age at the time of skin cancer is 8. The risk of skin cancer is estimated to be 2,000 times higher than the risk for the general population. Eight genes have been associated with xeroderma pigmentosum. Seven of them code for excision-repair proteins, and one (xeroderma pigmentosum variant) is a DNA polymerase that is required for accurate replication of damaged DNA. In contrast, Cockayne syndrome is associated with two genes, *CSA* and *CSB*, which are involved in transcription-coupled DNA repair. Trichothiodystrophy is caused by mutation of either *ERCC2/XPD* or *ERCC3/XPB*, which encode helicase subunits of the transcription factor II H complex. Neither Cockayne syndrome nor trichothiodystrophy is associated with an increased cancer risk.

Double-Strand Break Repair

Damage to DNA by radiation, chemicals (such as chemotherapy), and other insults produces double-strand breaks that are recognized and repaired by a coordinated response that involves the products of many tumor suppressor genes. Mutations of some of these genes cause inherited syndromes that have highly variable clinical manifestations. Ataxia telangiectasia is an autosomal-recessive disorder characterized by progressive cerebellar ataxia, telangiectasia, and immunodeficiency. Tumors, most commonly T-cell neoplasms, develop in more than one-third of homozygous individuals. The ataxia telangiectasia gene (*ATM*) encodes a large protein kinase with homology to PI3K. *ATM* is activated by serine phosphorylation in response to DNA

breaks and phosphorylates a number of downstream substrates with critical roles in DNA repair and checkpoint pathways including *CHK2, p53, BRCA1,* and *NBS1* (Fig. 2-24A).[90] Cells derived from patients with ataxia telangiectasia exhibit increased DNA damage after radiation therapy, as well as defects in normal cell cycle responses to DNA damage, called checkpoints.

Fanconi anemia (FA) is an autosomal-recessive disease characterized by developmental abnormalities, bone marrow failure, and susceptibility to cancers, particularly acute myeloid leukemia (AML), squamous cell cancer of the head and neck, gynecologic cancers, and esophageal cancer. The disease is typically fatal, and the mean survival is 16 years. Similar to ataxia telangiectasia, cells derived from patients with FA display abnormal chromosome breakage. However, FA cells are not hypersensitive to ionizing radiation; rather they are hypersensitive to DNA cross-linking by agents such as diepoxybutane and mitomycin C. Classic studies defined many distinct FA complementation groups, and 13 FA genes have now been cloned. Remarkably, many of these proteins (A, B, C, E, F, G, L, M) form a complex that catalyzes the monoubiquitination of two FA proteins: FANCD2 and the more recently discovered FANCI.[91,92] Monoubiquitinated FANCD2 and FANCI become localized to nuclear foci after DNA damage, and these foci also contain FANCD1 (identical with the *BRCA2* breast cancer gene) and other proteins previously discussed, including BRCA1 and NBS1 (Fig. 2-24B). The FA pathway is activated by and required for the cellular response to stalled replication forks.

The striking intersection of the BRCA1 and FA pathways underscores the central importance of this DNA damage sensing

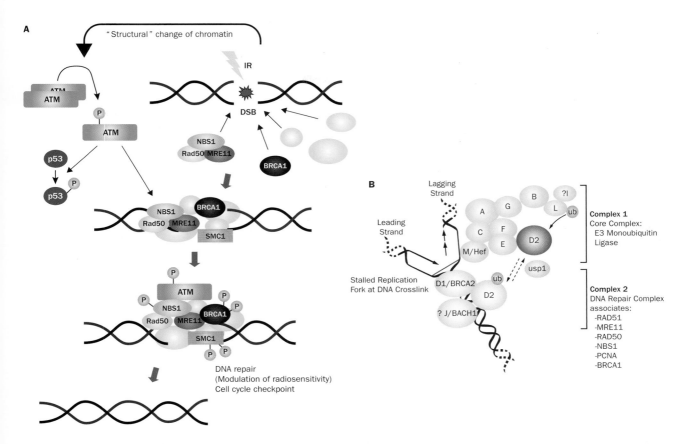

Fig. 2-24 Model for an ionizing radiation (IR)-induced signaling pathway.

(A) Chromatin structure changes caused by DNA breakage or other mechanisms lead to *ATM* autophosphorylation and activation. If DNA strand beaks are present, several proteins, including NBS1 and BRCA1, are recruited to the sites of the damage, independent of *ATM*. Activated *ATM* can phosphorylate substrates, such as *p53*, and if NBS1 and BRCA1 are localized to the DBA breaks, activated ATM is recruited. (B) Schematic interaction of the FA pathway. Protein complex 1 contains the A, B, C, E, F, G, L, M, and possibly I subunits. Protein complex 2 contains FANCD2-Ub, BRCA2, and possibly FANCJ. During S phase, when a replication fork encounters a DNA cross-link, the FA complex (complex 1) is activated. This activation leads to the monoubiquitination of FANCD2, which is then targeted to chromatin containing the cross-link. FANCD2-Ub then interacts with BRCA2 in complex 2, leading to repair of the cross-link possibly through HR and TLS. FANCD2 is deubiquitinated by USP1, thereby inactivating the pathway.

(A) *Reprinted from Cold Spring Harbor Press: Kitagawa R, Bakkenist CJ, McKinnon PJ, and Kastan MB. Phosphorylation of SMC1 is a critical downstream event in the ATMNBS1-BRCA1 pathway. Genes and Development. 2004;18:1423-1438. (B) Reprinted from Cold Spring Harbor Press: Kennedy, R., and D'Andrea, A. 2005. The Fanconi anemia/BRCA pathway: new faces in the crowd. Genes and Development. 2005;19:2925-2940.*

and repair mechanism in carcinogenesis. The NBS1 protein is another component of nuclear repair foci implicated in a chromosome breakage syndrome. Nijmegen breakage syndrome is an autosomal-recessive disease characterized by microcephaly, immunodeficiency, and increased frequency of hematopoietic cancers that is caused by mutations in the *NBS1* gene. *NBS1* forms a complex with MRE11 and RAD50, which binds to BRCA1 in nuclear foci. Deficiency of the NBS1 protein blocks the formation of the MRE11-NBS1-RAD50 complex, and this impairs the S-phase surveillance responses triggered by *ATM*. Accordingly, many of the symptoms of this disease are identical to symptoms of ataxia telangiectasia.

Mismatch Repair

DNA mismatch repair (MMR) corrects errors that occur during DNA replication, primarily single base mismatches or short insertions or deletions.[93] DNA mismatches are recognized and corrected by a complex of proteins that bind to the mismatch, identify the correct DNA strand, and then excise and repair the mismatch. Several of the proteins involved in MMR are tumor suppressors involved in HNPCC. Patients with HNPCC/Lynch syndrome develop colon cancer at an early age, as well as cancers in many other organ sites. The two most commonly mutated MMR genes in Lynch syndrome are *MSH2* and *MLH1*. *MSH2* is involved with the initial recognition of the mismatch, whereas *MLH1* helps determine which DNA strand contains the correct sequence. Mutations in other MMR genes are less commonly associated with HNPCC and include *MSH6*, *PMS1*, and *PMS2*. Patients with HNPCC inherit a nonfunctional MMR gene allele with subsequent loss of the remaining allele in a somatic cell that will ultimately give rise to a tumor. Importantly, impaired MMR causes a

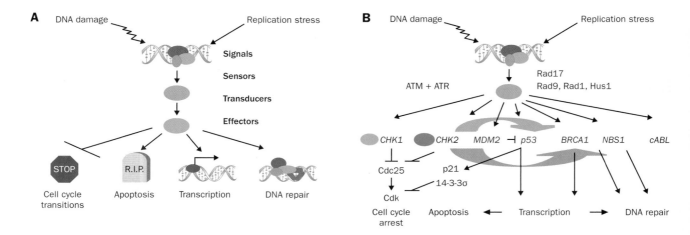

Fig. 2-25 Organization of DNA damage response pathways.

(A) A general outline of the DNA damage response signal-transduction pathway. Arrowheads represent activating events and perpendicular ends represent inhibitory events. Cell-cycle arrest is depicted with a stop sign, apoptosis with a tombstone. The DNA helix with an arrow represents damage-induced transcription, while the DNA helix with several oval-shaped subunits represents damage-induced repair. For the purpose of simplicity, the network of interacting pathways are depicted as a linear pathway consisting of signals, sensors/mediators, transducers, and effectors. (B) Organization of the mammalian DNA damage response pathway. Arrowheads represent positively acting steps while perpendicular ends represent inhibitory steps. Gene names are shown at the approximate positions where their encoded proteins function in the pathway. Although the general organization of the pathway is correct, some details are omitted, especially concerning the relationship between the ATR/ATM and Hus1/Rad17/Rad9/Rad1 proteins, which may participate in mutual regulation.

Adapted by permission from Macmillian Publishers Ltd: Zhou BB, Elledge SJ. The DNA damage response: Putting checkpoints in perspective. Nature. 2000;408(6811):433-439.

hypermutable phenotype, as evidenced by microsatellite instability, which is readily detected in tumors by PCR-based assays that reveal novel tumor-specific microsatellite fragments. Although microsatellite instability is the hallmark of HNPCC, it also is found in a subset of sporadic colon cancers. However, in these cases, *MLH1* is silenced by promoter hypermethylation rather than mutation.

CHECKPOINTS: CROSSROADS OF DNA REPAIR, CELL CYCLE REGULATION, AND GENETIC INSTABILITY

The fidelity of the enzymes that replicate DNA and segregate chromosomes is largely responsible for the accurate propagation of genetic information. However, these enzymes have an intrinsic error rate and the frequency of errors is increased by genotoxic insults, such as chemical mutagens and ionizing radiation. Normal cells continually monitor DNA replication and mitosis and stop the cell cycle if these do not occur correctly, allowing the damage to be repaired before proliferation resumes or initiating apoptotic and/or senescence responses. The pathways that link cell cycle progression to the accurate execution of prior cell cycle events are called checkpoints.[94]

Mammalian cells have checkpoints that operate in each phase of the cell cycle and are intricately interwoven with the cell cycle and DNA repair machinery.[95-97] Moreover, there is substantial overlap between the components of the various checkpoint pathways. The G1 and G2 checkpoints recognize DNA damage that occurs during these cell cycle phases and initiate responses leading to either cell cycle arrest or cell death. In addition to DNA damage, the S-phase checkpoint also

is activated by stresses that inhibit the proper function of the replication machinery.

Checkpoint pathways may be broadly viewed as being composed of sensors/mediators, signal transducers, and effectors (Fig. 2-25A). The sensors and mediators detect DNA damage and involve complexes (e.g., RAD9-HUS1-RAD1 and MRE1-RAD50-NBS1), as well as proteins that accumulate in DNA repair foci (e.g., BRCA1, claspin, and FANCD2). The DNA damage signal is then transmitted by signal transducing kinases that include ATM and ATR, and subsequently by downstream kinases, such as CHK1 and CHK2 (Fig. 2-25B). Finally, the transducing kinases activate effectors, such as p53 and Cdc25, directly affect the cell cycle machinery, and block cell division through inhibition of cyclin-CDK activity.

Checkpoint pathways are disrupted in most—and perhaps all—cancers. Impaired checkpoint function causes genetic instability, which drives tumor progression because the increased error rate allows mutations to accumulate in additional cancer genes. The p53 protein plays a central role in checkpoint pathways, and it is the most frequently mutated human tumor suppressor gene. Although *p53* is mutated in up to one-half of all spontaneous cancers, its role as a tumor suppressor first came to light in studies of patients with Li-Fraumeni syndrome, a rare autosomal disorder associated with the development of a wide variety of early-onset cancers, including soft tissue and bone sarcomas and breast, brain, and colon cancers. *p53* is a transcription factor that is activated by many triggers, including DNA damage and replication stress. When *p53* is activated by signals such as DNA damage, the outcome can be cell cycle

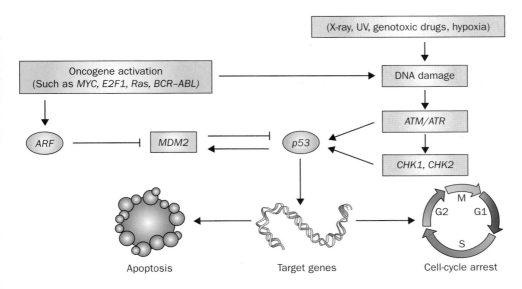

Fig. 2-26 The p53-MDM2-ARF network.

The activation of *p53* classically occurs in response to many other cellular stresses that produce DNA damage, including oncogene-induced stress. Depending on the nature of the inducing signal, these DNA-damage responses activate the kinase mutated in the ataxia telangiectasia syndrome *(ATM)* and/or the *ATM* and *Rad3*-related kinase (ATR). These kinases phosphorylate *p53* directly and also indirectly through the agency of the CHK kinases. These phosphorylations have an important role in increasing the transcriptional activity of *p53*. Target genes induced by *p53* can generate different biological outcomes depending on the tissue type and convergence of different activating signals. Sustained and increased signaling thresholds induced by mutated or overexpressed oncogenes activate the *ARF* promoter. Once expressed, the ARF protein interferes with the activity of *MDM2*, leading to *p53* stabilization and the triggering of a complex *p53*-dependent transcriptional program mediated by hundreds of target genes. *MDM2* is not only a negative regulator of *p53*-dependent transcription and turnover, but is also a canonical *p53*-activated gene that has a key role in negative-feedback regulation of the *p53* response.

Adapted by permission from Macmillan Publishers Ltd: Sherr CJ. Divorcing ART and p53: An unsettled case. Nat Rev Cancer. 2006;6(9):663-673.

arrest, apoptosis, or cellular senescence; these alternate outcomes depend on many factors.[98-100] *p53* largely accomplishes these outcomes by activating transcription of its target genes, although *p53* also may play a role independent of transcription. One critical *p53* target is the p21Cip CDK inhibitor; increased p21 abundance plays an essential role in G1 arrest signaled by *p53* after DNA damage. Tumors most commonly inactivate *p53* by loss of heterozygosity and intragenic point mutants that fall within critical *p53* functional domains, and a large number of *p53* mutations have been catalogued.

Another mechanism of *p53* loss in tumors involves the *MDM2* ubiquitin ligase (Fig. 2-26). *MDM2* expression is induced by *p53*, and it functions in a feedback loop to downregulate *p53* by catalyzing its ubiquitination. The normal *MDM2-p53* regulatory circuit is disrupted in many cancers. *MDM2* is overexpressed in a wide spectrum of neoplasms, and this leads to decreased *p53* abundance and function. A second mechanism that targets this pathway involves the *ARF* tumor suppressor. As discussed previously, *ARF* is encoded within the same gene as the p16Ink4a protein and is frequently deleted in cancers.[101] *ARF* normally binds to *MDM2*, which prevents *MDM2* from degrading *p53*. However, when *ARF* is deleted, *MDM2* activity is unrestrained, causing *p53* to be degraded. *ARF* expression is induced by oncogenes, such as *MYC*, and plays an important role in *p53* activation by oncogenic signaling. Thus, loss of *ARF* disables an important protective mechanism against oncogenic transformation.

There is enormous interest in developing cancer treatment strategies that target the *p53* pathway. In fact, studies in model systems demonstrating the antitumor activity of *p53* restoration in tumors has re-energized this active field.[102] Strategies that target the *p53* pathway range from peptides that restore *p53* function in cells with mutant *p53* proteins to recombinant adenoviruses (e.g., Onyx-015) that selectively kill cells with *p53* mutations. However, the scope of these approaches is too great to be covered in detail here, and many reviews address this large field.[103]

The mitotic or spindle assembly checkpoint ensures that chromosomes are equally segregated to daughter cells during mitosis, and it is the key safeguard against aneuploidy. The spindle apparatus is composed of tubulin and attaches to chromosomes through their kinetochores during mitosis. In a normal cell, the signal that activates the spindle checkpoint is generated by kinetochores that are unattached or have insufficient spindle tension, which delays mitosis and ensures that chromosome separation does not occur in situations where the daughter cells may receive an abnormal chromosome content because of misalignment (Fig. 2-27).[104] A number of spindle checkpoint proteins accumulate at the unattached kinetochore, including BUB1, BUBR1, MAD1, and MAD2. This complex prevents mitosis by sending a signal that inhibits the anaphase-promoting complex (APC), a RING-type E3 ubiquitin ligase that regulates mitotic entry and exit. Two critical APC targets that must be

Fig. 2-27 Mitotic checkpoint signaling.

(**A**) Unattached kinetochores are the signal generators of the mitotic checkpoint. They recruit mitotic checkpoint proteins, including Mad1, Mad2, BubR1, and Bub3, and convert them into inhibitors of APCCdc20. (**B**) Once all kinetochores have made productive attachments to spindle microtubules, production of the APC^{Cdc20} inhibitors is silenced.

Reprinted from Cancer Cell, *Volume 8(1). Weaver BAA, Cleveland DW. Decoding the links between mitosis, cancer, and chemotherapy: The mitotic checkpoint, adaptation, and cell death. Pages 7-12, copyright 2005. With permission from Elsevier.*

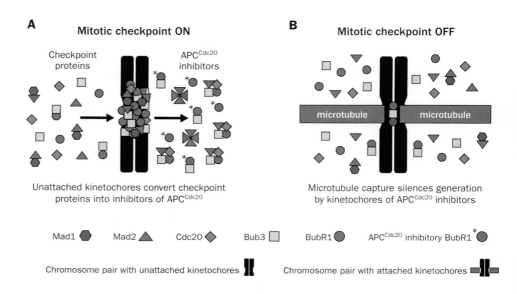

A Mitotic checkpoint ON

B Mitotic checkpoint OFF

Unattached kinetochores convert checkpoint proteins into inhibitors of APC^{Cdc20}

Microtubule capture silences generation by kinetochores of APC^{Cdc20} inhibitors

Mad1 ⬠ Mad2 △ Cdc20 ◇ Bub3 ☐ BubR1 ● APC^{Cdc20} inhibitory BubR1 ⊛

Chromosome pair with unattached kinetochores

Chromosome pair with attached kinetochores

degraded for mitosis to proceed are cyclin B and securins (the latter function to hold together sister chromatids). The spindle checkpoint thus prevents mitosis in the setting of an improperly attached spindle by blocking the degradation of APC substrates. A number of chemotherapeutic agents target the spindle apparatus (e.g., taxanes and vinca alkaloids) and trigger the spindle checkpoint in normal cells.

KEY POINTS

- Enzymes that promote protein degradation by the proteasome can function as tumor suppressors.
- Pharmacologic proteasome inhibitors are approved for the treatment of multiple myeloma.
- Genes that regulate cellular differentiation often are mutated in hematologic cancers.
- DNA repair pathways contain many tumor suppressor genes that are mutated in both familial and sporadic cancers.
- Mutations that disable different DNA repair pathways are associated with specific cancer syndromes.

MULTISTEP TUMORIGENESIS

Carcinogenesis is a multistep process, and the development of fully malignant cancers requires many independent events. Although the specific mutations that cause human cancers vary greatly between types of cancers and individuals, the broad consequences of these mutations are abnormal phenotypes that are shared by most cancers. Weinberg and Hanahan have proposed six "hallmarks of cancer" that they define as "distinctive and complementary capabilities that enable tumor growth and metastatic dissemination."[105] These include sustained proliferative signaling, evading growth suppressors, resisting cell death, enabling replicative immortality, inducing angiogenesis,

and activating invasion and metastasis. These capabilities can be acquired in different sequences, and in some cases, a single genetic mutation might provide more than one capability. This conceptualization provides an important framework within which to consider multistep carcinogenesis.

The first three of these "acquired capabilities" involve mutations within the mitogenic signaling, cell cycle, and cell death pathways that have been outlined previously. The fourth category involves the acquisition of cellular immortality in tumors. Normal cells are limited in the number of times that they can divide, even when they are provided with all of the normal mitogenic stimuli required for cell division. In contrast, many cancer cells can divide with apparently limitless potential. One fundamental mechanism that limits human cell division involves the ends of chromosomes, which are called telomeres. Telomeres normally protect the ends of chromosomes, and they shorten with each cell division. Thus the length of a cell's telomeres reflects the number of divisions it has undergone. Eventually the telomeres are shortened to the point where they can no longer protect the chromosome ends, which leads to a condition termed crisis and, ultimately, to cell death. Unlike normal cells, cancer cells maintain their telomere length during cell division. This usually results from expression of the enzyme telomerase that adds DNA back to the telomere. Telomerase activity can be detected in 85% to 90% of cancers, and the remaining tumors maintain their telomeres through a mechanism involving recombination.

The capability of induced angiogenesis reflects the fact that tumors often outgrow their blood supply and must actively recruit vasculature to grow. In normal tissues, the development of new blood vessels is highly regulated by both positive and negative signals. Tumor cells promote angiogenesis by upregulating the pathways that promote blood vessel formation (e.g., increased expression of growth factors such as vascular endothelial and fibroblast growth factors) and by reducing the activity of inhibitory pathways. Some of these pathways involve transcriptional networks under the control

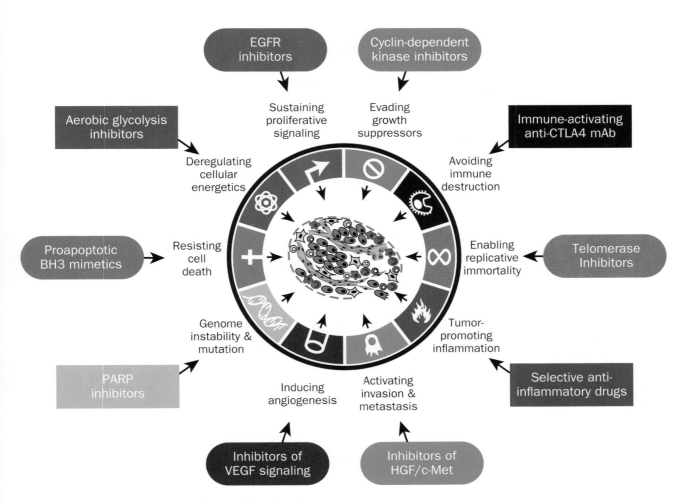

Fig. 2-28 Therapeutic targeting of the hallmarks of cancer.

Drugs that interfere with each of the acquired capabilities necessary for tumor growth and progression have been developed and are in clinical trials or in some cases approved for clinical use in treating certain forms of human cancer. Additionally, investigational drugs are being developed to target each of the enabling characteristics and emerging hallmarks, which also hold promise as cancer therapeutics. The drugs illustrated are examples of the deep pipeline of candidate drugs with different molecular targets and modes of action in development for most of these hallmarks.

Reprinted from Cell, Volume 144(5). Hanahan D, Weinberg RA. Hallmarks of Cancer: The Next Generation. Pages 646-674, copyright 2011. With permission from Elsevier.

of previously discussed genes, such as *VHL* mutations in renal cell carcinoma. The importance of these pathways in tumor cell growth has prompted the development of drugs that target angiogenesis.

The last of the six hallmarks—tissue invasion and metastasis—is the most heterogeneous and the least understood. It is, however, critically important because metastasis accounts for most cancer fatalities. Specific gene products are associated with the ability of tumor cells to metastasize to different organ sites, and other tissues, such as stroma and tumor-associated cell populations, also contribute to metastasis. Elegant animal models of metastasis, as well as transcriptional profiling of human cancers, are revealing that metastasis includes alterations in genes involved in processes such as cell adhesion, integrin signaling, growth factors, chemokine signal transduction, and extracellular proteolysis.

In addition to these six hallmarks, Weinberg and Hanahan outline two emerging hallmarks, and two enabling characteristics that make it possible for tumor cells to acquire the core

hallmarks. The two emerging hallmarks are deregulating cellular energetics and avoiding immune destruction. The concept that tumor cells reprogram their glucose metabolism toward glycolysis, even in the presence of oxygen, was first noted more than 50 years ago. However, during the past decade there has been an explosion of research into the significance and mechanisms of aerobic glycolysis in cancer, also known as the Warburg Effect. It is clear that energy reprogramming has critical roles in cancer cell growth and division. The second emerging hallmark reflects the large body of work that demonstrates the role of the immune system as an anticancer defect, and the molecular changes in cancer cells that allow them to evade immune destruction. Although many of the mechanistic underpinnings of the hallmark are poorly defined, the role of immunity in suppressing carcinogenesis is incontrovertible, and immunotherapies are a key component of current therapy for cancer in many organ sites.

The two enabling characteristics are properties of cancer cells that facilitate the acquisition of the hallmarks. The first of

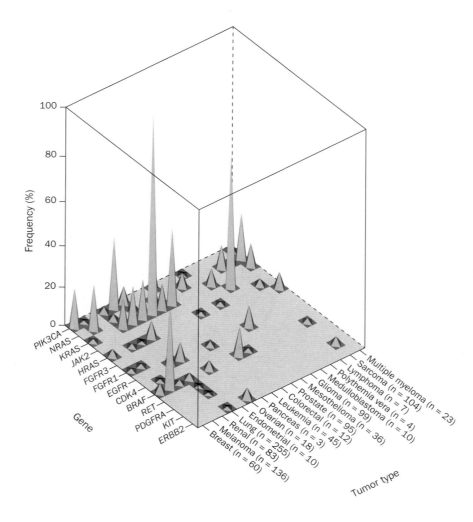

Fig. 2-29 Frequency of known oncogenic mutations in human cancers analyzed by high-throughput genotyping.

Frequencies (y-axis) were calculated as percentages of tumor samples (x-axis) from a given type that harbored an oncogene mutation (z-axis) compared with the total number of samples of that tumor type.

Reprinted by permission from Macmillian Publishers Ltd: Thomas RK, Baker AC, Debiasi RM, et al. High-throughput oncogene mutation profiling in human cancer. Nature Genetics. 2007;39(3):347-51.

KEY POINTS

- Checkpoints ensure the fidelity of cell division and protect against genomic instability.
- Many tumor suppressor genes and DNA repair proteins are intimately associated with checkpoint pathways.
- The loss of checkpoint functions causes genomic instability and fosters the accumulation of multiple mutations in cancer cells.
- *p53* is the most commonly mutated cancer gene, and it participates in diverse checkpoint responses. *p53* senses cellular stress and signals to pathways that regulate processes such as cell cycle progression and apoptosis.
- Tumorigenesis is a multistep process that requires the accumulation of multiple mutations. All tumors share a number of hallmarks that contribute to their malignant phenotype, but the specific molecular events that produce these phenotypes vary greatly among tumor types and individuals.

these characteristics is genomic instability, which (as discussed above) enables the acquisition of the multiple mutations required for multistep tumorigenesis. The second enabling characteristic is tumor-promoting inflammation, which reflects the rapidly advancing concept that inflammatory responses can actually facilitate tumor initiation and progression in some contexts.

One important aspect of the hallmark/enabling characteristics conceptualization is that it also provides a framework for understanding the development of mechanism-based targeted therapies, which target both hallmarks and enabling characteristics (Fig. 2-28).

MODERN ONCOGENOMICS
DETECTING ONCOGENE MUTATIONS AND THE DEVELOPMENT OF TARGETED CANCER THERAPY IN THE POST-GENOME ERA

A plethora of studies employing next-generation sequencing to study cancer genomes have been recently published or are nearing completion. Many of these studies used integrative approaches that incorporate many types of large-scale data to discover mutations in oncogenes and cancer pathways at an unprecedented rate. Although these approaches are in rapid evolution, they have already radically altered our understanding of the genomic

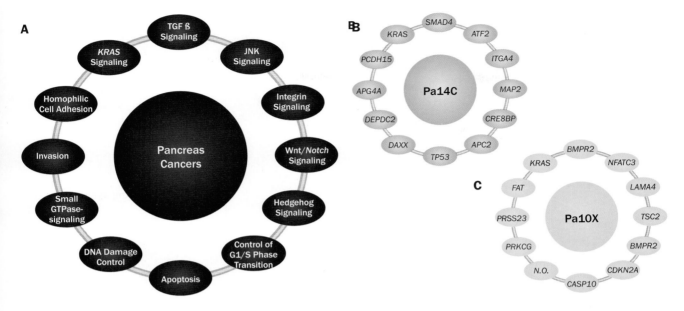

Fig. 2-30 Critical signaling pathways in pancreas cancer revealed by large-scale analyses.

(**A**) The 12 pathways and processes whose component genes were genetically altered in most pancreas cancers. (**B and C**) Two pancreas cancers (Pa14C and Pa10X) and the specific genes that are mutated in them. The positions around the circles in (**B**) and (**C**) correspond to the pathways and processes in (**A**). Several pathway components overlapped, as illustrated by the *BMPR2* mutation that presumably disrupted both the SMAD4 and Hedgehog signaling pathways in Pa10X. Additionally, not all 12 processes and pathways were altered in every pancreas cancer, as exemplified by the fact that no mutations known to affect DNA damage control were observed in Pa10X. N.O. indicates not observed.

From Jones S, Zhang X, Parsons DW. Core signaling pathways in human pancreatic cancers revealed by global genomic analyses. Science. 2008;321(5897):1801-1806.

landscape of cancers and have demonstrated the immediate effect of genome-scale analyses on oncology. Although many new studies will undoubtedly be published before this chapter is published, a few examples are briefly described in this section to illustrate the power and importance of these approaches.

High-throughput genotyping can detect the prevalence of many known oncogene mutations in primary cancers. In one study, mass spectrometry–based genotyping interrogated 238 known oncogene mutations in 1,000 human tumors. Although limited to known mutations, this approach revealed unexpected oncogene mutations in several tumor types and many co-occurring mutations (Fig. 2-29).[106] Because of their rapidity, high-throughput oncogene profiling approaches have the potential to guide therapeutic decisions that involve the use of agents that target specific pathways found to be mutated in a specific cancer.

Most current approaches to cancer genomics incorporate next-generation sequencing, and different strategies are used to achieve different goals. For example, when sequencing is limited to either known oncogenes or coding sequences (exomes, which compose only 5% of the total DNA), many tumors can be analyzed, which allows highly powered studies of genes and pathways that are targeted by mutations in cancers. Limited-sequencing approaches also provide rapid ways to characterize tumor genomes within time frames that allow treatment decisions to be made based on the presence of specific mutations, and this is critical to the success of targeted therapy. In contrast, whole-genome sequencing reveals genetic alterations in regions of DNA that cannot be assessed by limited approaches, and it may provide entirely

novel insight on the types of mutations that drive carcinogenesis. However, whole-genome approaches are more difficult to apply to large numbers of tumors, at least in the near future.

Two studies described an integrative approach that included sequencing of protein coding regions, SNP-based array analyses of DNA copy number, and next-generation sequencing of expressed mRNAs, to develop global views of the genes and pathways that are mutated in pancreas cancers and glioblastomas.[107,108] The use of these combined modalities helped distinguish mutations that likely played a causal role in tumorigenesis (driver mutations) from mutations that may be irrelevant (passenger mutations). In the case of pancreas cancer, these investigators found an average of 63 mutations per tumor in a group of 24 tumors, and these segregated into a core set of 12 signaling pathways that appear to be critical in pancreas cancer (Fig. 2-30). This study found that the isocitrate dehydrogenase gene, previously unrecognized as an oncogene, was mutated in 12% of glioblastomas. *IDH1* and *IDH2* mutations have subsequently been found in other cancers, including AML and chondrosarcoma. Importantly, *IDH1* mutations cause epigenetic dysregulation and DNA hypermethylation,[109] and pharmacologic IDH1 inhibitors are already demonstrating efficacy in experimental models.[110] A contemporaneous integrative genomics study of brain cancer was reported by The Cancer Genome Atlas (TCGA; a consortium sponsored by the National Institutes of Health), which examined DNA copy number, gene expression, and methylation aberrations in a group of 206 glioblastomas. In this case, the sequencing involved 600 genes with presumptive or

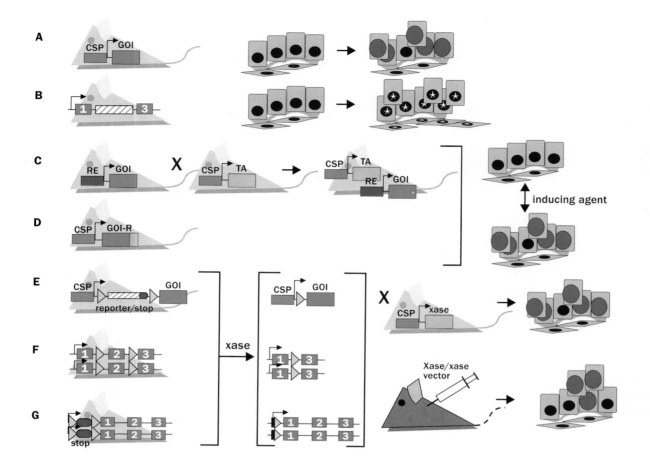

Fig. 2-31 Strategies for modeling cancer in the mouse.

Many of the current approaches for creating mice with specific genetic lesions and the resulting potential for cell specificity of alterations are diagrammed. Basic strategies are shown in (**A**) and (**B**), respectively. A gene of interest (GOI), for example an oncogene, can be expressed cell-specifically in transgenic mice using a cell-specific promoter (CSP) (**A**). Generally, expression is not achieved in every cell, but is usually widespread (as indicated by the light-blue nuclei). Standard targeting strategies in ES cells can be used to alter endogenous genes to create null (knock-out, as diagrammed in [**B**]) or other specific mutations (knock-in). In this case, a mouse strain is generated that carries the engineered alteration in every cell (designated by an asterisk); cell specificity of expression is dictated by the endogenous regulatory signals. Strategies in (**C–G**) offer conditional control of either transgene expression (**C–E**) or endogenous gene mutation (**F and G**). In (**C**), the GOI is regulated by transcriptional response elements (RE) of a transcriptional activator (TA) that is expressed in transgenic mice via a CSP. In this case, expression of the transgene is reversible, and the effects of expression or expression cessation can be assessed at specific times. Cell specificity is dictated by a CSP driving the TA. Activity of the transgenic protein can be regulated when using the strategy depicted in (**D**). In this case, the GOI is fused to a segment encoding a ligand-regulated protein domain. For example, the estrogen receptor ligand-binding domain has been used effectively to regulate transgenic proteins. Strategies in (**E–G**) utilize a recombinase (xase) and its cognate binding site (yellow triangles) to induce deletions resulting in expression of a transgene (**E**), an endogenous gene (**G**), or in a specific mutation (**F**). The recombinase can be introduced by crosses with transgenic mice expressing the xase cell specifically (as in [**A–C**]) or by limited introduction via injection into a specific organ. By introducing the xase somatically, it is possible to achieve the desired alteration in a limited number of cells so as to model the stochastic nature of events that produce cancer in humans.

Reprinted from Cell, Volume 108(2). Van Dyke T, Jacks T. Cancer modeling in the modern era: progress and challenges. Pages 135-44, copyright 2002. With permission from Elsevier.

known roles in cancer. In another integrated approach, limited sequencing of 1,507 coding genes was combined with CGH to study 441 tumors in multiple organ sites, which revealed more than 100 significantly mutated genes.[111] This study provided a broad overview of mutations across different types of cancers and identified several novel therapeutic targets.

TCGA studies of various important cancers are rapidly being completed. One TCGA study integrated genomic DNA copy number arrays, DNA methylation, exome sequencing, messenger RNA arrays, miRNA sequencing, and reverse-phase protein arrays to analyze a group of breast cancers and germ-line samples from 825 patients.[112] Only three genes demonstrated mutations in more than 10% of all breast cancers, but numerous subtype associations and novel mutations were found. A similar study used exome sequence, DNA copy number, promoter methylation, and messenger RNA and miRNA expression to analyze colorectal carcinomas and germ-line samples from 276 patients.[113] This study found 24 genes that were commonly mutated, amplifications of druggable targets and mutations in pathways that might be targeted by therapy, and these included *WNT, RAS, PI3K*, and *MYC*-related signaling. Another TCGA study sequenced the exomes of 316 high-grade serous ovarian adenocarcinomas and combined these data with mRNA expression, miRNA expression, promoter methylation, and DNA copy number.[71] This study revealed new approaches to tumor classification and prognosis, and well as mechanistic insights, such as the finding that 50% of the tumors had compromised homologous recombination pathways. Finally, a recent TCGA report used whole-genome sequencing (50 samples) and exome sequencing (150 samples) to comprehensively examine 200 adult AMLs.[114] This study found that AMLs contain fewer mutations than other adult cancers, with an average of 13 mutations per sample, only five of which involve recurrently mutated genes. At least one driver gene was identified in each AML sample, and these fell within nine distinct categories.

MOUSE MODELS OF HUMAN CANCER

Genetic techniques developed throughout the past 2 decades now make it possible to create mouse models that recapitulate sporadic human cancers with increasing fidelity. A complete review of mouse genetics is beyond the scope of this chapter, and several excellent reviews describe the various types of genetically engineered mice in detail.[115,116] However, the basic types of mouse models are reviewed here.

The first generation of genetically engineered mouse models involved expressing oncogenes from transgenes (that were injected into oocytes) or making "knockout" strains in which genes were inactivated by homologous recombination in mouse embryonic stem cells (Fig. 2-31). Hundreds of genes have been studied with these techniques, and they have led to important advances in understanding gene functions in development and tumorigenesis. In fact, these methods are still in wide use today. For example, mice containing a *MYC* transgene that mimics the translocation found in Burkitt lymphoma is used to study *MYC*-associated tumorigenesis and the development of therapeutic strategies targeting these neoplasms. However, these strategies affect gene expression early in development and, in the case of knockouts, affect every cell. These characteristics limit their ability to model human cancers, which sequentially acquire rare mutations in somatic cells. Moreover, many cancer genes are lethal when disrupted in the mouse germline, or they lead to rapidly developing neoplasms in one tissue that preclude studies of slower-growing cancers. More recent mouse genetic engineering strategies circumvent these problems by allowing mutations to be introduced in tissue-specific and temporally controlled manners.

Conditional expression strategies allow for either loss-of-function or gain-of-function mutations to be regulated in various ways. The most common strategies involve using recognition sites for site-specific recombinases that flank the gene region to be modified. Breeding these animals with mice that express the recombinase results in deletion of the intervening DNA segment, and this can lead to either gene deletion or activation, depending on the type of vector employed. Importantly, many mice strains that express the recombinase in specific tissues have been developed, and these allow the oncogene mutations to be tissue-restricted. However, in these cases, all of the cells in the target tissue contain the induced mutation. Strategies to restrict induced oncogenic mutations to only a subset of cells in a target tissue in adult mice include using viral gene therapy vectors to introduce recombinases to selected tissues (e.g., transbronchial delivery of adenovirus-Cre to pulmonary epithelial cells), or by developing gene-targeting vectors that require rare recombination events to express oncogenic mutants.[117] Another strategy for developing tissue-specific oncogene expression in mice involves engineering strains that express the receptor for avian retroviruses in selected tissues, thereby allowing avian retroviral vectors to introduce oncogenes in these specific tissues.[118]

The conditional nature of the systems described above involves restricting expression of the mutations to a subset of cells, but the mutation is expressed constitutively within the targeted cells or tissues. Other conditional systems allow control of the amount and timing of oncogene expression. One common method places the mutant protein under control of a transcriptional unit that can be regulated by tetracycline.[119] Thus, expression of the transgene can be turned off or on by administering doxycycline to the transgenic animals. Another approach involves fusing the test gene to a fragment of the estrogen receptor, which allows its activity to be regulated by estradiol administration. These strategies allow oncogenes to be temporally regulated and enable important studies determining the role of oncogene expression in tumor initiation and maintenance.

The current range of murine genetic engineering techniques now allows the development of meaningful models of human cancers that will be invaluable for investigating the mechanisms of tumorigenesis and will function as platforms for the development of cancer therapeutics. Importantly, multiple mutations can be combined by breeding to create strains that faithfully mimic the multistep nature of human cancers.

KEY POINTS

- Next-generation sequencing is revealing transformative and comprehensive insight on cancer genomics.
- These technologies may allow personalized and targeted cancer therapy strategies based on specific mutations detected in a patient's tumor cells.
- Gene targeting and transgenic methods are used to create murine models that mimic the genetic mutations found in human cancers. These models are invaluable for understanding the mechanisms underlying tumorigenesis and are used to determine the role of specific mutations in multistep tumorigenesis.

References

1. Alberts B, Johnson A, Lewis J, et al. *Molecular Biology of the Cell, 5th ed.* New York: Garland Science; 2008.

2. Lodish HF, Berk A, Kaiser CA, et al. *Molecular Cell Biology, 6th ed.* New York: W.H. Freeman; 2008.

3. Maston GA, Evans SK, Green MR. Transcriptional regulatory elements in the human genome. *Annu Rev Genomics Human Genet.* 2006;7:29-59. PMID: 16719718.

4. Näär AM, Lemon BD, Tjian R. Transcriptional coactivator complexes. *Ann Rev Biochem.* 2001;70:475-501. PMID: 11395415.

5. Perissi V, Jepsen K, Glass CK, et al. Deconstructing repression: evolving models of co-repressor action. *Nat Rev Genet.* 2010;11:109-123. PMID: 20084085.

6. Allis CD, Jenuwein T, Reinberg D. *Epigenetics.* Cold Spring Harbor, NY: Cold Spring Harbor Laboratory Press; 2007.

7. Jenuwein T, Allis CD. Translating the histone code. *Science.* 2001;293:1074-1080. PMID: 11498575.

8. Saha A, Wittmeyer J, Cairns BR. Chromatin remodelling: the industrial revolution of DNA around histones. *Nat Rev Mol Cell Biol.* 2006;7:437-447. PMID: 16723979.

9. Kouzarides T. Chromatin modifications and their function. *Cell.* 2007;128:693-705. PMID: 17320507.

10. Goll MG, Bestor TH. Eukaryotic cytosine methyltransferases. *Annu Rev Biochem.* 2005;74:481-514. PMID: 15952895.

11. Goldberg AD, Allis CD, Bernstein E. Epigenetics: a landscape takes shape. *Cell.* 2007;128:635-638. PMID: 17320500.

12. Suganuma T, Workman JL. Crosstalk among Histone Modifications. *Cell.* 2008;135:604-607. PMID: 19013272.

13. Laird PW. Cancer epigenetics. *Hum Mol Genet.* 2005;14 Spec No 1:R65-76. PMID: 15809275.

14. Bolden JE, Peart MJ, Johnstone RW. Anticancer activities of histone deacetylase inhibitors. *Nat Rev Drug Discov.* 2006;5:769-784. PMID: 16955068.

15. Oki Y, Issa JP. Review: recent clinical trials in epigenetic therapy. *Rev Recent Clin Trials.* 2006;1:169-182. PMID: 18473969.

16. Yang X, Lay F, Han H, et al. Targeting DNA methylation for epigenetic therapy. *Trends Pharmacol* Sci. 2010;31:536-546. PMID: 20846732.

17. Dieffenbach C, Dveksler, G. *PCR Primer: A laboratory manual, 2nd ed.* Cold Spring Harbor, NY: Cold Spring Harbor Laboratory Press; 2003.

18. Pray L. The biotechnology revolution: PCR and the use of reverse transcriptase to clone expressed genes. *Nature Education.* 2008;1:94.

19. Beaudet AL, Belmont JW. Array-based DNA diagnostics: let the revolution begin. *Annu Rev Med.* 2008;59:113-129. PMID: 17961075.

20. Shastry BS. SNPs in disease gene mapping, medicinal drug development and evolution. *J Hum Genet.* 2007;52:871-880. PMID: 17928948.

21. Wang Y, Armstrong SA. Genome-wide SNP analysis in cancer: leukemia shows the way. *Cancer Cell.* 2007;11:308-309. PMID: 17418407.

22. Mardis ER. The impact of next-generation sequencing technology on genetics. *Trends Genet.* 2008;24:133-141. PMID: 18262675.

23. Schuster SC. Next-generation sequencing transforms today's biology. *Nat Methods.* 2008;5:16-18. PMID: 18165802.

24. Meyerson M, Gabriel S, Getz G. Advances in understanding cancer genomes through second-generation sequencing. *Nat Rev Genet.* 2010;11:685-696. PMID: 20847746.

25. Bentley DR, Balasubramanian S, Swerdlow HP, et al. Accurate whole human genome sequencing using reversible terminator chemistry. *Nature.* 2008;456:53-59. PMID: 18987734.

26. Wang J, Wang W, Li R, et al. The diploid genome sequence of an Asian individual. *Nature.* 2008;456:60-65. PMID: 18987735.

27. Mendenhall EM, Bernstein BE. Chromatin state maps: new technologies, new insights. *Curr Opin Genet Dev.* 2008;18:109-115. PMID: 18339538.

28. Meissner A, Mikkelsen TS, Gu H, et al. Genome-scale DNA methylation maps of pluripotent and differentiated cells. *Nature.* 2008;454:766-770. PMID: 18600261.

29. Nature. Nature Encode Explorer. http://www.nature.com/encode/#/threads. Accessed May 14, 2014.

30. Bustin SA, Mueller R. Real-time reverse transcription PCR (qRT-PCR) and its potential use in clinical diagnosis. *Clin Sci (Lond).* 2005;109:365-379. PMID: 16171460.

31. Lutfalla G, Uze G. Performing quantitative reverse-transcribed polymerase chain reaction experiments. *Methods Enzymol.* 2006;410:386-400. PMID: 16938562.

32. Carlson JJ, Roth JA. The impact of the Oncotype Dx breast cancer assay in clinical practice: a systematic review and meta-analysis. *Breast Cancer Res Treat.* 2013;141:13-22. PMID: 23974828.

33. Warrington JA, Todd R, Wong D. *Microarrays and Cancer Research.* Westboro, MA: BioTechniques Press/Eaton Pub; 2002.

34. van 't Veer LJ, Dai H, van de Vijver MJ, et al. Gene expression profiling predicts clinical outcome of breast cancer. *Nature.* 2002;415:530-536. PMID: 11823860.

35. Alizadeh AA, Eisen MB, Davis RE, et al. Distinct types of diffuse large B-cell lymphoma identified by gene expression profiling. *Nature.* 2000;403:503-511. PMID: 10676951.

36. Glas AM, Floore A, Delahaye LJ, et al. Converting a breast cancer microarray signature into a high-throughput diagnostic test. *BMC Genomics.* 2006;7:278. PMID: 17074082.

37. Meister G, Tuschl T. Mechanisms of gene silencing by double-stranded RNA. *Nature.* 2004;431:343-349. PMID: 15372041.

38. Inui M, Martello G, Piccolo S. MicroRNA control of signal transduction. *Nat Rev Mol Cell Biol.* 2010;11:252-263. PMID: 20216554.

39. Shivdasani RA. MicroRNAs: regulators of gene expression and cell differentiation. *Blood.* 2006;108:3646-3653. PMID: 16882713.

40. Calin GA, Croce CM. MicroRNA signatures in human cancers. *Nat Rev Cancer.* 2006;6:857-866. PMID: 17060945.

41. He L, Thomson JM, Hemann MT, et al. A microRNA polycistron as a potential human oncogene. *Nature.* 2005;435:828-833. PMID: 15944707.

42. Bernards R, Brummelkamp TR, Beijersbergen RL. shRNA libraries and their use in cancer genetics. *Nat Methods.* 2006;3:701-706. PMID: 16929315.

43. Root DE, Hacohen N, Hahn WC, et al. Genome-scale loss-of-function screening with a lentiviral RNAi library. *Nat Methods.* 2006;3:715-719. PMID: 16929317.

44. Pinkel D, Albertson DG. Array comparative genomic hybridization and its applications in cancer. *Nat Genet.* 2005;37 Suppl:S11-S17. PMID: 15920524.

45. Walker JM. *The Protein Protocols Handbook, 3rd ed.* Totowa, NJ: Humana Press; 2009.

46. Peng J, Gygi SP. Proteomics: the move to mixtures. *J Mass Spectrom.* 2001;36:1083-1091. PMID: 11747101.

47. Srivastava S, Srivastava RG. Proteomics in the forefront of cancer biomarker discovery. *J Proteome Res.* 2005;4:1098-1103. PMID: 16083258.

48. Vogelstein B, Kinzler KW. *The Genetic Basis of Human Cancer, 2nd ed.* New York: McGraw-Hill Professional; 2002.

49. Weinberg RA. *The Biology of Cancer.* New York: Garland Science; 2007.

50. Look T. Genes altered by chromosomal translocations in leukemia and lymphomas. In Vogelstein B, Kinzler KW (eds). *The Genetic Basis of Human Cancer.* New York: McGraw-Hill Professional, 2002;57-92.

51. Look AT. Oncogenic transcription factors in the human acute leukemias. *Science.* 1997;278:1059-1064. PMID: 9353180.

52. Sankar S, Lessnick SL. Promiscuous partnerships in Ewing's sarcoma. *Cancer Genet.* 2011;204:351-365. PMID: 21872822.

53. Tomlins SA, Rhodes DR, Perner S, et al. Recurrent fusion of TMPRSS2 and ETS transcription factor genes in prostate cancer. *Science.* 2005;310:644-648. PMID: 16254181.

54. Hogarty MD. The metabolic & molecular bases of inherited disease. In Scriver C (ed). *The Metabolic and Molecular Bases of Inherited Disease, 8th ed.* New York: McGraw-Hill, 2001;597-610.

55. Sherr CJ. Principles of tumor suppression. *Cell.* 2004;116:235-246. PMID: 14744434.

56. Morgan DO. *The Cell Cycle: Principles of Control.* London Sunderland, MA: New Science Press Ltd.; 2007.

57. Finn RS, Slamon DJ. Monoclonal antibody therapy for breast cancer: herceptin. *Cancer Chemother Biol Response Modif.* 2003;21:223-233. PMID: 15338747.

58. Pritchard CC, Grady WM. Colorectal cancer molecular biology moves into clinical practice. *Gut.* 2011;60:116-129. PMID: 20921207.

59. Numico G, Silvestris N, Grazioso Russi E. Advances in EGFR-directed therapy in head and neck cancer. *Front Biosci (Schol Ed).* 2011;3:454-466. PMID: 21196389.

60. Sequist LV, Lynch TJ. EGFR tyrosine kinase inhibitors in lung cancer: an evolving story. *Annu Rev Med.* 2008;59:429-442. PMID: 17716025.

61. Campbell PM, Der CJ. Oncogenic Ras and its role in tumor cell invasion and metastasis. *Semin Cancer Biol.* 2004;14:105-114. PMID: 15018894.

62. Cox AD, Der CJ. Ras family signaling: therapeutic targeting. *Cancer Biol Ther.* 2002;1:599-606. PMID: 12642680.

63. Maurer G, Tarkowski B, Baccarini M. Raf kinases in cancer-roles and therapeutic opportunities. *Oncogene*. 2011;30:3477-3488. PMID: 21577205.

64. Altomare DA, Testa JR. Perturbations of the AKT signaling pathway in human cancer. *Oncogene*. 2005;24:7455-7464. PMID: 16288292.

65. Cully M, You H, Levine AJ, et al. Beyond PTEN mutations: the PI3K pathway as an integrator of multiple inputs during tumorigenesis. *Nat Rev Cancer*. 2006;6:184-192. PMID: 16453012.

66. Hollander MC, Blumenthal GM, Dennis PA. PTEN loss in the continuum of common cancers, rare syndromes and mouse models. *Nat Rev Cancer*. 2011;11:289-301.

67. Druker BJ. Imatinib as a paradigm of targeted therapies. *Adv Cancer Res*. 2004;91:1-30. PMID: 15327887.

68. Clurman B, Roberts J. Cell cycle control: an overview. In Vogelstein B, Kinzler KW (eds). *The Genetic Basis of Human Cancer*. New York: McGraw-Hill Professional, 2002;145-157.

69. Sherr CJ. The Pezcoller lecture: cancer cell cycles revisited. *Cancer Res*. 2000;60:3689-3695. PMID: 10919634.

70. Sherr CJ, Roberts JM. CDK inhibitors: positive and negative regulators of G1-phase progression. *Genes Dev*. 1999;13:1501-1512. PMID: 10385618.

71. Cancer Genome Atlas Research Network. Integrated genomic analyses of ovarian carcinoma. *Nature*. 2011;474:609-615. PMID: 21720365.

72. Hwang HC, Clurman BE. Cyclin E in normal and neoplastic cell cycles. *Oncogene*. 2005;24:2776-2786. PMID: 15838514.

73. Sherr CJ. The INK4a/ARF network in tumour suppression. *Nat Rev Mol Cell Biol*. 2001;2:731-737. PMID: 11584300.

74. Chu IM, Hengst L, Slingerland JM. The Cdk inhibitor p27 in human cancer: prognostic potential and relevance to anticancer therapy. *Nat Rev Cancer*. 2008;8:253-267. PMID: 18354415.

75. Schwartz GK, Shah MA. Targeting the cell cycle: a new approach to cancer therapy. *J Clin Oncol*. 2005;23:9408-9421. PMID: 16361640.

76. Danial NN, Korsmeyer SJ. Cell death: critical control points. *Cell*. 2004;116:205-219. PMID: 14744432.

77. Cory S, Adams JM. The Bcl2 family: regulators of the cellular life-or-death switch. *Nat Rev Cancer*. 2002;2:647-656. PMID: 12209154.

78. Wang S, Yang D, Lippman ME. Targeting Bcl-2 and Bcl-XL with nonpeptidic small-molecule antagonists. *Semin Oncol*. 2003;30(5 Suppl 16):133-142. PMID: 14613034.

79. Hershko A, Ciechanover A, Varshavsky A. Basic Medical Research Award. The ubiquitin system. *Nat Med*. 2000;6:1073-1781. PMID: 11017125.

80. Nakayama KI, Nakayama K. Ubiquitin ligases: cell-cycle control and cancer. *Nat Rev Cancer*. 2006;6:369-381. PMID: 16633365.

81. Kaelin WG. The von Hippel-Lindau tumor suppressor protein: roles in cancer and oxygen sensing. *Cold Spring Harb Symp Quant Biol*. 2005;70:159-166. PMID: 16869749.

82. Welcker M, Clurman BE. FBW7 ubiquitin ligase: a tumour suppressor at the crossroads of cell division, growth and differentiation. *Nat Rev Cancer*. 2008;8:83-93. PMID: 18094723.

83. Wood LD, Parsons DW, Jones S, et al. The genomic landscapes of human breast and colorectal cancers. *Science*. 2007;318:1108-1113. PMID: 17932254.

84. Clevers H. Wnt/beta-catenin signaling in development and disease. *Cell*. 2006;127:469-480. PMID: 17081971.

85. Kelly LM, Gilliland DG. Genetics of myeloid leukemias. *Annu Rev Genomics Hum Genet*. 2002;3:179-198. PMID: 12194988.

86. Maillard I, Fang T, Pear WS. Regulation of lymphoid development, differentiation, and function by the Notch pathway. *Annu Rev Immunol*. 2005;23:945-974. PMID: 15771590.

87. Weng AP, Ferrando AA, Lee W, et al. Activating mutations of NOTCH1 in human T cell acute lymphoblastic leukemia. *Science*. 2004;306:269-271. PMID: 15472075.

88. Aster JC, Pear WS, Blacklow SC. Notch signaling in leukemia. *Annu Rev Pathol*. 2008;3:587-613. PMID: 18039126.

89. de Boer J, Hoeijmakers JH. Nucleotide excision repair and human syndromes. *Carcinogenesis*. 2000;21:453-460. PMID: 10688865.

90. Kitagawa R, Kastan MB. The ATM-dependent DNA damage signaling pathway. *Cold Spring Harb Symp Quant Biol*. 2005;70:99-109. PMID: 16869743.

91. Grompe M, van de Vrugt H. The Fanconi family adds a fraternal twin. *Dev Cell*. 2007;12:661-662. PMID: 17488615.

92. Kennedy RD, D'Andrea AD. The Fanconi Anemia/BRCA pathway: new faces in the crowd. *Genes Dev*. 2005;19:2925-2940. PMID: 16357213.

93. Jiricny J. The multifaceted mismatch-repair system. *Nat Rev Mol Cell Biol*. 2006;7:335-346. PMID: 16612326.

94. Hartwell LH, Weinert TA. Checkpoints: controls that ensure the order of cell cycle events. *Science*. 1989;246:629-634. PMID: 2683079.

95. Hartwell L, Weinert T, Kadyk L, et al. Cell cycle checkpoints, genomic integrity, and cancer. *Cold Spring Harb Symp Quant Biol*. 1994;59:259-263. PMID: 7587077.

96. Gottifredi V, Prives C. The S phase checkpoint: when the crowd meets at the fork. *Semin Cell Dev Biol*. 2005;16:355-368. PMID: 15840444.

97. Lukas J, Lukas C, Bartek J. Mammalian cell cycle checkpoints: signalling pathways and their organization in space and time. *DNA Repair (Armst)*. 2004;3:997-1007. PMID: 15279786.

98. Zhou BB, Elledge SJ. The DNA damage response: putting checkpoints in perspective. *Nature*. 2000;408:433-439. PMID: 11100718.

99. Poyurovsky MV, Prives C. Unleashing the power of p53: lessons from mice and men. *Genes Dev*. 2006;20:125-131. PMID: 16418478.

100. Vogelstein B, Lane D, Levine AJ. Surfing the p53 network. *Nature*. 2000;408:307-310. PMID: 11099028.

101. Sherr CJ. Divorcing ARF and p53: an unsettled case. *Nat Rev Cancer*. 2006;6:663-673. PMID: 16915296.

102. Kastan MB. Wild-type p53: tumors can't stand it. *Cell*. 2007;128:837-840. PMID: 17350571.

103. Wiman KG. Strategies for therapeutic targeting of the p53 pathway in cancer. *Cell Death Differ*. 2006;13:921-926. PMID: 16557267.

104. Weaver BA, Cleveland DW. Decoding the links between mitosis, cancer, and chemotherapy: The mitotic checkpoint, adaptation, and cell death. *Cancer Cell*. 2005;8:7-12. PMID: 16023594.

105. Hanahan D, Weinberg RA. Hallmarks of cancer: the next generation. *Cell*. 2011;144:646-674. PMID: 21376230.

106. Thomas RK, Baker AC, Debiasi RM, et al. High-throughput oncogene mutation profiling in human cancer. *Nat Genet*. 2007;39:347-351. PMID: 17293865.

107. Parsons DW, Jones S, Zhang X, et al. An integrated genomic analysis of human glioblastoma multiforme. *Science*. 2008;321:1807-1812. PMID: 18772396.

108. Jones S, Zhang X, Parsons DW, et al. Core signaling pathways in human pancreatic cancers revealed by global genomic analyses. *Science*. 2008;321:1801-1806. PMID: 18772397.

109. Figueroa ME, Abdel-Wahab O, Lu C, et al. Leukemic IDH1 and IDH2 mutations result in a hypermethylation phenotype, disrupt TET2 function, and impair hematopoietic differentiation. *Cancer Cell*. 2010;18:553-567. PMID: 21130701.

110. Wang F, Travins J, DeLaBarre B, et al. Targeted inhibition of mutant IDH2 in leukemia cells induces cellular differentiation. *Science*. 2013;340:622-626. Epub 2013 Apr 4. PMID: 23558173.

111. Cancer Genome Atlas Research Network. Comprehensive genomic characterization defines human glioblastoma genes and core pathways. *Nature*. 2008;455:1061-1068. PMID: 18772890.

112. Cancer Genome Atlas Network. Comprehensive molecular portraits of human breast tumours. *Nature*. 2012;490:61-70. PMID: 23000897.

113. Cancer Genome Atlas Network. Comprehensive molecular characterization of human colon and rectal cancer. *Nature*. 2012;487:330-337. PMID: 22810696.

114. Cancer Genome Atlas Research Network. Genomic and epigenomic landscapes of adult de novo acute myeloid leukemia. *N Engl J Med*. 2013;368:2059-2074. PMID: 23634996.

115. Jonkers J, Berns A. Conditional mouse models of sporadic cancer. *Nat Rev Cancer*. 2002;2:251-265. PMID: 12001987.

116. Van Dyke T, Jacks T. Cancer modeling in the modern era: progress and challenges. *Cell*. 2002;108:135-144. PMID: 11832204.

117. Johnson L, Mercer K, Greenbaum D, et al. Somatic activation of the K-ras oncogene causes early onset lung cancer in mice. *Nature*. 2001;410:1111-1116. PMID: 11323676.

118. Fisher GH, Orsulic S, Holland E, et al. Development of a flexible and specific gene delivery system for production of murine tumor models. *Oncogene*. 1999;18:5253-5260. PMID: 10498877.

119. Gossen M, Bujard H. Studying gene function in eukaryotes by conditional gene inactivation. *Annu Rev Genet*. 2002;36:153-173. PMID: 12429690.

3

CLINICAL PHARMACOLOGY

Matthew P. Goetz, MD

Updates from 2012 ▶ Glucarpidase was approved as an orphan drug to treat patients with toxic levels of methotrexate in their blood (Widemann BC, *Pharmacotherapy* 2014).

Medical oncologists are responsible for administering anticancer therapies to patients with malignancies. Many of these drugs exhibit a narrow therapeutic window, meaning the difference between the toxic and therapeutic dose is small. Traditionally, researchers have developed antineoplastic agents to be delivered at the highest maximum doses to optimize the anticancer activity. However, the focus of drug development has shifted away from antineoplastic therapies that target DNA and toward molecules directed toward a specific molecular target, often a protein or pathway regulating cell growth or cancer progression. This class of drugs is commonly referred to as "targeted cancer therapies." Regardless of the agent, drug dosing requires a balance between the anticancer benefit and the known toxicities these agents cause on normal end-organ function. The purpose of this chapter is to review the fundamental principles of clinical pharmacology as they relate to the practice of oncology and to discuss the emerging area of pharmacogenomics, which refers to the relationship between specific DNA-sequence variation and drug effect.

PRINCIPLES OF CHEMOTHERAPY

Cytotoxic chemotherapy has been a relative success story. Cancers such as Hodgkin lymphoma, non-Hodgkin lymphomas, testicular cancer, germ cell tumors, leukemia, Wilms tumors, retinoblastomas, and others can be cured through the effective delivery of cytotoxic chemotherapy. These agents are now commonly administered in the adjuvant setting for breast, colon, ovarian, and lung cancers. In such cases, chemotherapy delivered after resection of the primary cancer can suppress or even eliminate the growth of occult cancer cells that have already metastasized, increasing overall survival. Additionally, chemotherapy sometimes is used in combination with radiation therapy. Combined-modality approaches (chemotherapy and radiation together) are used in many diseases to shrink the tumor burden to permit surgery, to control systemic disease, or both. Chemotherapy alone may also be used to shrink the tumor burden prior to surgery in some tumors.

Cytotoxic chemotherapy agents are most active during the cellular replication and division phases of the cell cycle. For most cancers, tumor turnover or replication takes days to weeks—not hours—creating an inherent problem between cell-cycle time and the exposure obtained with most cytotoxic chemotherapy agents, which is often only hours.[1] An understanding of this principle led to the introduction of combination chemotherapy, which was developed to provide maximal cell kill within the range of tolerable toxicity for each drug, for broad coverage in resistant cell lines within a heterogeneous tumor population, for prevention of drug resistance, and for stimulation of the cell cycle through cellular stress, thus increasing the pressure toward cell death (e.g., cisplatin and fluorouracil combinations).

Despite advances in the optimization of current cancer chemotherapy for patients with malignancies such as lymphoma and testicular cancer, classic anticancer agents that target DNA have not led to cures in most solid tumors. For example, combination chemotherapy delivered to patients with metastatic disease (e.g., metastatic breast cancer) confers little or no survival advantage compared with sequential chemotherapy. In these settings, sequential single-agent chemotherapy, with or without a biologically targeted agent, is a commonly accepted approach to treatment. In this setting, the balance between toxicity and efficacy is particularly important as these patients are likely to exhibit decreases in end-organ function resulting in alterations in metabolism.

KEY POINT

- Combination chemotherapy has become the standard of care for the majority of cancer therapy regimens in the adjuvant setting.

PHARMACOKINETICS

Pharmacokinetics is the relationship between time and plasma concentration following drug administration; it has been best described as "what the body does to the drug." An understanding of the pharmacokinetics of a chemotherapy drug is critical to the optimum administration of that drug. The measurement of pharmacokinetics is an outcome of most early-phase clinical trials.

From these studies, clinicians learn critical information:

- The range of tolerable doses
- The relationship between dose and exposure
- The relationship between drug exposure and toxicity
- The differences among patients between dose and exposure

The choice of drug administration route is based primarily on pharmacokinetic assessment of bioavailability—the ability of the drug to reach its target in an active form—and the formulation of an acceptable dose preparation for oral, intravenous, intramuscular, intrathecal, or subcutaneous use. Classically, oncologic drugs have been developed using the intravenous route, particularly for water-soluble compounds, because complete absorption is guaranteed. The method of administration also is highly dependent on the ability to formulate a compound into a satisfactory pharmacologic product that can be administered by the route of choice. Several common agents (e.g., paclitaxel) are poorly soluble and must be mixed in solvents, such as Kollipher

EL, formerly referred to as Cremophor EL, a proprietary castor oil and polyethylene glycol ether emulsifier. These agents can have their own toxicities, including the Kollipher-induced hypersensitivity reaction observed with paclitaxel administration.

Bioavailability is the fraction of an administered dose of unchanged drug that reaches the systemic circulation. By definition, when a drug is administered intravenously, its bioavailability is 100%. (Similar calculations can be made for intramuscular or subcutaneous dosing compared with intravenous dosing.) Bioavailability has become more important as more cytotoxic chemotherapy agents (e.g., capecitabine), as well as biologic agents, are developed for oral dosing. The oral route has the advantage of achieving a more prolonged exposure, thereby providing coverage throughout the cell cycle when toxicity allows. Agents with a high first-pass metabolism will, by nature, have poor oral bioavailability. Alterations in gastrointestinal tract absorptive capacity can alter oral bioavailability as well. Previous surgery, concomitant medications, malabsorption from other causes, and changes in motility, particularly with supportive care agents such as opiates, may alter absorption of an oral chemotherapy agent. Finally, the ingestion of drugs in either a fasting or a fed state can affect drug exposure. Therefore, when considering the administration of such drugs, it is necessary to account for these possible variations.

The study of pharmacokinetics is classically divided into four elements: absorption, distribution, metabolism, and excretion. Absorption is defined as 100% when agents are administered through an intravenous route but varies when other routes of administration are used. Distribution identifies what happens to a drug after its administration. Typically, drugs distribute from the plasma into extracellular and intracellular fluids. The distribution phase of pharmacokinetics may be the most complicated. In the simple two-compartment model, a drug is administered and enters into the plasma compartment, followed by a distribution and redistribution of the compound to the peripheral compartment. The drug concentration in this peripheral compartment is the critical value because this is where the drug-tumor interaction occurs. It is important to recognize that drug concentration in the peripheral compartment rarely is measured in clinical trials and is unknown for virtually all agents used today. The degree to which drugs distribute to the peripheral compartment alters their terminal half-life. Drugs that are more highly distributed to this compartment will have a longer terminal half-life.[2] This fact has important clinical ramifications for drugs such as methotrexate, which is the classic example of a drug distributing to the third space, such as pleural effusions or ascites. This scenario can lead to substantial and prolonged methotrexate-induced toxicity.

Metabolism of therapeutic agents is the area in which there has been the greatest increase in research and subsequent understanding during the past several decades (Table 3-1). In addition, cellular models have been developed that enable clinicians to define the metabolic pathways for many important chemotherapy agents. Hepatic enzymes responsible for phase I (oxidation, reduction, and hydrolysis) and phase II (conjugation) reactions prepare agents for their excretion by the liver

Table 3-1 Selected Drug-Metabolizing Enzymes of Importance in Oncology

Reaction	Substrates	Polymorphic*
Phase I Reactions		
Cytochrome P-450		
CYP1A1	Benzo(a)pyrene	×
CYP1A2	Theophylline, caffeine	×
CYP2B6	Cyclophosphamide	×
CYP2C8	Paclitaxel	×
CYP2C9	Phenytoin, warfarin	×
CYP2C19	Omeprazole, diazepam	×
CYP2D6	Tamoxifen, codeine, granisetron, many antidepressants	×
CYP2E1	Ethanol	×
CYP3A4/3A5	Etoposide, ifosfamide, docetaxel, irinotecan, bortezomib, imatinib, flutamide, exemestane, lapatinib, sunitinib, vinca drugs (e.g., vincristine vinorelbine, vindesine, and vinblastine)	
Ketoreductase	Anthracyclines	
Aldehyde dehydrogenases	Aldophosphamide	
Carboxylesterases	Irinotecan	
Dihydropyrimidine dehydrogenase	Fluorouracil	×
Cytosine deaminase	Cytarabine, gemcitabine	×
Phase II Reactions		
N-acetylation		
NAT2	Isoniazid	×
Glucuronidation		
UGT1A1	Bilirubin, SN-38	×
UGT2B7	Morphine, epirubicin, tamoxifen metabolites	×
Methyltransferases		
TPMT	Mercaptopurine, azathioprine	×

*Known genetic variants that influence enzyme activity.
Modified with permission from Ratain MJ. Pharmacology of cancer chemotherapy. In DeVita VT Jr, Hellman S, Rosenberg SA, eds. Cancer: Principles and Practice of Oncology, 6th ed. Philadelphia, Pa: Lippincott Williams & Wilkins; 2001:337.

or by the kidney. Hepatic and renal function are critical to the excretion of most cytotoxic chemotherapy agents. When choosing dosages for patients with cancer, clinicians typically have relied on hepatic enzyme function and serum creatinine levels as the primary means to assess end-organ function. However, other factors, such as age, sex, diet, and drug-drug interactions, can lead to clinically important variability in drug effect. For some drugs, genetic variation in genes that encode enzymes responsible for drug metabolism may substantially alter pharmacokinetics and, thus, drug effect.

KEY POINTS

- A broad understanding of the metabolism of cytotoxic and biologic agents is necessary.
- Bioavailability is an important consideration when using oral chemotherapy agents.
- Food can alter bioavailability and, thus, drug exposure.
- Drug-drug interactions are an important—but often unrecognized—factor influencing drug effect.

EXCRETION

There are two major routes of excretion: the kidneys and the biliary tract. Traditionally, chemotherapy agents were, and still generally are, administered using body surface area–adjusted doses. This method of dosing was originally used because of its relatively good correlation with creatinine clearance and glomerular filtration rate (GFR). However, for some agents, a more pharmacokinetically driven method of dosing has been developed based on the area under the curve (AUC). The classic example of this scenario is carboplatin; well-established formulae enable oncologists to determine a more accurate dose that is reflective of renal function. Many agents in current clinical practice must be adjusted for either renal or hepatic dysfunction (Table 3-2). Additional variables that affect excretion include enterohepatic circulation, wherein after biliary excretion, reabsorption of either the parent drug or its metabolites may take place in the small intestine.

Inulin clearance is regarded as the gold standard for measuring GFR. The classic method of inulin clearance can be cumbersome since it requires an intravenous infusion and timed urine collections. As a result, alternative measures for estimating GFR have been devised. The most frequently used equation for estimating GFR in adults is the Cockcroft-Gault equation, which was developed for estimating creatinine clearance; it has been tested extensively in its prediction of GFR.[3,4] Another equation for estimation of creatinine clearance, by Jelliffe, has been used extensively.[5] The Modification of Diet in Renal Disease equation provides estimates of GFR standardized for body surface area.[6] The abbreviated version is easy to implement since it requires only serum creatinine, age, sex, and race; however, no one formula for estimating GFR has yet proved superior for dosing carboplatin for optimum therapeutic index. Given new

Table 3-2 Drugs Requiring Dose Modification for Organ Dysfunction

Liver Dysfunction	Renal Insufficiency	Glomerular Filtration Rate of Less than 25%
Doxorubicin	Cisplatin	Cyclophosphamide
Epirubicin	Hydroxyurea	Ifosfamide
Dactinomycin	Etoposide	Bleomycin
Irinotecan	Pentostatin	Streptozotocin
Paclitaxel	Fludarabine	Daunorubicin
Thiotepa	Carboplatin	Idarubicin
Vincristine	Topotecan	Epirubicin
Vinorelbine	Capecitabine	Mercaptopurine
Vinblastine	Methotrexate	
Vindesine	Pemetrexed	
Cyclophosphamide	Bisphosphonates	
Ifosfamide		
Cytarabine		
Gemcitabine		
Etoposide		
Fluorouracil		
Docetaxel		

Modified from Cheson BD, ed. Oncology MKSAP, 2nd ed. *Philadelphia, PA: American College of Physicians, 1999.*

laboratory assays for creatinine, the relationship between current methods of GFR estimation and carboplatin safety/efficacy is the subject of ongoing investigation.

The clearance of an agent is an important aspect of accurate drug dosing. Clearance can be calculated by the dose divided by the AUC or dose rate divided by concentration at steady state. Few clinicians memorize the values of clearance for agents, but it is necessary to be aware of the variability in clearance. Most compounds used have a variation in clearance among patients of approximately 20% to 40%, although some agents have high variability (75% to 100%). Some of the important factors affecting variability in clearance include changes in end-organ function, drug-drug interactions, and genetic variation leading to alterations in enzymes that activate or clear a particular drug.

Variability in the metabolic or excretory organs because of dysfunction or the concomitant administration of medications that affect enzyme function is common and must be recognized. Many agents are highly protein-bound, and variability in the amount and function of proteins involved in drug metabolism will influence clearance. Genetic polymorphisms that lead to a reduction or an increase in the function of enzymes involved in the uptake, metabolism, and distribution of drugs can account for a substantial portion of the variability in drug-response phenotypes (toxicity and clinical response). Lastly, it is important to know which drugs form active metabolites (Table 3-3). Many agents, including cyclophosphamide, 5-fluorouracil, irinotecan,

and tamoxifen, are metabolized or activated before their full therapeutic effect is obtained.

In summary, when choosing a drug and a dose, it is critical that oncologists consider those factors known to affect the activation and/or clearance of a given drug, including 1) route of administration, recognizing those factors influencing absorption (e.g., gastric motility, food effect, prior surgery); 2) organ function; 3) drug-drug interactions; and 4) pharmacogenomics. After consideration of these factors, the clinician must develop a plan for careful monitoring of drug-response phenotypes, namely toxicity and response. Although classic toxicities, such as myelosuppression, are not commonly seen with newer targeted therapies that do not directly target DNA, substantial toxicity (e.g., trastuzumab- or sunitinib-induced cardiomyopathy) is not rare, and therefore, close observation is necessary.

Treatment of Patients with Toxic Drug Levels

For some chemotherapy drugs, the drugs may be intrinsically toxic to either the liver or kidneys. In this case, toxic levels of

Table 3-3 Oncology Drugs with Active Circulating Metabolites

Chemotherapy Drugs	Other Oncology Drugs
Alkylating Agents	**Analgesics**
Cyclophosphamide	Morphine
Ifosfamide	Codeine
Procarbazine	Hydrocodone
Dacarbazine	
Temozolomide	
Hexamethylmelamine	
Thiotepa	
Anthracyclines	
Doxorubicin	
Idarubicin	
Epirubicin	
Camptothecins	
Irinotecan	
Antimetabolites	
Tegafur, uracil, and fluorouracil (UFT)	
Methotrexate	
6-Mercaptopurine	
Antiestrogens	
Toremifene	
Tamoxifen	
Retinoids	
All-trans retinoic acid	

Reprinted with permission from DeVita VT Jr, Hellman S, Rosenberg SA, eds. Cancer: Principles and Practice of Oncology, 6th ed. *Philadelphia, Pa: Lippincott Williams & Wilkins; 2001.*

the drug can build up, leading to prolonged and severe adverse effects. Some drugs can be removed by dialysis; for other drugs, antidotes have been developed. Glucarpidase is a recent antidote approved to treat patients with toxic levels of methotrexate in their blood, defined as levels exceeding 1 μmol/L, as a result of reduced clearance because of renal impairment. Glucarpidase, a recombinant form of the bacterial enzyme carboxypeptidase G2, converts methotrexate into glutamate and 2,4-diamino-N(10)-methylpteroic acid, which are inactive metabolites that can be eliminated from the body via the nonrenal pathway.[7] Clinicians need to be aware that leucovorin should not be administered within 2 hours before or after a glucarpidase dose because leucovorin is a substrate for glucarpidase.

PHARMACOGENOMICS

Pharmacogenetics is the study of the role of genetic inheritance in the individual variation of drug response and toxicity. Pharmacogenomics is the term used to refer to the study of the relationship between specific DNA-sequence variation (either germ-line or somatic) and drug effect. Much of this genetic variation is in the form of single nucleotide polymorphisms—defined as variants with frequencies of 1% or greater—that can alter the amino acid sequence of the encoded protein, alter RNA splicing, or alter kinetics and catalysis of the protein.

Technologic advances now allow rapid and accurate assessment of tumor gene expression and function, both at the level of individual genes and by global gene analysis. In the latter example, massive parallel sequencing of the entire genome is now possible (see Chapter 2: Molecular Biology). This type of research has been critical in identifying specific biologic subsets of cancer that are more or less likely to relapse (prognostic) in the absence of systemic treatment, as well as the identification of genes or gene patterns associated with response (predictive to specific therapies or agents). In the case of breast cancer, many gene expression array tests are commercially available in which the expression patterns of a subset of genes important in proliferation identify tumors that are associated with a higher risk of recurrence (see Chapter 6: Breast Cancer).[8] This same technology may identify a subset of tumors more likely to benefit from chemotherapy.[9]

Mutations in genes that encode transmembrane receptor tyrosine kinases as well as proteins involved in downstream signaling cascades are important for response to tyrosine kinase inhibitors. In the case of drugs that target the epidermal growth factor receptor (EGFR), mutations that activate the EGFR tyrosine kinase domain lead to high response rates to the drugs gefitinib and erlotinib. Furthermore, in the case of colorectal cancer, mutations in the important oncogene *KRAS* are predictive of lack of response to the EGFR-inhibiting drugs panitumumab and cetuximab. In the latter example, retrospective studies have demonstrated that monoclonal antibodies that target EGFR appear to be effective only in tumors with wild-type *KRAS*.[10]

In the specialty of oncology, clinicians must take into account all sources of genetic variation that influence drug effect, including both tumor (somatic) and host (germ-line) genetic variation. The following sections will illustrate important examples wherein genetic variation at the level of both the tumor and the host lead to substantial changes in drug effect.

PHARMACOGENETICS

The promise of pharmacogenetics to individualize treatment according to gene sequence variation is well illustrated in the treatment of patients with cancer. Administration of "standard" doses of chemotherapy to patients with inherited deficiencies in enzymes responsible for their metabolism and disposition can result in marked, even lethal, toxicity. Conversely, patients who have increased enzymatic activity may be at risk for treatment failure—also an undesirable outcome when dealing with a potentially fatal illness. The traditional method by which individualized anticancer drug doses are developed and determined has involved the use of body surface area measurements and weight-based dosing.[11] However, multiple studies have indicated that dosing in this manner does not reliably account for the variability in exposure to most chemotherapy drugs.[12]

Examples of the role of pharmacogenetics have been clearly illustrated with both cytotoxic chemotherapy and with targeted therapies, including the two endpoints most important to patients with cancer: response and toxicity. Three examples illustrated in the following sections have led to relabeling or hearings by the U.S. Food and Drug Administration (FDA) to reflect the importance of pharmacogenetics.

TPMT AND THIOPURINES

The thiopurine drugs mercaptopurine and azathioprine (the latter of which is a prodrug that is converted to mercaptopurine in vivo) are purine antimetabolites used clinically to treat both pediatric and adult leukemia and as immunosuppressant agents.[13] Thiopurines are metabolized in part by S-methylation, catalyzed by the enzyme thiopurine S-methyltransferase (TPMT).[14,15] A group led by Richard M. Weinshilboum, MD, first identified three groups of patients on the basis of the level of TPMT activity in their red cells and found that the level of activity was inherited in an autosomal-codominant fashion.[14,16] Subsequently, it was shown that patients who received standard doses of thiopurines and who were homozygous for very low levels of TPMT activity or for no activity ($TPMT^L TPMT^L$) had greatly elevated concentrations of active drug metabolites, 6-thioguanine nucleotides, and a markedly increased risk of life-threatening, drug-induced myelosuppression.[17] As a result, the phenotypic test for the level of TPMT activity in red cells and, subsequently, DNA-based tests were among the first pharmacogenetic tests to be used in clinical practice. The result of *TPMT* gene resequencing has demonstrated that the most common variant allele responsible for low levels of activity among white populations encodes a protein with two alterations in the amino acid sequence as a result of single nucleotide polymorphisms.[18,19] These sequence changes result in a striking reduction in the quantity of TPMT,[18] at least in part because the variant protein is degraded rapidly.[13] A series of less frequent *TPMT* variant alleles also has been described.[16]

UGT1A1 AND IRINOTECAN

Irinotecan is metabolized in vivo to 7-ethyl-10-hydroxycamptothe-cin, SN-38 (Fig. 3-1), which is 1,000 times more potent as an inhibitor of topoisomerase I than the parent drug.[20-22] In humans, both gastrointestinal (e.g., diarrhea) and hematologic (e.g., neutropenia) toxicities are dose-limiting after the administration of irinotecan. SN-38 is inactivated by glucuronidation to form the glucuronide conjugate (SN38G) in a reaction catalyzed by the polymorphic hepatic enzyme uridine diphosphate glucuronosyl-transferase 1A1 (UGT1A1, Fig. 3-1).[23] A dinucleotide repeat polymorphism in the TATA box in the promoter for *UGT1A1* results in reduced hepatic *UGT1A1* expression and is considered the most common cause of Gilbert syndrome (mild unconjugated hyperbilirubinemia).[24-26] Patients homozygous for the *UGT1A1*28* polymorphism have substantially lower SN-38 glucuronidation rates and substantially higher rates of grade 4 or 5 neutropenia than those patients who do not carry this genetic variant.[27] The importance of *UGT1A1* pharmacogenetics in mediating irinotecan-related toxicity was recognized by the FDA when a black-box warning was applied to the irinotecan label to recommend a dose reduction for patients homozygous for the *UGT1A1* polymorphism. Recent studies have demonstrated that not only do patients homozygous for the *UGT1A1*28* polymorphism require lower doses of irinotecan, but patients who do not carry the genetic variant tolerate substantially higher doses of irinotecan.[28]

CYP2D6 AND TAMOXIFEN

Tamoxifen can be considered a prodrug that requires metabolic activation to elicit its pharmacologic activity. Tamoxifen undergoes activation to metabolites that are 100 times more potent suppressors of estradiol-stimulated breast cancer cell growth (4-OH tamoxifen and endoxifen) compared with tamoxifen or its primary metabolite, N-desmethyl tamoxifen. Endoxifen is the most abundant active metabolite in most individuals and results from the CY-P2D6-mediated oxidation of N-desmethyl tamoxifen (Fig. 3-2).[29] In separate studies of women treated with tamoxifen, genetic variation in *CYP2D6* and/or co-administration of CYP2D6 inhibitors were associated with a significant reduction in the mean plasma endoxifen concentrations, with the reduction in endoxifen concentrations directly related to inhibitor potency.[30,31] Multiple studies have evaluated whether genetic polymorphisms that alter CYP2D6 enzyme activity or the co-administration of CYP2D6 inhibitors are associated with disease recurrences, including conflicting data from large secondary analyses of prospective adjuvant tamoxifen trials including a meta-analysis of nearly 5,000 patients.[32-35] A secondary analysis of the prospective Austrian Breast and Colorectal Study Group 8 (ABCSG 8) trial demonstrated a significantly higher likelihood of recurrence or death for CYP2D6 poor metabolizers compared to extensive metabolizers in women treated with adjuvant tamoxifen for 5 years, but not in women receiving adjuvant anastrozole.[32] Clinicians should avoid the concurrent use of potent CYP2D6 inhibitors with tamoxifen. Ongoing prospective studies should provide definitive data as to the role of selecting hormone therapy according to *CYP2D6* genotype.

KEY POINT

■ Pharmacogenetics is the study of the role of genetic inheritance in individual variation in drug response and toxicity. FDA-recognized examples of oncologic drugs, wherein toxicity or response is influenced by pharmacogenetics, include the thiopurine drugs mercaptopurine and azathioprine *(TPMT)*, irinotecan *(UGT1A1)*, and tamoxifen *(CYP2D6)*.

PHARMACODYNAMICS

Pharmacodynamics is the study of the effects of drugs in the body, including the drug target. Pharmacodynamics is often summarized as the study of "what a drug does to the body." In early-phase clinical research, it is important to define the pharmacokinetic parameters of a given drug and to determine the effect of the drug on the tumor or on the target endpoints. These types of studies are best done in late phase I or early phase II clinical trials, in which the dose is fixed and the variability in target modulation can be assessed more easily. One of the greatest challenges in pharmacodynamic studies is selecting the endpoint. Ideally, endpoints are tumor-specific, but access to tumors may be difficult. Clinical trials may also be designed to study changes in a circulating blood factor to determine its correlation with disease endpoints. If such a relationship is determined in early phases of clinical research, this simplifies the clinical development pathway for a particular agent. Examples include tumor inhibition of phospho-ERK (MEK and phosphatidylinositide 3 kinase [PI3K] inhibitors), inhibition of phospho-Akt (PI3K inhibitors) and inhibition of retinoblastoma (Rb) phosphorylation (CDK4/6 inhibitors). Additionally, a drug may exhibit effects on normal tissue, which may be associated with efficacy. Examples include epidermal growth factor receptor inhibitors and skin rash (associated with a higher rate of tumor response) and aromatase inhibitor–induced arthralgias, associated with lower recurrence rates in the adjuvant treatment of estrogen receptor–positive breast cancer.

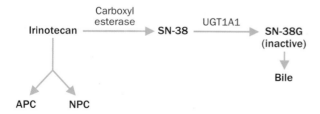

Fig. 3-1 Metabolic pathway of irinotecan, a prodrug that is activated by carboxylesterase to the active metabolite SN-38.

SN-38 is glucuronidated by uridine diphosphate glucuronosyltransferase 1A1 (UGT1A1), forming the inactive metabolite SN-38 glucuronide (SN-38G), which is eliminated by the bile.

Abbreviations: APC, aminopentanecarboxylic acid; NPC, 7-ethyl-20-(4-amino-1-piperidino) carbonyloxycamptothecine.

Reprinted with permission from Goetz MP, Ames MM, Weinshilboum RM. Primer on Medical Genomics: Part XII : Pharmacogenomics—General Principles with Cancer as a Model. Mayo Clin Proc 2004; 79(3):376-384.

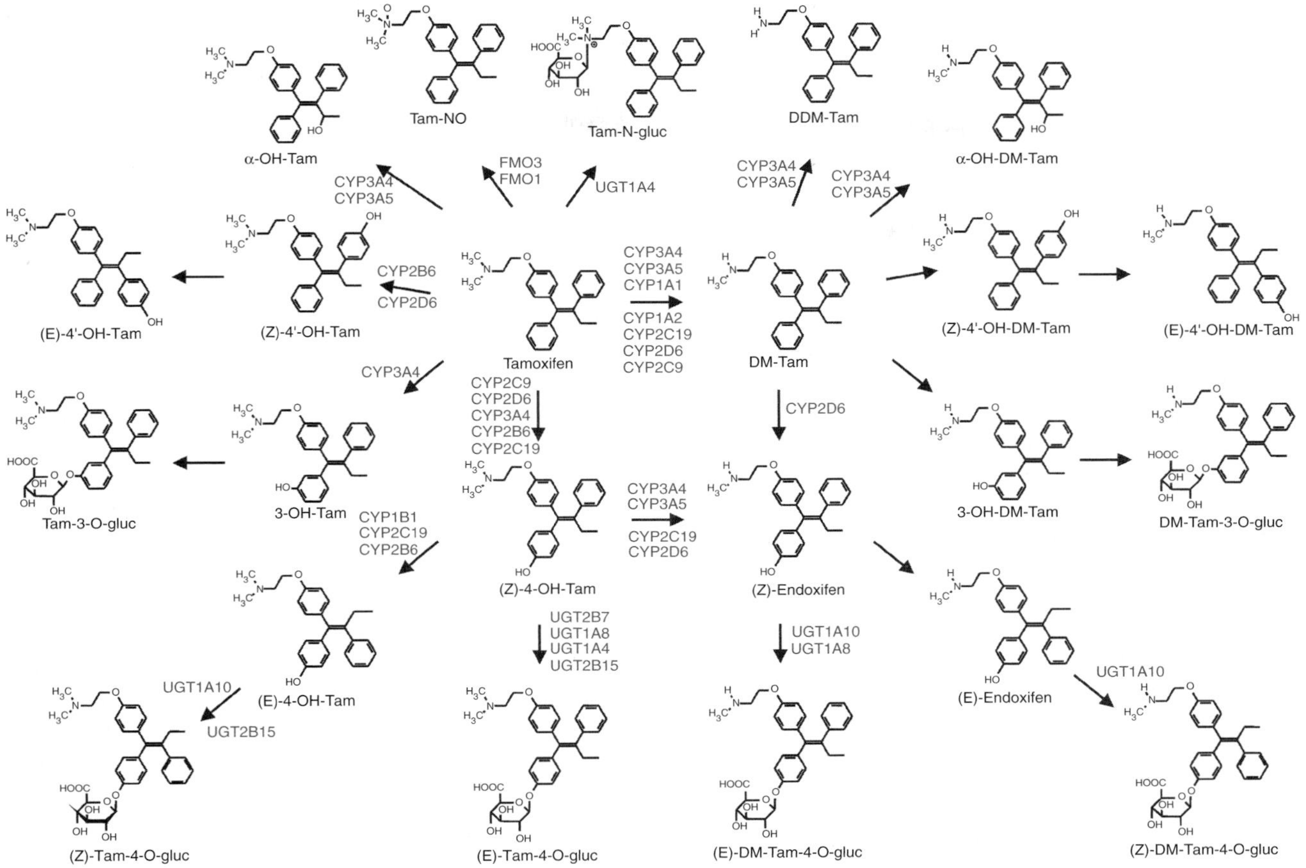

Fig. 3-2 Metabolism of tamoxifen.

Reprinted by permission from Macmillan Publishers Ltd: Clinical Pharmacology & Therapeutics, 89(5):708-17, copyright (2011).

BIOLOGIC AGENTS AND PREDICTIVE BIOMARKERS

There are hundreds of novel biologic agents that are in development for the treatment of cancer. Many of these agents bind a particular receptor or protein within a tumor. Therefore, it would be expected that the expression of the target is critical when applying such an agent. Examples include HER2-targeting drugs such as lapatinib, trastuzumab, trastuzumab emtansine, pertuzumab, and lapatinib, which target the *HER2* oncogene as well as other critical members of the EGFR system (*HER1* and *HER3*). In the metastatic setting, expression or amplification of the HER2 receptor is critical for the activity of HER2-targeting drugs.[36] More recently, the FDA approved biologic agents along with a companion biomarker (vemurafenib and the BRAF V600 Mutation Test).

DRUG DEVELOPMENT: CLINICAL TRIAL DESIGN

The goals of clinical research are to expand knowledge about new anticancer agents through the conduct of well-designed clinical trials, to rapidly gain approval by regulatory bodies, and to obtain adequate clinical information for safe and effective drug delivery. The medical literature is focused on clinical research and clinical trial design, which makes the comprehension of trial design critical for practicing physicians (see Chapter 5: Clinical Trials and Biostatistics).

NONCLINICAL DRUG TESTING

New compounds are discovered primarily by two means. First, there is rational design of new therapeutic agents. When a target is known, drugs can be tailored to fit the target. Second, compounds are discovered as a result of high-throughput screening, in which multiple compounds with unknown activity are tested against a series of cancer cell lines. Those with the best activity are selected for further development. From either source, new agents with promise are tested in vitro to determine whether the drug can kill cancer cells. If successful, in vivo testing is performed to determine whether the drug kills cancer cells with acceptable toxicity to the host organism. During in vivo testing, the schedule and route of administration are investigated. Subsequently, drugs are formulated for a specific route of administration (e.g., oral or intravenous), and the administration schedule is again optimized (e.g., daily, weekly, or via infusion). Although schedules often are based on expected toxicities, mechanisms of action, and animal studies, patient and physician convenience is also a priority.

If the agent yields positive results in nonclinical testing, clinical trials are performed. Based on toxicology studies involving animals, a starting dose is determined for phase I clinical trials using one of two standard methods. The more common method is to take one-tenth of the lethal dose that kills 10% of the most sensitive animal species. An alternative strategy is to use one-third of the toxic dose-low (defined as the lowest dose of a substance at which any toxic effect is produced). Once the phase I dose has been selected and appropriate regulatory measures have been met, phase I clinical trials are then performed.

PHASE I TRIALS

The primary goal of a phase I clinical trial using classic cytotoxic chemotherapy has been to determine the maximum tolerated dose, the highest dose of a drug or treatment that does not cause unacceptable side effects. However, the maximum tolerated dose may not be the optimal dose, especially for those drugs that target a specific receptor or growth factor pathway. Instead, an important focus is to additionally determine a dose that modifies or alters the intended target, resulting in a measurable effect that may occur at doses below the maximum tolerated dose. Secondary goals are to determine the optimal administration schedule, the toxicity profile of the agent, and the pharmacokinetics and pharmacodynamics, as discussed previously, as well as to observe for any clinical activity. Typically, patients with cancer who enter phase I clinical trials have advanced cancer and their disease has not responded to standard therapy. To be eligible, patients must have a good performance status and relatively normal end-organ function so that adequate pharmacology can be determined.

Classic phase I design for cytotoxic chemotherapy agents has been developed largely empirically. In the classic design, three patients are treated per dose level. The first cohort is treated at a starting dose that is considered to be safe based on extrapolation from animal toxicologic data, and the subsequent cohorts are treated at increasing dose levels that have been fixed in advance. Cohorts of three patients are expanded if severe (grade 3 or 4) toxicities occur. Pharmacokinetic measurements are typically obtained for all patients, as are toxicity and tumor assessments. Historically, dose escalation using this trial design typically followed a modified Fibonacci sequence in which the dose increments become smaller as the dose increases (e.g., the dose first increases by 100% of the preceding dose, and thereafter by 67%, 50%, 40%, and 30% to 35% of the preceding doses).

In newer trial designs, fewer patients are treated at low, theoretically inactive, doses. One popular trial design is the accelerated titration design that typically employs "one patient per dose level" and in which drug doses are doubled until drug-related grade 2 (or greater) toxicity is seen. After this, the design reverts back to the classic "cohort of three" design. The purpose of this approach is to rapidly escalate and reduce the number of patients treated with non-efficacious doses. One negative aspect of this design is the limited pharmacokinetic and pharmacodynamic opportunities with only one patient per dose level.

In another design, dose assignment is pharmacokinetically driven. This design is based on the immediate readout of the pharmacokinetics in an individual, and subsequent doses are chosen based on what was found in preceding patients.

Typically, phase I clinical trials have been performed for patients with multiple tumor types; however, these trials may focus on a single tumor or a particular group of tumors known to express a particular receptor or mutation. A newer focus in phase I trials is to "query" the metastatic tumor for important mutations in genes and gene pathways that "activate" oncogenic pathways, with the goal of selecting the right agent. One example includes mutations in the p110-alpha subunit of PI3K, called *PIK3CA*, responsible for activation of the PI3K/AKT/mammalian target of rapamycin (mTOR) pathway, which can cause neoplastic transformation and promote cancer progression. A report demonstrated that, in a phase I population of patients, *PIK3CA* mutations were detected in 18% of tested patients and patients with *PIK3CA* mutations treated with PI3K/AKT/mTOR inhibitors demonstrated a higher response rate than patients without mutations.[37]

With agents that are not expected to be excessively toxic or when clinical effects are expected before toxic effects are likely to develop, there are other designs that can be used. The phase 0 design is one example in which a small number of patients are treated with the goal of determining early on whether a given drug will affect its intended target.

Phase I clinical trials involving combination agents have the added emphasis of evaluating the interaction between the two agents. This is particularly important when there might be a pharmacologic interaction resulting in a substantial change in the toxicity profile. Phase Ib clinical trials are dose-escalation trials in which some measure of clinical outcome is included.

Although investigators are discouraged from making definitive decisions regarding the efficacy of a given cancer drug tested in a phase I study, observed tumor activity in the phase I setting is usually the impetus for studying the drug in subsequent phase II studies.

PHASE II TRIALS

The primary goal of phase II clinical trials is to better determine the preliminary efficacy and toxicity of an agent. Although traditional phase II trials have used a single-arm design, researchers are increasingly utilizing randomized trial designs, which allow for preliminary comparisons of efficacy and toxicity. Typically, a fixed dose and schedule of the therapy are selected, and patients have only one tumor type and have similar characteristics, including similar exposure to previous therapies.

The choice of tumor type is based on preclinical and early clinical research, as well as the molecular biology of the mechanism of the agent's action. Many studies involve patients who have untreated metastatic cancer; however, some studies involve patients who have highly refractory tumors to quickly evaluate efficacy and to obtain regulatory approval. Phase II clinical research is typically the standard point at which decisions are made about the subsequent development of a given compound. If minimal or no clinical activity is observed or there is excessive or unmanageable toxicity in phase II studies, the development of the drug is usually not continued.

Although the classic statistical design for a phase II single-arm trial relied on drug response (complete or partial), newer targeted therapies are often cytostatic, and, therefore, time-to-disease-progression endpoints are now more commonly employed. Additionally, randomized phase II trials are sometimes performed to establish proof of efficacy of a biologic agent. The randomized phase II discontinuation design was used to test the drug sorafenib, contributing to the approval of sorafenib for the treatment of renal cell carcinoma. In this design, after a 12-week run-in period, patients with minimal tumor shrinkage (less than 25%) were randomly assigned to sorafenib or placebo for an additional 12 weeks; patients with 25% or less tumor shrinkage continued with the drug, while patients with 25% or more tumor growth discontinued treatment.[38,39] The study effectively demonstrated that sorafenib significantly prolonged progression-free survival compared with placebo.

PHASE III TRIALS

The goal of phase III clinical research is either to gain approval of a new agent by a regulatory body or to replace the current standard of care. These trials are typically large, ranging from as few as 300 patients to as many as several thousand patients. By definition, these trials are randomized clinical studies. The design and size of each trial hinges specifically on the selected endpoints. The gold-standard endpoint is survival, recognized by all regulatory agencies. However, survival endpoints may not be optimal for all cancers, especially those where multiple active agents are available to patients after the patient completes the clinical trial. For breast and colorectal cancers, the FDA now recognizes disease-free survival, defined as the time to the first event, where an event is as follows: relapse, a second primary cancer, or death. Additionally, response rate, time to disease progression, quality of life, and other nontraditional endpoints have been incorporated into phase III clinical trial designs and have provided support to the approval process of many new agents in oncology.

NEW MEDICINES AND NOVEL MECHANISMS OF ACTION

A growing understanding of the molecular, genetic, and biochemical changes that occur during the processes of carcinogenesis, progression, and metastasis has shifted oncology drug development away from traditional chemotherapeutic agents that target DNA, toward therapeutics that act on specific molecular targets that drive the growth of the cancer. These advances in drug development include drugs that target signal transduction (the HER receptor family, Ras, Raf, PI3K, and MEK kinases); oncogenic proteins, such as BCR/ABL cell-cycle regulating proteins (the cyclins, the cyclin-dependent kinases, and inhibitors of cyclin-dependent kinases); and proteins involved in the tumor angiogenesis, such as endothelial growth factor receptors. Although the scope of discovery is not possible to address here, there are several areas worth reviewing.

Tyrosine kinases, pathways controlling apoptosis, and cell cycling represent important cancer-specific targets and many of the genes involved in these pathways may exhibit activating oncogenic mutations that are potentially "druggable" (see Chapter 2: Molecular Biology). There are many agents that target these pathways and that are now approved for clinical use, including drugs that target the EGFR and its downstream pathways, e.g., trastuzumab and lapatinib (HER2-positive breast cancer) and erlotinib (*EGFR*-mutant lung cancers). Angiogenesis is an important target for many new cancer drugs, driven by the proof of principle that drug-induced inhibition of new blood vessel growth can halt the growth, survival, and metastatic spread of cancer. Bevacizumab, a vascular endothelial growth factor antagonist, prolongs the time to disease progression when administered with standard cytotoxic chemotherapies in colon, breast, lung, and ovarian cancers. However, its use has not led to improvements in overall survival in many tumor types, including breast. Additionally, the multityrosine kinase inhibitors sunitinib and sorafenib (which inhibit vascular endothelial growth factor receptor tyrosine kinases) have demonstrated significant antitumor activity in renal cell carcinoma, leading to FDA approval for the treatment of metastatic disease.

Immunotherapy is a third area in which important research is taking place (see Chapter 4: Biologic Therapy). Clinicians have known for many years that using nonspecific enhancers of the immune system, such as interleukin-2 (aldesleukin) and interferon, can generate immune responses that lead to clinical responses for patients with kidney cancer or melanoma. More recently, there has been increased interest in the development of immune-based therapy for more common solid tumors, such as cancers of the breast, lung, and gastrointestinal tract. Although no vaccine or immune therapy has been approved for clinical use for these cancers in the United States, many agents in this category are in phase II and early phase III clinical trials; it is hoped that, in time, these agents will change the practice of oncology.

KEY POINT

- Substantial gains have been realized in the development of drugs for novel targeted therapies, including (but not limited to) angiogenesis, signal transduction growth pathways, and immune stimulation.

References

1. DeVita VT, Lawrence TS, Rosenberg SA. *DeVita, Hellman, and Rosenberg's cancer: Principles and Practice of Oncology. 9th ed.* Philadelphia, PA: Lippincott Williams & Wilkins; 2011.

2. Li J, Gwilt P. The effect of malignant effusions on methotrexate disposition. *Cancer Chemother Pharmacol.* 2002;50:373-382. PMID: 12439595.

3. Cockcroft DW, Gault MH. Prediction of creatinine clearance from serum creatinine. *Nephron.* 1976;16:31-41. PMID: 1244564.

4. Gault MH, Longerich LL, Harnett JD, et al. Predicting glomerular function from adjusted serum creatinine. *Nephron.* 1992;62:249-256. PMID: 1436333.

5. Jelliffe RW. Estimation of creatinine clearance when urine cannot be collected. *Lancet.* 1971;1:975-976. PMID: 4102307.

6. Levey AS, Bosch JP, Lewis JB, et al. A more accurate method to estimate glomerular filtration rate from serum creatinine: a new prediction equation. Modification of Diet in Renal Disease Study Group. *Ann Intern Med.* 1999;130:461-470. PMID: 10075613.

7. Widemann BC, Schwartz S, Jayaprakash N, et al. Efficacy of glucarpidase (carboxypeptidase g2) in patients with acute kidney injury after high-dose methotrexate therapy. *Pharmacotherapy.* 2014;34:427-439. Epub 2013 Oct 17. PMID: 24132809.

8. Fan C, Oh DS, Wessels L, et al. Concordance among gene-expression-based predictors for breast cancer. *N Engl J Med.* 2006;355:560-569. PMID: 16899776.

9. Paik S, Tang G, Shak S, et al. Gene expression and benefit of chemotherapy in women with node-negative, estrogen receptor-positive breast cancer. *J Clin Oncol.* 2006;24:3726-3734. PMID: 16720680.

10. Karapetis CS, Khambata-Ford S, Jonker DJ, et al. K-ras mutations and benefit from cetuximab in advanced colorectal cancer. *N Engl J Med.* 2008;359:1757-1765. PMID: 18946061.

11. Gurney H. Dose calculation of anticancer drugs: a review of the current practice and introduction of an alternative. *J Clin Oncol.* 1996;14:2590-2611. PMID: 8823340.

12. Baker SD, Verweij J, Rowinsky EK, et al. Role of body surface area in dosing of investigational anticancer agents in adults, 1991-2001. *J Natl Cancer Inst.* 2002;94:1883-1888. PMID: 12488482.

13. Lennard L. The clinical pharmacology of 6-mercaptopurine. *Eur J Clin Pharmacol.* 1992;43:329-339. PMID: 1451710.

14. Weinshilboum RM, Sladek SL. Mercaptopurine pharmacogenetics: monogenic inheritance of erythrocyte thiopurine methyltransferase activity. *Am J Hum Genet.* 1980;32:651-662. PMID: 7191632.

15. Woodson LC, Weinshilboum RM. Human kidney thiopurine methyltransferase. Purification and biochemical properties. *Biochem Pharmacol.* 1983;32:819-826. PMID: 6838629.

16. Raftogianis RB, Wood TC, Weinshilboum RM. Human phenol sulfotransferases SULT1A2 and SULT1A1: genetic polymorphisms, allozyme properties, and human liver genotype-phenotype correlations. *Biochem Pharmacol.* 1999;58:605-616. PMID: 10413297.

17. Lennard L, Van Loon JA, Weinshilboum RM. Pharmacogenetics of acute azathioprine toxicity: relationship to thiopurine methyltransferase genetic polymorphism. *Clin Pharmacol Ther.* 1989;46:149-154. PMID: 2758725.

18. Szumlanski C, Otterness D, Her C, et al. Thiopurine methyltransferase pharmacogenetics: human gene cloning and characterization of a common polymorphism. *DNA Cell Biol.* 1996;15:17-30. PMID: 8561894.

19. Tai HL, Krynetski EY, Schuetz EG, et al. Enhanced proteolysis of thiopurine S-methyltransferase (TPMT) encoded by mutant alleles in humans (TPMT*3A, TPMT*2): mechanisms for the genetic polymorphism of TPMT activity. *Proc Natl Acad Sci U S A.* 1997;94:6444-6449. PMID: 9177237.

20. Kaneda N, Nagata H, Furuta T, et al. Metabolism and pharmacokinetics of the camptothecin analogue CPT-11 in the mouse. *Cancer Res.* 1990;50:1715-1720. PMID: 2306725.

21. Kawato Y, Aonuma M, Hirota Y, et al. Intracellular roles of SN-38, a metabolite of the camptothecin derivative CPT-11, in the antitumor effect of CPT-11. *Cancer Res.* 1991;51:4187-4191. PMID: 1651156.

22. Rivory LP, Riou JF, Haaz MC, et al. Identification and properties of a major plasma metabolite of irinotecan (CPT-11) isolated from the plasma of patients. *Cancer Res.* 1996;56:3689-3694. PMID: 8706009.

23. Iyer L, King CD, Whitington PF, et al. Genetic predisposition to the metabolism of irinotecan (CPT-11). Role of uridine diphosphate glucuronosyltransferase isoform 1A1 in the glucuronidation of its active metabolite (SN-38) in human liver microsomes. *J Clin Invest.* 1998;101:847-854. PMID: 9466980.

24. Beutler E, Gelbart T, Demina A. Racial variability in the UDP-glucuronosyltransferase 1 (UGT1A1) promoter: a balanced polymorphism for regulation of bilirubin metabolism? *Proc Natl Acad Sci U S A.* 1998;95:8170-8174. PMID: 9653159.

25. Bosma PJ, Chowdhury JR, Bakker C, et al. The genetic basis of the reduced expression of bilirubin UDP-glucuronosyltransferase 1 in Gilbert's syndrome. *N Engl J Med.* 1995;333:1171-1175. PMID: 7565971.

26. Monaghan G, Ryan M, Seddon R, et al. Genetic variation in bilirubin UPD-glucuronosyltransferase gene promoter and Gilbert's syndrome. *Lancet.* 1996;347:578-581. PMID: 8596320.

27. Innocenti F, Undevia SD, Iyer L, et al. Genetic variants in the UDP-glucuronosyltransferase 1A1 gene predict the risk of severe neutropenia of irinotecan. *J Clin Oncol.* 2004;22:1382-1388. PMID:15007088.

28. Toffoli G, Cecchin E, Gasparini G, et al. Genotype-driven phase I study of irinotecan administered in combination with fluorouracil/leucovorin in patients with metastatic colorectal cancer. *J Clin Oncol.* 2010;28:866-871. PMID: 20038727.

29. Stearns V, Johnson MD, Rae JM, et al. Active tamoxifen metabolite plasma concentrations after coadministration of tamoxifen and the selective serotonin reuptake inhibitor paroxetine. *J Natl Cancer Inst.* 2003;95:1758-1764. PMID: 14652237.

30. Borges S, Desta Z, Li L, et al. Quantitative effect of CYP2D6 genotype and inhibitors on tamoxifen metabolism: implication for optimization of breast cancer treatment. *Clin Pharmacol Ther.* 2006;80:61-74. PMID: 16815318.

31. Mürdter TE, Schroth W, Bacchus-Gerybadze L, et al. Activity levels of tamoxifen metabolites at the estrogen receptor and the impact of genetic polymorphisms of phase I and II enzymes on their concentration levels in plasma. *Clin Pharmacol Ther.* 2011;89:708-717. PMID: 21451508.

32. Goetz MP, Suman VJ, Hoskin TL, et al. CYP2D6 metabolism and patient outcome in the Austrian Breast and Colorectal Cancer Study Group trial (ABCSG) 8. *Clin Cancer Res.* 2013;19:500-507. PMID: 23213055.

33. Rae JM, Drury S, Hayes DF, et al. CYP2D6 and UGT2B7 genotype and risk of recurrence in tamoxifen-treated breast cancer patients. *J Natl Cancer Inst.* 2012;104:452-460. PMID: 22395643.

34. Regan MM, Leyland-Jones B, Bouzyk M, et al. CYP2D6 genotype and tamoxifen response in postmenopausal women with endocrine-responsive breast cancer: the breast international group 1-98 trial. *J Natl Cancer Inst.* 2012;104:441-451. PMID: 22395644.

35. Province MA, Goetz MP, Brauch H, et al. CYP2D6 genotype and adjuvant tamoxifen: meta-analysis of heterogeneous study populations. *Clin Pharmacol Ther.* 2014;95:216-227. Epub 2013 Sep 23. PMID: 24060820.

36. Seidman AD, Berry D, Cirrincione C, et al. Randomized phase III trial of weekly compared with every-3-weeks paclitaxel for metastatic breast cancer, with trastuzumab for all HER-2 overexpressors and random assignment to trastuzumab or not in HER-2 nonoverexpressors: final results of Cancer and Leukemia Group B protocol 9840. *J Clin Oncol.* 2008;26:1642-1649. PMID: 18375893.

37. Janku F, Wheler JJ, Westin SN, et al. PI3K/AKT/mTOR inhibitors in patients with breast and gynecologic malignancies harboring PIK3CA mutations. *J Clin Oncol.* 2012;30:777-782. PMID: 22271473.

38. Karrison TG, Maitland ML, Stadler WM, et al. Design of phase II cancer trials using a continuous endpoint of change in tumor size: application to a study of sorafenib and erlotinib in non small-cell lung cancer. *J Natl Cancer Inst.* 2007;99:1455-1461. PMID: 17895472.

39. Ratain MJ, Eisen T, Stadler WM, et al. Phase II placebo-controlled randomized discontinuation trial of sorafenib in patients with metastatic renal cell carcinoma. *J Clin Oncol.* 2006;24:2505-2512. PMID: 16636341.

4

PRINCIPLES OF BIOLOGIC THERAPY

Pierre L. Triozzi, MD

Updates from 2012

▶ The number of biologic agents approved for use in the treatment of cancer continues to increase. Another HER2 monoclonal antibody, pertuzumab, has been approved. This approval is unique in that it includes use in the neoadjuvant setting for breast cancer and in combination with the previously approved HER2 antibody trastuzumab (Gianni L, *Lancet Oncol* 2012).

▶ Novel monoclonal antibody constructs are being developed. Obinutuzumab, a CD20 monoclonal antibody that has been glycoengineered to directly mediate cell death and enhance antibody-dependent cellular cytotoxicity, has been approved for use in combination with chlorambucil for chronic lymphocytic leukemia (Goede V, *N Engl J Med* 2014).

▶ Ramucirumab, a monoclonal antibody that binds to vascular endothelial growth factor receptor-2, has been approved for gastric or gastroesophageal junction adenocarcinoma, and ado-trastuzumab emtansine, a HER2 antibody–cytotoxic drug conjugate, has been approved for breast cancer (Fuchs C, *Lancet* 2014; Verma S, *N Engl J Med* 2012).

▶ Immunotherapy has been the focus of much activity. Immune checkpoint mechanisms are increasingly being addressed therapeutically in a variety of cancers (Wolchok J, *N Engl J Med* 2013).

Biologic therapy, whether for neoplastic, infectious, immunologic, or other diseases, refers to the use of biologic products or substances that are made by living organisms, such as cytokines, antibodies, and cells. In the setting of cancer, these substances are administered primarily to generate or to restore host immune responses to tumors. The distinctions between biologic therapy and chemotherapy are, to some extent, being effaced. Biologic agents have been exploited to mediate nonimmunologic antitumor activities. Several nonbiologic agents are used to promote antitumor immune response, including cytotoxic and targeted chemotherapeutics. Nonetheless, biologics are characterized by unique effects. Since the introduction of interferons (IFNs) more than 25 years ago, progress in biologic therapy for cancer has been rapid. Several cytokines have been approved by the U.S. Food and Drug Administration (FDA), and an increasing number of monoclonal antibodies are being used clinically. Cellular therapy is practiced in the setting of hematopoietic stem cell transplantation (HSCT), and a cell-based vaccine approach has also been approved. This chapter will focus on the immunology, pharmacology, and toxicology, as well as the spectrum of antitumor activity, of biologic therapy in clinical use. More detailed review of the clinical application of specific agents is provided in site-specific chapters.

IMMUNE RESPONSE

The immune system protects against microbial pathogens while simultaneously maintaining tolerance to "self." This innate response forms the first line of defense. Innate immune cells (e.g., macrophages, dendritic cells, and natural killer [NK] cells) express receptors (e.g., toll-like receptors, [TLR]) with which they recognize conserved molecular patterns, such as unmethylated CpG DNA motifs, found on microbes but not on human tissues. Stimulation through these receptors triggers a cascade of events that include the production of cytokines, activation of cellular cytotoxicity, increase in nitric oxide synthesis, and activation of the complement system. These events promote the elimination or lysis of microbial pathogens, as well as promote recruitment and activation of other immune cells.

Microbial/cellular fragments produced by the destruction affected by innate response are taken up by antigen-presenting cells (e.g., macrophages, dendritic cells, and B cells), which process the fragments and present these to generate "adaptive" immune effectors, namely, T cells and antibody-producing B cells. These cells express highly diverse antigen-specific receptors—the T-cell antigen receptors (TCR) and the B-cell antigen receptors (BCR)—generated by random rearrangement of the TCR and immunoglobulin (Ig) gene segments, respectively. The adaptive response allows generation of extremely diverse T and B cell repertoires that, compared with the innate response, provides a more specific, but also broader and more flexible, repertoire of responses that includes "memory."

Immune responses are highly regulated. The generation of a productive response requires that a number of immunologic "checkpoints" be passed. A key step in the generation of adaptive immunity is the presentation of antigens by antigen-presenting cells to T helper cells, which promote cellular effectors (e.g., cytolytic T lymphocytes [CTL]) or humoral effectors (e.g., antibodies) through the production of specific cytokines. Both stimulatory and inhibitory signals are generated. Regulatory cells and cytokines also serve to suppress the immune response to maintain tolerance to self and limit immune-mediated damage to normal tissues.

KEY POINTS

- Cells of both the antigen-nonspecific innate and antigen-specific adaptive response have been implicated in antitumor immunity.
- Specific immunity to tumors requires uptake of tumor antigens by antigen-presenting cells and presentation to T helper cells, which coordinate the generation of cellular and/or humoral responses.
- Immune responses are highly regulated. The generation of a productive response requires that a number of immunologic checkpoints be passed.

IMMUNE CELLS

A wide variety of hematologic (and nonhematologic) cells are important in innate and adaptive immunity. The following are considered to play prominent roles in antitumor immune responses.

T Cells

T cells play a central role in the adaptive immune responses as effectors and as regulators. The signaling complex of T cells includes the TCR dimer, the accessory molecules CD4 or CD8, and the CD3 signal transduction module. Unlike antibodies, which can react to intact proteins, T cells, through the TCR, only react to peptide fragments of antigens that are noncovalently complexed with major histocompatibility complex (MHC) molecules, which are integral membrane glycoproteins. There are two types of MHC molecules. Class I MHC (e.g., human leukocyte antigen type A2 [HLA-A2]) is expressed on all cell types and serves as the antigen-presenting molecule for CD8+ T cells. Class II MHC (e.g., HLA-DR) is recognized by CD4+ T cells and is present primarily on antigen-presenting cells but also can be present on other cells, including tumor cells. Polymorphisms within MHC molecules determine whether a peptide fragment will complex with the MHC molecule and, thus, whether a T cell from an individual will respond to a specific epitope of an antigen, resulting in the phenomenon referred to as MHC restriction. Whether T cells are activated during their "priming phase" not only requires the presentation of the antigen within the context of an MHC molecule and stimulation through the CD3 module, but also "costimulatory" signals. Activation is regulated by "co-inhibitory" signals. The CD28 family of receptors, which include the stimulatory receptor CD28 and the inhibitory receptors CTL antigen-4 (CTLA-4) and programmed death 1 (PD-1), interacting with the B7 family of ligands, which include B7-1, B7-2, programmed death ligands 1 (PD-L1, B7-H1), and 2 (PD-L2; B7-DC), are of central importance. Several other receptor-ligand interactions can be involved. Other molecules, such as adhesion molecules, also are required for effective activation. In part, the role of these checkpoints is to suppress unwanted and harmful self-directed immune activities (Fig. 4-1).

Cytolytic T Lymphocytes

CTL are primarily CD8+ T cells and, thus, recognize antigens presented within the context of MHC class I. Two mechanisms are involved in their cytolytic effector activity. The predominant mechanism is granule exocytosis and the release of perforin and granzymes. The second mechanism is mediated by the death activator, Fas ligand, which is expressed on the cell surface of CTL. Both mechanisms cause cells to undergo apoptosis (programmed cell death; Fig. 4-2). When appropriately activated, these cells also produce cytokines, such as IFN-gamma (IFN-γ), which also can mediate antitumor effects. CTL can move to another cell and, by reorienting their granules to another region of contact, destroy it. In this manner, CTL can kill many tumor cells, resulting in a very robust, as well as a very specific, response that is considered to play a central role in immune-mediated tumor rejection. Tumor-infiltrating

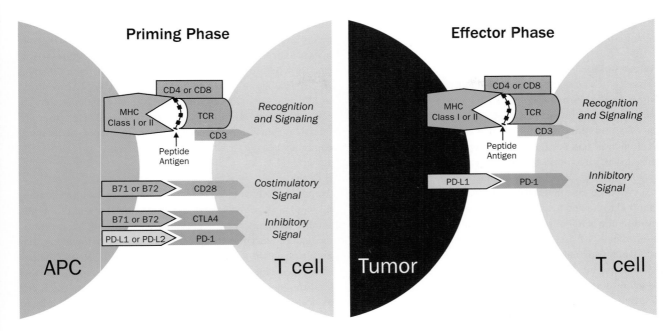

Fig. 4-1   Regulation of T-cell priming and effector function.

During the priming phase of T-cell activation, antigens are presented to the T-cell receptor (TCR) as peptide fragments within major histocompatibility complex (MHC) molecules on antigen-presenting cells (APC). The primary costimulatory signal is delivered through the CD28 receptor on the T cell after engagement of its ligands, B7-1 or B7-2, on the APCs. Fully effective engagement is also dependent upon the interaction of several other molecules, such as adhesion molecules (not shown). Failure of the costimulatory B7/CD28 complex to be engaged results in either a non-activating T-cell event and/or anergy. Engagement of the cytolytic T lymphocytes antigen (CTLA)-4 receptor (CD152) on the T cell by the same B7-1 or B7-2 ligands results in inhibition of the response. Engagement of the programmed death (PD)-1 receptor with one of its two ligands, PD-L1 and PD-L2, on APCs also results in inhibition of the response. PD-L1 is also expressed by tumors. During the effector phase, engagement of PD-1 on the activated T cell by PD-L1 on the tumor results in inhibition of T-cell function.

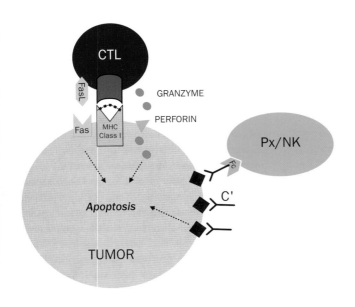

Fig. 4-2   Mechanisms of cell killing by cytolytic T lymphocytes and antibody.

After attaching to the major histocompatibility complex (MHC)-peptide complex, cytolytic T lymphocytes (CTL) discharge cytoplasmic granules containing perforin and granzymes by exocytosis. Perforin molecules insert themselves into the plasma membrane of target cells, which enables granzymes to enter the cell. Granzymes are serine proteases that, once inside the cell, activate caspases that cause the cells to undergo apoptosis. When CTL bind to their target, they also upregulate Fas ligand (FasL) on their surface, which binds with the Fas receptor on the surface of the target cell leading to its death, also by apoptosis. Antibody recognizes antigen in its native conformation. After binding, a complement reactive site on the antibody is activated that sets into motion a cascade of reactions, including the activation of many molecules of the complement system, which in turn activate increasing amounts of enzymes resulting in complement-mediated cytotoxicity (CMC). A product of the complement cascade also strongly activates phagocytosis by macrophages and neutrophils. These phagocytes (Px) and also natural killer (NK) cells bind their Fc receptor (CD16) to the antibody and destroy the antibody-bound cell (antibody-dependent cellular mechanisms). Antibody-recognizing cell surface molecules that regulate cell signaling/growth can directly elicit apoptosis.

Abbreviations: C', complement.

CD8+ lymphocytes can be associated with improved clinical outcome.[1]

T Helper Cells

T helper cells secrete cytokines that regulate all immune cells. They are essential in generating CTL, regulating B-cell antibody production, and activating phagocytes. Most T helper cells express CD4 and, thus, recognize antigens expressed by class II MHC. Depending on the nature of the peptide and the activation status of the antigen-presenting cells, either a cellular immune response mediated by CTL and by macrophages, referred to as a Th1 response, or a humoral immune response mediated by an antibody, referred to as a Th2 response (which also includes activation of eosinophils), is promoted. Predominant cytokines produced in a Th1-associated response are IFN-γ and interleukin-2 (IL-2). Predominant cytokines produced in a Th2-associated response are IL-4 and IL-5. The requirement for CD4+ T cells in antitumor response has been largely attributed to providing help to naive CD8+ T cells, leading to their differentiation and activation into tumor-specific CTL. Cytokines produced by T helper cells also may mediate antitumor effects by activating macrophages and NK cells. T helper cytokines (e.g., IFN-γ) also may directly suppress tumor growth.

Regulatory T Cells

Regulatory T cells (Treg) are subsets of T lymphocytes capable of discriminating self-antigens from nonself-antigens. In healthy individuals, Treg cells serve as a checkpoint and maintain tolerance by suppressing expansion of effector cells directed against self-antigen. Treg cells that express CD4, CD25, and FOXP3 (a forkhead family transcriptional regulator) play a central role in maintaining immune self-tolerance. The mechanism of suppression of self-reactive lymphocytes is not clear, but does appear to involve direct cell-cell contact and the production of IL-10 and of transforming growth factor-beta (TGF-ß). Given that many tumor-associated antigens are normal self-constituents, Treg cells that are CD4+, CD25+, FOXP3+ engage in the maintenance of self-tolerance and may impede tumor-reactive T cells. Their role in cancer, however, is not established. The prognostic significance of intratumoral Treg cells is unclear. In some cancers, such as breast, there are data that intratumoral Treg cells confer a poorer prognosis;[2] in colorectal cancer (CRC), a better prognosis.[3]

Natural Killer Cells

NK cells are a relatively small population (less than 10%) of circulating lymphocytes and are distinct from T and B cells. They are part of the innate response. Although their cytotoxic mechanisms are similar to those of CTL, NK cells do not require recognition of MHC molecules and, thus, killing by NK cells is designated non–MHC-restricted lysis. In fact, class I MHC molecules send a negative regulatory signal through receptors on the NK cells (killer inhibitory receptors [KIR]) that inhibit their lytic function. Conversely, loss of class I MHC on tumor cells may result in NK cell killing of cells that could otherwise escape T cell recognition. Also in contrast to CTL, NK cells express Fc receptors and thus can mediate antibody-dependent cellular cytotoxicity (ADCC) mechanisms. When activated, NK cells also produce IFN-γ. Although NK cells do not require activation for lytic activity, the stimulation of NK cells with IFNs and IL-2 markedly enhances their antitumor activity. In contrast to CTL, which can kill multiple cells, there is evidence that NK cells must rearm themselves in response to IL-2 before they are effective against new targets. Furthermore, there is no memory component to the response.

B Cells

Antibody-producing B cells are involved in adaptive immunity and also serve as antigen-presenting cells. The BCR binds soluble antigens, which are then internalized by receptor-mediated endocytosis and processed into peptide fragments that are displayed at the cell surface within class II MHC. T helper cells specific for this structure (i.e., with a complementary TCR) bind the B cell and secrete cytokines that stimulate the B cell to proliferate into cells with identical BCR, and ultimately to differentiate into plasma cells that secrete antibodies (i.e., the soluble version of the BCR). In contrast to T cells, which recognize only processed peptide antigen, antibodies produced by B cells recognize the intact protein antigen in its native conformation. Antibodies also can recognize polysaccharides and nucleic acids. Antigen-binding specificity is encoded by three complementarity-determining regions, whereas the Fc-region is responsible for binding to serum proteins (e.g., complement) or to cells. Cytotoxicity is mediated by complement-mediated cytotoxicity (CMC) or, for IgG in particular, ADCC mechanisms. Central to CMC is the ability of the antibody to redistribute the target on the cell membrane into large glycolipoprotein microdomains known as lipid rafts. Antibodies also can directly mediate antitumor effects by interacting with cell surface receptors that regulate cell growth (Fig. 4-2). Although cellular immune responses appear to be central in the generation of effective antitumor immunity, there is a substantial body of data to indicate that antibodies also are important. Furthermore, the antitumor effects of antibodies have been validated by the clinical efficacy of monoclonal antibodies specific for tumor-associated molecules.

Dendritic Cells

Dendritic cells are a widely distributed, heterogeneous population of antigen-presenting cells that are derived from bone marrow progenitors and circulate in the blood as immature precursors prior to migration into peripheral tissues. Within different tissues, dendritic cells differentiate and become active in the taking up and processing of antigens. Dendritic cells function at the intersection of the innate and adaptive immune responses. Upon stimulation provided by microbes (through TLR), cytokines, and/or T-cell signals (e.g., CD40 ligand), dendritic cells undergo further maturation and migrate to secondary lymphoid tissues where they present antigen to T cells. The nature of the immune response elicited depends on a variety of factors, including the mode and duration of activation and the cytokine microenvironment. Two distinct lineages have been described in humans. Myeloid dendritic cells (mDC) express the receptor for granulocyte-macrophage colony-stimulating factor (GM-CSF) and other myeloid markers. mDC reside in tissues and are the most efficient antigen-presenting cells, particularly with regard to the primary activation of naive T cells. They stimulate tumor-reactive CTL through an IL-12–dependent mechanism. Plasmacytoid dendritic cells (pDC) lack myeloid cell markers and express the receptor for IL-3 (CD123). They reside in peripheral blood, and following viral encounter, they secrete large amounts of IFN-alfa (IFN-α), a cytokine with immunomodulatory as well as antiviral properties. Their role in antitumor immunity is less clear.

Macrophages

Macrophages, which derive from peripheral blood monocytes, are widely dispersed throughout the body and mediate a variety of functions. Macrophages are specialized phagocytes. Phagocytosis is mediated through surface receptors for complement and other opsonins and through the uptake of particles into phagosomes that then fuse with cytoplasmic lysosomes. Macrophages express Fc receptors for Ig and can mediate antibody-dependent cellular uptake and cytotoxicity mechanisms. Similar to dendritic cells, macrophages function at the intersection of the innate and adaptive immune responses and can process and present particles captured within MHC molecules to activate specific T- and B-cell effector mechanisms. Macrophages also are potent secretory cells. They are major producers of the proangiogenic vascular endothelial growth factor (VEGF). Distinct activation states of macrophages have been described. "M1" macrophages produce high levels of inducible nitric oxide synthase, IL-12, and tumor necrosis factor (TNF), whereas "M2" macrophages produce arginase, IL-10, TGF-ß, and prostaglandin E2. M1 macrophages are potent effector cells that kill tumor cells by nitric oxide and TNF, whereas M2 macrophages limit Th1 immune responses and promote angiogenesis, processes that promote tumor growth. Whereas M2 macrophages are associated with a decrease in survival in patients with cancer, M1 macrophages have been associated with an improved survival.[4,5]

Myeloid-Derived Suppressor Cells

A number of investigations have identified immature myeloid cell populations present in tumors and lymphoid organs, referred to as myeloid-derived suppressor cells (MDSCs), which inhibit T-cell functions and play a role in tumor-associated immune suppression. They have been described in patients with many types of solid tumors.[6-8] Human MDSCs are still poorly defined but have been reported to lack the expression of markers of mature myeloid and lymphoid cells (i.e., lineage negative) and HLA-DR. MDSC do express the common myeloid marker CD33. The precise nature of this regulatory cell population and whether they are precursors of granulocytes, macrophages, or dendritic cells appear to depend on the tumor and tumor-derived factors of the hosts. This highly plastic population suppresses T-cell functions through different molecular pathways, mostly

involving arginase metabolism products, inducible nitric oxide synthase, reactive oxygen species, and/or production of soluble inhibitory factors such as TGF-ß, IL-10, prostaglandin E2, and nitric oxide.

KEY POINTS

- T cells recognize antigen presented to the T-cell antigen receptors as peptide fragments within major histocompatibility complex molecules. T-cell activation not only requires stimulation through the T-cell antigen receptor, but also through immune costimulatory receptors.
- T helper cells promote T helper cell type 1 (Th1)–associated cytolytic T lymphocytes through the production of cytokines, such as interferon-gamma and interleukin (IL)-2, and promote Th2-associated antibody through production of cytokines, such as IL-4 and IL-5.
- Cytolytic T lymphocytes kill tumors by apoptosis through granule exocytosis and Fas-mediated mechanisms.
- B cells produce antibodies that recognize antigens in their native conformation. The two principal ways antibodies can react against tumors are by complement-mediated and antibody-dependent cellular mechanisms.
- Dendritic cells are the most efficient antigen-presenting cells.
- Several lymphoid and myeloid cell populations act to suppress immune responses.

IMMUNE SURVEILLANCE

The existence of cancer immune surveillance—that the innate and adaptive immune system continually recognizes and removes malignant cells that arise during one's life—has been difficult to prove. Immune surveillance has been demonstrated in animal models. Although direct evidence is lacking, several lines of evidence support the view that immune responses can recognize and eliminate human tumors. Individuals with suppressed immune systems, such as organ transplant recipients or patients affected with primary or acquired immunodeficiency disorders, have an increased risk of malignancy. The rare spontaneous regression of cancer has been associated with brisk infiltrations of immune cells, suggesting a role for immune surveillance in cancer control. Brisk lymphocytic infiltration in tumor specimens is an independent positive prognostic factor for some cancers, such as melanoma and ovarian cancer.[9,10] Likewise, the natural occurrence of a humoral immune response to a tumor-associated antigen is associated with a favorable clinical outcome in some cancers, such as breast cancer.[11] Human T cells that accumulate within the mass of a tumor can be shown in some instances to proliferate in response to autologous tumor cells in vitro. Finally, a variety of immunotherapy modalities have produced objective tumor responses in patients. Treatment of patients with melanoma using CTL that have been expanded ex vivo can result in substantial tumor regression. Furthermore, T cells sensitized to peptide fragments of melanoma antigens can induce tumor regressions, as can blocking the negative T-cell regulator CTLA-4 with ipilimumab.[12]

Effective surveillance requires that the tumor express determinants capable of being recognized by the immune system (i.e., tumor antigens). Numerous tumor-associated antigens, such as carcinoembryonic antigen (CEA) and prostate-specific antigen (PSA), have been defined with antibodies and applied in diagnosis and in monitoring response to therapy. Whether these antigens can serve as targets for tumor rejection and for the cellular response that appears to be necessary is not clear. As outlined previously, antigens that are recognized by the T cells differ substantially from those defined by antibodies. To function as a T-cell rejection antigen, the tumor must express the associated peptide determinant in the context of MHC molecules. Failure of antigen processing or binding to MHC molecules or inadequate expression of costimulatory or adhesion molecules may lead to poor immunogenicity. Several types of antigens that can potentially serve as tumor rejection antigens have been identified by a variety of techniques (Table 4-1). Oncofetal, cancer-testis (a group of oncofetal antigens), and differentiation/lineage-specific antigens are expressed by normal adult tissues and, therefore, are not tumor-specific. In contrast to those that are overexpressed and not mutated (e.g., HER2), oncogenes/tumor suppressors that are mutated (e.g., p53) can be considered tumor-specific. Many of these antigens have been targeted in vaccine approaches.

KEY POINTS

- Although direct evidence for immune surveillance of tumors in humans is lacking, several lines of evidence, including clinical responses with pharmacologic modulation of the immune response, support its existence.
- A variety of antigens that can potentially function as tumor rejection antigens have been identified. Most are not tumor-specific.

Table 4-1 Examples of Tumor Antigens

	Example	Associated Malignancies (examples)
Oncofetal	CEA	Colorectal, breast, non-small cell lung cancers
	Beta-hCG	Colorectal, pancreas, non-small cell lung cancers
Cancer-testis	MAGE	Melanoma, lung, bladder, liver cancers
	NY-ESO	Melanoma, lung, bladder, liver cancers
Oncogene/tumor suppressor	HER2	Breast cancer
	p53	Multiple
	RAS	Multiple
	BCR-ABL	Chronic myeloid leukemia
Differentiation/ lineage-specific	Prostate-specific antigen (PSA)	Prostate cancer
	Prostatic acid phosphatase	Prostate cancer
	gp100	Melanoma
	Tyrosinase	Melanoma
	MART/Melan-A	Melanoma
	Ig (idiotype)	B-cell malignancies
Aberrantly glycosylated molecules	MUC1 (mucin)	Pancreas, breast cancers
	GM2 (ganglioside)	Melanoma, neuroblastoma
	GD2 (ganglioside)	Melanoma, neuroblastoma
Viral	E6, E7 (HPV)	Cervix cancer
	EBNA (Epstein-Barr virus)	Burkitt lymphoma, nasopharyngeal carcinoma

IMMUNE ESCAPE

Although immune checkpoints are a necessary function, tumors can co-opt these mechanisms and "escape" immune responses. Because most of the tumor antigens identified are nonmutated self-antigens, a high degree of immunologic tolerance exists that limits the generation of immune effectors. As noted, Treg cells engaged in the maintenance of self-tolerance may impede tumor-reactive T cells. Tumors are heterogeneous, and the repertoire of tumor antigens on cells of one tumor may be variable, even within the same patient. Downregulation of MHC class I molecules and other

components of the antigen-presentation process can occur. Tumors also do not normally express the ligands recognized by innate immune cells that microbes express (the "danger" hypothesis), nor do they express the costimulatory ligands necessary to stimulate adaptive T cells. Membrane-associated factors expressed by tumor cells also have been identified that directly inhibit T-cell function. These include PD-L1, which engages a co-inhibitory receptor on activated T cells (PD-1). Antibody blockade of PD-L1 and PD-1 has demonstrated therapeutic activity in patients with several types of cancer.[13,14] The expression of Fas ligand by some tumor cells may help to maintain a state of immune privilege by inducing apoptosis of Fas-sensitive T and NK effector cells—the "Fas counterattack." There also is evidence that the expression of anti-apoptotic molecules by the tumor that block perforin or death receptor–dependent cytotoxicity can result in escape despite the expression of the target antigen. In addition, tumor-associated factors, such as tumor-associated mucins, have been shown to reduce binding of antibodies to tumor cell surfaces.

Tumor cells and the surrounding stroma may release a number of suppressive cytokines and other soluble factors, such as prostaglandin E2, that are not conducive to antitumor immunity. Cancer-associated factors have been shown to inhibit the production and stimulatory capacity of dendritic cells.[15] The infiltration of pDCs with T-cell suppressive activities has been implicated in cancer progression.[16] The T-helper cell response also may be skewed toward a Th2 phenotype, which inhibits Th1 response and the cellular immunity that is critical in mediating tumor rejection.[17] TGF-ß is produced not only by host cells but also by tumors, and can inhibit the differentiation of T cells into CTL and T helper cells. By producing cytokines (e.g., GM-CSF), cancers can promote the infiltration of M2-polarized macrophages and MDSCs that can inhibit T-cell function. Down-regulation of the T-cell surface glycoprotein CD3 zeta chain of the TCR complex and impairment of function have been shown for T cells isolated from patients with cancer.[18]

Tumors are characterized by significant molecular instability as well as by clonal heterogeneity. As tumors develop, the immune system places cancer cells under selective pressure; it detects those that are more antigenic and susceptible to immune effectors. The resistant cells escape and, in turn, will proliferate and spread to distant sites. Loss of tumor antigens in humans after immunotherapy has been reported.[19] This phenomenon, called immune editing, has been implicated in the resistance of tumors to immunotherapies, analogous to the selective pressure induced by chemotherapy and the development of drug resistance.

KEY POINTS

- The ability of cancer to evade the immune response is aided by the fact that most tumor antigens are self-proteins, which impede the generation of immunity through toleragenic mechanisms, such as the elaboration of regulatory T cells.
- Cancer evasion of the immune system results not only from immunosuppressive factors secreted by or expressed on the tumor, but also from the ability of the tumor to modulate antigen expression and to develop mechanisms of resistance to immune effectors.

IMMUNE SUBVERSION

Although effective antitumor immunity has been demonstrated in experimental systems and in some patients, immune responses are abundantly present in tumor-bearing hosts that provide no apparent protection to the host and may contribute to the oncogenic process. Not only can tumors escape immune response, they can exploit or subvert the immune response to promote their growth, invasion, and metastasis. Local tumor growth within the stroma is promoted by angiogenesis. Immune cells, including macrophages, T cells, and neutrophils, fully participate in tumor angiogenesis by secreting cytokines, such as IL-1, IL-8, and VEGF, which directly affect endothelial cell functions, including endothelial cell proliferation, migration, and activation. Not only do macrophages produce angiogenic factors, they also produce proteases that degrade the extracellular matrix—matrix metalloproteinases. Hence, macrophages can promote tumor cell invasion and metastasis. Accumulating data show that many tumor cells express chemokine receptors and respond to chemokine gradients in vitro. Experimental studies in vivo also have indicated that certain chemokines can serve as tissue-specific attractant molecules for tumor cells, promoting tumor-cell migration/metastasis to particular sites. Several cytokines produced by immune cells have been shown to transmit cell growth signals in tumor cells and directly promote tumor cell growth; TGF-ß, TNFα, and IL-6 are able to promote the growth of some tumors (while suppressing the growth of others).

KEY POINTS

- Tumors can subvert the immune response by stimulating the production of immune cell factors that promote angiogenesis, invasion, and metastases.
- Immune cell cytokines also may function as tumor growth factors.

BIOLOGIC AGENTS

Many cytokines, monoclonal antibodies, and cell therapies for cancer have been developed and are applied clinically. The immune response can be activated to mediate tumor destruction through one of several mechanisms. These include increasing immune effectors and modifying tumor cells to increase their susceptibility to immune effectors. A major strategy is to block one or more of the negative immunoregulatory host checkpoints. The elimination of cells or cytokines that promote immune escape may permit a more effective and persistent immune response to a tumor. This approach cannot be effective unless there is a simultaneous positive immune response to the tumor. This may occur naturally, as is observed in select patients (e.g., patients with malignant melanoma). Alternatively, it may have to be induced, for example, by a cancer vaccine. There are two general immunotherapy approaches. "Active" approaches attempt to stimulate (in vivo) an intrinsic immune response to the tumor, either nonspecifically with cytokines or specifically with antibody or vaccine approaches. "Passive" or "adoptive" approaches involve the preparation of antibodies and immune cells outside the body (ex vivo) followed by administration to patients.

Table 4-2 **Examples of Cytokines Involved in Immune Regulation**

Group	Function	Receptor	Examples
Hematopoietic	Leukocyte proliferation, differentiation, and activation	■ Multimers with Trp-Ser-X-Trp-Ser motif ■ Signals primarily by receptor-associated JAK and STAT	IL-2, IL-3, IL-4, IL-6, IL-7, IL-11, IL-12, G-CSF, GM-CSF
Interferon	Inhibit virus replication	■ Two polypeptide chains with tandem fibronectin domains ■ Signals primarily by JAK-STAT	Interferon-alfa, interferon-beta, interferon-gamma
TNF	Inflammation and other biologic processes	Four extracellular domains activate caspases that mediate apoptosis ("death receptor") or pathways that promote cell survival and inflammation	TNF-alpha
Chemokine	Attract leukocytes to inflammatory sites	Seven transmembrane helices interact with G proteins	MIP-1-alpha, IL-8
IL-1	Inflammation and hematopoiesis	■ Extracellular Ig domain and cytosolic Toll-IL-1 receptor (TIR) domain ■ TIR activates signaling pathways	IL-1-beta
Growth factor	Growth and differentiation of nonimmune cells	Multimeric complexes with intrinsic tyrosine or serine/threonine kinase activities	TGF-beta, VEGF

Abbreviations: G-CSF, granulocyte colony-stimulating factor; GM-CSF, granulocyte-macrophage colony-stimulating factor; Ig, immunoglobulin; IL, interleukin; JAK, Janus tyrosine kinase; MIP, macrophage inflammatory protein; STAT, signal transducer and activator of transcription; TGF, transforming growth factor; TNF, tumor necrosis factor; VEGF, vascular endothelial growth factor.

Biologic agents can mediate antitumor effects by non-immune effector mechanisms. Some biologics are administered not to promote antitumor responses, but rather to address the complications of therapy and progressing cancer. These include hematopoietic growth factors. They also include cytokines that are produced by nonimmune cells and that do not directly activate antitumor immune effector mechanisms. For example, human recombinant keratinocyte growth factor (palifermin) is used to decrease the risk of severe mucositis associated with stem cell transplantation preparative regimens. Denosumab is a fully human monoclonal antibody that targets RANK ligand, a protein that acts as the primary signal to promote bone removal by osteoclasts. It is used for the prevention of skeletal-related events in patients with bone metastases and myeloma, as well as in the management of giant cell tumor of bone, osteoporosis, and rheumatoid arthritis.

Although the distinctions between biologic therapy and chemotherapy are being effaced, differences still exist. The pharmacokinetics of biologic agents are quite variable. Elimination half-lives for most cytokines are measured in minutes to hours, and for most antibodies in days to weeks. Infused cells can persist for months. Unlike chemotherapy, which acts directly on the tumor, cancer immunotherapies exert their effects on the immune system and demonstrate kinetics that involve generating an antitumor immune response. The approach to assessing and managing response and toxicity also can differ. Immunotherapy may induce novel patterns of antitumor response not adequately assessed by Response Evaluation Criteria in Solid Tumors (RECIST) or World Health Organization (WHO) criteria. New immune-related response criteria designed to more comprehensively capture all response patterns are under investigation.[20] As the goal of many approaches is to break immune tolerance, toxicity and evidence of autoimmunity is predicted and has been associated, in some studies, with clinical benefit. The removal of negative immunoregulatory mechanisms, in particular, does carry risk for autoimmune disease.

CYTOKINES

Cytokines are a diverse group of small proteins released by immune and nonimmune cells distributed throughout the body. Cytokines play integral roles in innate and adaptive immunity as effector and regulatory molecules. They also play an integral role in a variety of other biologic processes. Cytokines, which are active at very low concentrations, may act locally (autocrine or paracrine) or at a distance (endocrine). They are characterized by pleiotropy (one cytokine, multiple effects), redundancy (multiple cytokines, one effect), and synergy (the sum of the response together is greater than the sum of the individual responses). The administration of a cytokine will initiate a cascade of cytokine production and both stimulatory (amplification) and inhibitory/antagonistic effects. Cytokines act on their target cells by binding specific membrane receptors that contain cytokine-specific and signal-transducing subunits. They can be divided into groups based on function. For example, chemokines are cytokines that are chemoattractants or based on cellular source, and lymphokines are cytokines produced by lymphocytes. Study of the structure and function of cytokine receptors, however, has led to the improved understanding of cytokine action and a more useful classification (Table 4-2). Cytokines can lead to tumor destruction by one of two general mechanisms.

They can function indirectly and enhance the activity of antitumor cellular or humoral immune effector mechanisms. They also can interact directly with tumor cells; cytokines, such as TNF-ß, IFN-α, IFN-γ, IL-4, and IL-6 have been shown to initiate tumor cell apoptosis or cell cycle arrest. Recombinant cytokines in clinical use are displayed in Table 4-3.

KEY POINTS

- Cytokines can function indirectly and can enhance the activity of antitumor immune effectors.
- Cytokines, such as the interferons, have been shown to directly inhibit tumor cell growth.

INTERFERONS

IFN-α and IFN-ß (referred to as type I IFNs), which are produced by many cell types, and IFN-γ (referred to as type II IFN), which is produced primarily by lymphocytes, mediate a wide variety of biologic effects. A diversity of genes, at least a few hundred, are transcriptionally induced by IFNs. IFNs, type I in particular, inhibit virus replication in infected cells. IFNs affect nearly all phases of the innate and adaptive immune responses. All enhance class I MHC and thereby promote CD8+ CTL responses; IFN-γ is capable of inducing class II MHC. IFNs enhance NK cell cytotoxicity, upregulate Fc receptors, and promote ADCC mechanisms. They regulate the balance between Th1 and Th2 cells, promoting, for the most part, Th1 responses. In addition to affecting humoral immunity by modulating T helper cells, IFNs can have a direct effect on B cells, including regulating proliferation and Ig production. IFN-γ also plays an important role in macrophage activation. The immune effects elicited can be antagonistic (e.g., the stimulatory effect of NK cells may be offset by the upregulation of MHC class I molecules on the tumor). A role for immunomodulation is supported in one study by the appearance of autoantibodies or clinical manifestations of autoimmunity in patients with melanoma manifesting improved survival with IFN-α treatment.[21] IFNs can directly inhibit the growth of tumor (and normal) cells. The relative sensitivity to cell-cycle arrest or to apoptosis-inducing effects varies with the cell and with the type of IFN. IFNs have antiangiogenic activity, which is supported by the success of IFN-α-2 in treating hemangiomas and Kaposi sarcoma, which are angioproliferative diseases.

Among the more than 20 known IFNs, only IFN-α-2 has been extensively and clinically evaluated for cancer. Two recombinant IFN-α-2 preparations have been approved: IFN-α-2a and IFN-α-2b. A variety of doses have been applied. High-dose regimens apply more than 10 million international units (MIU), intermediate-dose regimens use 5 to 10 MIU, and low-dose regimens use 3 MIU or less. IFN has been administered by a variety of routes (e.g., intravenous, subcutaneous, and intratumoral) and by a variety of schedules. The plasma half-life is approximately 4 hours, and IFNs are usually administered either daily or three times per week. A pegylated form of IFN-α-2 has resulted in high

Table 4-3 Recombinant Cytokines in Clinical Use for Cancer

Cytokine	Effects	Cancer Indications
Interferon-alfa PEG-interferon alfa	- Immune (upregulate MHC, activate NK cells) - Antiangiogenesis - Direct antiproliferative	Melanoma, hairy cell leukemia, chronic myeloid leukemia, follicular lymphoma, Kaposi sarcoma, renal cell carcinoma
Aldesleukin (IL-2)	Activate cytotoxic T lymphocytes and NK cells	Melanoma, renal cell carcinoma
Sargramostim (GM-CSF)	Stimulates the development and function of neutrophils, monocyte-macrophages, and dendritic cells	Shorten chemotherapy-induced neutropenia in elderly patients with acute myeloid leukemia, promote myeloid reconstitution after HSCT, mobilize stem cells
Filgrastim (G-CSF) Pegfilgrastim (G-CSF)	Stimulates the development and function of neutrophils	Shorten chemotherapy-induced neutropenia, promote myeloid reconstitution after HSCT, mobilize stem cells

Abbreviations: G-CSF, granulocyte-colony stimulating factor; GM-CSF, granulocyte macrophage-colony stimulating factor; HSCT, hematopoietic stem cell transplantation; MHC, major histocompatibility complex; NK, natural killer; PEG, pegylated.

serum levels with the advantage of once-weekly administration. There are four types of toxicity, including constitutional, neuropsychiatric, hepatic, and hematologic. Flu-like symptoms, such as fever, chills, and myalgia, are associated with the initiation of IFN therapy. These symptoms are generally not dose-limiting and usually disappear after 1 to 2 days of therapy, at most after 1 to 2 weeks. With continued administration, neuropsychiatric side effects, such as fatigue and depression, may develop and become limiting. The latter can be occasionally partially ameliorated with the serotonin reuptake family of antidepressants. Liver function tests should be checked. Granulocyte counts and, to a much lesser extent, lymphocyte and platelet counts decline. Treatment should be temporarily suspended if hepatic transaminases increase more than 5 times normal or if granulocytes decrease to less than 500 mm^3 and restarted at a lower dose when recovery is evident. Changes in these laboratory values are not a cause for treatment discontinuation unless they become severely abnormal (e.g., hepatic transaminases more than 10 times normal).

The pleiotropic effects of IFN have led to its evaluation in almost all malignancies. IFN-α has been approved for use in melanoma, hairy cell leukemia, chronic myeloid leukemia (CML), follicular lymphoma, and Kaposi sarcoma. It is also approved in combination with bevacizumab for use in patients with renal cell carcinoma (RCC). IFNs have demonstrated activity in cutaneous T-cell lymphoma and myeloma. For the most part, the use of IFN in cancers other than melanoma has been supplanted by more active drugs. The activity of IFN-α in metastatic melanoma, producing response rates of approximately 15%, resulted in its evaluation in the adjuvant setting for patients at high risk for disease recurrence after primary surgery. Randomized trials demonstrated significant improvement in disease-free survival; the effect on overall survival (OS) is less clear.[22] As a result of these studies, IFN-α, administered intravenously at high doses for the first month followed by 11 months of intermediate doses subcutaneously, has become a standard treatment for patients with melanoma who are free of disease after surgery but at high risk for systemic recurrence. Adjuvant pegylated IFN administered weekly subcutaneously for up to 5 years is an alternative.[23] IFN-α has been combined with chemotherapy in several studies in melanoma. These "biochemotherapy" programs yielded higher response rates for metastatic disease; OS rates, however, were not significantly improved compared with chemotherapy alone.[24] Novel applications of IFNs are being tested both in solid tumors and hematologic malignancies.

INTERLEUKIN-2

IL-2 is a T-cell growth factor. Antigen binding to the TCR stimulates the secretion of IL-2 and the expression of IL-2 receptors (CD25). The interaction between IL-2 and the IL-2 receptor stimulates the growth, differentiation, and survival of antigen-selected T cells. IL-2 is a major activator of CTL and NK cytotoxicity. Interest in IL-2 as a therapeutic agent for patients with cancer was initially driven by the observation that lymphokine-activated killer (LAK) cells (which are generated by culturing peripheral blood cells with IL-2 and which, for the most part, represent IL-2–activated NK cells) killed a broad range of tumor types. IL-2 is necessary for the development of memory T cells and indirectly regulates B cells and hematopoiesis. More recent studies have focused on the role of IL-2 in maintaining immunologic tolerance. IL-2 is required for the generation and maintenance of Treg cells, which, as noted, have been implicated in abrogating antitumor activity.[25] Furthermore, IL-2 is involved in activation-induced cell death, a process that leads to the elimination of self-reactive T cells.

Recombinant IL-2, aldesleukin, has been applied in a variety of doses, routes, and schedules. The plasma half-life is short—1 to 2 hours. The high-dose regimen that led to FDA approval in patients with metastatic melanoma and metastatic RCC applies 600,000 IU/kg to 720,000 IU/kg, three times daily as an intravenous bolus. The maximum number of doses that most patients can tolerate is 14. A rest period of 5 to 9 days between cycles is recommended. Because of toxicities, administration of high-dose aldesleukin requires particular expertise, and patients must be treated in a step-down situation or intensive care unit. These toxicities stem from capillary-leak syndrome,

which is characterized by increased vascular permeability and decreased microcirculatory perfusion and leads to interstitial edema and multiple organ failure. Administering aldesleukin in high doses is comparable to inducing a controlled state of septic shock with fever, hypotension, decreased renal function, hyperbilirubinemia, rash, and marked malaise. Lower-dose regimens administered subcutaneously are much better tolerated, but are of uncertain clinical benefit. Decisions regarding the relative benefits of aldesleukin must be influenced by evaluations of toxicity and quality of life associated with the different regimens and schedules.

Aldesleukin was approved as treatment for patients with metastatic RCC and melanoma on the basis of experience with the high-dose regimen. Objective responses occur in a minority of patients, approximately 15%. More importantly, in approximately 5% of all treated patients, the response is complete and sustainable for many months or even years without additional therapy. Although FDA approval was granted only to high-dose bolus aldesleukin, other regimens have efficacy for RCC. Lower-dose aldesleukin administered subcutaneously for RCC was associated with similar response rates in small nonrandomized studies, but has not been evaluated sufficiently to determine its effect on long-term outcome.[26] Lower-dose aldesleukin has produced disappointing response rates in melanoma. To exploit potentially synergistic antitumor effects, aldesleukin has been applied with IFN-α. Response rates were generally not higher than those achieved with either agent alone. In addition, aldesleukin has been incorporated into biochemotherapy regimens for metastatic melanoma, which have, as noted previously, increased the response rate.[27] The combination of aldesleukin with a cancer vaccine has shown promise in patients with melanoma.[28] IL-2–based regimens have demonstrated activity in a variety of other solid tumors, such as colon, pancreas, and hepatocellular cancers, as well as mesothelioma, but not at levels required for regulatory approval. Activity also has been observed in hematologic malignancies, including acute myelogenous leukemia (AML). Studies evaluating predictors of response to IL-2 and novel applications are in progress.

HEMATOPOIETIC GROWTH FACTORS
GRANULOCYTE-MACROPHAGE COLONY-STIMULATING FACTOR

GM-CSF is a hematopoietic factor that stimulates the development of neutrophils and monocyte-macrophages and promotes the proliferation and development of early erythroid, megakaryocytic, and eosinophilic progenitor cells. It is produced by endothelial cells and fibroblasts, as well as by T cells and monocyte-macrophages. GM-CSF produces a variety of effects on cells of the neutrophil and monocyte-macrophage lineages, including augmentation of monocyte-macrophage MHC class II expression and enhancement of granulocyte and macrophage cellular cytotoxicity and ADCC mechanisms. GM-CSF also serves as the principal mediator of the proliferation and differentiation of myeloid dendritic cells. It enhances dendritic cell antigen uptake, MHC, and costimulatory molecule expression, as well as the ability of dendritic cells to stimulate T cells. However,

GM-CSF has been shown to stimulate MDSCs and to promote angiogenesis by stimulating VEGF production.

Although recombinant GM-CSF (sargramostim) can be administered intravenously, subcutaneous administration is preferred. Because of the sensitivity of rapidly dividing myeloid cells, sargramostim is typically initiated 1 to 3 days after completion of chemotherapy and administered daily through post-nadir recovery, usually for 2 weeks. Sargramostim has been well tolerated. Side effects include pain and inflammation at the injection sites, bone pain, myalgia, arthralgia, and low-grade fever, which usually are not limiting. Nausea, fluid retention, dyspnea, pericarditis, pleuritis, pulmonary emboli, splenomegaly, and hypersensitivity reactions have been reported, but are rare.

Sargramostim is indicated for use after induction chemotherapy in patients with AML who are age 50 to 70 in order to shorten the time to neutrophil recovery. It also is indicated for use in mobilization and after transplantation of autologous peripheral blood progenitor cells, in myeloid reconstitution after autologous and allogeneic HSCT, and in HSCT failure or engraftment delay. As with the recombinant granulocyte (G)-CSF, sargramostim can be used for the prevention of febrile neutropenia in adults with nonmyeloid malignancies receiving myelosuppressive chemotherapy. There have been, however, fewer trials of sargramostim as primary prophylaxis for febrile neutropenia in this setting.[29]

The ability of GM-CSF to function as an immunoadjuvant and to stimulate dendritic-cell and tumor-specific T-cell responses has led to its evaluation in a number of clinical trials. A variety of cancer vaccine approaches that incorporate GM-CSF have been tested clinically.[30] There also is evidence that administering sargramostim as monotherapy has antitumor activity in patients with prostate cancer or melanoma, in whom increases in dendritic cells have been observed.[31-33] Adjuvant GM-CSF improves disease-free survival of patients with completely resected high-risk melanoma with minimal toxicity. OS improvement is smaller and does not achieve statistical significance.[34] The ability of sargramostim to activate ADCC also is being tested in clinical trials, in which it is being administered with monoclonal antibodies.[35]

GRANULOCYTE COLONY-STIMULATING FACTOR

G-CSF is a hematopoietic factor produced by macrophages, lymphocytes, fibroblasts, and endothelial cells. It induces the production and release of neutrophilic granulocytes in the bone marrow and enhances their functional capacity in the periphery. Moreover, G-CSF possesses essential neutrophil-activating functions, such as the oxidative burst, degranulation, phagocytosis, and chemotaxis. G-CSF markedly stimulates neutrophil ADCC mechanisms. As a regulator of neutrophil activity, G-CSF plays a role in innate immune responses. There is growing evidence that G-CSF also exerts immunoregulatory effects in adaptive immunity. G-CSF mediates anti-inflammatory reactions accompanied by Th2 differentiation and promotes tolerogenic antigen-presenting cell/T-cell interactions.

Recombinant G-CSF (filgrastim), which has a plasma half-life of 3.5 hours, is usually administered subcutaneously daily for as long as 2 weeks, until post-nadir neutrophil recovery is at normal or near-normal neutrophil levels. Because filgrastim stimulates myeloid cells to divide and because dividing cells are sensitive to cytotoxic chemotherapy, filgrastim should be administered no earlier than 24 hours after the administration of cytotoxic chemotherapy and no earlier than 24 hours before the administration of chemotherapy to lessen the risk for aggravating leukopenia. A pegylated form of recombinant G-CSF, pegfilgrastim, has a variable plasma half-life of 15 to 80 hours, which allows administration once per cycle rather than daily. Pegfilgrastim is administered as a single subcutaneous injection once per chemotherapy cycle. Pegfilgrastim should not be administered in the period between 14 days before and 24 hours after administration of cytotoxic chemotherapy. The safety data appear to be similar between filgrastim and pegfilgrastim. The most commonly observed adverse effects are mild to moderate bone pain after repeated administration and local skin reactions at the site of injection. Bone pain, reported in approximately 20% of patients, is rarely dose-limiting and can usually be controlled with analgesics; it is not an indication to discontinue therapy. Fever, diarrhea, edema, dyspnea, skin rash, splenomegaly (with rupture), and hypersensitivity reactions also may occur, but are very rare. The G-CSF receptor, through which filgrastim and pegfilgrastim act, has been found on tumor cell lines. The possibility that pegfilgrastim acts as a growth factor for any tumor type, including myeloid malignancies and myelodysplasia, diseases for which pegfilgrastim is not approved, cannot be excluded.

Filgrastim and pegfilgrastim are indicated to decrease the incidence of infection, as manifested by febrile neutropenia, in patients with nonmyeloid malignancies who are receiving myelosuppressive chemotherapy associated with a high incidence (20%) of severe neutropenia with fever.[29] In addition to the chemotherapy regimens, several other factors are considered

KEY POINTS

- Interferons can mediate direct and indirect antitumor effects. Clinical trials have established a number of indications for interferon-alfa, both in hematologic malignancies and in solid tumors. This includes patients with malignant melanoma who are free of disease but at high risk for systemic recurrence.

- Interleukin-2 was approved for metastatic renal cell cancer and melanoma on the basis of the experience with high-dose intravenous bolus of the agent, a regimen limited by toxicity.

- Hematopoietic factors, recombinant granulocyte colony-stimulating factor (CSF), and granulocyte-macrophage CSF, are commonly used for the prophylaxis of febrile neutropenia and in hematopoietic cell transplantation. Their ability to modulate antitumor immune responses is under investigation.

when assessing the risk of febrile neutropenia and whether to administer recombinant G-CSF in this setting. These include factors that are treatment-related (e.g., severe neutropenia with similar chemotherapy), patient-related (e.g., age older than 65, open wounds, and chronic lung or heart disease), and cancer-related (e.g., bone marrow involvement with tumor). Filgrastim also is used after induction or consolidation chemotherapy treatment for adults with AML, for patients with nonmyeloid malignancies who are undergoing myeloablative chemotherapy followed by HSCT, and for the mobilization of hematopoietic progenitor cells.

Recombinant G-CSF is indicated to reduce the magnitude and sequelae of neutropenia (e.g., fever, infections, and oropharyngeal ulcers) in symptomatic patients with congenital, cyclic, or idiopathic neutropenia.[29] The immunomodulatory effects of G-CSF, such as the ability to promote ADCC mechanisms and to promote T-cell tolerance in pathologic conditions associated with a Th1/Th2 imbalance, are under investigation.

MONOCLONAL ANTIBODIES

Adoptive therapy with monoclonal antibodies, which can mediate antitumor activities by a variety of mechanisms (Fig. 4-2), has been one of the major advances in cancer immunotherapy. Most of the approved antibodies in oncology are of the human IgG1 subclass, the subclass that is the most effective at engaging Fc receptors on NK cells and macrophages. The monoclonal antibodies used in initial clinical trials were mouse and usually generated a vigorous human–anti-mouse antibody response. Therapeutic monoclonal antibodies are either chimeric with the mouse variable fused to human constant ("ximab"; 65% to 90% human) chain, humanized with the mouse hypervariable/complementarity-determining regions grafted to human immunoglobulin ("zumab"; 95% human), or fully human ("umab"). Many of these antibodies have been effective as monotherapy. However, effectiveness often can be enhanced by their combined application with other treatment modalities. Antibodies naturally have long serum half-lives. However, limitations have been identified. Triggering of tumor antigen-specific cellular immunity by monoclonal antibody, in conjunction with immune escape mechanisms used by tumor cells, may contribute to the differential clinical responses to monoclonal antibody–based immunotherapy.[36] The antigenic heterogeneity of most tumors presents challenges, as do the small fraction of injected antibodies that actually bind to tumors and the inability of antibodies to penetrate into large tumor masses. Furthermore, binding of antibodies to circulating antigens also can limit delivery to the tumor. Although now rare, immune responses to the artificial humanized antibody can still be problematic. Whether they target tumor cell membrane determinants, factors involved in tumor progression, or immune checkpoints, monoclonal antibodies are mainstays of cancer therapy (Table 4-4).

RITUXIMAB

The first monoclonal antibody to receive FDA approval for therapeutic use was rituximab, a human/mouse chimeric IgG1

KEY POINTS

- The effectiveness of monoclonal antibodies has been established for both hematologic malignancies and solid tumors.
- Targets have included tumor cell membrane determinants, factors involved in tumor progression, and immune checkpoints.
- Monoclonal antibodies can mediate antitumor activity via immune mechanisms (e.g., antibody-dependent and complement-mediated cellular mechanisms) and by nonimmunologic mechanisms (e.g., direct induction of apoptosis).
- Although active as single agents, monoclonal antibodies are most often applied with chemotherapy or radiation therapy.
- Most monoclonal antibodies have been well tolerated. Infusion reactions and severe organ toxicities, however, can occur.

directed to CD20, a transmembrane protein expressed on malignant and normal B cells. CD20 is expressed on more than 90% of cells for B-cell non-Hodgkin lymphoma and, to a lesser degree, on chronic lymphocytic leukemia (CLL). CD20 function is not established. The intracellular portion of CD20 contains phosphorylation sites for signaling kinases. It may affect cell cycle through calcium channel regulation. The cytotoxic effects of rituximab appear to involve CMC, ADCC, and induction of apoptosis. Rituximab is a type I monoclonal antibody in that it redistributes CD20 into membrane lipid rafts considered central to CMC. The dosing of rituximab is dependent on the clinical setting. Rituximab usually is administered intravenously weekly for four or eight doses. Serum concentrations double from the first to the fourth infusion, and elimination plasma half-life increases from 3 to 9 days because of elimination of circulating CD20+ B cells and reduction/saturation of CD20-binding sites. Rituximab infusions are generally well tolerated. Infusion-related reactions occur in the majority of patients, usually mild to moderate flu-like symptoms, and premedication with acetaminophen and diphenhydramine is recommended. Severe infusion reactions, such as bronchospasm and hypotension, occur in 10% of patients and are usually reversible with appropriate interventions. Transient hypotension may occur; therefore, withholding antihypertensives 12 hours before infusion should be considered. To address infusion reactions, the initial infusion is administered slowly. If hypersensitivity or infusion-related events do not occur, the infusion rate is increased incrementally. Subsequent infusions also are administered more slowly, initially with incremental rate increases. The incidence of hypersensitivity reactions decreases markedly with subsequent infusions. Rituximab can elicit a tumor lysis syndrome. It also induces lymphopenia, which lasts for approximately 6 months with full recovery in 9 to 12 months. CD20 is not expressed on hematopoietic stem cells. Rituximab therapy also has been

TABLE 4-4 Unconjugated Monoclonal Antibodies in Clinical Use for Cancer

Antibody	Type	Target	Indication
Lymphocyte determinants			
Rituximab	Chimeric	▪ Binds CD20 ▪ Mediates CMC/antibody-dependent cellular mechanisms ▪ Direct antiproliferative	Follicular lymphoma, diffuse large B-cell lymphoma, chronic lymphocytic leukemia
Ofatumumab	Human	▪ Binds CD20 ▪ Mediates CMC/antibody-dependent cellular mechanisms ▪ Direct antiproliferative	Chronic lymphocytic leukemia
Obinutuzumab	Humanized	▪ Binds CD20 ▪ Mediates antibody-dependent cellular mechanisms ▪ Direct antiproliferative	Chronic lymphocytic leukemia
Alemtuzumab	Humanized	▪ Binds CD52 ▪ Mediates CMC/antibody-dependent cellular mechanisms	Chronic lymphocytic leukemia
Epidermal growth factor family			
Trastuzumab	Humanized	▪ Binds HER2 ▪ Mediates CMC/antibody-dependent cellular mechanisms ▪ Direct antiproliferative ▪ Antiangiogenesis	Breast, gastric, gastroesophageal cancers
Pertuzumab	Humanized	▪ Binds HER2 and blocks ligand-dependent heterodimerization of HER2 with other HER family members, including EGFR, HER3, and HER4 ▪ Direct antiproliferative effects ▪ Mediates CMC/antibody-dependent cellular mechanisms ▪ Antiangiogenesis	Breast cancer
Cetuximab	Chimeric	▪ Binds EGFR ▪ Mediates CMC/antibody-dependent cellular mechanisms ▪ Direct antiproliferative ▪ Antiangiogenesis	Colorectal, head and neck cancers
Panitumumab	Human	▪ Binds EGFR ▪ Mediates CMC/antibody-dependent cellular mechanisms ▪ Direct antiproliferative ▪ Antiangiogenesis	Colorectal cancer
Angiogenic factor			
Bevacizumab	Humanized	▪ Binds VEGF ▪ Antiangiogenesis	Colorectal, nonsquamous non-small cell lung cancer, renal cell carcinoma, glioblastoma
Ramucirumab	Human	▪ Binds VEGF receptor 2 ▪ Antiangiogenesis	Gastric or gastroesophageal junction adenocarcinoma
Immune checkpoint			
Ipilimumab	Human	▪ Blocks CTLA-4	Melanoma

Abbreviations: CMC, complement-mediated cytotoxicity; CTLA, cytolytic T lymphocytes antigen; EGFR, epidermal growth factor receptor; VEGF, vascular endothelial growth factor.

associated with reactivation of hepatitis and with progressive multifocal leukoencephalopathy.[37,38] When used in combination with a variety of chemotherapeutic regimens, rituximab does not add to the toxicity of chemotherapy, with the exception of a slightly higher rate of neutropenia. This does not, however, translate into a higher infection rate.[39]

Rituximab is approved to treat several CD20+ malignancies. It is approved as first-line treatment for patients with diffuse large B-cell, CD20+, non-Hodgkin lymphoma in combination with cyclophosphamide/doxorubicin/vincristine/prednisone (CHOP) or other anthracycline-based chemotherapy regimens. It is approved as first-line treatment for patients with low-grade or follicular B-cell, CD20+, non-Hodgkin lymphoma combined with cyclophosphamide/vincristine/prednisone (CVP) or after CVP chemotherapy. It is also approved as maintenance therapy for patients with previously untreated follicular CD20+ B-cell non-Hodgkin lymphoma in whom rituximab achieved a disease response in combination with chemotherapy. Rituximab is approved in combination with fludarabine and cyclophosphamide for the treatment of both previously untreated and previously treated patients with CLL. Response rates for retreatment of patients with non-Hodgkin lymphoma are comparable to first-line treatment, which is unique for cancer chemotherapy.[40] Rituximab is being incorporated into the therapy of other CD20+ B-cell malignancies, such as mantle cell lymphoma. Laboratory assays are being developed to identify patients who are likely to have a response to rituximab; including assays of Fc receptor polymorphisms and tumor apoptotic regulators.[41] In addition, rituximab is also approved to treat rheumatoid arthritis, Wegener granulomatosis, and microscopic polyangiitis and is active in other immune diseases, such as immune thrombocytopenic purpura, systemic lupus erythematosus, and myasthenia gravis, and organ transplant recipients.

OFATUMUMAB

Ofatumumab is a human IgG1 monoclonal antibody also targeted to the CD20 protein. Ofatumumab targets an epitope different from rituximab and most other CD20-directed antibodies. Ofatumumab binds to both the small and large loops of the CD20 molecule on B cells. Its location is in closer proximity to the membrane, which in theory allows for more effective complement deposition and subsequent B-cell killing. Like rituximab, ofatumumab is a type I monoclonal antibody that redistributes CD20 into lipid rafts. Preclinical data suggest improved CMC and ADCC compared with rituximab. Direct effects on B-cell proliferation have also been demonstrated.

Ofatumumab is administered as an intravenous infusion weekly for the first eight doses, then every 4 weeks for the remaining four doses. The first dose of ofatumumab is reduced (300 mg) to reduce the risk for serious infusion reactions; all subsequent doses are 2,000 mg. The elimination half-life is approximately 14 days. Infusion reactions can be problematic, and premedication with an oral or intravenous antihistamine, oral acetaminophen, and an intravenous corticosteroid is administered prior to each dose. The dose of corticosteroid administered prior to doses three to eight and 10 to 12 can be reduced

on the basis of the absence of infusional toxicity on preceding doses. In addition to infusion reactions, which occurred in 44% of patients with the first infusion and 29% with the second infusion, adverse reactions have included infections, neutropenia, and pyrexia. The most serious side effect of ofatumumab is an increased chance of infections, including progressive multifocal leukoencephalopathy. Patients at high risk for hepatitis B should be screened before being treated with ofatumumab. Patients with evidence of inactive hepatitis should be monitored for reactivation of the infection during and after completing treatment.

Ofatumumab is approved for treating CLL that is refractory to fludarabine and alemtuzumab.[42] The effectiveness is based on the demonstration of durable objective responses. No data yet demonstrate an improvement in disease-related symptoms or increased survival. It is also not yet known whether the increased CMC activity of ofatumumab relative to rituximab is clinically relevant, as there are currently no head-to-head clinical data available. Ofatumumab has also shown potential in treating follicular non-Hodgkin lymphoma and diffuse large B-cell lymphoma. It is also used to treat rheumatoid arthritis and multiple sclerosis.

OBINUTUZUMAB

Obinutuzumab is a humanized, type II CD20 monoclonal antibody that has been glycoengineered to reduce core fucosylation, conferring enhanced affinity for the human FcγRIIIa receptor on effector cells and, hence, enhanced ADCC. As a type II monoclonal antibody, obinutuzumab has lower capacity to relocalize CD20 into lipid rafts upon binding compared with the type I antibodies rituximab and ofatumumab, and is less potent in inducing CMC. It is, however, more potent in mediating cell adhesion and direct cell death. Obinutuzumab and rituximab bind adjacent and partially overlapping epitopes on CD20, but acquire different orientation upon binding, which most likely contributes to different biologic characteristics of type I and II antibodies. In preclinical studies, obinutuzumab showed superior induction of direct cell death and enhanced ADCC with less CMC compared with rituximab. Obinutuzumab has been approved for use in combination with chlorambucil for the treatment of patients with previously untreated CLL. The approval was based on demonstration of an improvement in progression-free survival (PFS) in a randomized, open-label, multicenter trial comparing obinutuzumab in combination with chlorambucil to chlorambucil alone in patients with previously untreated CD20+ CLL.[43]

The most common adverse reactions with obinutuzumab in combination with chlorambucil were infusion-related reactions, neutropenia, thrombocytopenia, anemia, pyrexia, cough, and musculoskeletal disorder. Hepatitis B virus reactivation and progressive multifocal leukoencephalopathy are risks. Patients should be advised of these risks and assessed for hepatitis B virus and reactivation risk. Obinutuzumab is administered by intravenous infusion during cycle one on a day 1, 2, 8, and 15 schedule. Cycles two to six are administered intravenously every 28 days. Premedication with a glucocorticoid, acetaminophen, and an antihistamine is recommended. Chlorambucil on the approved regimen is administered on days 1 and 15 of each cycle.

ALEMTUZUMAB

Alemtuzumab is a humanized IgG1 directed against CD52, a nonmodulating glycoprotein expressed on the surface of normal and malignant B and T cells, NK cells, monocytes, macrophages, and tissues of the male reproductive system. CD52 function is unknown. The cytotoxic effects of alemtuzumab are presumed to involve ADCC and CMC mechanisms.

Alemtuzumab is usually initiated at low intravenous daily doses, with gradual dose escalation until a maintenance dose is reached. The maintenance dose is administered three times per week for up to 12 weeks. There is a rise in serum concentration with repeated infusions that corresponds with the reduction in malignant lymphocytosis. If therapy is interrupted for 7 or more days, it must be reinstituted at lower doses with gradual dose escalation. The subcutaneous route of administration is gaining popularity because it is effective and has fewer side effects than intravenous infusions. Alemtuzumab administration can be limited by toxicity, which includes infusion-related toxicities such as hypotension, rigors, fever, dyspnea, bronchospasm, chills, and/or rash. Premedication with diphenhydramine and acetaminophen before infusion is recommended, as is hydrocortisone if infusion-related events occur. Alemtuzumab induces profound lymphopenia, and a variety of opportunistic infections have been reported. Severe and prolonged myelosuppression also can occur. Infection prophylaxis, trimethoprim-sulfamethoxazole for pneumocystis pneumonia, and famciclovir (or its equivalent) for herpetic infections are necessary and must be continued for 2 months after completion of therapy or until CD4 cell counts are greater than 200, whichever occurs later.

Alemtuzumab was initially approved for the treatment of B-cell CLL in patients who have been treated with alkylating agents and in whom fludarabine therapy elicited no response. As first-line treatment for patients with CLL, alemtuzumab demonstrated substantial improvement in PFS, time to alternative treatment, overall response rate, complete response, and minimal residual disease-negative remissions compared with chlorambucil in a randomized trial. Toxicity was predictable and manageable. Also noted was a trend toward improved response in patients with high-risk cytogenetic abnormalities.[44] This led to approval of alemtuzumab as a single agent for the treatment of B-cell CLL in the first-line setting.

Alemtuzumab also has demonstrated activity in T-prolymphocytic leukemia and in cutaneous T-cell lymphoma.[45,46] In addition, it is being used as an immunosuppressive agent for various autoimmune diseases, as part of the conditioning regimens for allogeneic HSCT to prevent graft-versus-host disease (GVHD), and for organ transplant recipients.

TRASTUZUMAB

The antibody with the greatest effect on solid tumors has been trastuzumab, a humanized IgG1 directed against the extracellular domain of HER2, also known as ErbB2, a member of the epidermal growth factor (EGF) family of receptor tyrosine kinases. It is overexpressed by breast and other cancers. Overexpression is implicated in the malignant transformation process and is an independent, adverse prognostic factor in breast cancer, which may predict for response to both chemotherapy and hormone agents. HER2 also is overexpressed by other carcinomas. Trastuzumab exerts antitumor effects by several mechanisms that are not yet completely understood. Immune effector mechanisms, namely ADCC and CMC mechanisms, are considered to be central. Trastuzumab has direct antiproliferative effects, which include cell-cycle arrest and/or induction of apoptosis; it markedly accelerates HER2 endocytosis and degradation. Trastuzumab also can mediate antiangiogenic effects, including the inhibition of VEGF production.

Trastuzumab is administered intravenously, and a loading dose is administered initially followed by weekly administration. Other regimens, such as a dosing of every 3 weeks, also have been effectively applied. Trastuzumab is generally well tolerated. Infusion reactions do occur, but premedication is usually not required. Cardiac dysfunction can be problematic and was observed in almost 30% of patients who received an anthracycline and cyclophosphamide; concurrent therapy with anthracyclines is not recommended. Cardiac dysfunction also has been observed in approximately 15% of patients receiving trastuzumab plus paclitaxel and in approximately 5% of patients receiving trastuzumab alone. Cardiac myocytes (transverse tubules) can express HER2. Patients should undergo monitoring for decreased left ventricular function before trastuzumab treatment, and frequently during and after treatment. There are reports of fatalities in patients with poor performance status and lung dysfunction.

Trastuzumab is approved for HER2-overexpressing breast and gastric/gastroesophageal cancers. In patients with metastatic breast cancer, trastuzumab is indicated in combination with paclitaxel for first-line treatment and as a single agent for the treatment of patients who have received one or more chemotherapy regimens for metastatic disease. Trastuzumab is indicated for adjuvant treatment of HER2-overexpressing node-positive breast cancer or node-negative breast cancer that is either hormone receptor–negative or manifests one high-risk feature. In this setting trastuzumab is administered as part of treatment regimens consisting of doxorubicin, cyclophosphamide, and either paclitaxel or docetaxel, or consisting of docetaxel and carboplatin. It is also indicated for adjuvant treatment as a single agent following multimodality anthracycline-based therapy. Trastuzumab is also approved to be used with other drugs to treat HER2-positive metastatic gastric or gastroesophageal junction adenocarcinoma. It is being evaluated in other cancers that overexpress HER2, such as non-small cell lung cancer (NSCLC), ovarian cancer, and pancreas cancer, and in combination with small molecule inhibitors of EGF receptor (EGFR) tyrosine kinases.

PERTUZUMAB

Pertuzumab targets the extracellular dimerization domain (subdomain II) of HER2 and thereby blocks ligand-dependent heterodimerization of HER2 with other HER family members, including EGFR, HER3, and HER4. Pertuzumab has been approved for use in combination with trastuzumab and docetaxel for the treatment of patients with HER2-positive metastatic breast cancer who have not received prior anti-HER2 therapy or chemotherapy for metastatic disease. The approval is based on a randomized, placebo-controlled trial in patients with HER2-positive metastatic breast cancer in which a statistically significant improvement in PFS was observed in patients in the pertuzumab group compared with patients in the placebo group.[47] It is also approved as a neoadjuvant treatment of breast cancer, in combination with trastuzumab and docetaxel, for patients with HER2-positive, locally advanced, inflammatory, or early-stage breast cancer larger than 2 cm in diameter, as part of a complete early breast cancer regimen also containing fluorouracil, epirubicin, and cyclophosphamide or carboplatin. Pertuzumab is the first drug approved in the neoadjuvant setting, based on its ability to produce pathologic complete responses, defined as the absence of invasive cancer in the breast and lymph nodes, in a phase II study involving women with early HER2-positive breast cancer randomly assigned to one of four neoadjuvant treatment regimens.[48]

Pertuzumab is administered intravenously; a loading dose is initially administered, followed by infusions every 3 weeks. The half-life is approximately 3 weeks. There are specific dosing recommendations for drugs, such as trastuzumab and docetaxel, when administered with pertuzumab. The most common adverse reactions observed in patients who received pertuzumab in combination with trastuzumab and docetaxel were diarrhea, alopecia, neutropenia, nausea, fatigue, rash, and peripheral neuropathy. Cardiac dysfunction can occur. Of note, pertuzumab in combination with trastuzumab and docetaxel was not associated with an increase in the incidence of symptomatic left ventricular systolic dysfunction or decreased left ventricular ejection fraction compared with placebo in combination with trastuzumab and docetaxel. Other significant adverse reactions reported with pertuzumab included infusion-associated reactions, hypersensitivity reactions, and anaphylaxis.

CETUXIMAB

As with HER2, overexpression by tumors of the EGFR, also known as ErbB1, confers a negative prognosis. Cetuximab is a human/mouse chimeric IgG1 to the extracellular domain of EGFR. It competitively inhibits the binding of EGF and other ligands, such as TGFα. It blocks activation of receptor-associated kinases, resulting in inhibition of cell growth, apoptosis, and decreased VEGF and matrix metalloproteinases production. EGFR is expressed in many normal epithelial tissues, such as skin, and is overexpressed in many different human carcinomas. In animal studies, cetuximab inhibited tumor cells that overexpress EGFR, as well as increased the activity of chemotherapy and radiation.

Cetuximab is administered intravenously; a loading dose is initially administered, followed by weekly infusions. The plasma half-life is approximately 5 days. Every-other-week infusions have also been used. Women have 25% lower clearance

than men; response and toxicity are similar. In general, cetuximab has been well tolerated. Infusion reactions do occur and can be severe, particularly with the initial infusions, and premedication with diphenhydramine is recommended. The most common side effect has been an acne-like skin rash, which develops in up to 75% of patients and likely represents the biologic effects of blocking EGFR that is present in the skin. The rash develops rapidly following cetuximab initiation, peaks between weeks 2 to 4, and thereafter tends to steadily abate in severity with continuation. The development of a rash has been associated with greater therapeutic effectiveness. Life-threatening toxicities, such as interstitial lung disease, have rarely been observed.

Cetuximab is indicated for use in colorectal and head and neck cancers in combination programs and as monotherapy. Cetuximab is indicated in combination with irinotecan for patients with EGFR-positive metastatic CRC refractory to irinotecan. It also is indicated for use as a single agent for patients who are unable to tolerate irinotecan-based chemotherapy. In a randomized study in which cetuximab was compared with best supportive care, cetuximab improved OS and PFS and preserved quality-of-life measures in patients with metastatic CRC in whom other treatments had failed.[49] The development of rash was associated with improved survival. The presence of mutations in the KRAS oncogene, which encodes a signal transducer that mediates response to stimulation of cell surface receptors, including EGFR, has been associated with lack of response.[50] KRAS testing is recommended for all patients with metastatic CRC who are candidates for anti-EGFR antibody therapy, and it is recommended that patients with KRAS mutations (in codon 12 or 13) should not receive anti-EGFR antibody therapy.[51] Cetuximab, in combination with radiation therapy, is indicated for the treatment of locally or regionally advanced squamous cell carcinoma of the head and neck, in which it was shown to improve OS compared with radiation alone.[52] As a single agent, it is indicated for the treatment of patients with recurrent or metastatic squamous cell carcinoma of the head and neck for whom prior platinum-based therapy failed. Cetuximab is being evaluated in other cancers that express EGFR, such as NSCLC and pancreas cancer, as well as in novel combination programs.

PANITUMUMAB

Panitumumab is a recombinant human IgG2 monoclonal antibody that also binds specifically to EGFR. IgG2 is less efficient than IgG1 in mediating ADCC. In contrast to cetuximab, panitumumab is fully human. The theoretical advantage conferred by this agent, compared with its chimeric counterpart, is that there is less potential for an antigenic response. The antitumor effects are considered to be identical to that of cetuximab.

Panitumumab is administered intravenously without a loading dose. The elimination plasma half-life is approximately 7 days, and panitumumab is administered every 14 days. As was predicted, the development of human antihuman antibodies has not been detected with treatment. Approximately 1% of patients exposed to panitumumab, however, experienced a severe infusion reaction, whereas approximately 3% of patients treated with cetuximab experienced severe infusion reactions. Other toxicities appear to be similar. Skin rash with variable presentation is common. Rare but serious adverse events, such as pulmonary fibrosis, have been observed. Anecdotal reports have suggested that patients considered intolerant to cetuximab may be safely treated with panitumumab.

Panitumumab monotherapy is approved for the treatment of EGFR-expressing metastatic CRC with disease progression on or following chemotherapy regimens containing fluoropyrimidine, oxaliplatin, and irinotecan. It was approved on the basis of a phase III trial in which patients were randomly assigned to receive either panitumumab plus best supportive care or best supportive care alone.[53] Effectiveness is based on PFS. There was no difference in OS between the two study arms. Patients who received best supportive care alone could cross over to treatment. No patients who had been previously treated with cetuximab were included, and it is unknown if there will be cross-resistance with panitumumab. Efficacy has been confined to patients whose tumors do not express KRAS mutations.[54] An association between the development of rash and response has also been suggested. A clinical trial comparing the efficacy of panitumumab and cetuximab is underway. Panitumumab is being studied in other cancers, such as RCC and NSCLC. Additionally, clinical trials are in progress to determine efficacy in combination with other chemotherapeutic agents and as a radiosensitizing agent.

BEVACIZUMAB

Bevacizumab is humanized IgG1 directed against VEGF. Often overexpressed by tumor cells as well as by tumor-associated macrophages, VEGF has proven to be a pivotal stimulator of endothelial cell development and angiogenesis. Bevacizumab binds one VEGF isoform and prevents the interaction with its receptors (Flt-1 and kinase insert domain receptor [KDR]) on endothelial cells. Bevacizumab has been shown to inhibit new blood vessel formation in in-vitro models and reduced tumor vascularity and progression in in-vivo animal tumor models. Bevacizumab has been shown to have a direct and rapid antivascular effect in the tumors of patients with CRC.[55]

Bevacizumab is administered intravenously every 14 days. The plasma half-life is approximately 20 days (free plus bound to circulating VEGF). After correcting for body weight, men have a higher bevacizumab clearance, as do patients with higher tumor burden. However, there is no evidence of decreased efficacy in men or in patients with higher tumor burden. Clinical toxicities include gastrointestinal perforations, wound healing complications, and hemorrhage. At least 28 days following major surgery must pass and the incision should be fully healed prior to administrating bevacizumab. Administration also should be suspended several weeks prior to elective surgery. In addition, hypertensive crisis, nephrotic syndrome, and congestive heart failure have been observed in patients who received bevacizumab. In addition, bevacizumab must be suspended in patients with gastrointestinal perforation, wound dehiscence, serious bleeding, nephrotic syndrome, or hypertensive crisis. The risk of continuation or temporary suspension in patients with moderate to severe proteinuria is unknown. Infusion reactions are relatively uncommon. Other rare complications, including a reversible posterior leukoencephalopathy syndrome, have been observed in patients treated with bevacizumab.[56]

Bevacizumab is indicated for the treatment of patients with CRC, NSCLC, RCC, and glioblastoma. Bevacizumab has demonstrated little single-agent antitumor activity. Combined with 5-fluorouracil–based chemotherapy, it is indicated as first- or second-line treatment of patients with metastatic CRC.[57] Combined with carboplatin and paclitaxel, it is indicated for first-line treatment of patients with unresectable, locally advanced, recurrent, or metastatic nonsquamous cell NSCLC.[58] Hemorrhagic complications are more common in patients with squamous cell histology than with adenocarcinoma. Significant improvements in response rate and survival have been observed when compared with chemotherapy alone in patients with metastatic CRC and NSCLC. Bevacizumab is also approved in combination with IFN-α for the treatment of patients with metastatic RCC. The approval was based on results from randomized trials that demonstrated an improvement in median PFS in patients treated with bevacizumab.[59,60] It is also approved as a single agent for patients with glioblastoma with progressive disease following prior therapy. The approval was based on durable objective response rates demonstrated in single-arm trials.[61,62] Currently, no data have shown whether bevacizumab improves disease-related symptoms or survival in patients who were previously treated for glioblastoma. Correlation of antitumor activity with measures of angiogenesis inhibition has been difficult to demonstrate clinically. Bevacizumab has also shown activity in breast, pancreas, prostate, ovarian, and head and neck cancers, as well as in several hematologic malignancies. In addition to promoting angiogenesis, VEGF has immunosuppressive effects, and the immunomodulatory effects of bevacizumab are under investigation.

RAMUCIRUMAB

Ramucirumab is a monoclonal antibody that binds to VEGF receptor-2 and blocks the activation of the receptor. It has been approved for use as a single agent for the treatment of patients with advanced or metastatic gastric or gastroesophageal junction adenocarcinoma with disease progression during or after prior treatment with fluoropyrimidine- or platinum-containing chemotherapy. This approval was based on improved OS demonstrated in a randomized trial in which ramucirumab was compared with placebo.[63] It is the first biologic treatment given as a single agent that resulted in survival benefits in patients with advanced gastric or gastroesophageal junction adenocarcinoma progressing after first-line chemotherapy. The most common adverse reactions of ramucirumab are hypertension and diarrhea. Other important risks include hemorrhage, arterial thrombotic events, infusion-related reactions, gastrointestinal perforation, impaired wound healing, clinical deterioration in patients with cirrhosis, and reversible posterior leukoencephalopathy. Ramucirumab is administered by intravenous infusion every 2 weeks. Before receiving each dose, patients should be treated with an intravenous histamine H_1-receptor antagonist to decrease the risk for infusion-related reactions. Patients who suffer a grade 1 or 2 infusion-related reaction should also be premedicated with acetaminophen and dexamethasone or its equivalent before each infusion, and the infusion rate should be slowed by 50%.

IPILIMUMAB

Ipilimumab blocks the effects of the negative T-cell regulator CTLA-4 (Fig. 4-1), which may in turn augment T-cell responses to tumor cells. It is the first drug to improve survival in metastatic melanoma. Improvements in median survival were observed in a phase III trial comparing ipilimumab, gp100 vaccine, and ipilimumab plus gp100 vaccine (approximately 10 months with ipilimumab or ipilimumab plus gp100 vaccine compared with 6 months with gp100 vaccine alone),[64] and in a phase III trial comparing ipilimumab plus dacarbazine (11 months) with dacarbazine (9 months).[65] The unique mechanism of action of ipilimumab makes assessment of response by conventional criteria difficult. Response rates have been low, on the order of 10% to 15%. Of note, patients on ipilimumab may have delayed response or durable stable disease even after apparent disease progression, and benefit from ipilimumab can occur after what would be considered progression with RECIST or WHO criteria. Therapeutic responses peak between 12 and 24 weeks, with slow responses continuing up to and beyond 12 months. There is a suggestion that durable responses are achievable, though data supporting this are still developing.

Ipilimumab is administered intravenously for 90 minutes every 3 weeks for four doses. Toxicity can be problematic. Immune-related adverse events (IRAEs), likely the result of breaking immune tolerance upon CTLA-4 blockade, have included colitis/diarrhea, dermatitis, hepatitis, and endocrinopathies. Colonic perforation can occur and patients with diarrhea have to be monitored carefully. Stevens-Johnson syndrome and toxic epidermal necrolysis can result. Liver and thyroid function tests must be evaluated at baseline and before each dose. Inflammatory myopathy, nephritis, and uveitis also have been reported occasionally. In the phase III trials, severe (grade 3 or higher) IRAEs were seen in 10% to 15% of patients treated with ipilimumab plus gp100 vaccine and ipilimumab alone. Toxicity was higher for patients treated with ipilimumab plus dacarbazine, with grade 3 or higher IRAEs in 38%. The types of adverse events were consistent with those seen in prior studies of ipilimumab; however, the rates of elevated liver-function values were higher and the rates of gastrointestinal events were lower than expected on the basis of prior studies. Side effects were generally reversible and manageable by following specific treatment guidelines that include symptomatic therapies or systemic corticosteroids. An FDA Risk Evaluation and Mitigation Strategy and algorithms for the management of adverse side effects have been developed. Doses are withheld for any moderate IRAE or for symptomatic endocrinopathy. For patients with complete or partial resolution of adverse reactions, and who are receiving less than 7.5 mg of prednisone or equivalent per day, ipilimumab can be resumed until administration of all four planned doses or 16 weeks from first dose, whichever occurs earlier. Ipilimumab must be permanently discontinued if moderate adverse reactions persist, if the corticosteroid dose cannot be reduced to 7.5 mg of prednisone or equivalent per day, if a full treatment course cannot be completed within 16 weeks from administration of first dose, or if any severe or life-threatening adverse reactions develop. Because of the mechanisms involved, as well as the pharmacokinetics of the antibody (elimination half-life of approximately 15 days), prolonged treatment of IRAEs is often necessary. The treatment of IRAEs with immunosuppressive agents, such as corticosteroids, does not appear to impair antitumor response. With proper monitoring and management of side effects, ipilimumab is a safe drug to administer.

Ipilimumab has been approved for the first- or second-line treatment of patients with metastatic malignant melanoma. Ipilimumab has also shown promising activity in patients with NSCLC, RCC, and castrate-resistant prostate cancer. Combination with anti-PD1 antibody has demonstrated considerable promise.[66] Combination studies with targeted agents are under investigation, as are biomarkers of response.

CELLULAR THERAPY

One method of dealing with immune cell deficiencies in patients with cancer is to infuse immune cells generated ex vivo. A variety of immune effector cells have been generated for adoptive cellular therapy and tested in clinical trials. Early efforts examined the infusion of LAK cells, which had little activity and required the coadministration of high-dose IL-2 to maintain their activity. Initial studies in patients with advanced melanoma and RCC demonstrated antitumor activity. Comparable results, however, were seen subsequently with IL-2 alone. Similarly, studies on the effects of the infusion of TIL, which were generated by culturing cells obtained from surgically excised tumors with IL-2 and other cytokines ex vivo, demonstrated antitumor activity when administered with IL-2.[67] Methods of generating antitumor CTL by culturing peripheral blood, lymph node cells, and TIL with cytokines and tumor antigens ex vivo have also been evaluated clinically. Response rates of 50% or more in patients with metastatic melanoma, accompanied by long PFS, have been observed in nonrandomized studies.[68] Gene-modified CTLs genetically engineered to express receptors that specifically recognize tumor antigen, called chimeric antigen receptor T cells, are also demonstrating promise.[69-71] Dendritic cells have also been generated ex vivo and applied in vaccine approaches, as have monocyte/macrophages.

SIPULEUCEL-T

Sipuleucel-T is an autologous cellular immunotherapy designed to stimulate an immune response to prostate cancer. It is approved for the treatment of asymptomatic or minimally symptomatic metastatic castrate-resistant (hormone-refractory) prostate cancer. Sipuleucel-T is manufactured from peripheral blood mononuclear cells (PBMCs) isolated during leukapheresis at weeks 0, 2, and 4. PBMCs are cultured ex vivo with PA2024, a fusion protein consisting of prostatic acid phosphatase (PAP) and GM-CSF for 2 days, and then infused back into the patient. The approach is designed for the GM-CSF portion of the fusion molecule to activate blood monocytes and dendritic cells to present PAP as a tumor antigen. The final cell product, however, includes a variety of leukocytes, including T and B cells. In randomized phase III trials, patients in the control arm received infusions of a product made without PA2024 culture. Median OS was improved in patients treated with sipuleucel-T (approximately 26 vs. 22 months for controls).[72] This response was achieved without decreased levels of PSA. Response rate and the time to objective disease progression were also not affected. Adverse events more commonly reported in the sipuleucel-T group were chills, pyrexia, headache, flu-like illness, myalgia, hypertension, hyperhidrosis, and groin pain. These events were generally mild or moderate in severity and generally resolved within 1 to 2 days. The mechanism of sipuleucel-T activity is not established. Cellular and humoral responses against PA2024 and PAP antigens have been observed to increase in patients treated with sipuleucel-T compared with controls.[72] Activation status of the antigen-presenting cells infused also increases.[73]

DONOR LYMPHOCYTE INFUSION

Cells infused in allogeneic HSCT represent an effective adoptive cellular therapy in clinical use. An allogeneic graft-versus-leukemia (GVL) effect, which is a restricted form of GVHD, has been suggested by the increased relapse rate for recipients of T-cell–depleted allografts, higher relapse rates after either syngeneic or autologous transplants, and the lower frequency of relapse in patients with more severe GVHD. Given these clinical observations, donor leukocyte infusion (DLI) was tested in patients whose malignancies relapsed following allogeneic transplant. Numerous reports have documented success of DLI in patients with CML; durable complete molecular remission was achieved in the majority of these patients. Patients with AML have experienced only modest response rates, and acute lymphoblastic leukemia rarely responds. DLI also can eradicate Epstein-Barr virus–associated post-transplant lymphoproliferative disease following allogeneic transplant. More recent studies have identified potential target antigens in patients with a disease response to DLI. The major drawback of DLI is GVHD, which is a major source of transplant-related mortality, and methods of promoting GVL over GVHD are under investigation. New approaches aimed at improving the efficacy of DLI currently being explored include priming of donor lymphocytes to

recipient tumor antigens ex vivo, and infusions of alloreactive NK cells. The effects of lymphocyte infusions in myeloablative and nonmyeloablative settings are also under investigation in solid tumors. Antitumor activity has been observed in patients with melanoma undergoing myeloablative and nonmyeloablative treatments prior to autologous TIL infusion.[74]

IMMUNOTOXINS AND RADIOIMMUNOCONJUGATES

Biologic agents have been used to deliver toxins or radiation to malignant cells, as opposed to activating host antitumor mechanisms. Denileukin diftitox is a recombinant immunotoxin consisting of IL-2 fused to the enzymatically active domains of diphtheria toxin. It is internalized into IL-2 receptor-bearing cells (CD25) by endocytosis. Diphtheria toxin is activated, inhibits protein synthesis, and leads to apoptosis. Denileukin diftitox is indicated for the treatment of patients with persistent or recurrent CD25+ cutaneous T-cell lymphoma.[75] Cytokine release may occur, the result of the killing of T cells, and can result in capillary leak syndrome.

Brentuximab vedotin is an antibody-drug conjugate approved to treat anaplastic large cell lymphoma and Hodgkin lymphoma. The compound consists of the chimeric monoclonal antibody brentuximab, which targets the cell-membrane protein CD30, linked to 3 to 5 units of the antimitotic agent monomethyl auristatin E (MMAE, designated "vedotin"). The antibody portion of the drug attaches to CD30 on the surface of malignant cells, delivering MMAE, which is responsible for the antitumor activity. Brentuximab vedotin is usually well tolerated, with manageable side effects including peripheral sensory neuropathy.[76] Ado-trastuzumab emtansine, which consists of trastuzumab linked to the cytotoxic agent mertansine, an antitubulin, has demonstrated activity in patients with breast cancer in whom prior treatment with trastuzumab failed. It has been approved for use as a single agent for the treatment of patients with HER2-positive metastatic breast cancer who previously received trastuzumab and a taxane, separately or in combination.[77] Although well-tolerated in clinical trials, thrombocytopenia has been reported, and liver and cardiac toxicity can develop. Two mouse monoclonal antibodies to CD20 conjugated to radioisotopes, [131]iodine-tositumomab and [90]yttrium-ibritumomab, have demonstrated clinical effectiveness in patients with lymphoma. Both are indicated for the treatment of patients with relapsed or refractory low-grade or follicular B-cell non-Hodgkin lymphoma, with or without transformation, including patients with rituximab-refractory disease. Toxicity is typically quite mild. The main side effect is reversible myelosuppression.[78,79]

References

1. Mahmoud SM, Paish EC, Powe DG, et al. Tumor-infiltrating CD8+ lymphocytes predict clinical outcome in breast cancer. *J Clin Oncol.* 2011;29:1949-1955. PMID: 21483002.

2. Bates GJ, Fox SB, Han C, et al. Quantification of regulatory T cells enables the identification of high-risk breast cancer patients and those at risk of late relapse. *J Clin Oncol.* 2006;24:5373-5380. PMID: 17135638.

3. Salama P, Phillips M, Grieu F, et al. Tumor-infiltrating FOXP3+ T regulatory cells show strong prognostic significance in colorectal cancer. *J Clin Oncol.* 2009;27:186-192. PMID: 19064967.

4. Steidl C, Lee T, Shah SP, et al. Tumor-associated macrophages and survival in classic Hodgkin's lymphoma. *N Engl J Med*. 2010;362:875-885. PMID: 20220182.

5. Ohri CM, Shikotra A, Green RH, et al. Macrophages within NSCLC tumour islets are predominantly of a cytotoxic M1 phenotype associated with extended survival. *Eur Respir J*. 2009;33:118-126. PMID: 19118225.

6. Zea AH, Rodriguez PC, Atkins MB, et al. Arginase-producing myeloid suppressor cells in renal cell carcinoma patients: a mechanism of tumor evasion. *Cancer Res*. 2005;65:3044-3048. PMID: 15833831.

7. Filipazzi P, Valenti R, Huber V, et al. Identification of a new subset of myeloid suppressor cells in peripheral blood of melanoma patients with modulation by a granulocyte-macrophage colony-stimulation factor-based antitumor vaccine. *J Clin Oncol*. 2007;25:2546-2553. PMID: 17577033.

8. Almand B, Clark JI, Nikitina E, et al. Increased production of immature myeloid cells in cancer patients: a mechanism of immunosuppression in cancer. *J Immunol*. 2001;166:678-689. PMID: 11123353.

9. Tuthill RJ, Unger JM, Liu PY, et al. Risk assessment in localized primary cutaneous melanoma: a Southwest Oncology Group study evaluating nine factors and a test of the Clark logistic regression prediction model. *Am J Clin Pathol*. 2002;118:504-511. PMID: 12375635.

10. Zhang L, Conejo-Garcia JR, Katsaros D, et al. Intratumoral T cells, recurrence, and survival in epithelial ovarian cancer. *N Engl J Med*. 2003;348:203-213. PMID: 12529460.

11. von Mensdorff-Pouilly S, Verstraeten AA, Kenemans P, et al. Survival in early breast cancer patients is favorably influenced by a natural humoral immune response to polymorphic epithelial mucin. *J Clin Oncol*. 2000;18:574-583. PMID: 10653872.

12. Mellman I, Coukos G, Dranoff G. Cancer immunotherapy comes of age. *Nature*. 2011;480:480-489. PMID: 22193102.

13. Brahmer JR, Tykodi SS, Chow LQ, et al. Safety and activity of anti-PD-L1 antibody in patients with advanced cancer. *N Engl J Med*. 2012;366:2455-2465. PMID: 22658128.

14. Hamid O, Robert C, Daud A, et al. Safety and tumor responses with lambrolizumab (anti-PD-1) in melanoma. *N Engl J Med*. 2013;369:134-144. PMID: 23724846.

15. Almand B, Resser JR, Lindman B, et al. Clinical significance of defective dendritic cell differentiation in cancer. *Clin Cancer Res*. 2000;6:1755-1766. PMID: 10815894.

16. Zou W, Machelon V, Coulomb-L'Hermin A, et al. Stromal-derived factor-1 in human tumors recruits and alters the function of plasmacytoid precursor dendritic cells. *Nat Med*. 2001;7:1339-1346. PMID: 11726975.

17. Rayman P, Wesa AK, Richmond AL, et al. Effect of renal cell carcinomas on the development of type 1 T-cell responses. *Clin Cancer Res*. 2004;10(18 Pt 2):6360S-6366S. PMID: 15448031.

18. von Bernstorff W, Voss M, Freichel S, et al. Systemic and local immunosuppression in pancreatic cancer patients. *Clin Cancer Res*. 2001;7:925s-932s. PMID: 11300493.

19. Maeurer MJ, Gollin SM, Martin D, et al. Tumor escape from immune recognition: lethal recurrent melanoma in a patient associated with downregulation of the peptide transporter protein TAP-1 and loss of expression of the immunodominant MART-1/Melan-A antigen. *J Clin Invest*. 1996;98:1633-1641. PMID: 8833913.

20. Hoos A, Eggermont AM, Janetzki S, et al. Improved endpoints for cancer immunotherapy trials. *J Natl Cancer Inst*. 2010;102:1388-1397. PMID: 20826737.

21. Gogas H, Ioannovich J, Dafni U, et al. Prognostic significance of autoimmunity during treatment of melanoma with interferon. *N Engl J Med*. 2006;354:709-718. PMID: 16481638.

22. Kirkwood JM, Manola J, Ibrahim J, et al. A pooled analysis of eastern cooperative oncology group and intergroup trials of adjuvant high-dose interferon for melanoma. *Clin Cancer Res*. 2004;10:1670-1677. PMID: 15014018.

23. Eggermont AM, Suciu S, Santinami M, et al. Adjuvant therapy with pegylated interferon alfa-2b versus observation alone in resected stage III melanoma: final results of EORTC 18991, a randomised phase III trial. *Lancet*. 2008;372:117-126. PMID: 18620949.

24. Atkins MB, Hsu J, Lee S, et al. Phase III trial comparing concurrent biochemotherapy with cisplatin, vinblastine, dacarbazine, interleukin-2, and interferon alfa-2b with cisplatin, vinblastine, and dacarbazine alone in patients with metastatic malignant melanoma (E3695): a trial coordinated by the Eastern Cooperative Oncology Group. *J Clin Oncol*. 2008;26:5748-5754. PMID: 19001327.

25. Ahmadzadeh M, Rosenberg SA. IL-2 administration increases CD4+ CD25(hi) Foxp3+ regulatory T cells in cancer patients. *Blood*. 2006;107:2409-2414. PMID: 16304057.

26. Yang JC, Sherry RM, Steinberg SM, et al. Randomized study of high-dose and low-dose interleukin-2 in patients with metastatic renal cancer. *J Clin Oncol*. 2003;21:3127-3132. PMID: 12915604.

27. Dutcher J. Current status of interleukin-2 therapy for metastatic renal cell carcinoma and metastatic melanoma. *Oncology (Williston Park)*. 2002;16(11 Suppl 13):4-10. PMID: 12469934.

28. Schwartzentruber DJ, Lawson DH, Richards JM, et al. gp100 peptide vaccine and interleukin-2 in patients with advanced melanoma. *N Engl J Med*. 2011;364:2119-2127. PMID: 21631324.

29. Smith TJ, Khatcheressian J, Lyman GH, et al. 2006 update of recommendations for the use of white blood cell growth factors: an evidence-based clinical practice guideline. *J Clin Oncol*. 2006;24:3187- 3205. PMID: 16682719.

30. Warren TL, Weiner GJ. Uses of granulocyte-macrophage colony-stimulating factor in vaccine development. *Curr Opin Hematol*. 2000;7:168-173. PMID: 10786654.

31. Rini BI, Weinberg V, Bok R, et al. Prostate-specific antigen kinetics as a measure of the biologic effect of granulocyte-macrophage colony-stimulating factor in patients with serologic progression of prostate cancer. *J Clin Oncol*. 2003;21:99-105. PMID: 12506177.

32. Spitler LE, Grossbard ML, Ernstoff MS, et al. Adjuvant therapy of stage III and IV malignant melanoma using granulocyte-macrophage colony-stimulating factor. *J Clin Oncol*. 2000;18:1614-1621. PMID: 10764421.

33. Daud AI, Mirza N, Lenox B, et al. Phenotypic and functional analysis of dendritic cells and clinical outcome in patients with high-risk melanoma treated with adjuvant granulocyte macrophage colony-stimulating factor. *J Clin Oncol*. 2008;26:3235-3241. PMID: 18591558.

34. Lawson DH, Lee SJ, Tarhini AA, et al. E4697: phase III cooperative group study of yeast-derived granulocyte macrophage colony-stimulating factor (GM-CSF) versus placebo as adjuvant treatment of patients with completely resected stage III-IV melanoma. *J Clin Oncol*. 2010; 28:15s (suppl; abstr 8504).

35. Cartron G, Zhao-Yang L, Baudard M, et al. Granulocyte-macrophage colony-stimulating factor potentiates rituximab in patients with relapsed follicular lymphoma: results of a phase II study. *J Clin Oncol*. 2008;26:2725-2731. PMID: 18427151.

36. Ferris RL, Jaffee EM, Ferrone S. Tumor antigen-targeted, monoclonal antibody-based immunotherapy: clinical response, cellular immunity, and immunoescape. *J Clin Oncol*. 2010;28:4390-4399. PMID: 20697078.

37. Yeo W, Chan TC, Leung NW, et al. Hepatitis B virus reactivation in lymphoma patients with prior resolved hepatitis B undergoing anticancer therapy with or without rituximab. *J Clin Oncol*. 2009;27:605-611. PMID: 19075267.

38. Carson KR, Evens AM, Richey EA, et al. Progressive multifocal leukoencephalopathy after rituximab therapy in HIV-negative patients: a report of 57 cases from the Research on Adverse Drug Events and Reports project. *Blood*. 2009;113:4834-4840. PMID: 19264918.

39. Kimby E. Tolerability and safety of rituximab (MabThera). *Cancer Treat Rev*. 2005;31:456-473. PMID: 16054760.

40. Davis TA, Grillo-López AJ, White CA, et al. Rituximab anti-CD20 monoclonal antibody therapy in non-Hodgkin's lymphoma: safety and efficacy of retreatment. *J Clin Oncol*. 2000;18:3135-3143. PMID: 10963642.

41. Cheson BD, Leonard JP. Monoclonal antibody therapy for B-cell non-Hodgkin's lymphoma. *N Engl J Med*. 2008;359:613-626. PMID: 18687642.

42. Wierda WG, Kipps TJ, Mayer J, et al. Ofatumumab as single-agent CD20 immunotherapy in fludarabine-refractory chronic lymphocytic leukemia. *J Clin Oncol*. 2010;28:1749-1755. PMID: 20194866.

43. Goede V, Fischer K, Busch R, et al. Obinutuzumab plus chlorambucil in patients with CLL and coexisting conditions. *N Engl J Med*. 2014;370:1101-1110. PMID: 24401022.

44. Hillmen P, Skotnicki AB, Robak T, et al. Alemtuzumab compared with chlorambucil as first-line therapy for chronic lymphocytic leukemia. *J Clin Oncol*. 2007;25:5616-5623. PMID: 17984186.

45. Dearden CE, Matutes E, Cazin B, et al. High remission rate in T-cell prolymphocytic leukemia with CAMPATH-1H. *Blood*. 2001;98:1721-1726. PMID: 11535503.

46. Lundin J, Hagberg H, Repp R, et al. Phase 2 study of alemtuzumab (anti-CD52 monoclonal antibody) in patients with advanced mycosis fungoides/ Sezary syndrome. *Blood*. 2003;101:4267-4272. PMID: 12543862.

47. Baselga J, Cortés J, Kim SB, et al. Pertuzumab plus trastuzumab plus docetaxel for metastatic breast cancer. *N Engl J Med*. 2012;366:109-119. PMID: 22149875.

48. Gianni L, Pienkowski T, Im YH, et al. Efficacy and safety of neoadjuvant pertuzumab and trastuzumab in women with locally advanced, inflammatory,

or early HER2-positive breast cancer (NeoSphere): a randomised multicentre, open-label, phase 2 trial. *Lancet Oncol.* 2012;13:25-32. PMID: 22153890.

49. Jonker DJ, O'Callaghan CJ, Karapetis CS, et al. Cetuximab for the treatment of colorectal cancer. *N Engl J Med.* 2007;357:2040-2048. PMID: 18003960.

50. Karapetis CS, Khambata-Ford S, Jonker DJ, et al. K-ras mutations and benefit from cetuximab in advanced colorectal cancer. *N Engl J Med.* 2008;359:1757-1765. PMID: 18946061.

51. Allegra CJ, Jessup JM, Somerfield MR, et al. American Society of Clinical Oncology provisional clinical opinion: testing for KRAS gene mutations in patients with metastatic colorectal carcinoma to predict response to anti-epidermal growth factor receptor monoclonal antibody therapy. *J Clin Oncol.* 2009;27:2091-2096. PMID: 19188670.

52. Bonner JA, Harari PM, Giralt J, et al. Radiotherapy plus cetuximab for squamous-cell carcinoma of the head and neck. *N Engl J Med.* 2006;354:567-578. PMID: 16467544.

53. Van Cutsem E, Peeters M, Siena S, et al. Open-label phase III trial of panitumumab plus best supportive care compared with best supportive care alone in patients with chemotherapy-refractory metastatic colorectal cancer. *J Clin Oncol.* 2007;25:1658-1664. PMID: 17470858.

54. Amado RG, Wolf M, Peeters M, et al. Wild-type KRAS is required for panitumumab efficacy in patients with metastatic colorectal cancer. *J Clin Oncol.* 2008;26:1626-1634. PMID: 18316791.

55. Willett CG, Boucher Y, di Tomaso E, et al. Direct evidence that the VEGF-specific antibody bevacizumab has antivascular effects in human rectal cancer. *Nat Med.* 2004;10:145-147. PMID: 14745444.

56. Gressett SM, Shah SR. Intricacies of bevacizumab-induced toxicities and their management. *Ann Pharmacother.* 2009;43:490-501. PMID: 19261963.

57. Hurwitz H, Fehrenbacher L, Novotny W, et al. Bevacizumab plus irinotecan, fluorouracil, and leucovorin for metastatic colorectal cancer. *N Engl J Med.* 2004;350:2335-2342. PMID: 15175435.

58. Sandler A, Gray R, Perry MC, et al. Paclitaxel-carboplatin alone or with bevacizumab for non-small-cell lung cancer. *N Engl J Med.* 2006;355:2542-2550. PMID: 17167137.

59. Escudier B, Bellmunt J, Négrier S, et al. Phase III trial of bevacizumab plus interferon alfa-2a in patients with metastatic renal cell carcinoma (AVOREN): final analysis of overall survival. *J Clin Oncol.* 2010;28:2144-2150. PMID: 20368553.

60. Rini BI, Halabi S, Rosenberg JE, et al. Phase III trial of bevacizumab plus interferon alfa versus interferon alfa monotherapy in patients with metastatic renal cell carcinoma: final results of CALGB 90206. *J Clin Oncol.* 2010;28:2137-2143. PMID: 20368558.

61. Friedman HS, Prados MD, Wen PY, et al. Bevacizumab alone and in combination with irinotecan in recurrent glioblastoma. *J Clin Oncol.* 2009;27:4733-4740. PMID: 19720927.

62. Kreisl TN, Kim L, Moore K, et al. Phase II trial of single-agent bevacizumab followed by bevacizumab plus irinotecan at tumor progression in recurrent glioblastoma. *J Clin Oncol.* 2009;27:740-745. PMID: 19114704.

63. Fuchs CS, Tomasek J, Yong CJ, et al. Ramucirumab monotherapy for previously treated advanced gastric or gastro-oesophageal junction adenocarcinoma (REGARD): an international, randomised, multicentre, placebo-controlled, phase 3 trial. *Lancet.* 2014;383:31-39. PMID: 24094768.

64. Hodi FS, O'Day SJ, McDermott DF, et al. Improved survival with ipilimumab in patients with metastatic melanoma. *N Engl J Med.* 2010;363:711-723. PMID: 20525992.

65. Robert C, Thomas L, Bondarenko I, et al. Ipilimumab plus dacarbazine for previously untreated metastatic melanoma. *N Engl J Med.* 2011;364:2517-2526. PMID: 21639810.

66. Wolchok JD, Kluger H, Callahan MK, et al. Nivolumab plus ipilimumab in advanced melanoma. *N Engl J Med.* 2013;369:122-133. PMID: 23724867.

67. Rosenberg SA, Dudley ME. Adoptive cell therapy for the treatment of patients with metastatic melanoma. *Curr Opin Immunol.* 2009;21:233-240. PMID: 19304471.

68. Weber J, Atkins M, Hwu P, et al. White paper on adoptive cell therapy for cancer with tumor-infiltrating lymphocytes: a report of the CTEP subcommittee on adoptive cell therapy. *Clin Cancer Res.* 2011;17:1664-1673. PMID: 21325070.

69. Porter DL, Levine BL, Kalos M, et al. Chimeric antigen receptor-modified T cells in chronic lymphoid leukemia. *N Engl J Med.* 2011;365:725-733. PMID: 21830940.

70. Robbins PF, Morgan RA, Feldman SA, et al. Tumor regression in patients with metastatic synovial cell sarcoma and melanoma using genetically engineered lymphocytes reactive with NY-ESO-1. *J Clin Oncol.* 2011;29:917-924. PMID: 21282551.

71. Morgan RA, Dudley ME, Wunderlich JR, et al. Cancer regression in patients after transfer of genetically engineered lymphocytes. *Science.* 2006;314:126-129. PMID: 16946036.

72. Kantoff PW, Higano CS, Shore ND, et al. Sipuleucel-T immunotherapy for castration-resistant prostate cancer. *N Engl J Med.* 2010;363:411-422. PMID: 20818862.

73. Sheikh NA, dela Rosa C, Frohlich MW. Sipuleucel-T treatment results in sequential ex vivo activation of APCs and T cells during the culture step — evidence for in vivo immunological priming. *Cancer Res.* 2010;70(8 suppl):5608.

74. Dudley ME, Yang JC, Sherry R, et al. Adoptive cell therapy for patients with metastatic melanoma: evaluation of intensive myeloablative chemoradiation preparative regimens. *J Clin Oncol.* 2008;26:5233-5239. PMID: 18809613.

75. Olsen E, Duvic M, Frankel A, et al. Pivotal phase III trial of two dose levels of denileukin diftitox for the treatment of cutaneous T-cell lymphoma. *J Clin Oncol.* 2001;19:376-388. PMID: 11208829.

76. Younes A, Bartlett NL, Leonard JP, et al. Brentuximab vedotin (SGN-35) for relapsed CD30-positive lymphomas. *N Engl J Med.* 2010;363:1812-1821. PMID: 21047225.

77. Verma S, Miles D, Gianni L, et al. Trastuzumab emtansine for HER2-positive advanced breast cancer. *N Engl J Med.* 2012;367:1783-1791. PMID: 23020162.

78. Kaminski MS, Zelenetz AD, Press OW, et al. Pivotal study of iodine I 131 tositumomab for chemotherapy-refractory low-grade or transformed low-grade B-cell non-Hodgkin's lymphomas. *J Clin Oncol.* 2001;19:3918-3928. PMID: 11579112.

79. Witzig TE, Gordon LI, Cabanillas F, et al. Randomized controlled trial of yttrium-90-labeled ibritumomab tiuxetan radioimmunotherapy versus rituximab immunotherapy for patients with relapsed or refractory low-grade, follicular, or transformed B-cell non-Hodgkin's lymphoma. *J Clin Oncol.* 2002;20:2453-2463. PMID: 12011122.

5

CLINICAL TRIALS AND BIOSTATISTICS

Barry E. Storer, PhD

Both the practicing oncologist and cancer researcher are well aware of the heterogeneity that appears in almost every dimension of the disease and its treatment: among types of cancer, among patients with cancer, and in the response of disease to treatment. Although this challenge can be met in part by gaining a better understanding of the underlying factors that affect the disease and its response to treatment, the complexity of the underlying biology makes it almost certain that randomness and unpredictability will continue to be a significant component of cancer research and treatment.

Statistics is the branch of mathematics that deals with the collection and analysis of data in the face of uncertainty and random variation. *Biostatistics* is a term commonly used to refer to statistical methods and applications related to medical research, although the distinction is not necessary and not used here. The term *biometry* more commonly refers to nonmedical biologic applications. Not surprisingly, statistics plays a significant role in medicine as a whole and in oncology in particular, and statistical concepts and ideas will be encountered repeatedly in the medical literature relevant to the oncologist. This chapter is intended to cover topics that an oncologist will encounter and need a basic understanding of in order to read and interpret current articles in medical journals. There is an assumption that the reader has had only minimal didactic exposure to statistical concepts and methods, and thus there is no intent to cover the "how" of statistics (i.e., no formulas or equations)—just the "what" and "why."

Of course, in a single chapter it is impossible to summarize in any depth or breadth an entire scientific discipline, even when focused on its application to clinical oncology, so there is necessarily a focus on topics that are either commonly encountered or frequently misunderstood. In addition to reviewing basic statistical concepts and analytic methods common in clinical research, the chapter includes a section on clinical trial design. Although perhaps not a purely statistical topic, clinical trials are an essential part of clinical research, and are the means by which one attempts to control systematic sources of variation. Properly designed clinical trials help one to isolate the random components of variation, which can then be quantified by appropriate statistical analysis. Taken together, proper design and analysis allow one to make an objective evaluation of treatment options, reflecting both the strengths and uncertainties in the evidence at hand.

BASIC CONCEPTS

In this section we review some basic statistical concepts, with a focus on terms and issues that commonly arise in the analysis of medical data, especially those that are most commonly misunderstood. We start with the notion of sample and population, for which basic *descriptive statistics* are relevant. Then we move to topics in *inferential statistics*, where one attempts to relate characteristics of the sample to characteristics of the population. This is the crux of using statistics

Table 5-1 Basic Descriptive Statistics

Statistic	Definition and Description
Mean	The average value of the sample
Median	The value dividing the ordered values of the sample in half; equivalent to the 50th percentile. For an odd sample size the median is the middle value; for an even sample size the median is the average of the two middle values.
Percentile	The value below or equal to which a specified percentage of ordered observations fall. Tertiles, quartiles, and quintiles are values dividing an ordered sample into thirds, fourths, and fifths, respectively.
Mode	The most frequent value in the sample. Not often used.
Standard deviation	A measure of the variation of a sample distribution, based on the average squared distance from the sample mean. Most of a sample from a normal distribution is contained within two standard deviations above and below the mean.
Standard error	A measure of variation of the sample mean, or other estimated parameter describing a distribution. Unlike the standard deviation, the standard error gets smaller with larger sample size.
Range	The difference between the maximum and minimum value. In practice the maximum and minimum are usually given, not the difference.

in medical research, and includes the concepts of hypothesis testing, p-values, and confidence intervals. Finally, we describe a somewhat different point of view relating to these concepts, that of Bayesian statistics.

SAMPLE AND POPULATION

Two terms that arise early in a discussion of statistics are the *sample* and the *population*. In general terms, the data that are generated in medical studies (for example, in a clinical trial), represent an observed sample from an idealized larger population, such as all patients with a particular diagnosis and stage of disease. The sample data are described and subjected to statistical analysis in hopes of making inference about the larger population from which they came. In practice, the sample is rarely drawn randomly from the population, but it is assumed that the behavior of the sample, and statistics calculated from it, are governed by *parameters* that characterize this hypothetical larger population.

A *statistic*, as compared with the discipline called statistics, is a quantity summarized from a set of data, for example, the mean or median. These are commonly referred to as descriptive statistics. They may describe quantitative variables, such as age or tumor size; ordinal variables, such as stage of disease; or categorical variables, such as sex or race.

Table 5-1 defines some common descriptive statistics. Most of these terms refer also to characteristics of a population, but

are considered here as statistics calculated from a sample of data. In some cases a simple description of the sample characteristics is all that is intended; however, a common use of sample statistics, either explicitly or implicitly, is to estimate their counterparts in a population. For example, the mean is a statistic computed from a sample. At least conceptually, the mean of the population from which the sample arose could be determined by enumerating and averaging all the values in the population. Instead, the sample mean (a statistic whose value varies from sample to sample) is used to estimate the population mean (a parameter with a fixed value). Such usage is a part of inferential statistics.

HYPOTHESIS TESTING

The two basic components of inferential statistics are *estimation*, which was noted above, and *hypothesis testing*. Whereas estimation attempts to ascertain the value of a population parameter, hypothesis testing attempts only to decide whether it has a particular value (or range of values). Many aspects of clinical trial design are framed in terms of hypothesis testing. This framework is sometimes somewhat artificial, but is often used to plan the size of clinical trials, and is the origin of many commonly encountered statistical terms.

The statistical hypothesis test involves three basic steps: (a) formulation of the *null hypothesis*, (b) collection and analysis of data, and (c) a decision to "reject" or "not reject" the null hypothesis. The term "not reject" is deliberately used here, rather than the term "accept," for reasons that are elaborated below. The null hypothesis is a semantic concept that is not at all the same as a scientific hypothesis. For example, in a trial of a new therapy, there is likely a scientific belief or hypothesis that the new therapy will be more effective than a standard therapy currently in use. However, the null hypothesis in such a setting would be just the opposite: that the new therapy has the same effectiveness as the standard. In the clinical trial setting, the desired scientific outcome is usually to reject the null hypothesis.

If one formulates the problem such that the only outcomes are to reject or not reject the null hypothesis, then there are two possible errors that can be made. One is that the null hypothesis is true and is incorrectly rejected (false positive); the other is that the null hypothesis is false and is incorrectly not rejected (false negative). The first of these is called type I error, and the rate of type I error is usually designated α; the second is called type II error, and the rate of type II error is usually designated β. The rate of type II error requires specification of exactly how the null hypothesis is false, which is referred to as the *alternative hypothesis*. It is more commonly specified by the probability of correctly rejecting the null hypothesis when a particular alternative to the null hypothesis is true; this is called *power* and is designated 1-β.

Hypothesis tests are carried out by calculating a *test statistic* from one or more samples. In years past, one then referred to a table of *critical values* for the test statistic, calculated from the theoretical distribution of the test statistic under the null hypothesis for a given sample size and type I error rate. If the test statistic was larger than the critical value (or smaller, depending on the type of statistic and test) then one rejected the null hypothesis. Although this can still be done, the computation of a test statistic now almost always involves the automatic computation of an associated *p-value*, whose use, and misuse, is discussed in the next section.

Table 5-2 defines some common statistical tests. These all relate to simple comparisons of a quantitative or categorical characteristic, between groups or within a group. We have included examples of both *parametric* and *nonparametric* tests. Parametric tests are derived using a specific assumption about the distribution of the data—for example: normal, binomial, or exponential—whereas nonparametric tests make fewer such assumptions. Although the latter feature is desirable, a nonparametric test will generally have somewhat less statistical power than a parametric test that is correctly matched to a specific distribution. Fortunately, these considerations usually become less important with increasing sample size, and the choice of a parametric or nonparametric test is not critical. More complex statistical methods which relate to other types of endpoints, or which consider multiple variables simultaneously, are described later in the chapter.

INTERPRETING P-VALUES AND CONFIDENCE INTERVALS

One of the most widespread, and possibly most often misunderstood, concepts related to the statistical analysis of medical data is the p-value. The p-value is calculated after data have been collected and measures the strength of the evidence against the null hypothesis. For a given statistical model and assumptions, the p-value is the probability, if the null hypothesis were true, that a result as different (or more different) from the one observed could be produced by chance alone. If the p-value is "small," then one can reasonably infer that chance is not a good explanation for the observed data under the null hypothesis, and that therefore it is a consequence of some systematic effect. Whether the systematic effect has been designed into the study, as in a randomized trial, or is a result of bias or selection factors is a different question.

What constitutes a small p-value? In the world of clinical research a p-value of less than 0.05 has become the universal standard for statistical significance. This number is arbitrary, but is as good as any other if one wants only to establish a minimum threshold of evidence for something that is being measured on a continuous scale. In the formal hypothesis testing paradigm, it is equivalent to rejecting the null hypothesis when the type I error rate is set at 5%. The major error of interpretation of the p-value involves outcomes where the p-value is "large." The fact that a result is not statistically significant only means that chance is at least a reasonable explanation for the observed data. It does not mean that it is the only explanation and that the null hypothesis is true. The 0.05 level of significance (or any other level) does not discriminate truth from falsehood, and the p-value is most certainly not the probability that the null hypothesis is true.

What, then, does a large p-value mean? In the absence of any other information, and assuming that the data arise from a properly designed study, the safest and most accurate interpretation is that "there are insufficient data to resolve the question." The

Table 5-2 **Basic Statistical Tests**	
Test	**Definition and Description**
Two-sample t	Used to compare means between two groups for a quantitative variable. Generally robust to small sample size and non-normal distributions, but sensitive to outlying values, which inflate estimates of variability.
Paired t	Used to compare paired quantitative data; for example, a quantitative characteristic measured before and after treatment in each patient. Same sensitivity to outlying values as the two-sample t-test.
Wilcoxon rank sum (Mann-Whitney)	A nonparametric alternative to the two-sample t-test. Less sensitive to outlying values than the two-sample t-test, although somewhat more conservative.
Wilcoxon signed rank	A nonparametric version of the paired t-test. Less sensitive to outlying values than the paired t-test, although somewhat more conservative.
Chi-squared	Used to compare proportions between two or more groups. Fairly robust to small sample sizes, unless there is imbalance between groups. The "continuity correction" sometimes applied to the chi-squared test is conservative and generally unnecessary.
Fisher's exact	Used to compare proportions with small sample size. A conservative test compared to the chi-squared.
McNemar's	Used to compare paired proportions; for example, a binary characteristic assessed before and after treatment in each patient. It is based only on the discordant pairs (where outcome is different) and is not used to assess concordance.

reality is that the p-value, whether small or large, actually carries very little information. It conveys no information about the direction or magnitude of an effect, no information about the uncertainty in the estimated effect, and no information about the clinical significance of the effect. Even a small p-value is no guarantee that an effect has clinical significance. In studies with a very large sample size, even a modest departure from the null hypothesis can be associated with a high degree of statistical significance, but the departure from the null hypothesis may have little practical meaning.

The quantity that contains this missing information is the *confidence interval*. The confidence interval contains the full range of null and alternative values with which the data are reasonably consistent. An interval with a 95% confidence level will be expected to contain the true value of an effect 95% of the time, and miss it 5% of the time. Of course, for any particular confidence interval it is unknown whether it does or does not contain the true value. In contrast, the p-value provides information only about a single value. Figure 5-1 shows a variety of

Fig. 5-1 Interpreting confidence intervals with respect to statistical and clinical significance.

Heavy blue lines illustrate 95% confidence intervals that could arise from a comparative clinical trial of an experimental therapy versus standard therapy. The vertical dashed line indicates exact equality between arms, with a blue area indicating a difference close to equality that is considered clinically insignificant. The green area indicates a difference between arms that would be considered a clinically significant benefit for the experimental arm; the yellow indicates clinically significant harm for the experimental arm. The determination of statistical significance (at the $\alpha = 0.05$ level) is based only on whether the confidence interval includes 0. The full range of the confidence interval must be examined to determine what conclusions are reasonable with respect to the clinical significance of the study.

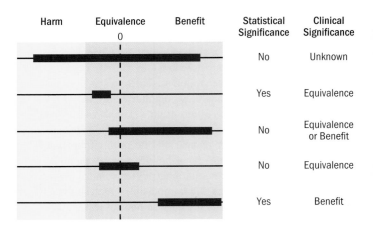

scenarios for the outcome of a statistical analysis and illustrates how confidence intervals relate to the concepts of statistical and clinical significance.

When a p-value is not less than 0.05, then the associated null value will be contained within the 95% confidence interval. The fallacy that this is therefore the true value is readily apparent, since the null value is only one among a range of possible values that could reasonably have produced the observed data.

SAMPLE SIZE AND POWER CALCULATIONS

The calculation of sample size for a clinical trial depends on a variety of factors, including the endpoint to be evaluated and the particular method of statistical analysis; however, all such calculations depend on the same basic considerations: the acceptable rates of type I and type II error (or power), a null hypothesis and the particular alternative to the null hypothesis for which power is calculated, and the variability of the outcome. In some cases, the latter is determined by the null hypothesis and a specified alternative, in other cases, it can vary independently. These factors influence the calculation of sample size or power in a reasonably intuitive way, summarized in Table 5-3.

The most common value specified for the α level is the ubiquitous 5%, especially in comparative clinical trials, and a common value for power is 80% or 90%, but of course these can vary depending on the situation at hand. The factor with the greatest influence in the design of a clinical trial is the particular alternative to the null selected for use in the calculations. This is frequently referred to as the *effect size* and specifies, for example, a difference in proportions, or a difference in means, or a hazard ratio that one is (scientifically) hypothesizing, or would be of interest. In most cases, a halving of the effect size used in the calculation results in roughly a 4-fold increase in the sample size requirement, all else being equal. Conversely, doubling the effect size results in roughly a 75% lower sample size. Thus, it is critically important to make realistic assumptions about the effect size for which a clinical trial is designed.

As noted above, the hypothesis testing framework is useful for formulating the calculation of power and sample size, but is an artificial and oversimplified view of the clinical trial as a whole. In the real world, interpreting a clinical trial and acting on its results is a far more complex undertaking than simply rejecting or not rejecting a statistical null hypothesis.

KEY POINTS

- Statistical significance and clinical significance are different concepts.
- Large p-values, by themselves, are not evidence for a lack of effect; they should generally be regarded as uninformative.
- Confidence intervals provide information about both statistical and clinical significance.
- Sample size requirements for comparative trials are extremely sensitive to the assumed effect size (difference in outcome between arms); for example, halving the effect size results in a 4-fold increase in the total number of patients required for a trial.

BAYESIAN STATISTICS

Most of the familiar statistical concepts and applications encountered in medical research are based on what is called the *frequentist* view of statistics and probability. In the frequentist perspective, probability is a quantity that, in principle, reflects the underlying long-term frequency with which an event will occur under repeated observation. This frequency is governed by unknown but fixed parameters that define a probability distribution. For example, the mean and standard deviation of a normal distribution determine how frequently, on average, a value from that distribution will exceed a certain value. The statistical procedures derived from this perspective are all based on relating observed data to the fixed parameters of the probability model generating the data.

*Bayesian** statistics also seek to relate observed data to the probability model generating the data. Although partly

---

* The term Bayesian derives from a basic theorem known as Bayes' rule, which was formulated by the Reverend Thomas Bayes in the mid-18th century.

Table 5-3 Factors Influencing Sample Size in a Comparative Study

Quantity	Effect
Type I error rate	Decreasing error rate increases sample size
Type II error rate	Decreasing error rate increases sample size
Effect size*	Smaller effect size increases sample size
Variability	Smaller variability decreases sample size

*Difference between null and alternative hypothesis values.

this is just a matter of mathematics, the Bayesian formulation allows the incorporation of a more subjective notion of probability—the notion of probability as a measure of the strength of one's belief in a single outcome, for example the probability that your team will win the Super Bowl this season, or that the moon is made of green cheese. It further allows the application of this view of probability to unknown parameters governing a probability distribution: for example, the probability that the response rate to a treatment exceeds a fixed value. This is not a meaningful concept in a frequentist framework, because the response rate is viewed as a fixed number.

The Bayesian approach to statistical inference involves three basic steps: (a) specification of a *prior distribution* for the unknown parameter, based on existing knowledge; (b) collection of data; and (c) use of the data to update the prior distribution, resulting in a *posterior distribution*. A simple example involves a card game such as poker. In a fair game, any particular hand of cards is presumed equally likely to be dealt to any particular player (the prior distribution). After the cards are dealt, one observes one's own hand and perhaps parts of the hands of other players (the data). This information can be used to recalculate the probability that other players hold particular hands, which are no longer equally likely (the posterior distribution).

Although the mathematical basis of Bayesian statistics is not in question, the first of the steps noted above is one that has the potential to generate controversy in applying Bayesian methods to medical research. This is because the prior distribution is allowed to incorporate subjective judgments about the quantity under investigation. Many statisticians argue that prior beliefs about an unknown quantity represent a form of bias that should be avoided in scientific research. Fortunately, it is possible to employ a Bayesian framework in a way that avoids this objection, by choosing a prior distribution that is said to be *uninformative* with respect to the quantity under study (also sometimes called a *flat prior*). Interestingly, and reassuringly, statistical procedures conducted within the latter framework are often very similar to, or even identical to, those conducted within a frequentist framework, and produce very similar results. They simply use different mathematical machinery and terminology.

Some clinical trial designs make use of Bayesian concepts and these are described briefly in the next section covering clinical trials. Although less common, some forms of data analysis may also employ Bayesian methods. In situations where Bayesian methods have been employed in the design or analysis of a research study, one should always be able to ascertain the nature of the prior distribution. If a subjective or *informative* prior distribution has been used, its rationale and appropriateness should be carefully considered, and it should be recognized that the choice of a prior distribution can influence the interpretation and conclusions of the study.

CLINICAL TRIAL DESIGN

Clinical trials are a fundamental part of the process of medical science leading to developing treatments for cancer, as well as its prevention and detection. In oncology, clinical trials have historically been classified according to the general phases of drug development. Though this classification by no means accounts for all of the clinical trials relevant to oncology, it is a useful starting point for describing the key elements of trial design, which necessarily vary according to the objectives of the trial. Phase I trials focus on toxicity, with a goal of determining a dose and treatment regimen that would have acceptable toxicity if the drug were effective. Phase II trials are then designed to provide a preliminary indication of whether that therapy is effective. The result is considered preliminary because the study is uncontrolled, uses a surrogate endpoint (such as tumor response instead of survival), or is not large enough to rule out chance effects. The phase III trial is typically a controlled, randomized trial large enough to distinguish chance effects from true treatment effects. It is also not uncommon to see trials that are classified in other ways: e.g., as phase I/II, phase Ib, or phase II/III. There is no single governing body for trial nomenclature and trial sponsors are free to attach whatever labels they wish to a particular study. Sometimes this is driven by regulatory or insurance considerations: for example, the U.S. Food and Drug Administration offers definitions of trial phases for studies it regulates, and insurers may decline coverage for patients participating in certain phases of trials.

PHASE I

The initial phase of human experimentation in the development of chemotherapeutic agents involves finding a dose that produces an acceptable level of toxicity. What is acceptable obviously depends on the disease in question: in diseases like cancer with significant morbidity and mortality, the acceptable level of toxicity may be quite high. Indeed, with cytotoxic drugs, the toxicity of the drug may be to some extent a measure of its potential efficacy. With newer cytostatic or targeted agents, however, the presumed correlation of toxicity and efficacy may not hold, and the design of appropriate phase I trials for such agents can be challenging.

Traditionally, the objective of a phase I trial is to determine the maximum dose of an agent, either alone or in combination with other agents, which will produce an acceptable level of toxicity when administered by a specific schedule and route.

This dose is usually referred to as the maximum tolerable dose (MTD) or the recommended phase II dose. For example, a simple definition of acceptable toxicity might be "toxicity of grade 4 or worse in not more than one out of six patients" where grade 4 toxicity is defined according to standard criteria. The toxicity that defines the MTD is said to be dose-limiting toxicity (DLT). Once an MTD is established, one presumes that this dose will be used in further evaluations of efficacy in phase II trials; however, this logical progression is complicated by the fact that patient populations in phase I and II trials are likely to be dissimilar.

Phase I Endpoints and Patient Population

Since agents or regimens being tested in phase I trials have unproven efficacy, ethical considerations necessarily limit the patient population that can be enrolled in phase I trials. Typically these are patients for whom multiple lines of therapy have failed and for whom no standard treatment options remain. The patient population is generally heterogeneous with respect to disease diagnosis, but may be restricted to specific cancers, depending on the type of agent being tested and its mechanism of action. For example, it would have been inappropriate to test a highly targeted agent like imatinib mesylate in cancers other than chronic myeloid leukemia.

The most important endpoint to specify in a phase I trial is the definition of DLT. Although certain definitions are relatively common, the definition can vary considerably and may be tailored to reflect toxicities expected on the basis of the mechanism of action of the agent. The most common standard for rating the severity of toxicities is the National Cancer Institute's (NCI's) Common Toxicity Criteria (CTC). This provides specific criteria for grading a wide range of toxicities on a numeric scale: 0 (none), 1 (mild), 2 (moderate), 3 (severe), 4 (life-threatening), 5 (fatal). Most definitions of DLT exclude grade 1 or 2 toxicities, and possibly some grade 3 toxicities if these are expected and manageable—for example, neutropenia or nausea/vomiting. Thus, a composite definition of DLT might be "grade 3 nonhematologic toxicity or grade 4 hematologic toxicity." One must also specify the time frame over which toxicities will be evaluated for purposes of the trial. This is typically a relatively short time, such as 4 weeks or one treatment cycle, and thus captures only acute toxicities. Toxicities that occur after the specified observation period are not reflected in the outcome of the phase I trial, but may influence how the agent is used in later phase II trials.

Phase I Design Options

Almost all phase I trials pre-specify the starting dose of the agent being tested and a sequence of doses to be tested subsequently. The initial dose level is generally derived either from animal experiments, if the agent in question is completely novel, or by conservative consideration of previous human experience, if the agent in question has been used before but with a different schedule, route of administration, or with other concomitant drugs. A common starting point based on the former is from one-tenth to one-third of the mouse LD_{10}, the dose that kills 10% of mice, adjusted for size of the animal on a per-kilogram basis or by another method. Subsequent dose levels are determined by increasing the preceding dose by decreasing fractions: for example, 100%, 67%, 50%, 40%, and 33% thereafter. Such sequences are often referred to as "modified Fibonacci." With some agents, particularly biologic agents, the dose levels may be determined by log (i.e., 10-fold) or half-log increases of the preceding dose.

Designs for phase I trials are constrained by the practical need to use relatively small numbers of patients and the ethical need to approach the MTD conservatively. By far the most common design option for phase I trials is the 3+3 design. This design, or minor variations on it, has been in use since the 1950s. Briefly, beginning at the first dose level, cohorts of three patients are entered. If all three patients receive the agent at the specified dose without DLT, then the next cohort of three patients is entered at the next higher dose level. If two of three patients experience DLT, then the toxicity associated with that dose is considered unacceptable, and the dose level below it (if any was tested) is considered the MTD. If one of three patients experiences DLT, then an additional cohort of three patients is entered at the same dose level. If no further DLT is seen, then escalation to the next dose level is permitted for the next cohort; otherwise the toxicity is considered unacceptable, and the dose level below it is considered the MTD.

If the starting dose is too low, and/or the spacing of doses is too small relative to the steepness of the dose-response curve, then large numbers of patients may be enrolled at doses without toxicity (and likely with no therapeutic benefit). To address this problem, an accelerated titration design may use only single patients at the initial dose levels. Escalation continues until a grade 2 toxicity is seen, and then a standard 3+3 design is implemented at the next lower dose level. Because dose escalation is permitted based on the experience of only one patient, such designs are usually restricted to situations where there is some human experience with the agent, and the toxicity profile is known to be manageable.

Another design option, based on a Bayesian approach, is referred to as the continual reassessment method (CRM). Though there are many variations in the details, the basic concept is to define the probability of DLT that is acceptable (for example, 20% or 33%), assume a simple mathematical model for a dose-response curve, and then, after each patient (or cohort of patients) has been treated, update the mathematical estimate of the dose-response curve and treat the next patient (or cohort) at the dose level where the estimated probability of DLT would be closest to the target. Although it is well recognized in the statistical literature that model-based designs can outperform the 3+3 design in many aspects, the 3+3 design remains by far the predominant design in practice, owing to its simplicity and transparency.

PHASE II

Trials falling under the umbrella of phase II can be highly variable in design. These can range from small, single-arm trials involving a dozen patients to double-blind, placebo-controlled trials involving 200 patients. Trials like the latter typically fall into the phase II category only because they use an endpoint or sample size that falls short of that required to get regulatory approval for a drug. Nevertheless, there are some typical features that characterize a phase II trial: the endpoints are primarily related to efficacy, rather than toxicity; the sample size is moderately small, often 25 to 50 patients; the efficacy endpoint is short-term and/or not definitive, such as tumor response; and the study relies on historical experience as context for judging whether the result is promising enough to carry forward to phase III. This is the type of trial that will be considered phase II for purposes of this discussion.

Phase II Endpoints and Patient Population

The general objective of a phase II trial is to evaluate the potential effectiveness of a drug or regimen in a specific patient population. The patient population is usually fairly narrowly defined (for example, patients with stage III estrogen receptor–negative breast cancer). Patients enrolled into phase II trials typically have experienced treatment failure with at least one or two standard therapies; however, in diseases with no effective therapy, or when adding a new agent to the standard of care, a phase II trial may be tenable in the first-line setting. Finally, there are cases in which the treatment being evaluated in a phase II study is not novel, but is being applied to a new patient population; for example, a different type of cancer, or a subtype of cancer defined by a genetic or other biologic marker.

As noted, the primary endpoint of a phase II trial is efficacy. The specific endpoint driving the trial design reflects a balance between the ability to assess it over a relatively short time frame (weeks or months) and its validity as a measure of true long-term benefit. For this reason, 5-year survival is almost never an endpoint for a phase II trial, although 6-month or 1-year survival might be. With cytotoxic agents, partial or complete tumor response is a common and accepted phase II endpoint; with cytostatic agents, stable disease or lack of progression might be included as a successful short-term response. There are a number of established schemes for defining tumor response. For solid tumors, the Response Evaluation Criteria in Solid Tumors (RECIST) is standard. Most response definitions for solid tumors are based on the size and presence of measurable lesions. Other criteria must be used for hematologic malignancies. Whatever criteria are used, the trial design must specify how and when response will be assessed. The assessment must be homogenous within the trial and also reasonably comparable to other trials or to whatever data are used as historical context to judge the outcome of the trial.

In addition to tumor response and survival, there has been growing interest in the use of tumor biomarkers or other biochemical measures to assess the effectiveness of therapy, for example, prostate-specific antigen (PSA) in prostate cancer, CA-125 in ovarian cancer, or carcinoembryonic antigen (CEA) in colon cancer. The interest in biomarkers correlates especially with the use of so-called targeted therapy, which may have very specific mechanisms of action that are measured by a variety of assays, possibly from blood or tumor samples that can be obtained quickly and easily, although the assays themselves may be neither inexpensive nor quick. Unfortunately, the valid use of biomarkers as surrogate endpoints requires specific criteria that may be difficult to validate. Notably, it is not sufficient to establish a correlation between the biomarker and outcome. A full discussion of these issues is beyond the scope of this chapter, but in general one should be cautious in evaluating claims of effectiveness based on biomarkers or other surrogate endpoints.

Phase II Design Options

We consider first the most common phase II paradigm, a simple single-arm trial using historical outcomes as a point of reference for the design and interpretation of the trial. Such a trial is often designed from a hypothesis testing point of view. For example, suppose that tumor response is the endpoint of choice, and that standard regimens have a response rate of approximately p_0, or otherwise that a regimen with a response rate of p_0 would be considered not worth further study. Conversely, suppose that p_1 is a response rate that would represent meaningful improvement over standard regimens, or otherwise that a regimen with a response rate of p_1 would be considered of interest for further study.

The hypothesis testing paradigm assumes that at the end of the trial, one will either (a) conclude that the true response rate for the regimen is greater than p_0 or (b) not conclude this. The design parameters must also include a specification of the false-positive (type I, or α) error rate and false-negative (type II, or β) error rate. The false-positive error rate is the probability of falsely concluding that the true response rate for the regimen is greater than p_0, when in fact it is equal to p_0. The false-negative error rate is the probability of falsely *not* concluding that the true response rate for the regimen is greater than p_0, when in fact it is equal to p_1. These error rates typically range from 5% to 20%. The possibility of relatively high error rates is accepted, because low error rates require a larger sample size for the trial; however, the major factor driving the sample size is the difference between p_0 and p_1: the larger the difference, the smaller the sample size required for a specified set of error rates. This fact often leads to unrealistic design assumptions, i.e., setting p_0 unrealistically low, or p_1 implausibly high.

Table 5-4 shows some possible trial designs under a variety of assumptions about p_0 and p_1, and allowable error rates. The value r is the minimum number of responses required in n patients in order to conclude (with specified type I error rate no greater than α) that the true response rate for the regimen is greater than p_0. A common misconception is that observing r responses allows one to conclude that the true response rate is at least p_1. That this is not the case is obvious from the fact that the observed minimum response rate required (that is, r/n) is less than p_1.

In some cases the endpoint of interest in a phase II trial may not be tumor response, but a time-to-event endpoint, such as overall survival or progression-free survival. For many cancer diagnoses, unfortunately, the median time to death or progression is measured in months or weeks. Thus, for example, if historical data suggest that the median progression-free interval with standard regimens is 3 months, this can be recast into the paradigm above by noting that this is equivalent to specifying

Table 5-4 Examples of Single-Stage Phase II Designs

Design Criteria				Resulting Design	
p_0	p_1	α	β	n	r
0.10	0.25	0.05	0.10	55	10
0.10	0.25	0.05	0.20	40	8
0.10	0.25	0.10	0.10	40	7
0.10	0.25	0.10	0.20	31	6
0.10	0.25	0.05	0.10	33	7
0.10	0.25	0.05	0.20	25	6
0.10	0.25	0.10	0.10	25	5
0.10	0.25	0.10	0.20	18	4
0.50	0.70	0.05	0.10	53	33
0.50	0.70	0.05	0.20	37	24
0.50	0.70	0.10	0.10	39	24
0.50	0.70	0.10	0.20	28	18

p_0, response rate under null hypothesis; p_1, response rate under alternative hypothesis; α, type I (false-positive) error rate if $p = p_0$; β, type II (false-negative) error rate if $p = p_1$; n, smallest sample size that satisfies design criteria; r, minimum number of responses required to reject null hypothesis and conclude $p > p_0$.

Table 5-5 Confidence Intervals for True Response Rates

Observed Rate = 0.10		95% CI	Observed Rate = 0.50		95% CI
n	r		n	r	
10	1	0.3, 44.5	10	5	18.7, 81.3
20	2	1.2, 31.7	20	10	27.2, 72.8
30	3	2.1, 31.7	30	15	31.3, 68.7
40	4	2.8, 23.7	40	20	33.8, 66.2
50	5	3.3, 21.8	50	25	35.5, 64.5
60	10	4.9, 17.6	60	50	39.8, 60.2

n, sample size; r, observed number of responses; CI, confidence interval for true response rate (Clopper-Pearson exact interval).

that the percent of patients alive and progression-free at 3 months, p_0, is 50%. With some simple assumptions about the distribution of progression times, a hypothetical improvement to the median progression-free interval can be converted to a value of p_1 at 3 months.

The hypothesis testing framework is useful for formulating the design and deciding on a sample size. In reality, however, it is rare that the hypothesis test is formally carried out at the end of the trial. Instead, one calculates an estimate and confidence interval for the response rate associated with the agent, and places this in context with a host of other factors before deciding whether further trials are warranted. The estimated response rate is relatively imprecise (Table 5-5), and actually provides only a rough indication of the response rate.

A common alternative to the simple single-stage design is a design that enrolls patients in two stages. The motivation for this alternative is simple. For example, consider the first scenario in Table 5-4, requiring 55 patients and 10 observed responses in order to reach a successful conclusion. Suppose that in a particular trial, after 25 patients have been treated, only two responses have been observed. Thus, in order to reach the target of 10 responses, eight responses must be observed in the final 30 patients, a seemingly unlikely scenario given what has been observed in the initial patients. Two-stage designs formalize the intuitive notion that the trial should be terminated early if the results are poorer than hoped for and there is little chance of a successful outcome to the trial. This is done by dividing the enrollment into two stages and specifying the minimum number of responses that must be observed in the first

stage before enrolling the second stage. For a given set of design parameters there are many two-stage designs that satisfy them. One common criterion for selecting a two-stage design is to use Simon's optimum design, which is the design that minimizes the average number of patients that would be enrolled if the true response rate was no better than the historical reference p_0. Table 5-6 shows Simon's optimal two-stage design for the same situations as in Table 5-4. Note that the maximum sample size for these designs is often only slightly larger than for a single-stage design, with error rates satisfying the same specifications. For example, the design for the first scenario requires (at most) 57 patients, compared with the 55 patients required with a single-stage design.

The term *optimum* relates to a mathematical criterion, which sometimes leads to a design with an imbalance in the sizes of the stages that seems impractical; for example, by assigning 70% of the enrollment to the first stage. In such cases there are almost always alternatives that are mathematically not quite optimal, but more appealing in terms of the split between stages, while still satisfying the other design parameters.

All of the designs considered thus far are single-arm, nonrandomized designs; however, some phase II trials enroll patients to more than one arm and use randomization for allocation to each arm. The reasons motivating randomized phase II designs are many, and sometimes somewhat controversial. In some cases, it is asserted that there is no intent to compare the arms: they are to be regarded as independent trials of different agents or regimens that happen to target the same patient population, and random assignment is simply a mechanism to ensure that the arms enroll patients with roughly similar characteristics.

The more classic setting of the randomized phase II trial is a case in which there are two or more variations of the same experimental agent, or two or more closely related experimental agents, and the desire is to "pick the winner" for subsequent study or for comparison against standard therapy in a phase III trial. For example, there might be two plausible doses of an agent or a gene vaccine carried in three possible vectors. In this

Table 5-6 Examples of Two-Stage Phase II Designs (Optimal Simon Design)

Design Criteria				Resulting Design			
				First Stage		Overall	
p_0	p_1	α	β	n_1	r_1	n	r
0.10	0.25	0.05	0.10	28	4	57	10
0.10	0.25	0.05	0.20	18	3	43	8
0.10	0.25	0.10	0.10	21	3	50	8
0.10	0.25	0.10	0.20	13	2	34	6
0.10	0.25	0.05	0.10	18	3	35	7
0.10	0.25	0.05	0.20	10	2	29	6
0.10	0.25	0.10	0.10	12	2	35	6
0.10	0.25	0.10	0.20	7	1	18	4
0.50	0.70	0.05	0.10	23	13	57	35
0.50	0.70	0.05	0.20	15	9	43	27
0.50	0.70	0.10	0.10	21	12	45	27
0.50	0.70	0.10	0.20	12	7	32	20

p_0, response rate under null hypothesis; p_1, response rate under alternative hypothesis; α, type I (false-positive) error rate if $p = p_0$; β, type II (false-negative) error rate if $p = p_1$; n_1, sample size for first stage; r_1, minimum number of responses required in first stage to enroll second stage; n, total sample size after both stages; r, total number of responses required to reject null hypothesis and conclude $p > p_0$.

Table 5-7 Minimum Sample Size (Per Arm) for "Pick the Winner" Randomized Phase II Designs

Difference (p_1-p_0)	Two Arms (p_0, p_1)		Three Arms (p_0, p_0, p_1)	
	1-β = 0.80	1-β = 0.90	1-β = 0.80	1-β = 0.90
0.10	45	92	78	134
0.15	22	43	37	61
0.20	13	25	22	35

1-β, probability that arm with highest true response rate has highest observed response rate; p_0, lower response rate; p_1, higher response rate.

of the response rate with the standard regimen, instead of relying on historical data. Nevertheless, if the results happen to be highly favorable for the regimen containing the experimental agent, it may be tempting to make an explicit statistical comparison between arms, as for a phase III trial, and claim it as equivalent to a phase III trial. Such selective comparisons inflate the type I error rate in ways that are difficult to correct for.

A final phase II design strategy that should be mentioned is an approach known as adaptive randomization. This may be applied in the setting described above, or the arms may involve quite distinct agents or regimens. The trial starts out by randomly assigning patients in equal proportion to each arm. As outcome data on these patients accumulate, the randomization scheme is altered so that it favors arms where the strength of the evidence that the response rate is greater than p_0 is greatest. Conversely, it disfavors arms where the strength of evidence is lowest, and ultimately may drop arms altogether if the strength of evidence falls too low. Such designs frequently are associated with Bayesian methods, though this is not an essential feature of the approach.

Although adaptive randomization seems like a highly rational way to select among competing experimental regimens, in practice it is often difficult to mount such a trial. The different agents likely have different sponsors and advocates, each of which naturally has a principal interest in their own agent, and a reluctance to cede control of its evaluation to an external process. Others have some ethical discomfort with the notion of unequal allocation based on evidence of efficacy, feeling that this violates the principle of *clinical equipoise* (that one truly is unable to say which treatment is better for the patient population to be enrolled).

Biases in Phase II Trials

Among all of the phases of therapeutic development, phase II is the most fraught with the potential for bias. The major source of bias is the absence of contemporaneous randomized comparison groups. Historical outcomes vary widely, for many reasons, and past experience may reflect many factors besides the agents being tested. These can include the eligibility criteria defining the patient population; the definition, timing, and methods used to assess outcome; standards of supportive care that vary by institution and over time; the use of surrogate endpoints; and, of course, simple random variation. Even in the

case there is a stated desire to compare the arms and pick the best one, but since both arms are experimental there is no need to control the false-positive (type I) error rate. That is, if the true response rate for two experimental arms is equivalent, there is no error in picking one over the other. This is in contrast to the prototypical phase III paradigm, in which concluding that the experimental arm is different from standard, when in fact they are equivalent, is considered an error.

In a pick-the-winner design, the arm that has the highest observed response rate at the end of the trial is selected for further study. The sole design consideration is that if the response rates in the two arms differ by a specified amount Δ, then the false-negative (type II) error rate should be no higher than β. Thus, Δ is a difference in response rates that is considered clinically important. If two arms differ by this amount or more, then the sample size should be large enough that the observed response rate in the better arm will be higher than that in the other arm, with probability 1-β. Table 5-7 provides some examples of design parameters for a randomized phase II trial and the sample size required for each.

Although the concept is statistically sound in principle, the randomized phase II design can be used in ways that compromise its validity. For example, suppose that the two arms are a standard regimen plus an experimental agent versus a standard regimen plus placebo. It may be asserted that the control arm is included simply to provide a more contemporaneous estimate absence of any systematic bias, itself an ideal unlikely achieved, the random outcomes observed in relatively small numbers of patients lead to many false conclusions. The most observable of these are false-positive results—agents that look promising in phase II trials often fail to be proven effective in phase III trials. Less observable, but just as unfortunate, are agents that are in truth effective but fail to show positive results in phase II trials.

PHASE III

The randomized clinical trial is the gold standard of clinical research, and this is the trial that is most often referred to as a phase III trial. The classic setting for the phase III trial is to compare an experimental therapy with a standard therapy. A common analogy applied to this setting is that of a legal trial. In a clinical trial one formulates a null hypothesis that the experimental treatment is equally effective as the standard (the defendant is innocent), though of course there must be some scientific basis to believe otherwise (the prosecution has evidence). In order to establish effectiveness (guilt), a trial is conducted that will lead to the rejection of the null hypothesis in a convincing way (beyond a reasonable doubt). As in a legal trial, failure to reject the null hypothesis (finding of not guilty) is not the same as establishing equivalence of the therapies (innocence).

Of course, randomized clinical trials don't always fit the classic paradigm of an experimental versus standard therapy, but the principles underlying the design and analysis will likely be equally applicable.

Basic Principles

The primary goal of a phase III trial is to provide a comparison of treatments that is free of the many biases that arise when trying to compare phase II trials conducted at different times, at different institutions, among different patient populations, etc. The accepted standard for ensuring freedom from bias is randomization. Randomization is not the only way to create comparable treatment groups, nor does randomization guarantee that the results of a particular trial are correct, but randomization does allow one to control and quantify the possibility of error.

The most common randomization strategy is equal allocation among all treatment arms. From the standpoint of statistical power this is the most efficient allocation, and also the one most compatible with the notion of clinical equipoise. A common variation of simple randomization is stratified randomization, which seeks to ensure even greater balance between arms by randomly assigning patients within strata defined by factors that strongly predict outcome. Additionally the randomization may be "blocked," which generally refers to a form of stratification designed to keep the number of patients allocated to each arm balanced over time. Stratification and blocking are most useful in small trials, in which random imbalances large enough to skew the composition of the treatment arms are not impossible. When the trials become larger (several hundred patients) these devices are largely superfluous, as it becomes highly unlikely the arms will become meaningfully imbalanced by chance.

Departures from equal allocation sometimes occur—for example, a 2:1 allocation between the experimental and control arm. Most commonly this is justified with the argument that this makes the trial more attractive to potential patients and their physicians, particularly when there is no way to get access to an experimental agent except through participation in the trial. However, this argument seems to presume that the experimental therapy is likely to be more effective than standard, which contradicts the principle of equipoise.

Other common, but by no means necessary, components of a phase III design include the use of a placebo, and the implementation of blinded (to the patient) or double-blinded (to both patient and physician) treatment assignments. Although randomization can help ensure that the treatment arms are balanced with respect to patient characteristics at the start of the trial, it cannot remove bias that arises after the trial starts, when differences arise between arms with respect to the conduct of the trial or the evaluation of trial data. This bias can be entirely unintentional and unconscious, but reflects behavior by either patients or physicians that compromises the benefits of randomization. The susceptibility of trials to bias can vary considerably depending on the endpoint in question. For example, placebo effects and ascertainment bias are probably unlikely to affect a trial where mortality is the primary endpoint. On the other hand, assessment of tumor response without blinding to treatment assignment could be subject to subtle bias, and studies with self-reported quality-of-life endpoints are obviously prone to placebo effects.

The use of placebo as the control arm in therapeutic oncology trials is extremely rare, since usually some form of therapy is available, even if ineffective. A placebo control is much more likely to be used in adjuvant trials, or trials of combination therapy where a new agent is being added to an existing combination. Though one may question the extent to which placebo effects play a role in such settings, if a placebo is feasible it adds credibility to a trial even if the likelihood of placebo effects is small. In some cases, of course, the nature of the treatments differs so much that neither placebos nor blinding are feasible.

The most acceptable primary analysis of a phase III trial is the intent-to-treat analysis. This analysis includes all patients enrolled onto an arm of a randomized trial, no matter what happens thereafter: for example, they are unable to receive the full course of treatment, they cross over to another treatment, etc. Since any of these contingencies can be related to the treatment itself and to the effectiveness of the treatment, an unbiased analysis must incorporate that information. For example, if a new drug is potentially effective but many patients won't take it because of side effects, then as a practical matter it may not be as effective as a drug with fewer side effects.

Nevertheless, alternative analyses may be undertaken that deviate from the intent-to-treat principle. These may involve analyzing a subset of patients (for example, those who received a minimum amount of therapy), or defining the treatment groups according to the treatment actually received instead of the treatment to which they were randomly assigned. These alternative analyses can be informative, but must be interpreted cautiously and are problematic when the results differ markedly from the intent-to-treat analysis.

Other subset analyses may be undertaken to evaluate whether the treatment difference, if any, varies according to other factors, such as disease stage, age, or the presence of a biomarker. Even if specified in advance, the results of such subset analyses must be interpreted cautiously. Phase III studies are almost never large enough to have reliable power in subsets of patients; conversely, examining many subsets of patients in a trial with an overall negative result can lead to spurious findings that are caused only by random fluctuation.

Interim Analysis

Randomized phase III trials can be large, expensive, and of several years' duration. For this reason, most phase III trials have a provision for interim analysis at one or more points in time, with the possibility of terminating the trial early. The indications for early termination can be varied and are generally specified in advance. These may include strong evidence that the experimental arm is better than the control arm, strong evidence that it is worse, or a determination that the trial will not be conclusive (futility).

There are a number of statistical approaches to interim analysis that codify the timing and nature of the analyses and the threshold required to terminate the trial early. In the case that the trial is to be stopped early because of evidence that the experimental arm is superior, there is a need to quantify and control the overall false-positive rate (type I error rate) for the trial as a whole. Because small sample sizes are subject to a large amount of random variation, the threshold for stopping a trial early generally involves a high degree of statistical significance, meaning type I error rates that are much lower than a standard 0.05 level of significance, for example as low as 0.001 or 0.0001.

Also, if some of the type I error rate is "spent" during interim analyses, then the significance level for the final analysis will be lower than nominal. The threshold significance levels at each of the interim analyses and final analysis comprise the stopping boundary.

In some cases, the data at an interim analysis contain little suggestion that there is a difference in outcome between arms, or indicate that the difference is much smaller than hypothesized when designing the trial. Based on the accumulated data and assumptions about the true treatment effect, it is possible to generate estimates of the probability that the trial will prove successful at demonstrating the superiority of the experimental arm. If this probability is too low, the trial may be terminated early so as to minimize unnecessary time and expense. This is referred to as stopping for futility. On the other hand, as noted above, the inability to demonstrate a difference is not the same as demonstrating equivalence. A trial that is terminated early for futility may be quite inconclusive. Therefore, in some cases it may be desirable to complete a trial that cannot demonstrate a treatment benefit, if completing the trial might allow one to make firm conclusions regarding the lack of benefit.

Although the interim analysis plan for a phase III trial should be pre-specified and an integral part of the trial design, the decision to stop a trial early involves complex and important issues which cannot be summarized in a simple statistical test. Typically, the results of an interim analysis will be reviewed by a Data and Safety Monitoring Board (DSMB). The role of the DSMB is to independently review the results of an interim analysis, consider the results in context with a host of other factors (which may be scientific, ethical, legal, or financial), and make a recommendation as to whether to continue the trial or not.

Equivalence and Noninferiority Designs

Although most phase III trials are undertaken with an underlying goal of demonstrating a difference between treatment arms, there are circumstances in which the goal is merely to demonstrate that one therapy is equivalent, or at least not inferior, to another. For example, a therapy that is less toxic, less inconvenient, or less expensive than another would be preferred if it was nearly equally effective.

It is impossible to design a trial to demonstrate that two therapies are exactly equivalent, and highly unlikely in truth that they are. Instead, one specifies the smallest difference that would be of practical clinical significance, for example a 5% difference in 1-year survival, and then designs a trial that has high power to reject the null hypothesis (low type II error rate) if such a difference truly existed. A successful trial from the standpoint of equivalence would then fail to reject the null hypothesis. Note that the concepts of a false-positive or a false-negative conclusion are in a way reversed from the usual design perspective, and the typical rates of type I and type II error employed in such designs might need to be reconsidered. Equivalence studies are notoriously large because the difference in outcome said to define equivalence is typically smaller than the difference hypothesized for a superiority trial, which dramatically affects the sample size. For example, as seen in Table 5-8, a trial with an equivalency

Table 5-8 **Required Sample Size (Per Arm) for Equivalence and Noninferiority Trials with a Binomial Endpoint (p_0 = 0.50, α = 0.05, and 1-β = 0.90)**

Allowable Difference (p_0-p_1)	Equivalence Design	Noninferiority Design
0.25	77	69
0.20	124	108
0.15	227	191
0.10	519	429
0.05	2,095	1,713

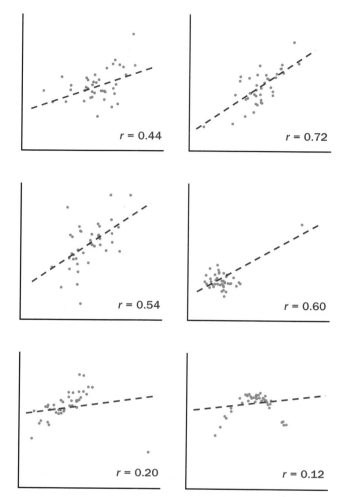

r = 0.44

r = 0.72

r = 0.54

r = 0.60

r = 0.20

r = 0.12

Fig. 5-2 Examples of linear correlation.

The six panels illustrate possible correlations between two variables, x and y. The dashed line indicates the least-squares line fit to the data, and r is the Pearson correlation coefficient.

threshold set at a 5% difference requires a sample size four times as large as a superiority trial powered to detect a 10% difference.

An alternative to an equivalency design that can require a somewhat smaller sample size is the noninferiority design. In this case one specifies an acceptable upper limit to inferiority of the new therapy compared to the old, i.e., how much worse it could be and still be considered acceptable. The trial is designed by formulating a null hypothesis that the new therapy has that level of inferiority, or worse, and then is powered to reject that null hypothesis for a specified alternative assumption (which might be equivalence, a lesser degree of inferiority, or even superiority). This usually results in a smaller sample size than an equivalence design, partly because it involves a one-sided hypothesis test, but often as a result of claiming a wider limit of acceptability for noninferiority than for equivalence.

CORRELATIVE STUDIES

Many studies in oncology are focused on evaluating the association between measureable attributes of a patient or the

patient's disease at a particular point in time and subsequent events or outcomes. These attributes may be measured before the start of treatment, possibly with a view toward predicting the therapy most likely to be effective, or after treatment has been initiated, with the intent of predicting whether the treatment is working. Although almost any clinical study is involved with evaluating association in the broad sense, the term *correlative study* most often refers to studies where the attribute being associated is not clinically apparent but must be assessed through some kind of test procedure, be it imaging, immunohistochemistry, gene expression, or any of a wide range of other procedures. Also bear in mind that a correlative study may or may not involve the analysis of *correlation*, which is a statistical term for a specific kind of association.

Correlative studies can be conducted during any of the phases of therapeutic development, and in fact are often explicitly incorporated as ancillary objectives in a therapeutic trial. They can also be conducted completely independently of therapeutic trials. The potential range of correlative studies is so broad that it is impossible to summarize succinctly the statistical methods or designs for such studies; this chapter first shows some examples of a basic measure of correlation and illustrates some general pitfalls in the evaluation of correlation. This chapter also discuss two important issues that can arise under the umbrella of correlative studies: the relationship between correlation and causation, and the issue of multiple comparisons.

Examples of Correlation

As noted above, correlation is a generic term that might describe almost any trial or analysis of association, but it may be helpful to consider a very basic notion of correlation that arises when both factors under study are measureable on a continuous scale, exemplified by the x-y scatterplot and sample correlation coefficient. The scatterplot is simply a visual representation of how one factor varies as a function of another. The Pearson correlation coefficient, r, is a measure of the *linear correlation* between the two variables: a value of +1 means perfect correlation, a value of 0 means no correlation, and a value of -1 means perfect inverse correlation. An associated value, r^2, ranges from 0 to 1 and is interpreted as the fraction of the variation in one variable that is explained by variation in another.* The degree of correlation is a function of three factors: (a) the magnitude of the association, i.e., whether the change in one variable is associated with a large or small change in the other; (b) the consistency of the relationship, i.e., whether the changes are consistent or highly variable; and (c) the linearity of the relationship. The first two factors pertain generally to any measure of correlation; the third is a consideration for Pearson's correlation coefficient r.

Figure 5-2 provides several examples of an x-y scatterplot, along with a fitted line and the value of r. The top panels illustrate how both the scatter and steepness of the association affect the degree of correlation. Moving from panel A to B, the data are just

---

* For r^2, variation is measured by the sum of squared deviations from the mean. There are many other measures of variation.

as variable, but there is an increase in the rate of change in y as a function of the change in x (slope), resulting in higher correlation. Moving to panel C, the slope stays the same as in panel B, but the variability increases, decreasing correlation. The bottom panels illustrate common pitfalls that arise in correlation studies: in panel D, the apparent correlation between x and y is based on a single point that is far away from the majority of data. Whether this represents a real biologic phenomenon would be debatable. Conversely, in panel E, an outlying observation obscures an apparent correlation in the majority of observations. Finally, in panel F, there is a clear relationship between x and y, but it is not a linear relationship and therefore is not reflected in r.

Correlation and Causation

One setting in which correlative studies have become common is the development of targeted therapies. These therapies are designed around specific attributes of tumors, which nominally can be quantified by measuring some biologic parameter. It may be possible to establish a clear correlation between this biomarker and prognosis; it may also be possible to establish that a targeted therapy has an effect on the biomarker in a direction that would imply a more favorable prognosis. Taking these two correlations together, it might appear that this is a clear indication that the therapy would be effective for that cancer, but this is not necessarily the case. Figure 5-3 indicates how this seeming contradiction can arise, when the biomarker is correlated with the disease process but is not part of the causal pathway related to the ultimate outcomes of interest.

A familiar analogy would be the association of elevated blood pressure and cholesterol with various forms of cardiovascular disease. Although there are many drugs that lower blood pressure and cholesterol, this does not guarantee that these drugs will be effective in lowering the risk of the correlated cardiovascular disease. In order for this to be true, the elevation of blood pressure or cholesterol must be part of the causal pathway to the cardiovascular event, not just a marker or symptom of the severity of the disease process. The same must hold true in order for the effect of a targeted therapy on a cancer biomarker to be considered an indicator of efficacy; that is, the biomarker must reflect at least part of the direct causal

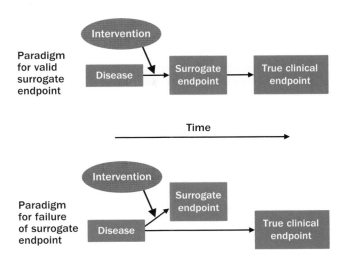

Fig. 5-3 Criteria for surrogate endpoints.
A schematic illustrating how a surrogate endpoint, or biomarker, may or may not be valid as a substitute for the true clinical endpoint. At the top, the surrogate endpoint is in the causal pathway of the disease process. An intervention that affects the surrogate endpoint should also affect the true clinical endpoint. At the bottom, the surrogate endpoint results from an independent causal pathway. It will be correlated with the clinical endpoint, but an intervention affecting the surrogate endpoint will have no effect on clinical outcome.

pathway by which growth or spread of the tumor has an effect on the survival of the patient.

Multiple Comparisons

Advances in technology have made it possible to assess hundreds, thousands, or even millions of potential markers within reasonable limits of expense and time. This is particularly true in the field of genomics, where single chips have the ability to simultaneously quantify the expression of 20,000 genes, or to genotype more than a million single nucleotide polymorphisms. Although there may be some sophisticated statistical methodology underlying the quantification of gene expression or assigning a genotype, the basic methodology for evaluating a correlation with outcome could be based on a simple t-test or chi-squared test, repeated thousands or hundreds of thousands of times.

From the hypothesis testing point of view, if each of these tests of association has a positive (type I) error rate set at conventional levels, such as 5%, then the number of false-positive correlations found will be enormous. For example, consider a gene expression study of 20,000 genes, to be correlated with tumor response in hopes of determining one or more markers that signal a high likelihood of treatment failure. Even if the 20,000 genes have been selected to represent a range of plausible causal pathways, only a small fraction of them are likely to be truly correlated with outcome. As an order of magnitude calculation, the number of false positives that will result from 20,000 hypothesis tests conducted with a 5% type I error rate is 1,000, which is far too many to represent practical progress.

Although it is obvious in this setting that some measure must be taken to decrease the number of false-positive correlations, it

KEY POINTS

- Common measures of correlation assess the linear correlation between variables. Lack of linear correlation does not necessarily mean that the variables are not related.
- Measures of correlation may be sensitive to a few outlying observations.
- Correlation, by itself, does not imply causation. Even though a biomarker may be correlated with both treatment and outcome, this is not sufficient to establish that the biomarker is a useful surrogate endpoint.

is not always clear what specific target to set. For example, if one insists that the rate of *any* false-positive correlation be 5%, then a simple, though conservative, method is to apply the Bonferroni correction, which divides the nominal single test error rate by the number of tests. In the example at hand, this would mean conducting each test with a type I error rate of 0.0000025. Although there are methods to make this conservative adjustment more accurate, it is not clear that this is even a reasonable goal. For example, it seems unreasonably conservative to demand that the rate of even a single false-positive result across 20,000 tests be only 5%. Unless the size of the study is increased, a reduction in the false-positive error rate by four orders of magnitude will increase the false-negative error rate, perhaps to the point that correlations of a plausible magnitude cannot be detected.

Another method of controlling false positives considers the error rate *among the tests that have been declared positive*, not among all tests. This is called the false discovery rate (FDR). With this approach, if there were 100 positive tests, an FDR of 5% would mean that, on average, 5 of the 100 would be false positives. Most researchers would consider such a result highly successful. In fact, 10 positive tests with an FDR of 20% to 30% could be considered an excellent result, and would greatly reduce the scale of the subsequent studies required to replicate and validate the findings. The FDR method is generally less conservative than a strict Bonferroni adjustment, though as noted above there are ways to calibrate the Bonferroni approach, for example through permutation, to make it more comparable to the FDR approach.

Although we have considered examples where the need to account for multiple tests is obvious, the problem of false positives remains even when dealing with five to 10 markers. Explicit accounting of the multiple tests is often omitted in such situations, but this does not obviate the need for independent replication and validation of any apparent correlation.

STATISTICAL ANALYSIS METHODS

This section discusses some of the more important and advanced statistical methods that are common in oncology studies. Of course, each of these is itself the subject of entire books, and thus only the most basic features of these methods can be covered. The greater part of the section is devoted to the analysis of survival or time-to-event data, which are ubiquitous in the evaluation of clinical research. Some other advanced methods that may be encountered are also covered.

A common feature of the analytic methods discussed here is that they can be extended to incorporate the simultaneous effects of multiple variables on outcome, referred to as *regression analysis*.* This is particularly important in comparative studies using retrospective or other nonrandomized data, or developing predictive models evaluating multiple, possibly correlated factors.

---

* Regression analysis involving multiple variables is frequently referred to as *multivariate* (or sometimes multivariable) analysis, in contrast to *univariate* analysis, which considers only one variable at a time.

SURVIVAL ANALYSIS

Because of the potentially long temporal course of the disease, a large part of the evaluation of cancer and its treatment involves extended periods of follow-up, often spanning many years. Measures of therapeutic efficacy or prognostic value are frequently defined by the percentage of patients alive at a particular time, or alive and free of recurrence at a particular time. Conversely, one might be interested in the median time to death, recurrence, or some other defining event. Very often it is not possible to follow all patients until the defining event occurs, or even until they have reached a specified length of follow-up.

The analysis of data related to the duration of time until an event is generically referred to as time-to-event analysis, or survival analysis. The methods employed in such analysis must take into account the fact that some patients will not be followed until the time of the event, but provide partial information about the length of that time, i.e., the length of time from the start of follow-up until the time of analysis. The truncation of follow-up prior to a defining event is called censoring. The fraction of event times that are censored may range from near 0, in settings where almost all patients die or have recurrent disease, to over 90% in settings with excellent survival.

The most common display of censored survival data is the survival curve. This is an estimate of the underlying survival function, $S(t)$, that defines the probability of surviving past time t, or more generally that the time to a defining event exceeds t. Although this is the way that data are visualized, the statistical analysis of such data is more often based on a related quantity called the hazard function, $\lambda(t)$, which is the underlying rate at which events occur among the population of patients at risk. This is feasible because there is a well-defined and fundamental mathematical relationship between the survival function and hazard function; intuitively, if the rate of events increases, then the probability of surviving without that event decreases.

The most common methods associated with displaying and analyzing time-to-event data are described below. There are two key assumptions underlying all of these methods. One is that the censoring of event times, if it occurs, is not related to the subsequent occurrence of the event, i.e., that the reason for censoring is uninformative with respect to what happens afterward. Another fundamental principle of survival analysis, since survival is a predictive quantity, is that only past information can be used in modeling and analyzing future events. An example in which the latter principle is violated would be the division of patients in to two groups, depending on whether they had a tumor response or not, and evaluating time to death from the time of initiation of therapy. The groups are therefore defined using future information, and unbiased predictions of survival after the start of therapy cannot use this information.

Kaplan-Meier Curves

The universal standard for providing estimates of survival curves is the Kaplan-Meier estimator (sometimes also called the product-limit estimator). This is typically plotted as a step function, with a step occurring at every unique death time. The calculation involved in the Kaplan-Meier estimator

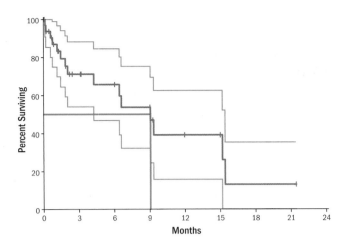

Fig. 5-4 A survival curve and related quantities.

The purple line is an example of a Kaplan-Meier curve for a group of 33 patients. At any point in time, the curve estimates the probability of surviving at least as long as that time. Gray lines indicate the limits of 95% confidence intervals for the survival probability calculated at each point in time. Tick marks indicate times at which surviving patients are last known alive. The green line indicates how median survival would be calculated: in this curve, the survival probability drops below 50% at 9 months.

is actually quite simple—the height of each step is the height of the curve at the previous step, multiplied by the fraction of patients at risk at the particular death time that survive beyond that time. The number of patients "at risk" at a particular point in time is the number of patients who have not died or been censored before that time. For example, suppose that the time until death or censoring is measured to the nearest week. If the estimated survival probability just before 14 weeks is 0.6, there are 10 patients who have not died or been censored before 14 weeks, and one patient dies at 14 weeks, then the height of the curve drops at that time from 0.6 to 0.6 × (9/10) = 0.54. In plots of Kaplan-Meier curves it is common to indicate points of censoring with tick marks, or to provide a table indicating the numbers of patients at risk at convenient benchmarks.

Because the Kaplan-Meier estimate is the product of fractions with increasingly smaller denominators, the precision of the estimate decreases over time. This is readily apparent if confidence bands are provided, as the confidence bands will grow increasingly wide over time. In almost all cases the confidence bands provided with a Kaplan-Meier curve are based on "pointwise" estimates of the variability of the survival estimate; it is usually not correct to infer that the bands contain the entirety of the true survival curve with the stated level of confidence. The step following the last observed death time is often extended out as far as the last censoring time, though technically the estimate is undefined after the last death. As noted above, the steps in the right-hand tail of the estimated curve grow larger as the number of patients at risk decreases. If the last patient under observation dies, then the estimated survival probability drops to 0 at that time point.

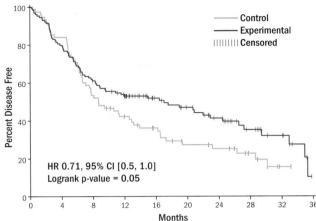

Fig. 5-5 Comparing survival curves.

The two curves represent a hypothetical comparison of disease-free survival for two treatments. The curves drop when a patient experiences relapse, or dies without relapse (treatment-related mortality).

Figure 5-4 illustrates a Kaplan-Meier curve in a relatively small sample of 33 patients, 15 of whom died. Tick marks indicate the points at which surviving patients are last known alive. The lighter gray bands indicate pointwise 95% confidence intervals for the survival probability. The green lines indicate how median survival is estimated from a Kaplan-Meier curve: this is the time at which the estimated survival probability first drops below 50%.

Although in the above discussion we have referred only to deaths, the Kaplan-Meier method readily encompasses the concept of event-free survival. For example, the estimate of disease-free survival counts both deaths and relapses as events, and the curve steps down whenever either event occurs, using the same calculation. The term "overall survival" is usually meant to refer to a survival curve that counts only deaths as events. The term "actuarial survival" is a misnomer—it refers back to a different method of estimating the survival curve (the actuarial, or life-table, method) that was used prior to the introduction of the Kaplan-Meier method but is now obsolete in the medical context. The Kaplan-Meier method should not be used when the intent is to estimate the probability of being free of a particular kind of event, for example a particular cause of death. This is a "competing risks" problem and requires the use of methods described below.

Comparing Kaplan-Meier Curves

The comparison of survival curves can be approached in several ways: (a) by comparing the estimated survival probability at a fixed point in time; (b) by comparing the time at which the estimated survival probability is a fixed value, usually the median; or (c) by comparing the survival curves across the entire period of follow-up. In general, the first two approaches should be avoided unless there is a very strong justification for focusing on a particular survival time or percentile. This is because the comparison clearly can vary depending on the point chosen.

The most common way to compare survival curves across time is with the log-rank statistic, as illustrated in Figure 5-5, which compares disease-free survival in a hypothetical clinical trial of an experimental versus control treatment. Perhaps somewhat surprisingly, this statistic is not based directly on the calculated survival estimates; rather, it is based on a comparison of the number of events *observed* to occur in one group to the number of events that would have been *expected* to occur in that group if the deaths occurred solely in proportion to the numbers of patients at risk. If this difference is too extreme (as reflected in a p-value) then it provides evidence that the underlying event rates in the groups are different. The standard log-rank test is most sensitive to situations where the event rates in the groups differ by the same ratio across time. There are weighted versions of this test that are appropriate if the differences are expected to occur primarily during the early or later periods of follow-up time; however, the intent to use a weighted log-rank should be specified prior to observing where the differences in event rates occur.

The comparison of survival curves is a special case of hazard ratio analysis, performed through Cox regression, which is discussed below. In fact, the log-rank test is also a test of the equality of hazard rates in the two groups. The result of the hazard ratio analysis is also provided in Figure 5-5, illustrating the notion that better survival is associated with a lower event rate for mortality.

Competing Risks and Cumulative Incidence

As noted above, when there are multiple types of events that define event-free survival, or multiple causes of death, then probabilities associated with a specific type of event or a specific cause of death should not be estimated by Kaplan-Meier methods. For example, suppose that one is interested in comparing breast cancer mortality, as opposed to all-cause mortality (the complement of overall survival), between two

treatment groups. The relevance of this comparison might be debated, since cause-of-death classification can be fairly subjective. A common but incorrect approach to this problem is to censor patients at the time of a non–breast-cancer death, and to plot the complement of the resulting Kaplan-Meier curve as a representation of cumulative breast cancer mortality over time. The problem with this approach is that patients who die of other causes are not even hypothetically at risk for future death from breast cancer—the implicit assumption that they are, which is appropriate for the standard types of censoring, results in an overestimation of the probability of breast cancer death.

The correct calculation of cumulative incidence in the competing risks setting must take into account the probability of remaining at risk (or event-free). When this is done, the sums of the cumulative incidence probabilities for each of the types of events is exactly the complement of the event-free survival probability. For example, at any point in time, the sum of (a) the overall survival probability, (b) the probability of breast cancer death, and (c) the probability of non–breast-cancer death will sum to 100%.

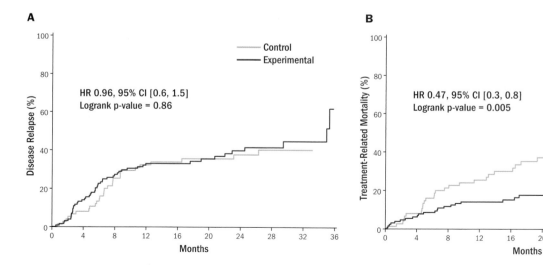

Fig. 5-6 Cumulative incidence curves and competing risks.

The data from Fig. 5-5 are decomposed into the two competing risks of relapse (**A**) and treatment-related mortality (**B**). Most of the improvement in disease-free survival in the experimental arm is attributable to a decrease in treatment-related mortality; there is not an observed difference in the rate of relapse between arms among those at risk for relapse.

Although we have emphasized that Kaplan-Meier methods are generally inappropriate for generating estimates of cumulative incidence in the presence of competing risks, the comparison of cumulative incidence curves is properly handled using the same log-rank statistic as for Kaplan-Meier curves, with events other than the type of interest being censored at the time of their occurrence. This seeming contradiction relates to the fact that in neither case is the log-rank statistic based directly on the estimates of the event probabilities themselves. Rather, it is based on the relative numbers of events that occur in each patient group, given the numbers of patients remaining at risk in each group over time. Thus it is appropriate, for this purpose, to censor patients that experience competing events at the time of the event, since they are no longer at risk for the event of interest.

Figure 5-6 illustrates competing risks analysis derived from the same data shown in Figure 5-5. Disease-free survival reflects two competing risks: relapse, and death without relapse, which perhaps reflects toxic complications of treatment. Panel A shows the cumulative incidence of relapse, and Panel B the cumulative incidence of treatment-related mortality. The sum of these two incidences, plus the event-free survival probability from Figure 5-5, will equal 100% at any point in time. The curves and the log-rank analysis clearly suggest that the improvement in disease-free survival associated with the experimental arm is based largely on a reduction in treatment-related mortality, with little apparent effect on relapse.

At the risk of making the issue seem overly complicated, it should be noted that in the competing risks setting, the results of statistical analysis may not always appear concordant with the visual interpretation of cumulative incidence curves. This is because incidence is a composite result of (a) the rate at which events occur among those at risk (the hazard rate), and (b) the size of the population at risk. For example, consider a setting where toxic regimens with potentially fatal complications are employed in a setting with high rates of relapse. The events of relapse and nonrelapse death constitute competing risks. Suppose that one regimen is much more effective than the other in preventing relapse, but has the same underlying toxicity, based on a hazard ratio analysis showing equivalent hazard rates for nonrelapse death in the two groups. In this case, the cumulative incidence of nonrelapse death will appear higher in the treatment group receiving the more effective therapy. This is because the effectiveness of the therapy in preventing relapse places more patients at risk for nonrelapse death.

The intent of the above example is not to imply that the hazard ratio analysis is correct, or that the cumulative incidence analysis is misleading. The important point is that competing risks should not be evaluated in isolation. Factors that influence one type of event may or may not influence another type, and an informed interpretation of data from a competing risks setting should consider each type of event. Further, a complete analysis should evaluate not only the underlying rates of the event types, which may be biologically more meaningful, but also the net outcome reflected in their cumulative incidence, which may bear on clinical interpretation.

Cox Regression

Although many clinical trials can be analyzed using only the methods above, there are many settings in which one wishes to incorporate more information about patient characteristics than just the treatment arm to which they were assigned. This is particularly true in nonrandomized comparisons, where patient groups may not be homogeneous with respect to factors known to affect outcome. Although accounting for these imbalances is in no way a substitute for randomization, it is nevertheless helpful to evaluate the extent to which patient characteristics influence the difference, or lack of difference, among treatment groups. In other cases the interest is not in comparing arms of a clinical trial, but in determining factors that are predictive of better or worse survival. This information is useful in designing trials, or simply in counseling patients about their likely prognosis.

Like other regression models, the Cox regression model relates patient characteristics, called covariates, to outcome. It is not the only model or method for doing this with time-to-event endpoints, but it is by far the most common regression model used in the context of medical research. As noted above, one of the fundamental quantities defining survival is the hazard function, $\lambda(t)$, which is the rate at which events occur among subjects at risk for the event. The Cox model, or proportional hazards model, assumes that covariates multiplicatively influence a "baseline" hazard function, $\lambda_0(t)$, which applies when the covariates have a specified baseline or reference value. For example, suppose that the reference value for patient sex is female. The hazard rate for females is thus $\lambda_0(t)$, and the hazard rate for males would be specified as $\lambda_0(t)e^{\beta male}$, so that the effect of being male is to multiply the hazard function by the quantity $e^{\beta male}$. The quantity β_{male} is a regression coefficient that captures the magnitude and direction of the effect. If $\beta_{male} > 0$, then $e^{\beta male} > 1$ and the effect of being male (relative to being female) is an increased hazard rate. Assuming that the hazard rate is for an untoward event, like mortality, this means a higher mortality hazard rate and poorer survival. If the coefficient is < 0, then the hazard multiplier is < 1 and this would yield a lower mortality hazard and better survival. Note that $e^{\beta male}$ is also the ratio of the hazard function for males to the hazard function for females at any point in time, and is called the *hazard ratio* (HR). Covariates need not relate to discrete groups, but can be defined quantitatively. For example, suppose that the reference value for patient age is 50 years. Then the multiplicative effect of age on the hazard function could be expressed as $e^{\beta age}$; for every year of age above 50 the hazard rate is multiplied by the quantity $e^{\beta age}$.

The basic regression model assumes that the covariates affect the hazard independently, i.e., that the effect of age is the same for males and females, but more complicated models can be constructed allowing interaction among covariates. Covariates for prognostic models are defined at the start of the survival period, but one can also allow the covariates to change over time, in which case they are called time-dependent covariates. The Cox regression model also extends directly to the analysis of cause-specific hazard rates found in the competing risks setting, by incorporating censoring for events of other types.

BINARY DATA ANALYSIS

In contrast to time-to-event analysis, there are occasions when the outcome of a clinical trial or other exercise may be summarized by the presence or absence of an event, outcome, or characteristic. This dichotomization of outcome is said to be binary data. Such data do not necessarily exclude aspects of time: for example, if outcome can be ascertained on all patients, then the occurrence of an event over a defined period of time can be a binary outcome. This is referred to as risk, but binary outcomes can refer to things other than risk. For example, two groups of patients with breast cancer might be compared with respect to the percentage of patients with estrogen receptor–positive disease. The same or similar statistical methods may be applied to both scenarios.

Chi-Squared Analysis

For basic statistical analysis of binary endpoints, for example comparing one or more groups in terms of the risk of an event or the percentage with a certain characteristic, the most common methodology is based on the chi-squared test (also mentioned in Table 5-1). For very small sample sizes, the accuracy of p-values from the chi-squared analysis may be in doubt, and Fisher's exact test is the most common alternative, although it is generally quite conservative.

Like the log-rank test for survival analysis, the basic methods associated with binary data provide a test of equality, but not necessarily a measure of effect. The most straightforward measure of effect is the simple difference in proportions. There are other common measures of effect associated with binary outcomes that must be used with some caution in typical applications involving clinical data. For example, if p is the risk of an event, then the odds of the event are $p/(1-p)$. Conversely, if ψ is the odds of an event, then the risk of the event is $\psi/(1+\psi)$. In certain epidemiologic settings, where p is small, then the ratio of the odds of an event between groups (*odds ratio*, or OR) will be approximately equal to the ratio of the risks (*relative risk*, or RR) and is a standard measure of association or effect. In clinical settings, however, the values of p associated with risk are not necessarily small. Although the same underlying statistical methods may be applicable, the OR in such settings may be unintuitive or even misleading. For example, consider a patient group with a risk of recurrence of 90% compared to another group with a risk of recurrence of 80%. The OR for risk of recurrence is 2.25, but clearly the risk of recurrence is not nearly doubled. Similar considerations apply when interpreting a hazard ratio in survival analysis. If the risk of an event is not too large, then a hazard ratio will approximate a risk ratio; however, the divergence between a risk ratio and a hazard ratio is not as dramatic as that between a risk ratio and an odds ratio. For example, a risk ratio of 2.0 (0.4/0.2, say) corresponds to an odds ratio of 2.67 and to a hazard ratio of 2.25 (under an exponential assumption).

Logistic Regression

The most common method for incorporating covariate effects into binary data analysis is logistic regression. The formulation of the underlying statistical model is not that dissimilar from Cox regression. If $\psi_0 = p_0(1 - p_0)$ is the odds of the event of interest for a specified baseline or reference value of the covariates (such as female sex), then the odds of the event for a male are specified as $\psi_0 e^{\beta male}$, so that the quantity $e^{\beta male}$ is the multiplicative effect on the baseline odds. It is also the OR for the risk of the event for males compared to females, although as noted one must be cautious in interpreting that as a risk ratio. Similarly, the multiplicative effect of a continuous covariate like age on the baseline odds (odds at age 50) would be expressed as $e^{(age-50)\beta age}$; for every year of age above 50 the odds of the event are multiplied by the quantity $e^{\beta age}$.

ANALYSIS OF RECURRENT EVENTS

In the discussion of survival analysis, we considered the time to an event that occurs only once, such as death, or that is generally only of interest the first time it occurs, such as relapse. Of course, patients whose disease relapses may be retreated, go into remission, and then experience relapse again, but this is usually a question for a different study. There are other events that may occur repeatedly over time, and where the rate of occurrence of such events is of interest. Examples of this relate commonly to the study of treatment complications, such as infection, seizure, or any sequelae that occur in distinct, well-defined episodes.

One technique for analyzing data of this kind involves what is called Poisson regression. This is related to the Poisson process, the classic example of which is the emission of particles in the process of radioactive decay. This is a stochastic event characterized by the fact that after one particle is emitted, the distribution of the time to the next particle is the same, regardless of how long the process has been going on. The rate of events over time is denoted λ, and over a period of the time, t, the number of events that occurs follows a Poisson distribution, which is characterized by its mean, equal to $\lambda \cdot t$. Poisson regression allows one to model the effect of covariates on λ in a manner analogous to that for Cox regression and logistic regression. For example, suppose that λ_0 is the rate of events for a specified baseline or reference value of the covariates (such as female sex), then the rate of events for a male are specified as $\psi_0 e^{\beta male}$ so that the quantity $e^{\beta male}$ is the multiplicative effect on the baseline rate, or the *rate ratio* (RR) for males relative to females. The same considerations apply to continuous covariates, such as age.

There are more complicated analytic strategies that can be applied when one is unwilling to assume that the event rate λ is constant over time; for example, by partitioning the time axis into intervals and modeling the counts in each interval separately. Cox regression also can be used to separately model the time to first event, time from first event to second event, time from second event to third event, etc.

LONGITUDINAL DATA ANALYSIS

There are many studies in which patients may be assessed repeatedly over extended periods of time. Data that arise from repeated measurement of the same patient over time are called *longitudinal data*, or sometimes *clustered data*. The distinction from the previous section is that the quantity under study is inherently measureable at any point in time. Common examples of such data would be quality-of-life assessments or the evaluation of biomarker levels over time.*

It is possible to do useful analysis of longitudinal data using very basic statistical methods, for example, by comparing groups at a fixed point in time, or by comparing one time to another. However, such methods may not allow one to evaluate the trajectory of the quantity under study as a whole, and do not fully accommodate common features of longitudinal data, such as missing data, variable times of assessment, and risk factors that also change over time. In order to analyze all of the data simultaneously, one must take into account the fact that repeated observations from the same patient are likely correlated. For example, one patient may report relatively high quality of life over the entire period of study, and another low quality of life, although both patients may experience a similar change over time.

Appropriately accounting for this within-patient correlation is not necessarily straightforward, and the methods involved may be quite complex and are beyond what can be presented in detail here. There are two fairly common approaches to handling longitudinal data analysis. Though the nomenclature may vary, one is generally referred to as a *linear mixed models* approach, the other as a *generalized estimating equation* (GEE) approach. The term "mixed" in the former case refers to the simultaneous estimation of parameters that model the mean effects (the effects of clinical interest) and parameters that model the within-patient correlation structure of the data. One must make explicit assumptions about the latter, and the results may be sensitive to that assumption. The GEE approach makes less explicit assumptions about the correlation structure. This is an advantage, particularly if one has no particular interest in the correlation structure itself, which is often the case when the interest is in comparing outcomes between groups or evaluating the effects of other factors on outcome.

SUMMARY

Statistical considerations are a key component in both the design and analysis of clinical research studies. Proper study design allows one to control the systematic and random factors that affect patient outcomes in clinical studies, and proper analysis allows one to make the best possible judgment as to which is more important. Few oncologists engaged in clinical research have sufficient statistical training or knowledge to do this on their own, which is why statisticians are in high demand in medical research and are considered a vital part of the research endeavor. Statisticians are also frequently engaged in evaluating research proposals for funding purposes and in reviewing research papers for publication in medical journals.

Although most clinical studies published in major medical journals have likely involved a statistician in both the conduct of the study and in the review of the article, it is still essential for the practicing oncologist to have some rudimentary familiarity with common statistical concepts and terminology, which has been the goal of this chapter. Such knowledge will enhance his or her ability to evaluate the medical literature, explain treatment options to patients, and make informed decisions about joining research studies available to the community.

Additional Reading

- Bailar JC, Hoaglin DC (eds). *Medical Uses of Statistics, 3rd ed.* Hoboken, NJ: John Wiley & Sons; 2009.
- Crowley J, Hoering A (eds). *Handbook of Statistics in Clinical Oncology, 3rd ed.* Boca Raton, FL: Chapman & Hall/CRC Taylor & Francis Group; 2012.
- Friedman LM, Furberg CD, DeMets DL. *Fundamentals of Clinical Trials, 2nd ed.* New York, NY: Springer-Verlag; 1998.
- Green S, Benedetti J, Smith A, et al. *Clinical Trials in Oncology, 3rd ed.* Boca Raton, FL: Chapman & Hall/CRC Taylor & Francis Group; 2012.
- Guyatt G, Jaeschke R, Heddle N, et al. Basic statistics for clinicians: 1. Hypothesis testing. *CMAJ.* 1995;152:27-32. PMID: 7804919.
- Guyatt G, Jaeschke R, Heddle N, et al. Basic statistics for clinicians: 2. Interpreting study results: confidence intervals. *CMAJ.* 1995;152:169-173. PMID: 7820798.
- Guyatt G, Walter S, Shannon H, et al. Basic statistics for clinicians: 4. Correlation and regression. *CMAJ.* 1995;152:497-504. PMID: 7859197.
- Jaeschke R, Guyatt G, Shannon H, et al. Basic statistics for clinicians: 3. Assessing the effects of treatment: measures of association. *CMAJ.* 1995;152:351-357. PMID: 7828099.
- Kelly WK, Halabi S, Schilsky R. *Oncology Clinical Trials: Successful Design, Conduct, and Analysis.* New York, NY: Demos Medical Publishing; 2010.
- Motulsky H. *Intuitive Biostatistics: A Nonmathematical Guide to Statistical Thinking, 3rd ed.* New York, NY: Oxford University Press; 2013.
- Piantadosi S. *Clinical Trials: A Methodologic Perspective, 2nd ed.* Hoboken, NJ: John Wiley & Sons; 2005.

---

* Pharmacokinetic data are a specialized case of longitudinal data. There are very specific methods for analyzing pharmacokinetics that are beyond the scope of this chapter.

6

BREAST CANCER

Beth Overmoyer, MD, and Eric Winer, MD

Risk factors/genetics

▶ There are now a number of multiplex test panels that assess both high- and moderate-penetrance genes for use in families who test negative for a known familial cancer syndrome, yet have characteristics suggestive of an inherited risk. The challenges of using these panels include a limited understanding of risk associated with moderate-penetrance genes and high prevalence of detecting variants of uncertain significance (Domchek SM, *J Clin Oncol* 2013).

Medical risk reduction (chemoprevention)

▶ IBIS-II supported the finding that aromatase inhibitors (AIs), in this case 5 years of anastrozole, reduced the risk of developing hormone receptor–positive invasive breast cancer and ductal carcinoma in situ by more than 50% (hazard ratio [HR] 0.47; $p < 0.0001$; Cuzick J, *Lancet* 2014).

Adjuvant systemic therapy

▶ The ATLAS and aTTOM studies demonstrated a reduced rate of systemic breast cancer recurrence and improved overall survival with 10 years of adjuvant tamoxifen use. The benefits were more robust during the later years and the absolute mortality reduction was 2.8% at 10 years after the start of treatment (Davies C, *Lancet* 2013; Gray RG, *J Clin Oncol* 2013).

▶ The phase II APT trial involved 406 patients with node-negative, HER2-positive breast cancer that measured 3 cm or smaller, treated with 12 weeks of standard paclitaxel and trastuzumab followed by 9 months of single-agent trastuzumab. The 3-year disease-free survival (DFS) was 98.7% at a median follow-up of 3.6 years, with two of the 10 DFS events being distant metastasis (Tolaney S, *SABCS* 2013).

Neoadjuvant systemic therapy

▶ The NeoSphere trial evaluated neoadjuvant therapy with four cycles of docetaxel combined with either trastuzumab alone, pertuzumab alone, or both agents, versus combination pertuzumab and trastuzumab without docetaxel (a nonchemotherapy arm). The combination pertuzumab and trastuzumab with docetaxel achieved the highest pathologic complete response rate at 39.3% compared with the other arms. Based upon these results, the U.S. Food and Drug Administration (FDA) issued an accelerated approval for the use of trastuzumab and pertuzumab in combination with taxane-based chemotherapy in the neoadjuvant setting for patients with stage II or III HER2-positive disease. In general, patients should receive an anthracycline postoperatively in this setting and also complete a total of 1 year of trastuzumab therapy. To date, the use of pertuzumab in the neoadjuvant or adjuvant settings has not been shown to improve disease-free survival or overall survival. This approach should be considered a promising option, but not a required standard of care (Gianni L, *Lancet Oncol* 2012).

Recurrent or metastatic disease

▶ CALOR (BIG 1-02/IBCSG 27-02/NSABP B-37) evaluated 162 patients with invasive breast cancer who developed an isolated local and/or regional ipsilateral recurrence following mastectomy or breast-conserving therapy. Patients received radiation therapy, endocrine therapy, or trastuzumab as appropriate, but were randomly assigned to receive chemotherapy or not. The 5-year disease-free survival was improved with chemotherapy (69%) compared with no chemotherapy (57%). The benefit was primarily seen in triple-negative breast cancer (TNBC; 67% vs. 35%, chemotherapy vs. no chemotherapy, respectively). The 5-year overall survival was comparable between the two groups; numerically higher in the chemotherapy group, but not statistically higher (88% vs. 76%, chemotherapy vs. no chemotherapy, respectively). Although this is a highly underpowered study, it does support the use of chemotherapy following local or regional disease recurrence in select circumstances (Aebi S, SABCS 2012).

▶ Three studies, SWOG 0226, FACT, and SoFEA, examined combination fulvestrant and AI versus AI alone in recurrent breast cancer. The benefit of combination fulvestrant and AI appears to be isolated to patients who have recurrent disease that is endocrine therapy–naive; a patient population that is rarely seen in the United States. For most patients, the standard practice remains the use of single-agent hormone therapy. Options for the treatment of hormone receptor–positive breast cancer progressing on a nonsteroidal AI include exemestane alone or fulvestrant alone (Mehta R, *N Engl J Med* 2012; Bergh J, *J Clin Oncol* 2012; Johnston S, *Lancet* Oncol 2013).

▶ The phase III BOLERO-2 trial demonstrated a superior median progression-free survival with combination everolimus (mTOR inhibitor) and exemestane compared with exemestane alone (10.6 months vs. 4.1 months, respectively; HR 0.36; p < 0.001) among postmenopausal women whose disease progressed or recurred while on a nonsteroidal AI. This study led to the 2012 FDA approval of everolimus in combination with exemestane in the treatment of estrogen receptor–positive, HER2-negative metastatic breast cancer following disease progression on either letrozole or anastrozole (Baselga J, *N Engl J Med* 2012).

▶ The CLEOPATRA trial was a phase III trial that randomly assigned patients to either pertuzumab, trastuzumab, and docetaxel (PTD) or trastuzumab and docetaxel with placebo (TD) as first-line therapy for HER2-positive metastatic breast cancer. The primary endpoint of progression-free survival was significantly improved among the patients receiving both HER2-targeting agents and docetaxel compared with TD (18.5 months vs. 12.5 months; HR 0.62; p < 0.001). The overall response rate was superior in the PTD arm (80.2% vs. 69.3%; p = 0.001), as was the overall survival, with a 34% reduction in the risk of death with PTD compared with TD (p = 0.0008). In June 2012, the FDA approved combination pertuzumab, trastuzumab, and either docetaxel or paclitaxel as the taxane backbone for first-line therapy of HER2-positive metastatic breast cancer (Baselga J, *N Engl J Med* 2012).

▶ Trastuzumab emtansine (T-DM1) is an antibody-drug conjugate of trastuzumab and the chemotherapy DM1. Both the EMILIA and TH3RESA studies demonstrated a superior progression-free survival compared with other HER2-targeted/chemotherapy combinations, and in the EMILIA trial there was also a statistically significant improvement in overall survival. T-DM1 offers an effective and tolerable option for treating HER2-positive disease that has progressed following trastuzumab and taxane chemotherapy (Verma S, *N Engl J Med* 2012; Wildiers H, presented at 2013 European Cancer Congress).

Breast cancer remains the most common malignancy diagnosed among women in the world. Approximately 1.38 million women worldwide were diagnosed with breast cancer in 2008, accounting for 23% of all new cancer cases.[1] The incidence rates are higher in economically developed regions, such as North America, western Europe, and Australia/New Zealand, and low in economically developing areas such as sub-Saharan Africa and Asia. The incidence rates of breast cancer in developed countries increased between 1980 and 1990 because of increased use of breast cancer screening and changes in reproductive factors. Since 2000, however, breast cancer incidence has decreased in these countries, which is attributed to the decline in the use of hormone replacement therapy (HRT).[2]

EPIDEMIOLOGY

Worldwide, breast cancer accounted for 14%, or 458,000, of the total cancer-related deaths in 2008.[1] Sixty percent of these deaths were found to occur in economically developing countries. Since 1990, the United States, United Kingdom, and France have experienced a reduction in breast cancer–related deaths, primarily thought to be due to improved early detection and more effective therapies. In contrast, changes in reproductive patterns, increased obesity, and decreased physical activity are thought to have contributed to a 2- to 3-fold increase in incidence of breast cancer in African and Asian countries.[3] This rise in incidence has translated into an increase in breast cancer–related deaths in developing countries.

In the United States, an estimated 234,580 new cases of invasive breast cancer were expected to be diagnosed in 2013, involving 2,240 men and 232,340 women.[4] It was estimated that 64,640 new cases of in situ breast cancer would be diagnosed in 2013. Breast cancer remains the most common malignancy among women in the United States (29%), and continues to be the second most common cause of cancer-related deaths among women, with lung cancer continuing to be first. Following an initial increase in incidence of localized (node-negative) and regional disease in the 1980s to 1990s, the incidence of each category has decreased by 2.3% and 2.8% per year, respectively. Between 1998 and 2007, the overall incidence of breast cancer has decreased by 0.5% per year; however, following a striking decrease in 2002 to 2003, the rate has remained relatively stable from 2003 to 2007. There has been no noticeable annual change in the 5% incidence of metastatic disease diagnosed at the time of presentation. The mortality from breast cancer has decreased by 34% from 1990 to 2008, with a greater effect seen among younger women.[4-6]

Race and ethnicity are important considerations in the evaluation of breast cancer incidence and mortality in the United States. The incidence of breast cancer is higher among white women compared with black women (e.g., 122 white women vs. 116 black women per 100,000 were diagnosed with breast cancer from 2003 to 2008). Some contributing factors to the higher incidence seen among white women include more frequent use of HRT and a more widespread use of screening mammography. This characteristic is reversed when mortality data are evaluated (e.g., 23 white women vs. 32 black women per 100,000 died of breast cancer from 2003 to 2008). Multiple factors play a role in this observation. Black women are often diagnosed at a more advanced stage of breast cancer, and there is a propensity for black women to develop unfavorable forms of breast cancer, which are high-grade, hormone receptor– and HER2-negative (i.e., triple-negative), and often have molecular profiling consistent with the basal-like subtype. Breast cancer–related incidence and death are lower among Asian, Native American, and Hispanic women living within the United States than in white women.[7]

RISK FACTORS

AGE AND GENDER

Older age and female gender are the most important risk factors for the development of breast cancer in the United States. Male breast cancer is rare, accounting for approximately 1% of all breast cancers.[1] Men are usually diagnosed after age 60, and the specific risk factors for this disease among men include genetic predisposition associated with *BRCA2* mutations, Klinefelter syndrome, testicular alterations that result in testosterone deficiency (such as undescended testes or testicular injury), and syndromes that increase the estrogen-to-testosterone ratio (such as obesity or hepatic cirrhosis).[8]

The risk of developing breast cancer among women in the United States is an estimated 1:8 (12%) over a normal lifespan (Table 6-1). Risk has been shown to increase by 8.5% per year from menarche to menopause, and then slows to 2.5% per year after menopause. From menarche to age 39, the risk of breast cancer developing is 1:202, from age 40 to 59 the risk is 1:26, from age 60 to 69 the risk is 1:28, and the risk from age 70 and older is an estimated 1:15.[4]

FAMILIAL FACTORS

A family history of breast and/or ovarian cancer is associated with a higher risk of developing breast cancer. Approximately 5% to 10% of all breast cancers are associated with highly penetrant mutations in genes, such as *BRCA1* and *BRCA2*. An additional 15% to 20% of women diagnosed with breast cancer have a positive family history, which may be a result of the inheritance of several low-penetrance genes that increase risk or, alternatively, shared environmental exposures. In some families, both the inheritance of low-penetrance genes and shared environmental factors may operate synergistically. Having first-degree relatives with breast cancer portends a 2-fold higher risk of developing breast cancer; however, this risk can increase to as high as 6- to 7-fold when there was a first-degree relative who was diagnosed at a young age, or when two first-degree relatives are affected.[9,10] Having a previous diagnosis of breast cancer is also associated with a higher risk of developing contralateral disease, which can be compounded when a family history of breast cancer is present.

Table 6-1 Established Risk Factors for Breast Cancer: Fixed Factors

Factor	Relative Risk
Gender (female vs. male)	100
Age (≤ 50 vs. > 50)	6.7
Endocrine factors	
Age of menarche (< 10)	1.4 to 1.9
Age at first birth (> 35)	1.7
Nulliparity	1.4
Age at menopause (> 55)	1.3
Benign breast disease	
ADH, LCIS	4.0 to 5.0
Family history	
First-degree relatives	2.0 to 7.0
BRCA1/BRCA2 mutation	10 to 30
p53 (Li-Fraumeni)	1.5 to 6.0
Cowden syndrome	2.0 to 4.0
Ethnicity (Ashkenazi Jewish)	1.4
Therapeutic radiation	35

Abbreviations; ADH, atypical ductal hyperplasia; LCIS, lobular carcinoma in situ.

GENETIC FACTORS

Hereditary breast cancer is characterized by the presence of high-penetrance genotypes, inheritance through maternal or paternal ancestry, and associations with other malignancies. Other malignancies that can be linked with a familial breast cancer syndrome include epithelial ovarian/fallopian tube/primary peritoneal cancer, pancreas cancer, aggressive prostate cancer, sarcoma, thyroid cancer, brain tumors, endometrial cancer, and diffuse gastric cancer. In general, the presence of an inherited predisposition to breast cancer can be connected with the following characteristics: onset of breast cancer at age 50 or younger, triple-negative breast cancer (TNBC; negative estrogen receptor [ER], negative progesterone receptor [PR], and negative HER2 overexpression), one or more primary breast cancers diagnosed at age 50 or younger, or one or more ovarian/fallopian tube/primary peritoneal cancers in a family, breast and ovarian cancer arising within a single individual, male breast cancer, family member with a known deleterious mutation in a susceptibility gene, a combination of breast cancer and one or more of the previously stated malignancies, and Ashkenazi Jewish ancestry.[11] The optimal individual to undergo genetic testing within a family is the youngest woman who carries the diagnosis of either ovarian or breast cancer. If a genetic linkage is not found in that individual, further testing among family members is usually not beneficial, unless there is a suspicion that the tested individual has a spontaneous breast cancer (phenocopy). In that setting, a second affected individual within the family should be tested.

Germ-line mutations in several genes have been identified as being associated with a high probability of developing breast and/or ovarian cancer, the most common genes being *BRCA1* and *BRCA2*. The transmission of mutations in *BRCA1* or *BRCA2* is autosomal-dominant. *BRCA1* and *BRCA2* function as tumor suppressor genes that protect chromosomal stability by enabling homologous recombination following double-strand DNA breaks. *BRCA2* binds directly to RAD51, an enzyme which is essential for homologous recombination. *BRCA2* is also the gene related to Fanconi anemia, and works in concert not only with RAD51 and *BRCA1*, but also PALB2 to facilitate recruitment of these enzymes to sites of DNA damage, resulting in repair.[12]

Mutations in *BRCA1* appear to be associated primarily with breast and ovarian cancer risk, which contrasts with *BRCA2* mutations that can be associated with other malignancies such as prostate cancer (relative risk [RR] 7.33 with age younger than 65), pancreas cancer (RR 3.51), malignant melanoma (RR 2.58), gallbladder and bile duct cancer (RR 4.97), and stomach cancer (RR 2.59).[13,14] The risk of developing male breast cancer before age 80 is approximately 7% among *BRCA2* mutation carriers.[15] Among women with *BRCA1* or *BRCA2* mutations, the risk of developing breast cancer over a lifetime is an estimated 50% to 75%. The risk of developing ovarian cancer is higher with a *BRCA1* mutation (30% to 40%) than with a *BRCA2* mutation (10% to 20%).[16] The development of contralateral breast cancer is also increased (RR 3.4 for *BRCA2* and RR 4.5 for *BRCA1*), although this risk is less pronounced among women older than age 50 (10.8%) compared with those patients who were diagnosed younger than age 30 (28.2%).[17] In addition, the use of more effective systemic

Table 6-2 Established Risk Factors for Breast Cancer: Modifiable Factors

Factor	Relative Risk
Exogenous hormones	
Oral contraceptive pills	0.9 to 1.0
Estrogen replacement (> 10 years)	1.1
Estrogen and progesterone	1.4 to 3.0
Obesity (BMI > 30)	2.5
Exercise (> 3 hours/week)	0.6
Alcohol use	1.1 to 2.2
Diet	1.0
Mammographic density	2.2 to 5.3

Abbreviation: BMI, body mass index.

therapies contributes to a reduction in the development of contralateral breast cancer.[13] Women with a *BRCA1* mutation can have a 1.6-fold higher risk of developing a contralateral breast cancer compared with women carrying a *BRCA2* mutation.

Approximately 2.5% of individuals of Ashkenazi Jewish ancestry carry one of three "founder" mutations in *BRCA1* (5382insC or 185delAG) or *BRCA2* (617delT), which account for 12% of breast cancers and 35% of ovarian cancers in this population. An additional 2% to 4% have nonfounder mutations; however, major gene rearrangements of *BRCA1* or *BRCA2* are rare among women with Ashkenazi Jewish ancestry.[18] Certain subtypes of breast cancer occur more commonly with specific genetic mutations. For example, *BRCA1* mutations are associated with TNBC, invasive lobular carcinoma seen in conjunction with a family history of diffuse gastric carcinoma can occur with mutations in the E-cadherin gene *CDH1*, and HER2-positive breast cancer is prevalent in the presence of *TP53* mutations (Li-Fraumeni syndrome).[19-21]

Li-Fraumeni syndrome is related to germ-line mutations in *p53*. These highly penetrant mutations are very rare (one in 5,000), and are associated with a 90% lifetime risk of developing a malignancy, which includes breast cancer in very young women (younger than age 30), sarcoma, leukemia, adrenocortical carcinomas, and brain tumors. Cowden syndrome is also a rare, autosomal-dominant syndrome; 80% of cases are caused by mutations in the *PTEN* tumor suppressor gene (located on chromosome 10q23). In this syndrome, breast cancer can occur in conjunction with thyroid, kidney, and endometrial cancer in addition to specific physical findings such as macrocephaly, hamartomas, autism, and trichilemmomas of the face, hands, and feet.[22] There are now a number of multiplex test panels that assess both high- and moderate-penetrance genes for use in families who test negative for a known familial cancer syndrome, yet have characteristics suggestive of an inherited risk. The challenges of using these panels include a limited understanding of risk associated with moderate-penetrance genes and high prevalence of detecting variants of uncertain significance.[23]

Table 6-3 Risk Factors Used in Risk Assessment Models

Modified Gail Model	Age, age at menarche, age at first live birth, number of breast biopsies, history of atypical hyperplasia, number of first-degree relatives with breast cancer, race
Claus Model	Age, affected first- and second-degree relatives with breast cancer, age of onset of breast cancer, ovarian cancer in a relative, paternal family history
BRCAPRO Model	Age, affected first- and second-degree relatives with breast cancer, age of onset of breast cancer in a relative, bilateral breast cancer in a relative, ovarian cancer in a relative, male breast cancer in a relative
International Breast Cancer Intervention Study (IBIS) Model (Tyrer-Cuzick Model)	Age, body mass index, age of menarche, age at first live birth, age at menopause, hormone replacement therapy use, number of prior breast biopsies, presence of atypical hyperplasia, lobular carcinoma in situ, number of first- and second-degree relatives with breast cancer, age of onset of breast cancer in a relative, bilateral breast cancer in a relative, ovarian cancer in a relative
Breast and Ovarian Analysis of Disease Incidence and Carrier Estimation Algorithm (BOADICEA)	Age, affected first-, second-, and third-degree relatives with breast cancer, age of onset of breast cancer in a relative, bilateral breast cancer in a relative, ovarian cancer in a relative, male breast cancer in a relative

REPRODUCTIVE/ENDOGENOUS HORMONES

Estrogens clearly play a role in breast cancer risk and development (Table 6-2). Increased levels of endogenous hormones are associated with an increased risk of developing disease among postmenopausal women.[24] A greater understanding of identifiable subtypes of breast cancer (i.e., hormone receptor–positive vs. triple-negative) has led to greater specificity in defining the role of reproductive risk factors. An early onset of menarche, late age of menopause, and nulliparity are all related to extended estrogen exposure and elevated risk of developing hormone receptor–positive disease.[25] In contrast, triple-negative disease is associated with increasing number of births, and is not associated with nulliparity or age at first full-term delivery.[26] Terminal differentiation of breast epithelium occurs following a full-term pregnancy. This pathologic change in breast parenchyma appears to be protective and associated with a reduction in breast cancer risk when first full-term pregnancy occurs at a younger age (younger than 30). Lactation may also convey protection; however, the duration of lactation required for this benefit is not well defined.

EXOGENOUS HORMONES

HRT in the form of combination estrogen and progesterone is associated with an increased risk of developing invasive breast cancer (hazard ratio [HR] 1.26); however, the risk returns to normal within 2 years after discontinuation of HRT.[27] The global cessation of combination HRT in 2002 was associated with an 8.6% reduction in the annual incidence of invasive breast cancer, primarily observed in hormone receptor–positive disease and in women older than age 50.[2] HRT has not been associated with an increased risk of developing ductal carcinoma in situ (DCIS). Breast cancer risk does not appear to be related to a limited duration of unopposed estrogen use (less than 10 years) or oral contraceptive use; however, oral contraceptive use may be associated with an increased risk in the presence of a BRCA mutation.[28,29]

RADIATION EXPOSURE

Low-level radiation exposure is associated with an increased risk of breast cancer as high as 3.6-fold, and can occur with multiple fluoroscopic examinations, frequent diagnostic radiographs for scoliosis, and, historically, as treatment for thymic enlargement, skin hemangiomas, and benign breast disease. Survivors of Hodgkin lymphoma and other hematologic malignancies who received therapeutic mediastinal or mantle-field radiation have a higher risk of developing breast cancer, which is dependent upon dose of radiation and the radiation field volume. The RR can range from 37 to 57, with a greater propensity of developing bilateral breast cancer. The risk is greatest when treatment occurred during active proliferation of breast tissue (i.e., between age 15 and 25). The median time to develop breast cancer following treatment is approximately 18 years; however, increased risk can be seen as early as 8 years following treatment, and the risk continues to increase over time, wherein the estimated cumulative incidence of breast cancer after 25 to 30 years of follow-up ranges from 12% to 26%. Use of lower doses of therapeutic radiation involving smaller volumes has resulted in lower risks of breast cancer.[30-32]

MAMMOGRAPHIC DENSITY

The determination of mammographic density is subjective, and reflects variation in breast tissue composition between radiodense areas related to a greater amount of epithelial or stromal tissue, and nondense areas that reflect the presence of fat. There is a linear trend associated with increasing mammographic density and risk of breast cancer, wherein women with greater than 75% breast density have a 4- to 6-fold higher risk of developing disease.[33] Exogenous hormone use, such as HRT or oral contraceptives, results in increased breast density, whereas endogenous hormone levels do not. Lower breast density may be a reflection of involution of the terminal duct lobule, which is a natural aging process of the breast and is associated with a lower incidence of developing breast cancer.[34]

BENIGN PROLIFERATIVE BREAST DISEASE

Pathologic changes within the breast have been shown to be independent risk factors for breast cancer. Benign proliferative lesions without atypia do not necessarily fall into this category, whereas benign proliferative breast disease with atypia, such as atypical ductal hyperplasia, atypical lobular hyperplasia, and lobular carcinoma in situ (LCIS), is associated with a 4-fold increased risk of developing breast cancer in either breast.[35] Lobular neoplasia (atypical lobular hyperplasia and LCIS) is associated with a 29% risk of developing breast cancer over 25 years. Thus, following the diagnosis by core biopsy, most individuals should undergo an excisional procedure to determine whether DCIS or invasive disease is present. The histologic type of atypical hyperplasia (i.e., ductal vs. lobular) does not affect risk, although the number of foci of atypia is associated with a higher incidence of risk.[36] Women younger than age 45 with atypical hyperplasia have a higher RR (6.76) of developing breast cancer. Interestingly, some data suggest that a family history of breast cancer does not appear to contribute to risk in the setting of benign proliferative disease.

BEHAVIORAL FACTORS

Consumption of one alcoholic beverage per day is associated with a 12% increased risk of breast cancer and has a linear correlation such that a 10% increase in risk is associated with every additional 10 g/day of alcohol (or 0.75 to 1 alcoholic beverage per day) consumed. The risk is independent of the type of alcohol consumed, and appears to be related to an increase in serum hormone levels.[37-39] Obesity increases the risk of breast cancer in postmenopausal women by more than 63% (body mass index [BMI], 30 to 40), but is inversely correlated with risk in premenopausal women.[40] However, when waist circumference is used as an indicator of body fat distribution, a larger waist circumference is associated with a greater incidence of premenopausal ER-negative breast cancer.[41] Waist circumference and BMI are markers of visceral adiposity associated with metabolic syndrome, a condition of hyperglycemia, hyperinsulinemia, and insulin resistance. The association of obesity with both increased breast cancer risk and mortality from breast cancer appears to be a result of the effects of obesity on increased production of estrogen, and insulin activation of tyrosine kinase growth receptor pathways.[42,43] Physical activity is inversely related to breast cancer risk, in that 4 to 7 hours per week of recreational exercise is associated with a 12% to 60% reduction in risk among both premenopausal and postmenopausal women. A number of epidemiologic observations suggest that the effects of exercise may be a result of weight control, hormonal effects, and/or changes in immune function.[44] Isoflavones (i.e., phytoestrogens most commonly found in soy), vitamin D, dairy products, and high-fat diets have unclear relationships to the incidence of breast cancer, and further investigation is warranted.[45]

RISK DETERMINATION MODELS

Several risk prediction models are available to predict the risk of developing breast cancer based upon family history and/or to determine the probability of carrying a BRCA mutation. The Claus Model includes first- and second-degree relatives with breast and/or ovarian cancer, and incorporates the age at diagnosis.[46] BRCAPRO,[47] the Tyrer-Cuzick Model (the International Breast Cancer Intervention Study [IBIS]),[48] and the Breast and Ovarian Analysis of Disease Incidence and Carrier Estimation Algorithm (BOADICEA) Model[49] all calculate risk based upon a probability of carrying a genetic mutation (Table 6-3).[50]

The modified Gail Model (cancer.gov/bcrisktool) is the most widely used risk assessment tool, which incorporates nongenetic factors such as current age, age at menarche, and age at first full-term pregnancy or nulliparity, number of breast biopsies and presence of atypical hyperplasia, number of first-degree relatives with breast cancer, and race. The original Gail Model was modified and validated to incorporate race as a risk factor, specifically assessing breast cancer risk in black women (Contraceptive and Reproductive Experience [CARE] Model).[51] The modified Gail Model is an excellent tool to determine risk on a population basis; however, the 5-year or lifetime risk of disease calculated for an individual woman is not robust.[52] This model will also underestimate risk if there is a significant genetic predisposition. Prevention strategies are often considered when the modified Gail Model calculates a 5-year risk exceeding 1.67%; however, this calculation does not take into account other factors such as breast density or presence of LCIS, and may also underestimate the risk associated with atypia.[53]

PREVENTION

The current goal of breast cancer prevention is to reduce the risk of developing disease with minimal toxicity. Women with the following characteristics may consider risk-reducing surgery (RRS): women who have tested positive for a high-penetrance genetic mutation, women with a strong family history of breast cancer that is not associated with *BRCA*, and women with a strong family history who have not been tested for a genetic linkage. Surgical prevention of breast cancer specifically relates to bilateral risk-reducing mastectomy (RRM). In addition, there is a significant contribution to breast cancer risk reduction from risk-reducing bilateral salpingo-oophorectomy (RRSO). Both lifestyle and medical risk-reducing strategies can be discussed with women who have any degree of breast cancer risk.

RISK-REDUCING SURGERY

Because of the difficulty in detecting ovarian or fallopian tube cancer at an early stage, women with *BRCA* mutations are recommended to undergo RRSO by age 40 or at the completion of childbearing. This has been shown to decrease the risk of developing ovarian cancer by approximately 85% (HR 0.14), reduce the risk of developing a first diagnosis of breast cancer among both *BRCA1* and *BRCA2* mutation carriers (HR 0.63 and HR 0.36, respectively), and is associated with a lower breast cancer–specific mortality (HR 0.44), lower all-cause mortality (HR 0.40), and lower ovarian cancer–specific mortality (HR 0.21).[54] Subsequent to RRSO, there remains an elevated risk of developing primary peritoneal carcinoma among *BRCA* mutation carriers. There appears to be an age effect of RRSO on breast cancer risk, wherein women who undergo RRSO after age 50 do not obtain a significant reduction in risk of developing breast cancer. RRSO does not seem to affect the risk of developing contralateral breast cancer after a prior diagnosis of breast cancer. The concern about the adverse effect on mortality from inducing early menopause can be safely ameliorated with short-term HRT given until age 50, without an apparent compromise in the overall benefit of RRSO on breast cancer risk.[55]

Bilateral RRM has been shown to reduce the risk of developing breast cancer by more than 90%. Women at high or moderate risk of developing breast cancer (i.e., known genetic linkage or a significant family history without a known genetic predisposition) should have a discussion concerning prevention. Improvements in surgical technique appear to result in a greater risk reduction from RRM than previous data had demonstrated.[54,56,57] Skin-sparing mastectomy is as effective as total mastectomy (removing all breast tissue without axillary lymph node dissection), whereas the safety of nipple-sparing mastectomy is still being evaluated in this setting. Reconstructive surgery following mastectomies does not appear to increase breast cancer risk. In the absence of a *BRCA* mutation, prophylactic contralateral mastectomy performed following the diagnosis of invasive breast cancer has not been associated with an improvement in overall survival (OS).

MEDICAL RISK REDUCTION (CHEMOPREVENTION)

When used for the treatment of invasive breast cancer, endocrine therapy has resulted in a significant reduction in risk of developing contralateral breast cancer. The 15-year follow-up of the Early Breast Cancer Trialists' Collaborative Group (EBCTCG) overview analysis demonstrated a 39% reduction in the development of a primary contralateral breast cancer with 5 years of adjuvant tamoxifen use.[58] This observation prompted

several randomized trials examining the efficacy of selective estrogen receptor modulators (SERMs), such as tamoxifen, in reducing the risk of developing breast cancer among high-risk women. The National Surgical Adjuvant Breast and Bowel Project (NSABP) Breast Cancer Prevention Trial (BCPT) P-1 trial defined a high-risk cohort as pre- or postmenopausal women older than age 60, or women age 35 or older with a 5-year predicted risk of developing disease of 1.66% or higher as predicted by the Gail Model (see Risk Determination Models section), or women with a diagnosis of LCIS. The 13,388 women enrolled in the BCPT were randomly assigned to receive 20 mg of tamoxifen daily for 5 years or a placebo.[59] A 7-year follow-up report supported the earlier results, demonstrating that tamoxifen reduced the risk of developing invasive breast cancer by 43%. The incidence of ER-positive invasive breast cancer was reduced by 62%; tamoxifen use did not affect the risk of ER-negative breast cancer. The risk of developing noninvasive breast cancer (i.e., DCIS) was also reduced by 37%. All subtypes of risk groups achieved a benefit from tamoxifen.

These results were supported by several other randomized trials involving tamoxifen, including the International Breast Intervention Study-1 (IBIS-1) trial (34% risk reduction), the Royal Marsden Tamoxifen Prevention trial (39% risk reduction), and the Italian Randomized Tamoxifen Prevention trial (76%).[60-62] The eligibility requirements of these studies varied, as did the acceptance of concurrent HRT or bilateral oophorectomy among participants, making cross-study conclusions more difficult. In general, all studies demonstrated that tamoxifen reduced the risk of developing invasive breast cancer; however, the Royal Marsden study showed the benefit of risk reduction for ER-positive breast cancer occurred primarily after completing 5 years of tamoxifen, and the Italian trial only demonstrated a significant reduction in risk of ER-positive disease among women at very high risk. None of the studies demonstrated an effect on all-cause mortality.[63]

Both the prevention studies and the studies using tamoxifen for the treatment of breast cancer demonstrated an association between tamoxifen use and an increased incidence of endometrial cancer, thromboembolic phenomenon, cataracts, gynecologic and vasomotor symptoms (vaginal discharge and hot flashes), and possibly stroke. Tamoxifen also has been shown to reduce the incidence of bone fractures among postmenopausal women. The risk of endometrial cancer is increased with tamoxifen use (RR 3.3), which translates into a 1.6% risk with tamoxifen compared with a baseline 0.7% risk over 7 years.[59] The majority of the endometrial cancers were stage I adenocarcinomas found among women older than age 50, and were associated with postmenopausal vaginal bleeding. There are no data which support routine screening for endometrial cancer using transvaginal ultrasound or biopsy, unless abnormal vaginal bleeding is present.[61] The risk of thromboembolic events was also increased (RR 1.9), and was primarily venous (deep venous thrombosis, pulmonary embolism). The risk of stroke is not consistently increased among the tamoxifen studies, and this association is not supported by large population studies.

A second-generation SERM, raloxifene, was shown to reduce the incidence of invasive breast cancer by 69% to 72% when investigated as a treatment for osteoporosis in two clinical trials, the Multiple Outcomes Raloxifene Evaluation (MORE) and Continuing Outcomes Relevant to Evista (CORE) trials.[64] The use of raloxifene was not associated with an increased risk of endometrial cancer, which made it a promising SERM to use for breast cancer prevention among postmenopausal women. The NSABP Study of Tamoxifen and Raloxifene (STAR) trial compared the efficacy of 5 years of tamoxifen to raloxifene among postmenopausal women who met the same high-risk criteria defined in the BCPT.[65] The initial evaluation after a median follow-up of 4 years demonstrated no difference between the effects of the two SERMs in the development of invasive breast cancer among the 19,747 women enrolled in the STAR trial. However, after an extended follow-up of nearly 8 years, raloxifene retained 76% of the effectiveness of tamoxifen in reducing the risk of invasive cancer. Whereas the initial evaluation of the STAR trial showed no statistical effect of raloxifene on DCIS risk, the 8-year follow-up revealed raloxifene to be about 78% as effective as tamoxifen in reducing the risk of developing DCIS.[66] There was no difference in mortality outcome between the two SERMs. Raloxifene use was associated with significantly less toxicity compared with tamoxifen—specifically, fewer endometrial cancers and thromboembolic events. Thus, while raloxifene did not appear to decrease breast cancer risk as well as tamoxifen did, its better safety outcome makes it a reasonable chemoprevention alternative to tamoxifen in postmenopausal women.

A recent meta-analysis of the individual participant data from all randomized prevention trials involving SERMs, including arzoxifene and lasofoxifene (nine trials with 83,399 participants), revealed a 10-year cumulative incidence of developing breast cancer equaling 6.3% versus 4.2% among controls and participants, respectively.[67] The reduction in breast cancer was evident in years 0 to 5 (42%) and years 5 to 10 (25%). The increased risk of endometrial cancer was confined to tamoxifen use during years 0 to 5 (HR 1.64), and although venous thromboembolic events were increased overall, there was no effect on incidence of myocardial infarction, stroke, or transient ischemic attacks. SERM use had no effect on the risk of developing ER-negative breast cancer or on overall mortality.

Clinical trials exploring the efficacy of aromatase inhibitors (AIs) compared with tamoxifen for the treatment of early-stage breast cancer have shown a 48% relative reduction in risk of developing contralateral breast cancer with the use of an AI.[64] These data prompted the investigation of exemestane, a steroidal third-generation AI, in the prevention of invasive breast cancer among postmenopausal women at high risk. In addition, AIs have not been shown to increase the risk of endometrial or uterine cancer, nor are they associated with an increased risk of thromboembolic phenomenon. The general eligibility criteria for enrollment on the placebo-controlled National Cancer Institute of Canada Clinical Trials Group Mammary Prevention.3 (NCIC CTC MAP.3) trial were essentially the same as those used for the BCPT and STAR trial.[68] Ethical justification for this placebo-controlled trial stemmed from the lack of benefit in mortality seen with the use of U.S. Food and Drug Administration (FDA)–approved SERMs for prevention. The results of the MAP.3 prevention trial demonstrated a 65% reduction in the incidence of invasive breast cancer and a 73% reduction in the incidence of ER-positive invasive breast cancer among women taking 5 years of exemestane compared with placebo. Although adverse events were more common in the exemestane group (88% vs. 85%; p = 0.003), only arthritis and menopausal symptoms were statistically more frequent. The international, randomized, placebo-controlled trial known as IBIS-II supported the finding that AIs, in this case 5 years of anastrozole, reduced the risk of developing hormone receptor–positive invasive breast cancer and DCIS by more than 50% (HR 0.47; p < 0.0001) among postmenopausal women at high risk of developing breast cancer.[69] As was seen in the prevention studies using SERMs, anastrozole did not convey a risk reduction for ER-negative breast cancer, nor improved survival.

SUMMARY OF RECOMMENDATIONS FOR MEDICAL PREVENTION

Both tamoxifen and raloxifene have been approved by the FDA to be used in the prevention of breast cancer; however, raloxifene is only approved for use in postmenopausal women.[70] Tamoxifen (20 mg daily for 5 years) can be offered to premenopausal women at high risk of developing breast cancer. Postmenopausal women who lack a uterus can also be offered tamoxifen for risk reduction. The criteria for risk are described by the BCPT trial. Raloxifene (60 mg daily for 5 years) can be offered to postmenopausal women with an intact uterus who have a risk profile as described. Women can use raloxifene for longer than 5 years if the medication is used to treat osteoporosis; however, the studies examining its effect on breast cancer risk only used a 5-year duration of treatment.[64] Very few women with BRCA mutations have been specifically evaluated in the prevention trials; therefore, the role of primary medical prevention in this population is not well known. However, recent data suggest that tamoxifen can reduce the development of contralateral breast cancers in BRCA1 (42% risk reduction) or BRCA2 (52% risk reduction) mutation carriers following the diagnosis of breast cancer.[71] Extrapolating from these data, tamoxifen can be offered as a medical prevention strategy among BRCA-positive patients who have not been diagnosed with breast cancer, similar to high-risk women who are not mutation carriers. Although exemestane has been shown to reduce the risk of invasive breast cancer among high-risk postmenopausal women, it has not been FDA-approved for this indication as of June 2014 (Table 6-4). The use of other medications for breast cancer prevention (e.g., metformin, aspirin) remains investigational.

LIFESTYLE MODIFICATIONS
Physical Activity
A significant amount of data supporting lifestyle modification associated with a reduction in risk of developing breast cancer stems from extrapolation from studies that link lifestyle factors and risk of a second primary contralateral breast cancer or

Table 6-4 Breast Cancer Chemoprevention Trials

Trial	Patients	Comparison	RR	RR+
STAR[65]	19,747	Raloxifene vs. tamoxifen	1.24 (1.065-1.47)	NA
MAP.3[68]	4,560	Exemestane vs. placebo	0.35 (0.18-0.70)	0.27 (0.12-0.60)
IBIS II[69]	1,920	Anastrozole vs. placebo	0.50 (0.32-0.76)	0.42 (0.25-0.71)
Italian[62]	5,408	Tamoxifen vs. placebo	0.84 (0.60-1.17)	0.61 (0.38-0.99)
Royal Marsden[61]	2,471	Tamoxifen vs. placebo	0.78 (0.58-1.04)	0.48 (0.29-0.79)
IBIS[60]	7,145	Tamoxifen vs. placebo	0.73 (0.58-0.91)	0.66 (0.50-0.87)
BCPT P-1[59]	13,338	Tamoxifen vs. placebo	0.57 (0.46-0.70)	0.38 (0.28-0.50)

Abbreviations: RR, relative risk for invasive breast cancer; RR+, relative risk for estrogen receptor– and/or progesterone receptor–positive invasive breast cancer; NA, data not available for most recent evaluation.

systemic breast cancer recurrence. Moderate exercise for 2 to 3 hours per week has been reported to reduce breast cancer recurrence and all-cause mortality by approximately 40% to 67%.[72] Three prospective cohort studies have demonstrated that current total or recreational exercise can reduce the incidence of breast cancer by 20% to 30%, primarily among premenopausal women.[73] All types of activity appear to be beneficial, and are associated with a risk reduction when performed at any point in life. Some data endorse a greater benefit with activity if it is performed later in life (after age 50), is more vigorous, occurs more frequently and for a longer duration, and for postmenopausal women.[74] The biologic mechanism behind physical activity and risk reduction is unknown, although some studies support an interaction among estrogen, fasting insulin levels, insulin resistance, and lipid metabolism.[72] While it can be argued that the true effect of physical activity on breast cancer recurrence has not yet been conclusively proven, it has far-reaching benefits for improvement in overall health.

Diet and Weight Change

The correlation among alcohol consumption, obesity, and the risk of breast cancer is well established. However, the current data that support risk reduction as it applies to alcohol and obesity focus on avoidance of the exposure or attribute, rather than introducing specific interventions. The majority of studies have not conclusively supported a reduction in risk from an increased consumption of fruits and vegetables. Although a study from the Women's Health Initiative suggested a 9% reduction in risk when women consumed a low-fat diet, prospective studies evaluating dietary changes and effect on breast cancer risk have not been conclusive.[73,75] Vitamin supplements, specifically vitamin D and calcium, have not been shown to affect the development of breast cancer to date.[76] Ongoing studies are addressing this question.

SCREENING
AVERAGE RISK

Effective screening for breast cancer detects disease during the preclinical phase (i.e., prior to the development of symptoms)

KEY POINTS

- Risk-reducing bilateral salpingo-oophorectomy reduces the risk of developing ovarian cancer by 85% and reduces the risk of developing breast cancer by 40% to 60% for women who are *BRCA* mutation carriers, if performed before age 50.
- Bilateral risk-reducing mastectomy reduces the risk of developing breast cancer by more than 90% among women with *BRCA* mutations.
- Five years of tamoxifen or raloxifene reduces the risk of developing primarily estrogen receptor–positive invasive breast cancer by approximately 40%, but does not affect overall mortality.
- The aromatase inhibitor exemestane may be an option for breast cancer risk reduction in the future if it receives U.S. Food and Drug Administration approval.

and therefore has a favorable impact on breast cancer–related mortality based upon the premise that earlier-stage disease is associated with a more favorable prognosis. Decades of controversy have surrounded standard screening recommendations for breast cancer because the published randomized trials are plagued by inconsistent quality of imaging, flawed study design or execution, insufficient duration of follow-up, and problems regarding lead-time bias. Unfortunately, additional randomized trials will never be performed; we are limited by the current data at hand. There are continual updated examinations of these studies in order to determine the efficacy of screening mammography for average-risk women based on age and screening interval. For this reason, it is fair to review the most recent evaluation of screening recommendations.

Data from an evaluation of the randomized trials published in 2002 suggested a 22% reduction in breast cancer mortality among women older than age 50 undergoing mammographic screening. An updated evaluation of these randomized trials in 2009 demonstrated a 14% benefit among women age 50 to 59, and a 32% benefit among women between age 60 and 69.[77] The effect of mammographic screening on breast cancer mortality among women age 40 to 49 or older than age 70 is less robust. An evaluation of eight randomized trials demonstrated a 15% reduction in breast cancer mortality with screening among women age 39 to 49; however, no strong data exist that provide a statistical benefit with screening women older than age 70.

The optimal interval for mammographic screening is not known. Based on six modeling groups that estimated benefits, risks, and use of resources, biennial screening interval was found to be most favorable among all age groups.[78] The optimal starting age remains unclear and is based upon personal risk. The U.S. Preventive Services Task Force (USPSTF) recommends initiating biennial screening at age 50 and continuing until age 74.[79] The American Cancer Society (ACS) recommends continuation of screening after age 70 as long as significant comorbid conditions do not exist, life expectancy is appreciable, and the woman is a candidate for treatment.[80] The ACS also supports annual imaging beginning at age 40. This recommendation is generally accepted by many experts in the field.

The Digital Mammographic Imaging Screening Trial (DMIST) conducted by the American College of Radiology Imaging Network (ACRIN) compared digital images with film-screen mammographic images among 49,528 women.[81] Overall, there was no difference in diagnostic accuracy between digital and film-screen images; however, digital mammography was superior in the detection of malignancy among pre- or perimenopausal women, women younger than age 50, and women with dense breast tissue. This translated into an improved sensitivity of digital mammography over film-screen mammography by 3% to 24%. A population-based study of two-view film-screen mammography compared with digital imaging in Oslo confirmed a higher cancer detection rate with the use of digital mammograms, with a sensitivity of 77%, compared with 62% seen with film-screen mammograms.[82]

Digital breast tomosynthesis (DBT) mammography is a newer techonology enabling a 3-dimensional image of the breast, similar to computed tomography (CT).[83] Investigators have demonstrated a greater than 90% sensitivity using DBT, with a reduction in recall rates. Interpretation times are longer with DBT than with digital imaging, the amount of radiation is slightly greater than that of digital mammography, and a comparison study has not been performed to determine if DBT is truly superior to routine breast cancer screening.

Breast ultrasonography is a significant aid in the diagnosis of breast cancer. It can detect and define ambiguous lesions seen on mammography, and is vital in the characterization of palpable masses within the breast. Ultrasonography is used in directing fine needle aspirations (FNAs) or core needle biopsies of lymph nodes or breast masses. It is not an effective screening modality and the interpretation of imaging is highly dependent upon the skill of the operator. ACRIN performed a study of screening mammogram with ultrasound compared with mammography alone among women at higher risk of developing

breast cancer by virtue of increased breast density.[84] The addition of ultrasound imaging to mammography improved the screening sensitivity in this select patient population by 25%; however, this was achieved at a substantial cost associated with an increase in the rate of false-positive images.

Breast self-examination (BSE) has not been found to improve the detection of early-stage breast cancer on a population basis. Two population studies from Leningrad and Shanghai found no difference in the detection rate of cancer, the tumor characteristics, or breast cancer–related mortality when BSE is performed after instruction, compared with no BSE.[85,86] Clinical breast examinations also do not appear to have affected breast cancer detection or mortality from a population perspective.[87] However, numerous health organizations, including ACS and USPSTF, recommend clinical breast examination in conjunction with mammographic screening among women older than age 40.[80,88] Beginning at age 20, health care providers should encourage women to become familiar with their breasts and report any changes to a health care professional.

HIGH RISK

The routine use of magnetic resonance imaging (MRI) screening for the general population of asymptomatic women is not recommended by virtue of the high cost, limited access, and high false-positive rates associated with MRI. Given its substantial sensitivity, this modality is most optimal in screening a high-risk population. Among patients with *BRCA* mutations, screening mammography can miss more than 50% of all breast cancers. Supplementing mammography with MRI has been shown to improve the sensitivity from the 25% to 59% seen with mammography to 80% to 100% when MRI is added.[89] The specificity of combined mammogram and MRI is lower (73% to 93%) than the specificity of mammography alone. Annual MRI screening among *BRCA* carriers has been shown to detect more interval cancers and earlier-stage cancers (DCIS and stage I, 13.8% with MRI vs. 7.2% without MRI) compared with women not screened with MRI.[90] Adding annual MRI screening to mammography is associated with a 70% reduction in the incidence of lymph node–positive or large invasive breast cancers.

This impressive improvement in detection of earlier-stage disease in high-risk women prompted ACS to review and present recommendations for annual MRI screening in conjunction with mammography for specific high-risk groups.[80,91] Clear evidence exists to support the recommendation for annual MRI screening with mammography for *BRCA* carriers. First-degree relatives of a *BRCA* carrier who are untested are considered high-risk and should be offered annual MRI screening. Women with other inherited risk factors, such as Li-Fraumeni or Cowden syndrome, are also recommended to have MRI screening, as are women who received mantle radiation for the treatment of lymphoma prior to age 30. Caution must be used in recommending annual MRI screening for women whose estimated lifetime risk of developing breast cancer is greater than 20%, since ACS guidelines specifically state that this risk should be determined by calculations obtained using risk models that are dependent upon family history, such as BRCAPRO. The Gail

Model does not meet these criteria (see Risk Determination Models section). There is not enough evidence to date to support annual MRI screening for women with dense breast tissue or the diagnosis of LCIS, atypical ductal hyperplasia, or DCIS. In addition, data are insufficient to support routine MRI screening for all women who have a history of invasive cancer as their only risk factor.

Nuances of High-Risk Breast Cancer Screening

The majority of the data supporting recommendations for breast cancer screening among women at high risk due to hereditary factors stems from studies among *BRCA* carriers. However, the recommendations for screening apply to all of the hereditary breast cancer syndromes. In general, screening for hereditary breast cancer begins at age 25 and includes annual mammography and annual breast MRI with biannual clinical breast exams. Since an estimated 29% of *BRCA*-associated cancers present as "interval" cancers (i.e., cancers presenting during the interval following a normal mammogram), women will often have their breast imaging (mammogram and MRI) alternate every 6 months coincident with their clinical breast examination, although no data supports a superiority in this screening schedule over that of administration of both imaging modalities on the same occasion.[92] Women who received chest radiation treatment for lymphoma are screened in a similar fashion, beginning approximately 10 years after completing radiation.[93] Women with other characteristics associated with high risk (e.g., LCIS or familial risk) should continue with annual mammograms and biannual clinical breast examinations. Initiation of screening should begin approximately 10 years earlier than the age of the youngest woman in the family diagnosed with breast cancer, but not later than age 40.

DIAGNOSIS

Neither physical examination nor imaging can correctly identify whether a breast mass is malignant. Only 60% of the diagnoses of palpable breast masses by physical examination are correct. This reinforces the necessity of tissue biopsy for pathologic evaluation in order to confirm malignancy. Ultrasonography is usually the first diagnostic procedure performed to evaluate palpable breast masses in women younger than age 30. Diagnostic mammography is used for this purpose in women older than age 30. Diagnostic mammography differs from screening mammography by adding additional images to the standard two-view imaging used with screening, (i.e., craniocaudal and mediolateral oblique). If a suspicious finding is seen on a diagnostic mammogram, or if the palpable breast mass is mammographically occult, a targeted ultrasound is used to obtain specific characteristics that will differentiate a suspicious solid mass from a benign cyst.

Although an FNA of a palpable breast mass is less invasive than a core needle biopsy, FNA specimens often have insufficient tissue for analysis and cannot differentiate invasive from noninvasive carcinoma.[94] FNA of suspicious palpable axillary lymph nodes is acceptable given the limited variability of tissue present within a lymph node. It is also appropriate to use FNA in the evaluation of a simple cyst detected by ultrasound, since drainage of the cystic fluid without reaccumulation can imply a benign etiology and eliminate the need for further evaluation.

Core needle biopsies can be obtained via ultrasound guidance or stereotactically when suspicious calcifications are seen on mammography and do not have an associated density. The amount of tissue obtained by core needle biopsy is usually sufficient to characterize the lesion and perform immunohistochemical (IHC) analysis of hormone receptors (ER/PR) and HER2 protein status. This provides sufficient information about the cancer to allow the initiation of neoadjuvant systemic therapy, if needed, without compromising future treatment. Core biopsies also provide enough detail about the pathology to permit decisions concerning surgical options, such as the need for sentinel lymph node biopsy and breast conservation. The need to identify the site of biopsy is crucial; a radiolucent clip is placed in the breast as a locator. The specific aspects of the procedure of core needle biopsy are dependent upon location of the abnormality within the breast, the size of the abnormality, including extent of calcifications, and breast size. High-risk lesions, such as atypical ductal hyperplasia, require additional tissue excision in order to avoid missing an area of more malignant potential within the breast.

MRI imaging can also be used to evaluate the extent of disease within the breast following the detection of invasive breast cancer. A meta-analysis of 19 studies assessing the role of MRI in revealing multifocal or multicentric disease found a 16% incidence of additional disease within the affected breast.[95] This was associated with an 8.1% conversion from breast conservation to mastectomy, and an 11.3% need for additional surgery following wide excision. MRI is also able to detect multicentric DCIS, but is not very accurate in assessing noninvasive tumor size. Caution must be used when assessing the contralateral breast with MRI after the diagnosis of breast cancer. MRI has been shown to detect an occult contralateral malignancy in approximately 3% of patients, resulting in a high rate of biopsies and contralateral mastectomies, given the lack of evidence that these findings will result in a survival advantage.[96]

PROGNOSTIC INDICATORS

TUMOR/NODE/METASTASIS STAGING

The tumor/node/metastasis (TNM) system, under the direction of the American Joint Committee on Cancer and the Union for International Cancer Control, is the standard staging system used for cancer (Table 6-5).[97] With reference to breast cancer, this classification continues to focus entirely on anatomic criteria and a measurement of disease extent, which aids in grouping patients with generally similar prognoses who likely need similar therapy. To some degree, the TNM system enables clinical trial activity and the assessment of outcomes. The specific prognosis for an individual cannot be determined from the TMN staging system, but instead requires an analysis of the biology of the tumor. In some situations, the TNM situation can provide a great deal of information in and of itself. For example, the prognosis for stage 0 disease, or DCIS, can be applied from TMN staging, since biologic characteristics of DCIS have little effect on treatment recommendations to date. Another application of the TMN staging system to breast cancer is in differentiating stage IV or metastatic disease, which is incurable in almost all patients, from all other stages of disease, which are associated with a goal of cure following treatment.

ANATOMIC PROGNOSTIC INDICATORS

Prognostic features of breast cancer can be divided into two categories: anatomic features and biologic features. Data suggest that the biologic characteristics of this disease offer considerable information to aid in the decision-making process about systemic therapies.

Lymph Node Involvement

The most important anatomic prognostic indicator for localized breast cancer is the presence of tumor involvement within axillary lymph nodes. Intramammary lymph nodes are found within the breast parenchyma and are included in the axillary lymph node category when they contain breast cancer metastasis. The clinical detection of internal mammary lymph node involvement is associated with a greater risk of local disease recurrence as well as risk of distant metastasis, classifying the nodal involvement into an N2 category. Regardless of other characteristics of the breast cancer, the number of axillary lymph nodes involved with disease is linearly related to the risk of systemic recurrence and disease-specific survival.

The number of lymph nodes involved with metastasis can be grouped into three categories: one to three positive lymph nodes, four to nine positive lymph nodes, and 10 or more positive lymph nodes. The size of the tumor contributes to prognosis when zero to three lymph nodes are involved, whereas the prognosis is predominantly governed by the nodal involvement once four or more nodes are positive. In the absence of systemic

therapy, more than 70% of patients with 10 or more involved lymph nodes will develop systemic metastasis; approximately 60% will experience relapse with four to nine involved lymph nodes; 25% to 55% will experience relapse with one to three involved lymph nodes; and only 20% to 35% of patients without lymph node involvement will experience relapse within 20 years.[98] These data are based upon routine level I and level II axillary lymph node dissections (ALND), wherein at least six, and more often at least 10, lymph nodes were evaluated. For more than 10 years, the evaluation of the clinically negative ipsilateral axilla has been performed by sentinel lymph node biopsy, which usually identifies only one or two lymph nodes for intense histopathologic assessment. More recently, the American College of Surgeons Oncology Group (ACOSOG) Z0011 trial demonstrated the equivalence between a full node dissection and observation for women who have a positive sentinel biopsy.[99] These women had T1 or T2 tumors and only one or two positive sentinel lymph nodes treated with breast-conserving surgery. All patients received tangential whole-breast irradiation (WBI). The acceptance of this trial is largely related to an understanding that breast cancer treatment decisions can be made based on biologic characteristics of the tumor and do not require the quantification of the specific number of lymph nodes.

The size of the metastatic component within the axillary lymph node is also prognostically important. Macrometastasis (larger than 2 mm) and micrometastasis (larger than 0.2 mm or more than 200 cells, but none larger than 2 mm) are classified as positive nodal involvement. There is a greater risk for disease recurrence and death with macrometastatic disease compared with micrometastatic involvement.[100] Isolated tumor cell clusters (clusters of cells not larger than 0.2 mm, or fewer than 200 cells) found within a sampled axillary lymph node are believed to represent cancer cells in transit, and are associated with a prognosis comparable to lymph node–negative disease.

Tumor Size and Histology

Tumor size is one of the most important prognostic indicators for breast cancer and it refers to the invasive component, which is measured microscopically. The size of associated DCIS does not contribute to the risk of systemic disease, but may contribute to the risk of ipsilateral cancer recurrence following breast conservation. Larger sizes of invasive cancer are associated with a shorter recurrence-free survival and higher breast cancer–specific mortality. Multifocal (two or more foci of disease within one quadrant of the breast) or multicentric (two or more foci of disease in separate quadrants) disease occurs in 10% to 30% of cases and is associated with a higher risk of ipsilateral breast recurrence following breast conservation, and an increased frequency of positive lymph nodes.

The majority of invasive breast cancer is either infiltrating ductal carcinoma (IDC; 75%) or infiltrating lobular carcinoma (ILC; 10%), or a combination of both ductal and lobular features. ILC is often more difficult to detect mammographically, has an increased frequency of multifocality and indistinct borders, and has a higher incidence of bilateral breast involvement at the time of original diagnosis. However, the prognosis associated

Table 6-5 TNM Classifications and Staging System of the American Joint Committee on Cancer (AJCC)[97]

a. The stage of a multifocal cancer is based upon the size of the largest foci.

b. The pathologic staging after neoadjuvant therapy has a "y" preceding the TNM stage.

c. The nodal staging after surgical dissection is preceded by "p."

d. T1* includes T1mic

Primary Tumor (T)

TX	Cannot be assessed
T0	Tumor is not present
Tis	Carcinoma in situ
T1	≤ 2.0 cm
T1mi	≤ 0.1 cm
T1a	> 0.1 cm but ≤ 0.5 cm
T1b	> 0.5 cm but ≤ 1.0 cm
T1c	> 1.0 cm but ≤ 2.0 cm
T2	> 2.0 cm but ≤ 5.0 cm
T3	> 5.0 cm
T4	Any size tumor with extension through the chest wall (T4a) or skin ulceration/nodules (T4b) or both (T4c)
T4d	Inflammatory breast cancer

Regional Lymph Nodes (N)

NX	Cannot be assessed
N0	Nodal involvement absent
N0(i+)	Isolated tumor cells: size ≤ 0.2 mm or fewer than 200 cells
N1	Clinical: movable ipsilateral axillary lymph nodes
pN1mic	Micrometastasis: > 0.2 mm (or more than 200 cells) but ≤ 2.0 mm
pN1a	1 to 3 positive axillary lymph nodes; at least one > 2.0 mm
pN1b	Pathologically positive internal mammary lymph nodes
pN1c	Criteria of both N1a and N1b
N2	Clinical: ipsilateral axillary lymph nodes that are fixed; or clinically apparent internal mammary lymph nodes in the absence of clinically positive axillary lymph nodes

Table 6-5 continued

pN2a	4 to 9 positive axillary lymph nodes; at least one > 2.0 mm
pN2b	Clinically apparent internal mammary lymph nodes in the absence of axillary lymph node involvement
N3	Clinical: ipsilateral infraclavicular lymph node involvement with or without axillary lymph node involvement; or clinically apparent internal mammary lymph nodes with axillary lymph node involvement; or involvement of ipsilateral supraclavicular lymph nodes
pN3a	≥ 10 positive axillary lymph nodes or infraclavicular lymph node involvement
pN3b	Positive axillary lymph nodes with clinical or pathologic involvement of internal mammary lymph nodes
pN3c	Ipsilateral supraclavicular lymph node involvement

Metastases (M)

M0	No clinical or radiographic evidence of distant metastasis
M1	Distant detectable metastasis as determined by classic clinical and radiographic means and/or histologically proven to be larger than 0.2 mm

AJCC Staging System

Stage	Tumor (T)	Node (N)	Metastasis (M)
0	Tis	N0	M0
IA	T1*	N0	M0
IB	T0-1*	N1mic	M0
IIA	T0-T1*	N1	M0
IIA	T2	N0	M0
IIB	T2	N1	M0
IIB	T3	N0	M0
IIIA	T0-2*	N2	M0
IIIA	T3	N1-2	M0
IIIB	T4	N0-2	M0
IIIC	Any T	N3	M0
IV	Any T	Any N	M1

The original source for this material is the AJCC Cancer Staging Manual, 7th Edition (2010) published by Springer Science and Business Media LLC, www.springerlink.com.

with ILC is comparable to IDC when viewed as an independent feature.[101] Rarer subtypes of IDC include pure tubular (1% to 4%), mucinous, medullary, papillary, and adenocystic. These subtypes have distinct pathologic criteria for classification, and are often associated with a more favorable prognosis, whereas the rare subtype of metaplastic carcinoma has an extremely unfavorable prognosis.[102]

Histologic Grade

The histologic grading system for breast cancer is a semiquantitative evaluation of morphologic features consisting of the percentage of tubular formation, degree of nuclear pleomorphism, and mitotic count within a predefined area.[103] There are three grades that reflect breast cancer differentiation based upon the scoring of these characteristics: low, intermediate, and high. Several grading systems have been accepted for breast cancer, namely the modified Bloom-Richardson system and the Nottingham system. These grading systems have been shown to be reasonably reproducible across pathologists, and have been validated in multiple studies demonstrating a correlation between disease-free survival (DFS) and breast cancer–specific survival with the tumor grade.[101,104] The histologic grade is an independent prognostic indicator that has been closely linked to the molecular biology of breast cancer.

Lymphatic Invasion

Tumor emboli present within lymphatic or vascular channels are associated with a less favorable prognosis, more so with regard to ipsilateral breast recurrence than systemic recurrence, although their presence does not preclude breast conservation. Dermal lymphatic involvement is present in 75% of patients with inflammatory breast cancer, which is associated with a poor prognosis and requires local treatment with mastectomy. An incidental finding of dermal lymphatic involvement in the absence of other clinical criteria defining inflammatory breast cancer may be associated with a higher risk of local disease recurrence.

Proliferation Rate

In the past, S-phase fraction and DNA flow cytometry were used to assess the proliferation rate of breast cancer. The complexity of the required technology to perform these analyses resulted in difficulties with quality control, and the clinical value of these indicators declined. Ki67 is a nuclear antigen specific for proliferating cells. IHC staining of the antigen is used as a marker of proliferation, with increased proliferation correlating with adverse prognostic indicators such as tumor size, nodal involvement, and histologic grade. The interpretation of the proliferation rate by Ki67 is subtle, and more data are required before it is widely accepted as an independent prognostic indicator.

MOLECULAR PROGNOSTIC AND PREDICTIVE MARKERS

We are gaining a greater understanding of the biology of breast cancer. The advantage of this information is to provide basic prognostic information, but more importantly, these features are most valuable in predicting response to targeted therapeutic intervention. The following sections provide more detail regarding molecular prognostic and predictive factors.

Hormone Receptors: Estrogen and Progesterone Receptors

The estrogen and progesterone receptors are weak prognostic indicators, but are highly predictive of response to endocrine therapy. The androgen receptor (AR) has more recently been a focus of interest; however, its utility remains investigational. The ER functions as a ligand-dependent transcription factor that regulates gene expression through interaction with hormone-response elements.[105] There are two isoforms of ER, alpha (ER-alpha) and beta (ER-beta). The IHC method of detecting functional ER measures ER-alpha levels. The PR also has two isoforms and regulates gene expression, although the IHC analysis of PR is essentially a functional assay, with a positive PR representing an active ER pathway, even if the ER itself is negative.

The majority of hormone receptor–positive breast cancers have functional ER and PR, whereas cancers that are ER-positive/PR-negative and ER-negative/PR-positive are less frequent but still respond to endocrine therapy, although to a lesser extent. Among all breast cancers, 55% are ER-positive/PR-positive, whereas ER-positive/PR-negative and ER-negative/PR-positive account for 16% and 4%, respectively.[106] There is a

proportional response to endocrine therapy with respect to the amount of hormone positivity observed with IHC. The criteria for positive receptor status remains controversial; however, data support efficacy with endocrine therapy in the setting of any percentage of positive hormone receptors, supporting the global use of endocrine therapy except when both the ER and PR are negative.[107]

The prognostic utility of hormone receptors is generally overshadowed by their frequent association with older patient age and lower tumor grade with negative lymph nodes. However, ER-positive/PR-positive disease is associated with a modestly superior disease-free interval, local recurrence rate, and OS compared with ER-negative/PR-negative disease, especially within the first 10 years following diagnosis. The single hormone receptor–positive subtypes (ER-positive/PR-negative and ER-negative/PR-positive) have outcomes that lie between the ER/PR-positive and ER/PR-negative subgroups. Whereas the risk of disease recurrence is greatest within the first 2 to 5 years with hormone receptor–negative disease and then dramatically declines, hormone receptor–positive breast cancer has a tendency toward a slower rise in risk of recurrence and a more gradual decline, so that late distant recurrences (more than 10 years after diagnosis) can happen.[108]

HER2

The *HER2* gene is a member of the epidermal growth factor receptor (EGFR) tyrosine kinase family that includes four transmembrane receptor proteins: EGFR-1, HER2, HER3, and HER4. Receptor activation, either through ligand binding or ligand-independent effects, results in dimerization of the receptor proteins, either homo- or heterodimerization, which stimulates cellular growth, cell survival, migration, and angiogenesis. Overexpression of the HER2 185-kd protein is a consequence of gene amplification, which occurs in approximately 20% of all breast cancers. This can be determined by either IHC analysis using anti-HER2 antibody staining with 0 or 1+ categorized as negative, 2+ as equivocal, and 3+ as positive.[109,110] Fluorescence in situ hybridization (FISH) classifies tumors as HER2-positive when the ratio of *HER2* gene copies to the centromeric portion of chromosome 17 (HER2:CEP17 ratio) is greater than or equal to 2.0. Up to 24% of breast cancers that are HER2 2+ by IHC have gene amplification and benefit from HER2-directed therapy; therefore, FISH analysis should be performed on all specimens that are IHC 2+. The effect of soluble levels of the HER2 extracellular domain, detected in the serum, remains controversial.

HER2 overexpression or amplification is a strong predictive factor for response to specific systemic therapies. HER2-positive status is predictive of increased efficacy with several chemotherapeutic agents, such as anthracyclines and taxanes.[111,112] It is also a marker of relative resistance to endocrine therapy.[113] Anti-HER2–directed therapy includes the use of trastuzumab, which is a humanized monoclonal antibody directed at the extracellular domain of the 185-kd protein; pertuzumab, another humanized monoclonal antibody directed at the extracellular dimerization domain of HER2; trastuzumab emtansine, an antibody-drug conjugate of trastuzumab and the microtubule inhibitor DM1; or lapatinib, which is the oral dual tyrosine kinase inhibitor (TKI) of both HER2 and EGFR-1.

HER2 status, in addition to being an excellent predictive factor, is also a modest prognostic indicator. It is correlated with a highly proliferative subtype of breast cancer, demonstrated by high-grade histology and lymph node involvement.[114] Independent of other prognostic indicators, including size, lymph node involvement, and hormone receptor status, HER2-positive disease that is not treated with anti-HER2 therapy is associated with a shorter disease-free survival and breast cancer–specific survival. However, the degree of HER2 positivity is not associated with prognosis, and higher levels of HER2 do not predict increased trastuzumab efficacy.

Intrinsic Molecular Subtypes

The use of whole-genome analysis has transformed the understanding of cancer in general, and specifically has resulted in the identification of molecular subtypes of breast cancer, known as "intrinsic subtypes," each with specific gene expression signatures and clinical characteristics. In addition to being prognostic for systemic disease recurrence, the intrinsic subtypes are now being established as prognostic indicators in terms of local disease recurrence following breast conservation or mastectomy.[115,116]

In general, the luminal subtype includes the hormone receptor–positive breast cancers (ER- and/or PR-positive), and is the most common subtype, with an incidence of approximately 67%.[117] The luminal A subtype expresses more ER-related genes, is often low-grade, has a low incidence of *p53* mutations, and is associated with the best overall prognosis in terms of DFS, OS, and local and regional disease relapse. Luminal B cancers express more proliferation- and HER2-related genes and fewer ER-related genes compared with luminal A cancers. Luminal B cancers are often higher grade and have a less favorable overall prognosis compared with luminal A. The luminal A category is often simplified as ER-positive and PR-positive, whereas the luminal B cancers are often ER-positive, PR-positive or -negative, and/or HER2-positive.[118]

The HER2 subtype does not express hormone receptors, but demonstrates overexpression of genes within the ERBB2 amplicon. These cancers are frequently HER2-positive, but are also ER/PR-negative, are more often high-grade, and are associated with more frequent *p53* mutations (40% to 80%).

The basal-like subtype has a gene expression profile that mimics basal epithelial cells by not expressing hormone-related or HER2-related genes. This subtype expresses proliferation-related genes and basal cytokeratins 5, 6, and 17, and has a greater propensity to be high-grade and contain *p53* mutations; thus, basal-like cancers are associated with the least favorable prognosis, with a high risk of systemic and local disease relapse and breast cancer–related death.[119] They are often classified as "triple-negative," meaning they usually, but not always, are negative for ER, PR, and HER2 overexpression. *BRCA1*-associated cancers are often basal-like, whereas *BRCA2* breast cancers include the entire spectrum of intrinsic subtypes, very much like

sporadic cancers. The true existence of a fifth intrinsic subtype, "normal breast," is controversial.

Not only are the individual molecular subtypes associated with prognosis, but they also provide predictive information about the efficacy of specific therapies. Basal-like cancers are often more sensitive to DNA-damaging chemotherapy agents, such as cisplatin, whereas luminal A cancers are treated very effectively with endocrine therapy alone. Luminal B cancers often benefit from the addition of chemotherapy to endocrine treatment. The basal-like subtype is also associated with a greater probability of achieving a pathologic complete response following neoadjuvant chemotherapy, whereas the luminal A and B subtypes are less likely to do so.[120] Routine use of molecular subtyping for clinical purposes is not yet feasible; however, with the extensive development of targeted therapy in a field increasingly focused on personalized medicine, molecular subtyping may play a larger role in the treatment of breast cancer in the future.

Gene Expression Signatures

Differential gene expression profiling for breast cancer (a way of putting into practice some molecular prognostic and predictive factors discussed above) has produced several validated tests to assess the risk of both local and systemic disease recurrence among breast cancers with a more favorable profile (i.e., hormone receptor–positive disease). They have not yet added substantial information about prognosis for the higher-risk subtypes, such as the HER2-positive or hormone receptor–negative breast cancers. The 70-gene signature was developed from the Netherlands Cancer Institute among women younger than age 55 with node-negative disease and tumor sizes smaller than 5 cm, and this group subsequently validated the signature in a group of young women (age younger than 53) with lymph node–positive or –negative disease.[121] Among the group with the poor prognostic signature, there was a 5-fold increase in the risk of systemic recurrence at 10 years compared with the group that had the good prognostic signature. This gene signature is known as "MammaPrint" (Agendia BV, Amsterdam, the Netherlands) and has been independently validated by the TRANSBIG consortium, which included older women (yet younger than age 60), all with lymph node–negative disease.[122] A prospective validation is ongoing in the MINDACT Trial (Microarray in Node-Negative Disease May Avoid Chemotherapy).[123]

The 21-gene recurrence score known as "Oncotype DX" (Genomic Health, Redwood City, California) was developed from patients with node-negative, ER-positive disease enrolled in the NSABP B-14 clinical trial which randomly assigned patients to tamoxifen adjuvant therapy or placebo.[124] This is the most widely used prognostic test in the United States because it uses paraffin-embedded breast tissue, whereas the 70-gene signature requires fresh, frozen samples. The recurrence score (RS) is used as a continuous function and assesses residual risk of systemic recurrence among women with ER-positive breast cancer treated with tamoxifen. The risk of recurrence is classified as low risk, intermediate risk, and high risk. The prognostic value of this model has also been validated among patients treated with AIs and combination chemotherapy for node-negative and node-positive disease. An ongoing validation trial, RxPonder (Refining Post-Surgical Therapy for Women with Lymph Node Positive Breast Cancer), will determine whether women with low recurrence scores can safely avoid chemotherapy in the setting of node-positive disease.[125]

Unlike the 70-gene signature, the 21-gene RS has established utility in predicting the benefit of chemotherapy when added to tamoxifen as adjuvant treatment. Those patients with low-risk disease (i.e., low RS) do not significantly benefit from chemotherapy when given in addition to tamoxifen in the setting of lymph node–negative disease, regardless of menopausal status; similar findings are observed in the setting of lymph node–positive disease in postmenopausal women.[126,127] The 21-gene RS has also been shown to predict risk of local disease recurrence (ipsilateral breast, chest wall, and regional nodal), regardless of administration of tamoxifen or chemotherapy.[128] A prospective clinical trial, TAILORx (the Trial Assigning Individualized Options for Treatment), will hopefully refine the utility of this test, especially among breast cancers classified as intermediate-risk.[129]

MULTIFACTOR PROGNOSTIC INDICES

There are several indices that incorporate the multiple prognostic indicators into a cohesive assessment. These models focus primarily on anatomic characteristics, and only include the traditional molecular variables such as hormone receptor and HER2 status. The Nottingham Prognostic Index (NPI) identifies three prognostic groups based on tumor size, lymph node status, and histologic grade.[130] Adjuvant! Online (www.adjuvantonline.com) is a web-based prognostic calculator that utilizes the same indicators as the NPI, plus patient age, comorbid conditions, lymph node status, and hormone receptor status. In addition to prognosis, Adjuvant! Online will provide an estimate of the benefit of treatment with endocrine therapy and/or chemotherapy; however, it does not include HER2 status or information about the effects of trastuzumab therapy on HER2-positive disease.[131]

TREATMENT OF EARLY-STAGE DISEASE: STAGE 0, I, II, III
INITIAL EVALUATION

The initial evaluation of women diagnosed with early-stage disease (stage I and II) includes a physical examination, breast imaging with mammography with or without ultrasound, baseline laboratory tests with a complete blood count, and liver function tests including an alkaline phosphatase test. Additional diagnostic testing should be individualized, especially the use of breast MRI (see Diagnosis section). Positron emission tomography (PET)/CT has not been shown to be beneficial in evaluating local disease (i.e., the primary breast cancer or axilla); however, it can be a useful tool for problem-solving, such as determining the extent of locoregional disease when stage III disease is present.[132] In the absence of symptoms, imaging studies are not required for patients with stage

I to IIB disease. Patients with stage III disease should generally have a CT of the chest and abdomen (with or without a CT of the pelvis) and bone scan. A PET/CT is another option, but this has not been shown to be superior to CT and bone scan for staging purposes. Genetic counseling should be provided for those patients with a significant family history of cancer or other characteristics that may suggest an inherited predisposition (see Risk Factors section).

STAGE 0: DUCTAL CARCINOMA IN SITU (TONOMO)

An appropriate definition of DCIS was accepted by the U.S. National Cancer Institute (NCI) during a State-of-the-Science conference, and can be described as a "complete replacement of normal ductal cells with a spectrum of abnormal cells confined to the ducts without invasion."[133] With the acceptance of mammographic screening in 1980, the incidence of DCIS has increased more than 7-fold, most commonly among women older than age 50, accounting for 25% of all breast cancers in the United States. Important features of DCIS include size, histologic subtype (comedo, micropapillary or papillary, cribriform, and solid), cytologic or nuclear grade (low, intermediate, or high), presence of central necrosis, and ER status. A multigene assay, the Oncotype DX DCIS (Genomic Health, Redwood City, California), has been validated as a prediction tool for recurrence risk among patients with DCIS treated with breast-conserving surgery without whole-breast radiotherapy; however, its utility in clinical practice has yet to be defined.[134]

An estimated 15% to 50% of DCIS will ultimately progress to invasive disease if left intact, either by direct transformation or developing in parallel from a single progenitor cell.[135] The exact biologic mechanism is not known, nor can we distinguish which subset of DCIS will progress to invasive breast cancer; therefore, by definition, we overtreat a proportion of women with DCIS in order to achieve the goal of preventing ipsilateral breast cancer, 50% of which will be invasive. The risk of local recurrence of DCIS or development of invasive cancer following simple mastectomy without ALND is approximately 1%, whereas the recurrence risk is 6% to 16% following treatment by surgical excision and whole-breast radiotherapy administered over 5 to 6 weeks. Both options are comparable with regard to disease-specific survival. Accelerated partial-breast radiation administered over 5 days remains investigational, but is being evaluated in a large randomized trial supported by the NCI (NSABP B-39).[136] Sentinel lymph node biopsy is not necessary when breast conservation is performed for DCIS; however, this procedure may be considered with mastectomy in the event of finding occult invasive disease within the breast, because a sentinel biopsy is not possible after the mastectomy has been performed.[137]

Approximately 50% of local recurrences following a diagnosis of DCIS are invasive. Overall, there is no difference in mortality between the local therapies, with the 10-year breast cancer survival following a diagnosis of DCIS equaling 96% to 98%. However, an ipsilateral development of invasive cancer is associated with a 2-fold greater mortality risk; this risk is not associated with a recurrence of DCIS.[136] The addition of tamoxifen (20 mg daily for 5 years) to breast conservation plus whole-breast radiotherapy (breast-conservation therapy [BCT]), contributes an additional 32% relative reduction in risk of local recurrence and a 53% reduction in risk of contralateral disease over the course of 15 years after diagnosis; however, the benefit of tamoxifen may be seen only with ER-positive DCIS and has not yet been associated with improved OS.[138] Further information on systemic therapy in addition to BCT is pending the analysis of NSABP B-35, which compares tamoxifen with anastrozole in ER-positive DCIS, and NSABP B-43, which compares two cycles of trastuzumab with placebo in HER2-positive DCIS.

STAGE I AND II DISEASE

In early-stage disease (i.e., stage I or II), the treatment approach focuses both on local disease control (breast and regional lymph nodes) and systemic disease control. Systemic treatment adds benefit to local disease control, and local therapies will reduce the risk of systemic recurrence. Thus, these therapies complement each other and are not mutually exclusive.[139] A meta-analysis from the EBCTCG reviewed 15-year survival data from 25,000 women and found that the addition of radiation therapy to the breast following breast conservation also resulted in a reduction in breast cancer mortality by approximately 5%.[140] Systemic therapy with tamoxifen reduces the relative incidence of ipsilateral breast recurrences by 50% in ER-positive disease, whereas chemotherapy also reduces the relative local recurrence rate by 33% regardless of hormone receptor status. Both endocrine therapy with tamoxifen or AIs and trastuzumab can safely be given concurrently with radiotherapy; however, chemotherapy is usually completed prior to starting radiation. The choices for both local and systemic therapies are based upon the prognostic indicators previously described, and treatment options have been outlined by several organizations to help guide decision-making.[141-143]

Local Disease Control

Breast Conservation Therapy. The Fisher hypothesis of breast cancer describes invasive breast cancer as a systemic disease at its inception. This theory differed from the Halstedian philosophy of direct nodal extension of disease beginning in the breast. Understanding the importance of systemic disease allowed Fisher and his colleagues at NSABP to design pivotal trials that resulted in limiting the extent of surgery in the treatment of early-stage breast cancer. NSABP B-04 found that after 25 years, there was no survival difference between radical mastectomy and simple mastectomy. These results were extended to NSABP B-06, which also demonstrated no significant difference in OS between total mastectomy and breast conservation.[144] A comparable survival outcome between mastectomy and BCT is also supported by several larger randomized trials. In general, radiation therapy to the conserved breast reduces the absolute risk of ipsilateral breast recurrence by 30% to 40%, down to a 5% to 7% risk of ipsilateral breast recurrence over approximately 10 years. Whereas modern systemic therapy has contributed to a further reduction in the risk of ipsilateral breast recurrence, the individual risk appears to

be intrinsic subtype–specific.[115] Based upon these results, options for local disease control in operable patients (stage I and II disease) include total mastectomy or breast conservation (lumpectomy) and whole-breast radiotherapy, with BCT being the preferred procedure. Sentinel lymph node biopsy is performed in both settings.

Optimal characteristics for breast conservation include the ability to resect the entire tumor with adequate negative surgical margins. Acceptable cosmetic outcome is important, and therefore the ability to adequately remove the cancer depends upon the size of the cancer and the size of the breast (see Neoadjuvant Systemic Therapy section below). The definition of adequate negative surgical margins is controversial, but in general, a negative margin greater than 2 mm is acceptable. The presence of an extensive intraductal component (EIC; defined as DCIS occupying at least 25% of an invasive carcinoma or a lesion that is predominantly DCIS with one or more foci of invasive disease) is not a contraindication to breast conservation as long as negative margins are obtained. There are a few relatively absolute contraindications to breast conservation for operable disease, and they include multicentric disease, prior radiation therapy, and connective tissue disease involving the skin (e.g., scleroderma).

As in stage 0 disease, patients with stage I or II invasive disease undergoing breast conservation should also receive tangential whole-breast irradiation (WBI) over a course of 5 to 6 weeks (25 fractions).[145] Often an additional 10 Gy to 16 Gy boost to the tumor bed is given over 1 week, so that the breast receives 45 Gy to 50 Gy of radiation and the tumor bed receives a total of 60 Gy. The boost has been shown to reduce the risk of local recurrence, specifically among women younger than age 50 and among those with high-grade invasive cancer.[146] A randomized trial compared local recurrence rates between standard WBI and accelerated hypofractionated WBI among 1,234 women with lymph node–negative disease.[147] Hypofractionated WBI delivers 42.5 Gy to the breast in 16 fractions over 22 days, without a boost. There was no difference in 10-year cumulative incidence of local recurrence between the standard and hypofractionated group (6.7% vs. 6.2%, respectively). However, high-grade cancers or subtypes of breast cancer associated with high-grade disease appear to have inferior local disease control when hypofractionated WBI is prescribed. The majority of ipsilateral recurrences develop in or near the tumor bed. Recurrences in other parts of the affected breast are rare (3% to 4%) and are believed to be new cancers rather than recurrences of the original cancer. This phenomenon has led to the concept of limiting radiation to the breast by using accelerated partial-breast irradiation, which remains controversial (see Stage 0 section).[148]

The potential morbidity associated with complete level I and II ALND is substantial, translating into acute complication rates of 20% to 30% and subsequent upper extremity lymphedema for up to 40% of patients. Sentinel lymph node dissection (SLND) is associated with fewer complications, and is the procedure of choice for the surgical evaluation of the clinically negative axilla. The sentinel lymph node is the first lymph node to receive lymphatic drainage from the breast cancer, and is the most likely site to contain metastatic involvement. Identification of the sentinel lymph node is made by lymphatic mapping using vital blue dye and/or radiolabeled colloid following preoperative lymphoscintigraphy, to document the drainage to the lymphatics. One or several "sentinel" lymph nodes are then dissected and intensively examined at two step-section levels of paraffin-embedded tissue, stained with hematoxylin and eosin. IHC staining for cytokeratins has limited utility and all therapeutic decisions should be based upon assessment with hematoxylin and eosin.[143,149] Based upon a review of 69 studies involving 8,059 patients comparing ALND with SLND, the false-negative rate of SLND is approximately 8%, and is comparable when used during breast conservation or mastectomy.[150]

If a sentinel lymph node cannot be identified or if the axilla is clinically positive, a complete level I and II ALND should be performed. Up to 48% of patients with a positive sentinel lymph node have further axillary lymph node involvement, which supported the recommendation for completing an ALND when the sentinel lymph node is positive.[150] The ACOSOG trial Z0011, however, found that a subset of patients treated with breast conservation and tangential WBI may achieve adequate disease control of the axilla without undergoing an ALND or receiving axillary radiotherapy.[99] Overall, 891 eligible patients had clinical T1 or T2 tumors with a clinically negative axilla (N0), and only one or two positive sentinel lymph nodes following SLND. There was no difference in axillary recurrence rate, DFS, or OS between the two groups; therefore, consideration can be made to avoid a complete ALND in the setting of one or two positive sentinel lymph nodes, but only when these strict criteria are present.[151] This approach has not been evaluated among patients having a mastectomy, receiving neoadjuvant therapy, or opting for breast conservation but not receiving WBI. In these individuals, complete ALND is still recommended following a positive sentinel lymph node.

In addition to WBI, treatment fields are added to control disease in the ipsilateral infraclavicular and supraclavicular areas when four or more axillary lymph nodes are positive, and are often considered when one to three lymph nodes are involved. The ipsilateral internal mammary lymph nodes are often treated in the setting of high-risk disease based upon the NCIC-CTG MA.20 clinical trial that randomly assigned 1,832 women to either WBI or WBI with regional lymph nodal irradiation (RNI).[152] Patients who received WBI and RNI attained a statistically significant improvement in locoregional (HR 0.59; p = 0.02) and distant DFS (HR 0.64; p = 0.002), with a non-statistically significant trend toward an improved OS (HR 0.76; p = 0.07). This improvement in disease control was obtained at a cost of increased toxicity including pneumonitis and lymphedema. The ultimate decision to include added radiation fields to WBI should be based upon individual risks and benefits.

There are special circumstances where the addition of radiation therapy following breast conservation may be avoided. Elderly women with favorable tumor characteristics may undergo breast conservation alone so long as they receive adequate endocrine therapy. A randomized trial of 636 women older than age 70 with ER-positive, pathologic T1 (2 cm or smaller), clinically N0 disease received breast conservation and tamoxifen with or without radiation therapy; at 10-year follow-up, there was no difference in DFS or OS.[153] At 10 years, the locoregional recurrence rate was 2% with radiation and 10% without radiation; however, only 6% of the overall deaths were related to breast cancer.

BCT remains an acceptable means of local therapy for women with *BRCA*-associated breast cancer, if the patient prefers this approach. A multi-institutional study of 655 women with *BRCA1* and *BRCA2* mutations treated with either BCT or mastectomy demonstrated a higher local recurrence rate with BCT; however, the majority of the ipsilateral breast recurrences were second cancers.[154] Systemic therapy reduced the incidence of local recurrences among those treated with BCT. There was no difference in breast cancer–specific survival or OS between those patients treated with BCT or mastectomy.

Total Mastectomy. Patients who are not candidates for BCT should undergo a total mastectomy and sentinel lymph node biopsy, with completion ALND if the sentinel lymph node is positive. The EBCTCG overview meta-analysis reviewed the outcome of 8,500 women enrolled in postmastectomy radiotherapy trials and demonstrated a 66% to 75% relative reduction in 5-year risk of local recurrence when the chest wall and regional lymph nodes (supraclavicular, infraclavicular, axillary, and internal mammary lymph node areas) were treated.[140] The absolute reduction in local recurrences among patients with lymph node–positive disease was 17%. This translated into a 5% reduction in 15-year breast cancer mortality risk and a 4% reduction in overall mortality. The proportional benefit was similar regardless of patient age, tumor characteristics, or whether systemic therapy was given. For this reason, consideration should be given for postmastectomy radiation therapy (PMRT) following the completion of adjuvant chemotherapy when four or more axillary lymph nodes are involved, when there is clinical evidence of internal mammary lymph node involvement, or in the setting of positive surgical margins. There remains some controversy about the absolute efficacy of PMRT when one to three axillary lymph nodes are involved, or when the tumor size is 5 cm or larger and the lymph nodes are negative. Recommendations for treatment should be based upon other adverse characteristics such as lymphovascular involvement, triple-negative tumor status, young age, or close surgical margins (smaller than 1 mm).[155] The risk of locoregional disease recurrence is greatest within the first 5 years, and radiation can safely be given concurrently with endocrine therapy or trastuzumab, but radiation is not recommended to be administered with concurrent chemotherapy. PMRT is also beneficial in the treatment of locally advanced disease (e.g., tumor invading the chest wall or skin involvement). The optimal sequence of treatment in this setting is usually systemic therapy followed by surgery, then radiation (see Stage III Disease, Neoadjuvant Systemic Therapy section). The use of modern treatment planning has resulted in less toxicity to the heart, great vessels, and lungs.

Adjuvant Systemic Therapy. The decision to add systemic therapy to the local treatment of breast cancer is based upon the risk of distant metastasis and the benefit of therapies to reduce that risk. The features described in the Prognostic Indicators section are utilized to determine risk of distant recurrence. In addition, age itself is a relatively independent prognostic feature in that younger women (younger than age 50) are at higher risk of both local and systemic disease recurrence, and the threshold for offering adjuvant therapy is often reduced in this setting. Relatively few clinical trials have included a substantial number of women older than age 70. In this patient population, the decision to administer adjuvant therapy is highly dependent upon treatment-associated toxicity and the presence of comorbid conditions.

In general, breast cancer that is T larger than 0.5 cm, N0, has a high enough risk of systemic recurrence to warrant consideration of adjuvant treatment (Fig. 6-1). Those cancers that are T 0.5 cm or smaller, N0, may not necessarily gain a clinical benefit from systemic therapy from the standpoint of reducing the risk of distant disease; however, if the cancer is hormone receptor–positive, adjuvant endocrine therapy is often considered to reduce the risk of both systemic and local disease recurrence. The lower level of toxicity associated with adjuvant endocrine therapy makes this decision somewhat easier. Aside from these generalizations as to who would benefit from adjuvant therapy, the specific choice of treatment is based upon the molecular profile of the cancer, namely the hormone receptor status (ER and/or PR), and the HER2 status. A collaborative meta-analysis of adjuvant therapy in early-stage breast cancer has been performed every 5 years by the EBCTCG since 1985.[58,156] These overview analyses lend support to current adjuvant therapy recommendations; however, the specific treatments are based upon individual clinical trial outcomes.

HORMONE RECEPTOR–POSITIVE DISEASE
Endocrine Therapy

Endocrine therapy reduces the risk of systemic recurrence and increases OS among all women with hormone receptor–positive (ER and/or PR) breast cancer, regardless of age, menopausal status, nodal involvement, tumor size, HER2 status, or use of chemotherapy. For this reason, endocrine therapy should be used as adjuvant therapy for almost all women with hormone receptor–positive disease. An exception to this involves older women with favorable breast cancer prognoses, especially with comorbid medical conditions. A commonly used adjuvant endocrine therapy is tamoxifen, which is effective in both pre- and postmenopausal women when given for 5 years. The EBCTCG meta-analysis showed that 5 years of tamoxifen reduces the relative risk of distant recurrence by approximately 41% and reduces the relative risk of dying by 34% (Table 6-6).[58]

Recent studies continue to support longer duration of endocrine therapy for adjuvant treatment. The ATLAS (Adjuvant Tamoxifen: Longer Against Shorter) trial randomly assigned 12,894 women with ER-positive disease to continue tamoxifen use for an additional 5 years (10 years total), or discontinue tamoxifen after 5 years of treatment.[157] Continued tamoxifen

A

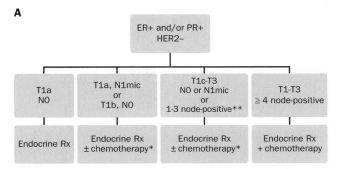

* Recurrence Score may help with decision-making in appropriate patients
** Many oncologists still consider chemotherapy + endocrine therapy as standard for all node-positive disease

B

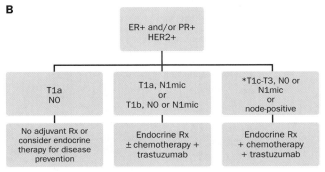

* Clinical trials did not include T1c, N0, therefore chemotherapy and trastuzumab may be omitted in selected patients, yet the majority should receive the combination

C

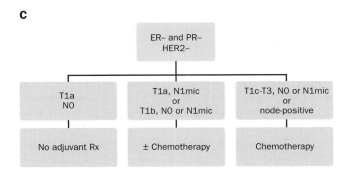

D

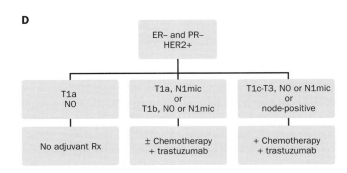

Fig. 6-1 Guidelines for adjuvant systemic therapy.

Guidelines for adjuvant systemic therapy for (**A**) hormone receptor–positive, HER2-negative disease (**B**) hormone receptor–positive, HER2-positive disease (**C**) hormone receptor–negative, HER2-negative, and (**D**) hormone receptor–negative, HER2-positive disease.

Abbreviations: ER, estrogen receptor; PR, progesterone receptor.

Table 6-6 Benefit of Adjuvant Endocrine Therapy in Hormone Receptor–Positive Disease

Study	Endocrine Therapy/Duration	RR recurrence	RR mortality
Primary therapy			
EBCTC[58]	Tamoxifen (5 yr)	0.61 (0.57-0.65)	0.70 (0.64-0.75)
ATAC[160]	Anastrozole vs. tamoxifen (5 yr)	0.90 (0.82-0.99)	1.00 (0.89-1.12)
BIG 1-98[161]	Letrozole vs. tamoxifen (5 yr)	0.88 (0.78-0.99)	0.81 (0.69-0.94)
Sequential therapy			
BIG 1-98	Tamoxifen/letrozole vs. letrozole	1.05 (0.84-1.32)	1.13 (0.83-1.53)
	Letrozole/tamoxifen vs. letrozole	0.96 (0.76-1.21)	0.90 (0.65-1.24)
Extended therapy			
NCIC CTG MA.17[169]	Tamoxifen × 5 yr followed by letrozole × 5 yr	-0.68 (0.55-0.83)	0.98 (0.78-1.22)
ATLAS[157]	Tamoxifen (10 yr)	0.84 (0.76-0.94)*	0.93 (0.86-1.00)*

Abbreviations: RR, relative risk; yr, years.
*Comparing 5 years versus 10 years of tamoxifen use.

use reduced the rate of recurrence and improved OS, though the benefits were more robust during the later years; the absolute mortality reduction was 2.8% at 15 years following diagnosis (i.e., 10 years after the second 5-year period of treatment). These results are supported by the aTTom (Adjuvant Tamoxifen Treatment Offers More) trial, which randomly assigned 6,953 women with ER-positive early-stage breast cancer to 5 additional years of tamoxifen, or to discontinue tamoxifen after 5 years of treatment.[158] This trial also demonstrated an improved breast cancer recurrence rate and OS, specifically seen after 10 years of treatment. Prolonged tamoxifen use was associated with an increased incidence in pulmonary embolism (HR 1.87) and endometrial cancer (HR 1.74), with a 3.1% cumulative risk of endometrial cancer after 5 years of tamoxifen, translating into an absolute increase in endometrial cancer mortality equaling 0.2%.[157] Though these data support increased efficacy of prolonged tamoxifen use, the decision must be weighed against potential adverse outcomes on an individual basis. For patients with early-stage disease (e.g., stage I) who are at low risk of disease recurrence, the potential toxicities may outweigh the benefits.

Significant research has been invested to determine the mechanism of tamoxifen resistance in hormone receptor–positive disease. Tamoxifen undergoes activation via the cytochrome p450 2D6 enzyme (CYP2D6), to metabolites that are 100 times more potent suppressors of estradiol-stimulated breast cancer cell growth (4-OH-tamoxifen and endoxifen) compared with

tamoxifen or its primary metabolite, *N*-desmethyl tamoxifen. Patients who carry genetic variants of CYP2D6 are classified as poor metabolizers who produce low amounts of endoxifen. This raised concern about a potential relationship between poor metabolizers and tamoxifen resistance, with the corollary that poor metabolizers should not be treated with tamoxifen, nor should medications that affect CYP2D6 activity be prescribed concurrently with tamoxifen. A retrospective analysis of 1,325 patients treated with adjuvant tamoxifen from 1986 to 2005 demonstrated a worse DFS among those patients with a CYP2D6 genotype consistent with a poor or intermediate metabolizer of tamoxifen compared with patients having a CYP2D6 genotype of an extensive metabolizer (HR 1.29), but there was no difference in OS.[159] Two subsequent randomized trials comparing adjuvant tamoxifen to an AI (Arimidex, Tamoxifen Alone or in Combination [ATAC][160] and Breast International Group [BIG] 1-98[161]) did not find any association between CYP2D6 genotype and disease outcome with the treatment of tamoxifen. These results were confirmed by a case-control study of 11,251 women registered with the Danish Breast Cancer Cooperative Group.[162] No association was found between CYP2D6 inhibition by genotype or medication and disease outcome with tamoxifen treatment. Because of this ongoing controversy, ASCO guidelines do not support routine testing of CYP2D6 as an instrument to help guide adjuvant endocrine therapy choices; however, ongoing prospective studies should provide more definitive data for decision-making in the future.[163]

The role of ovarian suppression as adjuvant therapy in premenopausal women remains uncertain. The EBCTCG meta-analysis evaluating women younger than age 50 found that ovarian ablation improves DFS by 11% and improves OS by approximately 5%; however, this benefit was not significant when chemotherapy was administered, most likely because of chemotherapy-induced amenorrhea. There did appear to be a greater effect among women younger than age 40.[58] A meta-analysis of 16 trials involving 11,906 premenopausal women using luteinizing hormone-releasing hormone (LHRH) agonists to induce ovarian suppression did not demonstrate a significant benefit when used alone; however, the addition of an LHRH agonist to chemotherapy, with or without tamoxifen, resulted in a 13% reduction in risk of recurrence and a 15% reduction in risk of dying, both of borderline significance.[164] Because of the variability in study design and consequent outcomes, tamoxifen alone continues to be the standard endocrine therapy for premenopausal women.[165] Outcomes are awaited from the Suppression of Ovarian Function Trial (IBCSG 24-02/BIG 2-02) that has evaluated the potential of added benefit from ovarian suppression to tamoxifen in this setting.

Although tamoxifen retains its efficacy in postmenopausal women, AIs (i.e., inhibitors of the enzyme that converts androgens to estrogens) should be considered for the treatment of postmenopausal women, either following 5 years of tamoxifen, following 2 to 3 years of tamoxifen, or as initial therapy for 5 years. New data supporting the use of 10 years of tamoxifen, however, has made this an option for women who are not candidates for AIs. AIs are not effective in pre- or perimenopausal women, and should not used for adjuvant therapy in this group of patients. It is important to remember

Table 6-7	**Adjuvant or Neoadjuvant Chemotherapy Options**
HER2-Negative Disease	Doxorubicin/cyclophosphamide × 4 cycles[173]
	Docetaxel/cyclophosphamide × 4 cycles[174]
	Cyclophosphamide/methotrexate/5-fluorouracil × 6 cycles[173]
	Dose-dense doxorubicin/cyclophosphamide × 4 cycles followed by dose-dense paclitaxel × 4 cycles[185]
	Doxorubicin/cyclophosphamide × 4 cycles followed by 12 weeks of paclitaxel[184]
	Docetaxel/doxorubicin/cyclophosphamide × 6 cycles[179]
HER2-Positive Disease	Doxorubicin/cyclophosphamide × 4 cycles followed by 12 weeks of paclitaxel and trastuzumab followed by trastuzumab (over a 40-week duration)[190]
	Docetaxel/carboplatin/trastuzumab × 6 cycles followed by trastuzumab (over a 34-week duration)[198]
	Adjuvant chemotherapy (various) followed by 1 year of trastuzumab[191]
	Paclitaxel and trastuzumab weekly × 12 weeks followed by trastuzumab × 9 months[201]
	Neoadjuvant only: pertuzumab, trastuzumab, and taxane (either paclitaxel or docetaxel) × 12 weeks total followed by doxorubicin/cyclophosphamide × 4 followed by trastuzumab (over a 40-week duration)[223]

that chemotherapy-induced amenorrhea can be transient, and therefore endocrine therapy should be based upon the menopausal status prior to treatment. There are three third-generation AIs: anastrozole, letrozole (nonsteroidal inhibitors), and exemestane (a steroidal inhibitor). They all appear to be comparable in efficacy and have similar side effect profiles (i.e., involvement of the musculoskeletal system, including arthralgias, myalgias, and reduction in bone density).

An analysis of 12 trials evaluating the efficacy of AIs used as adjuvant therapy can be divided into three cohorts: 5 years of primary therapy, switching to an AI after 2 to 3 years of tamoxifen, and extended therapy with an AI following 5 years of tamoxifen.[166] When compared with 5 years of tamoxifen, the use of an AI as primary therapy was associated with 29% proportional reduction in risk of recurrence, whereas switching from 2 to 3 years of tamoxifen to an AI resulted in a 40% proportional reduction in risk of recurrence.[167] This translated into a 5% absolute reduction in disease recurrence with the use of an AI compared with tamoxifen alone.

Three studies demonstrated a modest benefit in risk of disease relapse, all utilizing a switch to an AI following tamoxifen; two studies switched to an AI after 2 to 3 years of tamoxifen,

and one study switched following 5 years of tamoxifen. In longer follow-up, one trial, the Intergroup Exemestane Study (IES), revealed a small improvement in OS.[168] Three trials of extended endocrine therapy (i.e., an AI for 3 to 5 years following 5 years of tamoxifen) also demonstrated an added reduction in disease recurrence; however, only one (NCIC CTG MA.17[169]) demonstrated a modest improvement in OS. In general, postmenopausal women should receive treatment with an AI during their first 5 years of adjuvant therapy, with the optimal strategy being either initially using an AI as primary endocrine therapy, or switching from tamoxifen after 2 years to an AI for an additional 3 years. Women who are cannot tolerate an AI after 2 years of treatment may switch to tamoxifen for the remaining 3 years without compromising their outcome. There are no data supporting an extended duration of AI treatment for longer than 5 years, although the results of two clinical trials (IBCSG 35-07 and NSABP B-42) will provide important insights on that question.

Chemotherapy

Adjuvant chemotherapy reduces the risk of relapse early in the disease course (within the first 5 years) and can benefit hormone receptor–positive disease in many cases (Table 6-7). Over the past several years there has been a decrease in the use of chemotherapy for hormone receptor–positive (and HER2-negative) disease, stemming from recognition that, on average, chemotherapy is less beneficial in this large patient subgroup than in those with HER2-positive or triple-negative disease. Nevertheless, there are many patients with hormone receptor–positive disease who obtain a sizeable benefit from the administration of chemotherapy in addition to endocrine therapy. Chemotherapy can be considered when the tumor size is larger than 0.5 cm regardless of nodal status, or when there is lymph node involvement regardless of tumor size. Factors which prompt the use of chemotherapy are a high histologic grade, a moderate to large disease burden, and a high RS determined by Oncotype DX.[126] In this setting, chemotherapy is given first, then endocrine therapy. The role of the RS in assessing the added benefit from chemotherapy to endocrine therapy in lymph node–positive disease is less certain, although it can be helpful in postmenopausal patients.[127]

There are several appropriate chemotherapy regimens used for adjuvant treatment in HER2-negative disease (see HER2-Positive Disease section). Some principles for administering adjuvant chemotherapy are as follows[58]:

- The administration of full-dose chemotherapy is vital and should be administered based upon actual height and weight.
- Most studies involve women younger than age 70; therefore, administration of chemotherapy in elderly patients is based upon individual risk/benefit ratios.
- There is no apparent added benefit of dose escalation compared with standard-dose chemotherapy in adjuvant treatment.
- Polychemotherapy is preferred and is associated with greater benefits in women younger than age 50, with higher-risk disease (node-positive), and with hormone receptor–negative disease.

In general, multidrug regimens containing anthracyclines and taxanes are appropriate for higher-risk disease (i.e., node-positive or node-negative with large tumor size [T2 or higher]), whereas shorter and less complex regimens are usually used for smaller node-negative tumors, and selected node-positive tumors. The choice of regimen is dependent upon the overall risk of disease recurrence and the relative reduction of risk with the administration of chemotherapy, balanced by the toxicity of the drugs. In hormone receptor–positive disease, anthracycline-containing chemotherapy reduces the relative risk of recurrence by 36% and reduces the relative risk of death by 35% when added to tamoxifen.[55] In hormone receptor–positive breast cancer, the addition of taxanes to anthracycline-based regimens reduces the relative recurrence risk by an additional 26% and reduces relative mortality risk by an additional 23%.[170] Chemotherapy regimens that are appropriate for use as adjuvant therapy in both hormone receptor–positive and –negative disease are outlined below.

TRIPLE-NEGATIVE DISEASE

Adjuvant endocrine therapies are not effective without the presence of their target, as in ER- and/or PR-negative disease. In addition, trastuzumab, the humanized monoclonal antibody against the HER2 protein, is not effective in HER2-negative disease. For this reason, chemotherapy is the mainstay of adjuvant treatment for TNBC (ER/PR-negative and HER2-negative), a subtype of breast cancer that lacks a specific therapeutic target. TNBC only accounts for approximately 10% to 15% of all breast cancer, is more common among young and/or black women, and is usually high-grade. Unlike other subtypes of breast cancer, the biology of TNBC is such that its prognosis does not correlate as closely with tumor size or nodal involvement.[171] For example, a study suggested that once one axillary lymph node is involved, additional axillary nodal involvement does not affect the poor prognosis associated with node-positive TNBC. In addition, node-negative TNBC with tumor size greater than 0.5 cm (T1b or higher) has a high enough risk of disease recurrence and death to warrant a discussion of adjuvant chemotherapy.[172]

As stated previously, the efficacy of chemotherapy is greater in TNBC, where the risk of systemic recurrence is greatest within the first 2 to 3 years, compared with hormone receptor–positive disease, where the risk of recurrence continues for at least 10 to 15 years. In the adjuvant setting, however, the chemotherapy regimens recommended for treatment are identical for both TNBC and hormone receptor–positive cancer.

The addition of anthracyclines to methotrexate-containing regimens in adjuvant therapy improves the proportional reduction in risk of recurrence by 12% and death by 15%.[58] These data support the use of anthracyclines for adjuvant treatment, the most commonly used combination regimen being doxorubicin and cyclophosphamide (AC) for four cycles. AC has been found to be comparable to six cycles of cytoxan, methotrexate, and 5-fluorouracil (CMF), which is less commonly used today, given the preference for using anthracyclines.[173] A smaller randomized trial compared four cycles of AC with four cycles of another two-drug regimen, docetaxel and cyclophosphamide, among women with stage I to III breast cancer.[174] After a 7-year follow-up, there was a 6% improvement in DFS and a 5% improvement in OS with the docetaxel/cyclophosphamide regimen. Although the trial was relatively small in size, these data suggest that the two regimens are comparable. Docetaxel/cyclophosphamide was associated with less cardiotoxicity and a lower risk of treatment-induced leukemia compared with AC, but both of these toxicities are very rare. NSABP B-49 is a complicated study evaluating the efficacy and toxicity of six cycles of docetaxel/cyclophosphamide compared with multiple anthracycline-containing regimens. The results of this ongoing study should offer greater insight into the relative toxicities of anthracycline- versus nonanthracycline-containing adjuvant therapy regimens.

The question of duration of therapy was addressed by CALGB 40101, which evaluated 3,171 patients with primarily lymph node–negative disease (94% vs. 6% with one to three lymph nodes involved), and randomized their treatment to either four or six cycles of AC or single-agent paclitaxel.[175] Both regimens were administered every 2 weeks, with no difference in outcome (relapse-free survival or OS) between four or six cycles of treatment.

Based upon a meta-analysis of 13 randomized trials involving 22,453 women, the addition of taxanes to anthracycline-containing regimens resulted in a 17% reduction in the relative risk of relapse, and a 15% relative reduction in risk of death at 5 years. This translates into a 5% absolute improvement in DFS and a 3% improvement in OS.[176] This relative benefit is constant, regardless of the type of taxane used (paclitaxel or docetaxel), patient age, or number of lymph nodes involved. There is a suggestion that the addition of a taxane in sequence may offer a greater advantage compared with regimens where the taxane is combined with the anthracycline; however, only a small number of trials provide evidence for this suggestion.

Initial adjuvant taxane studies demonstrated superior DFS and OS when four cycles of paclitaxel were administered following four cycles of AC, compared with four cycles of AC alone (Cancer and Leukemia Group B [CALGB] 9344[177]), and similar results were seen when three cycles of docetaxel were given following three cycles of 5-fluorouracil, epirubicin, cytoxan (FEC), compared with six cycles of FEC (National Federation of French Cancer Centres [FNCLCC] PACS 01 trial[178]). Two concurrent studies compared six cycles of 5-fluorouracil, doxorubicin, and cyclophosphamide (FAC) with six cycles of docetaxel, doxorubicin, and cyclophosphamide (TAC) in both node-positive breast cancer (Breast Cancer International Research Group [BCIRG] 001[179]) and high-risk node-negative disease (Spanish Breast Cancer Research Group, GEICAM 9805[180]). Both studies demonstrated superiority of TAC in reducing the relative risk of recurrence by 30%, but only the node-positive study found a 30% relative reduction in risk of death.

Comparing the two strategies of adding taxanes to anthracycline-containing regimens, BCIRG 005 did not demonstrate a difference between six cycles of TAC and four cycles of AC followed by four cycles of docetaxel. NSABP B30, however, found a superior DFS and OS with four cycles of AC followed by four cycles of docetaxel compared with four cycles of TAC or four cycles of docetaxel/doxorubicin.[181,182] Neutropenia is associated with the combination regimens more frequently, whereas neuropathy and nail changes are more common with the sequential therapies. NSABP B-38 expanded this concept by comparing six cycles of TAC with two regimens: either four cycles of AC followed by four cycles of paclitaxel given every 2 weeks, or with this regimen when gemcitabine was added to the paclitaxel arm.[183] The additional chemotherapy (gemcitabine) did not add benefit; however, six cycles of TAC was comparable in DFS and OS with four cycles of AC followed by four cycles of paclitaxel. Again, the toxicity profile differed between the two regimens, with neutropenic fever and diarrhea being more prevalent with TAC chemotherapy.

In an attempt to determine the optimal taxane and its optimal schedule for adjuvant therapy use, the Eastern Cooperative Oncology Group (ECOG 1199) compared docetaxel with paclitaxel, both given either weekly for 12 weeks or every 3 weeks for four cycles, after completing four cycles of AC in node-positive and high-risk node-negative disease.[184] Many consider paclitaxel, administered weekly for 12 weeks, to be better than the three other options of taxane administration.

An every-2-week schedule may be more optimal for chemotherapy administration in early-stage breast cancer, as compared with an every-3-week schedule. This is supported by a study in which 2,005 women with lymph node–positive disease were randomly assigned to receive AC for four cycles followed by paclitaxel for four cycles, given either every 3 weeks or every 2 weeks with cytokine support for neutropenia (CALGB 9741). Patients could also receive sequential single-agent chemotherapy with doxorubicin for four cycles, followed by paclitaxel for four cycles, followed by cyclophosphamide for four cycles; each drug was randomly given either every 3 weeks or every 2 weeks.[185] While there was no difference between the concurrent or sequential regimens, the dose-dense regimen (every-2-week administration) did result in a 26% relative reduction in risk of recurrence and a 31% relative reduction in risk of death. As expected, within the group receiving the superior dose-dense regimen, patients with TNBC fared better compared with patients with hormone receptor–positive disease in terms of improved reduction in risk of recurrence (32% vs. 19%, respectively); however, this was not statistically significant. A meta-analysis of randomized trials evaluating dose-dense adjuvant therapy confirms the CALGB 9741 findings of a 15% relative reduction in risk of recurrence and a 10% relative reduction in risk of dying.[186] TNBC again obtained greater efficacy compared with hormone receptor–positive disease.

HER2-POSITIVE DISEASE

HER2 is an important therapeutic target for the 15% to 20% of breast cancers that are classified as HER2-positive either by over-expression of the HER2 protein (3+ by ICH) or by *HER2* gene amplification (FISH ≥ 2.0). As stated previously, HER2 is an adverse independent prognostic indicator, and predicts benefit with trastuzumab, the humanized monoclonal antibody against the extracellular domain of HER2. Trastuzumab has limited efficacy as a single agent in metastatic disease, and has only been studied in combination with chemotherapy in the adjuvant setting. Patients with HER2-positive cancer that is node-positive, regardless of tumor size, or node-negative disease with tumor size larger than

1 cm (T1c or higher) should be offered combination chemotherapy and trastuzumab for adjuvant treatment. There have been several attempts at delineating the smallest tumor size in lymph node–negative, HER2-positive disease that will benefit from chemotherapy and trastuzumab. Several studies have demonstrated that T1a and T1b, HER2-positive, node-negative breast cancer has a substantial risk of recurrence and death.[187,188] Several other studies support the recommendation that HER2-positive, node-negative, T1b tumors be considered for trastuzumab-based therapy if other adverse characteristics are present (e.g., high grade, young age); however, the optimal chemotherapy to combine with trastuzumab in this group has not been determined. The role of trastuzumab-based therapy in patients with T1aN0 disease remains unknown.

Trastuzumab adds substantial efficacy in terms of improving DFS and OS when added to chemotherapy compared with chemotherapy alone in HER2-positive disease (Table 6-7). A meta-analysis of five adjuvant therapy studies involving 9,748 patients demonstrated a 38% reduction in the relative risk of recurrence and a 34% relative reduction in risk of dying from any cause.[189] The largest individual analysis combined two U.S. studies: the three-arm North Central Cancer Treatment Group (NCCTG) N9831, which randomly assigned 1,944 patients to chemotherapy (AC every 3 weeks for four cycles followed by weekly paclitaxel for 12 weeks), chemotherapy followed by 1 year of trastuzumab (sequential arm), or chemotherapy with 1 year of trastuzumab beginning with the paclitaxel (concurrent arm); and NSABP B-31, which randomly assigned 2,101 patients to chemotherapy (AC every 3 weeks for four cycles followed by paclitaxel every 3 weeks for four cycles) or chemotherapy and trastuzumab beginning with the paclitaxel.[190] Regardless of other patient or tumor characteristics, the addition of trastuzumab to chemotherapy resulted in a 48% relative improvement in DFS and a 39% relative improvement in OS.

The adjuvant trastuzumab studies explored various questions. The Herceptin Adjuvant (HERA) trial and the FNCLCC PACS-04 trial compared multiple types of adjuvant chemotherapy followed by 1 year of trastuzumab with chemotherapy alone.[191-193] The HERA trial demonstrated a significant improvement in DFS with trastuzumab, but no impact on OS, whereas the PACS-04 study failed to demonstrate any additional efficacy with the addition of trastuzumab. These results suggest an interaction between chemotherapy and trastuzumab wherein concurrent administration may be of greater benefit compared with sequential treatment. This concept was supported by an analysis of the NCCTG N9831 study comparing chemotherapy (AC every 3 weeks for four cycles followed by weekly paclitaxel for 12 weeks [ACT]) followed by 1 year of trastuzumab (sequential arm) or chemotherapy with 1 year of trastuzumab beginning with the paclitaxel (concurrent arm).[194] The concurrent administration of trastuzumab with paclitaxel was associated with a 23% reduction in risk of an event (p = 0.0216), compared with sequential trastuzumab administration, suggesting that combined chemotherapy and trastuzumab is more beneficial than sequential chemotherapy followed by trastuzumab.

The currently accepted duration of adjuvant trastuzumab is 1 year. The HERA trial randomly assigned patients receiving trastuzumab to 1 or 2 years of treatment, and found no difference in progression-free survival (PFS) or OS after an 8-year follow-up.[195] The reduction in risk of recurrence remained 24%, yet cardiac toxicity was greater with the 2-year duration. In contrast, the Finnish Breast Cancer Group's FinHer trial evaluated the added benefit of 9 weeks of trastuzumab to three cycles of docetaxel or vinorelbine followed by three cycles of FEC (without trastuzumab).[196] Patients receiving trastuzumab experienced a 35% improvement in distant DFS; however, this was not statistically significant. The large phase III trial involving 3,380 women (PHARE: Protocol for Herceptin as Adjuvant Therapy with Reduced Exposure) failed to demonstrate non-inferiority with a 6-month duration of trastuzumab compared with 12 months.[197] The current recommended duration of adjuvant trastuzumab remains 1 year, and it should be given concurrently with a taxane (but not with anthracyclines); it should be given concurrently with endocrine therapy in hormone receptor–positive disease.

In the adult heart, HER2 functions to modify cardiac muscle response to stress. In theory, trastuzumab can interfere with the ability of the heart to adjust to stress, resulting in cardiac damage. The addition of trastuzumab in the adjuvant studies resulted in less than 4% difference in congestive heart failure or death between the treatment arms, which was less than the early stopping rules required. However, 5% of patients experienced asymptomatic decreases in ejection fraction requiring discontinuation of trastuzumab. Risk of cardiac compromise was associated with advanced age, hypertension, and initial ventricular function.

Concern for cardiac toxicity prompted investigation into a nonanthracycline-containing trastuzumab regimen: taxotere, carboplatin, and trastuzumab (TCH) administered every 3 weeks for six cycles. BCIRG 006 compared this regimen with four cycles of AC every 3 weeks followed by four cycles of docetaxel alone or with 1 year of trastuzumab beginning with the docetaxel.[182,198] BCIRG 006 confirmed a benefit with the addition of trastuzumab to chemotherapy; there was a 3% absolute difference in DFS and a 1% difference in OS at 5 years favoring the AC/docetaxel/trastuzumab arm over the TCH arm. It should be noted, however, that the study was not designed to compare the two trastuzumab-containing arms and any conclusions about the benefits of one regimen over another should be considered exploratory. TCH was associated with significantly less cardiac toxicity (p < 0.001) and risk of secondary leukemia compared with the AC/docetaxel/trastuzumab regimen, making it an acceptable treatment alternative in select patients.

Doxorubicin/cyclophosphamide/paclitaxel/trastuzumab (ACTH) with concurrent trastuzumab administration is commonly chosen as treatment for a patient who is at substantial risk of disease recurrence and who does not have risk factors for cardiac toxicity.[159] For patients at lower risk of disease recurrence or with cardiac risk factors, TCH represents a reasonable alternative. Although the standard ACTH regimen prescribes AC administered every 3 weeks, there are safety data to support administering AC every 2 weeks for four cycles (dose-dense) rather than every 3 weeks prior to 12 weeks of paclitaxel and trastuzumab.[199] When trastuzumab is used as a single agent following chemotherapy, it is commonly given every 3 weeks.[200] Cardiac monitoring with an echocardiogram or nuclear ventriculogram should be performed every 3 months during adjuvant trastuzumab therapy.

Retrospective data suggest that small, node-negative HER2-positive breast cancers have a small but real risk of distant recurrence. Most of these patients were not eligible for enrollment in the pivotal adjuvant trastuzumab clinical trials and the use of any of the standard adjuvant regimens seemed excessive to many clinicians. In this setting, investigators at Dana-Farber Cancer Institute and a number of other major cancer centers sought to explore the efficacy of a trastuzumab-containing adjuvant therapy regimen that included a minimal amount of chemotherapy. The phase II APT trial (Adjuvant Paclitaxel and Trastuzumab) involved 406 patients with node-negative, HER2-positive breast cancers that measured 3 cm or smaller in size, though over 90% had tumors 2 cm or larger.[201] In this single-arm, multi-institutional study, patients received 12 weeks of standard paclitaxel and trastuzumab given at the doses prescribed in the ACTH regimen, followed by 9 months of single-agent trastuzumab. The 3-year DFS was 98.7% at a median follow-up of 3.6 years, with two of the 10 DFS events being distant metastasis. The regimen was well tolerated, with minimal neuropathy and cardiac compromise. These practice-changing results are being further explored in the ATEMPT trial, which involves patients with stage I HER2-positive breast cancer, randomly assigned to 12 weeks of paclitaxel/trastuzumab followed by trastuzumab for 9 months or 12 months of trastuzumab emtansine (T-DM1).

STAGE III DISEASE

Stage III disease is often classified as "locally advanced disease" and can be grouped into two general categories: patients with large tumors or multiple positive lymph nodes but who clearly have operable disease that can be primarily resected, and patients with inoperable disease by virtue of skin involvement, disease attachment to the chest wall, or extensive nodal involvement that precludes surgical resection (e.g., matted axillary lymph nodes or supraclavicular lymph node involvement). Patients with operable stage III disease can be treated in the same manner as patients with stage II disease; however, often the preferred method is to administer systemic therapy first (primary systemic therapy, preoperative, neoadjuvant) followed by surgery and radiation. Often this sequence is performed to improve surgical options by allowing the possibility of breast conservation. The sequence of treatment using neoadjuvant systemic therapy is required for the treatment of inoperable stage III disease in order allow definitive local therapy, determine disease response to systemic therapy, and to improve survival.

Locoregional Therapy

A meta-analysis of nine randomized trials involving 3,946 patients (including patients with stage II cancer) evaluated outcomes when the same systemic therapy was administered to patients with operable breast cancer, either preoperatively (neoadjuvant) or postoperatively (adjuvant), revealing no difference in mortality or distant disease recurrence.[202] Neoadjuvant systemic therapy is associated with considerable tumor shrinkage, allowing for a greater proportion of patients to achieve breast conservation.[203]

A greater risk of locoregional disease recurrence was found among patients who received radiation alone as local therapy, excluding surgery. Even in the setting of a complete clinical disease response to neoadjuvant systemic therapy, resecting the region of the primary tumor site with appropriate breast surgery is required for optimal local disease control.[203,204] Should an inadequate clinical response occur with neoadjuvant systemic therapy, radiation therapy to the breast and regional lymph nodes may then facilitate surgery. In this setting, which is relatively rare in clinical practice, mastectomy and ALND are performed following radiation therapy.

Breast conservation post-neoadjuvant systemic therapy requires radiation therapy; however, the criteria for PMRT in this setting is less well defined. An NCI Health Conference held in 2007 discussed the relevant issues related to locoregional disease control following neoadjuvant systemic therapy.[205] A review of the presented data suggested that the initial clinical stage and the final pathologic extent of disease were related to risk of local recurrence postmastectomy. Patients presenting with clinical stage IIB (T3N0) disease, clinical stage III disease, and those with positive lymph node involvement post-neoadjuvant systemic therapy benefit from PMRT.[206] The decision for PMRT is less well defined in patients who were treated with neoadjuvant systemic therapy and have disease that does not correspond to these categories. A 10% or greater risk of local recurrence often prompts the recommendation for PMRT. Regional nodal irradiation recommendations mimic those for treatment following breast conservation surgery.

The optimal management of the axilla in the setting of neoadjuvant systemic therapy remains complex and an area under investigation. The standard approach for a patient with a positive axilla confirmed by FNA at the time of diagnosis is to proceed to a complete ALND following neoadjuvant systemic therapy. A clinically negative axilla at the time of presentation may lead to an SNLD after systemic therapy. An SNLD post-neoadjuvant systemic therapy is acceptable, and has a similar identification and false-negative rate as seen prior to systemic therapy.[203,204] Neoadjuvant systemic therapy has been shown to convert 20% to 40% of positive lymph nodes into negative lymph nodes; therefore, if the sentinel lymph node was found to be negative after neoadjuvant systemic therapy, this procedure may save the patient from further axillary surgery.

Neoadjuvant Systemic Therapy

Chemotherapy. A pathologic complete response (pCR) has variable definitions in the literature; however, the consensus definition is absence of invasive carcinoma in the breast and axillary lymph nodes.[203] A pCR to neoadjuvant systemic therapy is associated with a more favorable outcome compared with residual disease in the breast and/or axilla.[207] NSABP B-18 and NSABP B-27 compared neoadjuvant chemotherapy to adjuvant chemotherapy

using chemotherapy regimens of AC alone or AC followed by docetaxel.[208] Both studies demonstrated a superior DFS and OS among the patients who achieved a pCR compared with those who did not, although the pCR rate was only 13% to 26%. In the final analysis, however, there remained no difference in overall DFS or OS when the chemotherapy was administered neoadjuvantly versus adjuvantly. This raises an important question about whether pCR is an adequate surrogate for disease outcome.

Although TNBC is associated with a less favorable overall prognosis, this subtype of breast cancer is more chemosensitive and has a greater propensity of achieving a pCR to neoadjuvant chemotherapy compared with hormone receptor–positive disease.[209] Patients with TNBC who achieve a pCR have a favorable OS that is similar to those patients with non-TNBC achieving a pCR.[210] Residual disease following neoadjuvant chemotherapy in TNBC and HER2-positive disease is associated with a worse DFS compared with other subtypes of breast cancer treated similarly.[211] In this way, neoadjuvant chemotherapy can be used as mechanism of evaluating tumor biology and disease resistance. When neoadjuvant chemotherapy is used, it should be administered as in the adjuvant setting and consist of anthracycline- and taxane-based regimens.[203] There is no established role for adjuvant chemotherapy once neoadjuvant chemotherapy is completed, assuming a complete course of therapy has been administered as neoadjuvant systemic therapy.

Endocrine Therapy. Neoadjuvant endocrine therapy is an acceptable treatment for postmenopausal women with hormone receptor–positive disease, although the pCR rate of 1% to 8% is lower than with chemotherapy.[203] At least five randomized trials (including patients with stage II disease) have demonstrated superiority with neoadjuvant AI treatment compared with tamoxifen.[212] The Immediate Preoperative Anastrozole, Tamoxifen, or Combined with Tamoxifen (IMPACT) trial compared neoadjuvant anastrozole, tamoxifen, and the combination of anastrozole and tamoxifen, and found a greater ability to achieve BCT with anastrozole compared with tamoxifen (46% vs. 22%).[213] A comparison of neoadjuvant letrozole with tamoxifen, performed by the Letrozole Neoadjuvant Breast Cancer Study Group, demonstrated a superior clinical response with letrozole (55% vs. 36%) and superior frequency of BCT (45% vs. 35%) but no difference in the low pCR rate.[214]

All three third-generation AIs appear to be equally effective as neoadjuvant therapy, and patients whose disease responds favorably after 4 to 12 months of neoadjuvant AI therapy have an excellent prognosis, despite the low pCR rate.[215] Surrogate markers of response offer prognostic information about a favorable outcome, including the hormone receptor status of residual disease (ER-negative is less favorable), and the Ki76 expression in residual tumor (low value is more favorable).[216] Patients who have a disease response to neoadjuvant endocrine therapy should continue on endocrine therapy postsurgery, as per adjuvant treatment recommendations.

Trastuzumab. Like TNBC, HER2-positive breast cancer is associated with a high probability of tumor response to neoadjuvant chemotherapy, and this response rate is increased substantially with the addition of HER2-directed treatment. Two studies evaluated neoadjuvant trastuzumab-containing regimens administering the trastuzumab with an anthracycline. These two randomized trials compared neoadjuvant chemotherapy with and without trastuzumab for HER2-positive disease (the MD Anderson trial and the Neoadjuvant Herceptin [NOAH] trial).[217] Both studies demonstrated a significant benefit with added trastuzumab in the pCR rate (20% to 40% actual improvement), and a 33% relative reduction in risk of recurrence and death. The cardiac event rate was 11%. Two additional studies, using epirubicin/cyclophosphamide (EC) every 3 weeks followed by a taxane with or without capecitabine, also initiated trastuzumab with the anthracycline and observed favorable pCR rates of 32% to 39%, with a less than 4% incidence of cardiac toxicity.[218,219] These studies provide short-term safety data for the combination of anthracycline chemotherapy and neoadjuvant trastuzumab. A recent randomized study which included trastuzumab in both arms failed to demonstrate an improvement in pCR with the use of concurrent anthracycline and trastuzumab treatment. Given this result and the lack of long-term safety data, the approach should not be considered in the course of routine clinical practice.[220]

In an attempt to add to the efficacy of trastuzumab administered neoadjuvantly, two phase III trials evaluated the role of lapatinib in this setting. The GeparQuinto (GBG 44) trial compared four cycles of EC followed by four cycles of docetaxel concurrent with either lapatinib or trastuzumab. Among the 620 randomly assigned patients, the pCR rate was significantly higher with trastuzumab compared with lapatinib (30.3% vs. 22.7%, respectively; p = 0.04).[221] No difference in pCR rate was demonstrated between the lapatinib-alone and trastuzumab-alone arms (24.7% vs. 29.5%) in a second complex trial involving 455 patients randomly assigned to 6 weeks of lapatinib alone, trastuzumab alone, or lapatinib combined with trastuzumab prior to continuing HER2-directed therapy with 12 weeks of paclitaxel (NeoALTTO).[222] Combination lapatinib and trastuzumab with paclitaxel resulted in a superior pCR rate of 51.3%.

The benefit seen with combined HER2-directed therapy prompted an evaluation of pertuzumab in the neoadjuvant setting. The NeoSphere trial was an open-label, phase II study that randomly assigned 417 patients to four cycles of docetaxel combined with either trastuzumab alone, pertuzumab alone, or both agents, versus combination pertuzumab and trastuzumab without docetaxel (a nonchemotherapy arm).[223] The combination pertuzumab and trastuzumab with docetaxel achieved the highest pCR rate, 39.3%, compared with the other groups. This trial, as well as other trials in the preoperative setting, combined with the survival advantage seen with pertuzumab in the metastatic setting, led to the FDA approval of this combination for neoadjuvant treatment of HER2-positive breast cancer. All patients in the NeoSphere trial also received adjuvant treatment with three cycles of FEC chemotherapy concomitant with trastuzumab, which was then continued to complete 1 year of trastuzumab therapy.

Based upon these results, a promising option for neoadjuvant systemic therapy of HER2-positive disease is a combination of trastuzumab and pertuzumab with a taxane-containing regimen. An anthracycline is often administered after surgery, and trastuzumab should be administered for a total of 1 year. The optimal chemotherapy regimen used in neoadjuvant systemic therapy with trastuzumab and pertuzumab is still unknown.

INFLAMMATORY BREAST CANCER

Inflammatory breast cancer (IBC) is a rare but virulent subset of disease that accounts for approximately 2% to 5% of all breast cancers. The diagnosis of IBC (T4d) is a clinical diagnosis in the setting of documented invasive breast cancer and is characterized by a rapid onset of clinical changes in the breast: skin erythema, warmth, edema (peau d'orange), breast enlargement, and pain, usually occurring within a 3-month time frame, but not present longer than 6 months. This type of breast cancer is designated as "inflammatory" because the clinical signs mimic mastitis; an empiric treatment with antibiotics often delays the diagnosis of cancer. These clinical criteria differentiate IBC from a neglected locally advanced breast cancer with secondary inflammatory characteristics, which is associated with a more favorable prognosis. A discrete mass is frequently absent, and pathologically, tumor emboli are seen within dermal lymphatics in 75% of cases.[224] The classical physical findings of the breast are a result of damage of the dermal lymphatics caused by tumor emboli, and the corresponding palpable finding is known as ridging. Patients with IBC are often younger at the age of diagnosis (age 45 to 57), are often black, and, by definition, present with inoperable disease.[225] Breast imaging with mammography usually finds asymmetrical increased density throughout the affected breast, associated with skin thickening and axillary adenopathy. MRI is more sensitive and specific in finding breast masses and confirming disease response to neoadjuvant chemotherapy compared with mammography.[226]

Although the complete spectrum of intrinsic subtypes is seen in IBC, there is a propensity for the disease to segregate into the more proliferative HER2-positive and triple-negative molecular subtypes. Patients with IBC have as high as a 2-fold increased risk of dying of disease compared with patients diagnosed with noninflammatory locally advanced breast cancer, with OS rates being consistently less than 50%. Approximately 20% to 40% of patients with IBC have evident metastatic disease at the time of presentation.[227] Given the high risk of developing metastatic disease, a trimodality approach to treatment is appropriate: neoadjuvant chemotherapy (regardless of hormone receptor status) followed by mastectomy and radiation therapy. This treatment sequence allows for real-time assessment of the antitumor efficacy of the primary systemic therapy by evaluating the pathologic disease response at the time of mastectomy.

The optimal neoadjuvant chemotherapy regimen for IBC has not been defined; the neoadjuvant systemic therapy should include the standard neoadjuvant chemotherapy regimens outlined previously for noninflammatory breast cancer. Both prospective and retrospective studies support the use of combination anthracycline- and taxane-based regimens. The addition of conventional taxanes to anthracycline regimens has resulted in an improved pCR rate and improved OS.[228] The prognosis of HER2-positive IBC has greatly improved in the era of HER2-directed therapy. HER2-positive IBC should be treated with a standard trastuzumab-based neoadjuvant regimen, as previously described. Given the recent FDA accelerated approval of pertuzumab in the neoadjuvant setting, it is prudent to include this agent as well.

IBC appears to have a unique molecular profile characterized by overexpression of the epithelial adhesion protein E-cadherin, overexpression of the *RhoC* oncogene, and a high frequency of *p53* gene mutations, in addition to a loss of expression of *WISP3*, which has growth and angiogenesis inhibitory functions.[229] A greater understanding of the molecular biology of IBC is needed in order to decipher the pathophysiology of the disease and to develop rationally designed and more effective therapies.

There is a direct correlation between systemic disease control and local disease control with IBC. The goal of neoadjuvant chemotherapy is to render the breast operable. Breast conservation is contraindicated, as is SLND. A total mastectomy with level I and II ALND results in optimal surgical control. Radiation therapy follows, although the optimal radiation dose and sequence is not well established. The chest wall and regional lymph nodes (supraclavicular, infraclavicular, internal mammary) are included in the treatment field and often the cumulative radiation dose is 66 cGy. Reconstruction of the breast is best deferred in order to avoid delays in delivering optimal local therapy for IBC. If the neoadjuvant chemotherapy results in an inadequate response in the breast, radiation can be administered prior to mastectomy.[230] Hormone receptor–positive IBC is treated similarly to noninflammatory breast cancer, with endocrine therapy given following chemotherapy.

RECURRENT OR METASTATIC DISEASE
LOCOREGIONAL RELAPSE

Locoregional disease relapse can be defined as breast cancer recurrence in the ipsilateral breast following BCT, chest wall recurrence following mastectomy (with or without prior radiation), or a regional nodal recurrence. Isolated locoregional recurrences that occur within the first 5 years after diagnosis are treated with curative intent, although this event is associated with a poorer prognosis than recurrences which occur later. Those recurrences that develop after 5 years usually represent de novo second primary tumors and have a more favorable outcome compared with earlier recurrences within the proximity of the original tumor, which represent disease that is resistant to radiation and systemic therapy. The treatment of locoregional recurrences requires a multidisciplinary approach.

Historically, ipsilateral breast tumor recurrence (IBTR) following BCT was associated with a 3- to 4-fold increase in risk of systemic metastasis. The NSABP reviewed five of its more recent adjuvant studies involving 2,669 women treated with breast-conserving surgery, radiation therapy, and systemic treatment, and found that patients who experienced an IBTR had a 2.72-fold greater risk of developing distant disease at 5 years and a 2.58-fold greater risk of death compared with those who did not have disease recurrence.[231] Patients experiencing a chest wall recurrence following mastectomy fared worse, with a 6.68-fold greater risk of distant recurrence at 5 years and a 5.85-fold greater risk of death. IBTRs are treated with a total mastectomy, since repeat radiation treatment is contraindicated. A level I and II ALND should be performed if not performed originally.

As in IBTR, chest wall recurrences postmastectomy occur most frequently within the first 5 years post-treatment, and rarely occur after 10 years. The majority of chest wall recurrences develop in the proximity of the mastectomy incision, whereas fewer recurrences develop in the regional lymph node areas (in order of decreasing frequency: supraclavicular, axillary, internal mammary). A review of 11,452 women treated with standard locoregional therapy for early-stage breast cancer at the European Institute of Oncology demonstrated a shorter DFS and OS among those patients who developed regional lymph node recurrences compared with the DFS and OS associated with an IBTR or a chest wall recurrence.[232] The risk of subsequent distant disease and consequent adverse effect on OS decreased with time from the initial chest wall recurrence, whereas patients with regional lymph node recurrences remain, for a long time, at high risk of developing distant disease and having a shortened OS. The treatment of a chest wall recurrence requires a surgical excision with the goal of obtaining negative margins. The chest wall and supraclavicular lymph nodes should then receive standard radiation therapy if not given previously. Radiation alone may be able to be administered if surgical resection of the chest wall disease cannot be adequately performed.

Systemic therapy is often administered following completion of salvage local treatment for a locoregional recurrence, although some data support its efficacy. A review of three randomized trials exploring the benefit of subsequent systemic therapy following a locoregional recurrence was performed by the Cochrane Collaboration.[233] These studies demonstrated insufficient data to support an advantage with chemotherapy; however, there may be a favorable effect on DFS when endocrine therapy is administered in this setting. The effect of trastuzumab is unknown. An international trial, CALOR (Chemotherapy as Adjuvant for Locally Recurrent Breast Cancer; BIG 1-02/IBCSG 27-02/NSABP B-37) enrolled 162 out of a planned 977 patients with invasive breast cancer who developed an isolated local and/or regional ipsilateral recurrence following mastectomy or BCT.[234] Patients received radiation therapy, endocrine therapy, or trastuzumab as appropriate, but were randomly assigned to receive chemotherapy or not. The 5-year DFS was improved with chemotherapy (69%) compared with no chemotherapy (57%). The benefit was primarily seen in TNBC (67% vs. 35%, chemotherapy vs. no chemotherapy). The 5-year OS was comparable between the two groups; numerically higher in the chemotherapy group, but not statistically higher (88% vs. 76%, chemotherapy vs. no chemotherapy, respectively). Although this is a highly underpowered study, it does support the use of chemotherapy following local or regional disease recurrence in select circumstances.

SYSTEMIC DISEASE

Metastatic breast cancer is an extremely heterogeneous entity, with treatment options dependent upon location of metastasis and number of sites involved, presence or absence of hormone receptors and HER2 overexpression, an assessment of disease responsiveness to systemic therapy based on characteristics such as disease-free interval, and an estimation of the need for rapid disease response to therapy. Given the diverse presentation of metastatic disease and the wide range of therapeutic possibilities, the goal of this section is to provide a guide for approaching treatment options rather than providing specific treatment recommendations. As with adjuvant therapy for early-stage disease, there are options for treatment outlined by several organizations to help guide decision-making.[141,235]

The overall goal of treating metastatic breast cancer is to slow the progression of disease, improve quality of life, and prolong survival without causing significant treatment-associated toxicity. Metastatic breast cancer is a chronic disease; sequential therapy is a mainstay of treatment. The incorporation of new therapies over the recent decades has resulted in a gradual improvement in OS by 1% to 2% per year.[236] The benefits of individual regimens are often comparable in first-line or subsequent-line treatment; therefore, the optimal sequence of therapies has not yet been determined.[237]

Once metastatic disease is diagnosed, the extent of disease should be determined by radiographic imaging. The most common initial sites of metastasis include bone, liver, and lung, which can be imaged by conventional CT and bone scan. PET imaging can complement these studies, especially in the setting of lytic bone metastases which may be underestimated by bone scan. Central nervous system disease is less likely to be present at the initial presentation of metastatic disease; MRI of the brain can be deferred until symptoms arise. The molecular subtypes of breast cancer have a predilection for metastasizing to specific sites, which may affect the decision to image these areas. HER2-positive disease and TNBC are associated with a higher frequency of brain metastasis (23% and 24%, respectively) compared with the hormone receptor–positive group (10%).[238] Bone metastases are more common among the hormone receptor–positive subtype (68%), whereas TNBC is associated with a high frequency of metastasis to lung (40%). Discordance of hormone receptor and HER2 status between the primary tumor and the metastatic disease can occur in approximately 10% of cases. A biopsy of the initial metastatic site is warranted to determine receptor status and to confirm the presence of metastatic breast cancer rather than another malignancy, either primary or metastatic.

The measurement of circulating extracellular domain of HER2 does not serve as a surrogate marker for HER2 status of the tumor, and should only be obtained in clinical trials.[239] Other serum markers, such as the MUC-1 assays, CA 27.29 or CA 15-3, and the carcinoembryonic antigen levels, should not be used in nonmetastatic settings, but can complement the interpretation of imaging studies in metastatic disease. Changes in these assays, by themselves, should not dictate changes in therapy. The application of circulating tumor cells in the interpretation of disease response and management of therapy for metastatic disease remains investigational.

Hormone Receptor–Positive Disease

In the setting of ER- and/or PR-positive metastases that are not associated with rapidly progressing disease or visceral crisis, endocrine therapy should generally be the first treatment approach. Sequential treatment with single-agent endocrine therapy is appropriate; however, the likelihood of disease response and duration of response becomes smaller/shorter with each change in regimen. At the time of cancer progression, a switch to chemotherapy is always an option. Virtually all patients with metastatic hormone receptor–positive breast cancer ultimately receive chemotherapy. The decision to switch to chemotherapy is based on the likelihood of a response to additional hormone therapy, as well as all of the considerations outlined above. Chemotherapy should be given if the disease is rapidly progressing or in the setting of visceral crisis.

The choice of endocrine therapy is dependent upon the menopausal status of the patient, the type of prior endocrine therapy used for adjuvant treatment, and the duration between adjuvant endocrine therapy and disease recurrence. There is an association between response to endocrine therapy and the strength of ER and PR expression. In the setting of hormone receptor–positive metastatic disease, disease response is important, but clinical benefit (defined as the percentage of complete and partial disease responses plus stable disease exceeding 6 months) may supersede disease response.

Historically, ovarian suppression has been effective therapy in premenopausal women with hormone receptor–positive metastatic disease. The use of an LHRH agonist (medical oophorectomy) in the metastatic setting has resulted in similar outcomes to that of surgical ovarian ablation. Tamoxifen has also been found to be equally as effective as ovarian ablation, regardless of the degree of circulating estrogen levels. A meta-analysis of four randomized trials involving 506 premenopausal women compared an LHRH agonist alone with an LHRH agonist and tamoxifen in combination, and found a 22% reduction in the risk of death and a 30% reduction in the risk of disease progression/death with the combination.[240] Patients whose disease initially responds to combination ovarian suppression and tamoxifen can subsequently be treated in a similar fashion to postmenopausal women; however, ovarian suppression should continue throughout the duration of such endocrine therapy.

In postmenopausal women, third-generation AIs have been shown to be superior to tamoxifen in first-line therapy of hormone-responsive metastatic disease, with an 11% reduction in risk of death.[241,242] On an individual basis, selective AIs were found to be superior to tamoxifen in terms of overall disease response rate, time to treatment failure, and clinical benefit; the third-generation AIs are the recommended first-line endocrine therapy for postmenopausal women, unless disease progression occurred on adjuvant AI therapy.[242-244] In that case, tamoxifen or fulvestrant should be used as first-line therapy; otherwise, tamoxifen is usually considered standard second-line endocrine therapy. There are some data that suggest that switching from a nonsteroidal AI (letrozole or anastrozole) to a steroidal AI (exemestane) can result in a modest disease response, suggesting a component of non–cross-reactivity.[245]

Fulvestrant is an analog of 17-beta estradiol, which causes ER disruption and degradation when it binds to the ER, leading to inhibition of estrogen signaling and consequent cellular growth. Unlike other endocrine therapies, fulvestrant is given by monthly intramuscular injections, and early studies demonstrated the need to use a loading dose in order to obtain steady state drug concentrations within 1 month of administration. The First-Line Treatment for Advanced Breast Cancer (FIRST) study demonstrated a superior time to tumor progression compared with anastrozole in the first-line setting, although the clinical benefit and overall response were comparable.[246] The Comparison of Faslodex in Recurrent or Metastatic Breast Cancer (CONFIRM) trial demonstrated a dose relationship with fulvestrant on PFS as well as OS, supporting the results of the FIRST trial (which also administered fulvestrant as a 500-mg intramuscular monthly dose).[247,248] Fulvestrant is also an acceptable second- or third-line therapy. Other endocrine therapy options for third- and fourth-line treatment include megestrol acetate (progestins), fluoxymesterone (androgens), or relatively high doses of estrogen.

Three studies in postmenopausal women investigated combination AI with fulvestrant as endocrine therapy for recurrent hormone receptor–positive breast cancer. All studies utilized the lower dosing regimen for fulvestrant; a 250-mg intramuscular injection monthly. SWOG 0226 randomly assigned 694 patients to first-line therapy with anastrozole versus anastrozole and fulvestrant, with cross-over to fulvestrant being encouraged after disease progression on anastrozole alone.[249] Approximately 60% of the patients enrolled had not been exposed to prior adjuvant endocrine therapy. With a 35-month median follow-up, the primary endpoint of PFS was in favor of combination endocrine therapy compared with AI therapy alone (15 vs. 13.5 months, respectively; p = 0.007). The OS was also superior with combination therapy; the median OS was 47.7 months with the combination compared with 41.3 months with AI alone (p = 0.049). These data contrast with the FACT trial (Fulvestrant and Anastrozole Combination Therapy), which also randomly assigned 514 patients to first-line therapy with anastrozole plus fulvestrant versus anastrozole alone.[250] Unlike the patient population in SWOG 0226, two-thirds of the patients enrolled had received adjuvant tamoxifen. No difference was seen in the primary endpoint of time to progression (10.8 months with combination vs. 10.2 months with AI), or with median OS (37.8 months vs. 38.2 months, respectively).

The phase III SoFEA (the Study of Faslodex with or without Concomitant Arimidex vs. Exemestane following Progression on Nonsteroidal Aromatase Inhibitors) trial examined patients with disease progression on a nonsteroidal AI, and randomly assigned 723 patients to fulvestrant/placebo, fulvestrant/anastrozole, or fulvestrant/exemestane.[251] There was no difference in PFS or OS among the three groups. These studies support the recommendation that options for the treatment of hormone receptor–positive breast cancer progressing on a nonsteroidal AI include exemestane alone or fulvestrant alone. The benefit of combination fulvestrant and AI appears to be isolated to patients who have recurrent disease that is endocrine therapy–naive; a patient population that is rarely seen in the United States given the high frequency of adjuvant endocrine therapy use.

A major signaling pathway involved in the development of endocrine resistance is the phosphoniositide-3-kinase (PI3-kinase)-Akt-mTOR pathway.[252] Inhibition of this pathway can occur by targeting mTOR with the rapamycin analogs everolimus and temsirolimus. The efficacy of adding mTOR inhibitors to endocrine therapy is thought to be a result of the reversal of endocrine resistance as evidenced by two trials in metastatic breast cancer, TAMRAD (Tamoxifen Plus Everolimus) and BOLERO-2 (Breast Cancer Trials of Oral Everolimus-2). TAMRAD was a phase II trial involving 111 postmenopausal women whose disease was previously treated with an AI either in the adjuvant (41%) or metastatic (67%) setting.[253] The primary endpoint of clinical benefit rate, defined as all patients with either a complete or partial disease response or stable disease at 6 months, was achieved in 61% of patients receiving combination everolimus and tamoxifen compared with 42% treated with tamoxifen alone (exploratory p = 0.045). A greater difference in benefit from combination therapy was seen among patients with secondary hormone resistance (74% vs. 48%), defined as disease relapse during or within 6 months of completing adjuvant or metastatic AI therapy, compared with those having primary hormone resistance (46% vs. 36%), defined as disease relapse after 6 months of completing adjuvant AI or responding to AI treatment for metastatic disease for 6 months or longer.

The results of the phase III BOLERO-2 trial further supported the hypothesis that everolimus is effective in overcoming endocrine resistance. In the trial, 724 postmenopausal women whose disease progressed or recurred while on a nonsteroidal AI were randomly assigned 2:1 to receive either combination everolimus and exemestane, or exemestane alone.[254] The median PFS was improved with combination therapy from 4.1 to 10.6 months (HR 0.36; p < 0.001). The added toxicity from everolimus included stomatitis and pneumonitis. This study led to the 2012 FDA approval of everolimus in combination with exemestane in the treatment of ER-positive, HER2-negative metastatic breast cancer following disease progression on either letrozole or anastrozole.

Table 6-8 Metastatic Chemotherapy Options[141,142]

HER2-Negative Disease	**Single Agent**	Paclitaxel weekly
		Doxorubicin or pegylated liposomal doxorubicin
		Docetaxel every 21 days
		Nab-paclitaxel (weekly or every 21 days)
		Capecitabine
		Gemcitabine
		Vinorelbine
		Eribulin
		Ixabepilone
		Carboplatin
		Cisplatin
	Combination	Ixabepilone/capecitabine
		Gemcitabine/paclitaxel
		Docetaxel/capecitabine
HER2-Positive Disease	Pertuzumab, trastuzumab, and taxane (first-line only)	
	T-DM1	
	Paclitaxel weekly and trastuzumab	
	Vinorelbine and trastuzumab	
	Gemcitabine and trastuzumab	
	Capecitabine and lapatinib	

Chemotherapy

Chemotherapy is the mainstay of treatment for metastatic hormone receptor–negative breast cancer. It is also indicated in hormone receptor–positive breast cancer for the treatment of rapidly progressing metastatic disease, disease that is associated with visceral crisis, and hormone-refractory disease defined as the development of metastasis within 1 year of beginning adjuvant endocrine therapy or progression of metastatic disease after one or more lines of endocrine therapy (Table 6-8). Sequential use of single-agent chemotherapy is recommended, except in the setting of visceral crisis or rapidly progressive disease that requires prompt cytoreduction.[255] In that setting, the swift tumor response occurring with combination chemotherapy outweighs the added toxicity associated with these regimens.

Anthracyclines and taxanes are considered the most active chemotherapies for metastatic breast cancer, although the increased use of both drugs in adjuvant treatment has prompted the development of other non–cross-reacting agents. Single-agent anthracyclines such as doxorubicin and pegylated liposomal doxorubicin (PLD) are associated with an approximately 35% to 40% response rate for first-line therapy; PLD is associated with a safer cardiac profile.[256]

Among the taxanes, the most commonly used single-agent drugs include paclitaxel, docetaxel, and nab-paclitaxel, which are associated with an approximately 40% response rate for anthracycline-resistant disease treated in the first-line setting. The optimal schedule varies by taxane, with paclitaxel administered weekly, docetaxel given every 3 weeks, and nab-paclitaxel effective either weekly or every 3 weeks.[257] A randomized trial involving 799 patients compared the PFS of first-line therapy with weekly paclitaxel, nab-paclitaxel, or ixabepilone.[258] Ninety-eight percent of the patients also received concurrent bevacizumab. In two sequential interim analyses, the comparison of ixabepilone to paclitaxel crossed the futility boundary, and subsequently, the comparison of nab-paclitaxel crossed the futility boundary. Therefore, neither ixabepilone nor nab-paclitaxel is likely to be superior to paclitaxel as first-line chemotherapy for metastatic breast cancer, and the toxicity profile of paclitaxel was superior. The PFS associated with paclitaxel, nap-paclitaxel, and ixabepilone was 10.6 months, 9.6 months, and 7.6 months, respectively.

The development of taxane resistance is becoming more common with the general use of taxanes in the adjuvant setting. Several mechanisms of resistance exist, including overexpression and increased activity of the p-glycoprotein drug efflux pump, the development of mutations in the tubulin genes, or alterations in tubulin expression. Several chemotherapeutic agents have been developed in an attempt to overcome these various mechanisms of resistance. Other microtubule-targeting agents, such as the epothilones (e.g., ixabepilone) or the halichondrin B analog eribulin, have demonstrated antitumor efficacy as second-line or more distant therapies in the setting of both anthracycline- and taxane-resistant disease.[259] The Eisai Metastatic Breast Cancer Study Assessing Physician's Choice versus E7389 (EMBRACE) trial involved 762 women who had received between two and five prior chemotherapeutic regimens for metastatic disease, including anthracyclines and taxanes.[260] These patients were randomly assigned to single-agent eribulin or the treatment of physician's choice. Patients treated with eribulin achieved a significant improvement in median OS (13.1 vs. 10.6 months; p = 0.041).

Other effective single-agent chemotherapies available for the treatment of patients pretreated with anthracyclines and taxanes resulted in response rates of about 30% and include antimetabolites such as capecitabine (a 5-fluorouracil analog), the nucleoside analog gemcitabine, or the vinca alkaloid vinorelbine. The platinum salts, such as cisplatin or carboplatin, are DNA-damaging agents which appear to be more effective in the treatment of TNBC.

Combination chemotherapy usually results in superior overall response rates of 60% to 75% compared with single-agent chemotherapy, yet the added benefit of prolonging OS remains unclear.[255] Combination regimens, including docetaxel/capecitabine and gemcitabine/paclitaxel, have demonstrated a 3-month improved OS compared with single-agent therapy (capecitabine or paclitaxel); however, the lack of a prescribed cross-over design compromises the interpretation of these results. Combination ixabepilone/capecitabine demonstrated improved PFS in highly pretreated patients and specifically seemed to benefit the TNBC subtype.

The decision to use combination chemotherapy rather than sequential single-agent chemotherapy depends upon the need to obtain a rapid disease response and an assessment of the toxicity associated with the choices of treatment. Combination chemotherapy is associated with greater toxicity, with each individual drug allied with a specific spectrum of side effects. The anthracyclines contribute to cardiac toxicity based upon cumulative dosing and should be avoided in the setting of hyperbilirubinemia. Vinorelbine, ixabepilone, and taxanes increase peripheral neuropathy, with the duration and severity of symptoms dependent upon individual risks (e.g., diabetes mellitus) and choice of drug. Caution must be used when platinum agents are administered in the setting of renal failure, and ixabepilone should be avoided in hepatic dysfunction.

The optimal duration of chemotherapy administration for metastatic disease remains unknown. Multiple studies investigating this issue have used regimens that are considered obsolete by today's standards. In general, the continuation of chemotherapy may result in prolonged DFS, especially in the first-line setting, but this has not yet translated into a substantial improvement in OS. For this reason, the duration of treatment needs to be tailored to each individual patient, taking into account the toxicity of treatment, control of disease-related symptoms, and quality of life.[261] Patients whose disease is responding well to chemotherapy without significant toxicity do not need to stop after a proscribed number of cycles, whereas chemotherapy "holidays" are appropriate for patients who require time to recover from toxicity and whose disease is not responsive to less-toxic targeted therapy, such as endocrine therapy or HER2-directed therapy. Patients with hormone receptor–positive or HER2-positive disease whose disease achieves an adequate response can safely discontinue chemotherapy and begin a targeted treatment, such as endocrine therapy or single-agent trastuzumab, allowing for a break from chemotherapy-related toxicity.

HER2-Positive Disease

Pertuzumab and trastuzumab both target the extracellular domain of HER2; however, trastuzumab binds to subdomain IV and disrupts ligand-independent downstream signaling, whereas pertuzumab binds to subdomain II which blocks dimerization of HER2 and subsequent ligand-dependent signaling. The CLEOPATRA (Clinical Evaluation of Pertuzumab and Trastuzumab) trial assessed the added benefit of pertuzumab to combination docetaxel and trastuzumab for first-line treatment of metastatic HER2-positive breast cancer.[262] This phase III trial randomly assigned 808 patients to either pertuzumab/ trastuzumab/docetaxel (PTD) or trastuzumab/docetaxel with placebo (TD). The primary endpoint, PFS, was significantly improved among the patients receiving both HER2-targeting agents and docetaxel compared with TD (18.5 vs. 12.5 months, respectively; HR 0.62; p < 0.001). A 6-month improvement in PFS was also seen in the subgroup that had been exposed to adjuvant trastuzumab. The overall response rate (ORR) was superior in the PTD arm (80.2% vs. 69.3%; p = 0.001), as was the OS, with a 34% reduction in the risk of death with PTD compared

with TD (p = 0.0008).[263] In June 2012, the FDA approved combination pertuzumab, trastuzumab, and either docetaxel or paclitaxel as the taxane backbone for first-line therapy of HER2-positive metastatic breast cancer.

Single-agent trastuzumab administered in the metastatic setting results in an ORR of 15% to 26%. The addition of chemotherapy to trastuzumab for first-line treatment improves the ORR to 60% to 70%, regardless of the type of chemotherapy administered (e.g., vinorelbine, docetaxel, weekly paclitaxel, or combination taxane/carboplatin). Early studies evaluating the efficacy of early administration of combination trastuzumab and chemotherapy in metastatic disease demonstrated an improvement in OS, specifically 1-year OS. The dramatic disease response observed when trastuzumab was added to chemotherapy for the treatment of metastatic HER2-positive disease prompted oncologists to empirically continue trastuzumab when progressive disease dictated a change in chemotherapy. The GBG 26/ BIG 3-05 study subsequently confirmed the benefit of continuing trastuzumab with alternative chemotherapy following disease progression with combination chemotherapy/trastuzumab.[264] In this trial, 156 patients were randomly assigned to receive capecitabine alone or capecitabine with continued trastuzumab following disease progression on first-line trastuzumab or trastuzumab plus chemotherapy. The continuation of trastuzumab with capecitabine resulted in an improvement in PFS, but not OS, whereas further evaluation allowing for cross-over and effects of third-line therapy resulted in the longest OS (27 months) with continued administration of trastuzumab.

Lapatinib is a dual TKI of EGFR-1 and HER2, and is also effective in the treatment of HER2-positive metastatic breast cancer, either when administered alone, in combination with trastuzumab, or in combination with capecitabine.[265] Combination lapatinib/capecitabine following disease progression on trastuzumab resulted in a doubling of the time to tumor progression compared with capecitabine alone, but only a trend in improved OS, likely because of cross-over effects.

T-DM1 is an antibody-drug conjugate of trastuzumab and the chemotherapy DM1, a derivative of maytansine, which causes microtubule inhibition. The EMILIA study evaluated the impact of T-DM1 on PFS and OS compared with combination lapatinib and capecitabine among 991 patients with HER2-positive metastatic breast cancer whose disease had progressed following treatment with trastuzumab and a taxane.[266] Treatment with T-DM1 resulted in a 12.8% improvement in ORR, a 3-month improvement in PFS, and a 32% reduction in the risk of death compared with lapatinib and capecitabine, resulting in the FDA approval of T-DM1 in 2013. The differences in PFS and OS in favor of T-DM1 were both highly statistically significant. T-DM1 was also less toxic than capecitabine/lapatinib. A second trial, the TH3RESA study, involved 602 patients with recurrent HER2-positive breast cancer who were randomly assigned to T-DM1 or the treatment of physician's choice.[267] Approximately 30% of the patients enrolled had received more than five prior regimens for recurrent disease. The primary endpoint was PFS and was in favor of T-DM1, with an HR of 0.53 (p < 0.0001). The superiority of T-DM1 was also seen among patients who had received prior trastuzumab. Based upon the consistent results from EMILIA and TH3RESA studies, T-DM1 offers an effective and tolerable option for treating HER2-positive disease which has progressed following trastuzumab and taxane chemotherapy.

Approximately 45% of HER2-positive breast cancer is also hormone receptor–positive, which allows targeting therapy for both to be incorporated into the treatment of metastatic disease. Cross-talk exists between HER2 and the ER, resulting in relative resistance to endocrine therapy alone. The addition of trastuzumab to anastrozole, and lapatinib to letrozole, substantially improved PFS and clinical benefit compared with endocrine treatment alone in patients with hormone receptor–positive, HER2-positive metastatic disease; however, an OS advantage was not seen, likely because of cross-over design.[268]

KEY POINTS

- Metastatic breast cancer is considered to be incurable; therefore, the goal of treatment is to control disease progression and improve quality of life.
- The choice of systemic therapy is based upon the hormone receptor and HER2 status, as well as the extent of metastatic disease, effect of disease on the patient's quality of life (i.e., performance status), and the pace of the metastatic disease.
- Endocrine therapy is the initial treatment for hormone receptor–positive metastatic disease unless visceral crisis or extensive visceral involvement is present.
- Sequential single-agent chemotherapy is preferable to combination chemotherapy unless a rapid disease response is needed.
- Combination pertuzumab, trastuzumab, and taxane therapy is the recommended first-line treatment for HER2-positive metastatic disease.
- The antibody-drug conjugate T-DM1 is an effective treatment for recurrent HER2-positive disease after progression on trastuzumab.

Bone-Modifying Agents

Approximately 65% to 80% of patients with metastatic breast cancer will develop bone involvement, most commonly among the hormone receptor–positive subtype. Bone involvement is associated with a more favorable prognosis than visceral metastases. Patients are at higher risk of skeletal-related events (SRE) or other complications occurring over time, such as pathologic fracture, cord compression, pain, hypercalcemia, and the need for surgical interventions, such as kyphoplasty and vertebroplasty. Metastatic breast cancer to bone is treated with appropriate systemic therapy. Palliative radiation therapy to specific sites of disease can reduce the morbidity associated with pain and fracture, as well as control disease that may compromise the spinal cord.

Metastatic breast cancer to bone can produce osteoblastic or osteolytic bone lesions, both of which are associated with activation of osteoclasts. Breast cancer cells involving the bone can also secrete cytokines that stimulate receptor activation of nuclear factor kappa B ligand (RANKL) secretion by osteoblasts, which mediates osteoclast survival. Bisphosphonates are pyrophosphate analogs which are internalized by osteoclasts, disrupting function and resulting in apoptosis. Approved bisphosphonates (pamidronate, zoledronic acid) have been shown to reduce the incidence of SREs, the time to the occurrence of SREs, and pain.[269] Denosumab, a humanized monoclonal antibody to RANKL, delayed the advent of SREs by 18% over zoledronic acid among 2,046 women with metastatic breast cancer.[270] Zoledronic acid use was associated with renal compromise, whereas hypocalcemia was more common with denosumab. Both drugs are associated with a 2% incidence of osteonecrosis of the jaw; ideally, physicians should avoid administering these agents to patients, for an undefined period of time, before/after any dental procedure that involves manipulation of the bone. The optimal duration of treatment with either a bisphosphonate or denosumab is unknown, since the therapeutic intervals in published studies vary from 3 months to 34 months. These agents should be considered once lytic bone metastases are diagnosed (see Chapter 20: Symptom Management). The optimal dosing interval is also not known—the current recommendations are monthly.

Investigation is ongoing to determine the role of bisphosphonates given in the adjuvant setting in an attempt to reduce the development of metastatic disease. Conflicting data exists, with the Adjuvant Zoledronic Acid to Reduce Recurrence (AZURE) trial exhibiting no effect of zoledronic acid on DFS among 3,360 patients with early-stage disease who were treated with chemotherapy, whereas the Austrian Breast and Colorectal Cancer Study Group (ABCSG)-12 study revealed a 36% reduction in risk of disease recurrence among 1,803 premenopausal women treated with ovarian suppression and endocrine therapy, and randomly assigned to zoledronic acid or no treatment.[271,272] A meta-analysis of 13 studies investigating the role of adjuvant bisphosphonates showed no effect on DFS or OS; however, there was a suggestion of improved DFS and a reduction in risk of death among postmenopausal women.[273] Although the data are intriguing, the administration of bisphosphonates in the adjuvant setting for the express purpose of reducing risk of disease recurrence remains investigational.

KEY POINTS

- Bisphosphonates or denosumab should be given when lytic bone metastases are present.
- Renal function should be monitored with bisphosphonate use.

SPECIAL CIRCUMSTANCES

MALE BREAST CANCER

The biology of male breast cancer is similar to that seen among postmenopausal women; the majority of the disease is of ductal origin (85% to 95%) and is hormone receptor–positive.[274] Male patients with breast cancer are usually diagnosed at a later disease stage compared with female patients. Local therapy is often mastectomy because of anatomic constraints, although BCT can be offered if standard criteria for BCT are met (see Stage I and II, Local Disease Control section). Recommendations for local disease treatment should be governed by the same criteria outlined for breast cancer in women.

Adjuvant therapy also should be administered using the same criteria as that for women. Tamoxifen, however, is the mainstay of endocrine therapy in ER- and/or PR-positive male breast cancer. Little data exist supporting the use of AIs with or without LHRH agonists for adjuvant treatment among men. Biologically, AIs may increase the amount of circulating testosterone levels, thus increasing the availability of substrate to convert to estrogen. For this reason, AI use may be best administered with medical (LHRH agonist) or surgical orchiectomy. In the metastatic setting, there are case reports of responses with an AI alone and with an AI combined with a LHRH agonist. Although most clinicians favor the combination in this setting, and this is supported by biologic data, it is not unreasonable to start with an AI and follow closely.

The benefit of adjuvant chemotherapy seems to be limited to young men with high-risk characteristics associated with their breast cancer.

ELDERLY PATIENTS

There has been a dramatic increase in breast cancer in older adults in the United States, with an expected increase to 72 million adults older than age 65 by 2030. Since more than one-half of all breast cancer diagnoses occur among older women, there is an expectation that this population will become more prevalent in the realm of oncologic care. The current life expectancy of a women age 70 is 16 years, which is sufficient time for a high-risk breast cancer to recur. An assessment of comorbidities is essential, since more than 50% of patients older than age 50 have at least one comorbidity, and this percentage increases to 66% among patients older than age 75. Comorbidity is an independent predictor of worse survival; however, among healthy elderly women, newer chemotherapy regimens, given without dose reduction, impart the same relative benefit as in younger women.[275] Older women are more susceptible to the toxicity associated with chemotherapy. Hematologic toxicity is more common, often leading to dose reductions of chemotherapy which may compromise outcome. Women older than age 65 have a 26% higher risk of developing congestive heart failure associated with anthracycline use.[276] An adequate interpretation of chemotherapy benefit among high-risk elderly women is difficult to make given the fact that women older than age 65 comprise 8% of enrollment onto clinical trials. CALGB 49907 enrolled 633 women older than age 65 in a randomized trial of adjuvant therapy with capecitabine compared with AC

or CMF.[277] Two-thirds of the women were older than age 70, and 5% were older than age 80. The standard regimens of AC and CMF were associated with a 50% lower risk of recurrence or death compared with the "less toxic" oral capecitabine regimen. These data continue to support the benefit of standard chemotherapy in healthy elderly women without significant comorbidities.

PHYLLODES TUMOR

Phyllodes tumors of the breast are similar to fibroadenomas in that they contain both stromal and epithelial components. They are classified as benign, borderline, or malignant. Their prognosis, however, seems to depend more on the status of surgical margins following resection. The greatest risk of recurrence is local, although metastasis can occur, primarily to the lungs. The primary treatment of a phyllodes tumor is surgical, either with excision or mastectomy, both requiring generous negative margins (greater than 1 cm). ALND is not indicated, nor is routine adjuvant systemic therapy or radiotherapy. Because this tumor acts primarily like a stromal malignancy, options for the treatment of metastatic disease can be based upon therapies for soft tissue sarcomas.

SURVEILLANCE AND SURVIVORSHIP

With the increasing ability to detect earlier-stage breast cancer and the greater efficacy of adjuvant therapy, more women with breast cancer are expected to live long and prosperous lives following their diagnosis and treatment. Consequently, surveillance plans and survivorship issues play a large role in ongoing patient care. The primary goal of surveillance after completion of adjuvant therapy is to detect a new and curable cancer at an early stage (Table 6-9). Routine history and physical examinations and annual mammographic screening are important features of follow-up. ASCO recommendations for surveillance include a history and physical every 3 to 6 months for the first 3 years, then every 6 months for the next 2 years, then annually.[278] When breast conservation is used for local therapy, mammographic imaging of the affected breast should occur 6 months after the completion of radiation therapy (which is often approximately 1 year following diagnosis), and then continue annually once mammographic stability is observed.

The use of nonbreast imaging, tumor markers, or laboratory tests among asymptomatic patients has not been found to

Table 6-9 ASCO Recommendations for Follow-Up Care of Patients with Primary Breast Cancer

Mode of Surveillance	Summary of Recommendations
Recommended breast cancer surveillance	
History/physical examination	Every 3 to 6 months for the first 3 years after primary therapy; every 6 to 12 months for years 4 and 5; then annually
Patient education regarding symptoms of recurrence	Physicians should counsel patients about the symptoms of recurrence, including new lumps, bone pain, chest pain, abdominal pain, dyspnea, or persistent headaches; helpful websites for patient education include www.cancer.net and www.cancer.org
Referral for genetic counseling	Criteria include: Ashkenazi Jewish heritage; history of ovarian cancer at any age in the patient or any first- or second-degree relatives; any first-degree relative with a history of breast cancer diagnosed before age 50; two or more first- or second-degree relatives diagnosed with breast cancer at any age; patient or relative with diagnosis of bilateral breast cancer; and history of breast cancer in a male relative
Breast self-examination	All women should be counseled to perform monthly breast self-examination
Mammography	First post-treatment mammogram 1 year after the initial mammogram that leads to diagnosis but no earlier than 6 months after definitive radiation therapy; subsequent mammograms should be obtained as indicated for surveillance of abnormalities
Coordination of care	Continuity of care is encouraged and should be performed by a physician experienced in the surveillance of patients with cancer and in breast examination, including the examination of irradiated breasts; if follow-up is transferred to a primary care physician (PCP), the PCP and the patient should be informed of the long-term options regarding adjuvant hormone therapy for the particular patient; this may necessitate referral for oncology assessment at an interval consistent with guidelines for adjuvant hormone therapy
Pelvic examination	Regular gynecologic follow-up is recommended for all women; patients who receive tamoxifen should be advised to report any vaginal bleeding to their physicians
Breast cancer surveillance testing: not recommended	
Routine blood tests	Complete blood counts and liver function tests are not recommended
Imaging studies	Chest x-ray, bone scans, liver ultrasound, computed tomography (CT) scans, fluorodeoxyglucose positron emission tomography (FDG-PET) scans, and breast magnetic resonance imaging (MRI) are not recommended
Tumor markers	CA 15-3, CA 27-29, and carcinoembryonic antigen testing are not recommended
FDG-PET	FDG-PET scanning is not recommended for routine breast cancer surveillance
Breast MRI	Breast MRI is not recommended for routine breast cancer surveillance; MRI may be considered on an individual basis for high-risk women

be beneficial, and has been shown to adversely affect quality of life.[279] Most breast cancer recurrences are found between office visits; therefore, it is crucial to focus on patient education concerning signs and symptoms of disease recurrence. Once symptoms occur, appropriate imaging should be performed. The surveillance time should also be used to ensure that appropriate referrals for genetic counseling are made (see Screening section).

Clinical outcomes have been shown to be identical when patients continue their post-treatment surveillance with their oncologist or their primary care provider. This emphasizes the need to understand other women's health issues in addition to breast cancer. Understanding potential long-term complications of treatment is also important. Chemotherapy-induced amenorrhea or ovarian suppression can result in the onset of menopausal symptoms at an earlier-than-expected age. Hot flashes can often be controlled with venlafaxine or gabapentin, whereas the use of intravaginal estrogens to improve

vaginal dryness and sexual dysfunction requires ongoing discussions with patients. The use of AIs can adversely affect bone density, which should be closely monitored. Awareness of potential cardiac toxicity from anthracyclines and trastuzumab, and treatment of chronic neuropathy from taxanes, may require the involvement of cardiologists and neurologists, respectively. Focusing on good health activities, such as exercise and maintaining a normal BMI, appear to favorably impact the risk of disease recurrence. Cognitive dysfunction associated with cancer therapy is a subject of ongoing investigation. The psychosocial ramifications following the diagnosis and treatment of breast cancer cannot be minimized and may require ongoing support and therapy.

FUTURE DIRECTIONS

The improved understanding of the biology of breast cancer and the mechanisms associated with therapeutic resistance has resulted in improved OS of both early-stage and metastatic disease. A greater awareness of the molecular subtypes has enabled the development of targeted treatments, and has established the benefit of certain chemotherapies for each specific subtype. For example, the use of PARP inhibitors may result in improved disease response in patients with *BRCA*-related breast cancer, and DNA-damaging agents seem to be preferentially active in TNBC. Intense investigation is ongoing to find the optimal means of overcoming drug resistance in advanced disease. PI3 kinase inhibitors, AKT inhibitors, and other innovative agents are actively being investigated in this setting.

References

1. Jemal A, Bray F, Center MM, et al. Global cancer statistics. *CA Cancer J Clin.* 2011;61:69-90. PMID: 21296855.

2. Ravdin PM, Cronin KA, Howlader N, et al. The decrease in breast-cancer incidence in 2003 in the United States. *N Engl J Med.* 2007;356:1670-1674. PMID: 17442911.

3. Porter P. "Westernizing" women's risks? Breast cancer in lower-income countries. *N Engl J Med.* 2008;358:213-216. PMID: 18199859.

4. Siegel R, Naishadham D, Jemal A. Cancer statistics, 2013. *CA Cancer J Clin.* 2013;63:11-30. PMID: 23335087.

5. Siegel R, Ward E, Brawley O, et al. Cancer statistics, 2011: the impact of eliminating socioeconomic and racial disparities on premature cancer deaths. *CA Cancer J Clin.* 2011;61:212-236. PMID: 21685461.

6. American Cancer Society. Breast Cancer Facts & Figures 2009-2010. www.cancer.org/acs/groups/content/@nho/documents/document/f861009final90809pdf.pdf. Accessed September 19, 2012.

7. Chlebowski RT, Chen Z, Anderson GL, et al. Ethnicity and breast cancer: factors influencing differences in incidence and outcome. *J Natl Cancer Inst.* 2005;97:439-448. PMID: 15770008.

8. Johansen Taber KA, Morisy LR, Osbahr AJ 3rd, et al. Male breast cancer: risk factors, diagnosis, and management (Review). *Oncol Rep.* 2010;24:1115-1120. PMID: 20878100.

9. Rebora P, Czene K, Reilly M. Timing of familial breast cancer in sisters. *J Natl Cancer Inst.* 2008;100:721-727. PMID: 18477799.

10. Pharoah PD, Day NE, Duffy S, et al. Family history and the risk of breast cancer: a systematic review and meta-analysis. *Int J Cancer.* 1997;71:800-809. PMID: 9180149.

11. U.S. Preventive Services Task Force. Genetic risk assessment and BRCA mutation testing for breast and ovarian cancer susceptibility: recommendation statement. *Ann Intern Med.* 2005;143:355-361. PMID: 16144894.

12. Tischkowitz M, Xia B. PALB2/FANCN: recombining cancer and Fanconi anemia. *Cancer Res.* 2010;70:7353-7359. PMID: 20858716.

13. Breast Cancer Linkage Consortium. Cancer risks in BRCA2 mutation carriers. *J Natl Cancer Inst.* 1999;91:1310-1316. PMID: 10433620.

14. Thompson D, Easton DF. Cancer incidence in BRCA1 mutation carriers. *J Natl Cancer Inst.* 2002;94:1358-1365. PMID: 12237281.

15. Liede A, Karlan BY, Narod SA. Cancer risks for male carriers of germline mutations in BRCA1 or BRCA2: a review of the literature. *J Clin Oncol.* 2004;22:735-742. PMID: 14966099.

16. Chen S, Parmigiani G. Meta-analysis of BRCA1 and BRCA2 penetrance. *J Clin Oncol.* 2007;25:1329-1333. PMID: 17416853.

17. Malone KE, Begg CB, Haile RW, et al. Population-based study of the risk of second primary contralateral breast cancer associated with carrying a mutation in BRCA1 or BRCA2. *J Clin Oncol.* 2010;28:2404-2410. PMID: 20368571.

18. Stadler ZK, Saloustros E, Hansen NA, et al. Absence of genomic BRCA1 and BRCA2 rearrangements in Ashkenazi breast and ovarian cancer families. *Breast Cancer Res Treat.* 2010;123:581-585. PMID: 20221693.

19. Kwon JS, Gutierrez-Barrera AM, Young D, et al. Expanding the criteria for BRCA mutation testing in breast cancer survivors. *J Clin Oncol.* 2010;28:4214-4220. PMID: 20733129.

20. Fitzgerald RC, Hardwick R, Huntsman D, et al. Hereditary diffuse gastric cancer: updated consensus guidelines for clinical management and directions for future research. *J Med Genet.* 2010;47:436-444. PMID: 20591882.

21. Masciari S, Dillon DA, Rath M, et al. Breast cancer phenotype in women with TP53 germline mutations: a Li-Fraumeni syndrome consortium effort. *Breast Cancer Res Treat.* 2012;133:1125-1130. PMID: 22392042.

22. Garber JE, Offit K. Hereditary cancer predisposition syndromes. *J Clin Oncol.* 2005;23:276-292. PMID: 15637391.

23. Domchek SM, Bradbury A, Garber JE, et al. Multiplex genetic testing for cancer susceptibility: out on the high wire without a net? *J Clin Oncol.* 2013;31:1267-1270. PMID: 23460708.

24. Key T, Appleby P, Barnes I, et al. Endogenous sex hormones and breast cancer in postmenopausal women: reanalysis of nine prospective studies. *J Natl Cancer Inst.* 2002;94:606-616. PMID: 11959894.

25. Yang XR, Chang-Claude J, Goode EL, et al. Associations of breast cancer risk factors with tumor subtypes: a pooled analysis from the Breast Cancer Association Consortium studies. *J Natl Cancer Inst.* 2011;103:250-263. PMID: 21191117.

26. Phipps AI, Chlebowski RT, Prentice R, et al. Reproductive history and oral contraceptive use in relation to risk of triple-negative breast cancer. *J Natl Cancer Inst.* 2011;103:470-477. PMID: 21346227.

27. Chlebowski RT, Kuller LH, Prentice RL, et al. Breast cancer after use of estrogen plus progestin in postmenopausal women. *N Engl J Med.* 2009;360:573-587. PMID: 19196674.

28. Marchbanks PA, McDonald JA, Wilson HG, et al. Oral contraceptives and the risk of breast cancer. *N Engl J Med.* 2002;346:2025-2032. PMID: 12087137.

29. Brohet RM, Goldgar DE, Easton DF, et al. Oral contraceptives and breast cancer risk in the international BRCA1/2 carrier cohort study: a report from EMBRACE, GENEPSO, GEO-HEBON, and the IBCCS Collaborating Group. *J Clin Oncol.* 2007;25:3831-3836. PMID: 17635951.

30. Ng AK, Travis LB. Radiation therapy and breast cancer risk. *J Natl Compr Canc Netw.* 2009;7:1121-1128. PMID: 19930978.

31. De Bruin ML, Sparidans J, van't Veer MB, et al. Breast cancer risk in female survivors of Hodgkin's lymphoma: lower risk after smaller radiation volumes. *J Clin Oncol.* 2009;27:4239-4246. PMID: 19667275.

32. Henderson TO, Amsterdam A, Bhatia S, et al. Systematic review: surveillance for breast cancer in women treated with chest radiation for childhood, adolescent, or young adult cancer. *Ann Intern Med.* 2010;152:444-455; W144-154.

33. McCormack VA, dos Santos Silva I. Breast density and parenchymal patterns as markers of breast cancer risk: a meta-analysis. *Cancer Epidemiol Biomarkers Prev.* 2006;15:1159-1169. PMID: 16775176.

34. Martin LJ, Boyd NF. Mammographic density. Potential mechanisms of breast cancer risk associated with mammographic density: hypotheses based on epidemiological evidence. *Breast Cancer Res.* 2008;10:201. PMID: 18226174.

35. Chuba PJ, Hamre MR, Yap J, et al. Bilateral risk for subsequent breast cancer after lobular carcinoma-in-situ: analysis of surveillance, epidemiology, and end results data. *J Clin Oncol.* 2005;23:5534-5541. PMID: 16110014.

36. Degnim AC, Visscher DW, Berman HK, et al. Stratification of breast cancer risk in women with atypia: a Mayo cohort study. *J Clin Oncol.* 2007;25:2671-2677. PMID: 17563394.

37. Smith-Warner SA, Spiegelman D, Yaun SS, et al. Alcohol and breast cancer in women: a pooled analysis of cohort studies. *JAMA.* 1998;279:535-540. PMID: 9480365.

38. Dorgan JF, Baer DJ, Albert PS, et al. Serum hormones and the alcohol-breast cancer association in postmenopausal women. *J Natl Cancer Inst.* 2001;93:710-715. PMID: 11333294.

39. Chen WY, Rosner B, Hankinson SE, et al. Moderate alcohol consumption during adult life, drinking patterns, and breast cancer risk. *JAMA.* 2011;306:1884-1890. PMID: 22045766.

40. Calle EE, Rodriguez C, Walker-Thurmond K, et al. Overweight, obesity, and mortality from cancer in a prospectively studied cohort of U.S. adults. *N Engl J Med.* 2003;348:1625-1638. PMID: 12711737.

41. Harris HR, Willett WC, Terry KL, et al. Body fat distribution and risk of premenopausal breast cancer in the Nurses' Health Study II. *J Natl Cancer Inst.* 2011;103:273-278. PMID: 21163903.

42. Gunter MJ, Hoover DR, Yu H, et al. Insulin, insulin-like growth factor-I, and risk of breast cancer in postmenopausal women. *J Natl Cancer Inst.* 2009;101:48-60. PMID: 19116382.

43. Key TJ, Appleby PN, Reeves GK, et al. Body mass index, serum sex hormones, and breast cancer risk in postmenopausal women. *J Natl Cancer Inst.* 2003;95:1218-1226. PMID: 12928347.

44. Gammon MD, John EM, Britton JA. Recreational and occupational physical activities and risk of breast cancer. *J Natl Cancer Inst.* 1998;90:100-117. PMID: 9450570.

45. Wei EK, Wolin KY, Colditz GA. Time course of risk factors in cancer etiology and progression. *J Clin Oncol.* 2010;28:4052-4407. PMID: 20644083.

46. Claus EB, Risch N, Thompson WD. Genetic analysis of breast cancer in the cancer and steroid hormone study. *Am J Hum Genet.* 1991;48:232-242. PMID: 1990835.

47. Euhus DM, Smith KC, Robinson L, et al. Pretest prediction of BRCA1 or BRCA2 mutation by risk counselors and the computer model BRCAPRO. *J Natl Cancer Inst.* 2002;94:844-851. PMID: 12048272.

48. Tyrer J, Duffy SW, Cuzick J. A breast cancer prediction model incorporating familial and personal risk factors. *Stat Med.* 2004;23:1111-1130. PMID: 15057881.

49. Antoniou AC, Pharoah PP, Smith P, et al. The BOADICEA model of genetic susceptibility to breast and ovarian cancer. *Br J Cancer.* 2004;91:1580-1590. PMID: 15381934.

50. Amir E, Freedman OC, Seruga B, et al. Assessing women at high risk of breast cancer: a review of risk assessment models. *J Natl Cancer Inst.* 2010;102:680-691. PMID: 20427433.

51. Gail MH, Costantino JP, Pee D, et al. Projecting individualized absolute invasive breast cancer risk in African American women. *J Natl Cancer Inst.* 2007;99:1782-1792. PMID: 18042936.

52. Rockhill B, Spiegelman D, Byrne C, et al. Validation of the Gail et al. model of breast cancer risk prediction and implications for chemoprevention. *J Natl Cancer Inst.* 2001;93:358-366. PMID: 11238697.

53. Pankratz VS, Hartmann LC, Degnim AC, et al. Assessment of the accuracy of the Gail model in women with atypical hyperplasia. *J Clin Oncol.* 2008;26:5374-5379. PMID: 18854574.

54. Domchek SM, Friebel TM, Singer CF, et al. Association of risk-reducing surgery in BRCA1 or BRCA2 mutation carriers with cancer risk and mortality. *JAMA.* 2010;304:967-975. PMID: 20810374.

55. Rebbeck TR, Friebel T, Wagner T, et al. Effect of short-term hormone replacement therapy on breast cancer risk reduction after bilateral prophylactic oophorectomy in BRCA1 and BRCA2 mutation carriers: the PROSE Study Group. *J Clin Oncol.* 2005;23:7804-7810. PMID: 16219936.

56. Rebbeck TR, Friebel T, Lynch HT, et al. Bilateral prophylactic mastectomy reduces breast cancer risk in BRCA1 and BRCA2 mutation carriers: the PROSE Study Group. *J Clin Oncol.* 2004;22:1055-1062. PMID: 14981104.

57. Guillem JG, Wood WC, Moley JF, et al. ASCO/SSO review of current role of risk-reducing surgery in common hereditary cancer syndromes. *J Clin Oncol.* 2006;24:4642-4660. PMID: 17008706.

58. Early Breast Cancer Trialists' Collaborative Group (EBCTCG). Effects of chemotherapy and hormonal therapy for early breast cancer on recurrence and 15-year survival: an overview of the randomised trials. *Lancet.* 2005;365:1687-1717. PMID: 15894097.

59. Fisher B, Costantino JP, Wickerham DL, et al. Tamoxifen for the prevention of breast cancer: current status of the National Surgical Adjuvant Breast and Bowel Project P-1 study. *J Natl Cancer Inst.* 2005;97:1652-1662. PMID: 16288118.

60. Cuzick J, Forbes JF, Sestak I, et al. Long-term results of tamoxifen prophylaxis for breast cancer---96-month follow-up of the randomized IBIS-I trial. *J Natl Cancer Inst.* 2007;99:272-282. PMID: 17312304.

61. Powles TJ, Ashley S, Tidy A, et al. Twenty-year follow-up of the Royal Marsden randomized, double-blinded tamoxifen breast cancer prevention trial. *J Natl Cancer Inst.* 2007;99:283-290. PMID: 17312305.

62. Veronesi U, Maisonneuve P, Rotmensz N, et al. Tamoxifen for the prevention of breast cancer: late results of the Italian Randomized Tamoxifen Prevention Trial among women with hysterectomy. *J Natl Cancer Inst.* 2007;99:727-737. PMID: 17470740.

63. Cuzick J, Powles T, Veronesi U, et al. Overview of the main outcomes in breast-cancer prevention trials. *Lancet.* 2003;361:296-300. PMID: 12559863.

64. Visvanathan K, Chlebowski RT, Hurley P, et al. American society of clinical oncology clinical practice guideline update on the use of pharmacologic interventions including tamoxifen, raloxifene, and aromatase inhibition for breast cancer risk reduction. *J Clin Oncol.* 2009;27:3235-3258. PMID: 19470930.

65. Vogel VG, Costantino JP, Wickerham DL, et al. Effects of tamoxifen vs raloxifene on the risk of developing invasive breast cancer and other disease outcomes: the NSABP Study of Tamoxifen and Raloxifene (STAR) P-2 trial. *JAMA.* 2006;295:2727-2741. PMID: 16754727.

66. Vogel VG, Costantino JP, Wickerham DL, et al. Update of the National Surgical Adjuvant Breast and Bowel Project Study of Tamoxifen and Raloxifene (STAR) P-2 Trial: Preventing breast cancer. *Cancer Prev Res (Phila).* 2010;3:696-706. PMID: 20404000.

67. Cuzick J, Sestak I, Bonanni B, et al. Selective oestrogen receptor modulators in prevention of breast cancer: an updated meta-analysis of individual participant data. *Lancet.* 2013;381:1827-1834. PMID: 23639488.

68. Goss PE, Ingle JN, Alés-Martínez JE, et al. Exemestane for breast-cancer prevention in postmenopausal women. *N Engl J Med.* 2011;364:2381-2391. PMID: 21639806.

69. Cuzick J, Sestak I, Forbes JF, et al. Anastrozole for prevention of breast cancer in high-risk postmenopausal women (IBIS-II): an international, double-blind, randomised placebo-controlled trial. *Lancet.* 2014;383: 1041-1048. PMID: 24333009.

70. Visvanathan K, Hurley P, Bantug E, et al. Use of pharmacologic interventions for breast cancer risk reduction: American Society of Clinical Oncology clinical practice guideline. *J Clin Oncol.* 2013;31:2942-2962. PMID: 23835710.

71. Phillips KA, Milne RL, Rookus MA, et al. Tamoxifen and risk of contralateral breast cancer for BRCA1 and BRCA2 mutation carriers. *J Clin Oncol.* 2013;31:3091-3099. PMID: 23918944.

72. Winzer BM, Whiteman DC, Reeves MM, et al. Physical activity and cancer prevention: a systematic review of clinical trials. *Cancer Causes Control.* 2011;22:811-826. PMID: 21461921.

73. Cummings SR, Tice JA, Bauer S, et al. Prevention of breast cancer in postmenopausal women: approaches to estimating and reducing risk. *J Natl Cancer Inst.* 2009;101:384-398. PMID: 19276457.

74. Friedenreich CM, Cust AE. Physical activity and breast cancer risk: impact of timing, type and dose of activity and population subgroup effects. *Br J Sports Med.* 2008;42:636-647. PMID: 18487249.

75. Prentice RL, Caan B, Chlebowski RT, et al. Low-fat dietary pattern and risk of invasive breast cancer: the Women's Health Initiative Randomized Controlled Dietary Modification Trial. *JAMA.* 2006;295:629-642. PMID: 16467232.

76. Chlebowski RT, Johnson KC, Kooperberg C, et al. Calcium plus vitamin D supplementation and the risk of breast cancer. *J Natl Cancer Inst.* 2008;100:1581-1591. PMID: 19001601.

77. Nelson HD, Tyne K, Naik A, et al. Screening for breast cancer: an update for the U.S. Preventive Services Task Force. *Ann Intern Med.* 2009;151:727-737, W237-242. PMID: 19920273.

78. Mandelblatt JS, Cronin KA, Bailey S, et al. Effects of mammography screening under different screening schedules: model estimates of potential benefits and harms. *Ann Intern Med.* 2009;151:738-747. PMID: 19920274.

79. U.S. Preventive Services Task Force. Screening for breast cancer: U.S. Preventive Services Task Force recommendation statement. *Ann Intern Med.* 2009;151:716-726, W-236. PMID: 19920272.

80. Smith RA, Brooks D, Cokkinides V, et al. Cancer screening in the United States, 2013: a review of current American Cancer Society guidelines, current issues in cancer screening, and new guidance on cervical cancer screening and lung cancer screening. *CA Cancer J Clin.* 2013;63:88-105. PMID: 23378235.

81. Pisano ED, Gatsonis C, Hendrick E, et al. Diagnostic performance of digital versus film mammography for breast-cancer screening. *N Engl J Med.* 2005;353:1773-1783. PMID: 16169887.

82. Skaane P, Hofvind S, Skjennald A. Randomized trial of screen-film versus full-field digital mammography with soft-copy reading in population-based screening program: follow-up and final results of Oslo II study. *Radiology.* 2007;244:708-717. PMID: 17709826.

83. Patterson SK, Noroozian M. Update on emerging technologies in breast imaging. *J Natl Compr Canc Netw.* 2012;10:1355-1362. PMID: 23138164.

84. Berg WA, Blume JD, Cormack JB, et al. Combined screening with ultrasound and mammography vs mammography alone in women at elevated risk of breast cancer. *JAMA.* 2008;299:2151-2163. PMID: 18477782.

85. Semiglazov VF, Moiseyenko VM, Bavli JL, et al. The role of breast self-examination in early breast cancer detection (results of the 5-years USSR/WHO randomized study in Leningrad). *Eur J Epidemiol.* 1992;8:498-502. PMID: 1397215.

86. Thomas DB, Gao DL, Self SG, et al. Randomized trial of breast self-examination in Shanghai: methodology and preliminary results. *J Natl Cancer Inst.* 1997;89:355-365. PMID: 9060957.

87. Saslow D, Hannan J, Osuch J, et al. Clinical breast examination: practical recommendations for optimizing performance and reporting. *CA Cancer J Clin.* 2004;54:327-344. PMID: 15537576.

88. Humphrey LL, Helfand M, Chan BK, et al. Breast cancer screening: a summary of the evidence for the U.S. Preventive Services Task Force. *Ann Intern Med.* 2002;137:347-360. PMID: 12204020.

89. Warner E, Messersmith H, Causer P, et al. Systematic review: using magnetic resonance imaging to screen women at high risk for breast cancer. *Ann Intern Med.* 2008;148:671-679. PMID: 18458280.

90. Warner E, Hill K, Causer P, et al. Prospective study of breast cancer incidence in women with a BRCA1 or BRCA2 mutation under surveillance with and without magnetic resonance imaging. *J Clin Oncol.* 2011;29:1664-1669. PMID: 21444874.

91. Saslow D, Boetes C, Burke W, et al. American Cancer Society guidelines for breast screening with MRI as an adjunct to mammography. *CA Cancer J Clin.* 2007;57:75-89. PMID: 17392385.

92. Robson M, Offit K. Clinical practice. Management of an inherited predisposition to breast cancer. *N Engl J Med.* 2007;357:154-162. PMID: 17625127.

93. Ng AK, Garber JE, Diller LR, et al. Prospective study of the efficacy of breast magnetic resonance imaging and mammographic screening in survivors of Hodgkin lymphoma. *J Clin Oncol.* 2013;31:2282-2288. PMID: 23610104.

94. Bassett L, Winchester DP, Caplan RB, et al. Stereotactic core-needle biopsy of the breast: a report of the Joint Task Force of the American College of Radiology, American College of Surgeons, and College of American Pathologists. *CA Cancer J Clin.* 1997;47:171-190. PMID: 9152175.

95. Houssami N, Ciatto S, Macaskill P, et al. Accuracy and surgical impact of magnetic resonance imaging in breast cancer staging: systematic review and meta-analysis in detection of multifocal and multicentric cancer. *J Clin Oncol.* 2008;26:3248-3258. PMID: 18474876.

96. Brennan ME, Houssami N, Lord S, et al. Magnetic resonance imaging screening of the contralateral breast in women with newly diagnosed breast cancer: systematic review and meta-analysis of incremental cancer detection and impact on surgical management. *J Clin Oncol.* 2009;27:5640-5649. PMID: 19805685.

97. American Joint Committee on Cancer. *AJCC Cancer Staging Manual, 7th ed.* Philadelphia: Lippincott Raven Publishers, 2010.

98. Quiet CA, Ferguson DJ, Weichselbaum RR, et al. Natural history of node-positive breast cancer: the curability of small cancers with a limited number of positive nodes. *J Clin Oncol.* 1996;14:3105-3111. PMID: 8955655.

99. Giuliano AE, Hunt KK, Ballman KV, et al. Axillary dissection vs no axillary dissection in women with invasive breast cancer and sentinel node metastasis: a randomized clinical trial. *JAMA.* 2011;305:569-575. PMID: 21304082.

100. Colleoni M, Rotmensz N, Peruzzotti G, et al. Size of breast cancer metastases in axillary lymph nodes: clinical relevance of minimal lymph node involvement. *J Clin Oncol.* 2005;23:1379-1389. PMID: 15735114.

101. Pestalozzi BC, Zahrieh D, Mallon E, et al. Distinct clinical and prognostic features of infiltrating lobular carcinoma of the breast: combined results of 15 International Breast Cancer Study Group clinical trials. *J Clin Oncol.* 2008;26:3006-3014. PMID: 18458044.

102. Rosen PP, Groshen S, Kinne DW, et al. Factors influencing prognosis in node-negative breast carcinoma: analysis of 767 T1N0M0/T2N0M0 patients with long-term follow-up. *J Clin Oncol.* 1993;11:2090-2100. PMID: 8229123.

103. Dalton LW, Page DL, Dupont WD. Histologic grading of breast carcinoma. A reproducibility study. *Cancer.* 1994;73:2765-2770. PMID: 8194018.

104. Rakha EA, El-Sayed ME, Lee AH, et al. Prognostic significance of Nottingham histologic grade in invasive breast carcinoma. *J Clin Oncol.* 2008;26:3153-3158. PMID: 18490649.

105. Osborne CK. Steroid hormone receptors in breast cancer management. *Breast Cancer Res Treat.* 1998;51:227-238. PMID: 10068081.

106. Rakha EA, El-Sayed ME, Green AR, et al. Biologic and clinical characteristics of breast cancer with single hormone receptor positive phenotype. *J Clin Oncol.* 2007;25:4772-4778. PMID: 17876012.

107. Harvey JM, Clark GM, Osborne CK, et al. Estrogen receptor status by immunohistochemistry is superior to the ligand-binding assay for predicting response to adjuvant endocrine therapy in breast cancer. *J Clin Oncol.* 1999;17:1474-1481. PMID: 10334533.

108. Hess KR, Pusztai L, Buzdar AU, et al. Estrogen receptors and distinct patterns of breast cancer relapse. *Breast Cancer Res Treat.* 2003;78:105-118. PMID: 12611463.

109. Wolff AC, Hammond ME, Schwartz JN, et al. American Society of Clinical Oncology/College of American Pathologists guideline recommendations for human epidermal growth factor receptor 2 testing in breast cancer. *J Clin Oncol.* 2007;25:118-145. PMID: 17159189.

110. Wolff AC, Hammond ME, Hicks DG, et al. Recommendations for human epidermal growth factor receptor 2 testing in breast cancer: American Society of Clinical Oncology/College of American Pathologists clinical practice guideline update. *J Clin Oncol.* 2013;31:3997-4013. PMID: 24101045.

111. Gennari A, Sormani MP, Pronzato P, et al. HER2 status and efficacy of adjuvant anthracyclines in early breast cancer: a pooled analysis of randomized trials. *J Natl Cancer Inst.* 2008;100:14-20. PMID: 18159072.

112. Hayes DF, Thor AD, Dressler LG, et al. HER2 and response to paclitaxel in node-positive breast cancer. *N Engl J Med.* 2007;357:1496-1506. PMID: 17928597.

113. Houston SJ, Plunkett TA, Barnes DM, et al. Overexpression of c-erbB2 is an independent marker of resistance to endocrine therapy in advanced breast cancer. *Br J Cancer.* 1999;79:1220-1226. PMID: 10098763.

114. Slamon DJ, Clark GM, Wong SG, et al. Human breast cancer: correlation of relapse and survival with amplification of the HER-2/neu oncogene. *Science.* 1987;235:177-182. PMID: 3798106.

115. Arvold ND, Taghian AG, Niemierko A, et al. Age, breast cancer subtype approximation, and local recurrence after breast-conserving therapy. *J Clin Oncol.* 2011;29:3885-3891. PMID: 21900114.

116. Voduc KD, Cheang MC, Tyldesley S, et al. Breast cancer subtypes and the risk of local and regional relapse. *J Clin Oncol.* 2010;28:1684-1691. PMID: 20194857.

117. Brenton JD, Carey LA, Ahmed AA, et al. Molecular classification and molecular forecasting of breast cancer: ready for clinical application? *J Clin Oncol.* 2005;23:7350-7360. PMID: 16145060.

118. Cheang MC, Chia SK, Voduc D, et al. Ki67 index, HER2 status, and prognosis of patients with luminal B breast cancer. *J Natl Cancer Inst.* 2009;101:736-750. PMID: 19436038.

119. Rakha EA, Reis-Filho JS, Ellis IO. Basal-like breast cancer: a critical review. *J Clin Oncol.* 2008;26:2568-2581. PMID: 18487574.

120. Parker JS, Mullins M, Cheang MC, et al. Supervised risk predictor of breast cancer based on intrinsic subtypes. *J Clin Oncol.* 2009;27:1160-1167. PMID: 19204204.

121. van de Vijver MJ, He YD, van't Veer LJ, et al. A gene-expression signature as a predictor of survival in breast cancer. *N Engl J Med.* 2002;347:1999-2009. PMID: 12490681.

122. Buyse M, Loi S, van't Veer L, et al. Validation and clinical utility of a 70-gene prognostic signature for women with node-negative breast cancer. *J Natl Cancer Inst.* 2006;98:1183-1192. PMID: 16954471.

123. Cardoso F, Van't Veer L, Rutgers E, et al. Clinical application of the 70-gene profile: the MINDACT trial. *J Clin Oncol.* 2008;26:729-735. PMID: 18258980.

124. Paik S, Shak S, Tang G, et al. A multigene assay to predict recurrence of tamoxifen-treated, node-negative breast cancer. *N Engl J Med.* 2004;351:2817-2826. PMID: 15591335.

125. Ramsey SD, Barlow WE, Gonzalez-Angulo AM, et al. Integrating comparative effectiveness design elements and endpoints into a phase III, randomized clinical trial (SWOG S1007) evaluating oncotypeDX-guided management for women with breast cancer involving lymph nodes. *Contemp Clin Trials.* 2013;34:1-9. PMID: 23000081.

126. Paik S, Tang G, Shak S, et al. Gene expression and benefit of chemotherapy in women with node-negative, estrogen receptor-positive breast cancer. *J Clin Oncol.* 2006;24:3726-3734. PMID: 16720680.

127. Albain KS, Barlow WE, Shak S, et al. Prognostic and predictive value of the 21-gene recurrence score assay in postmenopausal women with node-positive, oestrogen-receptor-positive breast cancer on chemotherapy: a retrospective analysis of a randomised trial. *Lancet Oncol.* 2010;11:55-65. PMID: 20005174.

128. Mamounas EP, Tang G, Fisher B, et al. Association between the 21-gene recurrence score assay and risk of locoregional recurrence in node-negative, estrogen receptor-positive breast cancer: results from NSABP B-14 and NSABP B-20. *J Clin Oncol.* 2010;28:1677-1683. PMID: 20065188.

129. Sparano JA, Paik S. Development of the 21-gene assay and its application in clinical practice and clinical trials. *J Clin Oncol.* 2008;26:721-728. PMID: 18258979.

130. Balslev I, Axelsson CK, Zedeler K, et al. The Nottingham Prognostic Index applied to 9,149 patients from the studies of the Danish Breast Cancer

Cooperative Group (DBCG). *Breast Cancer Res Treat.* 1994;32:281-290. PMID: 7865856.

131. Olivotto IA, Bajdik CD, Ravdin PM, et al. Population-based validation of the prognostic model ADJUVANT! for early breast cancer. *J Clin Oncol.* 2005;23:2716-2725. PMID: 15837986.

132. Hodgson NC, Gulenchyn KY. Is there a role for positron emission tomography in breast cancer staging? *J Clin Oncol.* 2008;26:712-720. PMID: 18258978.

133. Allegra CJ, Aberle DR, Ganschow P, et al. National Institutes of Health State-of-the-Science Conference statement: Diagnosis and Management of Ductal Carcinoma In Situ September 22-24, 2009. *J Natl Cancer Inst.* 2010;102:161-169. PMID: 20071686.

134. Solin LJ, Gray R, Baehner FL, et al. A multigene expression assay to predict local recurrence risk for ductal carcinoma in situ of the breast. *J Natl Cancer Inst.* 2013;105:701-710. PMID: 23641039.

135. Kuerer HM, Albarracin CT, Yang WT, et al. Ductal carcinoma in situ: state of the science and roadmap to advance the field. *J Clin Oncol.* 2009;27:279-288. PMID: 19064970.

136. Wapnir IL, Dignam JJ, Fisher B, et al. Long-term outcomes of invasive ipsilateral breast tumor recurrences after lumpectomy in NSABP B-17 and B-24 randomized clinical trials for DCIS. *J Natl Cancer Inst.* 2011;103:478-488. PMID: 21398619.

137. Virnig BA, Tuttle TM, Shamliyan T, et al. Ductal carcinoma in situ of the breast: a systematic review of incidence, treatment, and outcomes. *J Natl Cancer Inst.* 2010;102:170-178. PMID: 20071685.

138. Allred DC, Anderson SJ, Paik S, et al. Adjuvant tamoxifen reduces subsequent breast cancer in women with estrogen receptor-positive ductal carcinoma in situ: a study based on NSABP protocol B-24. *J Clin Oncol.* 2012;30:1268-1273. PMID: 22393101.

139. Buchholz TA, Tucker SL, Erwin J, et al. Impact of systemic treatment on local control for patients with lymph node-negative breast cancer treated with breast-conservation therapy. *J Clin Oncol.* 2001;19:2240-2246. PMID: 11304777.

140. Clarke M, Collins R, Darby S, et al. Effects of radiotherapy and of differences in the extent of surgery for early breast cancer on local recurrence and 15-year survival: an overview of the randomised trials. *Lancet.* 2005;366:2087-2106. PMID: 16360786.

141. Carlson RW, Allred DC, Anderson BO, et al. Invasive breast cancer. *J Natl Compr Canc Netw.* 2011;9:136-222. PMID: 21310842.

142. Theriault RL, Carlson RW, Allred C, et al. Breast cancer, version 3.2013: featured updates to the NCCN guidelines. *J Natl Compr Canc Netw.* 2013;11:753-760; quiz 761.

143. Goldhirsch A, Winer EP, Coates AS, et al. Personalizing the treatment of women with early breast cancer: highlights of the St Gallen International Expert Consensus on the Primary Therapy of Early Breast Cancer 2013. *Ann Oncol.* 2013;24:2206-2223. PMID: 23917950.

144. Fisher B, Anderson S, Bryant J, et al. Twenty-year follow-up of a randomized trial comparing total mastectomy, lumpectomy, and lumpectomy plus irradiation for the treatment of invasive breast cancer. *N Engl J Med.* 2002;347:1233-1241. PMID: 12393820.

145. Buchholz TA. Radiation therapy for early-stage breast cancer after breast-conserving surgery. *N Engl J Med.* 2009;360:63-70. PMID: 19118305.

146. Jones HA, Antonini N, Hart AA, et al. Impact of pathological characteristics on local relapse after breast-conserving therapy: a subgroup analysis of the EORTC boost versus no boost trial. *J Clin Oncol.* 2009;27:4939-4947. PMID: 19720914.

147. Whelan TJ, Pignol JP, Levine MN, et al. Long-term results of hypofractionated radiation therapy for breast cancer. *N Engl J Med.* 2010;362:513-520. PMID: 20147717.

148. Sanders ME, Scroggins T, Ampil FL, et al. Accelerated partial breast irradiation in early-stage breast cancer. *J Clin Oncol.* 2007;25:996-1002. PMID: 17350949.

149. Pugliese M, Stempel M, Patil S, et al. The clinical impact and outcomes of immunohistochemistry-only metastasis in breast cancer. *Am J Surg.* 2010;200:368-373. PMID: 20800716.

150. Lyman GH, Giuliano AE, Somerfield MR, et al. American Society of Clinical Oncology guideline recommendations for sentinel lymph node biopsy in early-stage breast cancer. *J Clin Oncol.* 2005;23:7703-7720. PMID: 16157938.

151. Caudle AS, Hunt KK, Kuerer HM, et al. Multidisciplinary considerations in the implementation of the findings from the American College of Surgeons Oncology Group (ACOSOG) Z0011 study: a practice-changing trial. *Ann Surg Oncol.* 2011;18:2407-2412. PMID: 21327455.

152. Whelan TJ, Olivotto IA, Ackerman JW, et al. NCIC-CTG MA.20: An intergroup trial of regional nodal irradiation in early breast cancer. *J Clin Oncol.* 2013;29 (suppl; abstr LBA1003).

153. Hughes KS, Schnaper LA, Bellon JR, et al. Lumpectomy plus tamoxifen with or without irradiation in women age 70 years or older with early breast cancer: long-term follow-up of CALGB 9343. *J Clin Oncol.* 2013;31:2382-2387. PMID: 23690420.

154. Pierce LJ, Phillips KA, Griffith KA, et al. Local therapy in BRCA1 and BRCA2 mutation carriers with operable breast cancer: comparison of breast conservation and mastectomy. *Breast Cancer Res Treat.* 2010;121:389-398. PMID: 20411323.

155. Zellars R. Post-mastectomy radiotherapy. *Clin Adv Hematol Oncol.* 2009;7:533-543. PMID: 19927981.

156. Early Breast Cancer Trialists' Collaborative Group (EBCTCG), Davies C, Godwin J, et al. Relevance of breast cancer hormone receptors and other factors to the efficacy of adjuvant tamoxifen: patient-level meta-analysis of randomised trials. *Lancet.* 2011;378:771-784. PMID: 21802721.

157. Davies C, Pan H, Godwin J, et al. Long-term effects of continuing adjuvant tamoxifen to 10 years versus stopping at 5 years after diagnosis of oestrogen receptor-positive breast cancer: ATLAS, a randomised trial. *Lancet.* 2013;381:805-816. PMID: 23219286.

158. Gray RG, Rea D, Handley K, et al. aTTom: Long-term effects of continuing adjuvant tamoxifen to 10 years versus stopping at 5 years in 6,953 women with early breast cancer. *J Clin Oncol.* 2013;31:5 (suppl).

159. Schroth W, Goetz MP, Hamann U, et al. Association between CYP2D6 polymorphisms and outcomes among women with early stage breast cancer treated with tamoxifen. *JAMA.* 2009;302:1429-1436. PMID: 19809024.

160. Rae JM, Drury S, Hayes DF, et al. CYP2D6 and UGT2B7 genotype and risk of recurrence in tamoxifen-treated breast cancer patients. *J Natl Cancer Inst.* 2012;104:452-460. PMID: 22395643.

161. Regan MM, Leyland-Jones B, Bouzyk M, et al. CYP2D6 genotype and tamoxifen response in postmenopausal women with endocrine-responsive breast cancer: the breast international group 1-98 trial. *J Natl Cancer Inst.* 2012;104:441-451. PMID: 22395644.

162. Lash TL, Cronin-Fenton D, Ahern TP, et al. CYP2D6 inhibition and breast cancer recurrence in a population-based study in Denmark. *J Natl Cancer Inst.* 2011;103:489-500. PMID: 21325141.

163. Visvanathan K, Chlebowski RT, Hurley P, et al. American society of clinical oncology clinical practice guideline update on the use of pharmacologic interventions including tamoxifen, raloxifene, and aromatase inhibition for breast cancer risk reduction. *J Clin Oncol.* 2009;27:3235-3258. PMID: 19470930.

164. LHRH-agonists in Early Breast Cancer Overview group, Cuzick J, Ambroisine L, et al. Use of luteinising-hormone-releasing hormone agonists as adjuvant treatment in premenopausal patients with hormone-receptor-positive breast cancer: a meta-analysis of individual patient data from randomised adjuvant trials. *Lancet.* 2007;369:1711-1723. PMID: 17512856.

165. Griggs JJ, Somerfield MR, Anderson H, et al. American Society of Clinical Oncology endorsement of the cancer care Ontario practice guideline on adjuvant ovarian ablation in the treatment of premenopausal women with early-stage invasive breast cancer. *J Clin Oncol.* 2011;29:3939-3942. PMID: 21900112.

166. Burstein HJ, Prestrud AA, Seidenfeld J, et al. American Society of Clinical Oncology clinical practice guideline: update on adjuvant endocrine therapy for women with hormone receptor-positive breast cancer. *J Clin Oncol.* 2010;28:3784-3796. PMID: 20625130.

167. Dowsett M, Cuzick J, Ingle J, et al. Meta-analysis of breast cancer outcomes in adjuvant trials of aromatase inhibitors versus tamoxifen. *J Clin Oncol.* 2010;28:509-518. PMID: 19949017.

168. Bliss JM, Kilburn LS, Coleman RE, et al. Disease-related outcomes with long-term follow-up: an updated analysis of the intergroup exemestane study. *J Clin Oncol.* 2012;30:709-717. PMID: 22042946.

169. Jin H, Tu D, Zhao N, et al. Longer-term outcomes of letrozole versus placebo after 5 years of tamoxifen in the NCIC CTG MA.17 trial: analyses adjusting for treatment crossover. *J Clin Oncol.* 2012;30:718-721. PMID: 22042967.

170. Berry DA, Cirrincione C, Henderson IC, et al. Estrogen-receptor status and outcomes of modern chemotherapy for patients with node-positive breast cancer. *JAMA.* 2006;295:1658-1667. PMID: 16609087.

171. Hernandez-Aya LF, Chavez-Macgregor M, Lei X, et al. Nodal status and clinical outcomes in a large cohort of patients with triple-negative breast cancer. *J Clin Oncol.* 2011;29:2628-2634. PMID: 21606433.

172. Park YH, Kim ST, Cho EY, et al. A risk stratification by hormonal receptors (ER, PgR) and HER-2 status in small (≤ 1 cm) invasive breast cancer: who might be possible candidates for adjuvant treatment? *Breast Cancer Res Treat.* 2010;119:653-661. PMID: 19957028.

173. Fisher B, Brown AM, Dimitrov NV, et al. Two months of doxorubicin-cyclophosphamide with and without interval reinduction therapy compared with 6 months of cyclophosphamide, methotrexate, and fluorouracil in positive-node breast cancer patients with tamoxifen-nonresponsive tumors: results from the National Surgical Adjuvant Breast and Bowel Project B-15. *J Clin Oncol.* 1990;8:1483-1496. PMID: 2202791.

174. Jones S, Holmes FA, O'Shaughnessy J, et al. Docetaxel With Cyclophosphamide Is Associated With an Overall Survival Benefit Compared With Doxorubicin and Cyclophosphamide: 7-Year Follow-Up of US Oncology Research Trial 9735. *J Clin Oncol.* 2009;27:1177-1183. PMID: 19204201.

175. Shulman LN, Cirrincione CT, Berry DA, et al. Six cycles of doxorubicin and cyclophosphamide or Paclitaxel are not superior to four cycles as adjuvant chemotherapy for breast cancer in women with zero to three positive axillary nodes: Cancer and Leukemia Group B 40101. *J Clin Oncol.* 2012;30:4071-4076. PMID: 22826271.

176. De Laurentiis M, Cancello G, D'Agostino D, et al. Taxane-based combinations as adjuvant chemotherapy of early breast cancer: a meta-analysis of randomized trials. *J Clin Oncol.* 2008;26:44-53. PMID: 18165639.

177. Henderson IC, Berry DA, Demetri GD, et al. Improved outcomes from adding sequential Paclitaxel but not from escalating Doxorubicin dose in an adjuvant chemotherapy regimen for patients with node-positive primary breast cancer. *J Clin Oncol.* 2003;21:976-983. PMID: 12637460.

178. Roché H, Fumoleau P, Spielmann M, et al. Sequential adjuvant epirubicin-based and docetaxel chemotherapy for node-positive breast cancer patients: the FNCLCC PACS 01 Trial. *J Clin Oncol.* 2006;24:5664-5671. PMID: 17116941.

179. Martin M, Pienkowski T, Mackey J, et al. Adjuvant docetaxel for node-positive breast cancer. *N Engl J Med.* 2005;352:2302-2313. PMID: 15930421.

180. Martín M, Seguí MA, Antón A, et al. Adjuvant docetaxel for high-risk, node-negative breast cancer. *N Engl J Med.* 2010;363:2200-2210. PMID: 21121833.

181. Eiermann W, Pienkowski T, Crown J, et al. Phase III study of doxorubicin/cyclophosphamide with concomitant versus sequential docetaxel as adjuvant treatment in patients with human epidermal growth factor receptor 2-normal, node-positive breast cancer: BCIRG-005 Trial. *J Clin Oncol.* 2011;29:3877-3884. PMID: 21911726.

182. Swain SM. Chemotherapy: updates and new perspectives. *Oncologist.* 2011;16 Suppl 1:30-39. PMID: 21278439.

183. Swain SM, Tang G, Geyer CE, Jr., et al. definitive results of a phase iii adjuvant trial comparing three chemotherapy regimens in women with operable, node-positive breast cancer: the NSABP B-38 trial. *J Clin Oncol.* 2013;31:3197-3204. PMID: 23940225.

184. Sparano JA, Wang M, Martino S, et al. Weekly paclitaxel in the adjuvant treatment of breast cancer. *N Engl J Med.* 2008;358:1663-1671. PMID: 18420499.

185. Citron ML, Berry DA, Cirrincione C, et al. Randomized trial of dose-dense versus conventionally scheduled and sequential versus concurrent combination chemotherapy as postoperative adjuvant treatment of node-positive primary breast cancer: first report of Intergroup Trial C9741/Cancer and Leukemia Group B Trial 9741. *J Clin Oncol.* 2003;21:1431-1439. PMID: 12668651.

186. Bonilla L, Ben-Aharon I, Vidal L, et al. Dose-dense chemotherapy in non-metastatic breast cancer: a systematic review and meta-analysis of randomized controlled trials. *J Natl Cancer Inst.* 2010;102:1845-1854. PMID: 21098761.

187. Banerjee S, Smith IE. Management of small HER2-positive breast cancers. *Lancet Oncol.* 2010;11:1193-1199. PMID: 21126688.

188. Untch M, Gelber RD, Jackisch C, et al. Estimating the magnitude of trastuzumab effects within patient subgroups in the HERA trial. *Ann Oncol.* 2008;19:1090-1096. PMID: 18296421.

189. Dahabreh IJ, Linardou H, Siannis F, et al. Trastuzumab in the adjuvant treatment of early-stage breast cancer: a systematic review and meta-analysis of randomized controlled trials. *Oncologist.* 2008;13:620-630. PMID: 18586917.

190. Perez EA, Romond EH, Suman VJ, et al. Four-year follow-up of trastuzumab plus adjuvant chemotherapy for operable human epidermal growth factor receptor 2-positive breast cancer: joint analysis of data from NCCTG N9831 and NSABP B-31. *J Clin Oncol.* 2011;29:3366-3373. PMID: 21768458.

191. Piccart-Gebhart MJ, Procter M, Leyland-Jones B, et al. Trastuzumab after adjuvant chemotherapy in HER2-positive breast cancer. *N Engl J Med.* 2005;353:1659-1672. PMID: 16236737.

192. Spielmann M, Roché H, Delozier T, et al. Trastuzumab for patients with axillary-node-positive breast cancer: results of the FNCLCC-PACS 04 trial. *J Clin Oncol.* 2009;27:6129-6134. PMID: 19917839.

193. Gianni L, Dafni U, Gelber RD, et al. Treatment with trastuzumab for 1 year after adjuvant chemotherapy in patients with HER2-positive early breast cancer: a 4-year follow-up of a randomised controlled trial. *Lancet Oncol.* 2011;12:236-244. PMID: 21354370.

194. Perez EA, Suman VJ, Davidson NE, et al. Sequential versus concurrent trastuzumab in adjuvant chemotherapy for breast cancer. *J Clin Oncol.* 2011;29:4491-4497. PMID: 22042958.

195. Goldhirsch A, Gelber RD, Piccart-Gebhart MJ, et al. 2 years versus 1 year of adjuvant trastuzumab for HER2-positive breast cancer (HERA): an open-label, randomised controlled trial. *Lancet.* 2013;382:1021-1028. PMID: 23871490.

196. Joensuu H, Bono P, Kataja V, et al. Fluorouracil, epirubicin, and cyclophosphamide with either docetaxel or vinorelbine, with or without trastuzumab, as adjuvant treatments of breast cancer: final results of the FinHer Trial. *J Clin Oncol.* 2009;27:5685-5692. PMID: 19884557.

197. Pivot X, Romieu G, Debled M, et al. 6 months versus 12 months of adjuvant trastuzumab for patients with HER2-positive early breast cancer (PHARE): a randomised phase 3 trial. *Lancet Oncol.* 2013;14:741-748. PMID: 23764181.

198. Slamon D, Eiermann W, Robert N, et al. Adjuvant trastuzumab in HER2-positive breast cancer. *N Engl J Med.* 2011;365:1273-1283. PMID: 21991949.

199. Dang C, Fornier M, Sugarman S, et al. The safety of dose-dense doxorubicin and cyclophosphamide followed by paclitaxel with trastuzumab in HER-2/neu overexpressed/amplified breast cancer. *J Clin Oncol.* 2008;26:1216-1222. PMID: 18323546.

200. Baselga J, Carbonell X, Castañeda-Soto NJ, et al. Phase II study of efficacy, safety, and pharmacokinetics of trastuzumab monotherapy administered on a 3-weekly schedule. *J Clin Oncol.* 2005;23:2162-2171. PMID: 15800309.

201. Tolaney SM, Barry WT, Dang C, et al. A phase II study of adjuvant paclitaxel (T) and trastuzumab (H) (APT trial) for node-negative, HER2-positive breast cancer (BC). Paper presented at: 36th Annual San Antonio Breast Cancer Symposium; December 2013; San Antonio, TX.

202. Mauri D, Pavlidis N, Ioannidis JP. Neoadjuvant versus adjuvant systemic treatment in breast cancer: a meta-analysis. *J Natl Cancer Inst.* 2005;97:188-194. PMID: 15687361.

203. Kaufmann M, Hortobagyi GN, Goldhirsch A, et al. Recommendations from an international expert panel on the use of neoadjuvant (primary) systemic treatment of operable breast cancer: an update. *J Clin Oncol.* 2006;24:1940-1949. PMID: 16622270.

204. Kaufmann M, von Minckwitz G, Bear HD, et al. Recommendations from an international expert panel on the use of neoadjuvant (primary) systemic treatment of operable breast cancer: new perspectives 2006. *Ann Oncol.* 2007;18:1927-1934. PMID: 17998286.

205. Buchholz TA, Lehman CD, Harris JR, et al. Statement of the science concerning locoregional treatments after preoperative chemotherapy for breast cancer: a National Cancer Institute conference. *J Clin Oncol.* 2008;26:791-797. PMID: 18258988.

206. Nagar H, Mittendorf EA, Strom EA, et al. Local-regional recurrence with and without radiation therapy after neoadjuvant chemotherapy and mastectomy for clinically staged T3N0 breast cancer. *Int J Radiat Oncol Biol Phys.* 2011;81:782-787. PMID: 21885207.

207. Carey LA, Metzger R, Dees EC, et al. American Joint Committee on Cancer tumor-node-metastasis stage after neoadjuvant chemotherapy and breast cancer outcome. *J Natl Cancer Inst.* 2005;97:1137-1142. PMID: 16077072.

208. Rastogi P, Anderson SJ, Bear HD, et al. Preoperative chemotherapy: updates of National Surgical Adjuvant Breast and Bowel Project Protocols B-18 and B-27. *J Clin Oncol.* 2008;26:778-785. PMID: 18258986.

209. Carey LA, Dees EC, Sawyer L, et al. The triple negative paradox: primary tumor chemosensitivity of breast cancer subtypes. *Clin Cancer Res.* 2007;13:2329-2334. PMID: 17438091.

210. Liedtke C, Mazouni C, Hess KR, et al. Response to neoadjuvant therapy and long-term survival in patients with triple-negative breast cancer. *J Clin Oncol.* 2008;26:1275-1281. PMID: 18250347.

211. von Minckwitz G, Untch M, Blohmer JU, et al. Definition and impact of pathologic complete response on prognosis after neoadjuvant chemotherapy in various intrinsic breast cancer subtypes. *J Clin Oncol.* 2012;30:1796-1804. PMID: 22508812.

212. Barnadas A, Gil M, Sánchez-Rovira P, et al. Neoadjuvant endocrine therapy for breast cancer: past, present and future. *Anticancer Drugs.* 2008;19:339-347. PMID: 18454044.

213. Smith IE, Dowsett M, Ebbs SR, et al. Neoadjuvant treatment of postmenopausal breast cancer with anastrozole, tamoxifen, or both in combination: the Immediate Preoperative Anastrozole, Tamoxifen, or Combined with Tamoxifen (IMPACT) multicenter double-blind randomized trial. *J Clin Oncol.* 2005;23:5108-5116. PMID: 15998903.

214. Eiermann W, Paepke S, Appfelstaedt J, et al. Preoperative treatment of post-menopausal breast cancer patients with letrozole: A randomized double-blind multicenter study. *Ann Oncol.* 2001;12:1527-1532. PMID: 11822750.

215. Ellis MJ, Buzdar A, Unzeitig GW, et al. ACOSOG Z1031: a randomized phase II trial comparing exemestane, letrozole, and anastrozole in postmenopausal women with clinical stage II/III estrogen receptor-positive breast cancer. *J Clin Oncol.* 2010;28:18s (suppl; abstr LBA513).

216. Chia YH, Ellis MJ, Ma CX. Neoadjuvant endocrine therapy in primary breast cancer: indications and use as a research tool. *Br J Cancer.* 2010;103:759-764. PMID: 20700118.

217. Petrelli F, Borgonovo K, Cabiddu M, et al. Neoadjuvant chemotherapy and concomitant trastuzumab in breast cancer: a pooled analysis of two randomized trials. *Anticancer Drugs.* 2011;22:128-135. PMID: 21218604.

218. Untch M, Rezai M, Loibl S, et al. Neoadjuvant treatment with trastuzumab in HER2-positive breast cancer: results from the GeparQuattro study. *J Clin Oncol.* 2010;28:2024-2031. PMID: 20308670.

219. Untch M, Fasching PA, Konecny GE, et al. Pathologic complete response after neoadjuvant chemotherapy plus trastuzumab predicts favorable survival in human epidermal growth factor receptor 2-overexpressing breast cancer: results from the TECHNO trial of the AGO and GBG study groups. *J Clin Oncol.* 2011;29:3351-3357. PMID: 21788566.

220. Buzdar AU, Suman VJ, Meric-Bernstam F, et al. Fluorouracil, epirubicin, and cyclophosphamide (FEC-75) followed by paclitaxel plus trastuzumab versus paclitaxel plus trastuzumab followed by FEC-75 plus trastuzumab as neoadjuvant treatment for patients with HER2-positive breast cancer (Z1041): a randomised, controlled, phase 3 trial. *Lancet Oncol.* 2013;14:1317-1325.

221. Untch M, Loibl S, Bischoff J, et al. Lapatinib versus trastuzumab in combination with neoadjuvant anthracycline-taxane-based chemotherapy (Gepar-Quinto, GBG 44): a randomised phase 3 trial. *Lancet Oncol.* 2012;13:135-144. PMID: 22257523.

222. Baselga J, Bradbury I, Eidtmann H, et al. Lapatinib with trastuzumab for HER2-positive early breast cancer (NeoALTTO): a randomised, open-label, multicentre, phase 3 trial. *Lancet.* 2012;379:633-640. PMID: 22257673.

223. Gianni L, Pienkowski T, Im YH, et al. Efficacy and safety of neoadjuvant pertuzumab and trastuzumab in women with locally advanced, inflammatory, or early HER2-positive breast cancer (NeoSphere): a randomised multicentre, open-label, phase 2 trial. *Lancet Oncol.* 2012;13:25-32. PMID: 22153890.

224. Hance KW, Anderson WF, Devesa SS, et al. Trends in inflammatory breast carcinoma incidence and survival: the surveillance, epidemiology, and end results program at the National Cancer Institute. *J Natl Cancer Inst.* 2005;97:966-975. PMID: 15998949.

225. Anderson WF, Chu KC, Chang S. Inflammatory breast carcinoma and noninflammatory locally advanced breast carcinoma: distinct clinicopathologic entities? *J Clin Oncol.* 2003;21:2254-2259. PMID: 12805323.

226. Le-Petross HT, Cristofanilli M, Carkaci S, et al. MRI features of inflammatory breast cancer. *AJR Am J Roentgenol.* 2011;197:W769-776. PMID: 21940550.

227. Chia S, Swain SM, Byrd DR, et al. Locally advanced and inflammatory breast cancer. *J Clin Oncol.* 2008;26:786-790. PMID: 18258987.

228. Cristofanilli M, Buzdar AU, Sneige N, et al. Paclitaxel in the multimodality treatment for inflammatory breast carcinoma. *Cancer.* 2001;92:1775-1782. PMID: 11745249.

229. Woodward WA, Cristofanilli M. Inflammatory breast cancer. *Semin Radiat Oncol.* 2009;19:256-265. PMID: 19732690.

230. Dawood S, Merajver SD, Viens P, et al. International expert panel on inflammatory breast cancer: consensus statement for standardized diagnosis and treatment. *Ann Oncol.* 2011;22:515-523. PMID: 20603440.

231. Wapnir IL, Anderson SJ, Mamounas EP, et al. Prognosis after ipsilateral breast tumor recurrence and locoregional recurrences in five National Surgical Adjuvant Breast and Bowel Project node-positive adjuvant breast cancer trials. *J Clin Oncol.* 2006;24:2028-2037. PMID: 16648502.

232. Montagna E, Bagnardi V, Rotmensz N, et al. Breast cancer subtypes and outcome after local and regional relapse. *Ann Oncol.* 2012;23:324-331. PMID: 21525402.

233. Rauschecker H, Clarke M, Gatzemeier W, et al. Systemic therapy for treating locoregional recurrence in women with breast cancer. *Cochrane Database Syst Rev.* 2001; CD002195. PMID: 11687148.

234. Aebi S, Gelber S, Lang I, et al. Chemotherapy prolongs survival for isolated local or regional recurrence of breast cancer: the CALOR trial (Chemotherapy as Adjuvant for Locally Recurrent Breast Cancer; IBCSG 27-02, NSABP B-27, BIG 1-02). Paper presented at: 36th Annual San Antonio Breast Cancer Symposium; December 2013; San Antonio, TX.

235. Cardoso F, Senkus-Konefka E, Fallowfield L, et al. Locally recurrent or metastatic breast cancer: ESMO Clinical Practice Guidelines for diagnosis, treatment and follow-up. *Ann Oncol.* 2010;21 Suppl 5:v15-19. PMID: 20555067.

236. Chia SK, Speers CH, D'yachkova Y, et al. The impact of new chemotherapeutic and hormone agents on survival in a population-based cohort of women with metastatic breast cancer. *Cancer.* 2007;110:973-979. PMID: 17647245.

237. Mauri D, Polyzos NP, Salanti G, et al. Multiple-treatments meta-analysis of chemotherapy and targeted therapies in advanced breast cancer. *J Natl Cancer Inst.* 2008;100:1780-1791. PMID: 19066278.

238. Kennecke H, Yerushalmi R, Woods R, et al. Metastatic behavior of breast cancer subtypes. *J Clin Oncol.* 2010;28:3271-3277. PMID: 20498394.

239. Harris L, Fritsche H, Mennel R, et al. American Society of Clinical Oncology 2007 update of recommendations for the use of tumor markers in breast cancer. *J Clin Oncol.* 2007;25:5287-5312. PMID: 17954709.

240. Klijn JG, Blamey RW, Boccardo F, et al. Combined tamoxifen and luteinizing hormone-releasing hormone (LHRH) agonist versus LHRH agonist alone in premenopausal advanced breast cancer: a meta-analysis of four randomized trials. *J Clin Oncol.* 2001;19:343-353. PMID: 11208825.

241. Mauri D, Pavlidis N, Polyzos NP, et al. Survival with aromatase inhibitors and inactivators versus standard hormonal therapy in advanced breast cancer: meta-analysis. *J Natl Cancer Inst.* 2006;98:1285-1291. PMID: 16985247.

242. Gibson L, Lawrence D, Dawson C, et al. Aromatase inhibitors for treatment of advanced breast cancer in postmenopausal women. *Cochrane Database Syst Rev.* 2009: CD003370. PMID: 19821307.

243. Bonneterre J, Buzdar A, Nabholtz JM, et al. Anastrozole is superior to tamoxifen as first-line therapy in hormone receptor positive advanced breast carcinoma. *Cancer.* 2001;92:2247-2258. PMID: 11745278.

244. Mouridsen H, Gershanovich M, Sun Y, et al. Phase III study of letrozole versus tamoxifen as first-line therapy of advanced breast cancer in postmenopausal women: analysis of survival and update of efficacy from the International Letrozole Breast Cancer Group. *J Clin Oncol.* 2003;21:2101-2109. PMID: 12775735.

245. Lønning PE, Bajetta E, Murray R, et al. Activity of exemestane in metastatic breast cancer after failure of nonsteroidal aromatase inhibitors: a phase II trial. *J Clin Oncol.* 2000;18:2234-2244. PMID: 10829043.

246. Robertson JF, Llombart-Cussac A, Rolski J, et al. Activity of fulvestrant 500 mg versus anastrozole 1 mg as first-line treatment for advanced breast cancer: results from the FIRST study. *J Clin Oncol.* 2009;27:4530-4535. PMID: 19704066.

247. Di Leo A, Jerusalem G, Petruzelka L, et al. Final analysis of overall survival for the Phase III CONFIRM tril: Fulvestrant 500mg versus 250mg. Paper presented at: 35th Annual San Antonio Breast Cancer Symposium; December 2012; San Antionio, TX.

248. Di Leo A, Jerusalem G, Petruzelka L, et al. Results of the CONFIRM phase III trial comparing fulvestrant 250 mg with fulvestrant 500 mg in postmenopausal women with estrogen receptor-positive advanced breast cancer. *J Clin Oncol.* 2010;28:4594-4600. PMID: 20855825.

249. Mehta RS, Barlow WE, Albain KS, et al. Combination anastrozole and fulvestrant in metastatic breast cancer. *N Engl J Med.* 2012;367:435-444. PMID: 22853014.

250. Bergh J, Jönsson PE, Lidbrink EK, et al. FACT: an open-label randomized phase III study of fulvestrant and anastrozole in combination compared with anastrozole alone as first-line therapy for patients with receptor-positive postmenopausal breast cancer. *J Clin Oncol.* 2012;30:1919-1925. PMID: 22370325.

251. Johnston SR, Kilburn LS, Ellis P, et al. Fulvestrant plus anastrozole or placebo versus exemestane alone after progression on non-steroidal aromatase inhibitors in postmenopausal patients with hormone-receptor-positive locally advanced or metastatic breast cancer (SoFEA): a composite, multicentre, phase 3 randomised trial. *Lancet Oncol.* 2013;14:989-998. PMID: 23902874.

252. Lauring J, Park BH, Wolff AC. The phosphoinositide-3-kinase-Akt-mTOR pathway as a therapeutic target in breast cancer. *J Natl Compr Canc Netw.* 2013;11:670-678. PMID: 23744866.

253. Bachelot T, Bourgier C, Cropet C, et al. Randomized phase II trial of everolimus in combination with tamoxifen in patients with hormone receptor-positive, human epidermal growth factor receptor 2-negative metastatic breast cancer with prior exposure to aromatase inhibitors: a GINECO study. *J Clin Oncol.* 2012;30:2718-2724. PMID: 22565002.

254. Baselga J, Campone M, Piccart M, et al. Everolimus in postmenopausal hormone-receptor-positive advanced breast cancer. *N Engl J Med.* 2012;366:520-529. PMID: 22149876.

255. Cardoso F, Bedard PL, Winer EP, et al. International guidelines for management of metastatic breast cancer: combination vs sequential single-agent chemotherapy. *J Natl Cancer Inst.* 2009;101:1174-1181. PMID: 19657108.

256. O'Brien ME, Wigler N, Inbar M, et al. Reduced cardiotoxicity and comparable efficacy in a phase III trial of pegylated liposomal doxorubicin HCl (CAELYX/Doxil) versus conventional doxorubicin for first-line treatment of metastatic breast cancer. *Ann Oncol.* 2004;15:440-449. PMID: 14998846.

257. King KM, Lupichuk S, Baig L, et al. Optimal use of taxanes in metastatic breast cancer. *Curr Oncol.* 2009;16:8-20. PMID: 19526080.

258. Rugo H, Barry WT, Moreno-Aspitia A, et al. CALGB 40502/NCCTG N063H: Randomized phase III trial of weekly paclitaxel (P) compared to weekly nanoparticle albumin bound nab-paclitaxel (NP) or ixabepilone (Ix) with or without bevacizumab (B) as first-line therapy for locally recurrent or metastatic breast cancer (MBC). *J Clin Oncol.* 2012;30(suppl; abstr CRA1002).

259. Overmoyer B. Options for the treatment of patients with taxane-refractory metastatic breast cancer. *Clin Breast Cancer.* 2008;8 Suppl 2:S61-70. PMID: 18637401.

260. Cortes J, O'Shaughnessy J, Loesch D, et al. Eribulin monotherapy versus treatment of physician's choice in patients with metastatic breast cancer (EMBRACE): a phase 3 open-label randomised study. *Lancet.* 2011;377:914-923. PMID: 21376385.

261. Gennari A, D'amico M, Corradengo D. Extending the duration of first-line chemotherapy in metastatic breast cancer: a perspective review. *Ther Adv Med Oncol.* 2011;3:229-232. PMID: 21957429.

262. Baselga J, Cortés J, Kim SB, et al. Pertuzumab plus trastuzumab plus docetaxel for metastatic breast cancer. *N Engl J Med.* 2012;366:109-119. PMID: 22149875.

263. Swain S, Kim SB, Cortes J, et al. Confirmatory overall survival (OS) analysis of CLEOPATRA: a randomized, double-blind, placebo-controlled Phase III study with pertuzumab (P), trastuzumab (T), and docetaxel (D) in patients (pts) with HER2-positive first-line (1L) metastatic breast cancer (MBC). Paper presented at: 35th Annual San Antonio Breast Cancer Symposium; December 2012; San Antonio, TX.

264. von Minckwitz G, Schwedler K, Schmidt M, et al. Trastuzumab beyond progression: overall survival analysis of the GBG 26/BIG 3-05 phase III study in HER2-positive breast cancer. *Eur J Cancer.* 2011;47:2273-2281. PMID: 21741829.

265. Oakman C, Pestrin M, Zafarana E, et al. Role of lapatinib in the first-line treatment of patients with metastatic breast cancer. *Cancer Manag Res.* 2010;2:13-25. PMID: 21188093.

266. Verma S, Miles D, Gianni L, et al. Trastuzumab emtansine for HER2-positive advanced breast cancer. *N Engl J Med.* 2012;367:1783-1791. PMID: 23020162.

267. Wildiers H, Kim SB, Gonzalez-Martin A, et al. T-DM1 for HER2-Positive MBC: Primary results for TH3RESA, a phase 3 study of T-DM1 vs treatment of physician's choice. Paper presented at: European Cancer Congress; October 2013; Amsterdam, Netherlands.

268. Glück S, Arteaga CL, Osborne CK. Optimizing chemotherapy-free survival for the ER/HER2-positive metastatic breast cancer patient. *Clin Cancer Res.* 2011;17:5559-5561. PMID: 21764887.

269. Van Poznak CH, Temin S, Yee GC, et al. American Society of Clinical Oncology executive summary of the clinical practice guideline update on the role of bone-modifying agents in metastatic breast cancer. *J Clin Oncol.* 2011;29:1221-1227. PMID: 21343561.

270. Stopeck AT, Lipton A, Body JJ, et al. Denosumab compared with zoledronic acid for the treatment of bone metastases in patients with advanced breast cancer: a randomized, double-blind study. *J Clin Oncol.* 2010;28:5132-5139. PMID: 21060033.

271. Coleman RE, Marshall H, Cameron D, et al. Breast-cancer adjuvant therapy with zoledronic acid. *N Engl J Med.* 2011;365:1396-1405. PMID: 21995387.

272. Gnant M, Mlineritsch B, Schippinger W, et al. Endocrine therapy plus zoledronic acid in premenopausal breast cancer. *N Engl J Med.* 2009;360:679-691. PMID: 19213681.

273. Ben-Aharon I, Vidal L, Rizel S, et al. Bisphosphonates in the adjuvant setting of breast cancer therapy--effect on survival: a systematic review and meta-analysis. *PLoS One.* 2013;8:e70044. PMID: 23990894.

274. Korde LA, Zujewski JA, Kamin L, et al. Multidisciplinary meeting on male breast cancer: summary and research recommendations. *J Clin Oncol.* 2010;28:2114-2122. PMID: 20308661.

275. Ring A, Reed M, Leonard R, et al. The treatment of early breast cancer in women over the age of 70. *Br J Cancer.* 2011;105:189-193. PMID: 21694726.

276. Muss HB, Berry DA, Cirrincione C, et al. Toxicity of older and younger patients treated with adjuvant chemotherapy for node-positive breast cancer: the Cancer and Leukemia Group B Experience. *J Clin Oncol.* 2007;25:3699-3704. PMID: 17704418.

277. Muss HB, Berry DA, Cirrincione CT, et al. Adjuvant chemotherapy in older women with early-stage breast cancer. *N Engl J Med.* 2009;360:2055-2065. PMID: 19439741.

278. Khatcheressian JL, Hurley P, Bantug E, et al. Breast cancer follow-up and management after primary treatment: American Society of Clinical Oncology clinical practice guideline update. *J Clin Oncol.* 2013;31:961-965. PMID: 23129741.

279. Hayes DF. Clinical practice. Follow-up of patients with early breast cancer. *N Engl J Med.* 2007;356:2505-2513. PMID: 17568031.

7

LUNG CANCER

Jonathan W. Riess, MD, MS, and David R. Gandara, MD

Updates from 2012

▶ Broad genomic sequencing of lung cancer by The Cancer Genome Atlas and others demonstrates great complexity in genomic derangement of lung cancer (Cancer Genome Atlas Research Network, *Nature* 2012).

▶ New actionable oncogenic driver subsets of non-small cell lung cancer (NSCLC), such as *ROS1*, have been identified (Bergethon K, *J Clin Oncol* 2012).

▶ The U.S. Food and Drug Administration approved afatinib for first-line treatment of patients with epidermal growth factor receptor (*EGFR*) mutation–positive NSCLC based on a trial showing improved progression-free survival compared to cisplatin/pemetrexed in *EGFR* mutation–positive NSCLC (Sequist LV, *J Clin Oncol* 2013).

▶ Standard-dose thoracic radiotherapy (60 Gy) is superior to higher-dose (74 Gy) radiotherapy when combined with chemotherapy in terms of overall survival and local-regional control for stage III NSCLC (Bradley JD, *J Clin Oncol* 2013).

▶ Crizotinib results in higher response rates and prolonged progression-free survival compared to chemotherapy with pemetrexed or docetaxel in treating advanced, anaplastic lymphoma kinase (*ALK*) fusion–positive NSCLC after first-line platinum-based chemotherapy (Shaw AT, *N Engl J Med* 2013).

▶ Carboplatin and pemetrexed yields superior survival outcomes compared to pemetrexed alone in patients with advanced NSCLC with a Zubrod performance status of 2 (Zukin M, *J Clin Oncol* 2013).

▶ Continuation maintenance pemetrexed improves overall survival compared with placebo after four cycles of cisplatin/pemetrexed (Paz-Ares L, *Lancet Oncol* 2012).

An estimated 228,520 new cases of lung cancer were expected in 2013, leading to approximately 159,480 deaths.[1] Although lung cancer accounts for approximately 15% of all cancer diagnoses, it is responsible for about 28% of all cancer deaths. Thus, unlike breast, colon, and prostate cancers, most patients (about 84%) who are diagnosed with lung cancer will die of the disease. Lung cancer is the leading cause of cancer deaths for both men and women.[2] More women die of lung cancer each year than of breast, cervix, and uterine cancers combined; more men die annually of lung cancer than of colorectal and prostate cancers combined. Further, nearly twice as many women in the United States die from lung cancer than from breast cancer. The incidence and death rates from lung cancer have been decreasing for men, and these numbers were rising for women until approximately 2000 and have since been leveling off.

Smoking is the major cause of lung cancer. Numerous epidemiologic and laboratory studies, as well as in vitro data, have tied the present pandemic of lung cancer to the carcinogenic effects of tobacco smoke. Some data suggest that women with lung cancer who smoke and who are taking hormone-replacement therapy experience a less favorable outcome than those who are not undergoing such therapy.[3]

The incidence of lung cancer, although declining for both white and black men, is approximately 20% higher for black men.[2] Race-related variances in lung cancer, however, are complicated by differences in socioeconomic status, which are associated with disparities in smoking rates, types of cigarettes smoked, and exposures to inhaled agents in the workplace.

In the United States, the most common form of lung cancer was squamous cell cancer until approximately 1987, when it was supplanted by adenocarcinoma. Small cell lung cancer once accounted for approximately 20% of all lung cancers; however, its incidence has been decreasing.[4] The incidence of large cell histology is also decreasing.

ETIOLOGY

Cigarette smoking is the most common cause of lung cancer and is responsible for approximately 85% of all cases. Other risk factors include occupational or environmental substances such as arsenic, chromium or nickel, radon, air pollution, radiation exposure, and environmental (secondhand) tobacco smoke.

The risk of lung cancer among cigarette smokers increases with the number of cigarettes smoked and the duration of smoking history, the latter of which is a stronger risk factor than the number of cigarettes smoked per day. A tripling of the number of cigarettes smoked per day is estimated to triple the risk of lung cancer, whereas a tripling of the duration of smoking is estimated to increase the risk 100-fold.[5] Of note, moderate- to high-intensity smoking (defined as 10 or more cigarettes per day) has dramatically decreased in the United States since the 1960s.[6] The risk of lung cancer decreases with smoking cessation, and it approaches that of the nonsmoking population after 10 to 15 years of abstinence; however, one study in women reported that even after 30 years, the risk was not as low as for the nonsmoking population.[7] It is estimated that approximately one-half of all lung cancers in the United States occur in former smokers. The risks associated with e-cigarettes and their role in tobacco control still require clarification.[8]

Passive smoking also is a risk factor; the risk of developing lung cancer for nonsmoking spouses of cigarette smokers is approximately 20% to 30% higher than the risk for nonsmoking spouses of nonsmokers.[5] It has been estimated that approximately 25% of lung cancer cases among never-smokers are caused by exposure to environmental tobacco smoke.[5] Nevertheless, data on molecular profiling of cancers from never-smoking patients show a very different pattern of abnormalities from those associated with smoking (p53 and particular KRAS mutations), with a high incidence of mutations in the epidermal growth factor receptor (EGFR) or anaplastic

lymphoma kinase (ALK) fusions, as described in this chapter. These data suggest that the proportion of patients with lung cancer attributed to secondhand smoke may have been overestimated.[9]

Cigarette smoke contains thousands of constituents, many of which are carcinogenic. Two of the major classes of nicotine-related inhaled carcinogens include the polycyclic aromatic hydrocarbons and N-nitrosamines, which are metabolized to nitrosamine ketone and N'-nitrosonornicotine. Both compounds are activated by the p450 enzyme system and exert carcinogenic effects through the formation of DNA adducts. The distribution of benzo(a)pyrene diol epoxide adducts along the exons of the TP53 gene occurs preferentially in codons 157, 248, and 273, which are the same mutational "hotspots" of TP53. Nitrosamine ketone has been postulated as one factor that leads to the increased incidence of adenocarcinomas, because it predominantly induces these tumors in mice.[5]

Smoking causes each of the four major subtypes of lung cancer, although the dose-response relationship is steepest with small cell lung cancer. Indeed, small cell lung cancer is almost exclusively found in smokers. Although nonsmokers are more likely to develop adenocarcinoma in situ (AIS) than the other subtypes of lung cancer, smoking is still the major risk factor for this form of the disease.

Cigar smoking also is associated with an increased risk of lung cancer, although the risk is not as high as with cigarette smoking, most likely because cigar smokers do not inhale as deeply as cigarette smokers. Similarly, risks related to pipe smoking also are lower because of differences in smoking frequency and depth of inhalation. Light cigarettes provide no benefit compared with other cigarettes; the lower tar and nicotine numbers on light cigarette packs and in advertisements are misleading because the low tar and nicotine levels recorded on smoking machines are artificial.[10]

Radon is a naturally occurring, chemically inert gas that is a decay product of uranium. The relative risk of lung cancer is increased for underground miners who are exposed to high levels of radon. For underground miners who smoke, the risk may exceed 10 times the risk for a nonsmoking miner. The relationship between indoor residential radon exposure and lung cancer risk is less defined, although it is estimated that between 2% to 10% of lung cancers may be caused by exposure to residential radon.[11] Asbestos and smoking are independent causes of lung cancer, but together they appear to act synergistically to increase the risk. High doses of radiation also have been associated with an increased risk of lung cancer. For example, an increased risk has been observed for patients with breast cancer, as well as for long-term survivors of Hodgkin and non-Hodgkin lymphomas, particularly if patients continue to smoke after completing radiation therapy.

HOST FACTORS

Genetic susceptibility to lung cancer has been postulated based on the fact that cigarette smoking causes lung cancer in a minority of people who smoke. Because many carcinogens in tobacco smoke, such as the polycyclic aromatic hydrocarbons, are metabolized by the p450 cytochrome system, differences in subtypes or polymorphisms of these enzymes have been proposed as one mechanism of lung cancer risk. Other enzymes that may increase risk for some individuals include differences in glutathione S-transferase—an enzyme that detoxifies reactive metabolites of polycyclic aromatic hydrocarbons—and enzymes that modulate DNA repair capacity.

Epidemiologic studies have shown that a family history of lung cancer is a predictor of increased risk. Familial aggregation of lung cancer has led to the hypothesis that there is a genetic susceptibility for lung cancer.[12] This may be related to inherited differences in carcinogen metabolism and activation and also to DNA repair capacity. For example, leukocyte DNA adduct levels have been associated with the risk of lung cancer, with an odds ratio (OR) of 1.86 (95% CI 0.88, 3.93), particularly for never-smokers (OR 4.04, 95% CI 1.06, 15.42).[13] Germ-line polymorphisms in genes with products that activate (cytochrome p450 1A1 [CYP1A1]) and detoxify (glutathione S-transferases M1 [GSTM1] and T1 [GSTT1]) chemical carcinogens found in tobacco smoke have been associated with a risk of lung cancer from environmental tobacco smoke that is substantially greater than the risk for individuals who are heterozygous or homozygous carriers of the wild-type GSTM1 allele.[14] However, some of the results from these studies are conflicting, suggesting that some polymorphisms may predict increased risks in specific ethnic populations, limiting generalizability. Thus, germ-line polymorphisms

should not be used to predict an individual person's lung cancer risk or be used for screening purposes. Genome-wide association studies (GWAS) have identified the N allele of the D398N polymorphism of the nicotinic acid/acetylcholine receptor as well as polymorphisms in the reverse transcriptase component of telomerase as potential increased risk factors for lung adenocarcinoma.[15] However, these results must also be interpreted with caution because the GWAS studies were not based on a functional hypothesis and these alterations may not represent drivers of carcinogenesis.

Additional factors associated with increased lung cancer risk include previous lung damage, such as chronic obstructive pulmonary disease, and fibrotic disorders that restrict lung capacity, such as pneumoconiosis. Diets deficient in vitamins A and C and beta-carotene intake also have been associated with increased risk, whereas fruit and vegetable consumption may be weakly protective.

Preclinical evidence suggested that higher dietary intake of retinol is associated with a decreased risk of lung cancer. Based on this evidence, three double-blind placebo-controlled chemoprevention trials were conducted involving beta-carotene, vitamin A, or one of their derivatives. A protective effect against lung cancer was not observed in any of the studies. Rather, beta-carotene supplementation was associated with an increased risk of lung cancer among high-risk populations of heavy smokers in two of the three trials.[16-18]

PATHOLOGY

More than 95% of lung cancers consist of one of the four major histologic types: squamous (or epidermoid), adenocarcinoma, large cell, or small cell. Small cell lung cancer has scant cytoplasm, small hyperchromatic nuclei with fine chromatin pattern, and indistinct nucleoli with diffuse sheets of cells, whereas non-small cell lung cancer (NSCLC) has abundant cytoplasm, pleomorphic nuclei with coarse chromatin pattern, prominent nucleoli, and glandular or squamous architecture. Other subtypes, which are rare and therefore less well studied, include carcinoid, large cell cancer with neuroendocrine features, and large cell neuroendocrine cancer.[19] Extremely rare primary tumors in the lung include sarcomas, cancers with sarcomatoid or sarcomatous elements (e.g., giant cell cancer, carcinosarcoma, pulmonary blastoma), and cancers of salivary gland type (e.g., mucoepidermoid cancer, adenoid cystic cancer).

Adenocarcinoma, large cell cancer, and squamous cell cancer are collectively known as NSCLC. They exhibit differences in sensitivity to chemotherapy and radiation therapy when compared with small cell cancer, which is described in detail further in the chapter. Other clinical differences between small cell cancer and NSCLC include the more rapid clinical course of small cell lung cancer and the enhanced association of small cell lung cancer with paraneoplastic syndromes and neuroendocrine features on pathologic examination. AIS (discussed in the following section) is a subtype of adenocarcinoma that has received considerable attention because of its tendency to occur in women and never-smokers.

PREINVASIVE LESIONS
Squamous Dysplasia
Squamous dysplasia may be mild, moderate, or severe, depending on the severity of the atypia and the thickness of the abnormality within the bronchial epithelium. There is increasing interest in using squamous dysplasia as an indicator of heightened risk when identifying patients for participation in chemoprevention studies.

KEY POINTS

- Pre-invasive lung cancer lesions include squamous dysplasia and atypical adenomatous hyperplasia.
- Unlike other lung cancers, adenocarcinoma in situ occurs more commonly in never-smokers, is seen in men and women with the same frequency, and is associated more commonly with *EGFR* mutations than other types of lung cancer.
- Pulmonary neuroendocrine tumors represent a spectrum of neoplasms characterized by the presence of neurosecretory granules on electron microscopic evaluation and a distinct immunohistochemical phenotype.

Atypical Adenomatous Hyperplasia
Atypical adenomatous hyperplasia is considered a precursor to adenocarcinoma and is usually identified incidentally, often at the time of resection. The lesions are typically small (a few millimeters) and consist of discrete but ill-defined bronchoalveolar proliferation in which the alveoli are lined by monotonous, slightly atypical cuboidal to low-columnar epithelial cells. Their prognostic significance is unclear.

NON-SMALL CELL LUNG CANCER
Although the natural history of the subtypes of NSCLC differs somewhat, when assessed on a stage-by-stage basis, histologic subtype is not a significant prognostic indicator. However, histologic subtype now has an influence on treatment selection, based on different chemosensitivity and safety profiles of squamous and nonsquamous tumors.

Adenocarcinoma
Adenocarcinoma is the most common histologic subtype in the United States and appears to be increasing, although the reason for this is unknown. It accounts for more than 50% of all NSCLC, has been associated with scarring, is more likely to be peripherally located than squamous cell or small cell cancer, and tends to metastasize frequently. It consists of four subtypes: acinar, papillary, AIS, and solid with mucous formation.

AIS (formerly known as bronchioloalveolar cancer) is defined as an adenocarcinoma of the lung that grows in a lepidic fashion along alveolar septae. In the 1999 World Health Organization/International Association for the Study of Lung Cancer (WHO/IASLC) classification, the lack of invasive growth was added as an essential criterion because data suggested that surgical resection might cure disease for such patients. Histologically, pure AIS is rare; more common is adenocarcinoma, mixed subtype, with both AIS features and invasive components. The tumor typically presents in one of two forms: mucinous and nonmucinous. Mucin-producing tumors (30% to 40%) tend to be multicentric, TTF-1–negative, and rarely harbor sensitizing *EGFR* mutations. Nonmucinous tumors (50% to 60%) tend to be solitary, TTF-1–positive, and have high rates of *EGFR* mutations. This form of lung cancer develops in never-smokers more than the other subtypes. Although the prognosis is excellent for patients with small, solitary nonmucinous tumors, the prognosis for patients with advanced AIS is comparable with prognoses for other lung adenocarcinomas. Of note, small lesions discovered on screening computed tomography (CT)—which are commonly found to have a ground glass appearance—are often AIS.

Squamous Cell Cancer
Squamous cell cancers account for approximately 25% of all NSCLC. These lesions tend to be located centrally and are more likely to cavitate than other histologic types. Squamous cell cancers, which most often occur in segmental bronchi and involve lobar and main-stem bronchi by extension, are recognized by the histologic features of intercellular bridging, squamous pearl formation, and individual cell keratinization. Because of increased rates of hemoptysis, antiangiogenic therapy (e.g., bevacizumab) is not used in the treatment of squamous cell NSCLC.

Large Cell Cancer
Large cell cancers account for approximately 10% of all lung cancers, and the incidence is decreasing. These tumors are typically poorly differentiated and comprise large cells with abundant cytoplasm and large nucleoli.

SMALL CELL LUNG CANCER
In the 1999 WHO/IASLC classification, small cell cancer is divided into two subtypes: so-called "pure" small cell lung cancer and combined histology lung cancer—the latter of which consists of elements of both NSCLC and small cell lung cancers. Histologically, the tumor is characterized by small cells with scant cytoplasm, finely granular nuclear chromatin, and absent or inconspicuous nucleoli. Nuclear molding and smearing of the nuclear chromatin may be present owing to crush artifact. Mitotic figures are common, and necrosis can be extensive. By electron microscopy, the cells may appear to have neuroendocrine granules. Clinically, these tumors tend to be centrally located, are often found submucosally, and are more commonly associated with paraneoplastic syndromes. Because of the rapid growth and proliferation of these tumors, the clinical course tends to be more rapid than that of NSCLC. However, small cell lung cancers also are more responsive to both chemotherapy and radiation therapy, although resistance usually develops.

OTHER PULMONARY NEUROENDOCRINE TUMORS

The normal lung contains neuroendocrine cells, but their significance is unclear. Neuroendocrine lung tumors represent a spectrum of pathologic entities, including typical carcinoid, atypical carcinoid, and large cell neuroendocrine cancer. Small cell lung cancer and large cell neuroendocrine cancer are high-grade neuroendocrine tumors, whereas typical carcinoid and atypical carcinoid are low and intermediate grades. Neurosecretory granules, particularly chromogranin A and synaptophysin, often are seen by electron microscopy. The presence of chromogranin, synaptophysin, and CD56 (neural cell adhesion molecule) may be detected by immunohistochemistry (IHC). Approximately 20% to 40% of patients with both typical and atypical carcinoids are nonsmokers, whereas virtually all patients with small cell lung cancer and large cell neuroendocrine cancer are cigarette smokers.

Carcinoid Tumors

Carcinoid tumors are low-grade malignant neoplasms of neuroendocrine cells, which are divided into typical and atypical types, with the latter possessing more malignant histologic and clinical features. Surgery is the primary treatment for typical carcinoid tumors. The prognosis is excellent for patients with typical carcinoids.

Compared with typical carcinoids, atypical carcinoids tend to be larger, have a greater number of mitoses, and are associated with necrosis. Patients also are more likely to have distant metastases at presentation, and survival is significantly reduced.

Large Cell Neuroendocrine Cancer

Large cell neuroendocrine cancer is a high-grade, non-small cell neuroendocrine cancer. These tumors are characterized by histologic features similar to small cell cancer but are formed by larger cells. Large cell neuroendocrine cancer is defined as a tumor with neuroendocrine morphologic characteristics, including organoid nesting, palisading, a trabecular pattern, and rosette-like structures. A mitotic count of 11 mitoses or more per 2 mm^2 is the main criterion for separating large cell neuroendocrine cancers and small cell lung cancers from atypical carcinoid tumors. The mitotic rates are usually high for both large cell neuroendocrine cancers and small cell lung cancers, with an average of 70 to 80 mitoses per 2 mm^2. Large cell neuroendocrine cancers are separated from small cell lung cancers by using the criteria listed in Table 7-1.[20]

Large cell cancers with neuroendocrine morphology are tumors that resemble large cell neuroendocrine tumors by light microscopy but lack proof of neuroendocrine differentiation by electron microscopy or IHC. The significance of this histology is unknown.

The prognosis for patients with large cell neuroendocrine cancer is worse than the prognosis for patients with atypical carcinoid and classic large cell cancer. Five-year survival is 21% for patients with large cell neuroendocrine cancer, 65% for atypical carcinoid, and 90% for typical carcinoid.[20]

Table 7-1 Characteristics of Large Cell Neuroendocrine Tumors that Distinguish Them from Small Cell Lung Cancers[20]

- Larger cell size
- Abundant cytoplasm
- Prominent nucleoli
- Vesicular or coarse chromatin
- Polygonal rather than fusiform shape
- Less prominent nuclear molding
- Less conspicuous DNA encrustation of blood vessel walls

BIOLOGY

Recent paradigm-changing studies have changed the perspective on NSCLC from being considered a single disease or a few histology-based subgroups to the current concept of a large number of molecularly defined subtypes (Fig. 7-1) of variable prevalence.[21] Further, recent publications from The Cancer Genome Atlas effort and other groups have revealed the impressive complexity of lung cancer, as demonstrated by both inter-patient and intra-patient tumor heterogeneity.[22,23] Recently, guidelines for molecular testing have been issued by multiple organizations, including the International Association for the Study of Lung Cancer, American Society of Clinical Oncology, and the National Comprehensive Cancer Network (NCCN). All recommend concurrent testing for *EGFR* mutations and *ALK* translocations in lung adenocarcinoma, large cell carcinoma, and NSCLC-not otherwise specified, with a turnaround time of less than 2 weeks. Testing for *EGFR* mutations and *ALK* translocations should be considered in squamous cell histology, particularly in patients with never- or light-smoking history, small biopsy specimens, or mixed histology.[24] The most common and clinically relevant molecularly defined subtypes are described in Fig. 7-1.

EPIDERMAL GROWTH FACTOR RECEPTOR

EGFR belongs to the HER/erbB family of growth factor receptors, which includes EGFR (HER1 or erbB1), HER2/neu (erbB2), HER3 (erbB3), and HER4 (erbB4). These cell-surface proteins consist of an extracellular ligand-binding domain, a transmembrane structure, and an intracellular tyrosine kinase domain. The binding of ligand to receptor activates receptor dimerization and tyrosine kinase autophosphorylation, initiating a cascade of intracellular events and leading to increased cell proliferation, angiogenesis, metastasis, and a decrease in apoptosis. Inappropriate activation of this receptor-signal transduction pathway can be caused by ligand or receptor overexpression, receptor mutation, binding of intracellular ligands, or dimerization with other receptors (heterodimerization or "receptor crosstalk"; Fig. 7-2).

Overexpression of EGFR (which can be demonstrated by IHC) has been found in as many as 70% of NSCLC and is an independent negative prognostic factor.[25] However, the most

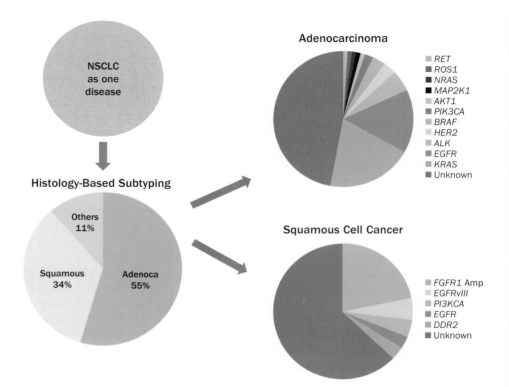

Fig. 7-1 Evolution of non-small cell lung cancer (NSCLC) subtyping from histologic- to molecular-based.

Abbreviations: Adenoca, adenocarcinoma; EGFR, epidermal growth factor receptor; HER2, human epidermal growth factor receptor 2; MAP2K1, mitogen-activated protein kinase kinase 1.

Adapted from Li T, Kung HJ, Mack PC, et al. Genotyping and genomic profiling of non-small-cell lung cancer: implications for current and future therapies. J Clin Oncol. 2013;31:1039-1049.

reliable biomarker to predict radiographic response to EGFR tyrosine kinase inhibitors is the presence of activating *EGFR* mutations. These mutations (detected by gene sequencing) hyperactivate the EGFR, rendering the cancer cell dependent upon EGFR for survival and progression ("oncogene addiction") and thus are exquisitely sensitive to EGFR inhibition. At diagnosis, these mutations appear mutually exclusive of *KRAS* and *ALK* aberrations and are associated with certain clinicopathologic features (women, East Asians, never- or light smokers, and adenocarcinoma histology [especially nonmucinous AIS]).

In NSCLC, activating mutations occur in the EGFR tyrosine kinase domain, centered around exons 18 to 21. Mutations in exons 19 and 21 (termed "classic" *EGFR* mutations) account for approximately 90% of *EGFR* mutations. Exon 19 mutations are most commonly in-frame deletions of amino acids 747 to 750. Exon 21 mutations are characteristically L858R substitutions. The presence of an *EGFR* activating mutation is both prognostic and predictive. Activating *EGFR* mutations are also associated with improved response to both conventional chemotherapy and EGFR tyrosine kinase inhibitors (TKIs). In NSCLC cases harboring classic *EGFR* mutations, EGFR TKIs yield response rates (RRs) higher than 60%—compared with RRs of approximately 10% in wild-type *EGFR* cases.

ANAPLASTIC LYMPHOMA KINASE

The *ALK* gene, which encodes a tyrosine kinase, was originally identified in a subset of anaplastic large cell lymphomas with a t(2;5)(p23;q35) translocation. In a rare subset (2% to

7% of cases) of NSCLC, chromosome 2p inversion results in fusion of the protein encoded by the echinoderm microtubule-associated protein-like 4 (*EML4*) gene with the intracellular signaling portion of the ALK receptor tyrosine kinase. Analogous to *EGFR* mutations, *EML4-ALK* fusions result in constitutive tyrosine kinase activity, dependence of the cancer cell on activated downstream mitogenic pathways, and sensitivity to ALK inhibition.[26]

Other genetic aberrations involving the *ALK* gene have been identified in anaplastic large cell lymphomas, inflammatory myofibroblastic tumors, and neuroblastomas. Efficacy of the ALK inhibitor crizotinib for treatment of some of these other conditions highlights the increasing recognition that a tumor's molecular characteristics—and not anatomic site or histology—may ultimately guide treatment selection in oncology.[27]

Phrases such as *"ALK* positivity," *"ALK* rearrangement," *"ALK* fusion," and *"ALK* translocation" are essentially synonymous and refer to the presence of the *EML4-ALK* translocation. Despite the rarity of this molecular aberration—because of the vast number of lung cancer cases worldwide—an estimated 40,000 such cases occur annually.[28] Similar to *EGFR* mutations, *EML4-ALK* translocations are associated with certain clinicopathologic features.[29,30] These include never or light smoking, adenocarcinoma histology (especially signet ring subtype), and younger age. In contrast to *EGFR* mutations, *ALK* translocations do not appear to have a clear association with patient sex or race/ethnicity. *ALK* translocations are typically mutually exclusive of *EGFR* and *KRAS* mutations,

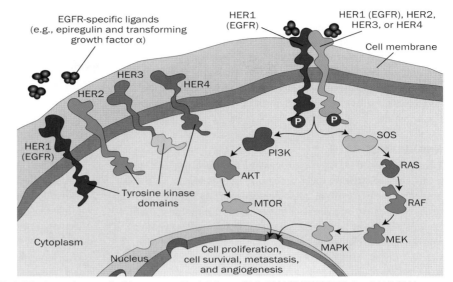

Fig. 7-2 Epidermal growth factor receptor (EGFR) signaling pathways.

Shown in the left portion of the figure are the four members of the ERBB (or HER) family of receptors. All four members of this family have tyrosine kinase domains in the cytoplasmic portion of the receptor. However, the tyrosine kinase domain of HER3 does not have catalytic activity. The right portion of the figure shows that binding of ligands to the HER family of receptors induces either homodimerization or heterodimerization of the receptors. Dimerization results in phosphorylation of the tyrosine residues of the EGFR kinase domain. The activated receptor may then phosphorylate a wide array of intracellular signaling cascades, such as the RAS–RAF–MEK–ERK and PI3K–AKT pathways, that induce cellular proliferation, angiogenesis, and metastases. EGFR amplification can obviate the requirement for ligand-induced dimerization.

Abbreviations: MTOR, mammalian target of rapamycin; P, phosphorylation; SOS, Son of Sevenless.

From N Engl J Med, Cataldo VD, Gibbons DL, Pérez-Soler R, et al, Treatment of non-small-cell lung cancer with erlotinib or gefitinib, 2011;364(10):947-55. Copyright © 2014 Massachusetts Medical Society. Reprinted with permission.

although they sometimes can occur together, particularly in the setting of acquired resistance to crizotinib.[31]

ALK rearrangements can be identified by IHC, fluorescence in situ hybridization (FISH), or polymerase chain reaction (PCR). Of these, FISH appears to be the most clinically applicable, although dual IHC and FISH may increase the detection of these cases.[30] *EML4-ALK* FISH employs differently labeled break-apart (split signal) probes on the 5' and 3' ends of the *ALK* gene. Normal *ALK* generates a fused (yellow) signal, whereas *ALK* rearrangements appear as separate red and green signals. The standard cutoff for a positive result is a split signal in more than 15% of cells examined.[32]

KRAS

RAS proteins are a family of guanine nucleotide-binding proteins that play an important role in the intracellular-signaling pathway. In response to the interaction between tyrosine kinase receptors and their ligands, RAS becomes activated in the triphosphate form, which leads to a cascade of downstream events responsible for the regulation of cell cycle and apoptosis, including the RAF-1/mitogen-activated protein kinase pathway and the RAC/RHO pathway. If mutated, the protein products of the mutated genes remain in an active state, resulting in a continuous "on" signal that causes uncontrolled cell growth.

KRAS mutations, which occur primarily in exons 12, 13, and 61, are found mostly in patients with lung adenocarcinomas (approximately 30%) and in smokers. At diagnosis, they are typically mutually exclusive of *EGFR* mutations and *ALK* translocations. *KRAS* mutations have been associated with poor prognosis and resistance to EGFR inhibitors.[33,34] Their effect on anti-EGFR monoclonal antibody therapy in NSCLC is not clear.

ROS1

ROS1 gene rearrangements are recently discovered oncogenic drivers present in about 2% of NSCLC tumors.[35] *ROS1* is an orphan tyrosine kinase of the insulin receptor family located on chromosome 6 and with sequence homology to ALK. Gene rearrangements of *ROS1* lead to constitutive activation of this tyrosine kinase. Like many oncogene-addicted lung cancers, *ROS1*-rearranged tumors commonly occur in young nonsmokers with lung adenocarcinoma histology. The ALK inhibitor crizotinib has activity in lung cancers with *ROS1* gene rearrangements, as evident from high RRs in early-phase clinical trials.[36]

RET

RET gene fusions have recently been identified in 1% to 2% of NSCLC.[37] Patients whose tumors harbor *RET* fusions can respond to RET inhibitors.[38] Clinical trials with RET inhibitors in patients with tumors harboring the *RET* fusion gene are underway.

HER2

HER2 mutations have been described in about 1% to 2% of NSCLC. HER2 can be amplified in lung cancer as it is in breast cancer, but the HER2 mutations found in NSCLC are distinct from HER2 amplification.[39] Responses to afatinib in patients with HER2-mutated lung cancer have been documented.[40]

OTHER MUTATIONS

The treatment paradigm for NSCLC has shifted over the past several years from a uniform chemotherapy approach to the identification and targeting of "actionable" driver mutations. This has led to the approval of erlotinib and afatinib for first-line treatment of patients with lung cancer with *EGFR*-activating mutations and of crizotinib for treatment of patients with *ALK* rearrangements. Molecular profiling of 1,000 patients with lung adenocarcinoma has identified other mutations that are being targeted in other clinical trials.[41] Mutations in *BRAF*, *PIK3CA*, *Akt*, and others have also been documented. Research is ongoing to determine whether these mutations are oncogenic drivers and to match such mutations to effective targeted therapeutics.

ANGIOGENESIS

Tumor angiogenesis is the process of proliferation and migration of endothelial cells to form new blood vessels, thus nourishing the tumor and giving it access for metastasis. This process is regulated primarily by vascular endothelial growth factor (VEGF)—a highly conserved, homodimeric glycoprotein. Once VEGF binds to its tyrosine kinase receptors (VEGFR1 [flt-1], VEGFR2 [flk-1/KDR], and VEGFR3 [flt-4]), the receptors dimerize, inducing intracellular signaling pathways and leading to endothelial cell proliferation and to the formation of new blood vessels. VEGF is overexpressed in different tumor types, including lung cancer. Both overexpression of VEGF and tumor microvessel density correlate with poor prognosis. Anti-VEGF antibodies suppress the growth of a variety of tumor cell lines in nude mice and inhibit angiogenesis in animal models of intraocular neovascularization. Bevacizumab, a monoclonal antibody to VEGF, has been approved for the treatment of patients with nonsquamous histology in combination with carboplatin/paclitaxel for first-line treatment of NSCLC (see Non-Small Cell Lung Cancer Treatment section).[42]

The major issues limiting the use and effect of antiangiogenic therapies are safety considerations and lack of predictive biomarkers. Bevacizumab and other antiangiogenic agents are associated with a distinct toxicity profile that reflects effects on normal vasculature and includes bleeding, clotting, hypertension, wound-healing complications, gastrointestinal perforation, and proteinuria. The mechanisms of these adverse events are diverse and not fully understood. Bleeding may be a result of vascular endothelial cell apoptosis or tumor detachment from blood vessels in response to VEGF-directed therapy.[45,46] Hypertension is thought to arise from reduced nitric oxide production because of VEGF inhibition, which promotes vasoconstriction.[47] Proteinuria may be a result of disruption of glomerular endothelial integrity or by glomerular basement membrane damage caused by hypertension.[48]

The identification of markers predictive of benefit from anti-VEGF monoclonal antibodies and VEGFR-directed TKIs has proven elusive. Emerging but unproven biomarkers include tumor microvessel density, serum VEGF, soluble VEGFR2 and VEGFR3, intracellular adhesion molecule and other angiogenic and inflammatory markers, VEGF and VEGFR polymorphisms, circulating endothelial cells, noninvasive imaging of perfusion and oxygenation, and development of on-treatment hypertension.[49-53]

DNA REPAIR ENZYMES

Excision repair cross-complementation group 1 protein (ERCC1) is a highly conserved excision nuclease within the nucleotide excision repair pathway, essential for repair of DNA adducts. Reduced DNA repair capacity has been associated with an increase in lung cancer risk.[54] Retrospective studies have suggested that decreased expression of ERCC1 is associated with an improved outcome with platinum-based therapy.[55] Presumably, patients with a high capacity to repair DNA adducts will be able to repair the adducts resulting from platinum therapy; thus, these patients experience a less favorable outcome than patients with a low expression of ERCC1. Patients unable to repair platinum-associated DNA adducts are predicted to fare better with platinum-based therapy than patients who are able to repair platinum-associated DNA adducts. Although intriguing, selecting therapy based on DNA repair enzymes has not been shown to be beneficial in prospective clinical trials of metastatic NSCLC. Assay reliability and variability has hindered the development of these enzymes as useful biomarkers and called into question previously positive retrospective results in the adjuvant setting.[56]

TUMOR SUPPRESSOR GENES

The *TP53* tumor suppressor is the most frequently mutated gene in cancer and is found in more than 50% of tumors. In lung cancer, loss of one *TP53* allele on chromosome 17p13 and mutational inactivation of the other allele occurs in more than 75% of small cell lung cancers and in 50% of NSCLC. Although *TP53* mutations are common in patients with lung cancer, their prognostic significance is unclear. The literature contains divergent results; some investigators report that the *TP53* mutation is a favorable prognostic factor, others consider it negative, and still others find that it has no prognostic significance.

LKB1 is another tumor suppressor inactivated or mutated in NSCLC. Inactivation of *LKB1* is present in about 19% of squamous lung cancer and 34% of lung adenocarcinoma. Inactivating mutations of *LKB1* contributes to lung cancer initiation, differentiation, and metastases.[57]

GENOMIC/PROTEOMIC PROFILING

Progress in the techniques for identifying proteins and genes over- and underexpressed in lung tumors has resulted in the ability to molecularly profile a tumor. For example, microarray techniques that profile the expression of thousands of genes can—in theory—simultaneously identify genetic signatures that may be able to identify patients with a favorable or unfavorable prognosis or patients likely to respond to a given therapy. A number of these genetic and protein signatures have been described, but they have not been validated as predictive markers in prospective clinical trials.[58-62] The serum proteomic VeriStrat test may help predict patients unlikely to benefit from EGFR TKIs after progression on first-line chemotherapy.[63]

CLINICAL PRESENTATION

Most patients with lung cancer present with symptomatic disease (Table 7-2). The most common symptoms are anorexia, fatigue, weakness, and cough. Patients with AIS may have bronchorrhea (large quantities of foamy sputum) and shortness of breath out of proportion to radiographic findings.

Metastatic disease at presentation is common in small cell lung cancer (75%) and adenocarcinoma (50%), and many metastatic sites are possible. Brain, bone, liver, and adrenal gland are the most common sites of metastatic disease.[64] Liver and bone marrow metastases develop in approximately 20% to 30% of patients, and brain metastases occur in approximately 20%.[65,66]

Paraneoplastic syndromes are caused by humoral factors produced by cancer cells that act at a distant site from both the primary site and its metastases or by cross-reactivity between host antitumor antibodies and normal tissues.[67] For all paraneoplastic syndromes, treatment of the underlying cancer is recommended. In addition, syndrome-specific therapies may be employed. The two most common paraneoplastic syndromes in patients with NSCLC are hypercalcemia and hypertrophic pulmonary osteoarthropathy. Although hypercalcemia is most often caused by diffuse skeletal metastases, it can be the result of ectopic production of a parathyroid hormone-related peptide or other humoral substances. Excessive production of corticotropin may result in Cushing syndrome with excess cortisol production, resulting in muscle weakness, weight loss, hypertension, hyperglycemia, and profound hypokalemia. This syndrome is most commonly found in small cell lung cancer.

Table 7-2	**Symptoms Associated with Lung Cancer**
Typical	▪ Cough ▪ Increased production of sputum ▪ Shortness of breath
Common	▪ Fatigue ▪ Weight loss ▪ Anorexia ▪ Low-grade fever
Less Common	▪ Chest pain (usually from a pleural-based lesion) ▪ Hemoptysis ▪ Hoarseness (secondary to laryngeal nerve involvement) ▪ Bone pain ▪ Pleural effusion
Infrequent	▪ Signs and symptoms consistent with obstruction of the superior vena cava, superior sulcus, or Pancoast tumors ▪ Pericardial tamponade ▪ Paraneoplastic syndromes ▪ Signs and symptoms consistent with brain metastases

As a result of the rapid tumor growth, the classical physical stigmata of Cushing syndrome are often absent.

Small cell lung cancer also is associated with paraneoplastic neurologic abnormalities. Central nervous system (CNS) paraneoplastic disorders include cerebellar degeneration, dementia, limbic encephalopathy, Lambert-Eaton syndrome, and visual paraneoplastic syndrome with optic neuritis and retinopathy.

Cerebellar degeneration is characterized by progressive cerebellar dysfunction with ataxia, dysarthria, hypotonia, and dementia. This syndrome is associated with four different antineuronal antibodies, the most common being an antibody against Purkinje cell proteins. Limbic encephalopathy is characterized by progressive dementia, hallucinations, depression, agitation, anxiety, or disturbances in affect. Paraneoplastic sensory neuropathy often is caused by an anti-Hu antibody and is associated with subacute distal sensory loss and the absence of deep tendon reflexes with normal muscle strength. Anti-Hu is a circulating polyclonal immunoglobulin G that reacts with CNS neurons, as well as the dorsal root and trigeminal ganglia. It can be associated with encephalopathy, autonomic neuropathy, and cerebellar degeneration.

Lambert-Eaton syndrome occurs in less than 1% of patients. It is caused by onconeural antibodies targeting presynaptic calcium channels and is characterized by proximal muscle weakness. Unlike myasthenia gravis, muscle strength tends to improve with repeated activity.

SCREENING

Most patients with lung cancer present with advanced disease, raising the question of the role of screening to detect these tumors at an earlier and theoretically more curable stage. The three screening interventions that have been explored for lung cancer include chest x-ray, cytologic analysis of sputum, and low-dose spiral CT. Although the role of screening patients at high risk for the development of early-stage disease was debated for many years, CT-based screening has been found to demonstrate a reduction in lung cancer mortality (Fig. 7-3).

Low-dose, noncontrast, thin-slice, helical, or spiral CT is a scan in which only the pulmonary parenchyma is examined, negating the use of intravenous contrast medium and the necessity of a physician's presence. This type of scan can usually be done quickly (within one breath) and involves low doses of radiation. In a nonrandomized, controlled study from the Early Lung Cancer Action Project, low-dose CT was shown to be more sensitive than chest x-ray for detecting lung nodules and lung cancer in early stages.[68]

The National Lung Screening Trial (NLST) was a randomized multicenter study comparing low-dose helical CTs with chest x-ray for the screening of older current and former heavy smokers for early detection of lung cancer.[69] From 2002 to 2004, more than 50,000 high-risk individuals from 33 U.S. centers were randomly assigned to receive three annual screenings with single-view posteroanterior chest x-ray or low-dose CT. The study enrolled individuals between ages 55 and 74 with at least a 30-pack per year smoking history (former smokers needed to have quit within the previous 15 years). Individuals with a prior lung cancer diagnosis, hemoptysis, unexplained weight loss of more than 15 pounds, or chest CT within 18 months before

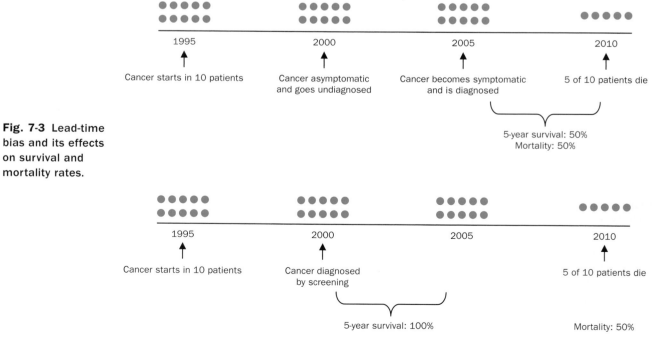

Fig. 7-3 Lead-time bias and its effects on survival and mortality rates.

enrollment were excluded. The rate of screening adherence exceeded 90%. The rate of positive screening tests was 24% with CT and 7% with chest x-ray. However, in both arms there was a false-positive rate of 93% to 96%. There were 247 deaths from lung cancer per 100,000 person-years in the CT group and 309 deaths per 100,000 person-years in the chest x-ray group, corresponding to a 20% relative reduction in lung cancer mortality ($p = 0.004$). CT was also associated with a 6.7% reduction in all-cause mortality ($p = 0.02$). Based on the NLST trial, the United States Preventive Services Task Force recently issued updated recommendations regarding lung cancer screening with low-dose CT for patients ages 55 to 80 with a 30 or greater pack per year smoking history and who are currently smoking or quit within the past 15 years. Although the NLST showed for the first time that CT-based screening reduced lung cancer mortality, numerous questions regarding implementation, cost, associated biomarkers to identify patients at highest risk, and management of false-positive tests remain and will be important topics for future studies (Table 7-3).

PROGNOSTIC FACTORS

Prognostic factors predict a patient's outcome independent of treatment. Favorable prognostic factors for both NSCLC and small cell cancers include stage, performance status (PS), lack of substantial weight loss (less than 5%), and female sex. Age is not an independent prognostic factor. "Fit" older patients tend to fare as well as their younger counterparts; further, older patients with good PS typically fare better than younger patients with poor PS. Histologic subtype also is not an independent prognostic factor for NSCLC, although adenocarcinoma is more likely to metastasize earlier than squamous cell. However, once metastasized, these two histologies have similar prognoses.

PREDICTIVE FACTORS

Predictive factors predict how a patient will fare with treatment. In lung cancer, *EGFR* mutation status is useful for predicting which patients are likely to derive the most benefit from EGFR TKIs, particularly responses and improved time to progression. However, this does not mean that patients with wild-type *EGFR* will not benefit from EGFR TKIs, especially in terms of disease control rate and progression-free survival (PFS).[70] It simply means that those with *EGFR* mutations are more likely to demonstrate higher objective RRs.

PREOPERATIVE EVALUATION FOR NSCLC

The suitability of the patient for a definitive resection depends on two factors: the stage of the lesion and the ability of the patient to withstand surgery. A detailed discussion of the preoperative evaluation and comorbid conditions are beyond the scope of this chapter; however, assessment of pulmonary reserve is discussed here.

MEDICAL ASSESSMENT OF PULMONARY RESERVE

Preoperative evaluation for a thoracotomy starts with spirometry. General guidelines are described here, although it should be emphasized that a certified general thoracic surgeon, working as part of a multidisciplinary thoracic oncology team, is best qualified to determine whether a patient is a surgical candidate. The forced vital capacity is the value that has been used most commonly to assess suitability for surgery; a predicted postoperative forced vital capacity of less than 1 L or a preoperative value of less than 2 L for a pneumonectomy or less than 1.5 L for a lobectomy usually suggests that the patient is at risk for perioperative complications. A diffusion capacity should be obtained if there is concern that the forced vital capacity may not be adequate or that the patient has signs or symptoms of interstitial lung disease. A low diffusion capacity (less than 50% predicted) suggests increased risk of postoperative morbidity or mortality.

Pulmonary status should be optimized as much as possible before surgery. Treatment of bronchitis with antibiotics, bronchodilators, and/or oral corticosteroids is helpful. The patient should quit smoking, if applicable, and preoperative training with incentive spirometry and weight reduction should be considered when appropriate.

NON-SMALL CELL LUNG CANCER

STAGING

The current (7th edition) tumor-nodes-metastasis (TNM) of the American Joint Committee on Cancer (AJCC) staging system is based on an analysis of more than 67,000 lung cases internationally (Tables 7-4 and 7-5). Key changes include several modifications to T and M descriptors, including tumor size cutoffs (tumors greater than 7 cm are now T3) and designations for intrapulmonary spread (T3 if intralobar; T4 if another lobe in the same lung; M1a if contralateral lung) and effusions (M1a). Certain stage groupings have also changed. T2bN0M0 cases (previously stage IB) are now stage IIA; T2aN1M0 (previously stage IIB) are now stage IIA; T4N0-1M0 (previously stage IIIB) are now stage IIIA.[71,72] It should be noted that a majority of cases analyzed were surgical, regardless of stage, and that some stage changes reflect a selected database.

OBTAINING A DIAGNOSIS

The diagnosis of lung cancer is most commonly made through cytologic or histologic evaluation of specimens

obtained by transbronchial biopsy or percutaneous needle biopsy. Although the disease is usually discovered on chest x-ray, CT of the chest and upper abdomen is necessary to evaluate the extent of the primary disease, mediastinal extension, or lymphadenopathy, as well as the presence or absence of other parenchymal nodules in patients for whom surgical resection is a consideration. Positron emission tomography (PET) is helpful primarily in detecting distant metastases, although they also assist in defining tumor size and in defining N2 stations appropriate for subsequent pathologic confirmation of cancer involvement. If a PET is done as part of the staging workup, a bone scan does not need to be performed. CT or magnetic resonance imaging (MRI) of the head is recommended for patients to be treated with curative intent or those with signs or symptoms suggestive of brain metastases.

Mediastinal nodal metastasis is a critical factor in determining tumor resectability (Table 7-4 and Fig. 7-4). Mediastinoscopy has long been considered the gold standard for mediastinal staging and has been recommended for mediastinal lymph nodes larger than 1 cm on CT, even if they are not 18-fluorodeoxyglucose (FDG)-avid on PET. Patients with a normal mediastinum on CT whose lymph nodes also appear negative on a PET may not need to undergo a preoperative mediastinoscopy, although the lymph nodes still must be sampled at the time of thoracotomy.

INVASIVE STAGING: MEDIASTINOSCOPY, CHAMBERLAIN PROCEDURE (ANTERIOR MEDIASTINOTOMY), ENDOBRONCHIAL ULTRASOUND, ENDOSCOPIC ULTRASOUND, AND TRANSTHORACIC AND TRANSBRONCHIAL BIOPSIES

Accurate staging of the mediastinum is critical for patients with NSCLC to guide optimal therapy. Clinical staging has been shown to differ markedly from pathologic staging at the time of resection.[73] In a review of numerous clinical trials, the performance of transthoracic, transbronchial, and endoscopic ultrasound-guided needle aspirations or biopsies was compared with mediastinoscopy for staging disease in the mediastinum.[73] Transthoracic and endoscopic needle aspirations had similar sensitivities to mediastinoscopies, although the transthoracic and endoscopic ultrasound needle aspirations were typically performed only for patients with enlarged nodes detected by CT, resulting in fewer false-negative results. However, mediastinoscopy has a higher negative predictive value. Mediastinoscopy does not provide access to Station 5 and 6 lymph nodes (aortopulmonary nodes), which provide lymphatic drainage for the left lung; assessment of these nodes typically requires a Chamberlain procedure (anterior mediastinotomy). Endobronchial ultrasound (EBUS) has emerged as an alternate means to evaluate the mediastinum. Thus far, EBUS appears accurate and safe. Although unlikely to completely replace mediastinoscopy, it may reduce the number of these more invasive procedures.[74]

Table 7-4 Definitions for Tumor, Node, and Metastasis (TNM) Descriptors[71]

T (Primary Tumor)

TX	Primary tumor cannot be assessed, or tumor proven by the presence of malignant cells in sputum or bronchial washings but not visualized by imaging or bronchoscopy
T0	No evidence of primary tumor
TIS	Carcinoma in situ
T1	Tumor ≤ 3 cm in greatest dimension, surrounded by lung or visceral pleura, without bronchoscopic evidence of invasion more proximal than the lobar bronchus (i.e., not in the main bronchus)
T1a	Tumor ≤ 2 cm in greatest dimension
T1b	Tumor > 2 cm but ≤ 3 cm in greatest dimension
T2	Tumor > 3 cm but ≤ 7 cm or tumor with any of the following features (T2 tumors with these features are classified T2a if ≤ 5 cm): • Involves main bronchus, ≥ 2 cm distal to the carina • Invades visceral pleura • Associated with atelectasis or obstructive pneumonitis that extends to the hilar region but does not involve the entire lung
T2a	Tumor > 3 cm but ≤ 5 cm in greatest dimension
T2b	Tumor > 5 cm but ≤ 7 cm in greatest dimension
T3	Tumor > 7 cm or one that directly invades any of the following: chest wall (including superior sulcus tumors), diaphragm, phrenic nerve, mediastinal pleura, parietal pericardium; or tumor in the main bronchus < 2 cm distal to the carina but without involvement of the carina; or associated atelectasis or obstructive pneumonitis of the entire lung or separate tumor nodule(s) in the same lobe
T4	Tumor of any size that invades any of the following: mediastinum, heart, great vessels, trachea, recurrent laryngeal nerve, esophagus, vertebral body, carina; separate tumor nodule(s) in a different ipsilateral lobe

N (Regional Lymph Nodes)

NX	Regional lymph nodes cannot be assessed
N0	No regional lymph node metastasis
N1	Metastasis in ipsilateral peribronchial and/or ipsilateral hilar lymph nodes and intrapulmonary nodes, including involvement by direct extension
N2	Metastasis in ipsilateral mediastinal and/or subcarinal lymph node(s)
N3	Metastasis in contralateral mediastinal, contralateral hilar, ipsilateral or contralateral scalene, or supraclavicular lymph node(s)

M (Distant Metastasis)

MX	Distant metastasis cannot be assessed
M0	No distant metastasis
M1	Distant metastasis
M1a	Separate tumor nodule(s) in a contralateral lobe; tumor with pleural nodules or malignant pleural (or pericardial) effusion*
M1b	Distant metastasis

*Most pleural (and pericardial) effusions with lung cancer are due to tumor. In a few patients, however, multiple cytopathologic examinations of pleural (pericardial) fluid are negative for tumor, and the fluid is nonbloody and is not an exudate. Where these elements and clinical judgment dictate that the effusion is not related to the tumor, the effusion should be excluded as a staging element and the patient should be classified as T1, T2, T3, or T4.

Copyright © 2007 by the International Association for the Study of Lung Cancer. Modified with permission from Goldstraw P, Crowley J, Chanksky K, et al. The IASLC Lung Cancer Staging Project: Proposals for the Revision of the TMN Stage Groupings in the Forthcoming (Seventh) Edition of the TNM Classification of Malignant Tumors. Journal of Thoracic Oncology. 2007;2:706-714.

Table 7-5 Stage Groupings by TNM Elements[71]

Stage Groups	Descriptors		
	T	N	M
IA	T1a,b	N0	M0
IB	T2a	N0	M0
IIA	T1a,b	N1	M0
	T2a	N1	M0
	T2b	N0	M0
IIB	T2b	N1	M0
	T3	N0	M0
IIIA	T1-3	N2	M0
	T3	N1	M0
	T4	N0,1	M0
IIIB	T4	N2	M0
	T1-4	N3	M0
IV	T$_{Any}$	N$_{Any}$	M1a,b

Clinical stage 5-year survival
IA 50%
IB 47%
IIA 36%
IIB 26%
IIIA 19%
IIIB 7%
IV 2%

Modified with permission from Goldstraw P, Crowley J, Chanksky K, et al. The IASLC Lung Cancer Staging Project: Proposals for the Revision of the TMN Stage Groupings in the Forthcoming (Seventh) Edition of the TNM Classification of Malignant Tumors. Journal of Thoracic Oncology. 2007;2:706-714.

Table 7-6 Comparison of Sensitivity and Specificity of PET and CT

	Sensitivity (%)	Specificity (%)	Accuracy (%)
Detection of Mediastinal Metastases[76]			
PET*	91	86	–
CT	75	66	–
Staging of Mediastinal Disease[77]			
PET	96	93	94
CT	68	65	66

*The sensitivity and specificity of PET for detecting distant metastases were 82% and 93%, respectively.

POSITRON EMISSION TOMOGRAPHY

PET, a metabolic imaging scan using FDG, is more sensitive, specific, and accurate than CT and has been shown to prevent unnecessary invasive procedures and/or "futile thoracotomies" in patients subsequently proven to be at a more advanced stage.[75]

In a prospective study, a standard approach to staging of NSCLC (CT, ultrasound, and bone scan) was compared with PET to determine which approach could more accurately detect metastases in mediastinal lymph nodes and distant sites.[76] Mediastinal involvement was confirmed histopathologically, and distant metastases were confirmed by other imaging tests. The results of PET and CT followed by pathologic staging were compared in a study involving 168 mediastinal nodes in 54 patients.[77] PET had higher sensitivity and specificity than CT in both studies (Table 7-6). However, the limitations of PET include the cost, availability, inability to detect lesions smaller than 8 mm, and lack of specificity, particularly for patients with inflammatory or granulomatous disease. Thus, PET cannot replace pathologic confirmation of malignancy because the scan can yield false-positive results when an inflammatory process is present and false-negative results when low-metabolic lung tumors, such as AIS, or carcinoid tumors are present.

Despite these problems, preoperative PET (in addition to a conventional workup) has been demonstrated to reduce the number of "futile" thoracotomies, as defined by benign disease, exploratory thoracotomy, pathologic stage IIIA (N2) or IIIB disease, postoperative relapse, or death within 12 months,[78] although it may not affect overall survival (OS).[79] PET also has been used to detect distant metastases; indeed, it is in this area that some investigators believe PET may have its primary role in staging.[75] Negative results of PET for patients without symptomatic disease probably obviates the need for bone imaging.[75] PET ultimately may be useful for judging response to therapy, because PET scans done early after treatment have been demonstrated to be better predictors of survival than CT, although this data needs to be confirmed in larger trials.[80]

NON-SMALL CELL LUNG CANCER TREATMENT

Treatment of NSCLC is specific to stage. Within a given stage category, a number of additional relevant factors enter therapeutic decision-making, including histology and molecular profiling for driver oncogenes. Of course, PS, comorbid conditions, and relevant social factors must also be taken into account.

STAGE I AND II DISEASE

Approximately one-third of all patients with lung cancer present with stage I or II disease. The treatment of choice is surgical resection, which can result in cure for many patients. The preferred surgical procedure is lobectomy, although for patients in whom disease crosses a major fissure or involves the proximal main-stem bronchus, pneumonectomy may be required. Lobectomy has traditionally been the procedure of choice, even for patients with small, peripheral lesions, because wedge resections have been shown to be associated with increased local recurrence and decreased survival.[81] Lobectomy should include resection of bronchial, hilar, and

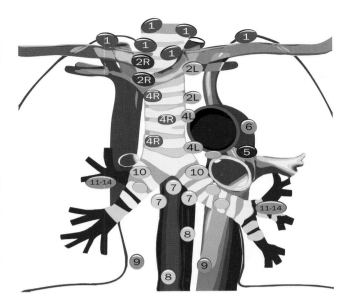

Fig. 7-4 Regional lymph node classification.

Supraclavicular nodes

1. Low cervical, supraclavicular and sternal notch nodes
From the lower margin of the cricoid to the clavicles and the upper border of the manubrium. The midline of the trachea serves as border between 1R and 1L.

Superior mediastinal nodes 2-4

2R. Upper paratracheal
From the upper border of manubrium to the intersection of caudal margin of innominate (left brachiocephalic) vein with the trachea. 2R nodes extend to the left lateral border of the trachea.

2L. Upper paratracheal
From the upper border of manubrium to the superior border of aortic arch. 2L nodes are located to the left of the left lateral border of the trachea.

3A. Prevascular
Nodes are not adjacent to the trachea like the nodes in Station 2, but they are anterior to the vessels.

3P. Prevertebral
Nodes not adjacent to the trachea like the nodes in Station 2, but behind the esophagus, which is prevertebral.

4R. Lower paratracheal
From the intersection of the caudal margin of innominate (left brachiocephalic) vein with the trachea to the lower border of the azygos vein. 4R nodes extend from the right to the left lateral border of the trachea.

4L. Lower paratracheal
From the upper margin of the aortic arch to the upper rim of the left main pulmonary artery.

Aortic nodes 5-6

5. Subaortic
These nodes are located in the aortopulmonary window lateral to the ligamentum arteriosum. These nodes are not located between the aorta and the pulmonary trunk but lateral to these vessels.

6. Para-aortic
These are ascending aorta or phrenic nodes lying anterior and lateral to the ascending aorta and the aortic arch.

Inferior mediastinal nodes 7-9

7. Subcarinal

8. Paraesophageal
Nodes below carina.

9. Pulmonary ligament
Nodes lying within the pulmonary ligaments.

Hilar, lobar, and (sub)segmental nodes 10-14
These are all N1 nodes.

10. Hilar nodes
These include nodes adjacent to the main stem bronchus and hilar vessels. On the right they extend from the lower rim of the azygos vein to the interlobar region; on the left, from the upper rim of the pulmonary artery to the interlobar region.

Reprinted with permission from Robin Smithuis; www.radiologyassistant.nl.

selected mediastinal nodes based on published guidelines (at least 4R and 7 for right-sided tumors; at least 5/6 and 7 for left-sided tumors). Research is ongoing regarding the management of the small, ground glass–appearing lesions discovered on low-dose, non–contrast-enhanced, thin-slice, helical CT. For example, because pure AIS does not feature lymphatic or hematogenous spread, it has been proposed that wedge resection without lymph node dissection may be adequate for localized tumors. For multifocal disease, some centers have performed lung transplantation, albeit with somewhat discouraging outcomes.[82]

In patients with medical contraindications to surgery but with adequate pulmonary function, conventional fractionated radiotherapy (e.g., 6,000 cGy or "rads" in 30 fractions of 200 cGy each) results in cure in about 20% of patients. Advances in imaging and radiation delivery have resulted in the use of stereotactic radiation for lung tumors. With this technology, radiation delivery to surrounding normal lung parenchyma is substantially less than that seen with conventional radiotherapy. It is therefore possible to administer much higher "ablative" doses of radiation with a small number of fractions (e.g., up to 2,000 cGy per fraction given every 2 to 3 days for

three fractions). To date, outcomes with this technique appear promising. In a multicenter phase II U.S. trial of patients with medically inoperable stage I NSCLC, the 3-year rate of primary tumor control was 98%, 3-year distant failure rate was 22%, 3-year disease-free survival (DFS) was 48%, and 3-year OS was 56%.[83]

Stereotactic radiation, which entails radiation to the primary tumor but not to the draining lymph nodes, is considered only for patients with clinical stage I (T1N0M0 or T2N0M0) disease. Because of toxicities, stereotactic radiation is usually not performed in situations where the tumor lies within 2 cm of the proximal bronchial tree. This technique is also usually restricted to tumors less than 5 cm in size.

In contrast to surgically resected early-stage tumors (see Adjuvant Chemotherapy section), the role of chemotherapy following radiation therapy for medically inoperable early-stage NSCLC is unclear.

The risk of developing second lung cancers is high (approximately 2% to 3% annually) for patients with resected stage I NSCLC. Vitamin A and one its derivatives (beta-carotene or cis retinoic acid) have been found to be ineffective as chemopreventive therapy and actually deleterious in current

- Treatment of stage I and II NSCLC involves surgical resection (if the patient is a candidate) or radiation therapy (if the patient is not a surgical candidate).
- Optimal management of Pancoast tumors consists of concurrent chemoradiation followed by surgical resection.
- Adjuvant chemotherapy consisting of a cisplatin-based combination is indicated for patients with stage II and IIIA disease after surgical resection. Though controversial, it should be discussed with patients with stage IB disease, particularly higher-risk stage IB such as those with larger tumors (larger than 4 cm). Cisplatin is the preferred platinum compound in this curative setting because it has been shown to be more effective than carboplatin-based regimens. Level 1 evidence from randomized trials suggests that the second drug should be vinorelbine or etoposide, although many clinicians extrapolate from the advanced disease setting and use other cisplatin-based doublets, which is supported by current National Comprehensive Cancer Network guidelines.
- Optimal treatment of "nonbulky" stage IIIA disease (e.g., small, single-station node) continues to evolve but optimally involves both systemic chemotherapy and local therapy (surgery and/or radiation). For patients with multistation N2 disease or bulky N2 nodes (3 cm or larger) concurrent chemotherapy plus radiation therapy is considered standard of care.
- For nonbulky N2 disease, a trimodality approach with chemoradiation followed by surgery can be considered, although patients requiring pneumonectomy (particularly right-sided pneumonectomy) had poor survival. Management decisions regarding stage IIIA NSCLC should be made in a multidisciplinary thoracic tumor board.
- Curative-intent treatment of stage IIIB NSCLC similarly involves combined-modality treatment with chemotherapy and radiation therapy. Evidence from randomized trials suggests that concurrent chemotherapy and radiation therapy will result in the best survival, albeit at an increase in toxicity.
- The optimal chemoradiation schedule remains debatable; there is Level 1 evidence for concurrent chemoradiation with full-dose cisplatin and etoposide, and Level 2 evidence (based on randomized phase II data) supporting weekly low doses of paclitaxel and carboplatin with concurrent radiation followed by consolidation paclitaxel and carboplatin.

smokers.[16-18] A study of secondary chemoprevention with selenium (Eastern Cooperative Oncology Group [ECOG] 5597) also did not demonstrate a reduction in the incidence of second primary cancers.[84]

Patients with peripheral chest wall invasion (T3N0; stage IIB) should have an en bloc resection of the involved ribs and underlying lung. Five-year survival rates as high as 50% have been reported.[85]

PANCOAST TUMORS

Pancoast, or superior sulcus tumors, in the upper lobe adjoining the brachial plexus are frequently associated with Horner syndrome (ptosis, miosis, and anhidrosis) or shoulder and arm pain; the latter is caused by rib destruction, involvement of the seventh cervical vertebra or T-1 nerve roots, or both. The Southwest Oncology Group (SWOG) intergroup phase II trial in patients with T3/4 N0/1 M0 superior sulcus NSCLC established current standard of care, consisting of cisplatin/etoposide and concomitant radiation therapy to 45 Gy followed by attempted surgical resection.[86] In those patients with available surgical specimens, 54 (65%) showed either a complete pathologic response or minimal microscopic disease on pathologic evaluation. The 2-year survival rate was 55% for all eligible patients and 70% for patients who had a complete resection.

Adjuvant Chemotherapy

The rationale for adjuvant chemotherapy in patients with early-stage lung cancer is based on the observation that distant metastases are the most common site of failure following potentially curative surgery. Interest in this treatment strategy grew after publication of a 1995 meta-analysis of more than 4,300 patients, in which those who received cisplatin-based regimens had an improved survival rate of approximately 5% at 5 years, with borderline statistical significance (p = 0.08).[87] Since that time, a number of randomized trials have evaluated the role of adjuvant chemotherapy following surgical resection of early-stage NSCLC (Table 7-7). In a pooled analysis of five of these trials, there was a 5.4% absolute survival benefit at 5 years (HR 0.89, 95% CI 0.82, 0.96; p = 0.005).[88] The Lung Adjuvant Cisplatin Evaluation study performed an individual patient meta-analysis of the five largest cisplatin-based adjuvant trials (ALPI, BLT, IALT, JBR.10, and ANITA). Importantly, the benefit of adjuvant chemotherapy varied considerably by disease stage. For stage IA NSCLC, adjuvant chemotherapy was associated with a trend toward worse survival (HR for death 1.40, 95% CI 0.95, 2.06). For patients with stage IB disease, the HR was 0.93 (95% CI 0.78, 1.10). In the Cancer and Leukemia Group B (CALGB) 9633 trial, patients with stage IB disease were randomly assigned to surgery alone or surgery followed by carboplatin/paclitaxel.[89] In long-term follow-up of this trial, only the subset of patients with tumors 4 cm or larger demonstrated a significant survival difference in favor of adjuvant chemotherapy (HR 0.69, 95% CI 0.48, 0.99; p = 0.04). The fact that this trial employed a carboplatin-based regimen

Table 7-7 Adjuvant Therapies Following Surgical Resection of Early-Stage Non-Small Cell Lung Cancer

Study (Stage)	Treatment	Patients	5-Year Survival (%)	Median Survival	Hazard Ratio	p-value
ECOG 3590 (II–IIIA)[203]	Surgery → radiation therapy vs. postop concurrent radiation therapy plus cisplatin and etoposide	242 246		39 months 38 months	0.92	0.56
ALPI (I–IIIA)[204]	Surgery vs. postop mitomycin, vindesine, and cisplatin	603 606	51 43		0.96	0.589
IALT (IB–IIIA)[92]	Surgery vs. postop cisplatin and etoposide, or vinca alkaloids	405 361	40 44.5		0.86	0.03
CALGB (IB)[89]	Surgery vs. postop carboplatin and paclitaxel	172 172	57 59		0.83	0.12
NCI-C (IB–II)[93]	Surgery vs. postop cisplatin and vinorelbine	241 241	54 69		0.80	0.03
ANITA (IB, II, IIIA)[91]	Surgery vs. postop cisplatin and vinorelbine	433 407	43 51	44 months 66 months	0.80	0.017

Abbreviations: ALPI, Adjuvant Lung Project Italy; ANITA, Adjuvant Navelbine International Trialist Association; CALGB, Cancer and Leukemia Group B; ECOG, Eastern Cooperative Oncology Group; IALT, International Adjuvant Lung Cancer Trial; NCI-C, National Cancer Institute of Canada; postop, postoperative.

further confounds interpretation, as cisplatin-paclitaxel was proven superior to carboplatin-paclitaxel in stage IV NSCLC, with median survivals of 9.8 months versus 8.5 months (p = 0.0019).[90] Given these data, whether patients with stage IB disease and tumors 4 cm or larger should be offered adjuvant chemotherapy remains controversial. In patients with resected stage IA NSCLC, there are no supporting data in favor of adjuvant chemotherapy, and some trials and meta-analyses even suggest a detrimental effect. The reason for a potentially negative effect in stage IA disease is speculative.

The role of adjuvant chemotherapy for resected stage II NSCLC is well established. In the Adjuvant Navelbine International Trialist Association (ANITA) trial, patients with stage IB to IIIA cancer were randomly assigned to surgery alone or surgery followed by four cycles of cisplatin/vinorelbine.[91] OS was significantly improved at 5 years (51% vs. 43%), although the survival benefit was limited to patients with stage II and IIIA disease. In a pooled analysis of cisplatin-based chemotherapy trials, there was a significant survival benefit (HR 0.83, 95% CI 0.73, 0.95) for stage II NSCLC. Accordingly, adjuvant chemotherapy is recommended following complete resection of stage II and stage III NSCLC.

The optimal regimen for adjuvant chemotherapy remains unclear. Almost all studies have employed cisplatin-containing doublets. The principal exception, CALGB 9633—which employed carboplatin/paclitaxel after resection of stage IB disease—did not meet statistical significance for OS (HR 0.83, 95% CI 0.6, 1.08; p = 0.12).[89] It is not known whether this result is because of the IB population, the relatively small sample size (344 patients), or the chemotherapy regimen. Nevertheless, cisplatin rather than carboplatin is recommended in the adjuvant, potentially curative, setting. Vinca alkaloids and

etoposide have been combined with cisplatin most commonly in adjuvant trials. In the International Adjuvant Lung Trial, patients with resected stage I to IIIA disease were randomly assigned to observation or chemotherapy (cisplatin plus etoposide, vinorelbine, vinblastine, or vindesine).[92] Although the study was terminated early because of slow accrual, there was a significant improvement in median survival, DFS, 5-year survival, and 5-year DFS in favor of the chemotherapy arm (HR for survival 0.86). A randomized trial by the National Cancer Institute of Canada (NCI-C JBR.10) randomly assigned 482 patients with stage IB or II disease to postoperative observation or vinorelbine and cisplatin. OS was significantly prolonged for the chemotherapy group compared with the observation group (94 vs. 73 months; HR for death 0.69; p = 0.04), as was relapse-free survival (not reached vs. 46.7 months; HR for recurrence 0.60; p < 0.001). Five-year survival rates were 69% and 54% for the two groups, respectively (p = 0.03).[93] Of note, this 15% absolute benefit at 5 years is among the highest in all adjuvant chemotherapy trials across cancer types. In the ANITA trial, 840 patients with postoperative stage I (T2N0), II, or IIIA disease were assigned to surgery alone or surgery followed by cisplatin/vinorelbine. Median survival was 65.8 months in the treatment arm and 43.7 months in the observation arm (HR 0.80, 95% CI 0.66, 0.96; p = 0.017). Survival at 2, 5, and 7 years was 68%, 51%, and 45% in the treatment arm, respectively, and 63%, 43%, and 37% in the observation arm, respectively. Five-year survival by stage I/II/IIIA was 62%, 52%, and 42%, respectively, in the treatment arm and 63%, 39%, and 26%, respectively, in the observation arm.[91] Given that there is no major difference in efficacy between various chemotherapy doublets in advanced disease, many clinicians extrapolate to earlier-stage disease and use other "third-generation" drugs (such as pemetrexed, docetaxel, and gemcitabine) in combination with cisplatin, albeit without Level 1 data. This approach is supported by current NCCN guidelines.

There is growing interest in the incorporation of molecularly targeted agents into the treatment of early-stage NSCLC. At this time, however, such an approach cannot be recommended outside of a clinical trial. In the NCI-C JBR.19 trial—which was terminated early when gefitinib lost its U.S. Food and Drug Administration (FDA) approval—administration of the EGFR inhibitor gefitinib after resection of stage I to III NSCLC did not improve OS. Surprisingly, in a subset analysis of patients with tumors harboring activating *EGFR* mutations, a population expected to derive particular benefit from such an approach, a detrimental effect from gefitinib was suggested.[94] The recently presented RADIANT trial showed a trend for improved disease-free survival with adjuvant erlotinib in stage IB to III disease in the subset of patients whose tumors harbored an *EGFR*-activating mutation.[94a] The use of antiangiogenic agents and ALK and EGFR inhibitors after surgery as an adjuvant treatment remains investigational.

Neoadjuvant Chemotherapy

The potential advantages of neoadjuvant chemotherapy include:

- Improved tolerability when administered before surgery (90% of patients will receive the planned dose preoperatively compared with 60% postoperatively);
- Micrometastases treated earlier rather than later; and
- Possible complete resection after downstaging with chemotherapy.

Two small randomized studies published in 1994 raised considerable interest in the role of neoadjuvant chemotherapy.[95,96] In these trials, each of which involved 60 patients, surgery alone was compared with surgery plus preoperative chemotherapy for stage IIIA disease. Both studies found improved survival for patients receiving neoadjuvant chemotherapy, although criticisms of these studies include their small size, imbalances between the two arms, and poor survival of the control arms.

In a larger randomized French trial, preoperative chemotherapy with mitomycin, ifosfamide, and cisplatin plus surgery was compared with surgery alone for 355 patients with resectable stage I (except T1N0), II, and IIIA (including N2) disease. The findings did not show a benefit with neoadjuvant chemotherapy.[97] A subset analysis suggested a survival advantage for neoadjuvant chemotherapy for N0 and N1 disease but not for N2 disease. A European intergroup study (Medical Research Council LU22/ Dutch Society of Physicians for Pulmonology and Tuberculosis 2/ European Organisation for the Research and Treatment of Cancer [EORTC] 08012) randomly assigned 519 patients to receive surgery alone or three cycles of platinum-based chemotherapy followed by surgery. There was no evidence of a benefit in survival (HR 1.02, 95% CI 0.80, 1.31; p = 0.86).[98]

Although Level 1 evidence supports the role of adjuvant chemotherapy, the exact role of neoadjuvant chemotherapy is less clear. Randomized trials have shown that patients tolerate preoperative chemotherapy better, dose delivery is better, and a higher percentage of patients complete preoperative versus postoperative therapy. Nevertheless, no studies have demonstrated a survival advantage for preoperative therapy.[99]

STAGE III DISEASE

Treatment of locally advanced NSCLC is one of the most controversial issues in the management of lung cancer. Treatment options include surgery or radiation therapy for local control plus chemotherapy to control micrometastases. Interpretation of the results of clinical trials involving patients with locally advanced disease has been clouded by a number of issues, including changing diagnostic techniques, different staging systems, and heterogeneous patient populations with tumors that range from nonbulky stage IIIA (clinical N1 nodes with N2 nodes discovered only at the time of surgery or mediastinoscopy) to bulky N2 nodes (enlarged adenopathy clearly visible on chest x-rays or multiple nodal level involvement) to clearly inoperable stage IIIB disease.

For some subsets of stage IIB (T3N0), IIIA (T3N1), or IIIA (T4N0±1) tumors, the outcome may be less related to the potential of micrometastatic disease and more to the location of the tumor and its resectability (e.g., superior sulcus, chest wall, proximal airway). For each location, a determination must be made on the basis of the potential of surgical resectability and the likelihood of distant metastases, as evidenced by mediastinal metastases.

Nonbulky Stage IIIA Disease

The optimal treatment for nonbulky stage IIIA typically consists of a local approach (surgery and/or radiation therapy) plus a systemic treatment (chemotherapy). Possible combinations include surgery followed by adjuvant chemotherapy (with or without thoracic radiation), neoadjuvant chemotherapy (or chemoradiation) followed by surgery, or concurrent or sequential chemotherapy and radiation.

The potential benefit of adding surgery to combined chemoradiation for stage IIIA has been evaluated in a randomized phase III intergroup trial (INT 0139).[100] This study randomly assigned 396 patients with stage T1-3N2M0 NSCLC to receive concurrent chemoradiation (45 Gy) plus two cycles of cisplatin/etoposide, followed by either surgical resection or continuation of radiation to 61 Gy total plus an additional two cycles of cisplatin/etoposide. Although PFS was significantly longer in the surgery arm (12.8 vs. 10.5 months; p = 0.02), there was no significant difference in OS (23.6 vs. 22.2 months; p = 0.24). There were more treatment-related deaths in the surgery arm (8% vs. 2%), with the majority of deaths among patients requiring pneumonectomy. However, the survival curves subsequently separated so that by the third year, 5-year OS rates were 27.2% compared with 20.3% (OR for 5-year survival 0.63, 95% CI 0.36, 1.10; p = 0.10). In the trimodality arm, more patients were alive without progression of disease (p = 0.008), but more patients died without progression (p = 0.021). Consistent with other trials, achievement of pathologic N0 status at the time of surgery was associated with improved clinical outcomes (median OS, 34 months).

Occasionally, despite preoperative staging, patients thought to have stage I or II disease are found to have N2 nodal involvement at the time of surgery. For these stage III patients, postoperative radiation therapy (PORT; 50 Gy to 54 Gy) may be considered, usually after completion of adjuvant chemotherapy. Based on the PORT meta-analysis, this approach reduces locoregional recurrence but does not prolong survival.[101]

Bulky Stage IIIA (N2) and Stage IIIB Disease

Bulky stage IIIA and stage IIIB tumors are typically considered unresectable, with the preferred treatment consisting of combined chemoradiation. Randomized studies have demonstrated an improvement in median and long-term survival with chemotherapy followed by radiation therapy compared with radiation therapy alone.[102,103]

The results from two randomized studies, one conducted in Japan and the other by the Radiation Therapy Oncology Group (RTOG), showed a survival advantage with concurrent chemoradiation compared with a sequential approach, albeit at the expense of increased toxicity. In the Japanese trial, two cycles of mitomycin-C, vindesine, and cisplatin (MVP) were given concurrently or sequentially with 56 Gy of radiation.[104] Patients in either arm who experienced a response received another two cycles of MVP after radiation therapy was completed. The RR and median survival were significantly improved with concurrent chemoradiation (84% vs. 66%, p = 0.0002; 17 vs. 13 months, p = 0.04). The confirmatory randomized RTOG 9401 trial also showed improved survival with concurrent cisplatin, vinblastine, and radiation therapy compared with sequential chemoradiation (median survival, 17 vs. 13 months; p = 0.08).[105]

Chemotherapy can be administered in either full systemic doses with radiation therapy, weekly radiosensitizing doses, or a combination of both. Although single-agent weekly carboplatin has not resulted in a survival benefit when administered with radiation therapy, preliminary results from phase I and II studies (Locally Advanced Multimodality Protocol) of weekly doses of paclitaxel (50 mg/m^2) and carboplatin (area under the curve [AUC] 2) with concurrent radiation therapy followed by consolidation paclitaxel and carboplatin proved promising.[106] However, a CALGB trial compared concomitant chemoradiotherapy, consisting of low-dose weekly carboplatin and paclitaxel, with induction therapy prior to the same concomitant chemoradiation regimen. Median survival with chemoradiation was 11.4 months compared with 14 months for induction chemotherapy followed by chemoradiation (p = 0.154). The median survival achieved in each of the treatment groups was low compared with other reports in the literature, possibly indicating that chemoradiation with induction chemotherapy followed by low-dose weekly carboplatin and paclitaxel is not optimal.

Thus, major questions remain unanswered regarding the best combination and scheduling of chemotherapy and radiation therapy. Although results from the Japanese trial demonstrated a slightly superior outcome with concurrent chemoradiation the mitomycin-based approach is not widely used in the United States. The RTOG trial involved an older chemotherapy regimen; none of the newer agents, such as carboplatin, paclitaxel, docetaxel, gemcitabine, and vinorelbine, have been tested in this context. SWOG 9504 demonstrated promising results with consolidation docetaxel following full-dose cisplatin/etoposide and concurrent radiation therapy, but these results were not confirmed in a randomized trial (Hoosier Oncology Group LUN 01-24).[107,108] Indeed, consolidation docetaxel after concurrent chemoradiation led to more febrile neutropenia, pneumonitis, and hospitalizations and cannot be recommended outside of a clinical trial. The efficacy of sensitizing doses of concurrent chemotherapy also has not been compared with full doses of chemotherapy in randomized trials. Thus, at this point, there is Level 1 evidence for concurrent chemoradiation therapy with full-dose cisplatin and etoposide, and Level 2 evidence (based on randomized phase II data) supporting weekly low doses of paclitaxel and carboplatin with concurrent radiation therapy followed by consolidation paclitaxel and carboplatin. A recent phase III trial (RTOG 0617) showed that standard 60 Gy thoracic radiotherapy is superior to 74 Gy radiation dose with chemotherapy in terms of OS and local-regional control for treatment of stage III NSCLC.[109] These results are not explained simply by an increase in toxicity.

Currently, there is no established role for molecularly targeted agents in the treatment of locally advanced NSCLC. In SWOG 0023, patients with stage III NSCLC whose disease had not progressed after concurrent chemoradiation (with cisplatin/etoposide) and consolidation docetaxel were randomly assigned to receive gefitinib or placebo maintenance therapy.[110] Unexpectedly, OS was significantly worse in the gefitinib arm (median, 23 vs. 35 months; p = 0.01), a result that remains largely unexplained. The antiangiogenic drug bevacizumab has been added to concurrent chemoradiation for stage III NSCLC. In small series, this combination was associated with substantial toxicities, including an increased incidence of tracheoesophageal fistulae, and should not be used with concurrent thoracic radiotherapy.[111]

Stage III Recommendations

Treatment of patients with stage III, N2 NSCLC is not standardized, as indicated in the previous discussion. Although results from ongoing or recently completed randomized studies are maturing, some general guidelines for treating a patient can be identified.

- Clinical N0 disease by CT and PET—A resection should be performed with mediastinal sampling or complete dissection at the time of surgery. If microscopic N2 (or N1) disease is detected at surgery, postoperative chemotherapy should be administered. For N2 disease detected at surgery, PORT can be considered.

- Nonbulky N2 by CT (e.g., one node measuring 1 cm to 2 cm) and/or by PET—The age, PS, and comorbid conditions of the patient should be considered. Level 1 evidence exists for a combined modality approach with chemotherapy and radiation therapy. If the patient is a surgical candidate, it is not unreasonable to have a discussion regarding the use of surgery plus preoperative chemotherapy and/or radiation therapy, stressing that the optimal treatment sequence has not been clearly identified. Some surgeons recommend resampling the mediastinal nodes after two cycles of the induction chemotherapy, rationalizing that if the N2 nodes remain positive following chemotherapy, a definitive resection should not be attempted, and the patient should proceed with definitive radiation therapy or with combined chemotherapy and radiation. Combined preoperative chemoradiation should be administered cautiously and only to the fit patient who will be undergoing resection by an experienced thoracic surgeon (given the high incidence of postoperative deaths). Particular caution should be exercised for patients undergoing a right-sided pneumonectomy. Overall, chemotherapy plus concurrent thoracic radiation therapy remains the standard of care in this setting.
- Bulky N2 nodes—Chemotherapy plus concurrent radiation therapy is indicated. The presence of pathologically involved N2 nodes should be confirmed when possible, because enlarged nodes detected by CT will be pathologically negative for approximately 30% of patients. The age, PS, and comorbid conditions of the patient must be considered. Concurrent chemoradiation provides a small survival benefit, albeit at the expense of enhanced toxicity, and thus should be reserved for patients with good PS. Weekly, low-dose, concurrent chemotherapy has not been compared with full-dose chemotherapy in randomized trials, although

it is often administered concurrently with radiation therapy if followed by two to three cycles of standard-dose chemotherapy.

STAGE IV DISEASE

Chemotherapy improves survival for patients with metastatic NSCLC (a 1-year survival rate of approximately 10% for untreated patients compared with 35% to 40% for treated patients). In addition, chemotherapy may reduce symptoms and improve quality of life; therefore, it is usually recommended for patients with good PS. Because chemotherapy is not curative, goals for treatment that should be discussed with the patient include palliation of symptoms and a modest improvement in survival.

The principal factors predictive of response to chemotherapy and survival are PS and bulk of disease. Favorable prognostic factors include no weight loss, female sex, normal level of serum lactate dehydrogenase, and no bone or liver metastases.

First-Line Treatment

Chemotherapy. Chemotherapy for metastatic NSCLC traditionally has consisted of a platinum-based two-drug "doublet" regimen. Results from randomized studies have shown an improvement in survival, symptomatology, and quality of life for patients treated with cisplatin-based therapy compared with patients receiving best supportive care. Median survival and 1-year survival rates have increasingly improved with use of second- and third-generation chemotherapy regimens (Table 7-8).

Until recently, findings from numerous randomized studies have not shown a clinically significant advantage of any platinum-based doublet regimen, although there are differences in toxicity, cost, schedule, and convenience. However, there are now data supporting different treatment approaches depending on histologic subtype of NSCLC, based on

Table 7-8 Survival Rates for Chemotherapy for Non-Small Cell Lung Cancer

	Chemotherapy Agents	Median Survival (months)	1-Year Survival (%)	2-Year Survival (%)
Best supportive care only		4–5	5–10	< 5
First-generation chemotherapy regimens	Cisplatin, vinblastine, mitomycin, vindesine	5–6	10–15	< 5
Second-generation chemotherapy regimens	Carboplatin, etoposide	6	20–25	< 10
Third-generation chemotherapy regimens	Paclitaxel and docetaxel, gemcitabine, vinorelbine, pemetrexed	8–9	35–40	10
Non-squamous histology (no hemoptysis)	Carboplatin and paclitaxel plus bevacizumab	12	50	20
Non-squamous histology	Cisplatin plus pemetrexed	12	50	20
EGFR mutations	EGFR TKI before or after doublet chemotherapy	18-27		

Abbreviations: EGFR, epidermal growth factor receptor; TKI, tyrosine kinase inhibitor.

efficacy (pemetrexed) and safety (bevacizumab). Pemetrexed is an inhibitor of thymidylate synthase and other folate-dependent enzymes, including dihydrofolate reductase and glycinamide ribonucleotide formyltransferase. A phase III trial of more than 1,700 patients who had not previously received chemotherapy has been reported, comparing pemetrexed/cisplatin with gemcitabine/cisplatin.[112] OS was the same between the two arms, with an improved toxicity profile in the pemetrexed arm. However, in a prespecified subset analysis, OS was statistically superior for cisplatin/pemetrexed compared with cisplatin/gemcitabine for patients with adenocarcinoma (12.6 vs. 10.9 months) and large cell carcinoma histology (10.4 vs. 6.7 months). Conversely, patients with squamous cell histology experienced a significant improvement in survival with cisplatin/gemcitabine compared with cisplatin/pemetrexed (10.8 vs. 9.4 months). This and other studies have led to approval of pemetrexed for the first-line, maintenance, and second-line treatment of non-squamous cell NSCLC. One proposed explanation for the differential pemetrexed sensitivity of squamous and nonsquamous NSCLC is higher expression and activity of thymidylate synthase in squamous tumors.[113]

Bevacizumab. Bevacizumab has been approved for the management of nonsquamous cell carcinoma based on results from the ECOG 4599 phase III trial of 878 patients randomly assigned to chemotherapy (paclitaxel and carboplatin) or to chemotherapy plus 15 mg/kg of bevacizumab every 3 weeks.[42] Median survival for patients who received chemotherapy plus bevacizumab was 12.3 months compared with 10.3 months for patients who received chemotherapy alone (HR 0.79; p = 0.003). Median duration of PFS for patients who received chemotherapy plus bevacizumab was 6.2 months compared with 4.5 months for those who received chemotherapy alone (HR 0.66; p < 0.001), with corresponding RRs of 35% and 15%, respectively (p < 0.001). However, because of the grade 3 to 4 bleeding episodes observed in the phase II study that preceded this one, it should be noted that eligibility to this study was restricted to patients with non-squamous cell carcinoma (because of higher levels of severe hemoptysis observed in squamous tumors) and no brain metastases, as well as no hemoptysis, bleeding disorders, or anti-coagulation requirement. Despite these restrictions, significant bleeding was more frequent for patients who received chemotherapy plus bevacizumab (4.4% vs. 0.9%; p = 0.001). There were 15 treatment-related deaths in the group of patients who received chemotherapy plus bevacizumab, including five as a result of pulmonary hemorrhage. Thus, the risks and benefits of bevacizumab should be clearly delineated to patients with advanced NSCLC.

A second randomized study of bevacizumab involving more than 1,000 patients has been conducted (the Avastin in Lung [AVAiL] trial).[114] Unlike the ECOG study, this study involved gemcitabine and cisplatin and randomly assigned patients to chemotherapy plus placebo, chemotherapy with 7.5 mg/kg of bevacizumab every 3 weeks, and chemotherapy with 15 mg/kg

of bevacizumab every 3 weeks. The study met its primary endpoint of PFS, with HRs of 0.75 and 0.82, respectively, for the low- and high-dose bevacizumab arms. However, the absolute benefit was modest (median PFS, 6.7 and 6.5 vs. 6.1 months), with no improvement in survival. It is unclear whether the lack of survival benefit is a result of the differences in chemotherapy doublets between the ECOG study and the AVAiL trial, differences in bevacizumab dose, or differences in study design, of which there were many.

Subsequent experience with bevacizumab and other anti-angiogenic agents in lung cancer and other malignancies has provided further insight into the nature of their vascular complications, in some instances suggesting that expanding patient eligibility for these agents may be feasible. Squamous cell tumors remain an absolute contraindication to bevacizumab. Although it has been proposed that squamous cell histology may be a surrogate marker of central tumor location and proximity to vascular structures, neither of these anatomic characteristics has emerged as an independent risk factor for severe pulmonary hemorrhage. In the AVAiL trial, central lesions (defined as tumors in which the center of the mass was within hilar structures) were present in 38% of patients and were not associated with increased rates of grade 3 to 4 pulmonary hemorrhage. The only potential radiographic risk factor identified to date is baseline tumor cavitation (OR 4.5, 95% CI 0.73, 28.33; p = 0.06).[115]

The FDA approval of bevacizumab for the treatment of glioblastoma has supported the concept of using bevacizumab in patients with intracranial malignancy. The phase II PASSPORT trial administered bevacizumab plus chemotherapy to 115 patients with brain metastases previously treated with radiation or surgery. No cases of CNS hemorrhage occurred.[116] The use of bevacizumab in patients receiving antiplatelet agents was evaluated in a pooled analysis of five randomized trials in NSCLC, colorectal cancer, and breast cancer, in which the concurrent administration of bevacizumab, chemotherapy, and low-dose prophylactic aspirin did not increase the risk of bleeding compared with chemotherapy and aspirin alone.[117] The use of bevacizumab in patients receiving therapeutic anticoagulation has not been described extensively. In the AVAiL trial, 86 patients who developed venous thromboembolism during the study were treated with full-dose anticoagulation. Once on a stable anticoagulation regimen, patients randomly assigned to receive bevacizumab were permitted to resume it. Patients on anticoagulants experienced higher bleeding rates than patients not using anticoagulants, regardless of whether they received bevacizumab.[118] As a result of these and other reports, bevacizumab is now being used in patients with previously treated brain metastases. Although not an absolute contraindication, given the limited data available, caution should be exercised before initiating bevacizumab in patients receiving anticoagulants.

EGFR Inhibitors. There are two main approaches to targeting EGFR: TKIs and monoclonal antibodies. TKIs (e.g., erlotinib, gefitinib) cross the cell membrane, binding to and inhibiting the function of the intracellular tyrosine kinase domain. Monoclonal antibodies bind to the extracellular domain of EGFR, interfering with ligand binding and receptor activation.

It is clear that EGFR TKIs provide superior radiographic RRs and PFS compared with conventional chemotherapy in patients with tumors harboring activating *EGFR* mutations (Table 7-9). Although no survival benefit has been observed in randomized studies, this has been postulated to be a result of crossover of patients on the chemotherapy arm to the EGFR TKI arm on progression. Importantly, clinicopathologic features appear insufficient to predict the presence of *EGFR* mutations. In the Iressa Pan-Asian Survival Study (IPASS) trial, only 60% of East Asian patients with adenocarcinoma who were never or former light smokers had *EGFR* mutations.[95] It should be noted that despite the emphasis on use of EGFR TKIs in *EGFR*-mutated cancers, randomized studies such as BR.21 have demonstrated benefit in PFS and OS in an unselected patient population in the second- and third-line settings.[70]

Afatinib is an irreversible EGFR inhibitor and an HER2 inhibitor recently approved by the FDA for first-line treatment of patients with metastatic NSCLC with tumors harboring *EGFR*-activating mutations.[119] Approval was based on afatinib improving median PFS compared to cisplatin/pemetrexed in patients with NSCLC with *EGFR*-mutated tumors (median PFS: 11.1 vs. 6.9 months; HR = 0.58, p < 0.001). Despite an initial dramatic response to EGFR inhibitors in patients with *EGFR*-mutated NSCLC, resistance generally develops 9 to 18 months later. Approximately one-half of these cases are associated with a secondary *T790M* mutation, which results in steric hindrance to EGFR TKI binding (analogous to the *T315I* mutation in chronic myeloid leukemia) and altered ATP handling.[120,121] Additional cases with secondary resistance appear because of overexpression of c-Met, a receptor tyrosine kinase that activates downstream components of the EGFR signal transduction cascade ("molecular crosstalk").[122] A subset of *EGFR*-mutated tumors can become resistant to EGFR TKI therapy by transforming into small cell lung cancer histology and may respond to small cell lung cancer type regimens.[123] Mutations in *PI3KCA* and HER2 amplification have also been implicated as resistance mechanisms. Therapeutic strategies to overcome these processes, including irreversible EGFR inhibitors and novel combination regimens, remain under investigation.

Although EGFR inhibitors improve PFS as first-line therapy for patients with tumors harboring activating *EGFR* mutations, it has not been shown that the order in which these patients receive EGFR inhibitors affects OS. In the IPASS trial, the gefitinib arm had clinically and significantly longer PFS as compared with the carboplatin/paclitaxel arm in *EGFR*-mutated tumors. Presumably because of the high proportion of crossover to gefitinib in the carboplatin/paclitaxel arm, there was no significant difference in OS. Similarly, a registry study of *EGFR*-mutated NSCLC from Spain has demonstrated no difference in OS between first- or second-line administration of EGFR inhibitors.[124] In the Northeast Japan Study Group 002 trial, 200 patients with *EGFR*-mutated tumors were randomly

assigned to carboplatin/paclitaxel or gefitinib. Gefitinib yielded superior PFS (10.8 vs. 5.4 months; HR 0.3, 95% CI 0.22, 0.41; p < 0.001) and radiographic RR (74% vs. 31%; p < 0.001). Although there was a numerical improvement in median OS (30.5 vs. 23.6 months), it was not statistically significant (p = 0.31).[125] A key observation from the IPASS trial is that, in patients with *EGFR* wild-type tumors, PFS with gefitinib in the first-line setting is substantially inferior to those with chemotherapy (HR 2.85, 95% CI 2.05, 3.98; p < 0.001), which is not the case in the second-line setting. A clinical trial in a predominantly European population that compared erlotinib to cisplatin-based doublet chemotherapy also showed much higher RRs and median PFS in patients with metastatic lung cancers harboring *EGFR* mutations (RR 58% vs. 15%, median PFS 9.7 vs. 5.2 months; p < 0.0001).[126]

Results combining EGFR inhibitors with cytotoxic chemotherapy are mixed. Four randomized trials (Iressa NSCLC Trial Assessing Combination Treatment [INTACT]-1, INTACT-2, Tarceva Lung Cancer Investigation [TALENT] and Tarceva Responses in Conjunction with Paclitaxel and Carboplatin [TRIBUTE]) failed to demonstrate a survival benefit, an outcome that has been attributed to enrollment of an unselected population and to potential pharmacodynamic interference between cytostatic EGFR TKIs and cell cycle–dependent chemotherapeutic agents.[127] Achieving pharmacodynamic separation by sequencing treatment to prevent G1-cell cycle arrest via EGFR inhibition from interfering with optimal chemotherapy effect was recently tested in the FASTACT-2 trial. In a predominantly Asian population enriched for *EGFR*-activating mutations, combination platinum and gemcitabine was intercalated separately from erlotinib. Compared to platinum/gemcitabine alone, this combination yielded improved PFS and OS (7.6 vs. 6 months, p < 0.0001; 18.3 vs. 15.2 months, p = 0.042). Patient benefit was primarily restricted to patients with tumors harboring *EGFR*-activating mutations (PFS 16.8 vs. 6.9 months, p < 0.0001) and OS (31.4 vs. 20.6 months, p = 0.009).[128]

In contrast to EGFR TKIs, the effect of anti-EGFR monoclonal antibodies in NSCLC does not appear to be associated with the presence of *EGFR* activating mutations. Nor is the effect associated with the presence of *KRAS* mutations, as has been shown in colorectal cancer.[129,130] Two phase III clinical trials incorporating anti-EGFR monoclonal antibodies have been performed. The BMS099 trial randomly assigned patients to platinum/taxane chemotherapy with or without cetuximab.[131] No difference in OS was noted. The First-line in Lung Cancer with Erbitux (FLEX) trial randomly assigned patients to cisplatin/vinorelbine with or without cetuximab.[132] The cetuximab-containing arm demonstrated a statistically significant improvement in OS (HR 0.87, 95% CI 0.76, 0.99; p = 0.04), with an increase in median OS from 10.1 months to 11.3 months. Whether differences in the chemotherapy regimen, geographic setting, or inclusion criteria (FLEX mandated *EGFR*-positive tumors, defined as at least one cell staining positive by IHC) underlie the different results of the BMS099 and FLEX trials is not known.

Table 7-9 Selected Phase III Trials of Epidermal Growth Factor Receptor (EGFR) Inhibitors for Non-Small Cell Lung Cancer (NSCLC)

Trial	Population	Line of Therapy	Treatment	Number of Patients	Primary Outcome(s)
RADIANT	*EGFR* FISH-positive stage IB-IIIA	Adjuvant	Adjuvant erlotinib × 2 yrs vs. placebo	973	DFS: 50.5 mos (EGFR FISH+ erlotinib) vs. 48.2 mos (placebo) (p = 0.32); 46.4 (EGFR-mut+ subset erlotinib) vs. 28.5 mos (placebo) (p = 0.039; not significant due to hierarchical testing)
NCI-C JBR.10[205]	Unselected stage IB-IIIA	Adjuvant	Adjuvant gefitinib vs. placebo	Closed after 500 (of 1,200 planned)	OS median survival: 5.1 yrs (gefitinib) vs. not reached (placebo) (p = 0.136)
Rigas et al.[206]	Unselected, unresectable stage III	Stage III maintenance	Chemoradiation (cisplatin/docetaxel) ± maintenance erlotinib	253	PFS: 13.5 mos (erlotinib) vs. 10.4 mos (placebo) (p = 0.12)
SWOG 0023[110]	Unselected, unresectable stage III	Stage III maintenance	Chemoradiation (cisplatin/etoposide) then consolidation docetaxel ± maintenance gefitinib	Closed after 243 (of 672 planned)	OS: 23 mos (gefitinib) vs. 35 mos (placebo) (p = 0.01)
RTOG 0617	Unselected, unresectable stage III	Stage III	Chemoradiation (carboplatin/paclitaxel) ± cetuximab	465	OS: 23.1 mos (cetuximab) vs. 23.5 mos (placebo) (p = 0.484)
TALENT[207]	Unselected stage IIIB-IV	First-line metastatic	Cisplatin/gemcitabine ± erlotinib	1,172	OS: 10.8 mos (chemo plus erlotinib) vs. 11.0 mos (chemo alone) (p = 0.49)
TRIBUTE[208]	Unselected stage IIIB-IV	First-line metastatic	Carboplatin/paclitaxel ± erlotinib	1,059	OS: 10.6 mos (erlotinib) vs. 10.5 mos (placebo) (p = 0.95)
INTACT-1[209]	Unselected stage IIIB-IV	First-line metastatic	Cisplatin/gemcitabine ± gefitinib	1,093	OS: 9.9 mos (gefitinib 500 mg/d) vs. 9.9 mos (gefitinib 250 mg/d) vs. 10.9 mos (placebo) (p = 0.46)
INTACT-2[210]	Unselected stage IIIB-IV	First-line metastatic	Carboplatin/paclitaxel ± gefitinib	1,037	OS: 8.7 mos (gefitinib 500 mg/d) vs. 9.8 mos (gefitinib 250 mg/d) vs. 9.9 mos (placebo) (p = 0.64)
IPASS[160]	East Asian nonsmokers or former light smokers with stage IIIB-IV adenocarcinoma	First-line metastatic	Gefitinib vs. carboplatin/paclitaxel	1,217	12-mo PFS: 24.9% (gefitinib) vs. 6.7% (carboplatin/paclitaxel) (p < 0.001)
WJTOG3405[211]	Stage IIIB-IV with *EGFR* mutations in Japan	First-line metastatic	Gefitinib vs. cisplatin/docetaxel	172	PFS: 9.2 mos (gefitinib) vs. 6.3 mos (cisplatin/docetaxel) (p < 0.001)
First-SIGNAL[212]	Korean never-smokers with IIIB-IV	First-line metastatic	Gefitinib vs. cisplatin/gemcitabine	313	OS: 20.3 mos (gefitinib) vs. 23.1 mos (cisplatin/gemcitabine) (p = 0.43)
NEJ002[125]	Stage IIIB-IV with *EGFR* mutations in Japan	First-line metastatic	Gefitinib vs. carboplatin/paclitaxel	200	PFS: 10.4 mos (gefitinib) vs. 5.5 mos (carboplatin/paclitaxel) (p < 0.001)
OPTIMAL[213]	Stage IIIB/IV with *EGFR* mutations in China	First-line metastatic	Erlotinib vs. gemcitabine/carboplatin	165	PFS: 13.1 mos (erlotinib) vs. 4.6 mos (gemcitabine/carboplatin) (p < 0.0001)

Table 7-9 **(continued)**

Trial	Population	Line of Therapy	Treatment	Number of Patients	Primary Outcome(s)
FLEX[132]	*EGFR*-positive stage IIIB-IV	First-line metastatic	Cisplatin/vinorelbine ± cetuximab	1,125	OS: 11.3 mos (chemo plus cetuximab) vs. 10.1 mos (chemo alone) (p = 0.04)
BMS099[131]	Unselected stage IIIB-IV	First-line metastatic	Carboplatin/taxane ± cetuximab	676	PFS: 4.4 mos (chemo plus cetuximab) vs. 4.2 mos (chemo alone) (p = 0.24) [Secondary endpoint, OS: 9.7 mos (chemo plus cetuximab) vs. 8.4 mos (chemo alone) (p = 0.17)]
SATURN[214]	Unselected stage IIIB-IV	First-line maintenance	4 cycles platinum doublet chemotherapy followed by maintenance erlotinib vs. placebo	889	6-mo PFS: 31% vs. 17% (p < 0.0001) [Secondary endpoint, OS: 12 mos (erlotinib) vs. 11 mos (placebo) (p < 0.05)]
ATLAS[215]	Non-squamous stage IIIB-IV	First-line maintenance	4 cycles platinum doublet chemotherapy followed by maintenance bevacizumab ± erlotinib	768	PFS: 4.8 mos (bevacizumab + erlotinib) vs. 3.7 mos (bevacizumab alone) (p = 0.001)
BR21[70]	Unselected stage IIIB-IV	Second- and third-line	Erlotinib vs. placebo	731	OS: 6.7 mos (erlotinib) vs. 4.7 mos (placebo) (p < 0.001)
ISEL[216]	Unselected stage IIIB-IV	Second-line	Gefitinib vs. placebo	1,692	OS: 5.6 mos (gefitinib) vs. 5.1 mos (placebo) (p = 0.09)
INTEREST[162]	Unselected stage IIIB-IV	Second-line	Gefitinib vs. docetaxel	1,466	OS: 7.6 mos (gefitinib) vs. 8.0 mos (docetaxel) (p > 0.05)
EURTAC[126]	Stage IV *EGFR*-mutation positive in Europe	First-line metastatic	Erlotinib vs. carboplatin/docetaxel or carboplatin/gemcitabine	174	PFS: 9.7 vs. 5.2 mos (p < 0.0001)

Abbreviations: BMS, Bristol-Myers Squibb; BR, Bronchus; chemo, chemotherapy; d, day; DFS, disease-free survival; First-SIGNAL, First-line Single agent Iressa versus Gemcitabine and cisplatin Trial in Never-smokers with Adenocarcinoma of the Lung; FLEX, First-line in Lung cancer with ErbituX; INTACT, Iressa NSCLC Trial Assessing Combination Treatment; INTEREST, Iressa NSCLC Trial Evaluating Response and Survival versus Taxotere; IPASS, Iressa Pan-Asia Study; ISEL, Iressa Survival Evaluation in Lung Cancer; mos, months; NCI-C, National Cancer Institute of Cancer; NEJ, North-East Japan; OS, overall survival; PFS, progression-free survival; RTOG, Radiation Therapy Oncology Group; SATURN, Sequential Tarceva in Unresectable NSCLC; SWOG, Southwest Oncology Group; TALENT, Tarceva Lung Cancer Investigation; TRIBUTE, Tarceva Responses in Conjunction with Paclitaxel and Carboplatin; WJTOG, West Japan Thoracic Oncology Group; yrs, years.

Crizotinib. In 2011, the FDA approved the ALK inhibitor crizotinib for the treatment of NSCLC harboring *EML4-ALK* fusions. The efficacy of crizotinib in *ALK*-positive NSCLC was initially seen in an expanded cohort of a multicenter phase I study.[133] Tumor specimens from approximately 1,500 patients with advanced NSCLC were screened for *ALK* translocations. A total of 82 patients, most of whom were treated previously, were enrolled. The radiographic RR was 57% and stable disease was 33%, yielding a clinical benefit rate of 90%. The estimated 6-month PFS rate was 72%. A retrospective analysis looked at outcomes of 82 patients who were *ALK*-positive and given crizotinib and compared them with 23 control patients who were *ALK*-positive (who did not receive crizotinib). Survival of 30 patients who were *ALK*-positive and given crizotinib in the second- or third-line setting was significantly longer than in 23 control patients who were *ALK*-positive and given any second-line therapy other

than crizotinib (median OS, not reached vs. 6 months; 1-year OS, 70% vs. 44%; and 2-year OS, 55% vs. 12%; p = 0.004).[134] A phase III clinical trial (PROFILE 1007) confirmed that crizotinib had a higher RR and PFS compared to investigators' choice of docetaxel or pemetrexed in patients with *ALK*-positive tumors whose disease progressed after first-line chemotherapy (overall RR 65% vs. 20%, median PFS, 7.7 vs. 3 months; p < 0.0001).[135] Results of an ongoing clinical trial (PROFILE 1014) comparing crizotinib to platinum/pemetrexed as first-line therapy for these patients are eagerly anticipated. It should be noted that FDA approval for crizotinib in *ALK*-rearranged NSCLC does not specify the line of treatment. A high RR in patients with NSCLC harboring a *ROS1* gene rearrangement (which shows sequence homology to *ALK*) has also been observed in clinical trials.[35]

In patients with tumors harboring *ALK* translocations or *EGFR* mutations treated with TKIs, occasionally progression occurs in limited sites, such as the CNS, while the remainder of the cancer remains controlled (oligoprogressive disease). In these situations, irradiating the site of progression, or resecting isolated brain metastasis, for example, and then continuing the TKI may result in a lengthening of clinical benefit.[136]

Older Patients. Treatment of patients 65 or older tends to be complicated by comorbid conditions and by patients taking multiple medications. However, studies show that fit older patients are likely to benefit as much from chemotherapy as their younger counterparts. Evidence from a phase III study in which patients older than 70 with advanced disease were randomly assigned to best supportive care or to weekly vinorelbine indicated that patients who received vinorelbine had better scores on quality-of-life scales than the control group, as well as fewer lung cancer–related symptoms; however, patients in the chemotherapy group experienced more severe toxicity-related symptoms.[137] There was a significant survival advantage for patients who received vinorelbine (median survival, 28 vs. 21 weeks). More recently, it has been shown that, despite increased toxicities, platinum-based doublet chemotherapy yields superior outcomes to single-agent chemotherapy in fit elderly individuals. In a phase III trial conducted by the Intergroupe Francophone de Cancérologie Thoracique, 451 previously untreated patients ages 70 to 89 (median 77) with ECOG PS of 0 to 2 were randomly assigned to carboplatin/paclitaxel or monotherapy with vinorelbine or gemcitabine. Twenty-seven percent of patients in each arm had an ECOG status of 2. Median OS was 10.3 months in the carboplatin/paclitaxel arm compared with 6.2 months in the monotherapy arm (HR 0.64, 95% CI 0.62, 0.78; p < 0.0001).[138] Subset analyses of other randomized trials show that the RR, toxicity, and survival for fit older patients receiving a platinum-based treatment for NSCLC appear to be similar to the same variables for younger patients; however, for patients 70 or older, comorbidity is greater and the frequency of leukopenia and neuropsychiatric toxicity are higher. Hence, advanced age alone should not preclude appropriate treatment.

Patients with Poor PS. The survival rates for patients with a poor PS (ECOG PS of 2, 3, or 4) are significantly shorter than the rates for patients with a good PS. Patients with a poor PS also are less likely to be able to tolerate treatment. Retrospective subset analyses suggest that patients with a PS of 2 may derive a modest benefit from chemotherapy. However, given the overall short survival—particularly for patients with a PS of 3 or 4—and the minimal benefit derived from chemotherapy, these patients probably should not be treated outside of a clinical study. A possible exception is patients with tumors harboring activating *EGFR* mutations or ALK fusion proteins, especially if poor PS is a result of the lung cancer. In general, EGFR and ALK inhibitors may be better tolerated than conventional chemotherapy and, in these patients, may result in rapid clinical and radiographic responses.

A recent clinical trial compared carboplatin (AUC 5) and pemetrexed to pemetrexed alone in patients with stage IV NSCLC with a Zubrod PS of 2. A substantial improvement in median OS with the combination compared to pemetrexed was observed (9.3 vs. 5.3 months; p = 0.001).[139]

Duration of Therapy and Maintenance Therapy. The role of maintenance treatment for patients with metastatic NSCLC remains under active investigation. Although results from earlier randomized studies did not show a survival difference with prolonged (more than six) cycles of chemotherapy compared with fewer (four to six) cycles (Table 7-10),[140,141] several more recent clinical trials challenged that paradigm. Two maintenance strategies have been investigated: so-called switch maintenance and continuation maintenance. The goal of continuation maintenance is to delay progressive disease by continuing an effective agent. Switch maintenance seeks to initiate a new second-line agent early to delay onset of progressive disease.

Three trials have been reported that suggest a benefit with prolonged-duration therapy.[142-144] In one study, patients who had stable or responding disease following their initial four cycles of gemcitabine/carboplatin were randomly assigned to receive maintenance docetaxel immediately following induction chemotherapy or at progression.[142] Median PFS for immediate docetaxel was significantly greater than for delayed docetaxel (5.7 vs. 2.7 months; p = 0.0001). Median OS for immediate docetaxel also was greater than for delayed docetaxel, although the difference was not significant (12.3 vs. 9.7 months; p = 0.0853). Interestingly, median OS for patients assigned to immediate docetaxel and those patients assigned to delayed docetaxel who received the specified therapy at the time of progression was identical. These findings raise the question of whether switch maintenance therapy may actually be similar to early use of second-line therapy at first sign of progressive disease. A second study investigating switch maintenance pemetrexed employed a slightly different trial design.[143] Six hundred thirty-three patients with stable or responding disease were randomly assigned in a 2:1 fashion to observation or pemetrexed following induction chemotherapy with platinum-based chemotherapy. Pemetrexed resulted in significantly better survival (13.4 vs. 10.6 months; HR 0.79, 95% CI 0.65, 0.95; p = 0.012) and PFS. The improvement in survival was observed primarily in patients with nonsquamous histology (15.5 vs. 10.3 months; OS HR 0.70; it was not the primary endpoint, but it was a preplanned secondary analysis). A third phase III study has examined the role of erlotinib maintenance therapy.[144] In the Sequential Tarceva in Unresectable NSCLC (SATURN) trial, 889 patients whose disease did not progress during first-line platinum-based chemotherapy were randomly assigned to erlotinib or placebo. There was a statistically significant improvement in PFS (HR 0.71, 95% CI 0.62, 0.82; p < 0.001) and OS (HR 0.81, 95% CI 0.70, 0.95; p = 0.009), with a median OS of 12 months (erlotinib) compared with 11 months (placebo).

Table 7-10 Selected Randomized Trials of Maintenance Therapy for Advanced Non-Small Cell Lung Cancer

Authors	Treatment Comparison	Type of Trial	Median Survival (months)	1-Year Survival (%)	p
Westeel et al.[140]	6 months of vinorelbine	Switch maintenance	13	53	Not significant
	Best supportive care		10	40	
Socinski et al.[141]	Four cycles of carboplatin plus paclitaxel	Continuation maintenance	7	28	Not significant
	Carboplatin plus paclitaxel until disease progression		9	35	
Smith et al.[217]	Three cycles of mitomycin-C, vindesine, and cisplatin	3 cycles vs. 6 cycles	6	22	Not significant
	Six cycles of same regimen		7	25	
Fidias et al.[142]	Four cycles of gemcitabine plus carboplatin, with docetaxel on disease progression	Switch maintenance	9.1	38	Not significant
	Four cycles of gemcitabine plus carboplatin, followed immediately by docetaxel for six cycles		11.9	48.5	
Ciuleanu et al.[143]	Four cycles of platinum-based therapy, followed by placebo	Switch maintenance	10.6		0.012
	Four cycles of platinum-based therapy, followed by pemetrexed		13		
Cappuzzo et al.[144]	Four cycles of platinum-based therapy, followed by placebo	Switch maintenance	11		0.0088
	Four cycles of platinum-based therapy, followed by erlotinib		12		
Paz-Ares et al.[145]	Four cycles of cisplatin and pemetrexed, followed by placebo	Continuation maintenance	11		0.0195
	Four cycles of cisplatin and pemetrexed, followed by pemetrexed		13.9		

A recently published phase III clinical trial (PARAMOUNT) randomly assigned patients with advanced nonsquamous NSCLC to four cycles of cisplatin and pemetrexed followed by observation versus continuation maintenance pemetrexed every 3 weeks until progression or intolerable toxicity. Continuation pemetrexed improved PFS, with a median PFS of 4.4 months compared with 2.8 months (HR 0.62, 95% CI 0.49, 0.79; p < 0.0001), and OS, with a median OS of 16.9 months compared with 14.0 months from induction (HR, 0.78; 95% CI 0.64, 0.96; p = 0.0195).[145]

Currently, switch-maintenance therapy with pemetrexed or erlotinib is FDA-approved, as is continuation maintenance with pemetrexed. This new treatment paradigm has raised many questions, including whether the apparent benefit is a result of the timing of therapy or rather higher rates of administering effective second-line agents, and how maintenance strategies should be implemented for patients receiving pemetrexed- or bevacizumab-containing first-line regimens. Several recently completed randomized studies examining these questions should help clarify these issues.

Number of Drugs. Although findings from numerous phase I and II studies have demonstrated the feasibility of triplet combinations, the results of most randomized trials have not demonstrated a survival advantage and have been at the expense of enhanced toxicity and cost. Thus, regimens that employ three cytotoxic drugs cannot be routinely recommended for patients with advanced NSCLC.

In randomized studies, single-agent paclitaxel, gemcitabine, or docetaxel was compared with double-agent cisplatin plus paclitaxel, gemcitabine, or docetaxel.[146-153] Findings from all of these trials showed a survival advantage for the two-drug regimens. These results can be interpreted either as demonstrating the advantages of cisplatin for the treatment of advanced

NSCLC or as evidence of the superiority of doublet compared with single-agent therapy.

Cisplatin versus Carboplatin. Meta-analyses have suggested that cisplatin may have a modest benefit in terms of survival compared with carboplatin for patients with advanced disease, albeit with a different toxicity profile.[154,155] In one direct comparison, a phase III trial of the Spanish Lung Cancer Group randomly assigned patients to receive either paclitaxel with cisplatin or carboplatin. Efficacy endpoints showed superiority of the cisplatin-based regimen with about a 1-month improvement in OS.[90] Although this difference may be of limited clinical consequence for patients with metastatic disease, it may be more important in the adjuvant setting where cure is the goal. In metastatic, incurable disease, carboplatin is acceptable as the toxicity profile of cisplatin with higher rates of renal insufficiency, neuropathy, and hearing loss that may impact quality of life.

Nonplatinum-based Regimens. Given the toxicities associated with cisplatin, there has been considerable interest in utilizing nonplatinum agents. In general, randomized studies have failed to show superiority of any nonplatinum regimen compared with platinum-based, third-generation regimens, although toxicities vary.[156] Consequently, nonplatinum regimens are uncommonly used in current practice.

KEY POINTS

- Cytotoxic chemotherapy improves survival and symptomatology for patients with metastatic NSCLC.
- Platinum-based doublet chemotherapy is considered standard of care and typically administered for four to six cycles for patients with good performance status (PS).
- Bevacizumab (15 mg/kg every 3 weeks) prolongs survival when administered with carboplatin/paclitaxel in eligible patients with advanced nonsquamous cell carcinoma in a large randomized trial.
- Fit elderly patients tolerate chemotherapy and derive the same survival benefit as their younger counterparts.
- Patients with advanced NSCLC with Zubrod PS 2 should be considered for carboplatin-based doublet chemotherapy.
- EGFR inhibitors should be considered standard of care in the first-line setting for patients with tumors harboring *EGFR*-activating mutations. Crizotinib is approved for the treatment of patients with *ALK*-positive NSCLC, regardless of the line of therapy.
- Maintenance therapy is an option to be discussed with patients with good progression-free survival who have had stable or responding disease to first-line doublet chemotherapy.

Second- and Third-Line Therapy

Currently, three agents—docetaxel, pemetrexed, and erlotinib—are approved for second-line therapy for advanced NSCLC. In two randomized trials, second-line docetaxel was evaluated for patients whose disease did not respond to first-line therapy. In one trial, docetaxel at a dose of 75 mg/m^2 significantly prolonged survival compared with best supportive care.[157] Although this dose of docetaxel resulted in an RR of only 7%, improved time to disease progression and survival was seen for patients treated with docetaxel. Moreover, docetaxel also improved quality of life and reduced weight loss and the need for pain medications. Previous exposure to paclitaxel did not affect response to docetaxel, suggesting non–cross-resistance between the two agents. In the second study, docetaxel was compared with either vinorelbine or ifosfamide.[158] Although OS was not significantly different among the three groups, the 1-year survival associated with docetaxel was significantly better than that associated with the control treatment (32% vs. 19%; p = 0.025).

A phase III study compared pemetrexed with docetaxel.[159] Although no difference in survival was observed (1-year survival of 29.7% in both arms), patients randomly assigned to receive docetaxel were more likely to have febrile neutropenia (12.7% vs. 1.9%; p = 0.001), infections (3.3% vs. 0%; p = 0.004), and hospitalizations for neutropenic fevers (13.4% vs. 1.5%; p = 0.001) than patients who received pemetrexed, resulting in the FDA's approval of pemetrexed as second-line therapy for NSCLC.

Erlotinib was approved in the United States for patients with NSCLC whose disease did not respond to taxane- and platinum-based treatment, based in large part on a randomized, placebo-controlled, double-blinded clinical trial conducted by the NCI-C (BR21). In BR21, patients with stage IIIB or IV NSCLC and a PS of 0 to 3 who had received one or two prior chemotherapy regimens were randomly assigned in a 2:1 ratio to receive either 150 mg of oral erlotinib daily or placebo.[160] Median survival rates were 6.7 months and 4.7 months for erlotinib and placebo, respectively (HR 0.70; p < 0.001). The only predictive factor to survival benefit was smoking status, where current or former smokers had an HR of 0.9, and never-smokers had an HR of 0.4.

As discussed earlier, the optimal use of EGFR testing and the optimal administration of EGFR inhibitors remain areas of active investigation. The following points may be taken into consideration: in unselected patient populations, EGFR TKIs provide a survival benefit in second- and third-line therapy[70]; even in highly clinically enriched populations, *EGFR* mutations occur in only about 60% of patients, and *EGFR* mutations occur in up to 10% of patients lacking typical clinical predictors[160,161]; in patients with tumors harboring *EGFR* mutations, PFS is similar if an EGFR TKI is administered as first-, second-, or third-line therapy[124]; in the first-line setting, patients with *EGFR* wild-type tumors have superior PFS with conventional chemotherapy compared with EGFR TKIs[160]; and in the second-line setting, patients with *EGFR* wild-type tumors have similar outcomes with conventional chemotherapy and with

EGFR TKIs.[162] EGFR TKIs are generally well tolerated, with rash and diarrhea the principal toxicities. Interstitial pneumonitis occurs rarely in North American and western European populations.

ISOLATED BRAIN METASTASES

For patients with controlled disease outside of the brain who have an isolated cerebral metastasis in a resectable area, resection followed by whole-brain radiation therapy is superior to whole-brain radiation therapy alone and may improve survival. Another therapeutic option for tumors smaller than 3 cm in diameter is stereotactic radiosurgery, which uses a stereotactic fixation system and noncoplanar convergent beams that create a sharp peripheral dose fall-off along the edge of the target. Stereotactic radiosurgery spares the surrounding normal tissue, enabling the use of a single, large fraction of radiation. Survival is improved when administered with whole-brain radiation therapy.

PARANEOPLASTIC SYNDROMES

Humoral-associated hypercalcemia is most commonly associated with squamous cell cancers and least commonly with small cell lung cancer. Manifestations of hypercalcemia depend more on the rate of onset than on the degree of elevation and include mental status changes, polydipsia, gastrointestinal complaints, and nephrolithiasis. In addition to treatment of the malignancy, treatment includes intravenous hydration, administration of bisphosphonates, and calcitonin. Use of diuretics, which may exacerbate volume depletion, is discouraged. Hypertrophic pulmonary osteoarthropathy is characterized by clubbing of the digits and, when severe, painful periostitis of the long bones. Hypertrophic pulmonary osteoarthropathy is most common with adenocarcinoma, although it is not pathognomonic for cancer; it may also occur with other pulmonary diseases.

SMALL CELL LUNG CANCER

STAGING

Small cell lung cancer is usually classified as either limited or extensive stage because of the propensity of small cell lung cancer to metastasize quickly and the fact that micrometastatic disease is presumed to be present in all patients at diagnosis. Limited-stage disease is typically defined as being encompassed within one radiation port and is usually limited to the hemithorax and to regional nodes, including mediastinal and ipsilateral supraclavicular nodes. Extensive-stage disease is usually defined as disease that has spread outside those areas. Although small cell lung cancer is typically staged by the Veterans Administration staging system of limited versus extensive disease, current guidelines also recommend staging by the usual AJCC TNM staging system.

PROGNOSTIC FACTORS

As with NSCLC, the major pretreatment prognostic factors are stage of disease, PS, serum lactate dehydrogenase, and sex. If the patient's initial poor PS is the result of the underlying malignant disease, symptoms often disappear quickly with treatment, resulting in a net improvement in quality of life. However, major organ dysfunction from nonmalignant causes often results in an inability of the patient to tolerate chemotherapy.

PRETREATMENT EVALUATION

Common sites of metastases include the brain, liver, bone marrow, bone, and CNS. For this reason, a complete staging work-up consists of a complete blood cell count, liver function tests, CT with contrast of chest and upper abdomen, CT or MRI of the brain, and consideration of PET or bone scan. Bone marrow aspirate is not recommended unless an otherwise unexplained hematologic abnormality is present (e.g., nucleated red blood cells are seen on peripheral blood smear, neutropenia, thrombocytopenia).

This complete work-up should probably not be undertaken unless the patient is a candidate for combined-modality treatment with chest radiation and chemotherapy, the patient is being evaluated for a clinical study, or the information is helpful for prognostic reasons. If the patient is not a candidate for combined-modality treatment or a clinical study, it is usually appropriate to stop the staging at the first evidence of extensive-stage disease. In addition, because the chance of metastases to the bone marrow only is less than 10%, biopsy of bone marrow is usually unnecessary except in certain cases of limited-stage disease where demonstration of localized disease may be important for prognostic or psychosocial reasons or for clinical trial eligibility. A PET scan can provide useful information and can replace the bone scan.

TREATMENT

The cornerstone of treatment for patients with small cell lung cancer is combination platinum-based chemotherapy. Until recently, no clear survival advantage was demonstrated for any regimen. With standard chemotherapy—etoposide with either cisplatin or carboplatin—an overall RR of 75% to 90% and a complete RR of 50% for localized disease can be anticipated. For extensive-stage disease, an overall RR of approximately 50% and a complete or near-complete RR of approximately 25% are common. Tumor regressions usually occur quickly, often within the first two cycles of treatment, and provide rapid palliation of tumor-related symptoms. Despite these high RRs, median survival time remains approximately 14 months for limited-stage disease and 9 months for extensive-stage disease. Less than 5% of patients with extensive-stage disease survive more than 2 years. Although initial results of irinotecan plus cisplatin showed improved survival (compared with etoposide plus cisplatin) in a Japanese population, these results were not confirmed in U.S. studies.[163,164]

Dose Intensity. Dose intensity has been evaluated in a number of randomized studies. Most—although not all—failed to show a benefit in survival, regardless of whether the chemotherapy was delivered in higher doses or more frequently (dose density). In addition, a meta-analysis of chemotherapy dose intensity for small cell lung cancer in which doses not requiring bone marrow transplantation support were evaluated showed no consistent correlation between dose intensity and outcome.[165] The role of marrow-ablative doses of chemotherapy with subsequent progenitor cell replacement (e.g., autologous bone marrow transplantation) was evaluated in several phase I and II clinical trials, and results for survival were not promising. In a randomized phase III study comparing high-dose chemotherapy with conventional-dose chemotherapy,

the high-dose regimen with stem cell support prolonged relapse-free survival but not OS.[166]

Duration and Maintenance of Therapy. The findings from most randomized studies do not show a survival benefit for prolonged administration of chemotherapy or for consolidation chemotherapy. The results of several randomized studies have demonstrated no survival benefit for prolonged first-line treatment when compared with treatment initiated on relapse. The optimal duration of treatment for patients with small cell lung cancer is four to six cycles.

Second-Line Therapy. The chance of response to second-line agents correlates with when the relapse occurred following induction chemotherapy; patients who experience relapse more than 3 months after completing first-line chemotherapy are considered to have sensitive disease and are more likely to have a response than patients who experience disease progression during or within 2 to 3 months after receiving a first-line regimen (resistant disease). The only drug approved for second-line therapy for small cell lung cancer in the United States is topotecan, which is associated with a 20% to 40% RR for patients with sensitive disease and with a median survival of 22 to 27 weeks.[167] A phase III trial comparing the novel anthracycline amrubicin to topotecan as second-line treatment of small cell lung cancer showed no difference in OS, although PFS was modestly superior.[168] Temozolomide also has modest activity in second- or third-line treatment of extensive-stage small cell lung cancer, including patients with platinum-refractory disease and brain metastases. As in glioma, tumor *MGMT* methylation status may predict benefit.[169] For patients with refractory disease, the RR in phase II studies has ranged from 3% to 13%. Median survival is approximately 20 weeks. Patients with platinum-sensitive disease also may have a response to repeat treatment with the first-line regimen. Other drugs that have modest activity in phase II studies in the second-line setting include combination cyclophosphamide, doxorubicin, vincristine, and single-agent paclitaxel.

Older Patients. As is the case with NSCLC, treatment of older patients is often complicated by poor PS and comorbid conditions. However, unlike older patients with NSCLC, older patients with small cell lung cancer may not benefit from single-agent therapy. Two randomized studies in which single-agent etoposide was compared with standard combination chemotherapy were stopped early because the single-agent arm was associated with a shorter median and long-term survival and a decreased quality of life.[170,171] Therefore, the standard treatment of fit older patients remains combination chemotherapy administered on a 3-week schedule.

Chemotherapy Plus Radiation to the Thorax. Radiation therapy to the thorax in addition to chemotherapy is associated with a small but significant improvement in long-term survival for patients with limited-stage disease, providing an additional 5% improvement in 3-year survival compared with chemotherapy alone.[172] Chemotherapy given concurrently with thoracic radiation is superior to sequential chemoradiation in terms of survival; however, it is associated with substantially more esophagitis and hematologic toxicity. To decrease the morbidity associated with such treatment, as well as to improve overall outcome, investigative efforts have focused on optimizing the radiation fields, fractionation, and schedule. In one randomized study, twice-daily, hyperfractionated radiation was compared with a once-daily schedule; both were administered concurrently with four cycles of cisplatin and etoposide. Survival was significantly higher with the twice-daily regimen (median survival, 23 vs. 19 months; 5-year survival, 26% vs. 16%), albeit at the expense of more grade 3 esophagitis.[173] In another randomized trial, early administration of thoracic radiation as part of the combined-modality therapy for limited-stage disease was superior to late or consolidative thoracic radiation.[174] These data suggest that patients with good PS who have limited disease should receive concurrent chemoradiation, preferably administered twice daily in an accelerated, hyperfractionated approach. However, because of logistical considerations, once-daily radiation is the most commonly used treatment schedule in clinical practice.

Prophylactic Cranial Irradiation. Brain metastases are the first site of relapse for approximately one-third of patients who have relapsing small cell lung cancers. Another one-third of such patients will have both brain and systemic metastases as the first site of relapse; the remaining one-third will have systemic-only disease. Because of the morbidity associated with brain metastases, the role of prophylactic cranial irradiation has been studied in numerous randomized trials. These findings have generally demonstrated that prophylactic cranial irradiation decreases the risk of brain metastases by approximately one-half without enhanced neurotoxicities, including cognitive dysfunction, ataxia, and seizures. A meta-analysis of seven randomized trials concluded that prophylactic cranial irradiation increased 3-year survival, with a net gain of 5%.[175] Typically, in the United States, patients are administered 24 Gy in 12 fractions. However, the optimal dose and schedule are not clear; the meta-analysis demonstrated a trend toward improved control with higher doses.

Although prophylactic cranial irradiation had been typically reserved for patients with limited-stage disease for which a complete response is achieved with induction chemotherapy, a study from the EORTC showed a survival benefit for patients with extensive-stage disease who had a response to induction chemotherapy.[176] Patients with extensive-stage small cell lung cancer who had a response to chemotherapy were randomly assigned to undergo prophylactic cranial irradiation or no further therapy. Irradiation was associated with an increase in median OS from 5.4 months to 6.7 months and an improvement in the 1-year survival rate (27.1% vs. 13.3%) in the radiation group and control group, respectively, in addition to a lower risk of brain metastases (risk of metastases at 1 year, 14.6% vs. 40.4%). Thus, prophylactic cranial irradiation should be considered for all patients who have a complete or very good partial remission after induction therapy.

Treatment of Paraneoplastic Syndromes. In small cell lung cancer, the most common paraneoplastic syndrome is inappropriate secretion of antidiuretic hormone (SIADH), which occurs in up to 5% of patients. The hallmark of SIADH is euvolemic, hypotonic hyponatremia (in the absence of thyroid or adrenal dysfunction). Clinical features include confusion, seizures, and altered sensorium. In addition to treatment of the underlying malignancy, treatment includes fluid restriction, demeclocycline, and hypertonic saline in severe cases. Care must be taken to avoid overly rapid correction of hyponatremia, which could result in central pontine myelinolysis. Treatment of Lambert-Eaton syndrome and other neurologic paraneoplastic syndromes with corticosteroids, other immunosuppressive agents, intravenous gamma globulin, and plasmapheresis have been used with varying success as therapy.[67] Response to edrophonium is poor.[177]

PALLIATION FOR PATIENTS WITH LUNG CANCER

BISPHOSPHONATES

Bisphosphonates (zoledronate) have resulted in the reduction of skeletal-related complications such as pain, hypercalcemia, pathologic fractures, and spinal cord and nerve compression, as well as improvements in the quality of life for patients with metastatic bone disease who are likely to have a prolonged clinical course (Table 7-11).[178]

RANK-LIGAND INHIBITOR

The monoclonal antibody to receptor activator of nuclear kappa B (RANK) ligand denosumab was noninferior to zolendronate in delaying or preventing skeletal-related complications in patients with advanced cancer, including patients with lung cancer.[179] Incidence of osteonecrosis is similar to bisphosphonates.

RADIATION THERAPY

Palliative radiation therapy often is helpful for controlling pain related to bone metastases or for improving neurologic function for patients with brain metastases. Radiation therapy to the thorax may help control hemoptysis, superior vena cava syndrome, airway obstruction, laryngeal nerve compression, and other local complications.

CHEMOTHERAPY

Randomized trials involving patients with NSCLC and patients with small cell lung cancer have shown that chemotherapy reduces the incidence of cancer-related symptoms such as pain, cough, hemoptysis, and shortness of breath.

COLONY-STIMULATING FACTORS

Filgrastim, a granulocyte colony-stimulating factor, decreases the incidence of neutropenic fevers, the median duration of neutropenia, days of hospitalization, and days of antibiotic treatment for patients with extensive-stage small cell lung cancer. However, as discussed previously, the clinical benefit of maintaining a dose-intense approach for patients with

Table 7-11 Palliative Approaches for Complications of Lung Cancer	
Superior Vena Cava Syndrome	▪ Chemotherapy alone (mild symptoms) ▪ Concurrent chemoradiation therapy (severe symptoms) ▪ Radiation therapy to the thorax (patients with non-small cell lung cancer) ▪ Placement of stent
Pleural Effusion	▪ Intermittent thoracentesis ▪ Pleurodesis ▪ Long-term catheter drainage ▪ Systemic chemotherapy
Bronchial Obstruction	▪ High-dose endobronchial radiation therapy ▪ Placement of stent ▪ Nd-YAG endobronchial laser therapy ▪ Electrocautery ▪ Photodynamic therapy
Cachexia	▪ Megestrol acetate (160 mg to 800 mg daily)
Bone Metastases	▪ Bisphosphonates (zoledronate) ▪ RANK-ligand inhibitor (denosumab)
Brain Metastases	▪ Corticosteroids ▪ Resection or stereotactic radiation and whole-brain radiation (for isolated brain metastases for patients with non-small cell lung cancer) ▪ Whole-brain radiation therapy (for multiple metastases)

this disease has not been established. In addition, caution must be exercised when using myeloid growth factors for patients receiving combined-modality treatment that consists of both chemotherapy and radiation therapy to the thorax, as this combination has been associated with an increase in thrombocytopenia.[180]

SUPERIOR VENA CAVA SYNDROME

Superior vena cava syndrome occurs when the superior vena cava becomes obstructed either directly by a tumor or by metastases to regional lymph nodes. Common symptoms include distension of the collateral veins over the anterior chest wall and neck; swelling and puffiness of the neck, face, throat, eyes, and arms; headache; and cyanosis. Although once thought to represent a medical emergency, in almost all cases, the symptoms are mild enough that treatment can be delayed until a histologic diagnosis has been determined. Radiation therapy is used to treat patients with NSCLC or other less chemosensitive tumors, whereas patients with extensive-stage small cell lung cancer and mild symptoms often may be treated with chemotherapy alone. Concurrent

chemoradiation therapy usually is necessary for patients with both small cell lung cancer and NSCLC who present with severe symptoms. Other options include the placement of vascular stents, although the literature regarding their role is relatively sparse.

PLEURAL EFFUSION

Palliative thoracentesis should be performed for patients who are symptomatic from pleural effusions, and management with intermittent thoracentesis can frequently be effective if the effusion does not re-accumulate quickly. When re-accumulation is rapid, pleurodesis may be considered. The two most common methods of a pleurodesis are through a chest tube or via thoracoscopy. Common sclerosing agents include doxycycline, talc, and bleomycin; talc is the most effective. Unfortunately, the procedure is effective in only about 50% of cases and is associated with discomfort and a prolonged hospital stay. For these reasons, long-term drainage through a semi-permanent catheter is being used more frequently. Systemic chemotherapy often reduces the effusion for patients with small cell lung cancer.

KEY POINT

▪ Every attempt should be made to palliate the symptoms of patients with lung cancer. In addition to systemic anticancer therapies, these include multidisciplinary management of painful bone metastases, dyspnea caused by pleural effusions, and maintenance of adequate analgesia.

THYMIC MALIGNANCIES

The thymus contains two major cell populations: epithelial cells and lymphocytes. A number of different tumors can arise in the thymus, including thymomas, Hodgkin and non-Hodgkin lymphomas, carcinoid tumors, and germ-cell neoplasms. Thymomas are malignant neoplasms originating within the epithelial cells of the thymus, which often contain admixtures of lymphocytes.[181] Thymic cancers also are tumors of the thymic epithelium, but they are associated with a paucity of lymphocytes and are more aggressive.

Although some subtypes of thymoma may have more invasive potential, prognosis is more commonly associated with the invasiveness of the tumor. Most thymomas are well encapsulated, but they are considered malignant because of their invasive potential. Cytokeratin is a useful diagnostic marker to distinguish thymomas from non–epithelial cell malignancies.

Thymomas are the most common anterior mediastinal tumors in adults, representing approximately 20% to 30% of all anterior mediastinal tumors. Although they usually present in the fourth and fifth decades of life, cases have been reported from infancy into the ninth decade. At presentation, one-third of patients have an asymptomatic anterior mediastinal mass on chest x-ray; one-third have local symptoms such as cough, superior vena cava syndrome, and dysphagia; and one-third have myasthenia gravis. Distant metastases are uncommon, with the most common metastatic site being the pleura.

A number of paraneoplastic syndromes have been associated with thymomas. Myasthenia gravis—an autoimmune disorder caused by circulating acetylcholine-receptor antibodies resulting in acetylcholine-receptor deficiency at the motor end plate—occurs in approximately one-third of patients with thymoma, although it is rarely seen with thymic cancers. Surgical removal of all thymic tissue, not just tumor tissue, usually results in an attenuation of the severity of myasthenia gravis, although complete disappearance of all symptoms of the disorder is uncommon. Patients should have their serum anti-acetylcholine receptor antibody levels measured prior to surgery to determine whether they have myasthenia gravis (to avoid respiratory failure during surgery).

Approximately two-thirds of patients with myasthenia gravis will have thymic lymphoid hyperplasia, and 10% to 15% will have thymoma. Myasthenia gravis is characterized by diplopia, dysphagia, weakness of the ocular muscles, and easy limb fatigability (proximal > distal). Interestingly, thymomas associated with myasthenia gravis tend to be less aggressive, and histologically, they tend to have a larger lymphocyte-to-epithelial-cell ratio. Other paraneoplastic syndromes include pure red cell aplasia, vasculitides, as well as hypogammaglobulinemia and other autoimmune disorders. Thymectomy may result in normalization of the bone marrow for up to 40% of patients with pure red cell aplasia, although the procedure rarely results in a return to normal immunoglobulin levels for patients with immunodeficiency.

The Masaoka staging for thymoma is based on encapsulation of the tumor and invasion into surrounding organs and distant sites outside the chest (Table 7-12). Important prognostic factors include WHO histologic grade, complete resection status, and size.[181,182] Negative prognostic factors include:

- Tumor size greater than 10 cm
- Tracheal or vascular compromise
- Age younger than 30
- Presence of hematologic paraneoplastic syndromes
- Extent of the surgical resection

The treatment of choice for thymomas is resection. Long-term survival for patients with encapsulated, noninvasive (stage I) tumors is excellent, approaching 90% to 95% at 10 years. The role of postoperative radiation after an R0 resection is controversial, but sometimes employed for completely resected stage II to IV thymomas. Adjuvant PORT should be considered for all patients with invasive disease.[182] For patients in whom complete resection is not possible because of extensive invasion, debulking with a subtotal resection followed by radiation therapy may result in improved survival. One small study suggested that chemotherapy plus radiation therapy may be more beneficial than either treatment alone.[183]

The optimal management of incompletely resected or unresectable thymomas is controversial. Achieving a complete (R0) resection is an important prognostic indicator. Thymomas are usually chemosensitive tumors; thus, debulking with chemotherapy for inoperable or locally advanced tumors to attempt to increase the potential for R0 (complete) resection is sometimes employed. Given the small number of patients, no randomized trials have been performed to identify the best chemotherapy regimen for inoperable or recurrent thymomas. Comparing RRs across single-arm trials, anthracycline-containing regimens have increased RRs.[184] Commonly used regimens include cisplatin/doxorubicin/cyclophosphamide,[185] etoposide/ifosfamide/cisplatin,[186] and cisplatin/etoposide.[187]

Thymic carcinomas are aggressive and characterized by a high degree of histologic anaplasia and architectural atypia. A number of different subtypes have been described, although more than half are undifferentiated. These tumors often metastasize to regional lymph nodes and distant sites; thus, they have a worse prognosis than thymomas, with 5-year survival rates of 20% to 30%. Responses to carboplatin and paclitaxel have been described.[188]

Table 7-12 Modified Masaoka Clinical Staging of Thymoma[182]

Masaoka Stage	Diagnostic Criteria
Stage I	Macroscopically and microscopically completely encapsulated
Stage II	(A) Microscopic transcapsular invasion (B) Macroscopic invasion into surrounding fatty tissue or grossly adherent to but not through mediastinal pleura or pericardium
Stage III	Macroscopic invasion into neighboring organs (i.e., pericardium, great vessels, lung) (A) Without invasion of great vessels (B) With invasion of great vessels
Stage IV	(A) Pleural or pericardial dissemination (B) Lymphatic or hematogenous metastasis

KEY POINTS

- Thymomas are often encapsulated, well differentiated, and associated with paraneoplastic syndromes, such as myasthenia gravis.
- The optimal treatment of thymomas is thymectomy and complete surgical resection, in which case the survival is excellent.
- The most important prognostic factors after resection are Masaoka stage, histology, complete resection status, and size.
- Thymic carcinomas are more aggressive than thymomas.
- Regimens incorporating anthracyclines increase response rates in thymoma.

MESOTHELIOMA

Mesothelioma arises from mesothelial cells, the cells that form the serosal lining of the pleura, pericardium, and peritoneal cavities. Although benign mesotheliomas have been described, most are malignant neoplasms with an aggressive clinical course.[189]

Malignant mesotheliomas are rare, with approximately 2,500 new cases diagnosed annually in the United States. Although approximately 80% are associated with exposure to asbestos, only approximately 5% of asbestos workers are diagnosed with mesothelioma. In contrast to lung cancer and asbestosis, smoking does not increase the risk of mesothelioma. Unlike asbestosis, in which there is a dose–response relationship, this association does not exist for mesothelioma, with the exception of chrysotile asbestos, which may be oncogenic only at high doses.

The various types of asbestos are divided into two major groups: serpentine, represented by chrysotile, the most common form of asbestos in the Western world; and rod-like amphiboles, which include crocidolite, the most oncogenic type of asbestos.

Carcinogenic effects of asbestos appear to result from its physical properties rather than from its chemical structure, with long, rod-like fibers of narrow diameter being more likely to induce tumors in laboratory animals. It is postulated that chrysotile asbestos fibers are less carcinogenic because the fibers can be partially digested and removed from the lung, whereas amphibole asbestos is more resistant to solubilization by cellular enzymes and accumulates in the lungs. The fibers cause mutagenic changes by several different mechanisms, including direct physical effects on chromosomes; the production of hydroxyl radicals and superoxide anions leading to DNA strand breaks and deletions; stimulation of EGFR autophosphorylation, activation, and signal transduction; and increased production of inflammatory cytokines. The expression of the Simian virus 40 large-tumor antigen in mesothelioma cells and not nearby normal cells, as well as the capacity of antisense T-antigen treatment to arrest mesothelioma cell growth in vitro, suggest that Simian virus 40 also may be a contributing factor to the development of mesothelioma, particularly for patients exposed to asbestos. Mesothelioma also has been associated with Thorotrast exposure and radiation.

Three histologic variants of mesothelioma have been described: epithelial, which is the most common form and is associated with the best prognosis; sarcomatoid; and mixed. To distinguish mesotheliomas from metastatic adenocarcinomas, the periodic acid-Schiff stain is frequently used before and after diastase digestion. Neutral mucopolysaccharides that are strongly positive to periodic acid-Schiff stain are found in intracellular secretory vacuoles and in intra-acinar vacuoles in most adenocarcinomas but are rarely found in most mesotheliomas. In addition, IHC staining for CD15, Ber-EP-4, TTF1, and carcinoembryonic antigen are usually absent in mesotheliomas but positive in most adenocarcinomas, whereas mesothelioma is characterized by staining for calretinin, Wilms tumor antigen (WT1), vimentin, CK5/6, mesothelin, or HBME-1 (an anti-mesothelial cell antibody).[190]

Mesothelioma most commonly develops in the fifth to seventh decade, and it affects men and women in a 5:1 ratio. The onset of disease occurs 20 to 50 years after exposure. Family members also are at higher risk of mesothelioma, presumably because of exposure to asbestos fibers brought home on the clothing and bodies of individuals who work with asbestos.

The typical presentation consists of dyspnea or chest wall pain secondary to a pleural effusion. Sixty percent of mesotheliomas occur on the right side, and bilateral involvement of the chest wall is present at the time of diagnosis in less than 5% of cases. Repeated cytologic examination of pleural fluid may be negative, necessitating either a thoracoscopy or thoracotomy, despite the risk of seeding the biopsy site or surgical scar with tumor. Serum mesothelin-related peptide is a serum marker that may be predictive of disease recurrence after surgical resection.[191] Osteopontin is a glycoprotein that binds integrin and CD44 receptors, and it may distinguish patients with mesothelioma from those with benign disease.[166] Fibulin-3 levels in pleural fluid and plasma have also recently emerged as a diagnostic and prognostic marker with potentially better sensitivity, specificity, and reproducibility than osteopontin.[192]

Mesotheliomas tend to be locally invasive. For approximately 20% of patients, a chest wall mass develops over tracts resulting from thoracentesis, chest tubes, or thoracotomy. Direct involvement of the ribs, diaphragm, pericardium, and vertebrae is common. Although various staging classifications have been described, the most recent staging system proposed by the International Mesothelioma Interest Group emphasizes the importance of the local extent of the tumor and node involvement.[193]

Evaluation of surgical resectability often includes echocardiogram to delineate cardiac involvement and MRI to delineate diaphragmatic involvement, in addition to chest CT and PET. The choice of surgical resection for mesothelioma is controversial. Extrapleural pneumonectomy results in a lower local recurrence rate and has traditionally been considered the procedure of choice, although no conclusive OS benefit has been demonstrated. Extrapleural pneumonectomy includes en bloc resection of the parietal pleura, lung pericardium, and diaphragm. Given the extent of the resection and long duration of anesthesia needed, this procedure should be reserved for patients younger than 65 who are in good health.

Treatment of resectable mesothelioma traditionally consists of a trimodality approach. The best results have been described in a retrospective series reported by Sugarbaker et al in which median survival was 19 months for 176 patients treated with extrapleural pneumonectomy (EPP), four to six cycles of adjuvant chemotherapy, and adjuvant radiation therapy to the ipsilateral hemithorax and mediastinum.[194] Patients with pure epithelial type and no node involvement had a significantly better outcome than patients with sarcomatoid/mixed histology or node involvement. Two- and 5-year survival for the 103 patients with epithelial cell–type tumors were 38% and 15%, respectively, compared with 16% at 2 years, with no 5-year survival for the 74 patients with sarcomatous or mixed cell types. Indeed, given the poor outcomes noted with sarcomatoid tumors, in some centers the presence of this histology guides treatment away from aggressive surgical intervention.

A large retrospective review suggested that pleurectomy with decortication may also provide long-term benefit.[195] A small randomized trial called Mesothelioma and Radical Surgery Feasibility Study showed a trend toward a survival benefit for 26 patients who did not undergo an EPP compared with the 24 patients who did (14.4 months for the EPP group vs. 19.5 months for the no-EPP group; HR 1.90, 95% CI 0.92, 3.93; exact p = 0.082).[196]

The role of preoperative (neoadjuvant) chemotherapy is also being explored. A multicenter phase II trial of neoadjuvant pemetrexed and cisplatin followed by EPP and hemithoracic radiation had a median survival in the overall population of 16.8 months (77 patients) and of 29 months for patients completing all therapy (40 patients; 2-year survival of 61%).[197]

For patients with unresectable disease, effusions may be controlled by thoracoscopy with talc pleurodesis. Pleurectomy with decortication, although rarely curative, also can be used to control effusions. Smaller doses of radiation (21 Gy in three fractions) may prevent seeding of the surgical wound by mesothelioma cells.

The prognosis is poor for patients who have unresectable disease at presentation, with a median survival of approximately 12 months. Single-agent chemotherapy yields RRs of 5% to 20%, with the most active agents being pemetrexed, gemcitabine, doxorubicin, and cisplatin.[198,199] Combination chemotherapy, which is usually cisplatin-based, typically yields an RR of 15% to 20%. Although single-agent gemcitabine is associated with an RR of 12% or less, findings from a phase II study of gemcitabine plus cisplatin showed a 48% RR.[200] The best results have been reported with pemetrexed and cisplatin. A phase III study in which cisplatin was compared with cisplatin plus pemetrexed demonstrated a 9-month median survival for patients treated with cisplatin alone and a 12-month survival

for patients treated with the combination (p = 0.02), making this regimen the standard of care for patients with advanced mesothelioma. RRs were 41.3% and 16.7% in the pemetrexed/cisplatin arm and control arms, respectively.[201]

Acknowledgment

The authors thank Dr. David E. Gerber and Dr. Joan H. Schiller, who authored this chapter in the previous edition of ASCO-SEP.

References

1. Siegel R, Naishadham D, Jemal A. Cancer statistics, 2013. *CA Cancer J Clin.* 2013;63:11-30. PMID: 23335087.

2. Ibid.

3. Chlebowski RT, Schwartz AG, Wakelee H, et al. Oestrogen plus progestin and lung cancer in postmenopausal women (Women's Health Initiative trial): a post-hoc analysis of a randomised controlled trial. *Lancet.* 2009;374:1243-1251. PMID: 19767090.

4. Govindan R, Page N, Morgensztern D, et al. Changing epidemiology of small-cell lung cancer in the United States over the last 30 years: analysis of the surveillance, epidemiologic, and end results database. *J Clin Oncol.* 2006;24:4539-4544. PMID: 17008692

5. Alberg AJ, Samet JM. Epidemiology of lung cancer. *Chest.* 2003;123 (1 Suppl):21S-49S. PMID: 12527563.

6. Pierce JP, Messer K, White MM, et al. Prevalence of heavy smoking in California and the United States, 1965-2007. *JAMA.* 2011;305:1106-1112. PMID: 21406647.

7. Ebbert JO, Yang P, Vachon CM, et al. Lung cancer risk reduction after smoking cessation: observations from a prospective cohort of women. *J Clin Oncol.* 2003;21:921-926. PMID: 12610194.

8. Bullen C, Howe C, Laugesen M, et al. Electronic cigarettes for smoking cessation: a randomised controlled trial. *Lancet.* 2013;382:1629-1637. PMID: 24029165.

9. Copas JB, Shi JQ. Reanalysis of epidemiological evidence on lung cancer and passive smoking. *BMJ.* 2000;320:417-418. PMID: 10669446.

10. U.S. Department of Health and Human Services. The Health Consequences of Smoking: The Changing Cigarette—A Report of the Surgeon General. profiles.nlm.nih.gov/ps/access/NNBBSN.pdf. Accessed July 23, 2012.

11. Catelinois O, Rogel A, Laurier D, et al. Lung cancer attributable to indoor radon exposure in france: impact of the risk models and uncertainty analysis. *Environ Health Perspect.* 2006;114:1361-1366. PMID: 16966089.

12. Gorlova OY, Weng SF, Zhang Y, et al. Aggregation of cancer among relatives of never-smoking lung cancer patients. *Int J Cancer.* 2007;121:111-118. PMID: 17304511.

13. Peluso M, Munnia A, Hoek G, et al. DNA adducts and lung cancer risk: a prospective study. *Cancer Res.* 2005;65:8042-8048. PMID: 16140979.

14. Bennett WP, Alavanja MC, Blomeke B, et al. Environmental tobacco smoke, genetic susceptibility, and risk of lung cancer in never-smoking women. *J Natl Cancer Inst.* 1999;91:2009-2014. PMID: 10580025.

15. Marshall AL, Christiani DC. Genetic susceptibility to lung cancer–light at the end of the tunnel? *Carcinogenesis.* 2013;34:487-502. PMID: 23349013.

16. Omenn GS, Goodman GE, Thornquist MD, et al. Effects of a combination of beta carotene and vitamin A on lung cancer and cardiovascular disease. *N Engl J Med.* 1996;334:1150-1155. PMID: 8602180.

17. The effect of vitamin E and beta carotene on the incidence of lung cancer and other cancers in male smokers. The Alpha-Tocopherol, Beta Carotene Cancer Prevention Study Group. *N Engl J Med.* 1994;330:1029-1035. PMID: 8127329.

18. Menkes MS, Comstock GW, Vuilleumier JP, et al. Serum beta-carotene, vitamins A and E, selenium, and the risk of lung cancer. *N Engl J Med.* 1986;315:1250-1254. PMID: 3773937.

19. Travis WD. Pathology of lung cancer. *Clin Chest Med.* 2002;23:65-81, viii. PMID: 11901921.

20. Moran CA, Suster S, Coppola D, et al. Neuroendocrine carcinomas of the lung: a critical analysis. *Am J Clin Pathol.* 2009;131:206-221. PMID: 19141381.

21. Li T, Kung HJ, Mack PC, et al. Genotyping and genomic profiling of non-small-cell lung cancer: implications for current and future therapies. *J Clin Oncol.* 2013;31:1039-1049. PMID: 23401433.

22. Cancer Genome Atlas Research Network, Weinstein JN, Collisson EA, et al. The Cancer Genome Atlas Pan-Cancer analysis project. *Nat Gen.* 2013;45:1113-1120. PMID: 24071849.

KEY POINTS

- Approximately 80% of pleural mesotheliomas are associated with exposure to asbestos, including indirect exposure.
- The epithelial histologic form of mesothelioma is associated with a better prognosis than the sarcomatoid or mixed histology forms.
- A trimodality approach consisting of surgery, chemotherapy, and radiation therapy should be considered for younger patients with good performance status, particularly patients with negative mediastinal nodes and the epithelial variant.
- First-line chemotherapy for patients with mesothelioma consists of cisplatin and pemetrexed.

23. Cancer Genome Atlas Research Network. Comprehensive genomic characterization of squamous cell lung cancers. *Nature.* 2012;489:519-525. PMID: 22960745.

24. Ettinger DS, Akerley W, Borghaei H, et al. Non-small cell lung cancer, version 2.2013. *J Natl Compr Canc Netw.* 2013;11:645-653. PMID: 23744864.

25. Rusch V, Klimstra D, Venkatraman E, et al. Overexpression of the epidermal growth factor receptor and its ligand transforming growth factor alpha is frequent in resectable non-small cell lung cancer but does not predict tumor progression. *Clin Cancer Res.* 1997;3:515-522. PMID: 9815714.

26. Gerber DE, Minna JD. ALK inhibition for non-small cell lung cancer: from discovery to therapy in record time. *Cancer Cell.* 2010;18:548-551. PMID: 21156280.

27. Butrynski JE, D'Adamo DR, Hornick JL, et al. Crizotinib in ALK-rearranged inflammatory myofibroblastic tumor. *N Engl J Med.* 2010;363:1727-1733. PMID: 20979472.

28. Palmer RH, Vernersson E, Grabbe C, et al. Anaplastic lymphoma kinase: signalling in development and disease. *Biochem J.* 2009;420:345-361. PMID: 19459784.

29. Shaw AT, Yeap BY, Mino-Kenudson M, et al. Clinical features and outcome of patients with non-small-cell lung cancer who harbor EML4-ALK. *J Clin Oncol.* 2009;27:4247-4253. PMID: 19667264.

30. Rodig SJ, Mino-Kenudson M, Dacic S, et al. Unique clinicopathologic features characterize ALK-rearranged lung adenocarcinoma in the western population. *Clin Cancer Res.* 2009;15:5216-5223. PMID: 19671850.

31. Doebele RC, Pilling AB, Aisner DL, et al. Mechanisms of resistance to crizotinib in patients with ALK gene rearranged non-small cell lung cancer. *Clin Cancer Res.* 2012;18:1472-1482. PMID: 22235099.

32. Camidge DR, Kono SA, Flacco A, et al. Optimizing the detection of lung cancer patients harboring anaplastic lymphoma kinase (ALK) gene rearrangements potentially suitable for ALK inhibitor treatment. *Clin Cancer Res.* 2010;16:5581-5590. PMID: 21062932.

33. Zhu CQ, da Cunha Santos G, Ding K, et al. Role of KRAS and EGFR as biomarkers of response to erlotinib in National Cancer Institute of Canada Clinical Trials Group Study BR.21. *J Clin Oncol.* 2008;26:4268-4275. PMID: 18626007.

34 Pao W, Wang TY, Riely GJ, et al. KRAS mutations and primary resistance of lung adenocarcinomas to gefitinib or erlotinib. *PLoS Med.* 2005;2:e17. PMID: 15696205.

35. Bergethon K, Shaw AT, Ignatius Ou SH, et al. ROS1 rearrangements define a unique molecular class of lung cancers. *J Clin Oncol.* 2012;30:863-870. PMID: 22215748.

36. Shaw AT, Camidge DR, Engelman JA, et al. Clinical activity of crizotinib in advanced non-small cell lung cancer (NSCLC) harboring ROS1 gene rearrangement. *J Clin Oncol.* 2012;30 (suppl; abstr 7508).

37. Wang R, Hu H, Pan Y, et al. RET fusions define a unique molecular and clinicopathologic subtype of non-small-cell lung cancer. *J Clin Oncol.* 2012;30:4352-4359. PMID: 23150706.

38. Drilon A, Wang L, Hasanovic A, et al. Response to Cabozantinib in patients with RET fusion-positive lung adenocarcinomas. *Cancer Discovery.* 2013;3:630-635. PMID: 23533264.

39. Mazières J, Peters S, Lepage B, et al. Lung cancer that harbors an HER2 mutation: epidemiologic characteristics and therapeutic perspectives. *J Clin Oncol.* 2013;31:1997-2003. PMID: 23610105.

40. De Grève J, Teugels E, Geers C, et al. Clinical activity of afatinib (BIBW 2992) in patients with lung adenocarcinoma with mutations in the kinase domain of HER2/neu. *Lung Cancer.* 2012;76:123-127. PMID: 22325357.

41. Kris MG, Johnson BE, Kwiatkowski DJ, et al. Identification of driver mutations in tumor specimens from 1,000 patients with lung adenocarcinoma: The NCI's Lung Cancer Mutation Consortium (LCMC). *J Clin Oncol.* 2011;29 (suppl; abstr CRA7506).

42. Sandler A, Gray R, Perry MC, et al. Paclitaxel-carboplatin alone or with bevacizumab for non-small-cell lung cancer. *N Engl J Med.* 2006;355:2542-2550. PMID: 17167137.

43. Omitted.

44. Omitted.

45. Ferrara N. VEGF: an update on biological and therapeutic aspects. *Curr Opin Biotechnol.* 2000;11:617-624. PMID: 11102799.

46. Hicklin DJ, Ellis LM. Role of the vascular endothelial growth factor pathway in tumor growth and angiogenesis. *J Clin Oncol.* 2005;23:1011-1027. PMID: 15585754.

47. Kamba T, McDonald DM. Mechanisms of adverse effects of anti-VEGF therapy for cancer. *Br J Cancer.* 2007;96:1788-1795. PMID: 17519900.

48. Kitamoto Y, Tokunaga H, Miyamoto K, et al. VEGF is an essential molecule for glomerular structuring. *Nephrol Dial Transplant.* 2002;17 Suppl 9:25-27. PMID: 12386279.

49. Dowlati A, Gray R, Sandler AB, et al. Cell adhesion molecules, vascular endothelial growth factor, and basic fibroblast growth factor in patients with non-small cell lung cancer treated with chemotherapy with or without bevacizumab--an Eastern Cooperative Oncology Group Study. *Clin Cancer Res.* 2008;14:1407-1412. PMID: 18316562.

50. Schneider BP, Wang M, Radovich M, et al. Association of vascular endothelial growth factor and vascular endothelial growth factor receptor-2 genetic polymorphisms with outcome in a trial of paclitaxel compared with paclitaxel plus bevacizumab in advanced breast cancer: ECOG 2100. *J Clin Oncol.* 2008;26:4672-4678. PMID: 18824714.

51. Mancuso P, Colleoni M, Calleri A, et al. Circulating endothelial-cell kinetics and viability predict survival in breast cancer patients receiving metronomic chemotherapy. *Blood.* 2006;108:452-459. PMID: 16543470.

52. Zhao D, Jiang L, Hahn EW, et al. Tumor physiologic response to combretastatin A4 phosphate assessed by MRI. *Int J Radiat Oncol Biol Phys.* 2005;62:872-880. PMID: 15936572.

53. Dahlberg SE, Sandler AB, Brahmer JR, et al. Clinical course of advanced non-small-cell lung cancer patients experiencing hypertension during treatment with bevacizumab in combination with carboplatin and paclitaxel on ECOG 4599. *J Clin Oncol.* 2010;28:949-954. PMID: 20085937.

54. Yu D, Zhang X, Liu J, et al. Characterization of functional excision repair cross-complementation group 1 variants and their association with lung cancer risk and prognosis. *Clin Cancer Res.* 2008;14:2878-2886. PMID: 18451256.

55. Olaussen KA, Dunant A, Fouret P, et al. DNA repair by ERCC1 in non-small-cell lung cancer and cisplatin-based adjuvant chemotherapy. *N Engl J Med.* 2006;355:983-991. PMID: 16957145.

56. Friboulet L, Olaussen KA, Pignon JP, et al. ERCC1 isoform expression and DNA repair in non-small-cell lung cancer. *N Engl J Med.* 2013;368:1101-1110. PMID: 23514287.

57. Ji H, Ramsey MR, Hayes DN, et al. LKB1 modulates lung cancer differentiation and metastasis. *Nature.* 2007;448:807-810. PMID: 17676035.

58. Ding L, Getz G, Wheeler DA, et al. Somatic mutations affect key pathways in lung adenocarcinoma. *Nature.* 2008;455:1069-1075. PMID: 18948947.

59. Weir BA, Woo MS, Getz G, et al. Characterizing the cancer genome in lung adenocarcinoma. *Nature.* 2007;450:893-898. PMID: 17982442.

60. Chen HY, Yu SL, Chen CH, et al. A five-gene signature and clinical outcome in non-small-cell lung cancer. *N Engl J Med.* 2007;356:11-20. PMID: 17202451.

61. Taguchi F, Solomon B, Gregorc V, et al. Mass spectrometry to classify non-small-cell lung cancer patients for clinical outcome after treatment with epidermal growth factor receptor tyrosine kinase inhibitors: a multicohort cross-institutional study. *J Natl Cancer Inst.* 2007;99:838-846. PMID: 17551144.

62. Kratz JR, He J, Van Den Eeden SK, et al. A practical molecular assay to predict survival in resected non-squamous, non-small-cell lung cancer: development and international validation studies. *Lancet.* 2012;379: 823-832. PMID: 22285053.

63. Lazzari C, Novello S, Barni S, et al. Randomized proteomic stratified phase III study of second-line erlotinib (E) versus chemotherapy (CT) in patients with inoperable non-small cell lung cancer (PROSE). *J Clin Oncol.* 2013;31 (suppl; abstr LBA8005).

64. Quint LE, Tummala S, Brisson LJ, et al. Distribution of distant metastases from newly diagnosed non-small cell lung cancer. *Ann Thorac Surg.* 1996;62:246-250. PMID: 8678651.

65. Barnholtz-Sloan JS, Sloan AE, Davis FG, et al. Incidence proportions of brain metastases in patients diagnosed (1973 to 2001) in the Metropolitan Detroit Cancer Surveillance System. *J Clin Oncol.* 2004;22:2865-2872. PMID: 15254054.

66. Tsuya, A, Kurata T, Tamura K, et al. Skeletal metastases in non-small cell lung cancer: a retrospective study. *Lung Cancer.* 2007;57:229-232. PMID: 17451841.

67. Pelosof LC, Gerber DE. Paraneoplastic syndromes: an approach to diagnosis and treatment. *Mayo Clin Proc.* 2010;85:838-854. PMID: 20810794.

68. Henschke CI, McCauley DI, Yankelevitz DF, et al. Early Lung Cancer Action Project: overall design and findings from baseline screening. *Lancet.* 1999;354:99-105. PMID: 10408484.

69. National Lung Screening Trial Research Team, Aberle DR, Adams AM, et al. Reduced lung-cancer mortality with low-dose computed tomographic screening. *N Engl J Med.* 2011;365:395-409. PMID: 21714641.

70. Shepherd FA, Rodrigues Pereira J, Ciuleanu T, et al. Erlotinib in previously treated non-small-cell lung cancer. *N Engl J Med.* 2005;353:123-132. PMID: 16014882.

71. Goldstraw P, Crowley J, Chansky K, et al. The IASLC Lung Cancer Staging Project: proposals for the revision of the TNM stage groupings in the forthcoming (seventh) edition of the TNM Classification of malignant tumours. *J Thorac Oncol.* 2007;2:706-714. PMID: 17762336.

72. Shepherd FA, Crowley J, Van Houtte P, et al. The International Association for the Study of Lung Cancer lung cancer staging project: proposals regarding the clinical staging of small cell lung cancer in the forthcoming (seventh) edition of the tumor, node, metastasis classification for lung cancer. *J Thorac Oncol.* 2007;2:1067-1077. PMID: 18090577.

73. Toloza EM, Harpole L, Detterbeck F, et al. Invasive staging of non-small cell lung cancer: a review of the current evidence. *Chest.* 2003;123 (1 Suppl):157S-166S. PMID: 12527575.

74. Ye T, Hu H, Luo X, et al. The role of endobronchial ultrasound guided transbronchial needle aspiration (EBUS-TBNA) for qualitative diagnosis of mediastinal and hilar lymphadenopathy: a prospective analysis. *BMC Cancer.* 2011;11:100. PMID: 21418631.

75. Toloza EM, Harpole L, McCrory DC. Noninvasive staging of non-small cell lung cancer: a review of the current evidence. *Chest.* 2003;123(1 Suppl):137S-146S. PMID: 12527573.

76. Pieterman RM, van Putten JW, Meuzelaar JJ, et al. Preoperative staging of non-small-cell lung cancer with positron-emission tomography. *N Engl J Med.* 2000;343:254-261. PMID: 10911007.

77. Gupta NC, Graeber GM, Bishop HA. Comparative efficacy of positron emission tomography with fluorodeoxyglucose in evaluation of small (<1 cm), intermediate (1 to 3 cm), and large (>3 cm) lymph node lesions. *Chest.* 2000;117:773-778. PMID: 10713005.

78. van Tinteren H, Hoekstra OS, Smit EF, et al. Effectiveness of positron emission tomography in the preoperative assessment of patients with suspected non-small-cell lung cancer: the PLUS multicentre randomised trial. *Lancet.* 2002;359:1388-1393. PMID: 11978336.

79. Fischer B, Lassen U, Mortensen J, et al. Preoperative staging of lung cancer with combined PET-CT. *N Engl J Med.* 2009;361:32-39. PMID: 19571281.

80. Mac Manus MP, Hicks RJ, Matthews JP, et al. Positron emission tomography is superior to computed tomography scanning for response-assessment after radical radiotherapy or chemoradiotherapy in patients with non-small-cell lung cancer. *J Clin Oncol.* 2003;21:1285-1292. PMID: 12663716.

81. Ginsberg RJ, Rubinstein LV. Randomized trial of lobectomy versus limited resection for T1 N0 non-small cell lung cancer. Lung Cancer Study Group. *Ann Thorac Surg.* 1995;60:615-622; discussion 622-623. PMID: 7677489.

82. Garver RI, Jr., Zorn GL, Wu X, et al. Recurrence of bronchioloalveolar carcinoma in transplanted lungs. *N Engl J Med.* 1999;340:1071-1074. PMID: 10194236.

83. Timmerman R, Paulus R, Galvin J, et al. Stereotactic body radiation therapy for inoperable early stage lung cancer. *JAMA.* 2010;303:1070-1076. PMID: 20233825.

84. Karp DD, Lee SJ, Shaw Wright GL, et al. A phase III, intergroup, randomized, double-blind, chemoprevention trial of selenium supplementation in resected stage I non-small cell lung cancer. *J Clin Oncol.* 2010;28:18s (suppl; abstr CRA7004).

85. Doddoli C, D'Journo B, Le Pimpec-Barthes F, et al. Lung cancer invading the chest wall: a plea for en-bloc resection but the need for new treatment strategies. *Ann Thorac Surg.* 2005;80:2032-2040. PMID: 16305839.

86. Rusch VW, Giroux DJ, Kraut MJ, et al. Induction chemoradiation and surgical resection for superior sulcus non-small-cell lung carcinomas: long-term results of Southwest Oncology Group Trial 9416 (Intergroup Trial 0160). *J Clin Oncol.* 2007;25:313-318. PMID: 17235046.

87. Chemotherapy in non-small cell lung cancer: a meta-analysis using updated data on individual patients from 52 randomised clinical trials. Non-small Cell Lung Cancer Collaborative Group. *BMJ.* 1995;311:899-909. PMID: 7580546.

88. Pignon JP, Tribodet H, Scagliotti GV, et al. Lung adjuvant cisplatin evaluation: a pooled analysis by the LACE Collaborative Group. *J Clin Oncol.* 2008;26:3552-3559. PMID: 18506026.

89. Strauss GM, Herndon JE, 2nd, Maddaus MA, et al. Adjuvant paclitaxel plus carboplatin compared with observation in stage IB non-small-cell lung cancer: CALGB 9633 with the Cancer and Leukemia Group B, Radiation Therapy Oncology Group, and North Central Cancer Treatment Group Study Groups. *J Clin Oncol.* 2008;26:5043-5051. PMID: 18809614.

90. Rosell R, Gatzemeier U, Betticher DC, et al. Phase III randomised trial comparing paclitaxel/carboplatin with paclitaxel/cisplatin in patients with advanced non-small-cell lung cancer: a cooperative multinational trial. *Ann Oncol.* 2002;13:1539-1549. PMID: 12377641.

91. Douillard JY, Rosell R, De Lena M, et al. Adjuvant vinorelbine plus cisplatin versus observation in patients with completely resected stage IB-IIIA non-small-cell lung cancer (Adjuvant Navelbine International Trialist Association [ANITA]): a randomised controlled trial. *Lancet Oncol.* 2006;7:719-727. PMID: 16945766.

92. Arriagada R, Bergman B, Dunant A, et al. Cisplatin-based adjuvant chemotherapy in patients with completely resected non-small-cell lung cancer. *N Engl J Med.* 2004;350:351-360. PMID: 14736927.

93. Winton T, Livingston R, Johnson D, et al. Vinorelbine plus cisplatin vs. observation in resected non-small-cell lung cancer. *N Engl J Med.* 2005;352:2589-2597. PMID: 15972865.

94. Goss GD, O'Callaghan C, Lorimer I, et al. Gefitinib versus placebo in completely resected non-small-cell lung cancer: results of the NCIC CTG BR19 study. *J Clin Oncol.* 2013;31:3320-3326. PMID: 23980091.

94a. Kelly K, Altorki NK, Spigel DR, et al. A randomized, double-blind phase 3 trial of adjuvant erlotinib (E) versus placebo (P) following complete tumor resection with or without adjuvant chemotherapy in patients (pts) with stage IB-IIIA EGFR positive (IHC/FISH) non-small cell lung cancer (NSCLC): RADIANT results. *J Clin Oncol.* 2014;32:5s (suppl; abstr 7501).

95. Rosell R, Gómez-Codina J, Camps C, et al. A randomized trial comparing preoperative chemotherapy plus surgery with surgery alone in patients with non-small-cell lung cancer. *N Engl J Med.* 1994;330:153-158. PMID: 8043059.

96. Roth JA, Fossella F, Komaki R, et al. A randomized trial comparing perioperative chemotherapy and surgery with surgery alone in resectable stage IIIA non-small-cell lung cancer. *J Natl Cancer Inst.* 1994;86:673-680. PMID: 8158698.

97. Depierre A, Milleron B, Moro-Sibilot D, et al. Preoperative chemotherapy followed by surgery compared with primary surgery in resectable stage I (except T1N0), II, and IIIa non-small-cell lung cancer. *J Clin Oncol.* 2002;20:247-253. PMID: 11773176.

98. Gilligan D, Nicolson M, Smith I, et al. Preoperative chemotherapy in patients with resectable non-small cell lung cancer: results of the MRC LU22/NVALT 2/EORTC 08012 multicentre randomised trial and update of systematic review. *Lancet.* 2007;369:1929-1937. PMID: 17544497.

99. Felip E, Rosell R, Maestre JA, et al. Preoperative chemotherapy plus surgery versus surgery plus adjuvant chemotherapy versus surgery alone in early-stage non-small-cell lung cancer. *J Clin Oncol.* 2010;28:3138-3145. PMID: 20516435.

100. Albain KS, Swann RS, Rusch VW, et al. Radiotherapy plus chemotherapy with or without surgical resection for stage III non-small-cell lung cancer: a phase III randomised controlled trial. *Lancet.* 2009;374:379-386. PMID: 19632676.

101. Postoperative radiotherapy in non-small-cell lung cancer: systematic review and meta-analysis of individual patient data from nine randomised controlled trials. PORT Meta-analysis Trialists Group. *Lancet.* 1998;352:257-263. PMID: 9690404.

102. Dillman RO, Seagren SL, Propert KJ, et al. A randomized trial of induction chemotherapy plus high-dose radiation versus radiation alone in stage III non-small-cell lung cancer. *N Engl J Med.* 1990;323:940-945. PMID: 2169587.

103. Sause WT, Scott C, Taylor S, et al. Radiation Therapy Oncology Group (RTOG) 88-08 and Eastern Cooperative Oncology Group (ECOG) 4588: preliminary results of a phase III trial in regionally advanced, unresectable non-small-cell lung cancer. *J Natl Cancer Inst.* 1995;87:198-205. PMID: 7707407.

104. Furuse K, Fukuoka M, Kawahara M, et al. Phase III study of concurrent versus sequential thoracic radiotherapy in combination with mitomycin, vindesine, and cisplatin in unresectable stage III non-small-cell lung cancer. *J Clin Oncol.* 1999;17:2692-2699. PMID: 10561343.

105. Curran WJ, Jr., Paulus R, Langer CJ, et al. Sequential vs. concurrent chemoradiation for stage III non-small cell lung cancer: randomized phase III trial RTOG 9410. *J Natl Cancer Inst.* 2011;103:1452-1460. PMID: 21903745.

106. Belani CP, Choy H, Bonomi P, et al. Combined chemoradiotherapy regimens of paclitaxel and carboplatin for locally advanced non-small-cell lung cancer: a randomized phase II locally advanced multi-modality protocol. *J Clin Oncol.* 2005;23:5883-5891. PMID: 16087941.

107. Gandara DR, Chansky K, Albain KS, et al. Long-term survival with concurrent chemoradiation therapy followed by consolidation docetaxel in stage IIIB non-small-cell lung cancer: a phase II Southwest Oncology Group Study (S9504). *Clin Lung Cancer.* 2006;8:116-121. PMID: 17026812.

108. Hanna N, Neubauer M, Yiannoutsos C, et al. Phase III study of cisplatin, etoposide, and concurrent chest radiation with or without consolidation docetaxel in patients with inoperable stage III non-small-cell lung cancer: the Hoosier Oncology Group and U.S. Oncology. *J Clin Oncol.* 2008;26:5755-5760. PMID: 19001323.

109. Bradley JD, Paulus R, Komaki R, et al. A randomized phase III comparison of standard-dose (60 Gy) versus high-dose (74 Gy) conformal chemoradiotherapy with or without cetuximab for stage III non-small cell lung cancer: Results on radiation dose in RTOG 0617. *J Clin Oncol.* 2013;31 (suppl; abstr 7501).

110. Kelly K, Chansky K, Gaspar LE, et al. Phase III trial of maintenance gefitinib or placebo after concurrent chemoradiotherapy and docetaxel consolidation in inoperable stage III non-small-cell lung cancer: SWOG S0023. *J Clin Oncol.* 2008;26:2450-2456. PMID: 18378568.

111. Spigel DR, Hainsworth JD, Yardley DA, et al. Tracheoesophageal fistula formation in patients with lung cancer treated with chemoradiation and bevacizumab. *J Clin Oncol.* 2010;28:43-48. PMID: 19901100.

112. Scagliotti GV, Parikh P, von Pawel J, et al. Phase III study comparing cisplatin plus gemcitabine with cisplatin plus pemetrexed in chemotherapy-naive patients with advanced-stage non-small-cell lung cancer. *J Clin Oncol.* 2008;26:3543-3551. PMID: 18506025.

113. Sigmond J, Backus HH, Wouters D, et al. Induction of resistance to the multitargeted antifolate Pemetrexed (ALIMTA) in WiDr human colon cancer cells is associated with thymidylate synthase overexpression. *Biochem Pharmacol.* 2003;66:431-438. PMID: 12907242.

114. Reck M, von Pawel J, Zatloukal P, et al. Phase III trial of cisplatin plus gemcitabine with either placebo or bevacizumab as first-line therapy for non-squamous non-small-cell lung cancer: AVAil. *J Clin Oncol.* 2009;27:1227-1234. PMID: 19188680.

115. Sandler AB, Schiller JH, Gray R, et al. Retrospective evaluation of the clinical and radiographic risk factors associated with severe pulmonary hemorrhage in first-line advanced, unresectable non-small-cell lung cancer treated with Carboplatin and Paclitaxel plus bevacizumab. *J Clin Oncol.* 2009;27:1405-1412. PMID: 19224857.

116. Socinski MA, Langer CJ, Huang JE, et al. Safety of bevacizumab in patients with non-small-cell lung cancer and brain metastases. *J Clin Oncol.* 2009;27:5255-5261. PMID: 19738122.

117. Scappaticci FA, Skillings JR, Holden SN, et al. Arterial thromboembolic events in patients with metastatic carcinoma treated with chemotherapy and bevacizumab. *J Natl Cancer Inst.* 2007;99:1232-1239. PMID: 17686822.

118. Leighl NB, Bennouna J, Yi J, et al. Bleeding events in bevacizumab-treated cancer patients who received full-dose anticoagulation and remained on study. *Br J Cancer.* 2011;104:413-418. PMID: 21245868.

119. Sequist LV, Yang JC, Yamamoto N, et al. Phase III study of afatinib or cisplatin plus pemetrexed in patients with metastatic lung adenocarcinoma with EGFR mutations. *J Clin Oncol.* 2013;31:3327-3334. PMID: 23816960.

120. Kosaka T, Yatabe Y, Endoh H, et al. Mutations of the epidermal growth factor receptor gene in lung cancer: biological and clinical implications. *Cancer Res.* 2004;64:8919-8923. PMID: 15604253.

121. Pao W, Miller VA, Politi KA, et al. Acquired resistance of lung adenocarcinomas to gefitinib or erlotinib is associated with a second mutation in the EGFR kinase domain. *PLoS Med.* 2005;2:e73. PMID: 15737014.

122. Engelman JA, Zejnullahu K, Mitsudomi T, et al. MET amplification leads to gefitinib resistance in lung cancer by activating ERBB3 signaling. *Science.* 2007;316:1039-1043. PMID: 17463250.

123. Sequist LV, Waltman BA, Dias-Santagata D, et al. Genotypic and histological evolution of lung cancers acquiring resistance to EGFR inhibitors. *Sci Transl Med.* 2011;3:75ra26. PMID: 21430269.

124. Rosell R, Moran T, Queralt C, et al. Screening for epidermal growth factor receptor mutations in lung cancer. *N Engl J Med.* 2009;361:958-967. PMID: 19692684.

125. Maemondo M, Inoue A, Kobayashi K, et al. Gefitinib or chemotherapy for non-small-cell lung cancer with mutated EGFR. *N Engl J Med.* 2010;362:2380-2388. PMID: 20573926.

126. Rosell R, Carcereny E, Gervais R, et al. Erlotinib versus standard chemotherapy as first-line treatment for European patients with advanced EGFR mutation-positive non-small-cell lung cancer (EURTAC): a multicentre, open-label, randomised phase 3 trial. *Lancet Oncol.* 2012;13:239-246. PMID: 22285168.

127. Pérez-Soler R, Chachoua A, Hammond LA, et al. Determinants of tumor response and survival with erlotinib in patients with non--small-cell lung cancer. *J Clin Oncol.* 2004;22:3238-3247. PMID: 15310767.

128. Wu YL, Lee JS, Thongprasert S, et al. Intercalated combination of chemotherapy and erlotinib for patients with advanced stage non-small-cell lung cancer (FASTACT-2): a randomised, double-blind trial. *Lancet Oncol.* 2013;14:777-786. PMID: 23782814.

129. Hanna N, Lilenbaum R, Ansari R, et al. Phase II trial of cetuximab in patients with previously treated non-small-cell lung cancer. *J Clin Oncol.* 2006;24:5253-5258. PMID: 17114658.

130. Pirker R, Pereira JR, von Pawel J, et al. EGFR expression as a predictor of survival for first-line chemotherapy plus cetuximab in patients with advanced non-small-cell lung cancer: analysis of data from the phase 3 FLEX study. *Lancet Oncol.* 2012;13:33-42. PMID: 22056021.

131. Lynch TJ, Patel T, Dreisbach L, et al. Cetuximab and first-line taxane/carboplatin chemotherapy in advanced non-small-cell lung cancer: results of the randomized multicenter phase III trial BMS099. *J Clin Oncol.* 2010;28:911-917. PMID: 20100966.

132. Pirker R, Pereira JR, Szczesna A, et al. Cetuximab plus chemotherapy in patients with advanced non-small-cell lung cancer (FLEX): an open-label randomised phase III trial. *Lancet.* 2009;373:1525-1531. PMID: 19410716.

133. Kwak EL, Bang YJ, Camidge DR, et al. Anaplastic lymphoma kinase inhibition in non-small-cell lung cancer. *N Engl J Med.* 2010;363:1693-1703. PMID: 20979469.

134. Shaw AT, Yeap BY, Solomon BJ, et al. Effect of crizotinib on overall survival in patients with advanced non-small-cell lung cancer harbouring ALK gene rearrangement: a retrospective analysis. *Lancet Oncol.* 2011;12:1004-1012. PMID: 21933749.

135. Shaw AT, Kim DW, Nakagawa K, et al. Crizotinib versus chemotherapy in advanced ALK-positive lung cancer. *N Engl J Med.* 2013;368:2385-2394. PMID: 23724913.

136. Weickhardt AJ, Scheier B, Burke JM, et al. Local ablative therapy of oligoprogressive disease prolongs disease control by tyrosine kinase inhibitors in oncogene-addicted non-small-cell lung cancer. *J Thorac Oncol.* 2012;7:1807-1814. PMID: 23154552.

137. Effects of vinorelbine on quality of life and survival of elderly patients with advanced non-small-cell lung cancer. The Elderly Lung Cancer Vinorelbine Italian Study Group. *J Natl Cancer Inst.* 1999;91:66-72. PMID: 9890172.

138. Quoix E, Zalcman G, Oster JP, et al. Carboplatin and weekly paclitaxel doublet chemotherapy compared with monotherapy in elderly patients with advanced non-small-cell lung cancer: IFCT-0501 randomised, phase 3 trial. *Lancet.* 2011;378:1079-1088. PMID: 21831418.

139. Zukin M, Barrios CH, Pereira JR, et al. Randomized phase III trial of single-agent pemetrexed versus carboplatin and pemetrexed in patients with advanced non-small-cell lung cancer and Eastern Cooperative Oncology Group performance status of 2. *J Clin Oncol.* 2013;31:2849-2853. PMID: 23775961.

140. Westeel V, Quoix E, Moro-Sibilot D, et al. Randomized study of maintenance vinorelbine in responders with advanced non-small-cell lung cancer. *J Natl Cancer Inst.* 2005;97:499-506. PMID: 15812075.

141. Socinski MA, Schell MJ, Peterman A, et al. Phase III trial comparing a defined duration of therapy versus continuous therapy followed by second-line therapy in advanced-stage IIIB/IV non-small-cell lung cancer. *J Clin Oncol.* 2002;20:1335-1343. PMID: 11870177.

142. Fidias PM, Dakhil SR, Lyss AP, et al. Phase III study of immediate compared with delayed docetaxel after front-line therapy with gemcitabine plus carboplatin in advanced non-small-cell lung cancer. *J Clin Oncol.* 2009;27:591-598. PMID: 19075278.

143. Ciuleanu T, Brodowicz T, Zielinski C, et al. Maintenance pemetrexed plus best supportive care versus placebo plus best supportive care for non-small-cell lung cancer: a randomised, double-blind, phase 3 study. *Lancet.* 2009;374:1432-1440. PMID: 19767093.

144. Cappuzzo F, Ciuleanu T, Stelmakh L, et al. Erlotinib as maintenance treatment in advanced non-small-cell lung cancer: a multicentre, randomised, placebo-controlled phase 3 study. *Lancet Oncol.* 2010;11:521-529. PMID: 20493771.

145. Paz-Ares L, de Marinis F, Dediu M, et al. Maintenance therapy with pemetrexed plus best supportive care versus placebo plus best supportive care after induction therapy with pemetrexed plus cisplatin for advanced non-squamous non-small-cell lung cancer (PARAMOUNT): a double-blind, phase 3, randomised controlled trial. *Lancet Oncol.* 2012;13:247-255. PMID: 22341744.

146. Wozniak AJ, Crowley JJ, Balcerzak SP, et al. Randomized trial comparing cisplatin with cisplatin plus vinorelbine in the treatment of advanced non-small-cell lung cancer: a Southwest Oncology Group study. *J Clin Oncol.* 1998;16:2459-2465. PMID: 9667264.

147. Sandler AB, Nemunaitis J, Denham C, et al. Phase III trial of gemcitabine plus cisplatin versus cisplatin alone in patients with locally advanced or metastatic non-small-cell lung cancer. *J Clin Oncol.* 2000;18:122-130. PMID: 10623702.

148. von Pawel J, von Roemeling R, Gatzemeier U, et al. Tirapazamine plus cisplatin versus cisplatin in advanced non-small-cell lung cancer: A report of the international CATAPULT I study group. Cisplatin and Tirapazamine in Subjects with Advanced Previously Untreated Non-Small-Cell Lung Tumors. *J Clin Oncol.* 2000;18:1351-1359. PMID: 10715308.

149. Gatzemeier U, von Pawel J, Gottfried M, et al. Phase III comparative study of high-dose cisplatin versus a combination of paclitaxel and cisplatin in patients with advanced non-small-cell lung cancer. *J Clin Oncol.* 2000;18:3390-3399. PMID: 11013280.

150. Le Chevalier T, Brisgand D, Douillard JY, et al. Randomized study of vinorelbine and cisplatin versus vindesine and cisplatin versus vinorelbine alone in advanced non-small-cell lung cancer: results of a European multicenter trial including 612 patients. *J Clin Oncol.* 1994;12:360-367. PMID: 8113844.

151. Lilenbaum RC, Herndon JE, 2nd, List MA, et al. Single-agent versus combination chemotherapy in advanced non-small-cell lung cancer: the cancer and leukemia group B (study 9730). *J Clin Oncol.* 2005;23:190-196. PMID: 15625373.

152. Georgoulias V, Ardavanis A, Agelidou A, et al. Docetaxel versus docetaxel plus cisplatin as front-line treatment of patients with advanced non-small-cell lung cancer: a randomized, multicenter phase III trial. *J Clin Oncol.* 2004;22:2602-2609. PMID: 15226327.

153. Negoro S, Masuda N, Takada Y, et al. Randomised phase III trial of irinotecan combined with cisplatin for advanced non-small-cell lung cancer. *Br J Cancer.* 2003;88:335-341. PMID: 12569373.

154. Ardizzoni A, Boni L, Tiseo M, et al. Cisplatin- versus carboplatin-based chemotherapy in first-line treatment of advanced non-small-cell lung cancer: an individual patient data meta-analysis. *J Natl Cancer Inst.* 2007;99:847-857. PMID: 17551145.

155. Hotta K, Matsuo K, Ueoka H, et al. Meta-analysis of randomized clinical trials comparing Cisplatin to Carboplatin in patients with advanced non-small-cell lung cancer. *J Clin Oncol.* 2004;22:3852-3859. PMID: 15326195.

156. D'Addario G, Pintilie M, Leighl NB, et al. Platinum-based versus non-platinum-based chemotherapy in advanced non-small-cell lung cancer: a meta-analysis of the published literature. *J Clin Oncol.* 2005;23:2926-2936. PMID: 15728229.

157. Shepherd FA, Dancey J, Ramlau R, et al. Prospective randomized trial of docetaxel versus best supportive care in patients with non-small-cell lung cancer previously treated with platinum-based chemotherapy. *J Clin Oncol.* 2000;18:2095-2103. PMID: 10811675.

158. Fossella FV, DeVore R, Kerr RN, et al. Randomized phase III trial of docetaxel versus vinorelbine or ifosfamide in patients with advanced non-small-cell lung cancer previously treated with platinum-containing chemotherapy regimens. The TAX 320 Non-Small Cell Lung Cancer Study Group. *J Clin Oncol.* 2000;18:2354-2362. PMID: 10856094.

159. Hanna N, Shepherd FA, Fossella FV, et al. Randomized phase III trial of pemetrexed versus docetaxel in patients with non-small-cell lung cancer previously treated with chemotherapy. *J Clin Oncol.* 2004;22:1589-1597. PMID: 15117980.

160. Mok TS, Wu YL, Thongprasert S, et al. Gefitinib or carboplatin-paclitaxel in pulmonary adenocarcinoma. *N Engl J Med.* 2009;361:947-957. PMID: 19692680.

161. Matsuo K, Ito H, Yatabe Y, et al. Risk factors differ for non-small-cell lung cancers with and without EGFR mutation: assessment of smoking and sex by a case-control study in Japanese. *Cancer Sci.* 2007;98:96-101. PMID: 17054433.

162. Kim ES, Hirsh V, Mok T, et al. Gefitinib versus docetaxel in previously treated non-small-cell lung cancer (INTEREST): a randomised phase III trial. *Lancet.* 2008;372:1809-1818. PMID: 19027483.

163. Noda K, Nishiwaki Y, Kawahara M, et al. Irinotecan plus cisplatin compared with etoposide plus cisplatin for extensive small-cell lung cancer. *N Engl J Med.* 2002;346:85-91. PMID: 11784874.

164. Hanna N, Bunn PA, Jr., Langer C, et al. Randomized phase III trial comparing irinotecan/cisplatin with etoposide/cisplatin in patients with previously untreated extensive-stage disease small-cell lung cancer. *J Clin Oncol.* 2006;24:2038-2043. PMID: 16648503.

165. Klasa RJ, Murray N, Coldman AJ. Dose-intensity meta-analysis of chemotherapy regimens in small-cell carcinoma of the lung. *J Clin Oncol.* 1991;9:499-508. PMID: 1847968.

166. Elias AD, Ayash L, Frei E, 3rd, et al. Intensive combined modality therapy for limited-stage small-cell lung cancer. *J Natl Cancer Inst.* 1993;85:559-566. PMID: 8384264.

167. von Pawel J, Schiller JH, Shepherd FA, et al. Topotecan versus cyclophosphamide, doxorubicin, and vincristine for the treatment of recurrent small-cell lung cancer. *J Clin Oncol.* 1999;17:658-667. PMID: 10080612.

168. Jotte R, Von Pawel J, Spigel DR, et al. Randomized phase III trial of amrubicin versus topotecan (Topo) as second-line treatment for small cell lung cancer (SCLC). *J Clin Oncol.* 2011;29 (suppl; abstr 7000).

169. Pietanza MC, Kadota K, Huberman K, et al. Phase II trial of temozolomide in patients with relapsed sensitive or refractory small cell lung cancer, with assessment of methylguanine-DNA methyltransferase as a potential biomarker. *Clin Cancer Res.* 2012;18:1138-1145. PMID: 22228633.

170. Souhami RL, Spiro SG, Rudd RM, et al. Five-day oral etoposide treatment for advanced small-cell lung cancer: randomized comparison with intravenous chemotherapy. *J Natl Cancer Inst.* 1997;89:577-580. PMID: 9106647.

171. Girling DJ. Comparison of oral etoposide and standard intravenous multidrug chemotherapy for small-cell lung cancer: a stopped multicentre randomised trial. Medical Research Council Lung Cancer Working Party. *Lancet.* 1996;348:563-566. PMID: 8774567.

172. Warde P, Payne D. Does thoracic irradiation improve survival and local control in limited-stage small-cell carcinoma of the lung? A meta-analysis. *J Clin Oncol.* 1992;10:890-895. PMID: 1316951.

173. Turrisi AT, 3rd, Kim K, Blum R, et al. Twice-daily compared with once-daily thoracic radiotherapy in limited small-cell lung cancer treated concurrently with cisplatin and etoposide. *N Engl J Med.* 1999;340:265-271. PMID: 9920950.

174. Murray N, Coy P, Pater JL, et al. Importance of timing for thoracic irradiation in the combined modality treatment of limited-stage small-cell lung cancer. The National Cancer Institute of Canada Clinical Trials Group. *J Clin Oncol.* 1993;11:336-344. PMID: 8381164.

175. Aupérin A, Arriagada R, Pignon JP, et al. Prophylactic cranial irradiation for patients with small-cell lung cancer in complete remission. Prophylactic Cranial Irradiation Overview Collaborative Group. *N Engl J Med.* 1999;341:476-484. PMID: 10441603.

176. Slotman B, Faivre-Finn C, Kramer G, et al. Prophylactic cranial irradiation in extensive small-cell lung cancer. *N Engl J Med.* 2007;357:664-672. PMID: 17699816.

177. Titulaer MJ, Wirtz PW, Willems LN, et al. Screening for small-cell lung cancer: a follow-up study of patients with Lambert-Eaton myasthenic syndrome. *J Clin Oncol.* 2008;26:4276-4281. PMID: 18779614.

178. Saba N, Khuri F. The role of bisphosphonates in the management of advanced cancer with a focus on non-small-cell lung cancer. Part 2: Clinical studies and economic analyses. *Oncology.* 2005;68:18-22. PMID: 15775689.

179. Henry DH, Costa L, Goldwasser F, et al. Randomized, double-blind study of denosumab versus zoledronic acid in the treatment of bone metastases in patients with advanced cancer (excluding breast and prostate cancer) or multiple myeloma. *J Clin Oncol.* 2011;29:1125-1132. PMID: 21343556.

180. Kelly K, Lovato L, Bunn PA, Jr., et al. Cisplatin, etoposide, and paclitaxel with granulocyte colony-stimulating factor in untreated patients with extensive-stage small cell lung cancer: a phase II trial of the Southwest Oncology Group. *Clin Cancer Res.* 2001;7:2325-2329. PMID: 11489808.

181. Thomas CR, Wright CD, Loehrer PJ. Thymoma: state of the art. *J Clin Oncol.* 1999;17:2280-2289. PMID: 10561285.

182. Wright CD. Management of thymomas. *Crit Rev Oncol Hematol.* 2008;65:109-120. PMID: 17570676.

183. Loehrer PJ Sr, Chen M, Kim K, et al. Cisplatin, doxorubicin, and cyclophosphamide plus thoracic radiation therapy for limited-stage unresectable thymoma: an intergroup trial. *J Clin Oncol.* 1997;15:3093-3099. PMID: 9294472.

184. Girard N, Lal R, Wakelee H, et al. Chemotherapy definitions and policies for thymic malignancies. *J Thorac Oncol.* 2011;6(7 Suppl 3):S1749-S1755. PMID: 21847058.

185. Loehrer PJ Sr, Kim K, Aisner SC, et al. Cisplatin plus doxorubicin plus cyclophosphamide in metastatic or recurrent thymoma: final results of an intergroup trial. The Eastern Cooperative Oncology Group, Southwest Oncology Group, and Southeastern Cancer Study Group. *J Clin Oncol.* 1994;12:1164-1168. PMID: 8201378.

186. Loehrer PJ Sr, Jiroutek M, Aisner S, et al. Combined etoposide, ifosfamide, and cisplatin in the treatment of patients with advanced thymoma and thymic carcinoma: an intergroup trial. *Cancer.* 2001;91:2010-2015. PMID: 11391579.

187. Giaccone G, Ardizzoni A, Kirkpatrick A, et al. Cisplatin and etoposide combination chemotherapy for locally advanced or metastatic thymoma. A phase II study of the European Organization for Research and Treatment

of Cancer Lung Cancer Cooperative Group. *J Clin Oncol.* 1996;14:814-820. PMID: 8622029.

188. Eng TY, Fuller CD, Jagirdar J, et al. Thymic carcinoma: state of the art review. *Int J Radiat Oncol Biol Phys.* 2004;59:654-664. PMID: 15183468.

189. Carbone M, Kratzke RA, Testa JR. The pathogenesis of mesothelioma. *Semin Oncol.* 2002;29:2-17. PMID: 11836664.

190. Robinson BW, Lake RA. Advances in malignant mesothelioma. *N Engl J Med.* 2005;353:1591-1603. PMID: 16221782.

191. Robinson BW, Creaney J, Lake R, et al. Mesothelin-family proteins and diagnosis of mesothelioma. *Lancet.* 2003;362:1612-1616. PMID: 14630441.

192. Pass HI, Levin SM, Harbut MR, et al. Fibulin-3 as a blood and effusion biomarker for pleural mesothelioma. *N Engl J Med.* 2012;367:1417-1427. PMID: 23050525.

193. Rusch VW. A proposed new international TNM staging system for malignant pleural mesothelioma from the International Mesothelioma Interest Group. *Lung Cancer.* 1996;14:1-12. PMID: 8696713.

194. Sugarbaker DJ, Flores RM, Jaklitsch MT, et al. Resection margins, extrapleural nodal status, and cell type determine postoperative long-term survival in trimodality therapy of malignant pleural mesothelioma: results in 183 patients. *J Thorac Cardiovasc Surg.* 1999;117:54-63; discussion 63-65. PMID: 9869758.

195. Flores RM, Pass HI, Seshan VE, et al. Extrapleural pneumonectomy versus pleurectomy/decortication in the surgical management of malignant pleural mesothelioma: results in 663 patients. *J Thorac Cardiovasc Surg.* 2008;135:620-626, 626. e1-3. PMID: 18329481.

196. Treasure T, Lang-Lazdunski L, Waller D, et al. Extra-pleural pneumonectomy versus no extra-pleural pneumonectomy for patients with malignant pleural mesothelioma: clinical outcomes of the Mesothelioma and Radical Surgery (MARS) randomised feasibility study. *Lancet Oncol.* 2011;12:763-772. PMID: 21723781.

197. Krug LM, Pass HI, Rusch VW, et al. Multicenter phase II trial of neoadjuvant pemetrexed plus cisplatin followed by extrapleural pneumonectomy and radiation for malignant pleural mesothelioma. *J Clin Oncol.* 2009;27:3007-3013. PMID: 19364962.

198. Ong ST, Vogelzang NJ. Chemotherapy in malignant pleural mesothelioma. A review. *J Clin Oncol.* 1996;14:1007-1017. PMID: 8622005.

199. Vogelzang NJ. Emerging insights into the biology and therapy of malignant mesothelioma. *Semin Oncol.* 2002;29(6 Suppl 18):35-42. PMID: 12571809.

200. Byrne MJ, Davidson JA, Musk AW, et al. Cisplatin and gemcitabine treatment for malignant mesothelioma: a phase II study. *J Clin Oncol.* 1999;17:25-30. PMID: 10458214.

201. Vogelzang NJ, Rusthoven JJ, Symanowski J, et al. Phase III study of pemetrexed in combination with cisplatin versus cisplatin alone in patients with malignant pleural mesothelioma. *J Clin Oncol.* 2003;21:2636-2644. PMID: 12860938.

202. Mulshine JL, Sullivan DC. Clinical practice. Lung cancer screening. *N Engl J Med.* 2005;352:2714-2720. PMID: 15987920.

203. Keller SM, Adak S, Wagner H, et al. A randomized trial of postoperative adjuvant therapy in patients with completely resected stage II or IIIA non-small-cell lung cancer. Eastern Cooperative Oncology Group. *N Engl J Med.* 2000;343:1217-1222. PMID: 11071672.

204. Scagliotti GV, Fossati R, Torri V, et al. Randomized study of adjuvant chemotherapy for completely resected stage I, II, or IIIA non-small-cell Lung cancer. *J Natl Cancer Inst.* 2003;95:1453-1461. PMID: 14519751.

205. Goss GD, Lorimer I, Tsao MS, et al. A phase III randomized, double-blind, placebo-controlled trial of the epidermal growth factor receptor inhibitor gefitinib in completely resected stage IB-IIIA non-small cell lung cancer (NSCLC): NCIC CTG BR.19. *J Clin Oncol.* 2012;28:18s (suppl; abstr LBA7005).

206. Rigas JR, Carey MA, Rubin MS, et al. Efficacy of maintenance erlotinib versus placebo in patients with unresectable stage III non-small cell lung cancer (NSCLC) following concurrent chemoradiation (D0410, NCT00153803). *J Thorac Oncol.* 2009;4(9 Suppl 1):S371 (Abstract C6.1).

207. Gatzemeier U, Pluzanska A, Szczesna A, et al. Phase III study of erlotinib in combination with cisplatin and gemcitabine in advanced non-small cell lung cancer: the Tarceva Lung Cancer Investigation Trial. *J Clin Oncol.* 2007;25:1545-1552. PMID: 17442998.

208. Herbst RS, Prager D, Hermann R, et al. TRIBUTE: a phase III trial of erlotinib hydrochloride (OSI-774) combined with carboplatin and paclitaxel chemotherapy in advanced non-small-cell lung cancer. *J Clin Oncol.* 2005;23:5892-5899. PMID: 16043829.

209. Giaccone G, Herbst RS, Manegold C, et al. Gefitinib in combination with gemcitabine and cisplatin in advanced non-small-cell lung cancer: a phase III trial—INTACT 1. *J Clin Oncol.* 2004;22:777-784. PMID: 14990632.

210. Herbst RS, Giaccone G, Schiller JH, et al. Gefitinib in combination with paclitaxel and carboplatin in advanced non-small-cell lung cancer: a phase III trial--INTACT 2. *J Clin Oncol.* 2004;22:785-794. PMID: 14990633.

211. Mitsudomi T, Morita S, Yatabe Y, et al. Gefitinib versus cisplatin plus docetaxel in patients with non-small-cell lung cancer harbouring mutations of the epidermal growth factor receptor (WJTOG3405): an open label, randomised phase 3 trial. *Lancet Oncol.* 2010;11:121-128. PMID: 20022809.

212. Han JY, Park K, Kim SW, et al. First-SIGNAL: first-line single-agent iressa versus gemcitabine and cisplatin trial in never-smokers with adenocarcinoma of the lung. *J Clin Oncol.* 2012;30:1122-1128. PMID: 22370314.

213. Zhou C, Wu YL, Chen G, et al. Erlotinib versus chemotherapy as first-line treatment for patients with advanced EGFR mutation-positive non-small cell lung cancer (OPTIMAL, CTONG-0802): a multicentre, open-label, randomised, phase 3 study. *Lancet Oncol.* 2011;12:735-742. PMID: 21783417.

214. Cappuzzo F, Ciuleanu T, Stelmakh L, et al. Erlotinib as maintenance treatment in advanced non-small-cell lung cancer: a multicentre, randomised, placebo-controlled phase 3 study. *Lancet Oncol.* 2010;11:521-529. PMID: 20493771.

215. Miller VA, O'Connor P, Soh C, et al. A randomized, double-blind, placebo-controlled, phase IIIb trial (ATLAS) comparing bevacizumab (B) therapy with or without erlotinib (E) after completion of chemotherapy with B for first-line treatment of locally advanced, recurrent, or metastatic non-small cell lung cancer (NSCLC). *J Clin Oncol.* 2009;27 (suppl; abstr LBA8002).

216. Thatcher N, Chang A, Parikh P, et al. Gefitinib plus best supportive care in previously treated patients with refractory advanced non-small-cell lung cancer: results from a randomised, placebo-controlled, multicentre study (Iressa Survival Evaluation in Lung Cancer). *Lancet.* 2005;366:1527-1537. PMID: 16257339.

217. Smith IE, O'Brien ME, Talbot DC, et al. Duration of chemotherapy in advanced non-small-cell lung cancer: a randomized trial of three versus six courses of mitomycin, vinblastine, and cisplatin. *J Clin Oncol.* 2001;19:1336-1343. PMID: 11230476.

8

HEAD AND NECK CANCERS

Bhoomi Mehrotra, MD

Updates from 2012

▶ Two phase III trials comparing induction chemotherapy followed by chemoradiation therapy versus standard concomitant cisplatin and radiation therapy (RT) for definitive management of locally advanced head and neck squamous cell cancer failed to show an advantage for the induction approach (Haddad R, *Lancet Oncol* 2013; Cohen E, *J Clin Oncol* 2012).

▶ Ten-year follow-up results from Intergroup R91-11 showed that induction platinum plus 5-fluorouracil followed by RT and concomitant cisplatin/RT demonstrated similar efficacy for the endpoint of laryngectomy-free survival. Local-regional control and larynx preservation were substantially improved with concomitant cisplatin/RT compared with the induction arm or RT alone. Overall survival did not differ across the three arms (Forastiere AA, *J Clin Oncol* 2013).

▶ De-intensification protocols in the management of human papillomavirus–related oropharyngeal cancers should be considered investigational at this time.

▶ Sorafenib has been approved by the U.S. Food and Drug Administration (FDA) for the treatment of locally recurrent or metastatic, progressive, differentiated thyroid cancer that no longer responds to radioactive iodine treatment.

▶ Vandetanib and cabozantinib have been approved by the FDA for the treatment of symptomatic or progressive, locally advanced, or metastatic medullary thyroid cancers.

The term "head and neck cancer" refers to a heterogeneous group of malignant tumors arising from the epithelial lining of the upper aerodigestive tract. The specific primary sites are subdivided by anatomic boundaries: the lip and oral cavity, pharynx (nasopharynx, oropharynx, and hypopharynx), larynx, and the nasal cavity and paranasal sinuses (Table 8-1, Fig. 8-1). Squamous cell cancer variant is the most common histologic type, accounting for 85% to 95% of head and neck cancers. Etiologic factors include tobacco/alcohol use and viruses, such as the human papillomavirus (HPV) and the Epstein-Barr virus (Table 8-2). The other two anatomic sites included in the head and neck region are the thyroid and salivary glands. These cancers are most commonly histologic variants of adenocarcinoma.

EPIDEMIOLOGY

In 2010, head and neck cancers accounted for about 3% (52,000) of all estimated new cancers and about 2% (11,500) of all estimated cancer deaths in the United States.[1] Worldwide, head and neck cancer is a substantial public health concern, with an estimated 664,000 new cases

Table 8-1 Head and Neck Cancer: Primary Sites

Oral Cavity and Lip	■ Floor of mouth ■ Oral tongue ■ Buccal mucosa ■ Alveolar ridges ■ Hard palate ■ Retromolar trigone
Pharynx	■ Nasopharynx (includes superior surface of soft palate) ■ Oropharynx (includes inferior surface of soft palate, uvula, base of tongue, tonsil, posterior pharyngeal wall) ■ Hypopharynx (pyriform sinus, postcricoid, posterior wall)
Larynx	■ Supraglottic larynx (false cords, arytenoids, epiglottis) ■ Glottic larynx (includes commissures) ■ Subglottic larynx
Nasal Cavity and Paranasal Sinuses	■ Nasal cavity ■ Maxillary sinuses ■ Ethmoid sinuses ■ Frontal sinuses ■ Sphenoid sinuses

Table 8-2 Characteristics of Virus-Associated Head and Neck Cancers

	Human Papillomavirus	Epstein-Barr Virus
Anatomic site	Oropharynx	Nasopharynx
Anatomic subsite	Lingual and palatine tonsils	Fossa of Rosenmüller
Percent virus associated	60% to 70%	WHO I: 70% to 80% WHO II to III: 100%
Associated histopathology	Basaloid	Lymphoepithelioma
Viral transmission	Sexual	Oral
Viral genome	Episomal/integrated	Episomal/integrated
Viral oncogenes	*E6* and *E7*	*LMP-1* and *EBNA1*
Cofactors	Tobacco and alcohol	Diet and genetics
Clinical presentation	Unknown primary	Distant metastases
Prognosis controlled for stage	Improved	Improved

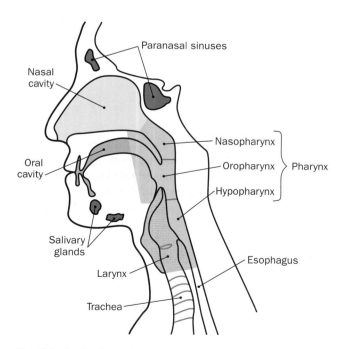

Fig. 8-1 Sagittal section showing head and neck cancer primary tumor sites.

Adapted from Vokes E, Weichselbaum R, Lippman S, Hong W. Head and Neck Cancer. N Engl J Med. 1993;328:184-194.

diagnosed in 2002 and 350,000 deaths.[2] Head and neck cancer affects men and women in a ratio of 2.5:1, although the ratio varies according to the primary site (e.g., 4:1 for cancer of oropharynx, 7:1 for cancer of the larynx). The median age of incidence is approximately 60. Oropharyngeal cancer incidence has dramatically increased from 1983 to 2002, predominantly in developed countries and at younger ages, likely as a result of a potential role for HPV infection, particularly among men.[3] The age-adjusted incidence and mortality are highest among black men, who generally present at a more advanced stage compared with white individuals. In addition, stage-specific survival rates also are lower for this racial group.

RISK FACTORS
TOBACCO AND ALCOHOL
Epidemiologic data document a multiplicative risk relationship between tobacco and alcohol. For example, the relative risk of oral and pharyngeal cancer is increased nearly 40-fold for patients with a pack-year history of more than 40 years who consume 30 or more alcoholic drinks per week.[4] Age at onset younger than 18 and duration of smoking of more than 35 years are prominent risk factors. Overall, an estimated 75% of head and neck cancers can be attributed to tobacco and alcohol use, highlighting the importance of tobacco and alcohol counseling in medical practice and as part of prevention strategies. The carcinogens that are found at high levels in tobacco that are considered directly mutagenic are benzopyrene and

nitrosamine 4-(methylnitrosamino)-1-(3-pyridyl)-1-butanone (NNK). The type of tobacco product used affects the distribution of observed primary sites. Smokeless tobacco and other orally chewed carcinogens, such as betel quid, a combination of betel leaf, lime, and areca nut that is commonly used in India and parts of Asia, are associated with the development of cancers of the oral cavity. Black, air-cured tobacco (as commonly found in cigars and pipe tobacco) is more irritating to the respiratory mucosa than blonde or flue-cured tobacco (more commonly found in cigarettes) and is associated with a higher risk of head and neck cancer.

KEY POINTS

- Tobacco and alcohol use are the major risk factors for squamous cell cancer of the head and neck, and the use of both results in a multiplicative increase in risk.
- There is evidence for a causal association between high-risk oncogenic human papillomavirus (HPV) and cancers of the lingual and palatine tonsils; these cancers are increasing in incidence in the United States.
- The survival prognosis is substantially better for HPV-positive cancers compared with HPV-negative cancers.
- The incidence of second primary cancers for patients with a history of squamous cell cancer of the head and neck is 3% to 7% annually, particularly for other sites of the lung, esophagus, head, and neck.

DIET

Because many patients with head and neck cancer are malnourished at the time of diagnosis, dietary deficiencies have been postulated as risk factors, and both laboratory and epidemiologic data suggest that vitamin A and its analogues may be protective. Plummer-Vinson syndrome, which is most commonly seen in women younger than age 50, is associated with iron-deficiency anemia, hypopharyngeal webs, dysphagia, and a higher risk of cancers of the postcricoid and hypopharynx.

OCCUPATIONAL EXPOSURE

Most tumors of the sinonasal tract originate in the maxillary sinus, and only 50% are of squamous cell histology. Of note, these cancers are associated with certain occupational exposures (e.g., nickel, radium, mustard gas, chromium, and byproducts of leather tanning and woodworking).

VIRUSES
Human Papillomavirus

HPV has emerged as an important cause of oropharyngeal cancer.[5] In the United States between 1984 and 1989, only 16% of oropharyngeal cancers were related to HPV compared to 73% of oropharyngeal cancers between 2000 and 2004, revealing a 4-fold increase over the past 2 decades.[6] This trend has

been a striking feature despite a decrease in tobacco use in the United States.[7] The rapid rise in the incidence of oropharyngeal cancers among men younger than age 60, with no or minimal use or history of alcohol or tobacco abuse, has been noted over the past decade.[8,9]

Genetic material from high-risk oncogenic strains (most commonly HPV types 16 and 18) is found in approximately 60% of oropharyngeal cancers arising from the palatine and lingual tonsils.[10] The transforming potential results from viral proteins E6 and E7 that inactivate the tumor suppressor proteins p53 and pRb, which results in loss of cell cycle regulation, cellular proliferation, and chromosome instability.[11] Recently, HPV 16 E6 seropositivity has been reported to be present more than 10 years before the diagnosis of oropharyngeal cancer.[12] These tumors are clinically and molecularly distinct from HPV-negative tumors. The histology of HPV-associated tumors frequently is basaloid or poorly differentiated squamous cell cancer, and the initial presentation often is as an unknown primary with a large cystic neck node(s). The verrucous cancer subtype of squamous cell cancer is strongly associated with HPV. Patients with HPV-associated tumors tend to be younger, have a history of minimal tobacco and alcohol exposure, and often a history of high-risk sexual behavior.

Patients with oropharynx carcinoma who are HPV-positive have higher survival rates compared with patients who are HPV-negative. A retrospective, multivariate analysis of the randomized, phase III Radiation Therapy Oncology Group (RTOG) 0129 trial, which was originally designed to compare accelerated-fractionation to standard-fractionation radiotherapy when delivered with concurrent cisplatin, was recently reported by Ang et al.[10] This analysis revealed significantly improved 3-year survival among patients who were HPV-positive compared with patients who were HPV-negative (84% vs. 57%, respectively).[10] Patients with HPV-positive tumors had a 58% reduction in risk of death compared with patients with HPV-negative tumors (hazard ratio [HR] 0.42, 95% CI 0.27 to 0.66). Patients with HPV-associated tumors also appear to have a lower risk of developing a second primary tumor.[13]

In a multicenter Eastern Cooperative Oncology Group (ECOG) study, patients with newly diagnosed stage III or IV head and neck squamous cell carcinoma (HNSCC) were treated with induction chemotherapy followed by chemoradiation; 60% of oropharynx primary tumors were found to be HPV-positive.[14] Two-year progression-free survival (PFS; 86% vs. 53%; p = 0.02) and overall survival (OS) rates (95% vs. 62%; p = 0.005)[14] also were significantly better for patients with HPV-associated cancer compared with HPV-negative cancers.

Another retrospective analysis of the Surveillance, Epidemiology, and End Results (SEER) data for patients with oropharyngeal cancer revealed a 4-fold higher survival in patients who were HPV-positive compared with patients who were HPV-negative (131 vs. 20 months).[6]

In situ hybridization, which is available at a limited number of referral centers, is considered the optimal test to confirm presence of HPV.[7] Expression of p16 is upregulated when HPV E7 oncoprotein degrades the retinoblastoma protein, whereas p16 expression in HPV-negative tumors is silenced by epigenetic promoter methylation or genetic mutation.[9] In RTOG 0129, analysis of tumoral p16 protein expression by immunohistochemistry performed numerically better than detection of HPV DNA in identifying the good prognostic group (HR 0.33, 95% CI 0.21 to 0.53). Thus, tumoral expression of p16 protein reflects biologically relevant HPV infection, is not genotype-specific, and is an excellent surrogate for HPV status.[15]

Epstein-Barr Virus

Nasopharyngeal and paranasal sinus cancers are not associated with tobacco or alcohol use; however, they are strongly associated with Epstein-Barr virus. Cancer of the nasopharynx is especially common among individuals from endemic areas in southern China and northern Africa, where World Health Organization (WHO) subtypes II (nonkeratinizing) and III (undifferentiated cancer), rather than type I (keratinizing), predominate. The Epstein-Barr viral genome can be found in nasopharyngeal cancer tissues and dysplastic lesions that progress to invasive disease. However, the exact role this virus plays in etiology is still being defined, and evidence of the Epstein-Barr virus can be found in nonmalignant nasopharyngeal tissue as well.

HEAD AND NECK CARCINOGENESIS
MOLECULAR PROGRESSION MODEL

A molecular progression model of multistep carcinogenesis has been elucidated for the transformation of normal mucosa to invasive squamous cell cancer.[16] The earliest genetic alteration noted during transition from normal mucosa to hyperplastic mucosa is the loss of genetic material from chromosome region 9p21 and inactivation of the *p16* tumor suppressor gene. The next step during transition from hyperplastic mucosa to dysplasia is the loss of 3p and 17p with inactivation of the *p53* gene. Transition from dysplasia to carcinoma in situ is associated with loss of chromosome regions 11q, 13q, and 14q; during transition to invasive squamous cell carcinoma, there is loss of chromosome regions 6p, 8p, and 4q.[16] More than one-half of patients with tobacco- and alcohol-associated HNSCC have disease with the *TP53* gene mutation and downregulation of p16 protein. In contrast, HPV-associated HNSCC characteristically demonstrates wild-type *TP53* and *RB1* genes and upregulation of p16 protein levels.

ORAL PREMALIGNANCY

Patients with head and neck cancer, specifically oral cancers, often have diffuse mucosal abnormalities related to tobacco (including marijuana), alcohol use, and betel quid chewing. Oral premalignancy, or intraepithelial neoplasia (IEN), is the precursor to invasive oral cancer. Understanding the stepwise molecular events that define the risk of progression to invasive disease and identifying potential targets for intervention are areas of intense research interest. The loss of genomic material–containing tumor suppressor genes (loss of heterozygosity [LOH] or allelic imbalance) of regions on chromosomes 3p, 9p, 11q, 17p, as well as p16 promoter hypermethylation and *p53* mutation, are steps in the progression of IEN to invasive cancer.[11]

Leukoplakia

Histologically, leukoplakia is the most common precancerous lesion in the oral mucosa. Clinically, it appears as white plaques distributed over the lip, buccal mucosa, floor of mouth, hard palate, tongue, and soft palate. The sites of leukoplakia at highest risk for severe (high-grade) dysplastic change or transformation to cancer are lesions located on the tongue, lip vermilion, and floor of mouth. Understanding the molecular events such as loss of 3p and/or 9p in the transformation of leukoplakia to invasive cancer may allow for stratification of patients by risk; this also may enable novel therapies to be tested in this population. There is no safe, effective systemic therapy for long-term use.

Erythroplakia

Clinically, erythroplakia presents as a red zone of mucosa clearly separated from the surrounding normal tissue by a distinct interface, and it occasionally has a pebbled or granular appearance. Erythroplakia may occur over the tongue, lower lip, floor of mouth, buccal mucosa, and oral commissure. Dysplasia is a common finding in most erythroplakic lesions, and the degree of dysplasia is increased compared to dysplasia associated with leukoplakia. The molecular changes noted with leukoplakia are also noted in the erythroplakia lesions.

FIELD CARCINOGENESIS AND SECOND PRIMARY TUMORS OF THE AERODIGESTIVE TRACT

Field carcinogenesis is a concept proposed in the 1950s that has been supported by many epidemiologic and molecular studies. Exposure to risk factors such as alcohol and tobacco results in carcinogen distribution over large areas in the upper aerodigestive tract, and the exposed mucosa (the "field") is a potential site for development of premalignant and invasive cancer. Given the central role of tobacco in the genesis of many head and neck cancers, medical comorbidity and synchronous or metachronous second primary tumors are common among these patients (3% to 7% per year, depending on whether tobacco use continues).[17] A tumor is considered synchronous if it occurred within 6 months of detection of the first primary tumor; a metachronous tumor is one that occurred more than 6 months after detection of the first primary. Geographically, these tumors should be separate and distinct with at least 1 cm of normal mucosa intervening. Synchronous lesions tend to present as premalignant mucosal lesions located in the head and neck, whereas metachronous lesions present as distinct tumors in the head and neck, lung, or esophagus.[18] Within the aerodigestive tract, the most frequent site of a second primary tumor is the lung, followed by the esophagus. The risk and distribution of second primary malignancies vary significantly according to the subsite of the index cancer. In a population-based cohort study of 75,087 patients with HNSCC in the SEER program, the risk of second primary tumors was highest for hypopharyngeal cancer and lowest for laryngeal cancer. Since the 1990s, during the HPV era, the risk for second primary tumors associated with oropharyngeal cancer has declined to the lowest risk level of any subsite. The most common second primary malignancy site for patients with oral cavity and oropharynx cancer was head and neck; for patients with laryngeal and hypopharyngeal cancer, the most frequent site was the lung.[19] A solitary pulmonary nodule is not rare in the work-up of a new pharyngeal or laryngeal cancer and should not be assumed to be a metastasis, particularly for a patient with an early-stage cancer. For example, a patient with early glottic cancer, no involved neck nodes, and a lung nodule is much more likely to have a second primary tumor than metastatic disease, mandating a curative treatment approach for both primaries.

PREVENTION AND CHEMOPREVENTION

Stopping the use of tobacco and alcohol (the two primary risk factors for HNSCC) is central to any prevention program. Counseling combined with the use of a pharmacologic intervention, such as a tapering nicotine patch, doubles success rates; however, very few smokers succeed in quitting on their first attempt. Important reasons for smoking cessation that clinicians can discuss with their patients include the fact that the rate of second primary tumors is higher among patients who continue to smoke and that continuing to smoke adversely influences the effectiveness and tolerance of cancer treatment.

PREVENTION TRIALS USING RETINOIDS

Testing of retinoids to halt or reverse the processes that ultimately lead to epithelial carcinogenesis began in the mid-1980s. Trials investigating 13-cis-retinoic acid (13cRA) in high and low doses for primary prevention of head and neck cancers demonstrated that high-dose 13cRA was able to reverse oral IEN for approximately two-thirds of premalignant lesions and was able to maintain the effect for the duration of treatment. However, intolerable side effects precluded chronic, long-term dosing.[20] As secondary prevention following curative treatment of early-stage head and neck cancer, placebo-controlled, randomized trials of isotretinoin have failed to demonstrate benefit for time to development of a second primary tumor, rate of second primary cancers, OS, and disease-free survival.[21-23]

No systemic therapy can be recommended, and patients with oral premalignant mucosal changes should be enrolled in clinical trials. Epidermal growth factor receptor (EGFR), which is dysregulated in the majority of premalignant and malignant lesions, appears to be a promising new target, and the role of cetuximab, an anti-EGFR monoclonal antibody, in secondary prevention is currently being explored. Another promising

target is the *p53* tumor suppressor gene. The pilot data from a trial evaluating ONYX-015, an adenovirus that lyses *p53*-deficient cells in a mouthwash formulation, reported 37% (7 out of 19 assessable patients) had histologic regression of a dysplastic lesion, and one had an improvement in grade of dysplasia.[24] The responses were transient. Future clinical application with this target would require a larger, randomized, phase II study.

CLINICAL PRESENTATION, DIAGNOSIS, AND STAGING

In general, cancers of the oral cavity, oropharynx, larynx, and hypopharynx are characterized by disease confined to the primary site with or without spread to regional nodes at the time of diagnosis and late metastatic spread. Less than 10% of patients have distant disease at presentation. Thus, initial disease staging and management focus on the extent of local-regional involvement and the effect of the choice of treatment on speech and swallowing function, as well as on the risk of recurrence.

PRESENTING SIGNS AND SYMPTOMS

Clinical signs and symptoms vary with the anatomic site affected. For example, patients with oral cavity cancer may present with mouth sores, a nonhealing ulcer, or pain. Symptoms of oropharyngeal cancer can range from sore throat to chronic dysphagia, persistent odynophagia, and otalgia. Patients with hypopharyngeal or supraglottic laryngeal cancer often seek medical attention at a later stage because of sore throat, hoarseness, difficulty swallowing, or neck mass as the initial presenting sign. Tumors of the glottic larynx tend to be diagnosed at an earlier stage than those of the supraglottic larynx or hypopharynx

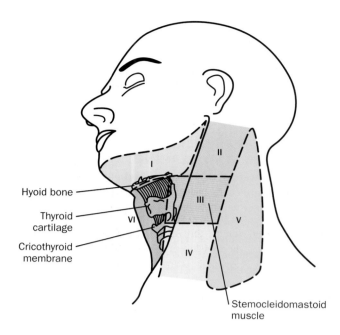

Hyoid bone

Thyroid
cartilage

Cricothyroid
membrane

Stemocleidomastoid
muscle

Fig. 8-2 Cervical lymph node levels.

*Reprinted from Shah JP, ed. Cancer of the Head and Neck. Hamilton, Ontario: BC
Decker Inc.; 2001.*

because hoarseness is an early symptom at the glottic subsite. The Eustachian tubes are frequently invaded by nasopharyngeal disease, leading to otitis media; for an adult patient, this mandates careful assessment of the nasopharynx. With more advanced tumors at this site, double vision may be the presenting symptom because of invasion of both the cavernous sinuses and the branches of the third, fourth, and particularly sixth cranial nerves, which track with these vascular structures.

Cervical Lymphadenopathy

The discovery of a painless lump in the neck is not an uncommon presenting complaint of a patient with head and neck cancer. The location of cervical adenopathy, denoted by dividing the neck into levels, may direct the physician to the primary site (Fig. 8-2). For example, cancers of the oral cavity typically spread to lymph nodes in the submental and submandibular areas (level I), laryngeal cancer spreads to the upper and mid-neck (level II and III), nasopharyngeal cancer spreads to the upper neck and posterior triangle (level II and V), and disease confined to the lower part of the neck or supraclavicular area should raise suspicion about a primary lesion below the clavicles or in the thyroid (level IV and V). Spread to the neck is uncommon for patients with primary cancers of the glottic larynx or paranasal sinus. Involvement of the neck nodes is prognostically important, reducing the cure proportion for a given tumor stage by approximately 50%.

DIAGNOSTIC EVALUATION

A comprehensive examination of the head and neck with the assistance of mirrors or fiber-optic scopes is central to the evaluation. Because lymph nodes track along the internal jugular vein,

examination of the neck for enlarged lymph nodes is facilitated by rotating the head toward the side being examined to promote relaxation of the sternocleidomastoid muscle on that side.

A commonly found mucosal lesion is leukoplakia (a white, hyperkeratotic patch, distinguishable from thrush in that it does not scrape off). The majority (approximately 80%) are benign lesions that can be observed without treatment. By contrast, erythroplakia presents as a red, velvety patch and is associated with a 90% incidence of severe dysplasia, carcinoma in situ, or invasive disease on microscopic examination.

Endoscopy

Examination under anesthesia often is necessary and important, especially for patients with tumors of the larynx or pharynx. The routine application of so-called triple endoscopy (laryngoscopy or pharyngoscopy with bronchoscopy and esophagoscopy added) to rule out synchronous tumors is controversial. If the primary site is known, the diagnostic yield of bronchoscopy or esophagoscopy is generally low. However, most clinicians agree these procedures are indicated for patients with evidence of diffuse mucosal abnormalities in the setting of a malignant neck node without a clear primary site, particularly when the lymph node is located in the lower part of the neck, which increases the likelihood of a lung or esophageal primary tumor. In addition, endoscopy has a low yield in nonsmokers, in whom a synchronous second primary cancer is less likely.

Imaging

Recommendations for imaging the primary site and the neck identify computed tomography (CT) or magnetic resonance imaging (MRI) for demarcating the extent of disease. A high-quality CT scan performed with contrast medium is less expensive than MRI and is sufficient for most cases. An extensive search for distant metastases for patients with head and neck cancer who do not have suspicious symptoms is not routinely done because the overall incidence of spread below the clavicles at the time of presentation is low (10% or less), particularly in the absence of lymph node involvement. Hence, performing positron emission tomography (PET)/CT or other body imaging is not cost-effective and should not be done routinely. A chest x-ray is performed to rule out a second primary lung cancer or to document chronic obstructive pulmonary disease, as well as to identify lung metastases.

A high-resolution CT scan is more sensitive than a chest x-ray for identifying a new primary site or metastases and could have a specific indication for the patient presenting with bulky N2 or N3 neck disease or a primary site of the hypopharynx, both of which are risk factors for metastatic spread. Formal imaging of the liver and bones should only be carried out if clinically indicated based on symptoms or a biochemical abnormality. By contrast, evaluation for metastatic disease with a body CT scan and bone scan, or by using 18-fluorodeoxyglucose (FDG)-PET/CT, is an appropriate part of the work-up for patients with nasopharyngeal cancer with lymph node involvement. In this setting, the incidence of distant metastases approaches 60%, and bone is the most common site of metastasis.

FDG-PET is appropriate when the primary site is unknown or to evaluate an equivocal finding on cross-sectional imaging; however, routine application of this test, particularly if disease management will not be affected, is expensive and not indicated. FDG-PET does not replace cross-sectional imaging of the primary site and neck and is best interpreted in the context of a separate or fused cross-sectional study performed with contrast. As with any diagnostic test, FDG-PET is not without fault. False-positive results can be related to dental disease or to an inflammatory process in the neck or elsewhere, and uptake by lesions smaller than 1 cm is inconsistent. FDG-PET with a fused contrast-enhanced CT scan may be useful for identifying spread to regional nodes in the N0 neck, the identification of which would alter radiation portals or the choice of neck dissection to be performed.[25-27] The sensitivity and specificity to detect nodal metastases is 90% and 94%, respectively.

Tissue Diagnosis

Histologic proof of cancer typically is obtained from a biopsy of the primary site, a neck node, or both. At least initially, needle aspiration of a lymph node is preferred to excisional biopsy, especially for an apparently malignant node with an occult primary lesion. This approach is both safe and feasible, and the theoretic risk of seeding malignant cells along the needle track has not been a problem in the clinic. Straightforward squamous cell cancers should pose few challenges to the cytopathologist; poorly differentiated tumors or lymphomas are more problematic. If an excisional biopsy is necessary, it ideally should be done to facilitate its incorporation into the definitive treatment of the patient. A surgeon capable of performing a neck dissection should be involved if squamous cell cancer is suspected.

STAGE CLASSIFICATION

The stage groupings for all primary sites are based on the tumor, node, and metastasis (TNM) classification of the American Joint Committee on Cancer (AJCC) and the Union for International Cancer Control (UICC). The TNM system is based on both clinical examination and radiographic information (Fig. 8-3). A few general rules of the clinical staging include:

- Primary tumors of the oral cavity and oropharynx that are 4 cm or larger are classified as T3; those with massive local invasion of adjacent structures are classified as T4.
- Vocal cord paralysis in the setting of a primary tumor of the larynx or hypopharynx indicates a T stage of no less than T3.
- For all primary sites except the nasopharynx, the nodal classifications are the same. In addition, the nasopharynx is one primary site for which an alternative staging system—the Ho staging system—is commonly used, particularly in Asia. Because definitions for component stages vary between the AJCC/UICC and Ho systems, these differences must be considered when reviewing the results of therapy.
- For all primary sites (Table 8-3) except the nasopharynx (Table 8-4), the TNM stage grouping is the same; clinical

lymph node involvement indicates an overall stage of at least stage III; the presence of distant metastases indicates stage IVC disease; and locally advanced resectable and unresectable stage IV disease (without distant metastases) are designated as IVA and IVB, respectively.
- The term "early-stage disease" refers to stage I and II disease and to low-volume stage III disease (e.g., T1 or T2 and N0 or N1); the term "locally advanced disease" refers to stage III and IV disease, specifically a large primary tumor (T3 or T4) or the presence of multiple or bulky neck nodes (N2 or N3). These designations correlate with the efficacy of single- or multimodality management.

A major modification to the sixth edition and reflected in the seventh edition of the AJCC/UICC TNM staging system (Table 8-3) was the division of T4 into T4a resectable (stage IVA) and T4b unresectable (stage IVB) categories. Stage IVC is metastatic disease. No changes were made to nodal classification staging: N1 is stage III, N2 is stage IVA, and N3 is stage IVB. For the nasopharynx, a T2a lesion is now considered T1, and stage IIA is now stage I. Similarly, a T2b lesion is considered T2 and stage IIB is now stage II. Retropharyngeal lymph node involvement (unilateral or bilateral location) is now considered N1.

Unresectable T4 Lesion

There is general agreement among surgeons regarding the following criteria for unresectability: base of skull involvement, fixation to the prevertebral fascia, carotid encasement, and involvement of the pterygoid musculature. Additional criteria that many would consider appropriate are the inability to perform an adequate reconstruction for a functional result, a low likelihood of achieving negative margins, and a requirement for total glossectomy. Assignment to the stage IVB category has implications for prognosis (i.e., less favorable) and treatment (i.e., primary surgical management not planned). For these primary sites, stage IVB disease now includes patients with T4b, any N category, and no metastasis (M0), or any T category and N3 (any neck node larger than 6 cm in greatest diameter). Stage IVC includes any T and N category, as well as M1 disease.

PRINCIPLES OF DISEASE MANAGEMENT

Historically, surgery and radiation therapy have been the central treatment modalities for head and neck cancers because they have curative potential. Management of the primary site and neck are separate but related concerns that influence decisions about which modality to use or the integration of combined-modality therapy. Although chemotherapy may enhance the effects of radiation therapy, chemotherapy by itself is not a curative modality. TNM stage groupings are helpful for defining prognosis and treatment options. Management of head and neck cancer is best served by multidisciplinary treatment planning that involves not only a surgeon, medical oncologist, and radiation oncologist, but also dentists, prosthodontists, nutritionists, audiologists, speech and swallowing therapists, physical and occupational therapists, and psychiatrists, as necessary. Plans for rehabilitation are an integral part of this process.

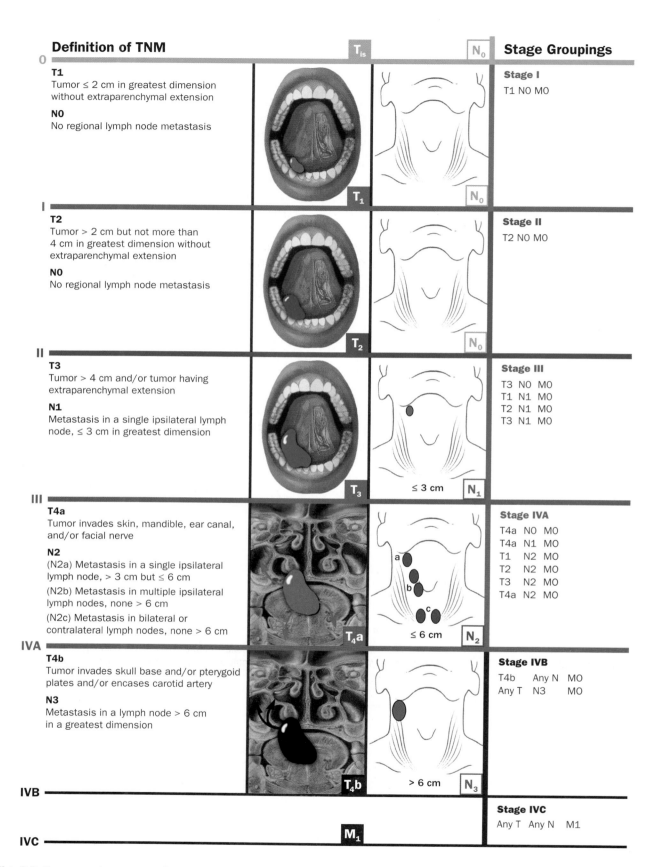

Definition of TNM

T1
Tumor ≤ 2 cm in greatest dimension without extraparenchymal extension

N0
No regional lymph node metastasis

T2
Tumor > 2 cm but not more than 4 cm in greatest dimension without extraparenchymal extension

N0
No regional lymph node metastasis

T3
Tumor > 4 cm and/or tumor having extraparenchymal extension

N1
Metastasis in a single ipsilateral lymph node, ≤ 3 cm in greatest dimension

T4a
Tumor invades skin, mandible, ear canal, and/or facial nerve

N2
(N2a) Metastasis in a single ipsilateral lymph node, > 3 cm but ≤ 6 cm

(N2b) Metastasis in multiple ipsilateral lymph nodes, none > 6 cm

(N2c) Metastasis in bilateral or contralateral lymph nodes, none > 6 cm

T4b
Tumor invades skull base and/or pterygoid plates and/or encases carotid artery

N3
Metastasis in a lymph node > 6 cm in a greatest dimension

Stage Groupings

Stage I
T1 N0 M0

Stage II
T2 N0 M0

Stage III
T3 N0 M0
T1 N1 M0
T2 N1 M0
T3 N1 M0

Stage IVA
T4a N0 M0
T4a N1 M0
T1 N2 M0
T2 N2 M0
T3 N2 M0
T4a N2 M0

Stage IVB
T4b Any N M0
Any T N3 M0

Stage IVC
Any T Any N M1

Fig. 8-3 Tumor, node, metastasis (TNM) staging for all primaries except nasopharynx.
Reprinted with permission from Rubin P, Hansen J. TNM Staging Atlas. Philadelphia, PA: Lippincott Williams & Wilkins; 2007.

Table 8-3 American Joint Committee on Cancer Staging: Lip and Oral Cavity, Oropharynx, Hypopharynx, and Larynx

Primary Tumor (T)	Tx	Primary tumor cannot be assessed
	T0	No evidence of primary tumor
	Tis	Carcinoma in situ
Lip and Oral Cavity	T1	Tumor 2 cm or less in greatest dimension
	T2	Tumor greater than 2 cm but less than 4 cm in greatest dimension
	T3	Tumor greater than 4 cm in greatest dimension
	T4	(lip) Tumor invades through cortical bone, inferior alveolar nerve, floor of mouth, or skin of face (i.e., chin or nose)
	T4a	(oral cavity) Tumor invades adjacent structures (e.g., through cortical bone, into deep [extrinsic] muscle of tongue [genioglossus, hyoglossus, palatoglossus, and styloglossus], maxillary sinus, skin of face)
	T4b	Tumor invades masticator space, pterygoid plates, or skull base and/or encases internal carotid artery
Oropharynx	T1	Tumor 2 cm or less in greatest dimension
	T2	Tumor greater than 2 cm but less than 4 cm in greatest dimension
	T3	Tumor greater than 4 cm in greatest dimension
	T4a	Tumor invades the larynx, deep/extrinsic muscle of tongue, medial pterygoid, hard palate, or mandible
	T4b	Tumor invades lateral pterygoid muscle, pterygoid plates, lateral nasopharynx, or skull base or encases carotid artery
Hypopharynx	T1	Tumor limited to one subsite of hypopharynx and 2 cm or less in greatest dimension
	T2	Tumor invades more than one subsite of hypopharynx or an adjacent site, or measures greater than 2 cm but less than 4 cm in greatest diameter without fixation of hemilarynx
	T3	Tumor greater than 4 cm in greatest dimension or fixation of hemilarynx
	T4a	Tumor invades thyroid/cricoid cartilage, hyoid bone, thyroid gland, esophagus, or central compartment soft tissue
	T4b	Tumor invades prevertebral fascia, encases carotid artery, or involves mediastinal structures
Larynx—Supraglottis	T1	Tumor limited to one subsite of supraglottis with normal vocal cord mobility
	T2	Tumor invades mucosa of more than one adjacent subsite of supraglottis or glottis or region outside the supraglottis (e.g., mucosa of base of tongue, vallecula, medial wall of pyriform sinus) without fixation of the larynx
	T3	Tumor limited to larynx with vocal cord fixation and/or invades any of the following: postcricoid area, pre-epiglottic tissues, paraglottic space, and/or minor thyroid cartilage erosion (e.g., inner cortex)
	T4a	Tumor invades through the thyroid cartilage and/or invades tissues beyond the larynx (e.g., trachea, soft tissues of neck including deep extrinsic muscle of the tongue, strap muscles, thyroid, or esophagus)
	T4b	Tumor invades prevertebral space, encases carotid artery, or invades mediastinal structures
Glottis	T1	Tumor limited to the vocal cord(s) with normal mobility
	T2	Tumor extends to supraglottis and/or subglottis, and/or with impaired vocal cord mobility
	T3	Tumor limited to the larynx with vocal cord fixation and/or invades paraglottic space, and or minor thyroid cartilage erosion
	T4a	Tumor invades through the thyroid cartilage and/or invades tissues beyond the larynx (e.g., trachea, soft tissues of neck including deep extrinsic muscle of the tongue, strap muscles, thyroid, or esophagus)
	T4b	Tumor invades prevertebral space, encases carotid artery, or invades mediastinal structures

Table 8-3 **continued**

	NX	Regional lymph nodes cannot be assessed		
Regional Lymph Nodes (N)	N0	No regional lymph node metastasis		
	N1	Metastasis in a single ipsilateral lymph node, 3 cm or less in greatest dimension		
	N2	Metastasis in a single ipsilateral lymph node, greater than 3 cm but less than 6 cm in greatest dimension, or in multiple ipsilateral lymph nodes, none greater than 6 cm in greatest dimension, or in bilateral or contralateral lymph nodes, none greater than 6 cm in greatest dimension		
	N2a	Metastasis in a single ipsilateral lymph node, greater than 3 cm but less than 6 cm in greatest dimension		
	N2b	Metastasis in multiple ipsilateral lymph nodes, none greater than 6 cm in greatest dimension		
	N2c	Metastasis in bilateral or contralateral lymph nodes, none more than 6 cm in greatest dimension		
	N3	Metastasis in a lymph node, greater than 6 cm in greatest dimension		
Distant Metastasis (M)	MX	Distant metastasis cannot be assessed		
	M0	No distant metastasis		
	M1	Distant metastasis		
Stage Grouping	Stage 0	Tis	N0	M0
	Stage I	T1	N0	M0
	Stage II	T2	N0	M0
	Stage III	T3	N0	M0
		T1	N1	M0
		T2	N1	M0
		T3	N1	M0
	Stage IVA	T4a	N0	M0
		T4a	N1	M0
		T1	N2	M0
		T2	N2	M0
		T3	N2	M0
		T4a	N2	M0
	Stage IVB	T4b	Any N	M0
		Any T	N3	M0
	Stage IVC	Any T	Any N	M1

The original source for this material is the AJCC Cancer Staging Manual, 7th Edition (2010) published by Springer Science and Business Media LLC, www.springerlink.com.

NEWLY DIAGNOSED T1 OR T2, N0 OR N1, AND M0 (STAGES I, II, AND LOW-BULK III) DISEASE

Single-modality treatment with surgery or radiation is typically used for previously untreated stage I, II, or low-bulk stage III disease—essentially, a small primary tumor with or without a single ipsilateral node measuring 3 cm or less in diameter. Cure rates for this group are quite favorable, ranging from 52% to 100%, depending on the primary site. Strategies to decrease the morbidity associated with treatment and to prevent second primary tumors have been research priorities. The chosen modality depends on local expertise, anticipated functional outcome, and patient preference. For example, a T1N0M0 tumor of the glottic larynx can be managed with surgery or radiation.

The 5-year OS rates associated with primary surgery (e.g., cordectomy and hemilaryngectomy) and primary radiation therapy (with salvage surgery as necessary) have been comparable (approximately 90%).[28] A cordectomy requires less time than radiation therapy and initially is cheaper, but repeat procedures may be necessary and could lead to a related decrease in function. Radiation therapy is associated with excellent control rates and voice function outcome, but it requires a 6-week course and initially may be more expensive.

NEWLY DIAGNOSED, HIGHER-VOLUME STAGE III AND STAGE IVA AND IVB DISEASE

If a higher-volume stage III or a stage IV tumor is resectable, the standard approach is surgery followed by adjuvant

Table 8-4 **American Joint Committee on Cancer Staging: Nasopharyngeal Carcinoma**

	WHO Classification	Former Terminology		
Classification of Nasopharyngeal Carcinoma	Type I: Squamous cell carcinoma	Squamous cell carcinoma		
	Type II: Nonkeratinizing carcinoma	Transitional cell carcinoma		
	Without lymphoid stroma	Intermediate cell carcinoma		
	With lymphoid stroma	Lymphoepithelial carcinoma (Regaud)		
	Type III: Undifferentiated carcinoma	Anaplastic carcinoma		
	Without lymphoid stroma	Clear cell carcinoma		
	With lymphoid stroma	Lymphoepithelial carcinoma (Schminke)		
Primary Tumor (T)	TX	Primary tumor cannot be assessed		
	T0	No evidence of primary tumor		
	Tis	Carcinoma in situ		
	T1	Tumor confined to the nasopharynx, extends to oropharynx and/or nasal cavity without parapharyngeal extension		
	T2	Tumor with parapharyngeal extension		
	T3	Tumor involves bony structures and/or paranasal sinuses		
	T4	Tumor with intracranial extension and/or involvement of cranial nerves, infratemporal fossa, hypopharynx, orbit, or masticator space		
Regional Lymph Nodes (N)	NX	Regional lymph nodes cannot be assessed		
	N0	No regional lymph node metastasis		
	N1	Unilateral metastasis in lymph node(s), 6 cm or less in greatest dimension, above the supraclavicular fossa		
	N2	Bilateral metastasis in lymph node(s), 6 cm or less in greatest dimension, above the supraclavicular fossa		
	N3	Metastasis in a lymph node(s) 6 cm or greater and/or to supraclavicular fossa		
	N3a	Greater than 6 cm in dimension		
	N3b	Extension to the supraclavicular fossa		
Distant Metastasis (M)	MX	Distant metastasis cannot be assessed		
	M0	No distant metastasis		
	M1	Distant metastasis		
Stage Grouping	Stage 0	Tis	N0	M0
	Stage I	T1	N0	M0
	Stage II	T1	N1	M0
		T2	N0	M0
		T2	N1	M0
	Stage III	T1	N2	M0
		T2	N2	M0
		T3	N0	M0
		T3	N1	M0
		T3	N2	M0
	Stage IVA	T4	N0	M0
		T4	N1	M0
		T4	N2	M0
	Stage IVB	Any T	N3	M0
	Stage IVC	Any T	Any N	M1

Abbreviation: WHO, World Health Organization.

The original source for this material is the AJCC Cancer Staging Manual, 7th Edition (2010) published by Springer Science and Business Media LLC, www.springerlink.com.

radiation therapy with or without concurrent chemotherapy based on pathologic risk features (see Principles of Surgery section), or combined chemotherapy and radiotherapy if organ preservation is desirable. If unresectable, the approach is radiation and concomitant chemotherapy. Cure rates are less favorable for this group, ranging from 10% to 65%, depending on the primary site and disease extent. Data from randomized trials support integrated chemotherapy and radiation as standard treatment options for patients with advanced, resectable cancers of the larynx and hypopharynx (with the intent of avoiding total laryngectomy) and for patients with cancers of the oropharynx when a nonsurgical approach is chosen. For patients with advanced tumors of the oropharynx, nasopharynx, or unresectable squamous cell cancers of the upper aerodigestive tract, combined-modality therapy improves survival compared with radiation alone (Table 8-5).[29-38] When primary chemotherapy and radiation therapy are used, surgery is reserved for persistent disease or for recurrence of resectable disease.

For locally advanced, resectable cancers of the oral cavity, primary surgical management with appropriate reconstruction and/or postoperative radiation therapy is the mainstay of treatment because anticipated functional outcomes are favorable.

Table 8-5 Concurrent Chemoradiotherapy Standard of Care

Organ Preservation	Regimen
Larynx	RT/cisplatin[28,29]
Oropharynx	RT/carboplatin/5-FU[30,31]
Nasopharynx	RT/cisplatin followed by cisplatin/5-FU[32]
Unresectable disease	RT/cisplatin[33]
Postoperative adjuvant	RT/cisplatin[34-38]

Abbreviations: 5-FU, 5-fluorouracil; RT, radiotherapy.

RECURRENT DISEASE WITHOUT A SURGICAL OR RADIATION OPTION, OR M1 DISEASE

For patients who receive chemotherapy, but for whom surgery or radiation therapy is not an option (including patients with distant metastases), disease is generally not curable, and the median survival ranges from 5 to 9 months for various available standard drugs. The identification of more effective chemotherapy and integration of targeted agents has been a research priority for this patient population.

PRINCIPLES OF SURGERY
SURGERY OF THE PRIMARY TUMOR

Complete removal of the tumor with negative margins defines an adequate surgical resection. Depending on the primary site and the size of the tumor, complete surgical extirpation may necessitate removal of key structures, such as the larynx, eye, or mandible. The potential adverse effect on cosmesis and function underscores the importance of rehabilitation as part of the treatment strategy. A variety of skin and bone flaps, as well as customized obturators and prosthetics, successfully address many defects that arise from surgery. Function-preserving procedures are applicable for selected patients in whom negative margins are achieved as uninvolved structures necessary for function are preserved. Examples include various subtotal laryngectomy procedures, for which adding a postoperative course of radiation therapy often compromises the functional outcome. Thus, all of these factors must be considered when deciding the best therapeutic option for each patient.

As the spectrum of reconstructive options increases, defining precise, reproducible criteria for tumor unresectability remains a challenge and complicates interpretation of the literature. A patient with an unresectable tumor should be distinguished from a patient with disease that is clearly resectable, but for whom there are medical contraindications to surgery (i.e., medically inoperable).

SURGERY OF THE NECK

Different types of neck surgery or dissection are used to address suspected or proven disease in the cervical lymph nodes. This is performed up-front or following completion of chemoradiation at the discretion of treating physicians. A comprehensive neck dissection involves the en bloc removal of all five lymph node levels (Fig. 8-2). Three important structures are potentially jeopardized by this procedure: the sternocleidomastoid muscle, the internal jugular vein, and the spinal accessory nerve. If none of these structures are spared, the procedure is considered a radical neck dissection, which also is associated with the highest likelihood of postoperative shoulder pain and weakness. Different types of comprehensive neck procedures that spare one, two, or three of these structures ("modified-radical neck dissections") may be performed for select patients, without compromising disease control. Comprehensive neck dissections generally are done with therapeutic intent, such as when cancerous lymph nodes are suspected or known to be present. In other settings, selective neck dissections are used, whereby fewer than five lymph node levels are removed. Selective procedures usually are performed electively in part to improve staging precision (such as when there are no palpable lymph nodes, but the estimated risk of occult metastases exceeds 15% to 20%, and negative findings on specimen analysis may obviate the need for postoperative radiation therapy). Additionally, PET imaging may prove useful in the post-treatment assessment of patients with node-positive disease who were treated with chemoradiotherapy and for whom a planned neck dissection is being considered.[39] Although the management of the clinically negative neck for patients with initial N2 or N3 neck disease is still controversial, the negative predictive value of FDG-PET and fused CT performed at least 8 weeks following completion of radiotherapy is high (94% to 100%) for patients with a negative clinical exam.[40,41] This suggests that such patients can be safely watched rather than moving forward with the planned neck dissection. Of note, all post-treatment assessments should be performed between 8 and 10 weeks after completion of all treatment.

PRINCIPLES OF RADIATION THERAPY

The curability of head and neck cancer with radiation therapy is inversely related to tumor bulk. The rate of disease control with radiation alone decreases with increasing T stage. This finding explains why radiation can be used as a single modality to treat early-stage disease but is generally applied as an adjunct to surgery or combined with chemotherapy for more advanced tumors.

RADIATION DOSE AND FRACTIONATION

The dose of radiation necessary to sterilize squamous cell cancer varies with the fractionation size and schedule used. Standard, once-daily fractionation consists of 2.0 Gy per day with a total dose of 70 Gy or greater to the primary site and gross adenopathy, and 50 Gy or greater to uninvolved nodal stations at risk. When given postoperatively, the total dose to the primary site and involved nodal stations is 60 Gy or greater, and the dose to uninvolved nodal stations at risk is 50 Gy or greater. Postoperative radiation generally begins 4 to 6 weeks after surgery. The delivery of radiation requires careful treatment planning. In particular, the spinal cord must be blocked to prevent radiation-induced cervical myelopathy.

Potential improvements in the therapeutic index of radiation for head and neck cancer may be achieved by altering the radiation fractionation (more than one fraction per day, often with change in the fraction size). The results of randomized trials have established the therapeutic benefits of an altered-fractionation strategy, particularly with regard to local-regional control. In one seminal study by the RTOG,[42] more than 1,000 previously untreated patients with stage II, III, or IV HNSCC were randomly assigned to four different radiation-only treatment arms: standard fractionation, 2 Gy daily, and 70 Gy over 7 weeks; hyperfractionation, 1.2 Gy twice daily, and 81.6 Gy over 7 weeks; accelerated fractionation with a split, 1.6 Gy twice daily, and 67.2 Gy over 6 weeks; and accelerated fractionation with a concomitant boost, 1.8 Gy daily, 1.5 Gy daily as a boost for the last 12 days only, and 72 Gy over 6 weeks.

With a median follow-up of 41.2 months among surviving patients, the hyperfractionation and concomitant boost arms yielded significantly improved local-regional control (p = 0.045 and p = 0.050, respectively), as well as a trend toward improvement in disease-free survival (p = 0.067 and p = 0.054, respectively). More acute toxicity, but not late effects, was seen in the three altered-fractionation groups. Although no significant differences in OS were demonstrated, a meta-analysis known as MARCH indicated a significant improvement in absolute survival at 5 years with altered-fractionation approaches (3.4%; HR 0.92, 95% CI 0.86 to 0.97; p = 0.003). This assessment included 15 randomized trials involving 6,515 patients that compared conventional radiotherapy with hyperfractionated or accelerated radiotherapy, or both.[43] The benefit was significantly higher with hyperfractionated radiotherapy than with accelerated radiotherapy (8% vs. 2% at 5 years, respectively). Altered-fractionation programs are increasingly being incorporated into standard practice for patients who can tolerate the added local-regional toxicity and also are being investigated in combination with concurrent chemotherapy.

With recent advances in technology, improved planning and delivery of radiotherapy has helped overcome some of the major side effects of conventional radiotherapy. Intensity-modulated

---

KEY POINTS

- Cells of both the antigen-nonspecific innate and antigen-specific adaptive response have been implicated in antitumor immunity.
- Specific immunity to tumors requires uptake of tumor antigens by antigen-presenting cells and presentation to T helper cells, which coordinate the generation of cellular and/or humoral responses.
- Immune responses are highly regulated. The generation of a productive response requires that a number of immunologic checkpoints be passed.

radiotherapy, a technique that is gaining popularity, delivers therapeutic radiation doses specifically around the tumor and the at-risk lymph nodes. The advantages of this technique are that the surrounding normal tissue can be spared and that anatomic structures (e.g., the pharyngeal constrictor muscles necessary for swallowing and the salivary glands) can be preserved.

RADIATION-RELATED TOXICITY

Radiation at the doses outlined previously is associated with predictable acute mucosal and skin toxicities. More aggressive dosing and fractionation schedules and the addition of concurrent chemotherapy generally increase the severity of these acute toxicities. Depending on the amount of salivary tissue included in the radiation portal, xerostomia and loss of taste are common. Because adequate saliva is an important component of oral hygiene, careful dental assessment is necessary before the start of radiation therapy, followed by ongoing dental prophylaxis and fluoride treatments. Pain management, nutritional support, swallowing evaluation and therapy, and aggressive oral care are required. Other potential complications include hypothyroidism, especially for patients receiving treatment to the larynx and pharynx; Lhermitte syndrome, a self-limited, shock-like sensation extending down the spine and extremities with neck flexion; long-term induration and fibrosis; and osteoradionecrosis of the mandible.

Some degree of xerostomia is common for patients. Pilocarpine (a cholinomimetic, muscarinic agent) and amifostine (a thiol with chemoprotectant and radioprotectant properties) are both approved for this indication. Amifostine is only approved for use with postoperative adjuvant radiotherapy and not in the definitive setting.

More effective therapies are needed to address xerostomia. In a prospective, randomized, double-blind, placebo-controlled trial of patients who received at least 40 Gy of radiation to the head and neck, oral pilocarpine (5 mg three times daily) improved salivary production and symptoms of dry mouth compared with placebo.[44] Amifostine was evaluated in a multicenter, open-label, randomized trial involving patients who received definitive radiotherapy or postoperative adjuvant radiotherapy with total radiotherapy doses of at least 40 Gy.[45] Patients were assigned to either radiation alone (cumulative dose of 50 Gy to 70 Gy) or to the same radiation dose with amifostine (200 mg/m^2 intravenously daily 15 to 30 minutes before radiation).[45] The incidence of grade 2 or higher acute and chronic xerostomia (as defined by RTOG Acute/ Late Morbidity Scoring Criteria) was significantly reduced in the amifostine arm (acute, 78% vs. 51%; p < 0.0001; chronic, 57% vs. 34%; p = 0.002), and median salivary production was significantly improved (0.10 vs. 0.26 g; p < 0.04). However, the frequency of mucositis was similar among the two groups. Nausea, vomiting, hypotension, and allergic reactions were significantly more common among patients treated with amifostine (p < 0.05), although grade 3 toxicities were infrequent (3% to 5% of patients). More convenient and better-tolerated ways to administer this drug (e.g., subcutaneous dosing) are being evaluated.

Conformal intensity-modulated radiation therapy (IMRT) also offers promise as a way to decrease the incidence and severity of xerostomia without compromising antitumor efficacy. The amount of salivary gland tissue included within the radiation portal can be reduced (defined as "salivary gland sparing"). Whether there is incremental benefit from the use of amifostine when IMRT is used is not known.

PRINCIPLES OF CHEMOTHERAPY

A number of drugs have activity against HNSCC, including methotrexate, cisplatin, carboplatin, fluorouracil (5-FU), paclitaxel, docetaxel, and ifosfamide. Gemcitabine, vinorelbine, bleomycin, topotecan, and irinotecan also are active but are used less frequently in current clinical practice. The reported response proportions vary with the setting (untreated or pretreated) and the drugs used (single-agent or combination). The best established and arguably most widely used treatment is a combination of cisplatin and infusional 5-FU, which will cause a complete plus partial response for 60% to 90% of previously untreated, advanced, local-regional tumors; clinical complete responses also are common (20% to 50%). By contrast, the activity of the same drug combination for recurrent disease is 30% to 40%, and complete responses are rare. Rates of complete and partial responses from single-agent therapy are approximately one-half of those observed with combination chemotherapy; these rates range from 13% to 31% for the previously listed drugs.

The use of chemotherapy for patients with potentially curable, advanced, local-regional disease is generally distinguished from the treatment of patients with incurable, recurrent, metastatic disease. For patients with potentially curable cancer, the chemotherapy literature can be divided into the following four groups:

- Induction or neoadjuvant chemotherapy administered for several cycles prior to definitive local therapy (surgery or radiation therapy);
- Concomitant chemotherapy and radiotherapy in the setting of locally advanced, unresectable disease;
- Organ-preservation techniques for patients with resectable cancers of the oropharynx, larynx, and hypopharynx; and
- Local curative therapy (surgery) followed by adjuvant chemotherapy and radiotherapy.

The goals of these multimodality approaches are to improve survival by reducing rates of local-regional recurrence and metastases, as well as to achieve preservation of the organ and its function without a decrement in the survival rates achievable with primary surgery. The latter specifically refers to preservation of the larynx for patients with primary cancers of the larynx or hypopharynx, and preservation of structures in the oropharynx for speech and swallowing function, such as the tongue.

INDUCTION CHEMOTHERAPY USING CISPLATIN AND 5-FU

Studies evaluating the integration of induction chemotherapy with local-regional treatment dominated the literature of head and neck cancer during the 1980s and early 1990s. The results of randomized, controlled trials evaluating two to four courses of cisplatin-based combination chemotherapy as induction followed by local therapy demonstrated a decrease in distant metastases in some trials, but no significant differences were observed in either local-regional control or OS when compared with the standard of care for most trials and meta-analyses.[46-49] This result was despite the high level of antitumor activity for cisplatin and infusional 5-FU in addition to the 85% complete and partial response rates.

A meta-analysis of 63 randomized trials of local-regional treatment with or without chemotherapy was performed using updated patient data.[49] In this comprehensive review, there was no significant survival benefit from the addition of induction chemotherapy (31 trials, 5,269 patients; HR 0.95, 95% CI 0.88 to 1.01; p = 0.10). A subgroup analysis focusing on trials in which induction cisplatin and 5-FU were used showed a significant survival benefit for this regimen (HR 0.88, 95% CI 0.79 to 0.97; p = 0.05).

Taken collectively, these data do not support a role in standard clinical practice for induction chemotherapy in the setting of planned surgery and radiation (with improvement in OS as the endpoint). However, trials that investigated the addition of a taxane (docetaxel or paclitaxel) to cisplatin and infusional 5-FU have stimulated much interest in the re-evaluation of induction chemotherapy. The approach likely will be of greatest research interest for patient populations at increased risk for distant metastatic disease (e.g., disease categories N2 to N3 and in selected primary sites) and for those in whom initial primary surgical treatment is not planned or feasible (i.e., unresectable disease or resectable disease with an organ-preservation endpoint).

INDUCTION CHEMOTHERAPY USING CISPLATIN AND 5-FU PLUS TAXANE

The results from three randomized, controlled trials comparing three or four cycles of induction docetaxel, cisplatin, and 5-FU with standard 100 mg/m² of cisplatin plus 1,000 mg/m² of continuous infusion 5-FU daily for 5 days have been published and presented at international meetings.[50-52] The TAX 323 trial enrolled more than 300 patients with locally advanced, unresectable disease. The control arm consisted of four cycles of the two-drug combination followed by radiotherapy, and the experimental arm consisted of four cycles of the three-drug combination (75 mg/m² of docetaxel; 75 mg/m² of cisplatin; 750 mg/m² per day of 5-FU continuous infusion for 5 days) followed by radiotherapy.[50] The response rate to the induction of the three-drug regimen was significantly higher compared with that of the two-drug regimen (68% vs. 54%; p = 0.006) as was OS (HR 0.73, 95% CI 0.57 to 0.94; p = 0.016). There also was less nonhematologic toxicity with the three-drug combination than with the two-drug combination; however, hematologic toxicity was more common with the three-drug regimen.

Similarly, the TAX 324 trial randomly assigned 501 patients with unresectable or resectable disease (all sites) to three cycles of standard cisplatin plus 5-FU or to combination docetaxel plus cisplatin and 5-FU (75 mg/m² of docetaxel; 100 mg/m² of cisplatin; 1,000 mg/m² per day of 5-FU continuous infusion for 4 days).[51] Definitive local therapy in both arms consisted of standard radiotherapy plus weekly carboplatin (area under the curve [AUC] = 1.5). OS was significantly improved for patients who received the three-drug therapy (HR 0.70, 95% CI 0.54 to 0.90; p = 0.0058).

The third trial was conducted by the European Groupe d'Oncologie Radiotherapie Tete et Cou (GORTEC) study group for organ preservation in patients with either cancer of the larynx or cancer of the hypopharynx.[52] In the trial, 220 patients were randomly assigned to receive standard cisplatin and 5-FU for three cycles (control) or combination docetaxel plus cisplatin and 5-FU for three cycles (dosing, same as TAX 323). More than one-half of the enrolled patients had a hypopharynx primary tumor and the stage of the primary tumor was T3 for the majority of patients. Following induction of both therapies, patients with responsive disease received 70 Gy of standard radiation; patients whose disease did not respond to chemotherapy underwent total laryngectomy followed by radiotherapy with or without additional chemotherapy. The three-drug therapy was shown to be statistically superior for the endpoints of response to the induction regimen (83% vs. 61%) and preservation of a functional larynx at 3 years (63% vs. 41%). More details of the patient population and outcomes are needed for interpretation of the results in the context of other larynx preservation trials for these two primary sites.

These three trials demonstrate that combination docetaxel plus cisplatin and 5-FU followed by radiotherapy alone or radiotherapy plus concurrent carboplatin is superior to cisplatin plus 5-FU followed by the same definitive local therapy. Also, the three-drug regimen administered in TAX 323 seems to have had an acceptable toxicity profile with lower rates of severe and life-threatening myelosuppression than those observed with the two-drug regimen.[50] A fourth phase III trial has been published in final form.[53] This trial compared induction paclitaxel plus cisplatin and 5-FU with induction cisplatin plus 5-FU in a heterogeneous population of patients with resectable and unresectable disease. Chemoradiation was planned following induction chemotherapy, but the actual treatment was not uniform. The taxane-containing treatment group experienced a higher overall response rate (80% vs. 68%); however, the difference in OS was not significant.

In addition to the above reviewed trials, a recently published meta-analysis of five randomized trials representing 1,772 patients that compared cisplatin plus 5-FU induction therapy versus a taxane plus cisplatin and 5-FU regimen confirmed the superiority of the taxane-containing induction regimen with a substantial reduction in progression, local-regional failure, and distant failure compared with cisplatin plus 5-FU.[54]

These data provided rationale for two recently presented phase III trials that compared induction chemotherapy with taxane plus cisplatin and 5-FU, followed by chemoradiation or radiation therapy alone compared with concomitant chemoradiation. Unfortunately, both of these trials were closed prematurely because of poor accrual.

The PARADIGM study randomly assigned 145 patients with locally advanced head and neck cancer to receive docetaxel, cisplatin, and 5-FU induction therapy followed by concurrent chemoradiation (with either docetaxel or carboplatin) versus cisplatin-based concurrent chemoradiotherapy alone (with two cycles of bolus cisplatin).[55] After a median follow-up of 49 months, the 3-year OS was 73% in the induction therapy followed by chemoradiation group and 78% in the chemoradiotherapy alone group (p = 0.77). More patients had febrile neutropenia in the induction therapy group.

The DeCIDE trial, which was presented at the 2012 ASCO Annual Meeting, was a phase III trial that randomly assigned 280 patients with N2 to N3 locally advanced head and neck cancer to receive two cycles of docetaxel, cisplatin, and 5-FU induction therapy, followed by chemoradiation therapy compared with chemoradiation therapy alone.[56] The concomitant therapy was similar in both arms and consisted of cisplatin, 5-FU, and hydroxyurea. With a minimum follow-up of 24 months, the OS was similar in both arms at 75% in the induction arm and 73% in the concomitant therapy alone arm (p = 0.70); however, the cumulative incidence of distant failure was higher in the concomitant therapy alone arm (19% vs. 10% in the induction therapy arm; p = 0.025). Grade 3 to 4 leukopenia and neutropenia was higher in the induction arm.

The PARADIGM and DeCIDE trials demonstrated better than expected survival outcomes in the control arm, and given poor accrual and premature closure, these studies were therefore underpowered to identify a difference in outcome. In addition, they both did not stratify for HPV status at study entry. Hematologic toxicity was higher in the induction arm. Therefore, at this time, although induction chemotherapy with a taxane plus cisplatin and 5-FU followed by chemoradiation remains a definite option, it cannot be concluded that it is superior to concomitant chemoradiation therapy alone in the management of locally advanced head and neck cancer.

The role of induction chemotherapy followed by surgery and postoperative radiation therapy was recently investigated in a phase III trial that evaluated 256 patients with locally advanced (stages III and IVa) oral squamous cell cancers.[57] Patients received two cycles of docetaxel, cisplatin, and 5-FU induction followed by surgery and postoperative radiation therapy compared with upfront surgery and postoperative radiation therapy. There was no increased perioperative morbidity noted with the induction arm. At a median follow-up of 30 months, there was no significant difference in OS between the two arms of the study. This approach of induction chemotherapy followed by surgery and postoperative therapy therefore cannot be considered as a standard treatment paradigm.

CONCOMITANT CHEMOTHERAPY AND RADIATION

Since the early 1990s, concomitant chemotherapy and radiation has progressively displaced induction chemotherapy followed by radiation in therapeutic investigations for patients with locally advanced HNSCC. The focus has been on drugs that show activity against the disease and radiation-enhancement properties (e.g., cisplatin and 5-FU). The two general strategies that can be identified amidst a broad spectrum of approaches are:

- Concomitant single-agent or combination chemotherapy with continuous-course radiation; or
- Combination chemotherapy with planned split-course radiation.

More recently, altered-fractionation approaches have become an added variable. Historically, the use of chemotherapy in this manner was applied to patients with unresectable disease and generally increased the severity of acute mucosal and skin toxicities, but also improved local-regional control compared with radiation alone. These encouraging efficacy results led to studies of other patient groups (e.g., resectable, organ-preservation intent, and poor-risk adjuvant).

A study first reported in 1992 was the turning point for the growing interest in concomitant chemoradiation for advanced head and neck cancer.[58] In this study, the investigators randomly assigned 157 patients with unresectable HNSCC to radiation alone (up to 70 Gy, conventional fractionation) or to a cisplatin plus 5-FU combination alternating with radiation (up to 60 Gy). The complete response rate (43%) and the survival rate (41%) in the group treated with chemoradiation were significantly superior to those in the radiation alone group (22% and 23%, respectively; p = 0.01).

Another trial randomly assigned 295 patients with unresectable HNSCC to one of three treatment groups: radiation alone (70 Gy, 2 Gy daily); the same radiation with concurrent cisplatin (100 mg/m^2) on days 1, 22, and 43; or split-course radiation (60 Gy to 70 Gy, 2 Gy daily) with three cycles of concurrent bolus cisplatin and infusional 5-FU. In the third arm, the option existed to pursue surgical resection after the second cycle of chemotherapy, if possible; resection was available for all three groups if feasible after the completion of treatment.[34] With a median follow-up of 41 months, there was a significant survival advantage at 3 years associated with concurrent cisplatin and radiation compared with radiation alone (37% and 23%; p = 0.014). The split-course concurrent regimen offered no survival advantage compared with the control groups (27%). Toxicity of grade 3 or higher was significantly more common with concurrent therapy (52% with radiotherapy alone vs. 89% with concurrent therapy; p < 0.0001). This trial established radiation with concurrent high-dose cisplatin as the standard of care for locally advanced unresectable head and neck cancer.

The meta-analysis by Pignon et al[49] that included the 1992 study and other trials of note highlights the favorable results seen with a concurrent approach in these early trials. Although substantial heterogeneity among trial designs was noted, the concurrent chemoradiation regimen was associated with an 8% absolute benefit in survival at 5 years compared with radiation alone (HR 0.81, 95% CI 0.76 to 0.88; p < 0.0001). An updated analysis of 87 trials involving more than 16,000 patients showed the same absolute benefit for survival with concomitant treatment (HR 0.81; p < 0.0001).[59]

The Meta-Analysis of Chemotherapy in Head and Neck Cancer (MACH-NC) examined randomized concurrent chemoradiation studies for patients with locally advanced HNSCC and was conducted with the intent of developing clinical recommendations.[60] With data from 1,514 patients in nine trials, the investigators found that platinum-based concurrent programs offered the greatest survival advantage compared with radiation alone (odds ratio [OR] 0.57, 95% CI 0.46 to 0.71; p < 0.00001). The investigators recommended that if concurrent therapy is pursued, a platinum-based regimen associated with a positive trial and a more favorable side-effect profile should be used. The MACH-NC analysis also confirmed that cisplatin-based chemoradiation provided the most substantial benefit in terms of survival and local-regional control.[61]

Once-daily fractionation radiation therapy for 7 weeks with high-dose cisplatin (100 mg/m^2 on days 1, 22, and 43) was compared with accelerated boost radiation therapy (42 fractions over 6 weeks) in combination with two cycles of cisplatin (100 mg/m^2 on days 1 and 22) in the RTOG 0129 trial.[10] There was no statistically significant difference in OS between the arm receiving three cycles or two cycles of high-dose cisplatin.

Carboplatin is an alternative to cisplatin, as a radiosensitizer, in patients with borderline renal function, poor performance status, or who cannot tolerate fluid boluses given with cisplatin.[51] Weekly carboplatin (AUC 1.5 to 2) has been considered acceptable if the patient is not a candidate for cisplatin.

The use of targeted therapies concurrent with radiotherapy is an area of great interest. EGFR is highly expressed in virtually all HNSCC, and expression is inversely associated with prognosis. Therefore, EGFR inhibitors have been the focus of most targeted therapy trials in head and neck cancer. Cetuximab was approved by the U.S. Food and Drug Administration (FDA) for use in combination with radiotherapy for patients with advanced head and neck cancer based on a multicenter trial published by Bonner and colleagues.[62] This important proof-of-principle trial randomly assigned patients with locally advanced squamous cell cancers of the oropharynx, larynx, and hypopharynx to treatment with radiotherapy alone (standard or altered fractionation schedules) or to the same radiotherapy with concurrent weekly cetuximab. Local-regional failure-free survival and OS rates were significantly improved with the addition of cetuximab. The median duration of local-regional failure-free survival was 24.4 months with cetuximab and 14.89 months with radiotherapy alone (p = 0.005). The 3-year survival rates were 57% with cetuximab compared with 44% for radiotherapy alone (p = 0.02). Cetuximab had no effect on distant metastases; the effect on local-regional control using standard definition (death censored, events defined as local and/or regional recurrence) was not reported. Whether this combination of radiotherapy plus a biologic therapy is as effective as the standard of chemoradiation is unknown; therefore, the exact role and indications for cetuximab with radiotherapy are not clear. The patient population was heterogeneous relative to resectability, primary site, and radiation schedule. Exploratory subset analyses suggested that benefit was limited to primary sites of the oropharynx and to treatment with altered-fractionation radiotherapy schedules, but the sample size was small and these analyses were unplanned.

At present, the only indication for cetuximab with radiotherapy in lieu of platinum-based chemotherapy is for the treatment of patients whose age, performance status, and/or extent of comorbid disease would preclude cisplatin or carboplatin use. Numerous trials are testing the addition of cetuximab or small molecule tyrosine kinase inhibitors (TKIs) to chemoradiation in various disease settings. One such trial, RTOG 0522, directly compared cisplatin and radiation with or without cetuximab.[63] After a median of 2.4 years, there was no statistically significant improvement in the 2-year PFS (64% vs. 63%; HR 1.05, 95% CI 0.84 to 1.29; p = 0.66) and OS (83% vs. 80%; HR 0.87, 95% CI 0.66 to 1.15; p = 0.17). Another recently reported randomized, phase II trial evaluated cisplatin and radiotherapy with or without erlotinib in locally advanced HNSCC.[64] In the trial, 200 patients were randomly assigned to receive cisplatin

100 mg/m^2 on days 1, 22, and 43 combined with 70 Gy of radiotherapy or the same chemoradiotherapy with 150 mg of erlotinib per day. With a median follow-up of 26 months, the complete response rates (40% vs. 52%; p=0.08) and PFS were similar (p = 0.71). Therefore, at this time the addition of cetuximab or small molecule TKIs to standard cisplatin and radiation is not supported, with the exception of a clinical trial setting.

Given the favorable prognosis of HPV-related oropharyngeal cancer, recent efforts have focused on attempts to de-intensify the definitive standard modalities of radiation and chemotherapy. The disease control rates for patients with HPV-positive low-risk disease (N0 to N2a or N2b with less than or equal to 10 pack-year smoking history) were similar for radiation therapy alone and chemoradiation therapy in a recently published retrospective series.[65] However, the rate of disease control was lower in the N2c subset managed by radiation therapy alone (73% vs. 92% for chemoradiation; p = 0.02). Besides T and N staging, stratification by smoking exposure may also help risk-stratify these patients. These data are considered exploratory and at this time any de-intensification approach, although attractive in reducing long-term toxicities, should be considered investigational.

In summary, concurrent chemoradiation leads to improved disease control compared with radiation alone for patients with unresectable HNSCC, and represents standard treatment for patients who are able to tolerate the anticipated added treatment-related toxicity. There also is a role for this approach in the organ-preservation and larynx-preservation setting and for advanced local-regional nasopharyngeal cancer. The data showing improvement are best established for platinum-based concurrent regimens; an advantage persists even when newer altered-fractionation approaches are employed.

ADJUVANT CHEMORADIATION

The results of two randomized, controlled trials have clarified the role of chemoradiation in the postoperative adjuvant setting when compared with radiotherapy alone. These studies, conducted by the European Organisation for Research and Treatment of Cancer (EORTC),[35] as well as the trial by the RTOG,[36] addressed the question of whether the addition of cisplatin to standard postoperative radiotherapy (based on pathologic criteria) would improve the outcome for patients. The experimental arms of both studies consisted of standard fractionation radiation with concurrent cisplatin (100 mg/m^2) on days 1, 22, and 43. The 5-year results of the EORTC study indicated significant improvement in PFS (47% vs. 36%; p = 0.04) and OS (53% vs. 40%; p = 0.02) in favor of concurrent cisplatin plus radiation. The findings of the RTOG study initially demonstrated a significant advantage with combined-modality adjuvant therapy for the first two outcomes, but not for OS (3-year survival, 56% vs. 47%; p = 0.09). In both studies, toxicity was greater with concurrent chemoradiation.

Although the treatment was very similar, the high-risk pathologic features were not uniform, and the study populations differed. The entry criteria for the RTOG study were the presence of multiple positive nodes, extracapsular extension of tumor, or a positive margin. In contrast, the EORTC trial defined

high-risk as having a positive margin, extracapsular extension of nodal disease, vascular embolisms, or perineural disease; for oral cavity or oropharynx primary sites, high-risk was defined as positive nodes at level IV or V. These differences may, in part, explain the variable outcome of the two trials. In an effort to reconcile these two trial results, a pooled analysis was performed, indicating that the subsets of patients in both trials who experienced a significant benefit from cisplatin added to radiotherapy had either microscopically involved margins or extracapsular extension of disease in neck nodes.[37] Therefore, the presence of either or both of these risk factors is considered a definite indication for adjuvant chemoradiation. Since these analyses were performed, the RTOG trial data have been re-analyzed with longer follow-up, and data now demonstrate a substantial advantage for chemoradiation in terms of improvement of local-regional control. The difference in disease-free survival is no longer significant.[38] These results underscore the importance of reporting mature outcome data, but do not change current treatment recommendations.

COMBINED MODALITY TREATMENT: ORGAN PRESERVATION

Initial organ preservation studies were designed around the use of induction chemotherapy for patients with resectable disease and subsequently have focused on concomitant chemoradiotherapy. A number of pilot studies established the feasibility of treatment with chemotherapy followed by radiation therapy, with surgery reserved for patients with disease at the primary site that did not respond to chemotherapy, patients with persistent disease after radiation, or patients experiencing local-regional recurrence. These trials yielded survival results comparable with historical controls and led to successful organ preservation for a substantial proportion of patients. Avoidance of total laryngectomy received the greatest attention in these early studies, and preservation of the larynx was the focus of three subsequent randomized trials.[48,66-68]

LARYNX AND HYPOPHARYNX ORGAN PRESERVATION

The Department of Veterans Affairs Laryngeal Cancer Study Group (VALCSG) conducted a seminal randomized trial in which induction cisplatin and 5-FU infusion (three cycles) followed by radiation therapy (with surgery reserved for patients whose disease had an inadequate response, disease persistence, or relapse) was compared with total laryngectomy followed by radiation therapy.[66,67] The 332 patients had advanced, resectable, T2 to T4 laryngeal cancer. There was no significant difference in survival between the groups with more than 10 years of follow-up subsequent to the original publication; total laryngectomy was avoided for approximately two-thirds of survivors who received combined chemotherapy and radiation. On multivariate analysis, T4 or N2 disease were both significant predictors of treatment failure, with 56% of T4 cases eventually requiring laryngectomy. The pattern of failure differed between the two treatment groups, with a substantial reduction in distant failure, but a higher rate of local failure for the patients randomly assigned to induction chemotherapy compared with those in the surgery control arm. Long-term quality-of-life outcomes also were assessed. Among the 46 long-term survivors surveyed, those who received induction chemotherapy plus radiation had significantly better quality-of-life scores (p < 0.05), better pain scores, and less depression. After 2 years, communication (speech) scores favored the induction chemotherapy group, but at longer follow-up the two treatment groups had similar speech scores.[69]

The EORTC performed a similar study involving patients with advanced, resectable (T2 to T4) cancer of the hypopharynx.[48] There was no difference in survival between the two groups; the 5-year estimate of successful larynx preservation (i.e., local control and no tracheostomy or feeding tube) was 35%. These two studies established induction cisplatin and infusional 5-FU followed by radiation (for the patients whose disease responded) as an alternative to initial surgical management. This combined-modality approach became a standard treatment option for patients with locally advanced, resectable laryngeal or hypopharyngeal cancer seeking to avoid total laryngectomy. Close monitoring for recurrence and timely integration of salvage surgery are important parts of these combined approaches and are necessary for survival to remain comparable with the survival rates associated with primary surgical management.

During the 1990s, interest shifted from induction chemotherapy to concomitant chemotherapy and radiation not only as definitive treatment for unresectable squamous cell cancers, but also for patients with resectable disease who chose organ preservation rather than initial surgery. Available data suggested that concomitant chemotherapy with radiation was more effective than the sequential administration of these modalities because of improvement in local-regional control. In one randomized study, primary radiation therapy (68 Gy to 72 Gy, 1.8 Gy to 2 Gy daily) was compared with the same radiation regimen plus concurrent daily cisplatin (20 mg/m² per day) and 5-FU (1,000 mg/m² per day) for 4 days starting on days 1 and 22. Enrolled patients had resectable, stage III or IV HNSCC.[70] Surgery was recommended for both groups if no response was evident at 50 Gy to 55 Gy, or for disease persistence or recurrence at the completion of treatment. Most of the 100 patients enrolled had primary lesions of the larynx, hypopharynx, or oropharynx. With a median follow-up of 5 years, survival with successful primary-site preservation was superior in the chemoradiation group (5-year rates were 34% vs. 42%, respectively; p = 0.004), albeit at the expense of greater acute hematologic toxicity, mucositis, cutaneous reaction, weight loss, and the need for a feeding tube during treatment. There was no significant difference in OS, which was attributed to effective salvage surgery and competing causes of death.[34]

Intergroup R91-11, a follow-up to VALCSG, addressed two questions unresolved in the prior trial, including the optimal sequencing of chemotherapy and radiotherapy (induction followed by radiation or concomitant chemoradiation) and the precise contribution of chemotherapy added to radiotherapy.[29] In the trial, 547 patients with T2 to low-volume T4, nonmetastatic,

squamous cell cancer of the larynx were randomly assigned to one of three treatment arms: radiation alone (70 Gy, 35 fractions); concomitant cisplatin (100 mg/m²) administered intravenously on days 1, 22, and 43 with the same radiation dose; or induction cisplatin plus 5-FU followed by radiation for patients who had a complete or partial disease response of the primary site. In all groups, laryngectomy was reserved for patients with insufficient response, suspected disease persistence, or local recurrence. A planned neck dissection was performed at approximately 8 weeks after completion of radiation in patients who had N2 or N3 disease at initial staging.

The results at 2 years showed significant improvement in the larynx preservation rate for the concomitant-treatment arm (88%) compared with the induction arm (75%; p = 0.005) and the radiation-alone arm (70%; p < 0.001). Local-regional control also was significantly better with concomitant treatment compared with the other two treatments (78% vs. 61% and 56%, respectively). Chemotherapy suppressed distant metastases, with rates of 8%, 9%, and 16% for concomitant, induction, and radiation-alone arms, respectively. Disease-free survival was significantly better in both the concomitant (61%) and the induction (52%) arms compared with the radiation-alone arm (44%); however, the OS rates did not differ among the three groups. Chemotherapy-related toxicities (grade 3 to 4 mucositis in the concomitant arm and grade 3 to 4 myelosuppression in the induction arm) were more common in the combination treatment groups than in the radiation-alone group, although rates for possible treatment-related deaths were not significantly different. Mature data (reported after a minimum follow-up of nearly 5 years and, more recently, 10.8 years) for all patients confirmed these results (Table 8-6).[71,27]

Laryngectomy-free survival is an endpoint that combines survival and a quality-of-life parameter and does not account for patients dying from other causes with an intact larynx. Although this would not be chosen as the primary endpoint in modern practice, laryngectomy-free survival was the endpoint used to generate the statistical hypothesis in 1990. In the initial 2-year data analysis of this endpoint, only the concomitant arm showed significant improvement when compared with radiation alone; however, in the mature analysis, both induction and concomitant arms reached statistical significance compared with radiation alone for laryngectomy-free survival. The importance of this finding for clinical practice is unclear because the larynx-preservation and local-control results were not different for patients treated with induction chemotherapy followed by radiotherapy or with radiotherapy alone; these results were inferior to the results with concomitant cisplatin and radiotherapy. Late toxicity did not differ across the three arms of the study. It is intriguing, however, that OS favored the induction arm numerically but not statistically by 11%. The clinical relevance of this finding and its rationale remain unclear at this time.

In summary, mature results from Intergroup R91-11 showed that induction platinum plus 5-FU followed by radiotherapy and concomitant cisplatin plus radiotherapy show similar efficacy for the endpoint of laryngectomy-free survival. Local regional control and larynx preservation were substantially

Table 8-6 RTOG 91-11 Results: 5- and 10-Year Outcomes

Treatment Arm	Time (years)	LFS (%)	LP (%)	DM (%)	DFS (%)	OS 5-Year (%)
Cis/5-FU followed by RT	5	44	71	14.7	37.7	58.1
	10	29	68	16.6	20.4	38.8
CRT	5	47	83.6	13.6	38	55.1
	10	24 (p = 0.68 vs. induction; p = 0.03 vs. RT alone)	81.7 (p = 0.005 vs. induction; p < 0.001 vs. RT alone)	16.1	21.6 (p = 0.04 vs. RT alone)	27.5 (p = 0.08 versus induction; p = 0.53 vs. RT alone)
RT alone	5	34	66	22	28	53.8
	10	17	64	24	14.8	31.5 (p = 0.29 vs. induction)

Abbreviations: 5-FU, 5-fluorouracil; cis, cisplatin; CRT, concomitant chemoradiation; DFS, disease-free survival; DM, distant metastases; LFS, laryngectomy-free survival; LP, larynx preservation; OS, overall survival; RT, radiotherapy; RTOG, Radiation Therapy Oncology Group.

improved with concomitant cisplatin plus radiotherapy compared with the induction arm or radiotherapy alone. OS did not differ significantly across the three arms.[71] For patients who wish to preserve their larynx, 100 mg/m^2 of daily cisplatin administered on days 1, 22, 43 during radiotherapy is the standard of care, with surgery reserved for patients with persistent or recurrent disease following treatment completion.

A randomized larynx preservation trial for patients with locally advanced, resectable cancer of the larynx or the hypopharynx is in progress by the EORTC. This trial will compare induction chemotherapy followed by radiotherapy with an alternating schedule of chemotherapy and radiotherapy. The preliminary results demonstrated no significant difference in rates for preservation of a functional larynx at 3 years and no difference in survival. Until further details of the trial are known, induction cisplatin plus 5-FU (as previously evaluated by the EORTC) remains the evidence-based recommendation of standard of care for locally advanced cancers of the hypopharynx.[72] However, based on the data involving combination docetaxel, cisplatin, and 5-FU as induction therapy, it would be appropriate to substitute this triple-drug regimen for cisplatin plus 5-FU for this treatment sequence.

OROPHARYNX ORGAN PRESERVATION

Given the results of these larynx-preservation studies, the concomitant chemoradiation approach also has been of investigational interest for locally advanced, resectable tumors of other primary sites for which surgical management may lead to substantial cosmetic or functional morbidity. GORTEC[31,32] reported a noteworthy site-specific trial in which 226 patients with stage III or IV squamous cell cancer of the oropharynx were randomly assigned to either radiotherapy alone (70 Gy, 35 fractions) or to the same radiation program with concomitant bolus doses of carboplatin (70 mg/m^2 daily for 4 days) and 5-FU (600 mg/m^2 as a daily 24-hour infusion for 4 days) starting on days 1, 22,

and 43. Concomitant treatment yielded a better 3-year survival rate (51% vs. 31%; p = 0.02) and disease-free survival (42% vs. 20%; p = 0.04), albeit at the expense of greater toxicity. Mucositis, related weight loss, and the need for a feeding tube, as well as hematologic toxicity, occurred more frequently in the chemoradiation group. Therefore, this treatment approach is considered an evidence-based standard treatment option and is particularly applicable for the management of T3 to T4 or N2 to N3 disease located at the base of tongue or tonsils.

Available data indicate that concomitant chemoradiation is feasible for oropharynx cancer, and disease-control outcomes compare favorably with those obtained historically with primary surgical management. However, a series of site-specific, direct, randomized comparisons with standard surgery and postoperative radiation therapy are lacking for this malignancy. Nonetheless, most head and neck oncologists believe the evidence is sufficiently compelling to support the use of concomitant chemoradiation in standard practice as initial management for advanced oropharyngeal cancer, even if resectable. For other sites of advanced resectable disease, especially the oral cavity (for which good reconstructive options exist), primary surgical management is better established and remains the standard of care.

In general, for patients with locally advanced squamous cell cancer of the larynx, hypopharynx, or oropharynx, concomitant chemoradiation yields better disease control compared with radiation alone, albeit at the expense of greater acute toxicity. This is the preferred organ preservation approach for cancer of the larynx and oropharynx. It must be emphasized that successful application of a chemoradiation strategy for organ preservation requires a team approach that includes not only the head and neck surgeon, radiation oncologist, and medical oncologist, but also a nutritionist, oncology nurse, and social worker. Close monitoring with comprehensive head and neck examinations and timely integration of salvage surgery, when necessary, are part of the treatment plan and are necessary to avoid compromising survival. The evaluation of functional and quality-of-life outcomes is another parameter for assessing the overall benefit of organ preservation therapies and will be an important factor in comparing therapeutic approaches.

Survivorship is an important area that needs attention. Studies involving survivors of head and neck cancer have mainly focused on the social supports, tobacco and alcohol use, functional status, and depression, and how these factors influence quality of life.[73-75] Chronic pain, xerostomia, impairments of speech and swallowing, alterations of taste and smell, and poor cosmesis are some of the long-term sequelae associated with treatment for head and neck cancer. These variable long-term factors can have a profound psychosocial effect on cancer survivors and their families. Fortunately, advances in reconstructive techniques and organ preservation strategies are having a positive effect on quality of life relative to the functional and cosmetic consequences of radical local therapies of the past. Nevertheless, quality of life and survivorship issues must be a focus of future research and an integral component of those efforts.[76]

NASOPHARYNGEAL CANCER

Cisplatin-based concurrent chemoradiation is the cornerstone of therapy for newly diagnosed, advanced, local-regional nasopharyngeal cancer. Although this treatment is widely used, disagreements arise regarding the role of adjuvant chemotherapy in this setting. The clinical behavior of nasopharyngeal cancer varies somewhat according to its histologic subtype.

WHO type I (squamous cell cancer) is more common in the United States than in regions endemic for Epstein-Barr virus and has a local-regional behavior similar to that of other head and neck cancers. WHO types II (nonkeratinizing cancer) and III (undifferentiated cancer), both of which can occur with lymphoid stroma ("lymphoepithelioma"; Table 8-4), predominate in endemic areas (such as southern China and northern Africa) and have a higher propensity for distant metastases. WHO types II and III are also more responsive to radiotherapy and chemotherapy than the differentiated squamous histology,

---

KEY POINTS

- WHO type I nasopharyngeal cancer (squamous cell cancer) is more commonly found in the United States, whereas WHO types II (nonkeratinizing cancer) and III (undifferentiated cancer) overwhelmingly predominate in endemic areas, such as southern China and northern Africa, and are associated with the Epstein-Barr virus. Types II and III are more responsive to chemotherapy and radiation therapy than type I.
- The standard of care (according to stage) is radiotherapy alone for stage I and IIA, and concurrent cisplatin and radiotherapy followed by three cycles of adjuvant cisplatin and 5-fluorouracil for stage IIB, III, IVA, and IVB nasopharyngeal cancer.

---

and more than 90% of cases are associated with the Epstein-Barr virus. Radiation is the historic mainstay of treatment for disease above the clavicles. The same drugs used in the management of squamous cell cancers arising from other sites in the head and neck, such as cisplatin, 5-FU, and the taxanes, are also active in nasopharyngeal cancer.

The management of locally advanced nasopharyngeal cancer was dramatically changed after the results of the Intergroup nasopharynx study were published.[33] In this trial, patients with stage III or IV nasopharyngeal cancer were randomly assigned to receive either radiation alone (70 Gy, 35 fractions for 7 weeks) or the same radiation schedule with three planned doses of concomitant cisplatin (100 mg/m^2) administered every 21 days, followed by three cycles of adjuvant cisplatin (80 mg/m^2) and 5-FU (1,000 mg/m^2 per day for 4 days). Most patients (91%) had stage IV disease, and WHO type I histology was more common compared with series from endemic areas. With a minimum follow-up of 5 years, OS was significantly improved for patients who had received combined-modality therapy (67% vs. 37%; p < 0.001), as was PFS (58% vs. 29%; p < 0.001). This occurred even though only 63% of patients received all three planned cycles of cisplatin during radiation and only 55% received all three cycles of adjuvant cisplatin and 5-FU.

The Intergroup study was criticized because the relative contributions of the concurrent and the adjuvant therapies could not be determined, and the trial results may be less applicable to endemic areas where WHO type I histologic subtypes are infrequent. However, subsequent randomized trials[77-79] in endemic areas and two meta-analyses[80,81] have confirmed the significant survival advantage afforded by concurrent platinum chemotherapy and radiation (as compared with radiation alone). By contrast, randomized trials of induction chemotherapy followed by radiation compared with radiation alone have shown no significant improvement in OS,[82-85] although some reported improved relapse-free survival. Two meta-analyses of trials that compared any sequence of chemotherapy and radiotherapy with radiotherapy alone have been published. The meta-analysis reported by Huncharek et al[80] was a pooled analysis of the published results of six randomized trials involving 1,500 patients. Investigators reported that at 4 years, chemotherapy improved PFS by 34% and OS by 20%. The second meta-analysis used updated individual patient data from eight randomized trials (1,753 patients with locally advanced disease), spanning from 1966 to 2003.[81] The effect on OS of adding chemotherapy to radiotherapy was an absolute survival benefit of 6% (56% to 62%) at 5 years (HR of death 0.82, 95% CI 0.71 to 0.94; p = 0.006). The effect observed on event-free survival was an absolute benefit of 10% (42% to 52%) at 5 years (HR of tumor failure [local, regional, or distant] or death 0.76, 95% CI 0.67 to 0.86; p < 0.0001). A significant interaction between the timing of chemotherapy and OS was observed, with the highest benefit resulting from concomitant administration of chemotherapy and radiotherapy (p = 0.005).

Based on these data as a whole, the survival benefit from cisplatin-based chemotherapy and radiation administered concomitantly seems clear and is the accepted standard of care within and outside of the United States. The benefit of adjuvant chemotherapy, theoretically used to suppress distant metastases common in nasopharyngeal cancer, is less widely accepted. Recently published, a trial by Chen et at[86] compared concurrent chemoradiation with or without adjuvant chemotherapy in 251 patients with nonmetastatic stage III or IV nasopharyngeal carcinoma. The primary endpoint was failure-free survival. After a median follow-up of 37.8 months, the estimated 2-year failure-free survival rate was 86% in the concurrent chemoradiation plus adjuvant chemotherapy arm and 84% in the concurrent chemoradiation only arm (p = 0.13). Based on these findings, the National Comprehensive Cancer Network guidelines were modified to include concurrent chemoradiation without adjuvant chemotherapy as an acceptable option. In the United States, the standard of care for treatment of patients with stage IIB, III, IVA (T4N0 to N2M0), and IVB (any TN3M0) nasopharyngeal cancer is radiotherapy (70 Gy) with concurrent high-dose cisplatin on days 1, 22, and 43, followed by three courses of adjuvant cisplatin and infusional 5-FU (dosing and schedule per the Intergroup trial published by Al-Sarraf).[33] Radiotherapy alone is indicated for stages I and IIA (N0 and no parapharyngeal space involvement).

Current areas of investigation in the management of nasopharyngeal cancer include the potential benefit of changing the sequencing of the three cycles of chemotherapy from adjuvant (after chemoradiation) to sequential (prior to chemoradiation) and the exploration of alternative cytotoxic regimens. The high risk of distant spread, coupled with the ability to successfully deliver all three cycles of adjuvant chemotherapy in only 55% of patients in the Intergroup trial, has motivated the investigation of sequential chemotherapy and chemoradiation. However, there is concern that this sequence of treatment might compromise the delivery of chemoradiation, the critical curative component of the treatment. The early results from several single-institution trials of sequential therapy have shown feasibility, as well as encouraging response and survival data. Rischin and colleagues[87] tested three cycles of induction epirubicin, cisplatin, and 5-FU followed by 60 Gy of radiotherapy and concurrent cisplatin (20 mg/m^2 daily for 5 days, administered on weeks 1 and 6) in 35 patients with stage III to IV nasopharyngeal cancer. All patients completed the induction phase, and 97% completed radiotherapy and cisplatin. It is noteworthy that the total dose of radiotherapy was lower than the standard dose and that two (rather than three) courses of cisplatin were administered concurrently with the radiotherapy. The OS at 4 years was 94%, and PFS was 81%. Chan and colleagues[88] evaluated induction carboplatin and paclitaxel followed by cisplatin (40 mg/m^2 per week) in 31 patients with stage III to IV nasopharyngeal cancer. All patients completed the induction phase, and 71% tolerated at least 6 weekly doses of cisplatin during radiotherapy. A preliminary report of the results at 2 years demonstrated an OS rate of 92% and a PFS rate of 78.5%. The preliminary results of a randomized, phase

II trial conducted by the same investigators were reported in 2005.[78] The two treatments were radiotherapy and cisplatin (40 mg/m^2 per week) with or without induction docetaxel and cisplatin. For 53 randomly assigned patients, major response to induction was observed in 86% of nasopharyngeal primary tumors and 80% of neck nodes; the complete response rate after cisplatin and radiotherapy was 96% at the primary site and 80% in regional nodes. In the chemoradiation arm, complete response was achieved for 84% at the primary site and for 64% of regional nodes. The numbers of patients in these trials was small, the enrolled population was from endemic areas, and the concurrent chemoradiation regimen that was used in the United States was not evaluated. However, the results appear promising, and this sequential approach warrants further study.

INCURABLE RECURRENT OR DISTANT METASTATIC DISEASE
Systemic Therapy

Disease that cannot be resected and has been previously irradiated or involves distant organs is considered incurable. Cisplatin, carboplatin, docetaxel, paclitaxel, 5-FU, and methotrexate are the most commonly used cytotoxic agents to treat recurrent or metastatic HNSCC. Activity also has been demonstrated for bleomycin, irinotecan, gemcitabine, capecitabine, oxaliplatin, cyclophosphamide, ifosfamide, pemetrexed, and, more recently, targeted drugs such as cetuximab. Randomized trials comparing combination chemotherapy and single-agent therapy show a near doubling of the response rate with platinum-based combinations, but unless a clinical complete response is achieved, the duration of response is brief (2 to 4 months) and does not have a significant effect on OS.[89-91]

Toxicity is generally greater when combination chemotherapy is used. As an example, one meta-analysis included all studies in which cisplatin and 5-FU, the historic gold-standard combination regimen, was compared with single-agent therapy.[92] A significant improvement in response was documented, which translated into only a 2-week difference in the median survival (OR 0.43, 95% CI 0.29 to 0.63). No formal quality-of-life data were available, but toxicity was greater for patients who received combination therapy. Numerous single agents have activity and can be used, but weekly methotrexate is the historic gold-standard because of its ease of administration, toxicity profile, and relative low cost.[93] Combination chemotherapy should be limited to patients with a good performance status (e.g., ECOG performance status of 0 to 1) who are better able to tolerate the added toxicity; for these individuals, the higher response rate may translate into better palliation, although there are no objective quality-of-life data to support this notion. Factors associated with poor response in this population are well known and include poor performance status, the presence of comorbidities, bulky local-regional disease or high tumor volume, and prior treatment for recurrent disease.

It was hoped that the introduction of the taxanes in the 1990s would result in improved survival for patients with recurrent disease, but this has not occurred. Two different weekly schedules of paclitaxel offered no advantage compared with weekly single-agent methotrexate.[94] Results from another study showed that paclitaxel plus cisplatin did not differ significantly from standard cisplatin plus 5-FU in terms of the median survival rate (9 vs. 8 months, respectively) and the 1-year survival rate (30% vs. 41%, respectively), although the paclitaxel regimen was generally better tolerated.[95]

Cetuximab is the only molecularly targeted drug to be approved for use in metastatic head and neck cancer; its indication is for platinum-refractory disease. Phase II trials of cetuximab alone or combined with cisplatin for patients who had experienced either stable or progressive disease as the best response to a standard platinum-based doublet were in the range of 10% to 13%.[96-98] In a randomized trial in which the combination of cisplatin and placebo was compared with cisplatin plus cetuximab for 123 patients, no significant difference was found in median PFS (2.7 vs. 4.2 months, respectively; p = 0.27), although the rate of major response (complete plus partial) was significantly higher for patients who received cisplatin plus cetuximab (10% vs. 26%, respectively; p = 0.03).[99]

A more recently published phase III trial by Vermorken et al randomly assigned 440 patients to either cisplatin plus 5-FU and cetuximab or cisplatin plus 5-FU as first-line treatment for patients with recurrent or metastatic HNSCC.[100] With a median follow-up of 19.1 months in the cetuximab group and 18.2 months in the chemotherapy-alone group, it was found that adding cetuximab to cisplatin and 5-FU significantly prolonged the median OS from 7.4 to 10.1 months (HR for death 0.80, 95% CI 0.64 to 0.99; p = 0.04), significantly prolonged the median PFS from 3.3 to 5.6 months (HR for progression 0.54; p < 0.001), and increased the response rate from 20% to 36% (p < 0.001). This is the first trial to show any improvement in OS when compared with the standard regimen of cisplatin plus 5-FU.

The small molecule TKIs gefitinib and erlotinib have modest activity in this setting (including responses for patients who received prior chemotherapy). In a phase II trial of 52 patients, administration of 500 mg per day of gefitinib resulted in an 11% major response rate.[101] For erlotinib, administration of 150 mg per day resulted in a 4% major response rate in a phase II trial of 115 patients.[102] Recently, a phase III trial evaluated the combination of docetaxel with or without gefitinib in 270 patients with recurrent or metastatic HNSCC. Although the addition of gefitinib to docetaxel was well tolerated, it did not improve outcomes.[103] Disease stabilization was similar, at approximately 50%. Combination trials with other agents directed at downstream targets of the EGFR pathway, such as the vascular endothelial growth factor (VEGF) inhibitor bevacizumab, are ongoing.[104] One phase II trial of erlotinib and bevacizumab resulted in a 17% response rate and median survival of 7.5 months for patients previously treated for recurrent disease.[105] A number of other multitargeted agents are entering clinical trials in head and neck cancer as well.

Re-Irradiation

Repeat radiation therapy is increasingly feasible with the greater availability of conformal technology. Building on the improved disease control seen with concurrent chemoradiation for untreated patients, this approach also has been investigated in the recurrent disease setting. Phase II trials suggest that for a proportion of patients (up to 25% in some studies), disease control is more durable than what would be anticipated with chemotherapy alone. This re-irradiation approach may represent a good option for select patients, but remains investigational. In one study, investigators reported the results with full-dose repeat radiation therapy with or without chemotherapy for 169 patients; 13 patients experienced complete remissions ranging from 12 months to 111 months.[106] Two successive phase II RTOG trials used split-course radiation and twice-daily fractionation at a total dose of 60 Gy.[107,108] The concurrent chemotherapy used in the first trial (R96-10) was 5-FU and hydroxyurea; the second trial (R96-11) utilized cisplatin and paclitaxel. At median follow-up of just under 2 years, the 2-year OS rates were 17%[96] and 25%,[108] respectively, suggesting that for a subset of patients, re-irradiation might provide a survival advantage over palliative chemotherapy alone. The two studies demonstrated feasibility of the approach when analyzed for factors that predicted a favorable survival outcome; an interval of at least 3 years from the original radiation was seen in R96-10, but not in R96-11. However, a phase III trial (R04-21) comparing re-irradiation and concurrent chemotherapy with chemotherapy alone was terminated because of poor accrual.[107] Quality-of-life and function data in addition to monitoring serious late effects (such as complications from vascular damage [stenosis and thromboembolism], osteoradionecrosis, and soft tissue necrosis) are critical assessments that were planned in addition to measurement of survival.

CANCER OF UNKNOWN PRIMARY SITE

Although for most patients the primary site will be found after comprehensive examination of the head and neck, assessment under anesthesia, and diagnostic imaging, a malignant neck lymph node without a clear primary tumor is a common occurrence in the head and neck. The location of the lymph node in the neck directs the examiner toward the likely potential primary sites, and PET scanning may be helpful. In recent years, FDG-PET has become an effective diagnostic tool in identifying the primary site for patients who present with cervical lymph node metastases with unknown primary. A meta-analysis of 16 studies revealed the overall sensitivity of FDG-PET was 88% and specificity was 75%.[109] FDG-PET is now considered part of the standard evaluation for squamous cell carcinoma of unknown primary.

A needle aspiration of the lymph node is the first choice for initial biopsy. If negative, repeat fine-needle aspiration with consideration of a core needle biopsy, if feasible, is appropriate. If the histologic diagnosis remains inconclusive, subsequent excisional biopsy should be performed in such a way that the incision can be incorporated into an appropriate neck dissection. Open biopsy done inappropriately may contaminate the surgical field and create a larger problem.

If pathologic findings from the neck indicate a diagnosis of squamous cell cancer and a primary lesion above the clavicles is suggested, especially if the lymph node is high in the neck, a comprehensive head and neck examination under anesthesia is the next step. Directed biopsies should be performed for suspicious mucosal areas, as well as locations known to be a source of occult tumors, such as the hypopharynx, base of the tongue, and nasopharynx. In addition, a bilateral tonsillectomy is recommended based on the increasing incidence of tonsillar cancers associated with HPV.[5] Of note, the skin, upper part of the esophagus, and lung are other potential sources of squamous cell cancer spread to the neck. If the findings on biopsy of the lymph node indicate an adenocarcinoma, the primary lesion sites such as the thyroid gland, salivary gland, or sites below the clavicles should be considered. Lymphoma is another important diagnostic possibility and may require a core needle biopsy for diagnostic purposes. Similarly, distinguishing lymphoma from anaplastic and undifferentiated or poorly differentiated cancers can be difficult based on cytologic analysis alone, and may require additional immunohistochemical studies or more tissue.

The treatment of patients with squamous cell cancer in a neck node of unknown primary site is controversial and evolving. Historically, either surgery or radiation was used to treat patients with low-bulk disease in a single lymph node, whereas both modalities were necessary for patients with more advanced disease. The extent of radiation to the putative primary sites requires clinical judgment regarding the likely source of the tumor because a larger portal will increase the morbidity associated with treatment. Findings from clinical series indicate that with longitudinal follow-up, the primary site will

ultimately be found for approximately 30% of patients. Long-term survival is better for patients in whom the primary lesion remains occult than for those in whom it does not. The mainstay of treatment is still a neck dissection followed by radiation with concomitant cisplatin when extracapsular extension of nodal disease is present. However, integrated concomitant chemoradiation is increasingly used for these patients based on the physician's impression of the likely primary site(s).

MALIGNANT LESIONS OF THE SALIVARY GLANDS

Cancers of the major salivary glands (parotid, submandibular, sublingual) and the minor salivary glands are uncommon, accounting for fewer than 10% of epithelial head and neck tumors. Tobacco and alcohol use are not risk factors for tumors of the salivary glands, but there may be an association with prior exposure to radiation. The WHO classification lists 24 different histologic subtypes of malignant epithelial salivary tumors. Their small numbers, as well as their histologic and prognostic heterogeneity, make them difficult to study; therefore, there are few adequately tested regimens in any one histology to guide the medical oncologist.

The most common types of salivary gland cancers are adenoid cystic carcinoma and adenocarcinoma, which originate from the intercalated ducts, and mucoepidermoid carcinoma, which originates from the secretory ducts. A histologic reading of high-grade mucoepidermoid or adenocarcinoma correlates with aggressive behavior and greater likelihood of eventual metastasis, whereas low-grade cancers of these histologies are more likely to be cured with initial local therapies. Adenoid cystic cancer is the most common tumor found in the minor salivary glands, is prone to neurotropic spread, and has the highest propensity of the different histologic subtypes for distant metastases, yet it can grow in a very indolent manner. Salivary duct carcinoma is an aggressive subtype of adenocarcinoma arising in the parotid with rapid appearance of metastases.

Surgery is the mainstay of treatment for all primary and recurrent resectable disease with adjuvant radiation, as indicated by the presence of adverse pathologic features.[110] There is a tendency among medical oncologists to recommend the addition of cisplatin or other chemotherapy as a radiosensitizer to improve local-regional control, but there are no data to support this. The role of systemic therapy is limited to the palliative management of metastases or locally recurrent disease that is no longer treatable by surgery or radiation.

Radiation-based therapy is used for unresectable tumors. Neutron beam therapy has shown promise in this setting, especially for adenoid cystic cancer. Concurrent chemotherapy with radiation is feasible—given the data from the management of squamous cell cancers of the upper aerodigestive tract—and not uncommonly applied for unresectable disease, although there are no data indicating improved efficacy with this approach compared with radiation alone.

The available data regarding the activity of different chemotherapy agents are limited and commonly include mixed histologic subtypes; most older reports are case series rather than true clinical trials. A trial of single-agent paclitaxel showed activity for patients with mucoepidermoid carcinoma and adenocarcinoma, but not for adenoid cystic carcinoma, emphasizing the importance of histology-specific trials.[111] The available data for other single agents and standard cytotoxic combinations were reviewed by Laurie and Licitra.[112] The most commonly used regimens include cyclophosphamide, doxorubicin, cisplatin, and 5-FU in various two- and three-drug combinations. Responses are reported for all three histologic types, but no one trial or case series included enough patients with a given histology for statistical confidence.

As a rule, mucoepidermoid cancer appears sensitive to the drugs used for HNSCC. Adenocarcinoma and adenoid cystic carcinoma may be more indolent; therefore, palliative chemotherapy should only be attempted for the symptomatic patient or when substantial tumor growth can be appreciated on serial imaging within a 6-month time frame. In this setting, doxorubicin, cisplatin, and 5-FU are often used as single agents; the combination of cyclophosphamide, doxorubicin, and cisplatin is also a frequently used regimen.[113] Even with combination chemotherapy, the rates of complete and partial responses will be low, and it is appropriate to consider investigational therapy. Epirubicin, mitoxantrone, and vinorelbine have demonstrated activity in adenoid cystic cancer,[114-116] but no such activity has been observed for paclitaxel.[111]

The search for molecular targets for which there are available therapies is the focus of investigation. It is reasonable to obtain a panel of immunohistochemical stains that might direct treatment. These markers may include c-kit, EGFR, BCL-2, HER2, and hormone receptors. The c-kit target is expressed in approximately 80% of adenoid cystic cancers, whereas EGFR expression is quite variable; the hormone receptors and HER2 are rarely expressed. Imatinib has been evaluated in adenoid cystic carcinoma in a phase II trial with no objective responses observed.[112] However, progressive disease was not an eligibility requirement, nor was the presence of c-kit mutations or high expression levels. Thus, further evaluation of imatinib may be warranted, but the data are insufficient to support a role for its use in adenoid cystic

carcinoma. Overexpression of EGFR is commonly seen in mucoepidermoid carcinoma, whereas c-kit, HER2, and hormone receptors are rarely expressed. In adenocarcinoma, c-kit is variably expressed depending on the histologic subtype; hormone receptor expression is rare, and EGFR expression is uncommon. With the proliferation of targeted agents, there is considerable interest in evaluating multitargeted agents, such as lapatinib (dual inhibitor of EGFR and HER2),[117] as well as agents that affect vascular endothelial cell proliferation, such as sorafenib and axitinib. Investigational agents for adenoid cystic carcinoma and the other salivary gland histologies are best evaluated in multicenter collaborations.

Microscopically, salivary duct carcinoma looks identical to ductal breast cancer, is commonly androgen receptor–positive, and may also overexpress HER2 and EGFR by immunohistochemistry. Responses have been reported to antiandrogen therapy.[118] A trial involving trastuzumab for patients with HER2-positive tumors is underway in the cooperative groups.

KEY POINTS

- Metastatic adenoid cystic cancer and adenocarcinoma are often characterized by an indolent natural history. Systemic treatment should be delayed until substantial tumor growth can be appreciated on serial imaging studies within a 6-month time frame.
- High-grade mucoepidermoid carcinoma responds to the same regimens used for squamous cell cancers from other sites.

THYROID CANCER

The American Cancer Society estimated 56,460 new cases of thyroid cancer in the United States and 1,780 deaths from the disease in 2012.[119] The incidence of this cancer continues to rise in the United States, with a 2.4-fold increase in incidence noted between 1973 (3.6 cases per 100,000 people) and 2002 (8.7 cases per 100,000 people); however, the mortality rate is stable at 0.5 deaths per 100,000 people.[120] This change in incidence is accounted for by an increase in papillary thyroid cancer, but not other histologic types. Nearly 90% of these cancers are subclinical or smaller than 2 cm in size, which suggests that earlier diagnosis may account for most of the observed change in incidence.

Thyroid cancers are classified based on the two main parenchymal cells of origin: the follicular cells involved in thyroid hormone production and the parafollicular cells that produce calcitonin. The former give rise to well-differentiated thyroid cancer (which constitutes 90% of thyroid malignancies) and to anaplastic thyroid cancer (1% to 2% of thyroid cancers); the latter give rise to medullary thyroid cancer (5% to 9% of thyroid cancers). The histologic subtypes within the well-differentiated thyroid cancer classification are papillary, mixed tumors with areas of papillary and follicular histologic features, follicular, follicular variant of papillary, and Hürthle cell.

ETIOLOGY

The only well-documented etiologic factor for thyroid cancer is radiation, with an inverse relationship between age of exposure and risk of developing a thyroid malignancy. When the thyroid gland of children younger than age 10 is exposed to ionizing radiation, it is highly vulnerable to developing thyroid cancer. The risk of developing thyroid cancer is much higher for individuals who have been exposed to radioactive iodine isotopes from nuclear reactor accidents and atomic bomb development testing, as well as for children and young adults who have received external radiotherapy for other cancers (e.g., Hodgkin lymphoma, neuroblastoma, or Wilms tumor) compared with individuals irradiated during childhood for benign conditions (as was common until 1960). Data from Chernobyl show that nearly all thyroid cancers developing in children after exposure to radioiodine fallout were well-differentiated papillary type, but had a higher rate of local invasion and lymph node involvement than usually observed for this histology. More than 90% of well-differentiated thyroid cancers, however, are unrelated to radiation exposure.

Familial syndromes should be suspected when there is a family history of thyroid cancer or a history of a familial syndrome associated with thyroid cancer. Approximately 5% of the differentiated thyroid cancers are associated with Gardner syndrome, familial adenomatous polyposis, Cowden syndrome, multiple endocrine neoplasia (MEN) variant of 2A, familial medullary thyroid carcinoma, and Carney complex.

CLINICAL PRESENTATION AND WORK-UP

The sporadic differentiated thyroid cancers are usually asymptomatic for long periods and usually present as a solitary nodule. The familial papillary thyroid cancers appear to be clinically more aggressive than the sporadic ones. The familial differentiated thyroid cancers are usually multifocal and bilateral, with a tendency to recur both locoregionally and in distant sites. Papillary thyroid cancer and its variants tend to recur locally in the regional lymph nodes, whereas follicular and Hürthle cell cancers tend to recur distantly, especially in bone and lung.

Various prognostic systems have been developed to assist in the risk classification of patients with differentiated thyroid cancer, with potential implications for management based on risk group. Several factors have been widely accepted as being associated with a poor prognosis: age older than 45, male sex, poorly differentiated histology, tumor size, and extrathyroid extension at diagnosis. In contrast, involvement of the regional lymph nodes is associated with greater risk of nodal recurrence but does not confer a worse prognosis for survival.[121] Overall, the 10-year survival rate for differentiated thyroid cancer is excellent (90%). Median age at diagnosis is 45, and median age at death is 75.[122]

Most thyroid cancers are detected as incidental thyroid nodules found on physical exam or by the patient presenting to the physician with a neck mass. The diagnostic evaluation should include a high-resolution ultrasound to aid in performing a fine-needle aspiration biopsy and to assess the number and characteristics of the nodules, including whether the nodules are solid or cystic. Fine-needle aspiration has high sensitivity and specificity and is the test of choice when evaluating solitary thyroid nodules.[123] Routine thyroid scanning with iodine-123 or technetium-99 is not recommended. This test provides information on whether a nodule is functional; however, the majority of benign and malignant nodules are "cold" or nonfunctioning, meaning that the test is nonspecific and not cost-effective. All patients with a thyroid nodule and suspected familial medullary thyroid cancer should have calcitonin level testing.

TREATMENT
Surgery

The mainstay of treatment is thyroid surgery; for differentiated thyroid cancer, levothyroxine suppression and administration of radioactive iodine are the standards. External beam radiotherapy and chemotherapy are reserved for palliation of refractory metastatic disease. The extent of initial surgical therapy is controversial. Many experts recommend removal of the entire thyroid, with the caveats that removal of only the affected lobe and the isthmus is necessary for patients with better risk (e.g., young patients with small tumors) and that total thyroidectomy is associated with a greater risk of complications, such as recurrent laryngeal nerve injury leading to vocal cord paralysis and hypocalcemia secondary to hypoparathyroidism.[124]

Radioactive Iodine

Although controversial, most U.S. physicians will administer a single dose of radioactive iodine to ablate any normal thyroid remnant and to destroy any microscopic deposits of the remaining thyroid cancer following a total thyroidectomy. It should be emphasized that use of iodinated contrast, an iodine-rich diet, and inadequate elevation of the level of thyroid-stimulating hormone (thyrotropin) can all undermine the effectiveness of radioactive iodine treatment. Human recombinant thyrotropin has replaced the need for a patient to be put into a hypothyroid state. Dosing strategies for radioactive iodine—ablative compared with higher therapeutic doses—are determined by the patient's prognostic risk, and they range from 50 mCi to 75 mCi for ablation of remnants following total thyroidectomy for low-risk patients, to 100 mCi to 150 mCi for the treatment of local-regional lymph nodes, and 150 mCi to 250 mCi for the treatment of lung and bone metastases.

Ablation of remnants enables improved surveillance because normal thyroid cells are also removed, which could cause false-positive results on whole-body scans or false-positive elevations of serum thyroglobulin. In the absence of all normal thyroid tissue, the serum thyroglobulin is a highly sensitive and specific tumor marker.[125] After total thyroidectomy and ablation of remnants, the serum thyrotropin level generally should be suppressed to below-normal levels with thyroxine because this hormone is a potential growth factor for microscopic cancer deposits.

Six to 12 months after initial therapy, measurement of the serum thyroglobulin while the patient is receiving suppressive doses of thyroxine should be performed. If the serum thyroglobulin is undetectable and the findings of ultrasound imaging of the neck are negative, an annual analysis of thyroglobulin levels and physical examination are sufficient for most low-risk patients. At 1 year after surgery and ablation, if there is no detectable level of serum thyroglobulin during treatment with suppressive doses of thyroxine, the thyroglobulin level should be determined after two doses of recombinant human thyrotropin. If the level rises above 2 ng/mL, a search for remaining disease is warranted. Diagnostic whole-body imaging with iodine scanning should be performed. If this is negative, FDG-PET scanning has been shown to be helpful for localizing disease in more than 60% of such cases.[126]

If metastases develop and concentrate, radioactive iodine is the treatment of choice. Complete response to treatment has been observed for 45% of patients with distant metastases, although a higher complete response rate has been noted for younger patients and those with small pulmonary metastases.[127] Chemotherapy is reserved for disease that is refractory to radioactive iodine. Some thyroid tumors grow very slowly, so a period of careful observation is reasonable before committing to treatment.

The best-studied single agent is doxorubicin, which has a 17% major response rate; when combined with cisplatin, a 26% response rate was reported in one trial.[128] Trials of other drugs such as cisplatin and paclitaxel have not yielded any improved response rates and were associated with increased toxicity.

MOLECULAR PATHWAYS IN THYROID CANCER

Interest in targeted therapies has been stimulated by the discovery of activating point mutations of the BRAF gene that occur early, are associated with more advanced disease at diagnosis,[129] and independently predict for recurrence. RET/PTC rearrangement is found in approximately 20% of adult sporadic papillary carcinomas.[130] Point mutations of the BRAF gene are found in 45% of thyroid papillary carcinomas.[131,132] BRAF serine-threonine kinase can lead to activation of the mitogen-activated protein kinase (MAPK) signaling pathway. Together, mutations involving one of these three genes (RET/PTC, BRAF, or RAS) are found in more than 70% of papillary carcinomas, and they rarely overlap in the same tumor. PAX8-PPAR-gamma rearrangement is found in about 35% of follicular carcinomas and a small number of Hürthle cell carcinomas.[133]

Clinical trials using such agents as sorafenib, which is an orally active inhibitor of VEGF receptor 1 through 3 and Raf kinases, have been conducted in metastatic thyroid cancers. The results of the phase III DECISION trial were presented at the 2013 ASCO Annual Meeting.[134] A total of 417 patients who had locally advanced or metastatic thyroid cancer that was refractory to radioactive iodine and had progression within the past 14 months were randomly assigned to receive 400 mg of oral sorafenib twice daily or matching placebo. Patients receiving placebo were allowed to receive open-label sorafenib upon progression. The primary endpoint was PFS. Tumor histology was 57% papillary, 25% follicular, and 10% poorly differentiated, and 96% of patients had metastatic disease. The most common site of metastatic disease was lung (86%), lymph nodes (~50%), and bone (~25%). Sorafenib treatment extended the median PFS to 10.8 months compared with 5.8 months with placebo treatment (p < 0.0001). Median OS had not been reached at the time of the presentation. The disease control rate (complete response plus partial response plus stable disease > 6 months) was 54% in the sorafenib arm compared with 38% in the placebo arm (p < 0.0001). Expected toxicities of sorafenib were reported, and the most common grade 3 to 4 toxicities included hand-foot syndrome, hypertension, and hypocalcemia. Based on the results of this study, the FDA approved sorafenib in November 2013 for the treatment of locally recurrent or metastatic progressive differentiated thyroid cancer that no longer responds to radioactive iodine.

Small molecule inhibitors of receptor tyrosine kinases also are under evaluation in differentiated thyroid cancer. One drug with activity is axitinib (AG-013736), which targets VEGF receptors 1 through 3, platelet-derived growth factor (PDGF) receptor B, and kit. A multi-institutional study assessed its safety and activity in 60 patients with radioactive iodine–resistant thyroid cancer of any histology.[135] The drug was given at a dose of 5 mg twice daily. Partial responses were observed in 30% of patients and stable disease lasting at least 16 weeks was reported in another 38%. Median PFS was more than 18 months.[136]

These results are more impressive when we consider that the majority of the patients were male and had metastatic disease, which are risk factors for poor prognosis. Common treatment-related adverse events were fatigue, diarrhea, nausea, anorexia, hypertension, stomatitis, weight decrease, and headache with very few high-grade events recorded.

Pazopanib is a potent small molecule TKI that targets all subtypes of the VEGF receptor without activity against the RET receptor, and has predominantly antiangiogenic activity. A phase II study with 37 evaluable patients with rapidly progressive, metastatic, radioiodine-resistant, differentiated thyroid cancer were treated with 800 mg of pazopanib administered once daily.[137] Partial response was seen in 49% (95% CI 35 to 68) and lasted longer than 1 year in 66% of the patients whose disease responded. The effect on survival was not clear. Dose reduction was required in 43%, despite which the above response was noted. The most common treatment-related adverse events were related to class effect, including hypertension, fatigue, diarrhea, bleeding tendencies, and skin and hair changes. Despite good clinical response, the effect on survival was not determined and must be clarified by controlled trials. Pazopanib appears to have promising activity in thyroid cancer, and trials are ongoing in medullary thyroid cancer and anaplastic thyroid cancer.

ANAPLASTIC THYROID CANCER

Unlike the case with differentiated thyroid cancer, the anaplastic or "giant cell" variant is associated with an extremely poor prognosis, with the best available therapy producing a median survival of less than 1 year. An association with prior well-differentiated thyroid cancer or benign thyroid nodule disease is not uncommon. Patients are older, generally age 60 to 70, and the distribution between the sexes is more balanced. Distinguishing the tumor from a large cell lymphoma of the thyroid is of fundamental importance. Clinically, anaplastic thyroid cancer is characterized by a rapidly growing mass in the thyroid that invades the trachea or larynx and causes symptoms of dysphagia, hoarseness, or hemoptysis. Twenty percent to 50% of patients have distant metastases at the time of presentation (most often pulmonary), and the remainder usually manifest metastases within 1 to 2 months of diagnosis. However, most deaths are a result of aggressive local-regional spread and upper airway respiratory failure. If resection is feasible, it should be pursued, although these tumors are typically unresectable at presentation, and the patient often requires an urgent tracheostomy. Initial external beam radiation-based therapy, both for definitive treatment and as an adjuvant (often with doxorubicin sensitization or doxorubicin and cisplatin), is commonly used and considered the standard of care. Chemotherapy alone has limited efficacy. Doxorubicin plus cisplatin is probably the most widely used combination.[138] Radioactive iodine generally plays no role in the treatment of these tumors. Combretastatin A4 phosphate is a novel drug whose precise mechanism of action is unknown; it has antitumor effects by binding tubulin and

disrupting vascular supply within tumors. In a phase I trial, in combination with paclitaxel, a single patient with anaplastic thyroid cancer had a complete response that lasted more than 30 months after treatment.[139] Preliminary data from a subsequent phase II study failed to obtain any objective responses; however, a number of patients achieved disease stabilization.[140] A randomized, open-label, controlled, phase II/III international trial to assess safety and efficacy of carboplatin and paclitaxel with or without combretastatin was reported at the 2011 ASCO Annual Meeting.[141] A total of 75 patients with anaplastic thyroid cancer were treated in this trial, with 51 patients treated in the combretastatin plus carboplatin and paclitaxel arm and 24 patients treated in the carboplatin plus paclitaxel arm. The median OS was 5.2 months (95% CI 3.1 to 9.0) in the experimental arm compared with 4.0 months (95% CI 2.8 to 6.2) in the control arm (HR 0.72, 95% CI 0.43 to 1.20). The 1-year survival was 25.5% (95% CI 15% to 38%) in the experimental arm compared with 8.7% in the control arm (95% CI 2% to 24%). Adverse events included grade 1 hypertension (31%), grade 3 hypertension (3.9%), QT prolongation (3.9%), and grade 1 reversible cardiac ischemia (3.9%). Deaths were primarily due to disease progression. These results suggest combretastatin improves OS and warrants a clinical trial to confirm its efficacy in combination with cytotoxic chemotherapy agents such as carboplatin and paclitaxel.

MEDULLARY THYROID CANCER

Medullary thyroid cancer is a neoplasm of the calcitonin-producing cells that reside in the thyroid. It constitutes approximately 5% to 9% of all thyroid cancers and is associated with a mutation in the RET proto-oncogene. Both sporadic and familial types occur. The sporadic form is more common (60% to 70% of cases) and tends to occur in an older age group than the familial form (40 to 45 vs. 15 to 25 years, respectively). Three distinct familial syndromes account for the remaining 30% to 40% of cases. The RET mutation is transmitted in the germ line, and familial medullary thyroid cancer may be part of MEN type 2A (medullary thyroid cancer, pheochromocytoma, and parathyroid hyperplasia) or type 2B (medullary thyroid cancer, pheochromocytoma, and intestinal and mucosal ganglioneuromatosis with characteristic marfanoid habitus); it also may be a familial form of medullary thyroid cancer not associated with MEN.

The clinical presentation of the sporadic type is usually a painless thyroid mass; however, high calcitonin levels may result in a watery secretory diarrhea as the primary symptom. The diagnosis is made based on a constellation of a thyroid mass, a high calcitonin level, and a fine-needle aspiration specimen that stains positive for calcitonin. Screening for pheochromocytoma (catecholamine excess) is important for the exclusion of a familial syndrome for a patient otherwise believed to have the sporadic type. CT and PET imaging are useful to detect metastases, but radioactive iodine scans are not useful. For the familial syndromes, a dominant inheritance pattern is recognized, and family members of patients with newly diagnosed cases of the disease should be screened for RET mutations because germ-line mutations are substantially higher than might be expected on the basis of family history alone. Total thyroidectomy often results in complete cures for young, at-risk family members (based on *RET* gene testing), even in the absence of clinically detectable thyroid abnormalities. Studies show that a minority of family members undergoing prophylactic thyroidectomy actually have histologically normal thyroid glands. More often there is evidence of C-cell hyperplasia and microscopic or macroscopic medullary thyroid cancer, which underscores the importance of operating early.

The treatment of choice for medullary thyroid cancer is a total thyroidectomy with bilateral central compartment node dissection and unilateral neck dissection (at the very least). The risk of multifocal disease is high for both familial and sporadic types. Radiation has disappointing efficacy for macroscopic disease, and postoperative radiation therapy is not routinely used. After resection of all disease in the neck, patients should be monitored with two tumor markers: calcitonin and carcino-embryonic antigen (CEA). The survival outcome has improved with genetic testing and prophylactic surgery. Ten-year survival rates are between 70% and 80% for combined series of familial and sporadic types.[142]

Vandetanib is an oral inhibitor that targets VEGF receptor, *RET*, and EGFR, and two important studies have demonstrated that vandetanib has clinically relevant antitumor activity in advanced medullary thyroid cancer with an acceptable safety profile.[143] In a randomized, phase III trial that evaluated 300 mg of vandetanib daily compared with placebo in 331 patients with advanced medullary thyroid cancer, a median follow-up of 24 months revealed a significant difference favoring vandetanib with prolongation of PFS compared with placebo (HR 0.46, 95% CI 0.31 to 0.69; p < 0.001). This study also revealed a significant difference with objective response rate, disease control rate, and biochemical response favoring vandetanib when compared with placebo.[143] Common adverse events (any grade) included diarrhea, rash, nausea, hypertension, and headache. OS data has not yet been reported. Based on the results of this study, the FDA granted approval for vandetanib for the treatment of symptomatic or progressive medullary cancer in patients with unresectable, locally advanced or metastatic disease in April 2011. QT prolongation, torsades de pointes, and sudden death are included in a boxed warning. Because of the risk of QT prolongation, vandetanib is only available through the FDA Vandetanib Risk Evaluation Mitigation Strategy Program. The recommended daily dose of vandetanib is 300 mg orally. The starting dose should be reduced to 200 mg in patients with moderate or severe renal impairment.

Cabozantinib is an oral TKI that targets MET, VEGF receptor 2, and *RET*. In a randomized, phase III double-blind, placebo-controlled, international trial, 330 patients with radiographic progression of metastatic medullary thyroid cancer were randomly assigned (2:1) to receive cabozantinib (140 mg per day) or placebo.[144] The primary endpoint was PFS. Patients treated with cabozantinib experienced a significant improvement in PFS of 11.2 months compared with 4.0 months for the placebo arm (p < 0.001). Response rates were 28% for cabozantinib and 0%

for placebo. Common cabozantinib-associated adverse effects included diarrhea, palmar-plantar erythrodysesthesia, decreased weight and appetite, nausea, and fatigue. Dose reductions were required in 79% of patients. On the basis of this study, the FDA approved cabozantinib for the treatment of progressive metastatic medullary thyroid cancer in November 2012.

Local recurrences are usually treated surgically. Metastatic disease (commonly to the mediastinum, lung, bone, and liver) often follows an indolent course, and in this case, observation is reasonable. The newly approved agents vandetanib and cabozantinib have not been directly compared with each other, and although both agents have been shown to decrease CEA and calcitonin levels and improve PFS, no OS benefit has been reported thus far. The choice of agent may therefore depend on the expected side effects of these agents, and the indications for starting therapy will need to be individualized and balanced with the toxicity profiles and quality-of-life outcomes. In a 2013 editorial, Haddad[145] supports using certain parameters such as calcitonin doubling time and the presence of symptomatic disease as important considerations prior to initiating these currently approved therapies.

Palliative surgery, including tumor debulking, or radiotherapy may be used as indicated for symptom control or to manage tumor encroachment on critical structures. Diphenoxylate, octreotide, and interferon alfa-2a may palliate the diarrhea that can occur. Doxorubicin, cisplatin, dacarbazine, 5-FU, streptozotocin, and somatostatin analogues have some reported activity; however, medullary thyroid cancer generally is resistant to standard cytotoxic agents, making investigational therapy appropriate.[146]

References

1. Jemal A, Siegel R, Xu J, et al. Cancer statistics, 2010. *CA Cancer J Clin.* 2010;60:277-300. PMID: 20610543.

2. Parkin DM, Bray F, Ferlay J, et al. Global cancer statistics, 2002. *CA Cancer J Clin.* 2005;55:74-108. PMID: 15761078.

3. Chaturvedi AK, Anderson WF, Lortet-Tieulent J, et al. Worldwide trends in incidence rates for oral cavity and oropharyngeal cancers. *J Clin Oncol.* 2013;31:4550-4559. PMID: 24248688.

4. Blot WJ, McLaughlin JK, Winn DM, et al. Smoking and drinking in relation to oral and pharyngeal cancer. *Cancer Res.* 1988;48:3282-3287. PMID: 3365707.

5. Gillison ML, Koch WM, Capone RB, et al. Evidence for a causal association between human papillomavirus and a subset of head and neck cancers. *J Natl Cancer Inst.* 2000;92:709-720. PMID: 10793107.

6. Chaturvedi AK, Engels EA, Pfeiffer RM, et al. Human papillomavirus and rising oropharyngeal cancer incidence in the United States. *J Clin Oncol.* 2011;29:4294-4301. PMID: 21969503.

7. Pierce JP, Messer K, White MM, et al. Prevalence of heavy smoking in California and the United States, 1965-2007. *JAMA.* 2011;305:1106-1112. PMID: 21406647.

8. Chaturvedi AK, Engels EA, Anderson WF, et al. Incidence trends for human papillomavirus-related and -unrelated oral squamous cell carcinomas in the United States. *J Clin Oncol.* 2008;26:612-619. PMID: 18235120.

9. Marur S, D'Souza G, Westra WH, et al. HPV-associated head and neck cancer: a virus-related cancer epidemic. *Lancet Oncol.* 2010;11:781-789. PMID: 20451455.

10. Ang KK, Harris J, Wheeler R, et al. Human papillomavirus and survival of patients with oropharyngeal cancer. *N Engl J Med.* 2010;363:24-35. PMID: 20530316.

11. Fakhry C, Gillison ML. Clinical implications of human papillomavirus in head and neck cancers. *J Clin Oncol.* 2006;24:2606-2611. PMID: 16763272.

12. Kreimer AR, Johansson M, Waterboer T, et al. Evaluation of human papillomavirus antibodies and risk of subsequent head and neck cancer. *J Clin Oncol.* 2013;31:2708-2715. PMID: 23775966.

13. Licitra L, Perrone F, Bossi P, et al. High-risk human papillomavirus affects prognosis in patients with surgically treated oropharyngeal squamous cell carcinoma. *J Clin Oncol.* 2006;24:5630-5636. PMID: 17179101.

14. Fakhry C, Westra WH, Li S, et al. Improved survival of patients with human papillomavirus-positive head and neck squamous cell carcinoma in a prospective clinical trial. *J Natl Cancer Inst.* 2008;100:261-269. PMID: 18270337.

15. El-Naggar AK, Westra WH. p16 expression as a surrogate marker for HPV-related oropharyngeal carcinoma: a guide for interpretative relevance and consistency. *Head Neck.* 2012;34:459-461. PMID: 22180304.

16. Haddad RI, Shin DM. Recent advances in head and neck cancer. *N Engl J Med.* 2008;359:1143-1154. PMID: 18784104.

17. Yamamoto E, Shibuya H, Yoshimura R, et al. Site specific dependency of second primary cancer in early stage head and neck squamous cell carcinoma. *Cancer.* 2002;94:2007-2014. PMID: 11932903.

18. Licciardello JT, Spitz MR, Hong WK. Multiple primary cancer in patients with cancer of the head and neck: second cancer of the head and neck, esophagus, and lung. *Int J Radiat Oncol Biol Phys.* 1989;17:467-476. PMID: 2674075.

19. Morris LG, Sikora AG, Patel SG, et al. Second primary cancers after an index head and neck cancer: subsite-specific trends in the era of human papillomavirus-associated oropharyngeal cancer. *J Clin Oncol.* 2011;29:739-746. PMID: 21189382.

20. Hong WK, Lippman SM, Itri LM, et al. Prevention of second primary tumors with isotretinoin in squamous-cell carcinoma of the head and neck. *N Engl J Med.* 1990;323:795-801. PMID: 2202902.

21. Pinto H, Li Y, Loprinzi C, et al. Phase III trial of low-dose 13-cis retinoic acid for prevention of second primary cancers in stage I-II head and neck cancer---an Eastern Cooperative Oncology Group study. *Proc Am Soc Clin Oncol.* 2001;20:(suppl abstr 886).

22. Khuri FR, Lee JJ, Lippman SM, et al. Randomized phase III trial of low-dose isotretinoin for prevention of second primary tumors in stage I and II head and neck cancer patients. *J Natl Cancer Inst.* 2006;98:441-450. PMID: 16595780.

23. Perry CF, Stevens M, Rabie I, et al. Chemoprevention of head and neck cancer with retinoids: a negative result. *Arch Otolaryngol Head Neck Surg.* 2005;131:198-203. PMID: 15781758.

24. Rudin CM, Cohen EE, Papadimitrakopoulou VA, et al. An attenuated adenovirus, ONYX-015, as mouthwash therapy for premalignant oral dysplasia. *J Clin Oncol.* 2003;21:4546-4552. PMID: 14597742.

25. Ng SH, Yen TC, Chang JT, et al. Prospective study of [18F]fluorodeoxyglucose positron emission tomography and computed tomography and magnetic resonance imaging in oral cavity squamous cell carcinoma with palpably negative neck. *J Clin Oncol.* 2006;24:4371-4376. PMID: 16983105.

26. Waldron, JN. Fluorodeoxyglucose positron emission tomography for the preoperative staging of oral cavity cancers: only one piece of the puzzle. *J Clin Oncol.* 2006;24:4367-4368. PMID: 16983103.

27. Kovács AF, Döbert N, Gaa J, et al. Positron emission tomography in combination with sentinel node biopsy reduces the rate of elective neck dissections in the treatment of oral and oropharyngeal cancer. *J Clin Oncol.* 2004;22:3973-3980. PMID: 15459220.

28. Hinerman RW, Mendenhall WM, Amdur RJ, et al. Early laryngeal cancer. *Curr Treat Options Oncol.* 2002;3:3-9. PMID: 12057082.

29. Forastiere AA, Goepfert H, Maor M, et al. Concurrent chemotherapy and radiotherapy for organ preservation in advanced laryngeal cancer. *N Engl J Med.* 2003;349:2091-2098. PMID: 14645636.

30. Forastiere A, Maor M, Weber R, et al. Long-term results of Intergroup RTOG 91–11: A phase III trial to preserve the larynx—Induction cisplatin/5-FU and radiation therapy versus concurrent cisplatin and radiation therapy versus radiation therapy. *J Clin Oncol.* 2006;24:18s (suppl; abstr 5517).

31. Calais G, Alfonsi M, Bardet E, et al. Randomized trial of radiation therapy versus concomitant chemotherapy and radiation therapy for advanced-stage oropharynx carcinoma. *J Natl Cancer Inst.* 1999;91:2081-2086. PMID: 10601378.

32. Denis F, Garaud P, Bardet E, et al. Late toxicity results of the GORTEC 94-01 randomized trial comparing radiotherapy with concomitant radiochemotherapy for advanced-stage oropharynx carcinoma: comparison of LENT/SOMA, RTOG/EORTC, and NCI-CTC scoring systems. *Int J Radiat Oncol Biol Phys.* 2003;55:93-98. PMID: 12504040.

33. Al-Sarraf M, LeBlanc M, Giri PG, et al. Chemoradiotherapy versus radiotherapy in patients with advanced nasopharyngeal cancer: phase III randomized Intergroup study 0099. *J Clin Oncol.* 1998;16:1310-1317. PMID: 9552031.

34. Adelstein DJ, Li Y, Adams GL, et al. An intergroup phase III comparison of standard radiation therapy and two schedules of concurrent chemoradiotherapy in patients with unresectable squamous cell head and neck cancer. *J Clin Oncol.* 2003;21:92-98. PMID: 12506176.

35. Bernier J, Domenge C, Ozsahin M, et al. Postoperative irradiation with or without concomitant chemotherapy for locally advanced head and neck cancer. *N Engl J Med.* 2004;350:1945-1952. PMID: 15128894.

36. Cooper JS, Pajak TF, Forastiere AA, et al. Postoperative concurrent radiotherapy and chemotherapy for high-risk squamous-cell carcinoma of the head and neck. *N Engl J Med.* 2004;350:1937-1944. PMID: 15128893.

37. Bernier J, Cooper JS, Pajak TF, et al. Defining risk levels in locally advanced head and neck cancers: a comparative analysis of concurrent postoperative radiation plus chemotherapy trials of the EORTC (#22931) and RTOG (# 9501). *Head Neck.* 2005;27:843-850. PMID: 16161069.

38. Cooper JS, Zhang Q, Pajak TF, et al. Long-term follow-up of the RTOG 9501/intergroup phase III trial: postoperative concurrent radiation therapy and chemotherapy in high-risk squamous cell carcinoma of the head and neck. *Int J Radiat Oncol Biol Phys.* 2012;84:1198-1205. PMID: 22749632.

39. Yao M, Smith RB, Graham MM, et al. The role of FDG PET in management of neck metastasis from head-and-neck cancer after definitive radiation treatment. *Int J Radiat Oncol Biol Phys.* 2005;63:991-999. PMID: 16099601.

40. Isles, MG, McConkey C, Mehanna HM. A systematic review and meta-analysis of the role of positron emission tomography in the follow up of head and neck squamous cell carcinoma following radiotherapy or chemoradiotherapy. *Clin Otolaryngol.* 2008;33:210-222. PMID: 18559026.

41. Ong SC, Schöder H, Lee NY, et al. Clinical utility of 18F-FDG PET/CT in assessing the neck after concurrent chemoradiotherapy for Locoregional advanced head and neck cancer. *J Nucl Med.* 2008;49:532-540. PMID: 18344440.

42. Fu KK, Pajak TF, Trotti A, et al. A Radiation Therapy Oncology Group (RTOG) phase III randomized study to compare hyperfractionation and two variants of accelerated fractionation to standard fractionation radiotherapy for head and neck squamous cell carcinomas: first report of RTOG 9003. *Int J Radiat Oncol Biol Phys.* 2000;48:7-16. PMID: 10924966.

43. Bourhis J, Overgaard J, Audry H, et al. Hyperfractionated or accelerated radiotherapy in head and neck cancer: a meta-analysis. *Lancet.* 2006;368:843-854. PMID: 16950362.

44. Johnson JT, Ferretti GA, Nethery WJ, et al. Oral pilocarpine for post-irradiation xerostomia in patients with head and neck cancer. *N Engl J Med.* 1009;329:390-395. PMID: 8326972.

45. Brizel DM, Wasserman TH, Henke M, et al. Phase III randomized trial of amifostine as a radioprotector in head and neck cancer. *J Clin Oncol.* 2000;18:3339-3345. PMID: 11013273.

46. Domenge C, Hill C, Lefebvre JL, et al. Randomized trial of neoadjuvant chemotherapy in oropharyngeal carcinoma. French Groupe d'Etude des Tumeurs de la Tete et du Cou (GETTEC). *Br J Cancer.* 2000;83:1594-1598. PMID: 11189100.

47. Licitra L, Grandi C, Guzzo M, et al. Primary chemotherapy in resectable oral cavity squamous cell cancer: a randomized controlled trial. *J Clin Oncol.* 2003;21:327-333. PMID: 12525526.

48. Lefebvre JL, Chevalier D, Luboinski B, et al. Larynx preservation in pyriform sinus cancer: preliminary results of a European Organization for Research and Treatment of Cancer phase III trial. EORTC Head and Neck Cancer Cooperative Group. *J Natl Cancer Inst.* 1996;88:890-899. PMID: 8656441.

49. Pignon JP, Bourhis J, Domenge C, et al. Chemotherapy added to locoregional treatment for head and neck squamous-cell carcinoma: three meta-analyses of updated individual data. MACH-NC Collaborative Group. Meta-Analysis of Chemotherapy on Head and Neck Cancer. *Lancet.* 2000;355:949-955. PMID: 10768432.

50. Vermorken JB, Remenar E, van Herpen C, et al. Cisplatin, fluorouracil, and docetaxel in unresectable head and neck cancer. *N Engl J Med.* 2007;357: 1695-1704. PMID: 17960012.

51. Posner MR, Hershock DM, Blajman CR, et al. Cisplatin and fluorouracil alone or with docetaxel in head and neck cancer. *N Engl J Med.* 2007;357:1705-1715. PMID: 17960013.

52. Pointreau Y, Garaud P, Chapet S, et al. Randomized trial of induction chemotherapy with cisplatin and 5-fluorouracil with or without docetaxel for larynx preservation. *J Natl Cancer Inst.* 2009;101:498-506. PMID: 19318632.

53. Hitt R, López-Pousa A, Martínez-Trufero J, et al. Phase III study comparing cisplatin plus fluorouracil to paclitaxel, cisplatin, and fluorouracil induction chemotherapy followed by chemoradiotherapy in locally advanced head and neck cancer. *J Clin Oncol.* 2005;23:8636-8645. PMID: 16275937.

54. Blanchard P, Bourhis J, Lacas B, et al. Taxane-cisplatin-fluorouracil as induction chemotherapy in locally advanced head and neck cancers: an individual

patient data meta-analysis of the meta-analysis of chemotherapy in head and neck cancer group. *J Clin Oncol.* 2013;31:2854-2860. PMID: 23835714.

55. Haddad R, O'Neill A, Rabinowits G, et al. Induction chemotherapy followed by concurrent chemoradiotherapy (sequential chemoradiotherapy) versus concurrent chemoradiotherapy alone in locally advanced head and neck cancer (PARADIGM): a randomized phase 3 trial. *Lancet Oncol.* 2013;14:257-264. PMID: 23414589.

56. Cohen E, Karrison T, Kocherginsky M, et al. DeCIDE: A phase III randomized trial of docetaxel (D), cisplatin (P), 5-fluorouracil (F) (TPF) induction chemotherapy (IC) in patients with N2/N3 locally advanced squamous cell carcinoma of the head and neck (SCCHN). *J Clin Oncol.* 2012;(suppl; abstr 5500).

57. Zhong LP, Zhang CP, Ren GX, et al. Randomized phase III trial of induction chemotherapy with docetaxel, cisplatin, and fluorouracil followed by surgery versus up-front surgery in locally advanced resectable oral squamous cell carcinoma. *J Clin Oncol.* 2013;31:744-751. PMID: 23129742.

58. Merlano M, Benasso M, Corvó R, et al. Five-year update of a randomized trial of alternating radiotherapy and chemotherapy compared with radiotherapy alone in treatment of unresectable squamous cell carcinoma of the head and neck. *J Natl Cancer Inst.* 1996;88:583-589. PMID: 8609658.

59. Pignon JP, le Maître A, Maillard E, et al. Meta-analysis of chemotherapy in head and neck cancer (MACH-NC): an update on 93 randomised trials and 17,346 patients. *Radiother Oncol.* 2009;92:4-14. Epub 2009 May 14. PMID: 19446902.

60. Browman GP, Hodson DI, Mackenzie RJ, et al. Choosing a concomitant chemotherapy and radiotherapy regimen for squamous cell head and neck cancer: A systematic review of the published literature with subgroup analysis. *Head Neck.* 2001;23:579-589. PMID: 11400247.

61. Bourhis J, Le Maître A, Baujat B, et al. Individual patients' data meta-analyses in head and neck cancer. *Curr Opin Oncol.* 2007;19:188-194. PMID: 17414635.

62. Bonner JA, Harari PM, Giralt J, et al. Radiotherapy plus cetuximab for squamous-cell carcinoma of the head and neck. *N Engl J Med.* 2006;354:567-578. PMID: 16467544.

63. Ang KK, Zhang QE, Rosenthal DI. A randomized phase III trial (RTOG 0522) of concurrent accelerated radiation plus cisplatin with or without cetuximab for stage III-IV head and neck squamous cell carcinomas (HNC). *J Clin Oncol.* 2011;29:15s (suppl; abstr 5500).

64. Martins RG, Parvathaneni U, Bauman JE, et al. Cisplatin and radiotherapy with or without erlotinib in locally advanced squamous cell carcinoma of the head and neck: a randomized phase II trial. *J Clin Oncol.* 2013;31:1415-1421. PMID: 23460709.

65. O'Sullivan B, Huang SH, Siu LL, et al. Deintensification candidate subgroups in human papillomavirus-related oropharyngeal cancer according to minimal risk of distant metastasis. *J Clin Oncol.* 2013;31:543-550. PMID: 23295795.

66. The Department of Veterans Affairs Laryngeal Cancer Study Group. Induction chemotherapy plus radiation compared with surgery plus radiation in patients with advanced laryngeal cancer. The Department of Veterans Affairs Laryngeal Cancer Study Group. *N Engl J Med.* 1991;324:1685-1690. PMID: 2034244.

67. Spaulding MB, Fischer SG, Wolf GT. Tumor response, toxicity, and survival after neoadjuvant organ-preserving chemotherapy for advanced laryngeal carcinoma. The Department of Veterans Affairs Cooperative Laryngeal Cancer Study Group. *J Clin Oncol.* 1994;12:1592-1599. PMID: 8040671.

68. Richard JM, Sancho-Garnier H, Pessey JJ, et al. Randomized trial of induction chemotherapy in larynx carcinoma. *Oral Oncol.* 1998;34:224-228. PMID: 9692058.

69. Terrell JE, Fisher SG, Wolf GT. Long-term quality of life after treatment of laryngeal cancer. The Veterans Affairs Laryngeal Cancer Study Group. *Arch Otolaryngol Head Neck Surg.* 1998;124:964-971. PMID: 9738804.

70. Adelstein DJ, Saxton JP, Lavertu P, et al. A phase III randomized trial comparing concurrent chemotherapy and radiotherapy with radiotherapy alone in resectable stage III and IV squamous cell head and neck cancer: preliminary results. *Head Neck.* 1997;19:567-575. PMID: 9323144.

71. Forastiere AA, Zhang Q, Weber RS, et al. Long-Term results of RTOG 91-11: a comparison of three nonsurgical treatment strategies to preserve the larynx in patients with locally advanced larynx cancer. *J Clin Oncol.* 2013;31:845-852. PMID: 23182993.

72. Lefebvre J, Horiot J, Rolland F, et al. Phase III study on larynx preservation comparing induction chemotherapy and radiotherapy versus alternating chemoradiotherapy in resectable hypopharynx and larynx cancers. EORTC protocol 24954-22950. *J Clin Oncol.* 2007;25:18s (suppl; abstr LBA6016).

73. Hassanein, KA, Musgrove BT, Bradbury E. Psychological outcome of patients following treatment of oral cancer and its relation with functional status and coping mechanisms. *J Craniomaxillofac Surg.* 2005;33:404-409. PMID: 16253509.

74. Duffy SA, Ronis DL, Valenstein M, et al. Depressive symptoms, smoking, drinking, and quality of life among head and neck cancer patients. *Psychosomatics.* 2007;48:142-148. PMID: 17329608.

75. Karnell LH, Christensen AJ, Rosenthal EL, et al. Influence of social support on health-related quality of life outcomes in head and neck cancer. *Head Neck.* 2007;29:143-146. PMID: 17111431.

76. Murphy BA, Ridner S, Wells N, et al. Quality of life research in head and neck cancer: a review of the current state of the science. *Crit Rev Oncol Hematol.* 2007;62:251-267. PMID: 17408963.

77. Chan AT, Teo PM, Ngan RK, et al. Concurrent chemotherapy-radiotherapy compared with radiotherapy alone in locoregionally advanced nasopharyngeal carcinoma: progression-free survival analysis of a phase III randomized trial. *J Clin Oncol.* 2002;20:2038-2044. PMID: 11956263.

78. Chan AT, Leung SF, Ngan RK, et al. Overall survival after concurrent cisplatin-radiotherapy compared with radiotherapy alone in locoregionally advanced nasopharyngeal carcinoma. *J Natl Cancer Inst.* 2005;97:536-539. PMID: 15812080.

79. Lin JC, Jan JS, Hsu CY, et al. Phase III study of concurrent chemoradiotherapy versus radiotherapy alone for advanced nasopharyngeal carcinoma: positive effect on overall and progression-free survival. *J Clin Oncol.* 2003;21:631-637. PMID: 12586799.

80. Huncharek M, Kupelnick B. Combined chemoradiation versus radiation therapy alone in locally advanced nasopharyngeal carcinoma: results of a meta-analysis of 1,528 patients from six randomized trials. *Am J Clin Oncol.* 2002;25:219-223. PMID: 12040275.

81. Baujat B, Audry H, Bourhis J, et al. Chemotherapy in locally advanced nasopharyngeal carcinoma: an individual patient data meta-analysis of eight randomized trials and 1753 patients. *Int J Radiat Oncol Biol Phys.* 2006;64:47-56. PMID: 16377415.

82. Chua DT, Ma J, Sham JS, et al. Long-term survival after cisplatin-based induction chemotherapy and radiotherapy for nasopharyngeal carcinoma: a pooled data analysis of two phase III trials. *J Clin Oncol.* 2005;23:1118-1124. PMID: 15657403.

83. Chan AT, Teo PM, Leung TW, et al. A prospective randomized study of chemotherapy adjunctive to definitive radiotherapy in advanced nasopharyngeal carcinoma. *Int J Radiat Oncol Biol Phys.* 1995;33:569-577. PMID: 7558945.

84. International Nasopharynx Cancer Study Group. Preliminary results of a randomized trial comparing neoadjuvant chemotherapy (cisplatin, epirubicin, bleomycin) plus radiotherapy vs. radiotherapy alone in stage IV (> or = N2, M0) undifferentiated nasopharyngeal carcinoma: a positive effect on progression-free survival. VUMCA I trial. *Int J Radiat Oncol Biol Phys.* 1996;35:463-469. PMID: 8655368.

85. Ma J, Mai HQ, Hong MH, et al. Results of a prospective randomized trial comparing neoadjuvant chemotherapy plus radiotherapy with radiotherapy alone in patients with locoregionally advanced nasopharyngeal carcinoma. *J Clin Oncol.* 2001;19:1350-1357. PMID: 11230478.

86. Chen L, Hu CS, Chen XZ, et al. Concurrent chemoradiotherapy plus adjuvant chemotherapy versus concurrent chemoradiotherapy alone in patients with locoregionally advanced nasopharyngeal carcinoma: a phase 3 multicentre randomised controlled trial. *Lancet Oncol.* 2012;13:163-171. PMID: 22154591.

87. Rischin D, Corry J, Smith J, et al. Excellent disease control and survival in patients with advanced nasopharyngeal cancer treated with chemoradiation. *J Clin Oncol.* 2002;20:1845-1852. PMID: 11919243.

88. Chan AT, Ma BB, Lo YM, et al. Phase II study of neoadjuvant carboplatin and paclitaxel followed by radiotherapy and concurrent cisplatin in patients with locoregionally advanced nasopharyngeal carcinoma: therapeutic monitoring with plasma Epstein-Barr virus DNA. *J Clin Oncol.* 2004;22:3053-3060. PMID: 15284255.

89. Forastiere AA, Metch B, Schuller DE, et al. Randomized comparison of cisplatin plus fluorouracil and carboplatin plus fluorouracil versus methotrexate in advanced squamous-cell carcinoma of the head and neck: a Southwest Oncology Group study. *J Clin Oncol.* 1992;10:1245-1251. PMID: 1634913.

90. Jacobs C, Lyman G, Velez-García E, et al. A phase III randomized study comparing cisplatin and fluorouracil as single agents and in combination for advanced squamous cell carcinoma of the head and neck. *J Clin Oncol.* 1992;10:257-263. PMID: 1732427.

91. Clavel M, Vermorken JB, Cognetti F, et al. Randomized comparison of cisplatin, methotrexate, bleomycin and vincristine (CABO) versus cisplatin and 5-fluorouracil (CF) versus cisplatin (C) in recurrent or metastatic

squamous cell carcinoma of the head and neck. A phase III study of the EORTC Head and Neck Cancer Cooperative Group. *Ann Oncol.* 1994;5: 521-526. PMID: 7522527.

92. Browman GP, Cronin L. Standard chemotherapy in squamous cell head and neck cancer: what we have learned from randomized trials. *Semin Oncol.* 1994;21:311-319. PMID: 7516093.

93. Colevas AD. Chemotherapy options for patients with metastatic or recurrent squamous cell carcinoma of the head and neck. *J Clin Oncol.* 2006;24:2644-2652. PMID: 16763278.

94. Vermorken JB, Catimel G, Mulder PD, et al. Randomized phase II trial of weekly methotrexate (MTX) versus two schedules of triweekly paclitaxel (Taxol) in patients with metastatic or recurrent squamous cell carcinoma of the head and neck (SCCHN). *Proc Am Soc Clin Oncol.* 1999;18:(suppl; abstr A1527).

95. Gibson MK, Li Y, Murphy B, et al. Randomized phase III evaluation of cisplatin plus fluorouracil versus cisplatin plus paclitaxel in advanced head and neck cancer (E1395): an intergroup trial of the Eastern Cooperative Oncology Group. *J Clin Oncol.* 2005;23:3562-3567. PMID: 15908667.

96. Vermorken JB, Trigo J, Hitt R, et al. Open-label, uncontrolled, multicenter phase II study to evaluate the efficacy and toxicity of cetuximab as a single agent in patients with recurrent and/or metastatic squamous cell carcinoma of the head and neck who failed to respond to platinum-based therapy. *J Clin Oncol.* 2007;25:2171-2177. PMID: 17538161.

97. Herbst RS, Arquette M, Shin DM, et al. Phase II multicenter study of the epidermal growth factor receptor antibody cetuximab and cisplatin for recurrent and refractory squamous cell carcinoma of the head and neck. *J Clin Oncol.* 2005;23:5578-5587. PMID: 16009949.

98. Baselga J, Trigo JM, Bourhis J, et al. Phase II multicenter study of the anti-epidermal growth factor receptor monoclonal antibody cetuximab in combination with platinum-based chemotherapy in patients with platinum-refractory metastatic and/or recurrent squamous cell carcinoma of the head and neck. *J Clin Oncol.* 2005;23:5568-5577. PMID: 16009950.

99. Burtness B, Goldwasser MA, Flood W, et al. Phase III randomized trial of cisplatin plus placebo compared with cisplatin plus cetuximab in metastatic/recurrent head and neck cancer: an Eastern Cooperative Oncology Group study. *J Clin Oncol.* 2005;23:8646-8654. PMID: 16314626.

100. Vermorken JB, Mesia R, Rivera F, et al. Platinum-based chemotherapy plus cetuximab in head and neck cancer. *N Engl J Med.* 2008;359:1116-1127. PMID: 18784101.

101. Cohen EE, Rosen F, Stadler WM, et al. Phase II trial of ZD1839 in recurrent or metastatic squamous cell carcinoma of the head and neck. *J Clin Oncol.* 2003;21:1980-1987. PMID: 12743152.

102. Cohen EE. Role of epidermal growth factor receptor pathway-targeted therapy in patients with recurrent and/or metastatic squamous cell carcinoma of the head and neck. *J Clin Oncol.* 2006;24:2659-2665. PMID: 16763280.

103. Argiris A, Ghebremichael M, Gilbert J, et al. Phase III randomized, placebo-controlled trial of docetaxel with or without gefitinib in recurrent of metastatic head and neck cancer: a eastern cooperative oncology group trial. *J Clin Oncol.* 2013;31:1405-1414. PMID: 23460714.

104. Seiwert TY, Haraf DJ, Cohen EE, et al. A phase I study of bevacizumab (B) with fluorouracil (F) and hydroxyurea (H) with concomitant radiotherapy (X) - B-FHX for poor prognosis head and neck cancer (HNC). *J Clin Oncol.* 2006;24:18s (suppl; abstr 5530).

105. Vokes EE, Cohen EEW, Mauer AM, et al. A phase I study of erlotinib and bevacizumab for recurrent or metastatic squamous cell carcinoma of the head and neck (HNC). *J Clin Oncol.* 2005;23:16s (suppl; abstr 5504).

106. De Crevoisier R, Bourhis J, Domenge C, et al. Full-dose reirradiation for unresectable head and neck carcinoma: experience at the Gustave-Roussy Institute in a series of 169 patients. *J Clin Oncol.* 1998;16:3556-3562. PMID: 9817275.

107. Spencer SA, Harris J, Wheeler RH, et al. RTOG 96-10: reirradiation with concurrent hydroxyurea and 5-fluorouracil in patients with squamous cell cancer of the head and neck. *Int J Radiat Oncol Biol Phys.* 2001;51:1299-1304. PMID: 11728690.

108. Horwitz EM, Harris J, Langer CJ, et al. Concurrent split course hyperfractionated radiotherapy (Hfx RT), cisplatin (DDP) and paclitaxel (P) in patients with recurrent previously irradiated squamous cell carcinoma of the head and neck (SCCHN): Update of RTOG 91-11. *J Clin Oncol.* 2005;23:16s (suppl; abstr 519s).

109. Rusthoven KE, Koshy M, Paulino AC. The role of fluorodeoxyglucose positron emission tomography in cervical lymph node metastases from an unknown primary tumor. *Cancer.* 2004;101:2641-2649. PMID: 15517576.

110. Spiro RH. Management of malignant tumors of the salivary glands. *Oncology (Williston Park).* 1998;12:671-680; discussion 683. PMID: 9597678.

111. Gilbert J, Li Y, Pinto HA, et al. Phase II trial of taxol in salivary gland malignancies (E1394): a trial of the Eastern Cooperative Oncology Group. *Head Neck.* 2006;28:197-204. PMID: 16470745.

112. Laurie SA, Licitra L. Systemic therapy in the palliative management of advanced salivary gland cancers. *J Clin Oncol.* 2006;24:2673-2678. PMID: 16763282.

113. Licitra L, Cavina R, Grandi C, et al. Cisplatin, doxorubicin and cyclophosphamide in advanced salivary gland carcinoma. A phase II trial of 22 patients. *Ann Oncol.* 1996;7:640-642. PMID: 8879381.

114. Jones AS, Phillips DE, Cook JA, et al. A randomised phase II trial of epirubicin and 5-fluorouracil versus cisplatinum in the palliation of advanced and recurrent malignant tumour of the salivary glands. *Br J Cancer.* 1993;67:112-114. PMID: 7678976.

115. Gedlicka C, Schüll B, Formanek M, et al. Mitoxantrone and cisplatin in recurrent and/or metastatic salivary gland malignancies. *Anticancer Drugs.* 2002;13:491-495. PMID: 12045460.

116. Airoldi M, Pedani F, Succo G, et al. Phase II randomized trial comparing vinorelbine versus vinorelbine plus cisplatin in patients with recurrent salivary gland malignancies. *Cancer.* 2001;91:541-547. PMID: 11169936.

117. Agulnik M, Cohen EW, Cohen RB, et al. Phase II study of lapatinib in recurrent or metastatic epidermal growth factor receptor and/or erbB2 expressing adenoid cystic carcinoma and non adenoid cystic carcinoma malignant tumors of the salivary glands. *J Clin Oncol.* 2007;25:3978-3984. PMID: 17761983.

118. Locati LD, Quattrone P, Bossi P, et al. A complete remission with androgen-deprivation therapy in a recurrent androgen receptor-expressing adenocarcinoma of the parotid gland. *Ann Oncol.* 2003;14:1327-1328. PMID: 12881399.

119. American Cancer Society. Thyroid Cancer. www.cancer.org/cancer/thyroidcancer/detailedguide/thyroid-cancer-key-statistics. Accessed October 17, 2012.

120. Davies L, Welch HG. Increasing incidence of thyroid cancer in the United States, 1973-2002. *JAMA.* 2006;295:2164-2167. PMID: 16684987.

121. Dean DS, Hay ID. Prognostic indicators in differentiated thyroid carcinoma. *Cancer Control.* 2000;7:229-239. PMID: 10832109.

122. Mazzaferri EL, Kloos RT. Clinical review 128: Current approaches to primary therapy for papillary and follicular thyroid cancer. *J Clin Endocrinol Metab.* 2001;86:1447-1463. PMID: 11297567.

123. Oertel YC, Oertel JE. Diagnosis of malignant epithelial thyroid lesions: fine needle aspiration and histopathologic correlation. *Ann Diagn Pathol.* 1998;2:377-400. PMID: 9930575.

124. Shah JP, Loree TR, Dharker D, et al. Lobectomy versus total thyroidectomy for differentiated carcinoma of the thyroid: a matched-pair analysis. *Am J Surg.* 1993;166:331-335. PMID: 8214286.

125. Mazzaferri EL, Robbins RJ, Spencer CA, et al. A consensus report of the role of serum thyroglobulin as a monitoring method for low-risk patients with papillary thyroid carcinoma. *J Clin Endocrinol Metab.* 2003;88:1433-1441. PMID: 12679418.

126. Larson SM, Robbins R. Positron emission tomography in thyroid cancer management. *Semin Roentgenol.* 2002;37:169-174. PMID: 12134369.

127. Schlumberger M, Challeton C, De Vathaire F, et al. Radioactive iodine treatment and external radiotherapy for lung and bone metastases from thyroid carcinoma. *J Nucl Med.* 1996;37:598-605. PMID: 8691248.

128. Shimaoka K, Schoenfeld DA, DeWys WD, et al. A randomized trial of doxorubicin versus doxorubicin plus cisplatin in patients with advanced thyroid carcinoma. *Cancer.* 1985;56:2155-2160. PMID: 3902203.

129. Xing M, Westra WH, Tufano RP, et al. BRAF mutation predicts a poorer clinical prognosis for papillary thyroid cancer. *J Clin Endocrinol Metab.* 2005;90:6373-6379. PMID: 16174717.

130. Nikiforov YE. RET/PTC rearrangement in thyroid tumors. *Endocr Pathol.* 2002;13:3-16. PMID: 12114746.

131. Cohen Y, Xing M, Mambo E, et al. BRAF mutation in papillary thyroid carcinoma. *J Natl Cancer Inst.* 2003;95:625-627. PMID: 12697856.

132. Kimura ET, Nikiforova MN, Zhu Z, et al. High prevalence of BRAF mutations in thyroid cancer: genetic evidence for constitutive activation of the RET/PTC-RAS-BRAF signaling pathway in papillary thyroid carcinoma. *Cancer Res.* 2003;63:1454-1457. PMID: 12670889.

133. Nikiforova MN, Lynch RA, Biddinger PW, et al. RAS point mutations and PAX8-PPAR gamma rearrangement in thyroid tumors: evidence for distinct molecular pathways in thyroid follicular carcinoma. *J Clin Endocrinol Metab.* 2003;88:2318-2326. PMID: 12727991.

134. Brose MS, Nutting C, Jarzab B, et al. Sorafenib in locally advanced or metastatic patients with radioactive iodine-refractory differentiated thyroid cancer: The phase III DECISION trial. *J Clin Oncol.* 2013;31(suppl; abstr 4).

135. Kim S, Rosen LS, Cohen EE, et al. A phase II study of axitinib (AG-013736), a potent inhibitor of VEGFRs, in patients with advanced thyroid cancer. *J Clin Oncol.* 2006;24:18s (suppl; abstr 5529).

136. Cohen EE, Rosen LS, Vokes EE, et al. Axitinib is an active treatment for all histologic subtypes of advanced thyroid cancer: results from a phase II study. *J Clin Oncol.* 2006;26:4708-4713. PMID: 18541897.

137. Bible KC, Suman VJ, Molina JR, et al. Efficacy of pazopanib in progressive, radioiodine-refractory, metastatic differentiated thyroid cancers: results of a phase 2 consortium study. *Lancet Oncol.* 2010;11:962-972. Epub 2010 Sep 17. PMID: 20851682.

138. Tennvall J, Lundell G, Hallquist A, et al. Combined doxorubicin, hyperfractionated radiotherapy, and surgery in anaplastic thyroid carcinoma. Report on two protocols. The Swedish Anaplastic Thyroid Cancer Group. *Cancer.* 1994;74:1348-1354. PMID: 8055459.

139. Dowlati A, Robertson K, Cooney M, et al. A phase I pharmacokinetic and translational study of the novel vascular targeting agent combretastatin a-4 phosphate on a single-dose intravenous schedule in patients with advanced cancer. *Cancer Res.* 2002;62:3408-3416. PMID: 12067983.

140. Cooney MM, Agarwala S, Wang D, et al. Phase II study of combretastatin A4 phosphate (CA4P) in patients with advanced anaplastic thyroid carcinoma (ATC). *J Clin Oncol.* 2006;24:18s (suppl; abstr 5580).

141. Sosa JA, Elisei R, Jarzab B, et al. A randomized phase II/III trial of a tumor vascular disrupting agent fosbretabulin tromethamine (CA4P) with carboplatin (C) and paclitaxel (P) in anaplastic thyroid cancer (ATC): Final survival analysis for the FACT trial. *J Clin Oncol.* 2011;29:15s (suppl; abstr 5502).

142. Kebebew E, Clark OH. Medullary thyroid cancer. *Curr Treat Options Oncol.* 2000;1:359-367. PMID: 12057161.

143. Wells SA Jr, Robinson BG, Gagel RF, et al. Vandetanib in patients with locally advanced or metastatic medullary thyroid cancer: a randomized, double-blind phase III trial. *J Clin Oncol.* 2012;30:134-141. PMID: 22025146.

144. Elisei R, Schlumberger MJ, Müller SP, et al. Cabozantinib in progressive medullary thyroid cancer. *J Clin Oncol.* 2013;31:3639-3646. PMID: 24002501.

145. Haddad RI. How to incorporate new tyrosine kinase inhibitors in the treatment of patients with medullary thyroid cancer. *J Clin Oncol.* 2013;31:3618-3620. PMID: 24002516.

146. Ball DW. Medullary thyroid cancer: therapeutic targets and molecular markers. *Curr Opin Oncol.* 2007;19:18-23. PMID: 17133107.

9

GASTROINTESTINAL CANCERS

Joleen M. Hubbard, MD, and Axel Grothey, MD

▶ Epidermal growth factor receptor (EGFR) antibodies have been shown to have no activity in the management of advanced gastroesophageal cancers (Lordick F, *Lancet Oncol* 2013).

▶ Ramucirumab as a single agent (vs. best supportive care) and in combination with paclitaxel (vs. paclitaxel alone) has been shown to improve survival as second-line therapy in advanced gastroesophageal cancers (Fuchs CS, *Lancet* 2013; Wilke H, *J Clin Oncol* 2013).

▶ In HER2-positive cancers, trastuzumab is the only active HER2-targeting agent, as trials investigating lapatinib were disappointing (Hecht JR, *J Clin Oncol* 2013; Bang YJ, *J Clin Oncol* 2013).

▶ S-1, an oral fluoropyrimidine, has shown superiority compared with gemcitabine as adjuvant therapy in resected pancreas cancer (Fukutomi A, *J Clin Oncol* 2013).

▶ Nab-paclitaxel plus gemcitabine has been established as one potential standard of care in the first-line treatment of patients with metastatic pancreas cancer (Von Hoff DD, *N Engl J Med* 2013).

▶ Screening colonoscopies have documented benefit on cancer-related mortality (Nishihara R, *N Engl J Med* 2013; Shaukat A, *N Engl J Med* 2013).

▶ The benefit of aspirin as secondary prophylaxis in patients with resected colorectal cancers appears to be linked to the presence of *PIK3CA* mutations (Liao X, *N Engl J Med* 2013; Domingo E, *J Clin Oncol* 2013).

▶ Capecitabine in combination with bevacizumab has emerged as one standard first-line treatment option in elderly patients with advanced colorectal cancer (Cunningham D, *Lancet Oncol* 2013).

▶ The induction-maintenance strategy in the management of colorectal cancers was validated by the results of the Dutch CAIRO-3 trial (Koopman M, *J Clin Oncol* 2013).

▶ Expanded *RAS* mutation testing beyond *KRAS* exon 2 (codons 12/13) should be considered standard of care before the use of EGFR antibodies in colorectal cancer (Douillard JY, *N Engl J Med* 2013).

▶ 5-fluorouracil/leucovorin/irinotecan/oxaliplatin plus bevacizumab should be considered as standard treatment options for *BRAF*-mutated colorectal cancer based on the phase III TRIBE study (Falcone A, *J Clin Oncol* 2013).

▶ Cisplatin/5-fluorouracil as a radiation sensitizer can be considered a second standard of care for anal cancer in addition to mitomycin/5-fluorouracil based on the findings of the phase III ACTII study (James RD, *Lancet Oncol* 2013).

All cancers of the digestive system combined make up more than 290,000 cases per year in the United States and are more common than breast cancer (234,580) and lung cancer (228,520).[1] Approximately 145,000 patients will die of gastrointestinal malignancies, with about one-third of these fatalities attributed to colorectal cancer. The spectrum of diseases encountered in this field varies from rather indolent malignancies, such as low-grade neuroendocrine tumors with overall survival measured in years, to very aggressive and rapidly fatal cancers, such as pancreas and hepatocellular carcinomas where in advanced stages survival is measured in months. Several cancers of the digestive tract are linked to hereditary syndromes that require genetic counseling of patients and family members. Advances in the development of medical therapies, which now routinely include targeted agents beyond conventional chemotherapy in most gastrointestinal malignancies, as well as the identification of specific biomarkers that allow tailoring medical therapy to subsets of patients with cancer, place significant demands on the medical oncologist. The complexity associated with the diagnosis and treatment of gastrointestinal cancers is further increased by the fact that most of these malignancies require multimodality management with close interaction of gastroenterologists, interventional radiologists, surgeons, radiation oncologists, and medical oncologists. Therefore, one of the key roles of the medical oncologist is to coordinate the multimodality team and counsel the patient on various potential, sometimes competing, treatment options for the disease.

ESOPHAGEAL CANCER

Esophageal cancers exhibit great variation in histology, geographic distribution, and incidence. Historically, the most common type of esophageal cancer was a squamous cell cancer of the upper to middle esophagus. However, during the past 2 to 3 decades, the incidence of squamous cell cancers has decreased, as the incidence of adenocarcinoma of the esophagus and gastroesophageal junction has increased rapidly. In the United States, esophageal cancers represent the fifth most common gastrointestinal cancer (after colorectal, pancreas, liver, and gastric cancers) and rank among the 10 most common cancers worldwide.[2,3] The incidence of esophageal cancers shows remarkable variation throughout the world, with a 60-fold difference between high- and low-incidence regions. Areas of high incidence include portions of Iran, Russia, and northern China where squamous cell cancers are more common.[4] The disease is less common in Japan, Europe, the United States, and Canada. In the United States, carcinoma of the esophagus is infrequent, constituting approximately 1% of all cancers and approximately 6% of gastrointestinal malignancies. During the last 2 decades, the incidence of adenocarcinoma of the distal esophagus and gastroesophageal junction has increased, parallel to the rise of gastroesophageal reflux disease (GERD) in the general population, most notably for patients with a high body mass index.[5,6] Squamous cell tumors are more likely to occur in patients who are black; these tumors are associated with achalasia, caustic injury, tylosis, Plummer-Vinson syndrome,

cigarette smoking, and excessive alcohol consumption. There also is an increased frequency of secondary aerodigestive tumors among patients with squamous cell cancers of the esophagus, likely as a result of tobacco exposure.

Adenocarcinomas of the distal esophagus and gastroesophageal junction more typically occur in metaplastic epithelium, a condition known as Barrett's esophagus.[5,6] This premalignant condition is characterized by the presence of columnar epithelium lining involving 3 cm or more of the distal tubular esophagus, in the presence or absence of hiatal hernia. The incidence of Barrett's esophagus is 10% to 20% among symptomatic patients who have endoscopy, and 30% to 50% for patients with peptic strictures. Risk factors for Barrett's esophagus include GERD, white or Hispanic race, male sex, advancing age, smoking, and obesity.[6,7] Although Barrett's esophagus is associated with chronic reflux disease, the true cause is unknown. Approximately 60% of cases of distal esophageal or gastroesophageal adenocarcinomas have evidence of Barrett's esophagus. In a nationwide population study from Denmark, the relative risk of adenocarcinoma among patients with Barrett's esophagus was 11.3 (95% CI 8.8, 14.4) compared with the risk in the general population.[8] The annual risk of esophageal adenocarcinoma was 0.12% (95% CI 0.09, 0.15). Detection of low-grade dysplasia on the index endoscopy was associated with an incidence rate for adenocarcinoma of 5.1 cases per 1,000 person-years. In contrast, the incidence rate among patients without dysplasia was 1.0 case per 1,000 person-years. Risk estimates for patients with high-grade dysplasia were slightly higher.

It is unclear if rigorous medical management of reflux disease with long-term proton-pump inhibitors can affect the natural history of the disease or the development of the subsequent malignant process. The typical treatment for patients with Barrett's esophagus is surveillance using upper endoscopy and biopsy to examine tissue for evidence of dysplasia.[7] High-grade dysplasia is an indication for more aggressive management, including surgical resection. Tumor markers, such as *TP53*, may be predictors of potential progression to malignant disease. There is an inverse association between *Helicobacter pylori* (*H. pylori*) infection and adenocarcinomas of the lower

---

KEY POINTS

- In the United States, incidence of esophageal squamous cell carcinoma is decreasing, and the incidence of adenocarcinomas is increasingly rapidly, likely as an effect of lifestyle changes.
- Combined-modality chemotherapy and radiation are standard neoadjuvant approaches to the treatment of esophageal cancer.
- Definitive chemoradiotherapy (without surgery) can be a valid treatment option, in particular for patients with squamous cell cancers of the esophagus.
- After trimodality therapy (chemoradiotherapy followed by surgery), adjuvant therapy is not standard of care.

esophagus, presumably a result of the reduced acidity associated with atrophic gastritis.[9] Infection with human papillomavirus (HPV) has been correlated with an increased incidence of squamous cell cancers of the upper esophagus.[10]

CLINICAL PRESENTATION AND DIAGNOSIS

The most common clinical presentation of esophageal cancer is dysphagia. Cachexia and substantial weight loss are complications of this presenting symptom, which cause many patients to be debilitated at the time of the diagnosis. Bleeding (hematemesis, tarry stools, and anemia) can be present as well.

Esophageal cancer should be suspected when a patient presents with dysphagia and weight loss. The history and physical examination are important elements to establish the diagnosis. Imaging techniques as well as an upper endoscopy are vital to the staging evaluation. Computed tomography (CT) of the thorax should be performed with tomographic slices through the liver to evaluate the extent of disease in the upper abdomen with special attention paid to potential liver metastases and celiac lymphadenopathy. To diagnose and carry out clinical staging of esophageal tumors, a thorough clinical examination with careful attention to the lymph nodes in the supraclavicular and axillary regions is essential. If needed, high-resolution ultrasound can help assess supraclavicular and axillary lymph nodes. In addition, an upper endoscopy should be performed to obtain a minimally invasive biopsy.

Imaging techniques, such as endoscopic ultrasound (EUS), have become more important in the evaluation and staging of esophageal cancer.[11] EUS, in the hands of a skillful sonographer, can accurately assess the depth of penetration in as many as 90% of tumors and determine involvement of mediastinal lymph nodes in nearly all patients. In addition, EUS allows the biopsy of suspicious lymph nodes to confirm the presence of lymph node metastases. Particularly in the era of preoperative chemotherapy and radiation, obtaining accurate staging with the use of EUS and CT has become a standard component when evaluating patients with esophageal cancer. Positron emission tomography (PET), preferably as a PET/CT scan, has become part of the routine pretreatment diagnostic work-up for patients with esophageal cancers. PET allows for the determination of lymph node status and the detection of occult sites of distant metastatic spread, and, therefore, may spare the patient the morbidity of an aggressive local-regional treatment approach.[12,13]

TREATMENT

The treatment of choice for patients with esophageal cancer had long been controversial, but accumulating evidence from meta-analyses and clinical trials has led to the establishment of a consensus regarding the practical management of esophageal cancers. The most frequently used initial treatment was primary surgical resection. However, the results of treatment with surgical resection alone have been discouraging, spawning a series of clinical trials to determine the efficacy of chemotherapy and radiation, in addition to surgical resection.

Surgery

The two most commonly used surgical techniques are transhiatal esophagectomy, which is generally reserved for patients with tumors of the lower esophagus, and a transthoracic approach (e.g., an Ivor-Lewis resection), which utilizes a combination of thoracotomy and laparotomy. The latter procedure is a more traditional operation for esophageal cancer. The results associated with both approaches are similar.[14,15] Reports suggest an increased retrieval rate of lymph nodes with an Ivor-Lewis approach.[16,17] Operative mortality rates should be less than 5% when the operation is performed by an experienced surgeon. Survival is poor for patients who have been treated with surgery only, with fewer than 10% to 15% of patients surviving 5 years.

The poor surgical outcome and the relatively advanced nature of disease at the time of diagnosis (stage II and III) in most cases led to investigations of combined-modality approaches for the treatment of patients with esophageal cancer. Use of chemotherapy alone did not result in a significant improvement in outcome. Similarly, radiation therapy alone for the treatment of esophageal cancer failed to yield a positive survival benefit. Radiation therapy, administered either before or after surgery, has been associated with shrinkage of the tumor, improvement in swallowing, and local-regional tumor control, but the combination has not been associated with a better survival rate compared with surgery alone.[18-20]

It is important to monitor and maintain patients' nutritional status when weight loss occurs and there is continued difficulty with alimentation before and during treatment. To palliate tumor-related esophageal obstruction and alleviate local swallowing dysfunction, there has been a shift away from surgical resection in favor of the use of newer techniques such as esophageal stents, laser therapy, endoscopic dilation, and gastric/jejunal tube feeding.

Combined-Modality Treatment

Combined-modality treatment involves both chemotherapy and radiation therapy and has been the focus of most of the research for esophageal cancer during the past 2 decades. The addition of chemotherapy is designed to treat micrometastases and enhance the local effects of radiation. An original landmark clinical trial, performed by Herskovic, was the first to demonstrate the benefit of combined-modality therapy.[18] In this trial, patients were randomly assigned to either radiation therapy alone or combined-modality radiation therapy and chemotherapy. More than 25% of patients were alive at 5 years in the group that received combined-modality therapy; none of the patients who received radiation therapy alone were alive at 5 years. The median survival was 14 months for combined-modality therapy compared with 9 months for radiation therapy alone.[21] The results of the study led to a series of trials designed to confirm this positive result. The purpose of these early studies was to determine if chemoradiotherapy could be used to replace surgery for patients who were not candidates for operation or to improve survival with preoperative chemoradiotherapy for surgical candidates. The chemotherapy agents historically administered with radiation were fluorouracil, a platinum drug (cisplatin or carboplatin), and/or mitomycin-C.[22] With these combinations, the pathologic complete response (CR) rate was approximately 25%. With newer chemotherapy agents, such as taxanes, the pathologic CR rate has increased.[23] Pathologic CR is now considered to be a good intermediate endpoint for efficacy in this clinical setting. Therefore, chemoradiotherapy alone can be considered a viable option for patients with localized esophageal cancer, in particular for patients who are not considered optimal candidates for surgery because of age or poor performance status. In addition, squamous cancers (mainly found in the middle and upper esophagus) appear to be more sensitive to chemoradiotherapy than adenocarcinomas and exhibit different tumor biology. Therefore, esophagectomy after chemoradiotherapy might not improve overall outcome after chemoradiotherapy in these patients.[24] This is especially important for cancers of the cervical esophagus, which can provide a surgical challenge. However, patients with a good performance status and in good physical condition for a surgical approach should still undergo surgery after chemoradiotherapy, rather than receiving chemoradiotherapy alone. A trial conducted in Germany randomly assigned patients with localized esophageal cancers to induction chemotherapy with 5-fluorouracil/leucovorin (5-FU/LV), etoposide, and cisplatin followed by either chemoradiotherapy (65 Gy) without surgery or chemoradiotherapy (40 Gy) followed by surgery.[25] The pathologically confirmed CR rate in the surgical arm was 33%. Although there was a significant difference in 2-year local failure rates (surgery vs. combined modality therapy: 33% vs. 58%, p = 0.003), there was only a paradoxical trend toward increased 3-year overall survival in favor of the surgery arm (31% vs. 24%), a result conceivably influenced by the relatively small number of patients (172) enrolled in the trial.

Perioperative chemotherapy alone, without radiation, has not been shown to have any benefit for patients with non-metastatic esophageal cancer. However, the Medical Research Council Adjuvant Gastric Infusional Chemotherapy (MAGIC) trial, which compared perioperative chemotherapy using epirubicin, cisplatin, and continuously infused 5-FU (ECF) with surgery alone for patients with gastric and gastroesophageal cancers, yielded a significant improvement in overall survival for patients who received perioperative chemotherapy (see the Gastric Cancer section for more on gastric and gastroesophageal junction cancers).[26] Twenty-six percent of patients in this trial had esophageal and gastroesophageal junction cancers, and multivariate subgroup analyses indicated a survival benefit from perioperative chemotherapy at least for gastroesophageal junction cancers. Thus, perioperative chemotherapy with a combination regimen such as ECF should be considered for patients with gastroesophageal junction cancers who are not optimal candidates for chemoradiotherapy. Trials comparing optimized perioperative chemotherapy with neoadjuvant chemoradiotherapy are highly warranted, but not planned at this point.

Patients are most commonly treated with either trimodality treatment using chemoradiotherapy and surgery, chemoradiotherapy alone, or chemotherapy including novel combinations of agents. The precise treatment algorithm is not well defined, and attempts to determine the optimum treatment method in randomized clinical trials have proven difficult. Various randomized trials were conducted to compare preoperative chemoradiotherapy with surgery alone, but results were conflicting. A meta-analysis, which included 18 randomized controlled trials with approximately 3,000 patients, found that trimodality therapy significantly improved 2-year survival (hazard ratio [HR] 0.81; p = 0.002; 13% absolute difference) and reduced locoregional recurrence when compared with surgery alone.[27,28] In the absence of medical contraindications, most patients in the United States with localized esophageal cancers are receiving neoadjuvant combined-modality therapy followed by surgery. This practice is so prevalent that clinical trials that try to enroll patients to a surgery-alone arm have had major accrual problems. The Cancer and Leukemia Group B (CALGB) 9781 trial was closed after only 56 of 500 planned patients were randomly assigned to surgery alone or to surgery and combination fluorouracil and cisplatin as radiosensitizing chemotherapy.[29] Despite this low accrual rate, the 5-year survival rate of patients receiving trimodality therapy was 39% compared with 16% for surgery alone. Median overall survival rates for the two groups were 4.5 years and 1.8 years, respectively. Most recently, data from a Dutch phase III trial confirmed the superiority of a neoadjuvant chemoradiotherapy approach compared with surgery alone in patients with localized esophageal cancer.[20] In this study, 363 patients were randomly assigned to receive chemoradiotherapy with a carboplatin/paclitaxel regimen and a relatively low radiation dose of 41.4 Gy followed by surgery or surgery alone. The neoadjuvant treatment led to a pathologic CR rate of 32.6%. The overall survival was significantly better (p = 0.011) in the group of patients treated with chemoradiotherapy (HR 0.67, 95% CI 0.50, 0.92). Median survival was 49 months in the neoadjuvant arm compared with 26 months in the surgery-alone arm. One-, 2- and 3-year survival rates were 82%, 67%, and 59% in the trimodality arm and 70%, 52%, and 48% in the surgery-alone arm. Importantly, the results appeared to be more convincing in squamous cell cancers than in adenocarcinomas. In a cross-trial comparison, the toxicity of the carboplatin/taxanes regimen was mild and appeared less severe than the toxicity seen with the 5-FU/platinum combination used in CALGB 9781. These results add further support for the use of trimodality therapy as standard of care for patients with localized esophageal cancers.

There are no convincing data that justify the routine use of adjuvant chemotherapy after surgery.[30] Similarly, radiation therapy has no role as the sole postoperative modality. Although no data support or refute combined-modality chemotherapy and radiation therapy after initial surgical resection, this technique is frequently employed in academic medical centers, in particular after R0 resection of patients with lymph node–positive disease.[31]

The intent of treatment for metastatic esophageal cancer is palliation. Many agents have demonstrated some activity in esophageal cancer, including fluoropyrimidines (fluorouracil and capecitabine), platinum agents, taxanes, irinotecan, mitomycin-C, anthracyclines, and, to a lesser extent, methotrexate, vinorelbine, and gemcitabine.[32] Treatment commonly is administered as a combination of two or three drugs or, less frequently, as single-agent therapy, depending on the patient's performance status. The utility of treatment regimens is similar to the experience in gastric cancer, especially with regard to adenocarcinomas of the gastroesophageal junction. In most clinical trials with single-agent therapy, the response rate has ranged from 10% to 40%. Combination regimens have yielded response rates as high as 50%. Palliation of dysphagia and bleeding is important and difficult to achieve. The liberal use of esophageal stents and local therapies, such as laser therapy and brachytherapy, as well as palliative radiation with or without chemotherapy can be very useful in this setting. The activity of novel targeted agents, such as epidermal growth factor receptor (EGFR) inhibitors and vascular endothelial growth factor (VEGF) inhibitors in combination with chemotherapy and/or with radiotherapy, is being investigated in ongoing clinical trials.[33] Initial results of a phase III trial that investigated the role of bevacizumab in advanced gastroesophageal and gastric cancers have been disappointing.[34] EGFR monoclonal antibodies added to chemotherapy even exhibit a detrimental effect on outcome.[35] Data from a second-line phase III trial comparing the VEGF receptor (VEGFR)-2 monoclonal antibody ramucirumab against best supportive care have shown improved survival in advanced gastroesophageal cancers.[35,36] Trastuzumab, the humanized monoclonal antibody against HER2, added to standard chemotherapy in HER2-overexpressing gastric and gastroesophageal cancers improved overall and progression-free survival as well as response rates compared with chemotherapy alone.[37] These data on novel biologic agents are discussed in detail in the Gastric Cancer section.

GASTRIC CANCER
EPIDEMIOLOGY AND ETIOLOGY
The incidence of gastric cancer has varied considerably during the last century. In the United States, where the incidence of gastric cancer has decreased approximately 75% during the last few decades, the incidence of gastroesophageal tumors has concomitantly increased.[6] Although gastric cancer incidence has significantly declined worldwide, it is still common in regions of the world where the storage of fresh foods and the quality of water are poor. Gastric cancer is a major health issue in Japan and has resulted in a unique effort to screen this population for early-stage disease. In Japan, gastric cancer is associated with a distinctly better prognosis than in Western cultures. The improved prognosis in Japan is often attributed to superiority of surgical techniques, but this hypothesis has not been universally accepted. The endoscopic screening programs in Japan also have conceivably contributed to an improved outcome through the detection of gastric cancer lesions at an earlier—and possibly more curable—stage. The lowest incidences for gastric cancer are in Western cultures and in people of higher socioeconomic status. Studies of migrant populations have supported evidence for the effect of environmental influences on the development of gastric cancer.[38] Together, these data support the concept that gastric cancer is strongly influenced by nutritional, socioeconomic, and medical factors rather than dominated by genetic predisposition. In the United States, gastric cancer develops twice as often in men than in women, is more frequent in black men than in white men, and its incidence increases with age starting in the fifth decade.[39] The mortality rate associated with gastric cancer has decreased for white men, paralleling the overall decline in the incidence of gastric cancer in this population. As mentioned previously, determining the reason for the considerable increase in the incidence of adenocarcinoma of the proximal stomach and distal esophagus remains a challenge for epidemiologists. Possible reasons for the increase include the prevalence of obesity, elevated body mass index with increased incidence of GERD, and increased calorie consumption.[40] Aspirin and other nonsteroidal anti-inflammatory agent use has been associated with a lower risk for cancer of the gastroesophageal junction and other gastrointestinal tumors.[41]

Factors associated with an increased risk for gastric cancer include nutritional factors such as high salt and nitrate intake, a diet low in vitamins A and C, the consumption of large amounts of smoked or cured foods, lack of refrigerated foods, and poor-quality drinking water.[42] Occupational exposure to rubber and coal also increases the risk. Cigarette smoking, *H. pylori* infection, Epstein-Barr virus, radiation exposure, and prior gastric surgery for benign ulcer disease also have been implicated as risk factors. Genetic risk factors include type A blood, pernicious

---

KEY POINTS

- The incidence of gastric cancer correlates with socioeconomic status and is clearly dependent on environmental factors.
- The worldwide incidence of gastric cancer is decreasing; however, there is an increase in more proximal and gastroesophageal cancers.
- Controversy surrounds the question of the best operation for gastric cancer, with data from Japanese studies suggesting a better result using a more aggressive, extensive lymph node dissection.
- Randomized trials have demonstrated a benefit for adjuvant chemoradiotherapy as well as for preoperative and postoperative chemotherapy and adjuvant chemotherapy without radiation for stages I to III gastric cancer, resulting in competing standards of care.
- Combination chemotherapy regimens have become more widely used for advanced disease, with some evidence to support benefit compared with single-agent therapy.
- The addition of trastuzumab to chemotherapy is standard of care in HER2-overexpressing metastatic gastric and gastroesophageal cancers.
- The VEGFR antibody ramucirumab has shown efficacy in second-line phase III trials in advanced gastric cancer.

anemia, a family history of gastric cancer, hereditary nonpolyposis colon cancer (HNPCC), and Li-Fraumeni syndrome. Gastric cancer precursor lesions include adenomatous gastric polyps, dysplasia, chronic atrophic gastritis, and intestinal metaplasia. Results from several studies have demonstrated an increased likelihood of *H. pylori* infection in patients with gastric cancer, particularly cancer of the distal stomach.[43,44] Although cancer does not develop in most people with *H. pylori* infections, the increased risk for patients who are infected has raised the issue of whether treatment of *H. pylori* might decrease the risk for gastric cancer. Although the role of *H. pylori* in gastric carcinogenesis is well defined, no definitive evidence shows that mass eradication could reduce incidence of gastric cancer.[45] A large Chinese study showed no benefit in the prevention of gastric cancer with the eradication of *H. pylori*.[46] By contrast, a meta-analysis suggested that eradication could indeed reduce the risk for gastric cancer.[47] At present, treatment of patients with this infection should be reserved for patients with demonstrated ulcers or GERD.

CLINICAL PRESENTATION AND DIAGNOSIS

The common presenting symptoms for gastric cancers are bleeding, hematemesis, pain, anorexia, and dyspepsia. The first clinical symptoms often are a result of metastatic spread inside the peritoneal cavity resulting in the formation of ascites and abdominal pain. The disease is most often diagnosed by upper endoscopy and direct biopsy or, less commonly, by CT. Biopsy should be performed for samples from any gastric ulcer because it is difficult to distinguish benign from malignant ulcers endoscopically. In areas of increased cancer incidence, such as Japan, mass screening programs have been successful in detecting gastric cancers in an early stage, with higher cure rates observed after resection. Staging includes chest x-ray, chest CT scans, and abdominal imaging to rule out metastasis and to determine surgical resectability. PET scans are not (yet) recommended as standard diagnostic procedure in view of limited sensitivity, but can be helpful to determine the resectability of gastric cancers in select cases.[48] The role of EUS is less clear in gastric cancer than in esophageal and gastroesophageal junction cancers.

TREATMENT

The only potentially curative treatment approach for patients with gastric cancer is surgical resection. The type of surgery performed in Asia differs from the type of resection performed in the United States. D2 resection, the standard surgery in Japan, involves the meticulous resection of all regional lymph nodes, whereas in the United States, D1 resection (removal of only perigastric lymph nodes) has long been the standard. Retrospective data suggest that the outcome for D2 resection is better than the outcome for D1 resections; however, the disparity might well be caused by a fundamental difference in the disease process itself, rather than the surgical technique. Randomized trials initially did not clearly demonstrate a survival benefit for patients undergoing a D2 compared with a D1 dissection.[49,50] After 15-year follow-up of a 1,078-patient randomized Dutch trial, however, D2 lymphadenectomy was associated with lower locoregional recurrence (12% vs. 22%) and gastric cancer–related death rates (37% vs. 48%) than D1 surgery.[51] Although D2 dissection was associated with increased operative morbidity, these data suggest that D2 lymphadenectomy should be considered surgical standard of care.

Early-Stage Disease

Patients with operable gastric cancer have a reasonable chance of being cured with surgery alone. Surgery cures 75% to 80% of patients with early-stage node-negative disease. However, for patients with stage III disease, the reported 5-year survival rates are 25% or less. There is extensive literature evaluating the use of postoperative chemotherapy for the adjuvant treatment of gastric cancer. Many phase III randomized clinical trials, the majority of which used "outdated" chemotherapy regimens, have shown no clear trend toward a benefit for chemotherapy alone (without concomitant radiation).[52] This postoperative nihilism was abandoned when a randomized phase III trial was presented in which adjuvant chemotherapy was combined with radiation therapy.[53] Patients with stages I to III gastroesophageal or gastric cancers were randomly assigned to either surgery alone or surgery followed by bolus 5-FU/LV-based chemotherapy (Mayo Clinic regimen) with sandwiched chemoradiotherapy (45 Gy) with bolus 5-FU/LV as a radiosensitizer. The results showed an approximate 20% improvement in survival for the group receiving the combined-modality therapy. The median overall survival in the surgery-only group was 27 months compared with 36 months in the chemoradiotherapy group; the HR for death in the surgery-only arm was 1.35 (95% CI 1.09, 1.66; p = 0.005); the HR for relapse was 1.52 (95% CI 1.23, 1.86; p < 0.001). The study has been criticized for the very low rate of D1 (or D2) lymph node dissection. In fact, less than 50% of patients underwent a D1 resection, which was mandated per protocol. In addition, only the rate of local recurrence, not the rate of distant metastasis, was reduced in the adjuvant chemoradiotherapy group, suggesting that the adjuvant therapy could have mainly compensated for inferior surgery. On the other hand, the survival benefit observed with postoperative therapy was maintained in all (preplanned) subgroup analyses. Although these trial results were met with skepticism elsewhere, they established a new standard of care for patients with this disease in the United States. A large CALGB-led Intergroup trial (C80101) tried to improve upon the results obtained with bolus 5-FU/LV plus radiation therapy by randomly assigning patients with resected gastric cancer to the standard "Macdonald" regimen[53] or chemoradiotherapy with ECF, a combination regimen of infusional 5-FU, cisplatin, and epirubicin.[54] The study did not demonstrate any difference in outcomes between the two arms, although it is of note that only one cycle of ECF was administered before and two cycles after standard 5-FU-based chemoradiotherapy in the experimental arm with not all patients being able to complete the whole duration of adjuvant therapy.

Perioperative chemotherapy with the ECF regimen administered before and after surgery for resectable gastric cancer also has shown a significant overall survival benefit compared with surgery alone in the MAGIC trial.[26] As compared with the surgery group, the perioperative chemotherapy group had a higher likelihood of overall survival (HR for death 0.75, 95% CI 0.60, 0.93; p = 0.009; 5-year survival rate, 36% vs. 23%) and of progression-free survival (HR for progression 0.66, 95% CI 0.53, 0.81; p < 0.001). It is of note that only about 55% of patients in the perioperative chemotherapy group actually received postresection therapy, which suggests that the main therapy component responsible for the improved outcome was the preoperative treatment phase.

The results of trials investigating the role of adjuvant chemotherapy without additional radiation therapy are mixed. An Italian trial using an intensified, ECF-based treatment regimen as adjuvant therapy after gastric cancer resection (and not preoperatively) did not demonstrate a benefit in outcome.[55] On the other hand, a Japanese phase III trial of S-1, an oral fluoropyrimidine, as adjuvant therapy after D2 resection of stage II or III gastric cancer demonstrated an overall survival benefit with a 3-year overall survival rate of 80.1% in the S-1 group and 70.1% in the surgery-only group (HR 0.68, 95% CI 0.52, 0.87, p = 0.003).[56] The improvement in overall survival was confirmed after 5-year follow-up.[57] Recently, a Korean phase III trial (CLASSIC) in 1,035 patients with D2-resected stage II/III gastric cancer identified adjuvant therapy with capecitabine plus oxaliplatin as superior to surgery alone with significant improvement in 3-year disease-free survival (DFS; 74% vs. 59%; HR 0.56, p < 0.0001).[58] Definitive overall survival data of this trial are pending. In addition to these individual trials a meta-analysis of 17 trials with 3,838 patients confirmed that adjuvant chemotherapy without radiation after gastric cancer resection was associated with a significant survival benefit with a HR of 0.82 (95% CI 0.79, 0.90, p < 0.001).[59]

Based on the aforementioned trials and meta-analyses, three different approaches toward the management of early-stage gastric cancer are considered standard of care and are used with varying frequency based on regional preferences: postoperative chemoradiotherapy (United States), pre- and postoperative chemotherapy (United Kingdom), or adjuvant chemotherapy alone after D2 resection (Asia).

Neoadjuvant chemotherapy has been shown to shrink primary tumors and regional lymph nodes in phase II clinical trials with intriguing results[60]; however, these small studies have not established any definitive role for preoperative neoadjuvant chemotherapy with or without radiation in facilitating resection of initially unresectable tumors.

ADVANCED DISEASE

The medical treatment of metastatic cancer of the stomach is primarily palliative and confers a moderate effect on overall survival. Multiple agents are active, including fluoropyrimidines (fluorouracil, capecitabine, and S-1), anthracyclines, platinum agents, taxanes (paclitaxel and docetaxel), irinotecan, and others, including trastuzumab for HER2-overexpressing gastric

cancers, and most recently, ramucirumab, a VEGFR2 antibody.[36] Combination regimens are associated with higher response rates and, according to a meta-analysis, also are associated with increased overall survival when compared with single-agent therapies.[61] Combinations including cisplatin and fluorouracil in various schedules were long considered the standard of care, with epirubicin commonly added to form a triple-drug regimen that was pioneered mainly in the United Kingdom.[62] A phase III trial involving 445 patients with gastric cancer demonstrated superiority of the addition of docetaxel to cisplatin and fluorouracil compared with cisplatin and fluorouracil alone, in terms of response rate (37% vs. 25%, p = 0.01), time to tumor progression (5.6 vs. 3.7 months, p < 0.001), and overall survival (9.2 vs. 8.6 months, p = 0.02).[63] However, the addition of docetaxel is associated with significant toxicities, most notably, a high rate of febrile neutropenia (30%); therefore, this regimen is not advisable for patients with gastric cancer who have a poor performance status. Another large randomized phase III trial including 1,002 patients tried to improve the ECF regimen by substituting oral capecitabine (X) for continuous-infusion fluorouracil and by using the non-nephrotoxic compound oxaliplatin (O) instead of cisplatin (C).[64] The combination of epirubicin, oxaliplatin, and capecitabine (EOX) was found to be less toxic and at least as active as the ECF combination, with all efficacy parameters trending toward superiority. Median survival times in the ECF (control arm), ECX, EOF, and EOX groups were 9.9 months, 9.9 months, 9.3 months, and 11.2 months, respectively; survival rates at 1 year were 37.7%, 40.8%, 40.4%, and 46.8%, respectively. In a secondary analysis, overall survival was longer with EOX than with ECF, with a HR for death of 0.80 in the EOX group (95% CI 0.66, 0.97; p = 0.02). Progression-free survival and response rates did not differ significantly between the regimens. Although these two trials investigated triplet combinations, the value of an anthracycline or taxane component in the treatment of advanced gastric cancer has repeatedly been questioned; thus, a fluoropyrimidine/platinum chemotherapy doublet is still considered standard of care by most experts.[65]

A third phase III trial compared cisplatin plus 5-FU with irinotecan plus 5-FU in 333 patients with advanced gastric cancer. No difference in outcome measures (response rate, progression-free, and overall survival) could be found, but the non-cisplatin, irinotecan-based regimen was found to be less toxic and, thus, could be an alternative for patients not considered candidates for a platinum-based treatment regimen.[66] Based on these trial data, a combination regimen with a platinum agent (cisplatin or oxaliplatin) plus fluoropyrimidine as a backbone, with or without the addition of epirubicin or docetaxel, can be considered first-line standard of care in the palliative treatment of advanced gastric cancer. Irinotecan has clearly demonstrated activity and could be integrated in a sequential treatment approach.

The role of targeted agents, in particular drugs targeting the VEGF and EGFR/HER2 system, has been investigated in several clinical trials.

The first targeted agent with documented efficacy in advanced gastric and gastroesophageal junction cancer was trastuzumab, the humanized monoclonal antibody against HER2. Based on the preclinical observations that about 20% of gastric cancers (and about 30% of gastroesophageal adenocarcinomas) overexpress HER2,[67] the phase III ToGA trial investigated whether the addition of trastuzumab to standard chemotherapy would extend survival in patients with advanced adenocarcinoma of the stomach or gastroesophageal junction.[37] Of 3,807 tumors from patients with gastric cancer tested, 810 (22.1%) were positive for HER2 overexpression using immunohistochemistry (IHC) and fluorescence in situ hybridization analysis. Eventually, 584 patients were randomly assigned to a fluoropyrimidine (5-FU 800 mg/m^2/day on days 1 to 5 or capecitabine 1,000 mg/m^2 twice daily on days 1 to 14 based on physician choice) plus cisplatin 80 mg/m^2 on day 1 with or without trastuzumab (8 mg/kg loading dose followed by 6 mg/kg) on day 1. Cycles were repeated every 3 weeks for six cycles, and trastuzumab was subsequently continued every 3 weeks until disease progression. In the study, 55% of patients were from Asia and 18% of patients had tumors originating in the gastroesophageal junction. The addition of trastuzumab to cisplatin/fluoropyrimidine increased median overall survival from 11.1 months to 13.8 months (HR 0.74, 95% CI 0.60, 0.91; p = 0.0046). In addition, secondary endpoints such as progression-free survival (6.7 vs. 5.5 months, p = 0.0002) and overall response rate (47.3% vs. 34.5%, p = 0.0017) were also improved in the trastuzumab arm. There were no significant differences in the toxicity between the two treatment arms. Asymptomatic decrease in ejection fraction occurred in 4.6% and 1.1% of patients in the trastuzumab and chemotherapy-alone arms, respectively. The ToGA trial was the first phase III trial to demonstrate a survival advantage with the addition of a biologic agent, trastuzumab, to standard chemotherapy in advanced gastric cancer. Combination therapies of trastuzumab added to standard chemotherapy have emerged as the standard of care in patients with metastatic, HER2-overexpressing gastric and gastroesophageal cancers. Further phase III trials are currently investigating the role of other EGFR/HER2 inhibitors such as lapatinib, cetuximab, and panitumumab in gastric cancer.

In contrast with the positive results for trastuzumab in HER2-overexpressing gastric cancers, two phase III trials of lapatinib, an oral HER2/EGFR kinase inhibitor, added to chemotherapy in first- (LOGIC) and second-line (TYTAN) failed to meet their primary endpoints.[68,69] In the second-line trial, however, the subgroup of patients with high HER2 expression by IHC 3+ exhibited a survival benefit with the addition of lapatinib to paclitaxel compared with placebo. It is unclear, however, if lapatinib will be further developed in gastric cancer given the fact that trastuzumab has become standard of care for HER2-positive gastroesophageal cancers.

Antibodies targeting the EGFR, a member of the HER family of receptor tyrosine kinases, such as cetuximab and panitumumab, have also been tested in randomized phase III trials, unfortunately with negative results. The EXPAND trial randomly assigned more than 900 patients with advanced gastroesophageal adenocarcinoma to capecitabine plus cisplatin with or without cetuximab.[70] Although the toxicity was increased in the cetuximab arm, no benefit in any outcome parameter was noted. The REAL-3 trial investigated the addition of panitumumab to EOX in 553 patients.[35] The dose of EOX had to be reduced after an interim toxicity analysis and the trial was eventually stopped when an interim efficacy analysis documented a detrimental effect in overall survival for the panitumumab-containing combination compared with the standard arm. The consistently negative data from these two large phase III trials confirm that there is no role for the use of EGFR monoclonal antibodies in advanced gastroesophageal adenocarcinoma.

Results of trials investigating angiogenesis inhibitors in gastric and esophageal cancers have demonstrated inconsistent results. In the first phase III trial, bevacizumab failed to demonstrate an overall survival benefit when added to cisplatin/fluoropyrimidine (mainly capecitabine) in patients with gastroesophageal junction and gastric adenocarcinomas.[34] However, the AVAGAST trial demonstrated increased response rates and longer progression-free survival for the bevacizumab-containing arm. Median overall survival was 12.1 months with bevacizumab plus fluoropyrimidine-cisplatin and 10.1 months with placebo plus fluoropyrimidine-cisplatin (HR 0.87, 95% CI 0.73, 1.03; p = 0.10). Both median progression-free survival (6.7 vs. 5.3 months; HR 0.80, 95% CI 0.68, 0.93; p = 0.0037) and overall response rate (46.0% vs. 37.4%; p = 0.0315) were significantly improved with bevacizumab compared with placebo. Preplanned subgroup analyses revealed regional differences in efficacy outcomes with a survival benefit for "Pan-American" patients, but not for patients from Asia who constituted the largest regional group, as expected. It has long been speculated that the biology of gastric cancers and the treatment approach toward these tumors differs greatly between Asian and non-Asian countries. Thus, one would have to be careful with the interpretation of global trials in this disease, which will invariably include a substantial number of Asian patients.

A second set of trials investigated ramucirumab, a VEGFR2 monoclonal antibody, in the second-line setting of advanced gastroesophageal cancer. The REGARD trial randomly assigned 472 patients after first-line fluoropyrimidine/platinum therapy in a 2:1 fashion to single-agent ramucirumab or placebo.[36] Median overall survival was 5.2 months for the ramucirumab arm and 3.8 months for the placebo arm (HR 0.776, 95% CI 0.603, 0.998; p = 0.047). Aside from a higher rate of hypertension, no relevant differences were seen in recorded side effects between ramucirumab and placebo. In comparison with the AVAGAST bevacizumab trial, REGARD enrolled fewer patients from Asian countries (15% vs. 49%) and included a higher percentage of gastroesophageal junction cancers (25% vs. 14%). Concerns have been raised regarding the placebo-control arm in the REGARD study given the convincing documentation of a survival benefit associated with second-line chemotherapy. The RAINBOW study addressed these concerns by randomly assigning 665 patients with advanced gastroesophageal cancer after first-line therapy with a platinum-fluoropyrimidine combination to weekly paclitaxel with or without ramucirumab.[71] The study met its primary endpoint of overall survival with an HR of 0.81 and a median difference of 2.2 months (9.6 vs. 7.4 months, p = 0.017). Progression-free survival and response rates were also improved in favor of the paclitaxel-ramucirumab combination. It is expected that ramucirumab will receive regulatory approval as a second-line therapy for metastatic gastroesophageal cancer in 2014.

The usefulness of second-line chemotherapy in the palliative management of gastric cancer had long been questioned. Eventually, three randomized trials of chemotherapy compared with best supportive care clearly demonstrated an improvement in overall survival with the use of second-line chemotherapy with either irinotecan or a taxane after failure of first-line fluoropyrimidine/platinum therapy.[72-74] A head-to-head comparison between two commonly used second-line therapies, paclitaxel and irinotecan, demonstrated similar efficacy for these approaches.[75]

Radiation therapy can be effective for metastatic disease (e.g., metastasis to bony structures for symptomatic control) and perhaps for unresectable, bleeding tumors in conjunction with chemotherapy, but it is rarely used to treat primary advanced unresectable gastric cancer.

Several novel agents are currently being investigated in advanced gastric cancer. The most promising early data have emerged from studies with drugs targeting the HGF/c-met ligand/receptor system.[76]

PANCREAS CANCER
EPIDEMIOLOGY AND ETIOLOGY

Cancer of the exocrine pancreas is a substantial health problem in the United States, with an annual incidence of 45,220 patients and an annual mortality of 38,460 cases in the United States, with almost all of those patients dying within 2 years of diagnosis.[1,77] It is estimated that more about 270,000 patients die of pancreas cancer each year worldwide.[3] The incidence of pancreas cancer increased until the late 1970s and then reached a plateau. The risk factors for pancreas cancer are largely unknown, although there is some suggestion of a link to tobacco exposure.[78,79] Data regarding coffee and excess alcohol consumptions are conflicting; therefore, they cannot be considered true etiologic factors. There is an association between pancreas cancer and diabetes; however, it is more likely that diabetes is an early manifestation of cancer and not necessarily a predisposing factor.[78,80] Chronic pancreatitis also may be a predisposing factor. Selective mutations of BRCA2, and, to a lesser degree, BRCA1 have been associated with familial pancreas cancer. Other less common genetic syndromes have been linked to pancreas cancer (e.g., hereditary pancreatitis, HNPCC, familial breast cancer with BRCA2 mutations, p16 mutations, Peutz-Jeghers syndrome, ataxia telangiectasia).[81] Approximately 10% to 20% of patients are thought to have a familial predisposition. There is no standard surveillance or screening for this disease. Most pancreas cancers harbor activating genetic mutations of the oncogene KRAS, which is integrated in signaling pathways of various receptor-kinases such as EGFR and the insulin-like growth factor receptor (IGFR)-I. In addition, most pancreas cancers show mutations in several tumor suppressor genes such as p53, DPC4, p16, and BRCA2.[81,82] A whole-genome

sequencing study in 24 pancreas cancers identified an average of 63 genetic alterations per cancer, the majority of which were point mutations.[83] Pancreatic adenocarcinomas arise from ductal epithelial cells. Pancreatic intraepithelial neoplasia, which are microscopic lesions of the pancreas, and intraductal papillary mucinous neoplasms and mucinous cystic neoplasms, which are both macroscopic lesions, are thought to be precursors of invasive ductal adenocarcinomas.[82,84]

KEY POINTS

- Pancreas cancer has the highest lethality of all the gastrointestinal malignancies.
- Diagnostic tests, such as PET and endoscopic ultrasound, do not replace the need for a biopsy to prove the diagnosis.
- Gemcitabine, as a single agent, has long been the standard of care for patients with advanced pancreas cancer; FOLFIRINOX is superior to gemcitabine in patients with good performance status who are considered candidates for more aggressive therapy.
- The addition of nab-paclitaxel to gemcitabine improves outcome compared with gemcitabine alone in advanced pancreas cancer.
- The best approach to adjuvant therapy (especially the role of radiation) is controversial.

CLINICAL PRESENTATION AND DIAGNOSIS

Symptoms associated with pancreas cancer at the time of presentation include either abdominal pain or jaundice. The disease typically is not diagnosed for several months after the initial presentation of vague abdominal symptoms or, quite commonly, back pain. The diagnosis is most often made with a CT scan, magnetic resonance imaging (MRI), or ultrasound. When evaluating patients with adult-onset diabetes without other risk factors, physicians should consider pancreas cancer as a possible diagnosis.[85] The most common diagnostic tests used for pancreas cancer are CT scan, MRI, EUS, and endoscopic retrograde cholangiopancreatography. Diagnostic tests, such as PET and EUS, may play a role in distinguishing cancer from other abnormalities and—most importantly—are used to adequately stage the disease, but do not replace a biopsy (e.g., EUS-guided) as a definitive diagnostic test.

TREATMENT

The treatment for resectable pancreas cancer is primarily surgery, although neoadjuvant treatment strategies with either chemoradiotherapy or chemotherapy alone have made inroads into clinical practice. For patients with tumors that appear resectable, which includes only approximately 20% to 25% of all pancreas cancers, surgery remains the only potentially curative treatment option. Tools such as EUS, MRI, and PET have improved the ability to determine which patients are candidates for surgery. In order to determine the resectability of a pancreas mass, a detailed evaluation of its spatial relationship to critical vascular structures, in particular, the superior mesenteric artery and celiac axis, has to be performed. Most patients with pancreas cancer are found to have unresectable disease either because of a locally advanced disease (involvement of critical vascular structures) or obvious metastatic disease (liver, peritoneal involvement) at the time of diagnosis. The 5-year survival rate for the minority of patients who are able to undergo resection is 5% to 25%.[86]

Adjuvant Therapy

The optimal adjuvant therapy after pancreas cancer resection is controversial, in particular, with regard to the value of radiation therapy. Based on a small randomized study (43 patients) conducted in the United States, approximately 30 years ago in which a significantly larger number of patients in the combined-modality group were alive at 1 year compared with the surgery-alone group, postoperative chemoradiotherapy with bolus fluorouracil became the standard of care in the United States.[87] Since then, the role of radiation in this context has been repeatedly challenged by European investigators,[88] culminating in a trial suggesting that the use of radiation conferred an adverse outcome compared with patients who received adjuvant chemotherapy alone.[89,90] The complex study design, concerns about the radiation protocol, and the questionable randomization strategy used in the study long prevented chemotherapy without radiation from becoming an accepted standard of care in the United States.

More recently, clinical trials have set somewhat competing standards for the adjuvant medical therapy of pancreas cancer. A German phase III trial (CONKO-1) including 364 patients demonstrated the superiority of adjuvant chemotherapy with gemcitabine compared with surgery alone for patients with resected pancreas cancer, regardless of whether a tumor-free resection margin could be obtained.[91,92] An update of this study demonstrated a significant improvement in 5-year overall survival of 20.7% (95% CI 14.7%, 26.6%) for gemcitabine compared with 10.4% (95% CI 5.9%, 15.0%) for surgery alone, and 10-year overall survival of 12.2% (95% CI 7.3%, 17.2%) compared with 7.7% (95% CI 3.6%, 11.8%).[93]

A large phase III trial mainly conducted in the United Kingdom, the ESPAC-3 trial, compared weekly gemcitabine to bolus 5-FU/LV (Mayo Clinic regimen) as adjuvant therapy in 1,088 patients with resected pancreas cancer.[94] Median survival was almost identical in both groups (5-FU/LV: 23.0 months vs. gemcitabine: 23.6 months, p = 0.39). More mucositis/stomatitis and diarrhea were seen with bolus 5-FU/LV; patients assigned to gemcitabine had more thrombocytopenia. Based on these data, both adjuvant gemcitabine or bolus 5-FU/LV can be considered as appropriate adjuvant chemotherapy for resected pancreas cancer.

Most recently, at the 2013 ASCO Annual Meeting data from a randomized phase III comparison of gemcitabine with S-1, an oral fluoropyrimidine not available in the United States but commonly used in Japan, in 385 patients with resected pancreas cancer were presented.[95] Although S-1 and gemcitabine had previously shown similar results in the advanced setting,[96] adjuvant S-1 was found to be superior to gemcitabine in preliminary analysis with a substantial improvement of overall survival (2-year overall survival rate 53% vs. 70%, HR 0.54, p < 0.0001) and relapse-free survival (median 11.2 vs. 23.2 months, HR 0.57, p < 0.0001). In Japan, S-1 has since emerged as the standard of care in adjuvant therapy of pancreas cancer. It is unclear if these results can be extrapolated to the population of Western countries in which, at this point in time, adjuvant gemcitabine remains the adjuvant standard of care.

To expand on the potential role of radiation therapy, a U.S. trial (Radiation Therapy Oncology Group, RTOG 9704) involving 451 patients documented an improved outcome for patients with pancreas head cancers (but not cancers of the pancreas body or tail) who received adjuvant gemcitabine followed by chemoradiotherapy with continuous infusion of fluorouracil (50.4 Gy, 5-FU at 250 mg/m^2/day) and subsequent gemcitabine monotherapy compared with postoperative fluorouracil-based chemoradiotherapy.[97] Patients with pancreas head tumors (388 patients) had a median survival of 20.5 months and a 3-year survival of 31% in the gemcitabine group compared with a median survival of 16.9 months and a 3-year survival of 22% in the fluorouracil group (HR 0.82, 95% CI 0.65, 1.03; p = 0.09). By design, this trial was not able to verify if radiation therapy is an essential component of adjuvant therapy in resected pancreas cancer. Thus, for the foreseeable future, the standards of care might differ between the United States and Europe, with adjuvant gemcitabine-based chemotherapy without radiation favored in Europe and combined-modality approaches favored in the United States. It should be noted, however, that the data from the CONKO-1 trial (with a more than doubling of long-term overall survival) have made inroads into U.S. practice standards.[98] The ongoing RTOG Intergroup phase III trial 0848 is currently evaluating the value of radiation therapy as adjuvant therapy for resected pancreas cancer.

Based on the convincing results in advanced pancreas cancer, a phase III trial investigating the efficacy of FOLFIRINOX (see Treatment of Metastatic Pancreas Cancer section) compared with gemcitabine as adjuvant therapy has been activated in France and Canada (NCT01526135). Similarly, an adjuvant phase III trial comparing gemcitabine to gemcitabine plus *nab*-paclitaxel will soon open.

Chemotherapy and Radiation for Locally Advanced Pancreas Cancers

Preoperative chemotherapy and radiation are used in some centers in a neoadjuvant fashion in upfront resectable pancreas cancers, and results of phase II trials regarding this treatment approach have been published.[99] For patients with initially unresectable cancers a "conversion approach" of chemotherapy with or without radiation is tolerable, with occasional tumor responses allowing subsequent surgical resection. No randomized trial has been conducted yet, so it is unclear if this approach is associated with a survival advantage. In addition, no clear definition of "borderline resectable" pancreas cancer has been established; although most surgeons consider abutment of major upper abdominal blood vessels the main criterion.[100]

For patients with locally advanced, unresectable disease, there are two treatment strategies: primary chemoradiotherapy or systemic chemotherapy. Most patients in the United States are currently treated with a combination of radiation therapy and chemotherapy. The standard regimen is infusional fluorouracil and radiation therapy, but the role of contemporary chemotherapy agents, including low-dose gemcitabine, capecitabine (an oral fluorouracil substitute), and targeted agents in combination with radiation therapy is now being explored. This approach may improve pain and prevent gastric or biliary obstruction. A randomized trial (E4201) validated this approach with a better outcome for patients receiving gemcitabine in combination with radiation therapy compared with gemcitabine alone in patients with localized, unresectable pancreas cancer.[101] The primary endpoint of the trial was survival, which was 11.1 months (95% CI 7.6, 15.5 months) and 9.2 months (95% CI 7.9, 11.4 months) for chemoradiotherapy and gemcitabine alone, respectively (one-sided p = 0.017). However, this trial only enrolled 74 of 316 planned patients with unresectable pancreas cancer, so the results are not necessarily definitive.

The other feasible strategy is to initiate systemic chemotherapy as primary therapy because the clinical benefit of gemcitabine-based therapy in this setting is well documented, even in the absence of significant tumor shrinkage. This approach has been found superior in a European phase III trial that included 119 patients and compared induction chemoradiotherapy (60 Gy, infusional 5-FU and intermittent cisplatin) followed by maintenance gemcitabine with gemcitabine alone for locally advanced unresectable pancreas cancer.[102] Interestingly, median overall survival was shorter in the chemoradiotherapy arm compared with gemcitabine alone (8.6 vs. 13 months, p = 0.03).

The role of radiation therapy as a component of the management of locally advanced pancreas cancers was further investigated by the international LAP-07 phase III trial presented at the 2013 ASCO Annual Meeting.[103] In this trial, patients were initially randomly assigned to gemcitabine with or without erlotinib. Patients with at least stable disease after 4 months underwent a second random assignment to either continue the same chemotherapy as in the first phase of the trial or proceed to chemoradiotherapy with capecitabine as radiation sensitizer. A total of 449 patients were randomly assigned up front; 269 patients (61% of the initial study cohort) were eligible for the second random assignment. One of the key findings of this study was that the addition of erlotinib to gemcitabine in this setting did not provide any benefit in overall survival. In fact, the overall survival trended toward a detriment effect in the erlotinib arm. Secondly, no survival benefit was observed with the switch from chemotherapy to consolidating chemoradiotherapy; the arms showed no difference in progression-free and overall survival. In conclusion, there appears to be no role for erlotinib in the management of locally advanced pancreas cancers. Chemoradiotherapy in patients after an induction chemo-

therapy phase can be considered in select patients, even though no survival benefit could be documented with this approach.

Based on the available data, chemoradiotherapy or chemotherapy alone can be used as initial treatment of patients with unresectable pancreas cancer without distant metastases. Chemoradiotherapy might be preferred for patients with poorly controlled pain from local tumor invasion in view of the well-documented analgesic effect of radiation therapy. Whether the high antitumor activity of FOLFIRINOX (see Treatment of Metastatic Pancreas Cancer section) with documented response rates greater than 30%[104] or gemcitabine plus *nab*-paclitaxel can emerge as the preferred neoadjuvant treatment in select patients is the focus of ongoing studies.

Other palliative means to treat patients in this setting include biliary stenting, intraoperative or external beam radiation therapy, and celiac axis nerve blocks. Aggressive management of symptoms, such as pain, anorexia, and obstruction, should be the primary focus of palliative treatment. Some patients require the placement of a duodenal stent for relieving gastric-outlet obstruction.[105] It is noteworthy that in this context the routine preoperative placement of biliary stents in patients with biliary obstruction and operable pancreas head cancers was associated with an increase in surgical complications when compared with upfront surgery without prior biliary drainage.[106] Thus, routine preoperative biliary drainage in patients undergoing subsequent surgery for cancer of the pancreas head is not recommended.

Treatment of Metastatic Pancreas Cancer

Regarding advanced metastatic disease, several agents, such as fluoropyrimidines, gemcitabine, irinotecan, platinum compounds, and taxanes, have minor to moderate single-agent activity in pancreas cancer. In the mid-1990s, gemcitabine was tested against single-agent intravenous fluorouracil (administered without leucovorin as short-term infusion, thus not optimally administered) in a randomized clinical trial with 126 patients.[107] Gemcitabine was found to be superior to fluorouracil regarding clinical benefit, with more patients (24% vs. 5%) experiencing a reduction of pain as well as improvements in appetite and weight. There were few clinical responses in either arm (less than 10%), but the median survival (5.65 vs. 4.4 months, p = 0.0025) and the 1-year survival rate (18% vs. 2%) were better for patients treated with gemcitabine. Subsequently, a plethora of clinical trials have tried to outperform gemcitabine monotherapy, with all studying gemcitabine compared with gemcitabine plus another agent. In phase III trials, agents added to gemcitabine consisted of several conventional chemotherapy drugs, such as fluorouracil, cisplatin, oxaliplatin, irinotecan, or pemetrexed. Novel biologic agents also were used, such as matrix metalloproteinase inhibitors, farnesyltransferase inhibitors, or the VEGF inhibitor bevacizumab and the EGFR antibody cetuximab. All of these trials failed to lead to improvements in overall survival.[108]

Subsequently, two phase III trials showed small survival benefits of similar magnitude when another agent was used in combination with gemcitabine. In the first trial, the combination of gemcitabine with erlotinib, an EGFR tyrosine kinase inhibitor, was found to significantly increase progression-free survival (HR 0.77, 95% CI 0.64, 0.92; p = 0.004) and overall survival (HR 0.82, 95% CI 0.69, 0.99; p = 0.038), albeit only with a median overall survival improvement of about 2 weeks.[109] No increase in response rate was noted. Nevertheless, based on these data, erlotinib obtained approval from the U.S. Food and Drug Administration (FDA) for the treatment of advanced pancreas cancer in conjunction with gemcitabine. The second trial, a phase III trial comparing gemcitabine with or without capecitabine, initially demonstrated moderate benefits regarding response rates as well as progression-free and overall survivals.[110] However, only in a combined analysis of two similar trials was the addition of capecitabine to gemcitabine found to be associated with improved overall survival (HR 0.86, 95% CI 0.75, 0.98; p = 0.02).[110] A meta-analysis of 15 randomized trials involving 4,465 patients that compared gemcitabine alone with gemcitabine plus either a platinum compound or fluoropyrimidine demonstrated a survival benefit for patients with good performance status who received combination chemotherapy (HR 0.76, 95% CI 0.67, 0.87; p < 0.0001). By contrast, application of combination chemotherapy to patients with an initially poor performance status appeared to be ineffective (HR 1.08, 95% CI 0.90, 1.29; p = 0.40).[111]

A new standard of care in the palliative therapy of pancreas cancer was defined by the results of a French study of 342 patients comparing gemcitabine with FOLFIRINOX, a combination of standard modified FOLFOX6, a well-known regimen established in colorectal cancer with full-dose irinotecan (180 mg/m²) in an every-2-week schedule.[104] The median overall survival was an unprecedented 11.1 months in the FOLFIRINOX group compared with 6.8 months in the gemcitabine group (HR 0.57, 95% CI 0.45, 0.73; p < 0.001). Median progression-free survival was 6.4 months in the FOLFIRINOX group and 3.3 months in the gemcitabine group (HR 0.47, 95% CI 0.37, 0.59; p < 0.001). The objective response rate was 31.6% for FOLFIRINOX compared with 9.4% for the gemcitabine group (p < 0.001). More adverse events were noted in the FOLFIRINOX group; 5.4% of patients in this group had febrile neutropenia. These results established FOLFIRINOX as new standard of care in patients with advanced pancreas cancer, good performance status, absence of biliary obstruction, and no infectious complications. The usefulness of FOLFIRINOX as adjuvant and neoadjuvant therapy as well as a backbone for the addition of targeted agents is currently being investigated in clinical trials.

A potentially competing standard first-line therapy to FOLFIRINOX in patients with good performance status was established when the addition of nab-paclitaxel to gemcitabine was found to be superior to gemcitabine alone in a phase III trial of 861 patients with metastatic pancreas cancer.[112] The median overall survival was 8.5 months in the nab-paclitaxel-gemcitabine group compared with 6.7 months in the gemcitabine group (HR 0.72, 95% CI 0.62, 0.83; p < 0.001). The median progression-free survival was 5.5 months in the nab-paclitaxel-gemcitabine group compared with 3.7 months in the gemcitabine group (HR 0.69, 95% CI 0.58, 0.82; p < 0.001);

the response rate according to independent review was 23% compared with 7% in the two groups (p < 0.001). Neutropenia, febrile neutropenia (3% vs. 1%), neuropathy, and fatigue were significantly higher in the nab-paclitaxel arm. Subsequently, nab-paclitaxel received regulatory approval as a component of gemcitabine-based first-line therapy of pancreas cancer.

Based on these studies, several first-line regimens can be considered appropriate treatment options for patients with metastatic pancreas cancer. With all caveats surrounding cross-trial comparisons, the outcomes data associated with FOLFIRINOX appear to be stronger than the nab-paclitaxel-gemcitabine results. On the other hand, the side effect profile seems to favor the nab-paclitaxel-gemcitabine combination. It is unlikely that a direct head-to-head comparison between these two regimens will ever be performed; the available data will need to suffice to inform clinical practice. It could be reasonable to establish a three-tier approach toward metastatic pancreas cancer. Otherwise healthy, younger patients in good performance status could preferentially be treated with FOLFIRINOX first-line and potentially nab-paclitaxel-gemcitabine second-line. Patients with poor performance status, advanced age, and significant comorbidities could still be considered candidates for gemcitabine as a single agent. In between these extremes lies a group of patients who could be considered for nab-paclitaxel-gemcitabine as first-line therapy. It will be interesting to see how these treatment standards will be adopted in clinical practice in the future.

The role of second-line therapies after failure of gemcitabine-based first-line approaches is not very well validated. In view of the commonly rapid progression of disease and deterioration of patients' performance status, randomized trials in second-line therapy are difficult to conduct. A German phase III trial randomly assigned 46 patients with advanced pancreas cancer who had received first-line gemcitabine to weekly infusional 5-FU/LV with biweekly oxaliplatin or best supportive care. The oxaliplatin-based therapy was able to confer a significant overall survival benefit (4.8 vs. 2.3 months, HR 0.45, p = 0.008).[113] Second-line treatment options should be considered for patients with good performance status after progression on first-line therapy.

So far, agents targeting VEGF (bevacizumab) and EGFR (cetuximab) have failed to demonstrate activity in metastatic pancreas cancer.[114-116] Studies utilizing other targeted agents including hedgehog inhibitors and IGFR inhibitors have also not lived up to their initial promise. Other agents of interest currently undergoing investigation in clinical trials include JAK-2 inhibitors, PI3K, MEK, and BRAF inhibitors as well as immune modulators and vaccines.

CANCERS OF THE LIVER AND BILIARY TREE
EPIDEMIOLOGY AND ETIOLOGY
Primary hepatobiliary cancers, which include hepatocellular cancers, cholangiocarcinomas, and gallbladder cancers, represent the highest global incidence of solid organ tumors and are responsible for about 1 million deaths annually, although

Table 9-1 Risk Factors for Hepatocellular Cancer

Hepatitis B and C

Excessive alcohol consumption

Autoimmune hepatitis

Primary biliary cirrhosis

Androgenic steroids

Aflatoxins

Tobacco

Nitrosylated compounds

Thorotrast

Hemochromatosis

Alpha-1 antitrypsin deficiency

Wilson disease

Porphyria

Glycogen storage disease

they are uncommon in Western cultures (particularly hepato-cellular cancers).[3] The risk factors for hepatocellular cancer are well known (Table 9-1). Hepatitis B infection accounts for about 60% of the total liver cancer in developing countries and for about 23% of cancer in developed countries; the corresponding percentages for hepatitis C virus infection are 33% in develop-ing countries and 20% in developed countries.[117] In the United States and several other low-risk Western countries, alcohol-related cirrhosis and possibly non-alcoholic fatty liver disease associated with obesity are thought to account for the majority of liver cancer.[118]

HEPATOCELLULAR CANCER
CLINICAL PRESENTATION AND DIAGNOSIS

Hepatocellular carcinoma is graded as well differentiated, moderately well differentiated, and poorly differentiated. The most important pathologic issue is the distinction between the fibrolamellar variant and the more traditional hepatocel-lular cancer. Fibrolamellar cancer is generally seen in younger patients, is much more likely to be resectable, and is less com-monly associated with infection or cirrhosis.[119] In contrast, traditional hepatocellular cancer is found more often in men older than 65. Less than 25% of the tumors are resectable, often because of underlying liver disease and inadequate he-patic reserve.[120] The predominant reason for non-resectability is the multifocal nature of the disease in the liver and late de-tection, the latter of which is because of the long asymptom-atic latency until diagnosis. Patients at high risk for the disease, such as patients with chronic hepatitis, are often monitored with imaging tests, which are often not very useful because of the similarity in appearance between cirrhotic and cancerous livers. Frequently, biopsies are required to distinguish cancer from cirrhosis. Likewise, the alpha-fetoprotein (AFP) tumor marker is not always helpful to distinguish between the two

diseases. Data suggest that an elevated subfraction of AFP, the lens culinaris agglutinin-reactive fraction of AFP (AFP-L3%), is a more reliable indicator for the presence of a hepatocellular carcinoma in patients with hepatitis C-related cirrhosis than is the total AFP.[121]

TREATMENT

The treatment of choice for patients with hepatocellular cancer is surgical resection. However, resection is not possible in most cases. Attempts at administration of systemic chemotherapy have been unsuccessful at generating radiographic responses, with almost no suggestion of improvement in survival. None-theless, hepatic arterial infusions of chemotherapy as well as chemoembolization (transcatheter arterial chemoemboliza-tion) have proved to be useful and have been associated with improved outcome in randomized trials.[122] Local ablative treatments are generally reserved for unresectable, localized disease. These approaches include alcohol injection and ra-diofrequency ablation. Percutaneous ablation achieves CR in more than 80% of tumors smaller than 3 cm in diameter, but in only 50% of tumors of 3 cm to 5 cm in size.[123] Although these response rates are high, it is unclear whether these techniques result in a survival benefit. A pooled analysis of eight compara-tive studies suggested that radiofrequency ablation was supe-rior to other locally percutaneous ablative techniques.[124]

Liver transplantation represents the ultimate local therapy for unresectable hepatocellular cancer. For patients with sub-stantial cirrhosis, liver transplantation provides an excellent option for early-stage tumors because the procedure is thera-peutic for the cancer and for the underlying pathology. Once patients have passed the high-risk peritransplant phase, the prognosis is similar to that for patients who have had resection of more localized disease.[125] Patients with known extrahepatic disease are not candidates for liver transplantation.

Based on repeated unfavorable results, no standard sys-temic chemotherapy has emerged for advanced unresectable disease. Single-agent anthracyclines and fluoropyrimidines have been most widely used in clinical trials and clinical prac-tice, but reported response rates and times to tumor progres-sion vary considerably.[126] Combination regimens are associated with higher response rates but do not necessarily translate into better overall outcome. A recent Chinese phase III trial comparing standard doxorubicin to FOLFOX4 noted a benefit in progression-free survival and a trend toward improved out-come in overall survival with FOLFOX (median overall survival, 6.40 vs. 4.97 months; HR 0.80, 95% CI 4.23, 6.03; p = 0.07), but the overall results were disappointing.[127]

Current trials are focusing on targeted therapies, such as angiogenesis and signal transduction inhibitors, either as sin-gle agents, in combination with chemotherapy, or with other biologic agents, in particular, sorafenib since it was established as standard first-line therapy. Sorafenib, an oral inhibitor of VEGFR and Raf, plus placebo was compared with placebo alone in a phase III trial (SHARP) of 602 patients with unresectable hepatocellular cancer.[128] In this trial, sorafenib was associ-ated with significant prolongation of time to radiologic tumor

Table 9-2 Child-Pugh Scoring System*

Measure	1 Point	2 Point	3 Point
Total bilirubin (μmol/L [mg/dL])	< 34 (< 2)	34 to 50 (2 to 3)	> 50 (> 3)
Serum albumin (g/dL)	> 3.5	2.8 to 3.5	< 2.8
Prothrombin time/international normalized ratio (PT/INR)	< 1.7	1.71 to 2.30	> 2.30
Ascites	None	Mild	Moderate to severe
Hepatic encephalopathy	None	Grade I to II (or suppressed with medication)	Grade III to IV (or refractory)

*The score employs five clinical measures of liver disease. Each measure is scored 1 to 3, with 3 indicating most severe derangement. Chronic liver disease is classified into Child-Pugh class A to C, by the added score from this table (A: 5 to 6, B: 7 to 9, C: 10 to 15).

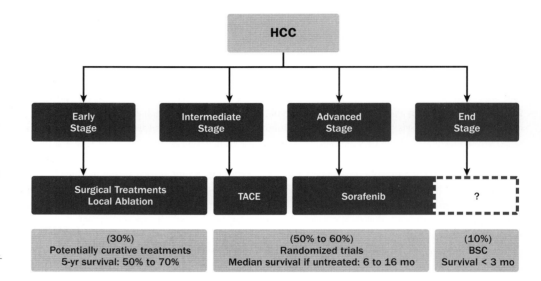

Fig. 9-1 Hepatocellular cancer (HCC) treatment algorithm.

Abbreviations: TACE, transcatheter arterial chemoembolization; yr, year; mo, months; BSC, best supportive care.

Reprinted with permission from Elsevier. Llovet JM, Burroughs A, Bruix J. Lancet. Hepatocellular carcinoma. 2002; 362(9399):1907-1917.

progression (5.5 vs. 2.8 months, p = 0.000007) and overall survival (10.7 vs. 7.9 months, p = 0.00058). Based on these data, sorafenib has emerged as a new standard therapy for advanced, unresectable hepatocellular carcinoma and has received approval by regulatory agencies. It is unclear at this point if the observed efficacy of sorafenib is more related to its VEGFR- or its Raf-inhibitory capacity. Interestingly, a large phase III trial comparing sorafenib with sunitinib, another oral multikinase inhibitor with significant antiangiogenic activity, clearly demonstrated the superiority of sorafenib.[129] The superiority was especially pronounced in patients with hepatitis C-associated hepatocellular carcinoma. Since the SHARP trial only included patients classified as Child-Pugh A (Table 9-2), questions have been raised regarding the activity and tolerability of sorafenib in patients with more severe liver dysfunction. In clinical practice, only patients with Child-Pugh A and perhaps B7 scores should be routinely considered for sorafenib therapy.

Clinical trials using VEGF and other kinase inhibitors (e.g., HGF/c-met targeting agents) for hepatocellular cancer with or without other targeted agents or chemotherapy are un-

derway, even though several studies with initially promising agents like the bFGF/VEGF inhibitor brivanib have already found to be negative.

A potential treatment algorithm for hepatocellular cancer is outlined in Fig. 9-1.[120]

BILIARY CANCERS

Cancers of the extrahepatic bile duct and gallbladder are relatively rare, with only 10,310 cases diagnosed annually in the United States, resulting in approximately 3,230 annual deaths.[1] The low mortality of biliary cancers can be explained by the fact that about 50% of gallbladder cancers are incidental findings on cholecystectomy, which—commonly diagnosed in an early stage—can have an excellent prognosis (3-year overall survival, 70% to 100%). It is important to note, though, that when a gallbladder cancer is found after laparoscopic cholecystectomy, re-resection of the adjacent liver segment and lymphadenectomy is indicated for all disease except stage I.[130,131]

Unfortunately, U.S. statistics do not give specific numbers for intrahepatic cholangiocarcinomas, but subcategorize them under "hepatobiliary tumors," so that the actual incidence of biliary cancers is definitely higher, perhaps approaching the incidence of esophageal cancers, with about 15,000 cases per year.[132] Because of the location of these tumors, they are frequently difficult to resect; therefore, specialized surgical intervention should always be sought. Cholangiocarcinoma is most common in women older than 50, and long-term survival is highly dependent on the effectiveness of surgical therapy. Conditions that are associated with an increased risk include primary sclerosing cholangitis (with an increased incidence in patients with inflammatory bowel disease), choledochal cysts, and other hepatic infections.[133] Gallstones also increase the risk for cancers of the gallbladder.

Cholangiocarcinomas typically present with jaundice, with a mass evident on CT or ultrasound, or are visualized endoscopically. The primary treatment is surgical resection, if possible. The cure rate for patients with early-stage disease ranges from 60% to 70%; however, for patients with more advanced disease, the 5-year survival rate is only 10% to 25%.[134,135] Thus, the role of either preoperative or postoperative radiation and chemotherapy may be important. Although the role of radiation therapy—either alone or in combination with chemotherapy—has been evaluated in several studies, no substantial benefit has been seen.[136,137] Adjuvant therapy is often used for patients with positive margins (chemoradiotherapy) or for patients with positive lymph nodes (chemoradiotherapy and/or chemotherapy), but there is no clear standard of care in this area because of the lack of adequately powered randomized trials in this rare malignancy. Based on Surveillance, Epidemiology, and End Result (SEER) data for patients with resected gallbladder cancer between 1995 and 2005, a web-based nomogram predicting the benefit of adjuvant chemoradiotherapy was developed for this patient group that can serve as a guideline in the absence of definitive phase III data in this setting.[138]

The effectiveness of systemic chemotherapy alone in advanced cancers is poor, with response rates ranging from 10% to 40% for both single-agent and combination chemotherapy regimens.[134] Although the surgical approach toward intra- and extrahepatic cholangiocarcinomas and gallbladder cancers differs, systemic chemotherapy does not currently distinguish between these cancers. Most of the regimens used are gemcitabine- or fluoropyrimidine-based and follow treatment strategies established in pancreas cancer. A pooled analysis of clinical trials in biliary cancers documented higher response rates and longer time to tumor progression for gemcitabine-based combination regimens with fluoropyrimidines and with platinum agents than for gemcitabine alone.[134]

The results of this pooled analysis were confirmed by a standard-setting phase III trial that randomly assigned 410 patients with advanced biliary tract cancers to receive gemcitabine 1,000 mg/m^2 on days 1, 8, and 15 every 4 weeks for six cycles or gemcitabine 1,000 mg/m^2 plus cisplatin 25 mg/m^2 on days 1 and 8 every 3 weeks for eight cycles.[139] The addition of low-dose cisplatin did not result in significant differences in grade 3 or 4 toxicities. Progression-free survival was 8.4 months in the gemcitabine/cisplatin arm and 6.5 months in the gemcitabine-only arm (HR 0.72, 95% CI 0.57, 0.90; p = 0.003). This translated into an overall survival benefit of 11.7 months in the gemcitabine/cisplatin arm compared with 8.3 months in the gemcitabine-only arm (HR 0.70, 95% CI 0.54, 0.89; p = 0.002). This trial established a new standard of care in the treatment of advanced biliary cancers, gemcitabine/cisplatin, which can now serve as the backbone for the addition of targeted agents in future trials.

The role of photodynamic therapy for superficial, hilar cholangiocarcinomas is not well defined, but sustained palliation of biliary drainage has been reported.[140] Chemoembolization or radioembolization techniques have been used for unresectable cholangiocarcinomas with dominating liver involvement, but should not yet be considered standard of care because of the paucity of available data.[141]

COLORECTAL CANCER
EPIDEMIOLOGY AND ETIOLOGY

Colorectal cancer is diagnosed in approximately 142,820 patients in the United States every year. Among all cancers, it is the second leading cause of death in the United States, with about 50,830 deaths, affecting both men and women equally.[1] Colorectal cancer is both sporadic and familial. The incidence of colorectal cancer is higher in developed countries than in developing countries. In the last decade, there has been a decrease in the incidence of colorectal cancer in the United States.[1] Findings from epidemiologic studies indicate that during the last 2 decades, the anatomic distribution of colorectal cancer may have shifted from the distal colon to the proximal end. These results indicate strong environmental associations for colorectal cancer. The amount of fat intake relative to dietary fiber has long been believed to have an effect on colorectal cancer. Findings from case-controlled studies demonstrate that intake of fiber-rich foods (at least 13 g per day of dietary fiber) is strongly associated with a low risk of colorectal cancer. Other etiologic factors include the content and quality of bile acids, as well as vitamin and mineral intake, with calcium appearing to play a critical role. Folate has long been thought to be able to work as a chemoprotectant against colorectal cancer, but data from a prospective study failed to demonstrate a protective effect against the development of colorectal adenomas.[142] However, data from prospective, interventional studies indicate that the association among dietary fiber, calcium, fat intake, and colorectal cancer is not clear.[143,144] Additional environmental factors include the intake of alcohol and tobacco, hormone replacement in women (protective), total calorie consumption, and physical activity as it relates to obesity.[145-148] Interestingly, there has been an increased recognition that the regular use of nonsteroidal anti-inflammatory agents including aspirin and cyclooxygenase-2 inhibitors, such as celecoxib, may have a protective effect against colorectal adenomas and colorectal cancer,[41,149-152] but likely not against cancer occurring in the context of nonpolyposis familial predisposition such as Lynch syndrome.[153]

FAMILIAL SYNDROMES: FAP AND HNPCC

There are two common inherited forms of colorectal cancer, HNPCC (Lynch I and Lynch II syndromes) and the familial adenomatous polyposis (FAP) syndrome (Table 9-3). These two recognized genetic syndromes are distinct in molecular biology and in clinical characteristics.

The first syndrome to be recognized was FAP, which is caused by an inherited mutation in the FAP coli (*APC*) gene, a key regulator of the *wnt*-signaling pathway. Mutations of the *APC* gene lead to the formation of a dysfunctional protein, which prevents it from binding beta-catenin so that beta-catenin can then activate the transcription of various oncogenes. Patients with mutated *APC* have hundreds to thousands of colonic polyps, predisposing them to malignant tumors at a young age. Although FAP represents a small percentage (approximately 0.5% to 1%) of the overall number of cases of colorectal cancer, *APC* (or beta-catenin) mutations activating the *wnt*-signaling pathway have been found in the majority (80% to 85%) of sporadic colorectal cancers. Further gene expression studies along the adenoma-carcinoma sequence have provided an important genetic model in which specific genetic mutations leading to invasive colorectal cancers have been clearly elucidated (Fig. 9-2).[154]

HNPCC is an inherited autosomal-dominant disease with high penetrance. Patients who inherit a mutant of this gene class develop colorectal cancers at a young age. In addition, for patients with type II HNPCC (Lynch II syndrome), other cancers develop including ovarian, pancreas, breast, biliary, endometrial, gastric, genitourinary, and small bowel

Table 9-3 **Factors that Increase the Risk of Colon Cancer**
Polyposis Syndromes
■ Familial polyposis
■ Peutz-Jeghers syndrome
■ Juvenile polyposis
Nonpolyposis Syndromes
■ Hereditary nonpolyposis colorectal cancer (HNPCC)
Other
■ Inflammatory bowel disease
■ Prior colon cancer
■ Prior polyps
■ First-degree relative diagnosed when younger than age 50
■ Western diet
■ Alcohol consumption
■ Sedentary lifestyle
■ Obesity
■ Diabetes

primaries. Approximately 5% of all colorectal cancers are attributed to this inherited syndrome. The Amsterdam Criteria and Bethesda Criteria are used to classify patients with this disease (Table 9-4). The genetic abnormality of microsatellite instability (MSI) is common in HNPCC cancers and is caused by mutations in a group of genes that code for DNA mismatch repair enzymes, including *MSH-2*, *MLH-1*, *PMS-1*, *PMS-2*, and *MSH-6*.[155] The defect in mismatch repair allows spontaneous genetic mutations to accumulate in colonic mucosa, which predisposes for the development of dysplasia, and eventually, for invasive cancers. The term "microsatellite instability" denotes that with reduced or absent DNA repair activity, the length of repetitive DNA sequences varies (becomes instable) upon DNA replication. Apart from the hereditary HNPCC forms, approximately 10% to 15% of sporadic colon cancers also carry mutations (or gene promoter methylations) in the mismatch repair enzymes and, thus, are characterized as

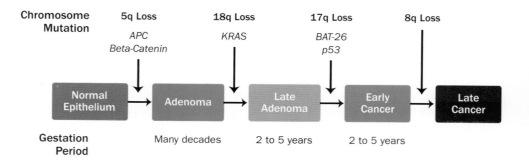

Fig. 9-2 A genetic model showing specific genetic mutations that lead to invasive colorectal cancers.

having MSI.[156] Depending on how much the DNA repair capacity is affected in standardized polymerase chain reaction (PCR) tests, MSI-high or MSI-low (as well as microsatellite-stable [MSS] tumors) are distinguished. IHC for protein products hMLH1 and hMSH2 provides a rapid, cost-effective, sensitive (92.3%), and specific (100%) method for screening for DNA mismatch repair defects. In a comparative study, the predictive value of normal IHC for an MSS/MSI-L phenotype was 96.7%, and the predictive value of abnormal IHC was 100% for an MSI-H phenotype.[157] Clinically, patients with these tumors do not present with premalignant polyps; rather, cancers develop quickly from macroscopically normal mucosa. This issue is critical because the screening used for patients with HNPCC must be different. HNPCC is clinically associated with an early onset age, a proximal tumor location, mucinous histology, and a higher grade at the time of diagnosis. Interestingly, the prognosis for patients with this type of cancer is better, independent of stage, when compared with that for patients with MSS tumors. The improvement is seen despite an apparent lower responsiveness to fluorouracil-based chemotherapy.[156,158-162] Other polyposis and colorectal cancer syndromes also exist (Table 9-5). Since the identification of Lynch syndrome in patients with colorectal cancer has significant implications for the choice of therapy and for screening recommendations for family members, universal testing of all patients with colorectal cancer using MSI analysis of IHC for mismatch repair enzyme expression in tumor tissue has been recommended.[163] Current guidelines published by the National Comprehensive Cancer Network (www.nccn.org, Colon v3.2014) suggest that Lynch syndrome screening should be considered for patients with colorectal cancer at age 70 or younger and also those older than 70 who meet the Bethesda guidelines.

Inflammatory bowel disease, particularly ulcerative colitis, is associated with an increased risk for colon cancer, estimated to be 5% to 10% by 20 years after the time of diagnosis; it also is associated with a high incidence of synchronous cancers, affecting 10% to 20% of cases.[164] Crohn's disease also may have a role in increasing colorectal cancer, particularly cancer in the ileocolic region. However, in the absence of colonic involvement by Crohn's disease, there is no increased risk for colon cancer.

Table 9-4 Clinical Criteria to Determine Likelihood of Hereditary Nonpolyposis Colorectal Cancer (HNPCC)

Amsterdam Criteria (all criteria must be met)

- Three or more family members with colorectal cancer, at least two of whom must be first-degree relatives (i.e., parent, sibling, or child)
- Family members from at least two successive generations are affected
- Development of colorectal cancer occurred before age 50 in at least one family member
- Familial adenomatous polyposis is excluded

Bethesda Criteria (any criterion is sufficient)

- Cancer in a family that fulfills the Amsterdam criteria
- Development of two HNPCC-related (extracolonic) cancers in one individual (i.e., endometrial, small intestine, ovarian, or gastric cancer)
- Development of colorectal cancer in an individual who has a first-degree relative with colorectal cancer and/or HNPCC-related extracolonic cancer and/or colorectal adenoma, with one of the cancers diagnosed before age 45 and the adenoma diagnosed before age 40
- Colorectal or endometrial cancer diagnosed before age 45
- Right-sided colorectal cancer with an undifferentiated pattern on histopathologic evaluation, diagnosed before age 45
- Signet ring cell-type colorectal cancer diagnosed before age 45
- Adenoma diagnosed before age 40

Table 9-5 Polyposis and Colorectal Cancer Syndromes

Syndrome	Number of Colon Polyps	Extracolonic Manifestations
Familial adenomatous polyposis	> 100, diffuse	Small-bowel adenoma and adenocarcinoma, gastric adenoma and cancer, fundic gland polyps, adrenal adenomas and cancers, thyroid cancer, and desmoid tumor
Gardner's syndrome	> 100, diffuse	Epidermoid cysts, desmoid tumors, osteomas, and fibromas
Turcot syndrome	> 100, diffuse	Brain tumors
Flat adenoma syndrome	1 to 100, right-sided	Fundic gland polyps and periampullary cancer
Discrete adenomas	1 to 10	None
Hereditary nonpolyposis colon cancer	1 to 10	Cancers of the endometrium, stomach, biliary tree, and small bowel; transitional cell cancer of the ureter and renal pelvis
Peutz-Jeghers syndrome	1 to hundreds, diffuse	Ovarian and testicular tumors

Modified with permission from Cheson BD, ed. Oncology MKSAP, 2nd ed. Philadelphia, Pa: American College of Physicians; 1999:160.

The risk for the development of a subsequent cancer is 3% for patients with a history of adenomatous polyps.

SCREENING

The screening tests for colorectal cancer include digital rectal examination, fecal occult blood testing (FOBT), fecal immunochemical test (FIT), sigmoidoscopy, colonoscopy, and air-contrast barium enema. The FIT is done essentially the same way as the traditional guaiac FOBT, but it does not require drug or dietary restrictions. The most recent technique, virtual CT colonography, is a new tool that reliably visualizes polyps and cancer in a non-endoscopic way, but which still requires a standard bowel preparation.[165] Each of these tools, with the exceptions of digital rectal examinations and virtual CT colonography (for paucity of prospective data), has been shown to have a positive effect on colorectal cancer–related mortality. However, there is still a poor compliance rate with these tests, with fewer than 30% of patients ever undergoing any screening procedures. For many years, the guidelines for standard screening options varied according to different medical societies, with a general shift away from emphasizing sigmoidoscopy in favor of colonoscopy, particularly in light of the observed shift toward more proximal colon cancers. The obvious advantages of colonoscopic screening are that the entire large bowel and distal ileum can be assessed and that immediate intervention, such as biopsy and polypectomy, is possible. The results of studies have demonstrated that although sigmoidoscopy in conjunction with annual FOBT (better: FIT[166]) is an effective means of reducing the mortality related to colon cancer, approximately 8% of distal cancers and all proximal cancers (approximately 40% to 50% of all colorectal cancers) will be missed. Therefore, the most common recommendation from various organizations is for colonoscopy to be performed every 5 to 10 years for a patient with average risk, starting at age 50 (see Chapter 1: Epidemiology and Prevention for more information). In March 2008, the American Cancer Society, the American College of Radiology, and the U.S. Multi-Society Task Force on Colorectal Cancer (a group that comprises representatives from the American College of Gastroenterology, American Gastroenterological Association, and American Society for Gastrointestinal Endoscopy) released the first-ever joint consensus guidelines for colorectal cancer screening.[167] The guidelines added two new tests to the list of recommended options, stool DNA (sDNA) and CT colonography, and for the first time included a preference for screening tests that can not only detect cancer early but also detect precancerous polyps, as those tests provide a greater potential for cancer prevention through polyp removal. Two recent studies confirmed the long-term reduction in colorectal cancer mortality by population screening with either FOBT or endoscopy.[168,169] Table 9-6 lists the recommendations of the joint task forces.

Screening should be more regular for patients at high risk, including those with inherited syndromes, inflammatory bowel disease, and previous adenomatous polyps or colorectal cancer. Individuals with HNPCC should have

Table 9-6 Screening Guidelines for Colon and Rectal Cancer (released March 2008)[124]

Beginning at age 50, both men and women at average risk for developing colorectal cancer should use one of the screening tests below. The tests that are designed to find both early cancer and polyps are preferred if these tests are available and the person is willing to have one of these more invasive tests.

Tests to Detect Polyps and Cancer

- Flexible sigmoidoscopy every 5 years*
- Colonoscopy every 10 years
- Double contrast barium enema every 5 years*
- Computed tomography (CT) colonography (virtual colonoscopy) every 5 years*

Tests to Primarily Detect Cancer

- Fecal occult blood test (FOBT) every year*†
- Fecal immunochemical test (FIT) every year*†
- Stool DNA test (sDNA), interval uncertain*

People should talk to their doctor about starting colorectal cancer screening earlier and/or being screened more often if they have any of the following colorectal cancer risk factors:

- Personal history of colorectal cancer or adenomatous polyps
- Personal history of chronic inflammatory bowel disease (Crohn's disease or ulcerative colitis)
- Strong family history of colorectal cancer or polyps (cancer or polyps in a first-degree relative [parent, sibling, or child] discovered younger than 60, or in two or more first-degree relatives of any age)
- Known family history of hereditary colorectal cancer syndromes such as familial adenomatous polyposis (FAP) or hereditary nonpolyposis colon cancer (HNPCC)

*Colonoscopy should be done if test results are positive.
†For FOBT or FIT used as a screening test, the take-home multiple sample method should be used. A FOBT or FIT done during a digital rectal exam in the doctor's office is not adequate for screening.

screening by total colonoscopy every 1 to 3 years beginning between ages 20 and 25 because of the lack of a visible premalignant lesion in this population and the higher risk for right-sided colon cancers.[170] Individuals with FAP should start screening colonoscopies as young as age 10. If a colon cancer or severe dysplasia is found in patients with inflammatory bowel disease, the general recommendation is for a near-total or a subtotal colectomy because of the high incidence of synchronous and metachronous cancers in this population.[171] Surgery can be less extensive for patients with sporadic cancers. For patients with type II HNPCC, a more extensive surgery can be recommended, particularly for women beyond childbearing age, for whom hysterectomy and oophorectomy should be considered.

TREATMENT FOR COLORECTAL CANCER

Early-Stage Colon Cancer (Stages 0, I, II, and III)

Nearly all patients with stage 0 disease (carcinoma in situ or intramucosal cancer) are cured by endoscopic resection alone, recognizing that the lymph nodes are not adequately assessed by this technique. The primary treatment for virtually all invasive non-metastatic colorectal cancers is surgery. Studies indicate that laparoscopic-assisted surgery for colon cancer provides the same outcomes for overall survival and rate of recurrence as open laparotomy.[172] Studies prospectively evaluating the role of laparoscopic-assisted surgery in rectal cancer are ongoing. Early outcomes parameter of a large, 1,103-patient European study did not demonstrate a difference between open and laparoscopic surgery for rectal cancer.[173]

Surgery alone is curative for more than 85% of patients who have stage I or early stage II disease. For patients with more advanced stage II disease (T4, N0), the 5-year survival rate is approximately 70% to 75%; for stage III disease (positive lymph nodes), the 5-year survival rate is 30% to 50% with surgical resection alone.

Prognostic and predictive factors. Other factors beyond stage (Table 9-7) that adversely affect outcome include male sex, extent of local invasion (T4), undifferentiated histology, mucinous features, signet-ring features, lymphovascular invasion, and elevated levels of carcinoembryonic antigen (preoperatively).[174] Another important prognostic factor is the number of lymph nodes identified in the resected specimen, with a minimum number of 12 lymph nodes necessary for adequate staging. The prognosis for colon cancer for patients with HNPCC (and cancers with the defective mismatch-repair phenotype in general) is better than the prognosis for patients with sporadic tumors (or proficient mismatch repair phenotype), perhaps because the accumulation of genetic mutations in tumor cells do not allow for metastatic spread. Findings from retrospective studies indicate that tumor aneuploidy and S phase determined by flow cytometry are associated with a less favorable outcome, but these results have not reached a point where the techniques are applied routinely in clinical practice. Similarly, testing for MSI, TP53 expression, mutations in the DCC gene, KRAS, p16, loss of heterozygosity (LOH) at 18q, thymidylate synthase, and dihydropyrimidine dehydrogenase expression eventually may play roles when treating patients.[174] High tumor concentrations of thymidylate synthase may be predictive of poor outcome. The DCC gene mutation/LOH 18q may distinguish patients at higher risk for metastatic disease; therefore, candidates for adjuvant therapy, for example, in stage II colon cancer, may be identified. These issues are being investigated in large adjuvant clinical trials. After a genome-wide or a candidate-gene screening approach, gene signatures are currently being developed in colorectal cancer that could identify prognostic and predictive markers for the usefulness of adjuvant chemotherapy in patients with borderline indications.[175,176]

Adjuvant chemotherapy. Adjuvant chemotherapy was established as standard of care in the early 1990s from a trial in stage III colon cancer that used a combination of fluorouracil and levamisole administered for 12 months.[177] A 10% to 20% improvement in 5-year survival was documented for patients receiving postoperative adjuvant fluorouracil-based chemotherapy. Evidence from subsequent trials demonstrated that fluorouracil combined with leucovorin provided a superior outcome, with 6 months of therapy adequate to achieve this survival benefit.[178] For longer than a decade, the standard in adjuvant therapy remained unchanged because of the lack of novel agents with relevant activity in colorectal cancer. This changed when oxaliplatin, irinotecan, and the oral fluoroura-

Table 9-7 Staging, Incidence per Stage, and Treatment Recommendations for Invasive Colon Cancer

	Stage I	Stage II	Stage III	Stage IV
Staging	T1, N0, M0	A: T3, N0, M0	A: T1-2, N1/N1c, M0; T1, N2a, M0	A: Any T, Any N, M1a
	T2, N0, M0	B: T4a, N0, M0	B: T3-4a, N1/N1c, M0; T2/3, N2a, M0; T1-2, N2b, M0	B: Any T, Any N, M1b
		C: T4b, N0, M0	C: T4a, N2a, M0; T3-4a, N2b, M0; T4b, N1-2, M0	
Definition	Invades submucosa (T1) or muscular propria (T2)	Invades subserosa, nonperitonealized pericolic/perirectal tissues (T3) or penetrates to the surface of the visceral peritoneum (T4a) or directly invades into or is adherent to other organs or structures (T4b)	Involves 1-3 (N1-N1a: 1, N1b: 2-3) or more (N2-N2a: 4-6, N2b: > 6) lymph nodes; N1c for tumor deposits in subserosa, mesentery, or pericolic/perirectal tissue without lymph node metastasis	M1a: distant metastasis confined to one organ or site M1b: distant metastasis in more than one organ or site
Incidence	15%	25%	35%	25%
Usual treatment	Surgery	Surgery with or without chemotherapy	Surgery with chemotherapy	Chemotherapy with or without surgery

The original source for this material is the AJCC Cancer Staging Manual, 7th Edition (2010) published by Springer Science and Business Media LLC, www.springerlink.com.

cil prodrug capecitabine were utilized for the treatment of advanced colorectal cancer, with combination regimens of infusional fluorouracil plus either irinotecan and oxaliplatin demonstrating high antitumor efficacy.

Worldwide, six phase III trials were conducted to evaluate the value of these three novel chemotherapeutic agents in the adjuvant setting. To set the stage for the conduct and interpretation of these trials and their results, a large retrospective meta-analysis confirmed that, for adjuvant colon cancer, 3-year DFS can serve as an definitive surrogate marker for 5-year overall survival.[179] This finding had a major effect on clinical trial design and endpoint definition in subsequent studies regarding adjuvant colon cancer. Based on these findings, the FDA recognized 3-year DFS as an appropriate endpoint for full approval of a regimen for adjuvant colon cancer. Oxaliplatin was approved as part of adjuvant treatment for stage III colon cancer in 2004 based on this endpoint. One trial established 6 months of oral capecitabine as a safe and at least equally effective alternative to conventional intravenous bolus fluorouracil with leucovorin (Mayo Clinic regimen) for stage III colon cancer.[180] Two other trials confirmed the value of oxaliplatin as a component of adjuvant chemotherapy for stage II and III colon cancer.[181,182] The results of the pivotal Multicenter International Study of Oxaliplatin/5-Fluorouracil/Leucovorin in the Adjuvant Treatment of Colon Cancer trial clearly demonstrated that oxaliplatin plus infusional fluorouracil and leucovorin (FOLFOX) is superior to fluorouracil with leucovorin in terms of 3-year DFS.[181] In a subgroup analysis, only the increase in DFS for patients with stage III disease was statistically significant, providing an absolute benefit of approximately 8% to 10% (HR 0.76, 95% CI 0.62, 0.92). In unselected patients with stage II disease, the DFS benefit for FOLFOX compared with fluorouracil and leucovorin alone was approximately 3.5%, but it exceeded 5% for patients with stage II tumors with clinical high-risk features (undifferentiated tumors, T4, perforation, obstruction, fewer than 10 lymph nodes identified, and angiolymphatic invasion). An update demonstrated a significant improvement in 6-year (not 5-year) overall survival for patients with stage III, but not for patients with stage II, colon cancer when an oxaliplatin-based regimen was used as adjuvant therapy.[183] Results of the National Surgical Adjuvant Breast and Bowel Project (NSABP) C-07 trial further strengthened the role of oxaliplatin plus fluorouracil-based regimens in the adjuvant therapy of colon cancer.[182,184]

The third phase III trial in the sequence of studies comparing 5-FU/LV to a fluoropyrimidine-oxaliplatin combination as adjuvant therapy, the XELOXA trial (oxaliplatin plus capecitabine, XELOX, vs. bolus 5-FU/LV), confirmed the role of oxaliplatin as a component of adjuvant therapy in stage III colon cancer with significant improvements in DFS (HR 0.80, 95% CI 0.69, 0.93, p = 0.0045) and a trend toward improved overall survival at 5 years.[185] As in the MOSAIC trial, longer follow-up is likely needed to demonstrate improved overall survival because of the available active treatment options upon tumor recurrence that shift overall survival differences to a later time point.

Although irinotecan- and oxaliplatin-based regimens are thought to be equally effective as palliative therapy for advanced colorectal cancer, for unknown reasons, none of the three phase III trials using combination regimens of irinotecan, fluorouracil, and leucovorin demonstrated significantly superior efficacy regarding 3-year DFS when compared with fluorouracil and leucovorin alone.[186-188]

Based on these results, the standard adjuvant chemotherapy for stage III colon cancer is an oxaliplatin-containing regimen (FOLFOX, XELOX or bolus fluorouracil, folinic acid, and oxaliplatin [FLOX]) administered for 6 months. Capecitabine or fluorouracil and leucovorin should be reserved for patients who are not considered optimal candidates for oxaliplatin.

To mitigate the long-term neurotoxic side effects of oxaliplatin-based adjuvant therapy, the International Duration Evaluation of Adjuvant Chemotherapy (IDEA) collaboration was established to prospectively combine and analyze data from six randomized trials conducted around the world to answer whether a 3-month course of oxaliplatin-based adjuvant therapy is noninferior to the current standard 6-month treatment for patients with stage III colon cancer. More than 11,000 patients will be included in the final analysis, which is expected in 2015.[189]

Although the efficacy and tolerability of adjuvant FOLFOX was long considered similar both for patients younger and older than age 70,[190] more recent data with longer follow-up have now put this notion into question. Updated results from the MOSAIC trial did not document a significant improvement with the addition of oxaliplatin to 5-FU/LV for patients older than 70.[191] In addition, an analysis of pooled individual patient data from NSABP C-07 and MOSAIC demonstrated that only patients younger than age 70 had a statistically significant benefit in terms of DFS, overall survival, and time to tumor recurrence with the use of adjuvant FOLFOX compared with 5-FU/LV.[192] These findings can inform clinical practice and highlight the importance of careful risk/benefit assessment when adjuvant FOLFOX is offered to elderly patients.

For patients with stage II disease, the role of adjuvant chemotherapy remains controversial; the results from a series of clinical trials demonstrated a trend toward improved recurrence-free survival and overall survival (HR 0.80, 95% CI 0.56, 1.15). Findings from two pooled retrospective analyses showed conflicting results.[193,194] One analysis suggested a 30% risk reduction, translating into an approximate 8% absolute reduction in mortality, whereas a similar pooled data set showed no benefit from adjuvant chemotherapy. An analysis of Medicare data revealed that more than 50% of patients in the United States with stage II colon cancer receive postoperative adjuvant chemotherapy.[195] In view of these data, and the U.K. QUASAR trial, it appears that unselected patients with stage II colon cancer (i.e., not distinguished between high-risk and low-risk stage II) will have a 3% benefit in 3-year DFS and overall survival with fluorouracil and leucovorin as adjuvant chemotherapy.[196] It has to be kept in mind that the quality of lymph node assessment in the QUASAR trial did not meet current standards, with more than 60% of patients having fewer than 12 lymph nodes identified in resected specimens so that the inclusion of a certain percentage of stage III cancers in this analysis seems likely.[197] Current ASCO recommendations dating back to 2004 suggest that not all patients with stage II tumors should receive adjuvant chemotherapy, but that a discussion should be conducted with patients about their individual benefit/risk ratio when utilizing adjuvant chemotherapy in stage II colon cancer.[198] Efforts have been made to individualize the baseline prognosis and to predict the benefits of chemotherapy for patients with resected colon cancer.[199] As a result, there are two web-based tools available to provide data of this type: an adjuvant therapy calculator developed by the Mayo Clinic[200] and Adjuvant! Online. These tools can provide helpful information for clinical decision-making.[201,202]

The identification of prognostic factors might help distinguish patients at high risk for relapse and enrich the patient population with stage II disease, who will more likely benefit from adjuvant treatment. Apart from the clinical risk factors listed previously, molecular determinants of poor prognosis, such as MSS and LOH*18q*, are being evaluated in prospective clinical trials. Remarkably, consistent results from retrospective analyses of large adjuvant trials and pooled datasets confirmed that patients with stage II colon cancer and MSI-high tumors, which represent tumors of the deficient mismatch-repair phenotype, have excellent prognosis and do not need be treated with adjuvant chemotherapy.[162,197,203,204] Efforts are underway to develop a molecular profile of prognostic variables that could potentially guide adjuvant treatment decisions in stage II colon cancer.[197,205,206] These tests include gene expression signatures such as the Oncotype DX Colon[197] and ColoPrint[206] as well as molecular detection assays of micrometastasis in morphologically unaffected lymph nodes.[205] At this point, none of these assays is routinely recommended for use in clinical practice as a decision tool for adjuvant therapy in stage II colon cancer.

The role of novel targeted agents with clear efficacy in advanced colorectal cancer, such as bevacizumab, an antibody against VEGF, and cetuximab, an antibody against EGFR, have been investigated in the adjuvant setting in ongoing large phase III trials. The first trial in a human malignancy to test bevacizumab in the adjuvant setting, NSABP C-08 randomly assigned 2,710 patients with stage II (25%) and stage III (75%) colon cancer to receive modified FOLFOX6 every 2 weeks for 12 cycles, or modified FOLFOX6 using the same schedule plus bevacizumab given every 2 weeks on day 1 for a total of 1 year, meaning bevacizumab was continued for 6 months beyond the planned completion of chemotherapy.[207] After a median 35.6-month follow-up, 3-year DFS, the primary endpoint, was 77.4% for modified FOLFOX6 alone and 75.5% in the bevacizumab arm. These results were not statistically significant (HR 0.89, p = 0.15). A transient reduction in the rate of tumor recurrences was observed at 1 year, coinciding with the extended duration of bevacizumab in the experimental arm, but this effect was lost after discontinuation of the VEGF inhibitor. Almost identical observations were made in the international three-arm phase III AVANT trial that included a capecitabine/oxaliplatin plus bevacizumab experimental arm.[208] At this point, bevacizumab

plays no role in the adjuvant therapy of colon cancer outside of clinical trials.

The EGFR antibody cetuximab has also been tested as a component of adjuvant therapy in stage III colon cancer added to a modified FOLFOX6 backbone.[209] Initially conceived as a FOLFOX with or without cetuximab phase III trial in all patients with resected stage III colon cancer, the trial was eventually amended to enroll only patients with *KRAS* wild-type cancers.[210] Unfortunately, even in this preselected patient group that has shown to benefit from EGFR antibodies in the palliative setting, cetuximab failed to improve outcome measures. Indeed, cetuximab showed a trend toward a detrimental effect, in particular, in patients with *KRAS*-mutated cancers.[209] A similar European adjuvant study with cetuximab (PETACC-8) confirmed the lack of efficacy of cetuximab in the adjuvant setting when added to FOLFOX in *KRAS* wild-type colon cancers, although this trial did not suggest a detrimental effect.[211] The body of evidence confirms that EGFR antibodies do not enhance the efficacy of FOLFOX in the adjuvant setting.

KEY POINTS

- Screening for colorectal cancer, which can conceivably reduce the mortality of this disease, is underutilized. Screening endoscopy and fecal occult blood test/fecal immunochemical testing have been shown to reduce colorectal cancer mortality long-term.
- Specific genetic mutations have been identified that characterize familial and sporadic colorectal cancers.
- Adjuvant chemotherapy with an oxaliplatin-based regimen is the standard of care for stage III colon cancer; the role of adjuvant therapy in stage II colon cancer continues to be controversial. Patients with stage II colon cancer and mismatch repair deficiency have an excellent prognosis and do not require adjuvant therapy.
- After completion of adjuvant therapy, a discussion of lifestyle changes should be held with the patient.
- Neoadjuvant chemoradiotherapy followed by total mesorectal excision is the standard treatment approach for stages II and III rectal cancer.
- Patients with stage IV disease have a curative chance if their metastases are amenable to complete surgical resection.
- Various conventional cytotoxic drugs (fluoropyrimidines, oxaliplatin, and irinotecan) and targeted agents (bevacizumab, aflibercept, regorafenib, as well as cetuximab and panitumumab in *RAS* wild-type cancers) have shown proof of efficacy for metastatic colorectal cancer.
- Expanded *RAS* mutation testing for mutations in *KRAS* and *NRAS* exons 2, 3, and 4 can be considered mandatory before use of EGFR monoclonal antibodies.

After completion of adjuvant therapy, lifestyle changes should be discussed with the patient since there is growing evidence that certain interventions can improve outcomes in patients with resected early-stage colorectal cancer.[212] Increased exercise after diagnosis and avoidance of a Western pattern diet are associated with reduced risk for cancer recurrence and improved overall survival. Patients with class II and III obesity (body mass index ≥ 35 kg/m^2) have a modestly increased risk for recurrence. Regular use of aspirin or cyclooxygenase-2 inhibitors decrease recurrence rates and increase serum vitamin D levels. In contrast, change of weight after diagnosis or smoking status (never, past, or current) are not associated with outcomes after diagnosis. The role of aspirin in this setting deserves particular attention. Recent data from a large population cohort study[213] and an analysis of a prospective trial[214] demonstrated a profound effect of aspirin as secondary prophylaxis in patients with resected colorectal cancer harboring PIK3CA mutations (exon 9 and 20). PIK3CA mutations are found in about 12% of colorectal cancers, and aspirin could emerge as key component of post-resection therapy in these patients.

Advanced Colorectal Cancer (Stage IV)

The prognosis for patients with stage IV disease without specific therapy is poor, with a median survival of 5 to 6 months. However, a subset of patients with isolated sites of metastases is potentially curable with surgery (see section on Limited Hepatic or Pulmonary Metastasis). Nevertheless, for the majority of patients with metastatic disease, the goal of therapy is palliation using systemic medical therapy. For decades, standard first-line therapy consisted of fluorouracil plus leucovorin, with response rates of approximately 20% and a median survival of approximately 1 year. In the late 1990s and early 2000s, the addition of oxaliplatin and irinotecan to the backbone of fluorouracil and leucovorin resulted in an improvement in median survival to nearly 24 months when patients received active first-line and second-line therapy. The introduction of biologic agents, such as bevacizumab, cetuximab, and panitumumab, have further enhanced the efficacy of systemic medical therapy.[215] The emphasis of current advances in medical therapy focuses on the development of predictive biomarker signatures that can help guide treatment decisions for specific patient subpopulations.

The availability of various active agents for the treatment of metastatic colorectal cancer has resulted in an abundance of therapeutic options that now demands a goal-oriented, strategic approach to therapy to maximize patient benefit. When treating a patient with metastatic colon cancer, the first determination is whether a patient with stage IV disease is potentially curable by surgical resection of metastases either at the time of diagnosis or after downsizing initially unresectable metastases by neoadjuvant chemotherapy.[215] This will guide the choice and timing of chemotherapy because, in this scenario, the most appropriate treatment is conceivably the one that generates the highest response rates and carries the greatest potential to downsize metastases. If the patient does not appear curable, the main goals of systemic chemotherapy are to extend the duration of a patient's life and to maintain quality of life as long as possible. In this scenario, treatment regimens that offer the longest progression-free and overall survivals, as well as a favorable toxicity profile, are preferred.

Fluorouracil. Until 2000, standard first-line therapy for metastatic colon cancer was the fluoropyrimidine analog fluorouracil plus leucovorin as biomodulator and activator. Leucovorin forms a complex with fluorouracil that permits prolonged inhibition of the enzyme thymidylate synthase, a key factor in the DNA synthesis. Response rates of fluorouracil with leucovorin range from 15% to 25%. Fluorouracil has been given with leucovorin in varying schedules and doses. The most commonly used regimens in the United States included the Mayo Clinic regimen (425 mg/m^2 of fluorouracil and 20 mg/m^2 for leucovorin on days 1 to 5 every 4 to 5 weeks)[216] and the Roswell Park regimen (500 mg/m^2 of fluorouracil and 500 mg/m^2 of leucovorin administered weekly for 6 out of 8 weeks).[217] Although these regimens used fluorouracil exclusively as bolus administration, European protocols preferred to use fluorouracil in the form of protracted infusions (e.g., for 2 days in the French biweekly LV5FU2 regimen or for 24 hours in the German weekly Arbeitsgemeinschaft Internistische Onkologie [AIO] regimen).[218,219] The incorporation of the novel cytotoxic agents irinotecan and oxaliplatin into fluorouracil-based regimens has resulted in significantly improved efficacy. This has shifted the paradigm for front-line treatment from fluorouracil and leucovorin alone to combination regimens incorporating these newer cytotoxic agents.

Capecitabine. Capecitabine is an oral fluoropyrimidine, a prodrug of fluorouracil, which is metabolized to its active form in three enzymatic steps. Its efficacy is similar to bolus fluorouracil and leucovorin, with slightly higher response rates.[220] Common side effects of this drug include diarrhea and hand-foot syndrome. Capecitabine has been used as the backbone of combination regimens with both oxaliplatin and irinotecan, but overlapping toxicities (diarrhea) make a combination with irinotecan more difficult to tolerate than oxaliplatin. Other oral fluoropyrimidines, which have not been approved in the United States, include tegafur-uracil, S-1 (a prodrug of 5-FU), gimeracil (5-chloro-2,4 dihydropyridine), which inhibits dihydropyrimidine dehydrogenase enzyme activity, and oteracil (potassium oxonate). Although capecitabine has never been directly compared with infusional fluorouracil/leucovorin, oxaliplatin-based combination regimens with either capecitabine (CAPOX or XELOX) compared with infusional fluorouracil/leucovorin (FOLFOX) have shown to be of similar efficacy in the treatment of advanced colorectal cancer.[221-223] It is of note, though, that patients in the United States do not tolerate the capecitabine doses used in European or Asian trials, presumably as a result of the higher nutritional folate intake in the United States.[224,225] Dose-reducing capecitabine by about 20% in combination regimens with oxaliplatin, however, does not appear to decrease the treatment efficacy, but greatly improves the side-effect profile of the treatment.[226]

Irinotecan. The first chemotherapy agent other than fluorouracil that improved survival for metastatic colon cancer—initially in second-line, later in first-line therapy—was irinotecan.[227-230] This compound has single-agent activity, which yields an approximate 15% response rate for patients with metastatic colon cancer refractory to fluorouracil.[227,229,231] In a landmark clinical trial, patients with fluorouracil-refractory metastatic colon cancer were randomly assigned to best supportive care or single-agent irinotecan. The results of the trial demonstrated that irinotecan offers an approximate 3-month survival advantage as well as an improvement in quality of life.[227] A second trial in the same second-line patient population found irinotecan superior to infusional 5-FU.[229] After this, three key trials were conducted to test the role of irinotecan in the front-line setting. In the United States, a three-arm trial was conducted to compare three treatment regimens: weekly bolus fluorouracil and leucovorin (Roswell Park regimen); weekly bolus fluorouracil and leucovorin plus irinotecan (IFL); and irinotecan alone.[230] The results of the trial revealed a longer than 2-month survival advantage (14.8 vs. 12.6 months, p = 0.04) and an almost doubling of response rate (39% vs. 21%, p < 0.001) for patients receiving the three-drug regimen compared to those receiving the bolus fluorouracil/leucovorin regimen. This study established the three-drug regimen as the then standard of care in the United States.

In Europe, two phase III trials were conducted in which fluorouracil was given as an infusion in combination with irinotecan, to form the FOLFIRI regimen. The results demonstrated a similar significant increase in response rate and time to disease progression for the three-drug regimen.[228,232] However, only the trial reported by Douillard et al[228] demonstrated significant prolongation of overall survival (17.4 vs. 14.1 months, p = 0.031), likely because of the limited availability of active second-line and third-line treatment options compared to the second European trial that was conducted later.[232] The main side effects of irinotecan are diarrhea, myelosuppression, and alopecia.

Oxaliplatin. Although oxaliplatin has very limited activity in colorectal cancer as a single agent, it shows enhanced clinical efficacy in combination with fluoropyrimidines, in particular with infusional fluorouracil and leucovorin. In three European phase III trials, combination protocols of infusional fluorouracil and leucovorin plus oxaliplatin (biweekly FOLFOX or weekly FUFOX) were compared with fluorouracil and leucovorin as first-line therapy for patients with advanced colorectal cancer.[233-235] In all three studies, a higher antitumor activity was noted for the combination regimens, with response rates of approximately 50% and progression-free survival in the range of 8 to 9 months. However, this higher efficacy did not translate into a significantly improved overall survival, most likely because of the availability of active salvage therapies for both treatment arms, which blurred the effects of the first-

line chemotherapy on the overall survivals in the trials. Of note, the median overall survival achieved with fluorouracil, leucovorin, and oxaliplatin ranged from 17.5 to 20 months, the longest overall survival reported in phase III trials for advanced colorectal cancer at that time. Because no overall survival benefit was achieved in these first-line trials, in 2000, the FDA did not approve oxaliplatin for colorectal cancer. The FDA approval of oxaliplatin in combination with fluorouracil and leucovorin in 2002 was based on the results of a second-line study that showed prolonged progression-free survival and increased response rates compared with infusional fluorouracil and leucovorin for patients who experienced disease progression while receiving IFL as first-line therapy.[236] It is of note that, in this trial, the arm with oxaliplatin as a single agent, without 5-FU, did not show any relevant tumor activity, which highlights that oxaliplatin needs to be combined with another agent, preferably a fluoropyrimidine. The key side effect and dose-limiting toxicity of oxaliplatin is neurotoxicity, which comes in two distinct forms: an acute, cold-triggered sensory neuropathy, which is temporary, rapidly reversible, and does not appear to cause structural nerve damage; and a chronic cumulative sensory neurotoxicity, which is related to the cumulative dose of oxaliplatin administered and constitutes the dose-limiting side effect of oxaliplatin.[237] Preliminary data initially suggested that the infusion of calcium/magnesium salts before and after oxaliplatin can potentially reduce the incidence and severity of chronic neurotoxicity,[238] but a larger, definitive trial showed no neuroprotective effect of intravenous calcium/magnesium.[239]

Comparing irinotecan- and oxaliplatin-based regimens. With its FDA approval in 2000, the combination regimen IFL emerged as standard first-line therapy for patients with advanced colorectal cancer in the United States. The encouraging results of trials conducted in Europe using oxaliplatin formed the rationale for the North Central Cancer Treatment Group (NCCTG)/ Intergroup trial N9741.[240] This pivotal and practice-changing trial compared FOLFOX and the non–fluorouracil-containing combination of irinotecan and oxaliplatin (IROX), as well as with standard combination IFL. The results of N9741 clearly demonstrated the superiority of FOLFOX compared with IFL as first-line therapy for colorectal cancer regarding response rate (45% vs. 31%, p = 0.002), progression-free survival (8.7 vs. 6.9 months, p = 0.0014), and overall survival (19.5 vs. 15.0 months, p = 0.0001). The toxicity profile likewise favored FOLFOX compared with IFL, with only neurotoxicity being more prevalent for patients receiving the oxaliplatin-based combination. Results for IROX were in between the two other arms (response rate, 35%; progression-free survival, 6.5 months; overall survival, 17.4 months), and, as such, FOLFOX emerged as new standard first-line therapy with rapid and widespread adaptation in the United States. It should be emphasized that N9741 did not directly compare oxaliplatin and irinotecan; rather, it compared two different combination regimens with different fluorouracil and leucovorin backbones. The higher efficacy and better tolerability observed with infusional fluorouracil and leucovorin may have contributed to the differences in efficacy between IFL and FOLFOX. Two smaller trials comparing FOLFOX and FOLFIRI with the same fluorouracil and leucovorin backbone failed to show significant differences in activity.[241,242] Although the small sample size of these trials might preclude wide-reaching conclusions, the choice between FOLFOX and FOLFIRI in the clinic should mainly be based on the expected side-effect pattern. Because the benefit of second-line therapy in colorectal cancer has been well established, patients should receive all active cytotoxic drugs in the course of their therapy to optimize outcome.[243] Combinations of 5-FU/LV, irinotecan and oxaliplatin (FOLFOXIRI) show high activity, but also increased toxicity.[244] The use of this triplet combination should be reserved for specific situations, for example, when substantial tumor shrinkage is a prerequisite for a surgical approach toward borderline resectable liver metastases.

Bevacizumab. An adequate blood supply is necessary for the rapid growth and development of tumors beyond the micrometastatic state of 1 to 2 mm in diameter. VEGF contributes to tumor growth by stimulating new tumor blood vessel growth (angiogenesis) and maintaining immature tumor vasculature. VEGF was initially characterized for its ability to induce vascular leakage and permeability (vascular permeability factor) and to induce vascular endothelial proliferation. VEGF is a member of a family of structurally related proteins. These proteins bind to the family of VEGF receptors, thereby stimulating various biologic processes. The most important interaction in the process of tumor-mediated angiogenesis is the binding of VEGF-A to VEGFR2. Antibodies directed at VEGF block VEGF interactions with its receptors, thus preventing VEGF signaling through both VEGFR1 and VEGFR2.[245]

Bevacizumab, a recombinant humanized monoclonal antibody to VEGF-A, has demonstrated clinical efficacy for the treatment of metastatic colorectal cancer. In a large phase III placebo-controlled trial with 813 patients, IFL was compared with IFL plus bevacizumab (5 mg/kg every 2 weeks) as first-line therapy for advanced colorectal cancer.[246] The addition of the anti-VEGF antibody led to significantly increased response rate (45% vs. 35%, p = 0.0036), progression-free survival (10.6 vs. 6.2 months, HR 0.54, p < 0.00001), and median overall survival (20.3 vs. 15.6 months, HR 0.66, p = 0.00004). This trial was the first phase III validation of an antiangiogenic agent as an effective treatment option in a human malignancy. Subsequently, bevacizumab also has been shown to enhance the efficacy of oxaliplatin-based regimens in first- and second-line settings, as well as in combination with fluorouracil and leucovorin alone or with irinotecan.[247-250] It is important to note that bevacizumab does not appear to have significant single-agent activity in metastatic colorectal cancer.[247] The main side effects observed with bevacizumab consist of hypertension (a class-effect of all agents targeting VEGF signaling), bleeding, gastrointestinal perforations (1.5% to 2% of patients), as well as arterial thrombotic events in approximately 4% to 5% of patients.[251] In addition to arterial thrombotic events, a meta-analysis identified a 33% higher incidence of venous thrombotic events in patients receiving bevacizumab compared with the non-bevacizumab control

arm in randomized trials,[252] although another, more recent analysis refuted this claim.[253] Based on its well-documented efficacy and relative moderate toxicity, bevacizumab has emerged as a standard component of first-line chemotherapy for advanced colorectal cancer.

Although most patients with metastatic colorectal cancer will tolerate and receive bevacizumab in the context of an irinotecan- or oxaliplatin-based combination regimen, it is unclear if specific subgroups, in particular elderly patients, could benefit from a bevacizumab-fluoropyrimidine combination alone. This question was addressed in the pivotal and practice-informing AVEX phase III trial.[254] In this study, 280 patients aged 70 and older (median age 76), who were not deemed to be candidates for oxaliplatin-based or irinotecan-based chemotherapy first-line regimens, were randomly assigned to capecitabine (1,000 mg/m^2 orally twice a day on days 1 to 14) alone or with bevacizumab (7.5 mg/kg intravenously on day 1), given every 3 weeks. Progression-free survival, the primary endpoint, was significantly longer with bevacizumab and capecitabine than with capecitabine alone (median 9.1 vs. 5.1 months, HR 0.53, 95% CI 0.41, 0.69; p < 0.0001). Although the study was underpowered to demonstrate a statistically significant improvement in overall survival, the median survival in the bevacizumab arm of 20.7 months (compared with 16.8 months for capecitabine alone) is remarkable given the age of the patient population and the limited postprogression therapies patients received. The combination of a fluoropyrimidine plus bevacizumab can be considered as an acceptable standard of care for elderly patients who are not considered for irinotecan or oxaliplatin, but have no contraindication against bevacizumab.

Initial reports suggested an over-additive activity when bevacizumab was combined with cetuximab in a salvage-therapy setting.[255] However, subsequent larger, randomized first-line trials suggested an antagonistic effect of the combination of EGFR antibodies with bevacizumab in the context of concurrent chemotherapy.[256,257] Thus, combinations of bevacizumab and EGFR antibodies should not be used in clinical practice.

It has been suggested that prolonged inhibition of the VEGF-mediated proangiogenic system is required to maximize treatment benefit for patients on anti-VEGF therapy, in particular, since the mechanism and onset of secondary resistance could differ between chemotherapy and bevacizumab.[258] The efficacy of prolonged VEGF inhibition with bevacizumab added to chemotherapy was highlighted by several randomized trials. A prespecified analysis of a large phase III trial (NO16966) adding bevacizumab to an oxaliplatin-based first-line regimen demonstrated that improvements in progression-free survival were greater in patients who received treatment until progression than in those who stopped therapy for other reasons.[249] Since the treatment-limiting toxicity of oxaliplatin-based first-line therapy is cumulative neurotoxicity, proactive strategies have to be employed to maximize treatment duration for patients who start palliative therapy with FOLFOX plus bevacizumab, the most commonly used first-line regimen in the United States. Therefore, induction-maintenance approaches with a limited number of oxaliplatin-containing treatment cycles up front and maintenance therapy with a fluoropyrimidine-bevacizumab combination can be considered a standard of care. This concept is supported by several prospective trials, most prominently by the recently presented Dutch CAIRO-3 study.[259] In this trial, 558 patients who had at least achieved stable disease after an 18-week (six cycles) induction therapy of XELOX plus bevacizumab were randomly assigned to a complete chemotherapy-free interval or maintenance therapy with low-dose continuous capecitabine (625 mg/m² twice daily) plus bevacizumab (7.5 mg/kg every 3 weeks). All prospectively defined outcomes parameters in this strategy trial were in favor of the maintenance therapy arm, even with a strong trend toward improved overall survival. Toxicity associated with maintenance was mild and manageable. Thus, an induction-maintenance approach with limited duration of oxaliplatin-based therapy and prolonged fluoropyrimidine/bevacizumab can be considered an optimized approach to maximize efficacy and limit toxicity in first-line palliative therapy of advanced colorectal cancer.

Further evidence supporting the concept of prolonged VEGF inhibition as an optimized treatment approach in colorectal cancer comes from the so-called ML18147 ("TML") phase III trial that tested the efficacy of bevacizumab beyond progression (BBP) added to chemotherapy in metastatic colorectal cancer.[260] A total of 820 patients who had received first-line palliative therapy with a bevacizumab-based combination were randomly assigned at progression to either continue bevacizumab with another investigator's choice chemotherapy backbone or stop bevacizumab. The primary endpoint of the study, improvement in overall survival, was reached with an HR of 0.81 (95% CI 0.69, 0.94) and a median improvement of 1.4 months (11.2 vs. 9.8 months, p = 0.0062). This effect was confirmed in all evaluated subgroups and supported by the results of progression-free survival, which demonstrated superiority for the BBP arm (HR 0.68, median 5.7 vs. 4.1 months, p < 0.0001). No increase in response rate was seen in the BBP group and the response rates seen in both arms in second-line therapy were low, around 4% to 5%. No new or unexpected safety issues emerged for bevacizumab.

Several other agents targeting various components of the VEGF-mediated signal transduction cascade have been developed and some have already demonstrated efficacy in clinical testing (see Novel Agents with Efficacy in Colorectal Cancer section).

Anti-EGFR antibodies: cetuximab and panitumumab. Both monoclonal antibodies against the EGFR, cetuximab and panitumumab, have single-agent efficacy in advanced colorectal cancer. Two U.S. phase II trials confirmed the activity of cetuximab for the treatment of patients who had experienced disease progression on prior irinotecan-based therapy.[261] The single-agent response rate of approximately 10% noted with cetuximab alone was in the same range as previously noted with FOLFOX in the same setting. A large international randomized phase III trial comparing cetuximab with cetuximab plus irinotecan confirmed the findings with almost identical results.[262] For patients who experienced progressive disease while receiving irinotecan-based therapy (with approximately

two-thirds of patients also refractory to oxaliplatin), cetuximab monotherapy induced responses for approximately 11% of patients. When irinotecan was added, response rate and time to progression were significantly increased (HR 0.54, 95% CI 0.42, 0.71; p < 0.001). These data served as the basis for the initial approval of cetuximab as a treatment option for patients with metastatic colorectal cancer who were pretreated with irinotecan-based regimens.

Single-agent panitumumab was tested against best supportive care in a large international phase III trial in an extensively pretreated population; cross-over was optional upon progression.[263] Panitumumab demonstrated similar single-agent activity to cetuximab, with an approximate 10% response rate when used as salvage therapy after failure of standard chemotherapy. In comparison with best supportive care, it significantly prolonged progression-free survival (HR 0.54, 95% CI 0.44, 0.66; p < 0.0001). Overall survival was not increased, presumably because 75% of patients crossed over from best supportive care to the panitumumab arm. Based on these data, panitumumab was approved as a single-agent salvage therapy option in the United States in 2006. A similar last-line trial comparing cetuximab with best supportive care (without cross-over) showed almost identical results in terms of response rate and progression-free survival, but also with survival benefit for the cetuximab arm.[264] Both antibodies have been tested as components of first-line therapy in combination with modern chemotherapy regimens, such as FOLFOX and FOLFIRI, the results of which are discussed below.[265-268] A phase III head-to-head comparison of both antibodies in a salvage therapy setting in 999 patients recently confirmed the superimposable efficacy of both agents.[269]

The main toxicities of anti-EGFR antibodies are skin rash, hypomagnesemia, diarrhea, and hypersensitivity reactions, which is particularly relevant for the chimeric antibody cetuximab.[251] Anaphylactic reactions to cetuximab have been correlated to the presence of preexisting serum IgE antibodies to an oligosaccharide, galactose-alpha-1,3-galactose, which is present on the Fab portion of the cetuximab heavy chain.[270] These antibodies have been found in up to 21% in individuals from Tennessee who had never been exposed to cetuximab, compared with only 0.6% of individuals from the Boston metropolitan region.[270] The reason for these geographic differences are not known, but it is conceivable that environmental influences with exposure to sensitizing antigens play a role.

Data from various clinical trials and translational studies now have opened the door toward individualized treatment approaches in colorectal cancer by identifying patients who are most likely to benefit from antibodies against the EGFR, cetuximab and panitumumab. It increasingly appears that patients with advanced colorectal cancer must have tumors with wild-type *KRAS* for EGFR antibodies to be effective (Fig. 9-3).[266,268,271-276] *KRAS* is a phosphorylated signal transducer that self-inactivates via intrinsic guanosine triphosphatase (GTPase) activity.[277] It is a homolog of the transforming gene Kirsten rat sarcoma-2 virus. Several *KRAS* oncogene mutations—in colorectal cancer mainly in codons 12 and 13 (exon 2)—that result in the production of proteins with reduced GTPase activity have been identified.

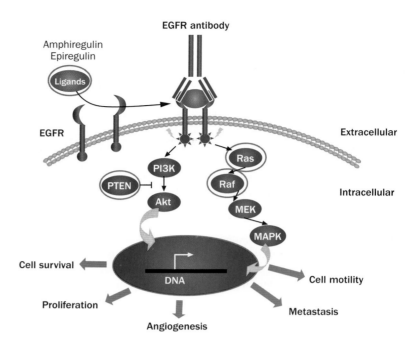

Fig. 9-3 The EGFR-signaling pathway and predictive biomarkers for the efficacy of EGFR antibodies.

Abbreviation: EGFR, epidermal growth factor receptor.

These *KRAS* mutations are among the most common oncogenic alterations in cancer. Four points are important to note with regard to *KRAS* mutations in colorectal cancer:

- *KRAS* mutations occur early in the adenoma–carcinoma sequence, leading to colorectal cancer, implying that the mutation can be found in all tumor cells derived from the initial malignant clone, in metastases as well as the primary tumor.[154,272]
- The determination of KRAS mutations is a yes/no binary decision; a tumor harbors either wild-type or mutated *KRAS*. No cut-off levels or subjective grades of expression levels have to be considered.
- The tests for *KRAS* mutation, whether mutation-specific PCR or gene sequencing is being used, are very robust, of high sensitivity and specificity, and can be obtained from formalin-fixed, paraffin-embedded tissue.
- The frequency of *KRAS* exon 2 mutations in colorectal cancer is about 40%.

In 2013, data emerged that beyond the current routinely tested *KRAS* exon 2 mutations (codon 12 and 13), lower frequency mutations in *KRAS* exon 3 and 4 and in *NRAS* also lead to resistance to EGFR monoclonal antibodies.[278,279] Thus, these mutations identify another 10% to 15% of patients beyond the 40% of patients identified with the conventional *KRAS* exon 2 mutations who have no benefit from cetuximab and panitumumab. In fact, results of the pivotal PRIME phase III trial in which patients were randomly assigned to first-line FOLFOX with or without panitumumab suggest that patients with tumors carrying these additional *RAS* mutations might actually experience a detrimental effect when treated with panitumumab.[278] A similar trend was observed for cetuximab added to FOLFIRI in the FIRE-3 trial that will be discussed in de-

tail in the following section.[279] It is conceivable that regulatory agencies and treatment guidelines will soon demand expanded *RAS* mutation testing before EGFR monoclonal antibodies are used in patients with colorectal cancer.

Further predictive biomarkers for the activity of EGFR antibodies in colorectal cancer have been identified in retrospective studies, in which the activity of cetuximab was correlated with the maintained expression of phosphatase and tensin homolog (PTEN) and higher levels of the EGFR ligands amphiregulin and epiregulin.[280-283]

BRAF encodes a protein GTPase downstream of *RAS*. Mutations in *BRAF*, which can be found in about 5% to 10% of patients with advanced colorectal cancer, are mutually exclusive with *KRAS* mutations[276] and have been consistently found to be associated with a very poor prognosis.[267,272,284] Even in the era of modern combination therapy, median survival of patients with *BRAF*-mutated stage IV colorectal cancer is only in the range of 12 to 14 months.[267] More recent data, however, suggest that an aggressive first-line treatment approach using a triplet chemotherapy combination (FOLFOXIRI) plus bevacizumab might at least partially counteract the poor prognosis of patients with *BRAF*-mutated colorectal cancers.[285,286] Thus, FOLFOXIRI plus bevacizumab could emerge as preferred treatment option in these patients.

The validity of *BRAF* mutations as a negative predictive marker for the activity of EGFR antibodies is unclear, but more recent data suggest that cetuximab and panitumumab might still have some, albeit attenuated, activity in *BRAF*-mutated colorectal cancers.[267]

With the proof of efficacy of two biologic therapeutic approaches in colorectal cancer, bevacizumab as a VEGF-targeting agent and cetuximab/panitumumab as EGFR antibodies, it appears logical to try to further enhance the efficacy of therapy by combining both approaches. Initial data for the combination of bevacizumab and cetuximab with or without irinotecan in a salvage therapy setting were promising,[255] so that several subsequent clinical trials investigated the combination of standard chemotherapy (FOLFOX, CAPOX, or FOLFIRI) plus bevacizumab with or without either cetuximab or panitumumab. The addition of an EGFR antibody to the bevacizumab-based combination therapy reduced progression-free survival in the intent-to-treat populations and not even the *KRAS* wild-type tumor population benefited from the intensified therapy.[256,257] In view of these findings, the combination of bevacizumab with EGFR antibodies should not be used in clinical practice outside of clinical trials.

Head-to-head comparison between EGFR monoclonal antibodies and bevacizumab. At the 2013 ASCO Annual Meeting, the first results of a phase III trial with a direct comparison between a cetuximab- and bevacizumab-containing first-line therapy were presented.[287] The FIRE-3 trial randomly assigned 592 patients with conventionally assessed *KRAS* exon 2 wild-type colorectal cancer to FOLFIRI plus cetuximab or FOLFIRI plus bevacizumab. The primary endpoint of the trial was investigator-assessed response rate with an expected difference in the intent-to-treat analysis of 12%. The primary endpoint was not reached in the intent-to-treat analysis (cetuximab 62%, bevacizumab 58%, p = 0.18). In addition, no difference in progression-free survival was noted (cetuximab 10.0 vs. bevacizumab 10.3 months), in fact, the progression-free survival curves were almost completely superimposable. Surprisingly, however, a statistically significant difference was found in overall survival with a difference in median overall survival of 3.7 months (28.7 vs. 25.0 months, HR 0.77, p = 0.017) in favor of FOLFIRI-cetuximab. The survival curves appeared to split at 24 months, meaning more than 12 months after the median progression-free survival has been reached. An updated analysis which accounted for additional mutations in *KRAS* exon 3 and 3 and *NRAS* mutations demonstrated an even larger difference in median overall survival (33.1 months for cetuximab vs. 25.6 months, HR 0.70; p = 0.011), again without statistically significant difference in response rate and progression-free survival.[279] As outlined above, in patients with tumors harboring the additional *KRAS* and *NRAS* mutations a detrimental effect might have been inflicted with the use of cetuximab.

Data from the larger U.S. Intergroup study CALGB/SWOG 80405, which compared chemotherapy (FOLFOX or FOLFIRI) with cetuximab or bevacizumab as first-line therapy in *KRAS* exon 2 wild-type colorectal cancer, and which was powered for an overall survival benefit of the cetuximab-based arm, are expected to be released in 2014.

Novel agents with efficacy in colorectal cancer. Since 2011, results of two phase III trials became available that demonstrated the efficacy of two novel agents in advanced colorectal cancer. Both agents gained U.S. regulatory approval in 2012.

VEGF-Trap (aflibercept) is a VEGF receptor decoy fusion protein that consists of extracellular domain components of VEGFR1 and VEGFR2 fused with the Fc region of IgG1. VEGF-Trap binds to the VEGF-A, VEGF-B, and PlGF ligands and prevents their interaction with VEGF receptors.[288] Aflibercept was tested in a second-line trial in patients in whom oxaliplatin-based first-line chemotherapy had failed.[289] About 1,200 patients were randomly assigned to FOLFIRI with aflibercept or placebo. The primary endpoint of improvement in overall survival was reached (13.5 vs. 12.1 months, HR 0.82, p = 0.0032) and was mirrored by improvements in progression-free survival (6.9 vs. 4.7 months, HR 0.758, p = 0.00007) and response rate (19.8% vs. 11.1%, p = 0.0001). It is of note, though, that only 30% of patients in this trial had access to front-line bevacizumab so that the data are largely based on a VEGF inhibitor–naive population. The FDA approved aflibercept in 2012 as a component of second-line therapy in combination with FOLFIRI.

The second novel agent with documented efficacy in advanced colorectal cancer is regorafenib, a small molecule inhibitor of multiple cell-signaling kinases.[290] After preliminary data suggesting a high disease control rate in patients with treatment-refractory colorectal cancer, regorafenib was investigated in a placebo-controlled randomized phase III trial in a salvage therapy setting. Efficacy results of the trial demonstrated a benefit in overall survival for patients receiving regorafenib compared with placebo (6.4 vs. 5.0 months, HR 0.77, p = 0.0052).[291] The activity of regorafenib was also reflected in an improvement of progression-free survival (1.9 vs. 1.7 months, HR 0.49, p < 0.000001). The most common severe toxicities observed with regorafenib were hand-foot skin reaction, fatigue, diarrhea, and hypertension. Regorafenib is FDA-approved as a salvage therapy option in patients with advanced colorectal cancer who have previously been treated with a fluoropyrimidine, oxaliplatin, irinotecan, a VEGF inhibitor, and—if *KRAS* wild-type—an EGFR monoclonal antibody.

An evidence-based treatment algorithm in the palliative management of colorectal cancer, including biologic agents based on molecular testing for *RAS* and *BRAF*, is outlined in Fig. 9-4.

Limited Hepatic or Pulmonary Metastasis

For the subgroup of patients with recurrent metastatic colon cancer confined to the liver, the roles of hepatic-directed chemotherapy and hepatic resection have become better defined. There is only one multicenter evaluation of potentially resectable liver metastases; the results showed an improved survival for patients undergoing resection compared with those who either had unresectable disease or had noncurative resection.[292] The survival advantage is clinically significant, with a near doubling of survival, to almost 37 months.[293] When pooling data for all patients who have a hepatic resection, the average 5-year survival rate is approximately 30%, with a less favorable prognosis for patients with multiple lesions, a short interval between the diagnosis of the primary tumor and recurrence, and presence of stage III disease at the time of initial diagnosis.[294-296]

Preoperative chemotherapy can be used to downsize initially unresectable metastases to make them amenable for a surgical approach. It has been shown that the overall survival

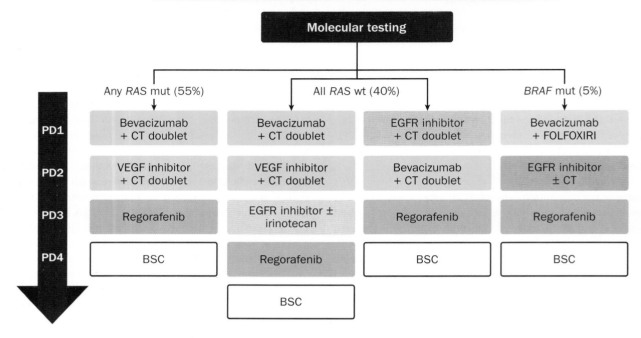

Fig. 9-4 Evidence-based treatment algorithm in the palliative management of colorectal cancer, including biologic agents based on molecular testing for *RAS* and *BRAF*.

VEGF inhibitor = bevacizumab or aflibercept.

Abbreviations: BSC, best supportive care; CT, chemotherapy; FOLFOXIRI, leucovorin/5-fluorouracil/oxaliplatin/irinotecan; mut, mutation; PD, progressive disease; wt, wild type.

of patients who undergo successful neoadjuvant therapy with subsequent R0 resection of liver metastases approaches the survival of patients with initially resectable metastases.[293,294] Thus, the initial therapeutic approach for a patient with limited metastatic disease should always include consideration of a potentially curative option.

The role of chemotherapy in the potentially curative management of metastatic colorectal cancer can be classified in three different categories:

- Neoadjuvant therapy for initially resectable metastases, mainly to obtain prognostic information, treat potentially disseminated micrometastases as early as possible, and test the chemotherapy sensitivity of the tumor;
- Conversion therapy for initially unresectable or borderline resectable metastases to allow for metastasectomy after tumor shrinkage; and
- Adjuvant therapy after curative resection of metastases.

To date, no studies have been conducted to establish the value of neoadjuvant therapy (vs. surgery alone or surgery plus postoperative therapy) for patients with resectable liver metastases. A European phase III trial in resectable, liver-limited metastatic colorectal cancer randomly assigned 364 patients to proceed to surgery directly or receive FOLFOX chemotherapy for 3 months followed by resection, and then again followed by 3 months of FOLFOX.[297] Patients meeting the eligibility criteria of the trial who received perioperative

chemotherapy had a significant improvement in 3-year progression-free survival compared with patients in the surgery-alone arm (36.2% vs. 28.1%; HR 0.77, p = 0.041). The study was not able to determine whether all patients with resectable liver metastasis should receive neoadjuvant chemotherapy. Any beneficial effects of chemotherapy in this situation will have to be balanced against potential side effects of therapy and, in particular, against the observed higher surgical morbidity after neoadjuvant therapy.[297,298] The likelihood of conversion therapy to eventually lead to liver resection has been correlated with the overall response rate observed with a specific treatment regimen.[244,299]

The data on adjuvant therapy after the resection of hepatic or pulmonary metastasis are limited. In one randomized clinical trial, half of the patients who had successful hepatic resection received both systemic and intrahepatic chemotherapy with floxuridine; the other half received only systemic chemotherapy.[300] The results demonstrated a survival advantage at 2 years for patients who received the intrahepatic chemotherapy combination. This approach has not gained widespread use worldwide because of its difficult drug-delivery process, its associated hepatic toxicities, and in view of the high activity of modern systemic combination chemotherapy. A pooled analysis of two small trials with a combined 278 patients that utilized adjuvant therapy after liver resection and a fluorouracil plus leucovorin regimen demonstrated a strong trend toward improved outcome with systemic adjuvant chemotherapy in this setting (progression-free survival: 27.9 vs. 18.8 months, HR 1.32, p = 0.058).[301] A trial demonstrated that the addition of irinotecan to infusional fluorouracil/leucovorin in the adjuvant setting did not improve outcome after liver resection, similar to the findings of lack of irinotecan efficacy for stage III colon cancer.[186]

The role of biologic agents (EGFR antibodies and VEGF inhibitors) in the context of preoperative and perioperative therapy for potentially resectable liver metastases is unclear. Initial data suggest some benefit for the addition of cetuximab to chemotherapy (FOLFOX or FOLFIRI) in this setting,[302] but more recent results from a randomized trial conducted in the United Kingdom suggested an unexplained detrimental effect when cetuximab was added to chemotherapy in the perioperative setting.[303] No randomized trial exists to test the role of bevacizumab in the context of liver resection. If bevacizumab is used in the preoperative setting it needs to be discontinued about 6 weeks before planned surgery to reduce the risk of wound healing complications.[304]

It is important to note that there are substantial data to support disease resection outside of the liver, with the lung being the next most common site for secondary resection. In contrast, the role of aggressive surgical approaches toward peritoneal carcinomatosis, commonly conducted in the context of hyperthermic intraperitoneal chemotherapy, is controversial.[305]

NEOADJUVANT AND ADJUVANT THERAPY FOR RECTAL CANCER

Cancers arising in the rectum are associated with a higher overall risk for recurrence than the recurrence risk associated with similar stages of colon cancer. The reason for local recurrence in rectal cancer is believed to be the anatomic location of the rectum and the challenge this presents to the surgeon, particularly surgeons practicing in low-volume hospitals. However, pre- and postoperative therapy can help decrease differences in local recurrence rates between hospitals.[306,307] There is increasing evidence to suggest that local excision should be restricted to patients with T1 stage rectal cancer without high-risk factors.[308] For all other stages, total mesorectal excision (TME) has emerged as the preferred surgical technique. This technique honors natural tissue planes and decreases the chance for local seeding and subsequent recurrence.[309] In combination with preoperative or postoperative chemoradiotherapy, 5-year local recurrence rates of less than 10% can be achieved.[307,310-312]

The recognition of the significant morbidity and the potential mortality associated with local relapse led to the use of both preoperative or postoperative radiation therapy as additional regional treatment options designed to reduce local recurrence. Two different approaches have been used in this regard: short-term, high-dose radiation commonly delivered as daily 5 Gy for 5 days (5 x 5) immediately before surgery, or prolonged combined-modality therapy with radiosensitizing chemotherapy administered parallel to radiation to a total dose of 50.4 Gy (45 + 5.4 Gy local boost) for 5 to 6 weeks followed by a 3- to 4-week interval before curative surgery.[310,312,313] It is important

to note that only the longer chemoradiotherapy approach has repeatedly been demonstrated to be able to downstage tumors and cause tumor shrinkage, which might allow sphincter-preserving surgery. Both treatment approaches, however, have been associated with a decrease in local-regional failure. Prevention of local recurrence has not uniformly been associated with improved overall survival. However, the results of one Swedish trial, in which 1,168 patients were randomly assigned to either 5 days of high-dose radiation therapy (to 25 Gy) in the week before surgery or to surgery alone, demonstrated a reduction in local recurrences (11% vs. 27%, p < 0.001) and a survival advantage at 5 years (58% vs. 48%, p = 0.004) for preoperative radiation therapy.[313] A subsequent Dutch trial, using the same radiation technique in combination with quality-controlled TME surgery, confirmed a low rate of local recurrence (at 2 years: 2.4% vs. 8.4%, p < 0.001), but failed to demonstrate a survival benefit.[310] However, it is of note that the local recurrence rate of tumors more than 10 cm from the anal verge was not significantly affected. Although the shorter, high-dose preoperative radiation strategy is most commonly used in Scandinavia and in other European countries, U.S. oncologists have historically preferred combined-modality therapy as preoperative or postoperative chemoradiotherapy. Findings from two studies of postoperative adjuvant chemoradiotherapy demonstrated that fluorouracil-based chemotherapy plus radiation was more effective than radiation or surgery alone in preventing both local and distant recurrence.[314,315] Results from another trial showed that prolonged infusion of fluorouracil was superior to bolus administration during radiation therapy, providing a 3-year DFS advantage.[316] This finding confirms that protracted delivery of chemotherapy sensitizing agents concomitant with radiation is the best way to deliver combined-modality therapy. In clinical practice, capecitabine administered twice daily parallel to radiation (common dose: 825 mg/m^2 twice daily on days of radiation) has become a widely used substitute for continuous infusion of fluorouracil. Two phase III studies confirmed the noninferiority of capecitabine as a radiosensitizer compared with protracted infusion of 5-FU as neoadjuvant therapy in rectal cancer.[317,318]

The long-standing question about whether preoperative or postoperative chemoradiotherapy delivers improved outcome was definitively answered by the results of a large German randomized trial that compared standard continuously infused fluorouracil plus radiation either before or after quality-controlled TME surgery.[312] Patients undergoing preoperative combined-modality therapy had a lower rate of local recurrence (at 5 years: 6% vs. 13%), lower rate of acute and chronic toxicities, and a significantly higher rate of sphincter preservation compared with postoperative chemoradiotherapy (p = 0.006). This trial established preoperative neoadjuvant chemoradiotherapy with fluorouracil as radiosensitizer as the new standard of care for stage II and III rectal cancers. Subsequent studies are trying to further improve the local control rate by incorporating additional radiosensitizing agents, such as oxaliplatin, and biologic agents into the preoperative treatment phase.[319-322]

Data question the potential role of oxaliplatin as radiosensitizer when added to fluoropyrimidines in the neoadjuvant chemoradiotherapy of rectal cancer.[317,323,324] Consistent results from Italian, French, and U.S. phase III trials found that the addition of oxaliplatin to fluoropyrimidine (5-FU or capecitabine) as a component of neoadjuvant chemoradiotherapy did not increase the rate of pathologic CR with the use of oxaliplatin, but significantly increased toxicity, mainly diarrhea. Only a German trial that used a slightly different schedule of oxaliplatin administration showed superiority of the oxaliplatin arm in terms of pathologic response.[325] However, the overwhelming body of evidence suggests that at this point in time, oxaliplatin should not be used as part of neoadjuvant chemoradiotherapy for rectal cancer outside of clinical trials even if the results of long-term efficacy parameters, such as local recurrence rate, DFS, and overall survival, are still pending.

Two smaller phase III trials compared neoadjuvant chemoradiotherapy after the Sauer protocol to short-course radiation therapy (5 x 5 Gy) as neoadjuvant treatment for localized rectal cancer.[326,327] Both trials demonstrated that both treatment approaches are valid options in the preoperative setting of rectal cancer with similar rates of local recurrence and overall survival.

Current studies are seeking to enhance the efficacy of preoperative therapy by adding biologic agents to a fluoropyrimidine backbone. In addition, studies are underway to compare systemic chemotherapy without radiation against standard chemoradiotherapy for patients with cancers of the mid- and upper rectum to spare them the short- and long-term toxicity of radiation therapy.

ANAL CANCERS
EPIDEMIOLOGY AND ETIOLOGY

Cancers of the anus are relatively uncommon in the United States; however, there is an increased incidence in certain populations, such as young men in whom genital viral infections have been implicated. The man-to-woman ratio is approximately 2 to 3.5. The most clear causal relationship for anal cancer is infection with HPV (mainly HPV 16). One large study found a strong positive correlation between the amount of sexual activity and the risk for anal cancer.[328] In addition, an association between venereal infection in both men and women was noted. Infection with HPV was presumed to be the etiologic cause. Although earlier studies suggested that anal-receptive intercourse was directly linked to an increased risk for anal cancer, this finding has not been confirmed in more recent larger scale trials. Cancers of the anal canal also have been associated with condylomata in both the general population and in homosexual men. In women with a history of genital warts, anal cancer was associated with seropositivity for herpes simplex virus type 1 and chlamydia trachomatis. For men with no history of genital warts, there was an association with gonorrhea. The association between AIDS and anal cancer has been known for some time, but the exact etiologic relationship has not been elucidated. The incidence of anal cancer in patients infected with HIV

is increased more than 40 times compared with the general population.[329] Further risk factors for anal cancers are smoking and chronic inflammation/fistulas in the context of inflammatory bowel disease.

The efficacy of a quadrivalent HPV vaccine (HPV 6, 11, 16, and 18) against anal intraepithelial neoplasia was prospectively investigated in a double-blind randomized study in 602 healthy homosexual men age 16 to 26.[330] The rate of grade 2 or 3 anal intraepithelial neoplasia related to infection with HPV 6, 11, 16, or 18 was reduced by 54.2% (95% CI 18.0, 75.3) in the intention-to-treat population and by 74.9% (95% CI 8.8, 95.4) in the per-protocol efficacy population. These intriguing findings, which could lead to a decrease in the incidence of anal cancers through HPV vaccination, prompted the Advisory Committee on Immunization Practices in October 2011 to recommend the routine use of the quadrivalent HPV vaccine in boys age 11 to 12.[331]

Most anal cancers are squamous cell cancers or cloacogenic cancers, with a few adenocarcinomas. In addition, melanoma accounts for a small percentage of cancers found in the anal canal. Tumors tend to spread by local extension but have the potential to metastasize. Involvement of the inguinal lymph nodes is found in as many as 63% of cases. The most important prognostic factors are the T stage (T1 is less than 2 cm, T2 is 2 to 5 cm, T3 is greater than 5 cm, and T4 is invasion into adjacent organs) and lymph node status. In a pooled analysis of four randomized trials with a total of 644 patients, tumor diameter greater than 5 cm and lymph node involvement were associated with poorer 5-year DFS (p < 0.0001) and 5-year overall survival (p = 0.0001). In stratified analyses, lymph node involvement had more adverse influence on DFS and overall survival than did tumor diameter. Patients with larger than 5-cm tumor and lymph node metastases had the worst DFS (only 30% at 3 years vs. 74% for the best group; < 5 cm primary and N0) and overall survival (only 48% at 4 years vs. 81% for the best group; < 5 cm primary and N0). Men had worse DFS (p = 0.02) and overall survival (p = 0.016).[332]

TREATMENT

In the distant past, treatment for patients with anal cancers was surgical resection using an anterior-posterior approach. This treatment option was curative for only approximately 50% of patients and was associated with a high morbidity rate. Today, the standard approach to treatment of anal cancers is combined-modality chemotherapy and radiation. Local excision is reserved for patients with small tumors that are well differentiated or are removed incidentally at the time of hemorrhoidectomy.

In initial chemoradiotherapy trials, combinations of fluorouracil and mitomycin-C with radiation yielded a high rate of response, including pathologic CR.[329,333] Eventually, it was recognized that surgical resection was not necessary, and it is used today only as salvage therapy for patients with local recurrences after radiation. The expectation for patients is that the CR rate with combined-modality therapy will be between 70% and 80%, with an overall 5-year survival rate of greater than 65%. However, a substantial number of patients will still experience either local relapse or metastatic disease. Treatment of disease in such patients is much more difficult. A phase III RTOG trial involving 682 patients with anal cancer that compared the role of mitomycin-C and fluorouracil with an intensified treatment approach consisting of induction chemotherapy with cisplatin and fluorouracil followed by cisplatin and fluorouracil during radiation therapy did not show superiority of the experimental arm.[334] In fact, both the 5-year local-regional recurrence rate (25% vs. 33%) and the distant metastasis rates (15% vs. 19%) trended in favor of the mitomycin-based treatment. The cumulative rate of colostomy was significantly better for mitomycin-based than for cisplatin-based therapy (10% vs. 19%; p = 0.02). An updated analysis with long-term follow-up identified the standard mitomycin-based arm as significantly superior in overall survival.[335] Results of a more recent phase III comparison between fluorouracil combined with either mitomycin or cisplatin parallel to upfront radiation therapy did not find a significant difference in outcome[336] so that the inferior results of the RTOG trial for the cisplatin arm could be related to the delay in radiation because of its initial induction chemotherapy component.

Thus, in clinical practice, the well-established combined-modality approach using fluorouracil and mitomycin-C plus radiation remains the standard of care. Cisplatin-fluorouracil can be used in patients with contraindication against mitomycin.

Intensity-modulated radiation therapy for anal cancer is currently being evaluated, in an effort to reduce acute and long-term toxicity from radiotherapy.[337] Further trials are evaluating the role of cetuximab and bevacizumab as components of multimodality therapy in local and metastatic anal cancers. It is of note in this context that anal cancers have a very low rate of KRAS mutations.[338]

For patients in whom disease is present in the inguinal lymph nodes at the time of diagnosis or in whom disease develops in those nodes metachronously, additional radiation therapy or node dissection may be beneficial, although the latter is used less frequently. Salvage radiation therapy may result in a cure for as many as 50% of patients who have an incomplete response to initial combined-modality therapy or for those who have a local relapse.[339] For patients who have metastatic disease, chemotherapy regimens used for other squamous cell cancers, such as fluorouracil, mitomycin-C, cisplatin, paclitaxel, and others (e.g., EGFR antibodies) should be considered, but such treatment is palliative at best.

KEY POINTS

- Anal cancers are often cured by chemoradiotherapy.
- A quadrivalent HPV vaccine has shown to reduce the incidence of anal intraepithelial neoplasia.

The treatment of anal cancer for patients with HIV is somewhat more complex. Standard aggressive combined-modality therapies should be used for patients with a CD4 count of more than $200/mm^3$ x 10^9/L who have no signs or symptoms of other HIV-related diseases. For patients with more severe HIV-related problems, reduced doses of radiation, chemotherapy, or both should be considered to maintain local disease control.[340]

PANCREATIC ENDOCRINE TUMORS AND NEUROENDOCRINE TUMORS, INCLUDING CARCINOIDS

Pancreatic endocrine tumors are a group of uncommon neoplasms that histologically share several key cytochemical features with melanoma, pheochromocytoma, carcinoid tumors, and medullary thyroid cancers. All amine precursor uptake and decarboxylation neoplasms have the capacity to synthesize and secrete polypeptide products that have specific endocrine hormone activity. Most behave in a malignant fashion. The types of tumors are characterized by the hormones they secrete, including gastrinomas, insulinomas, vasoactive intestinal peptide tumors (VIPomas), glucagonomas, somatostatinomas, growth hormone-releasing factor tumors, and adrenocorticotropic hormone tumors. Pancreatic endocrine tumors and carcinoids are considered either functional (if associated with a clinical syndrome because of the production of hormones) or nonfunctional (if hormones are not a substantial element of the presentation). Thus, it is important to note that the absence of detectable hormone production does not rule out the presence of a neuroendocrine tumor. The nomenclature and classification of neuroendocrine tumors are summarized in Table 9-8.[341]

PANCREATIC NEUROENDOCRINE TUMORS

The diverse clinical presentation of pancreatic neuroendocrine (or islet cell) tumors and their frequently silent and relatively benign pathologic presence makes an accurate determination of their true incidence difficult. Many pancreatic neuroendocrine tumors remain asymptomatic and undiagnosed. Most of these tumors appear in sporadic cases without substantial personal or family history. However, certain patient groups have clear evidence of an inherited predisposition to multiple neoplasias of the endocrine system that is manifested in an autosomal-dominant fashion with mutations in the tumor suppressor gene MEN1 that encodes the protein menin.[342] The syndrome first described (multiple endocrine neoplasia type 1 [MEN1], Wermer syndrome) is characterized by the presence of tumors of the pituitary gland and parathyroid gland, as well as neuroendocrine tumors of the pancreas.[343] Multiple endocrine neoplasia type 2, associated with mutations in the RET gene, typically does not involve pancreatic neuroendocrine tumors; rather, it expresses tumors of the parathyroid, pheochromocytoma, and medullary thyroid cancer.[344]

Table 9-8 Nomenclature and Classification of Neuroendocrine Tumors[341]

Differentiation and Grade	Mitotic Count (/10 HPF)*	Ki-67 Index (%)†	Traditional Classification	ENETS/WHO Classification
Well differentiated				
Low grade (grade 1)	< 2	< 2	Carcinoid, islet cell, pancreatic (neuro) endocrine tumor	Neuroendocrine tumor, grade 1
Intermodiate grade (grade 2)	2 to 20	3 to 20	Carcinoid, atypical carcinoid‡, islet cell, pancreatic (neuro)endocrine tumor	Neuroendocrine tumor, grade 2
Poorly differentiated				
High grade (grade 3)	> 20	> 20	Small-cell carcinoma	Neuroendocrine carcinoma, grade 3 small cell
			Large-cell neuroendocrine carcinoma	Neuroendocrine carcinoma, grade 3 large cell

*HPF, high-power field (x 40 magnification).

†MIB1 antibody.

‡The term atypical carcinoid only applies to intermediate-grade neuroendocrine tumors of the lung.

Abbreviations: ENETS, European Neuroendocrine Tumor Society; WHO, World Health Organization.

Modified from Kulke MH, Siu LL, Tepper JE, et al. Future directions in the treatment of neuroendocrine tumors: consensus report of the National Cancer Institute Neuroendocrine Tumor clinical trials planning meeting. J Clin Oncol. 2011;29:934–943. PMID: 21263089.

CARCINOID TUMORS

About two-thirds of carcinoid tumors occur within the gastrointestinal system, with the appendix being the most common primary location.[345] However, carcinoid tumors may occur throughout the body, including in the chest. Carcinoid tumors are members of the neuroendocrine tumor family and share cytochemical features with melanomas, pheochromocytomas, medullary thyroid cancers, and pancreatic endocrine tumors. Some undifferentiated, and often nonfunctional, carcinoids behave like small cell cancers and have a much more aggressive clinical behavior than common carcinoids, and share characteristics with small cell lung cancers, including their chemotherapy and radiation sensitivity.[346] The determination of cancer can be made only if invasion or distant metastases are found. The disease is most commonly diagnosed during routine appendectomy. Carcinoid tumors synthesize bioactive amine and peptides, including neuron-specific enolase, 5-hydroxytryptamine, synaptophysin, chromogranin A, and other peptides such as insulin, growth hormone, neurotensin, corticotropin, gastrin, pancreatic polypeptide, and calcitonin. More than 80% of patients with resectable primary tumors are disease-free at 20 years with similar overall survival rates for an age- and sex-matched cohort. Of those tumors with regional node metastasis, as many as 50% will recur longer than 10 years after diagnosis. Typically, the prognosis for patients with resectable carcinoid tumors is favorable.[347] It is important to recognize the long disease-free interval that can occur, which requires patients to have a longer period of follow-up than patients with other tumor types. It is also important to note that appendectomy is inadequate if the carcinoid tumor is larger than 2 cm and/or if lymphovascular invasion or involvement of the mesoappendix is present. In these cases, right hemicolectomy is indicated as definitive oncologic surgery.[348]

Carcinoid Syndrome

As with pancreatic neuroendocrine tumors, carcinoid tumors can manifest with signs and symptoms of abnormal hormone production, namely the malignant carcinoid syndrome. Flushing is the most common sign, followed by diarrhea, heart disease (valvular abnormalities), and bronchoconstriction. Diarrhea is not necessarily related to the flushing but appears to be caused by increased gastrointestinal motility as a direct consequence of hormone secretion. For intestinal carcinoids, the characteristic carcinoid syndrome only appears when liver metastases have been established and the biogenic amines can bypass the hepatic metabolic activity. When carcinoid syndrome is suspected, serologic testing should be done to measure 5-hydroxyindoleacetic acid (5-HIAA), 24-hour urine levels, serum serotonin levels, and/or serum chromogranin A. The cardiac disease associated with this condition typically involves abnormalities of the valves on the right side of the heart. Therefore, an echocardiogram is an important element in the evaluation of patients with prolonged disease courses. Novel imaging techniques, including octreotide scanning—a nuclear medicine test specifically designed for the detection of carcinoid tumors—have become more common. Individuals with positive findings on an octreotide scan are more likely to benefit from therapy with octreotide. The most common imaging techniques are CT and MRI, with the latter showing the greatest sensitivity for detection of intrahepatic metastases. PET scans commonly are ineffective because of the low proliferative and low metabolic activity of differentiated carcinoids. Selective sampling of blood through venous catheterization sometimes can be helpful, but this technique is rarely used.

TREATMENT OF PANCREATIC NEUROENDOCRINE TUMORS AND CARCINOID TUMORS

Surgery is the main treatment for these tumors. Most tumors are easily resectable or are found incidentally during operations for other indications. Even when lymph nodes are involved, patients may live for long periods without apparent recurrence, but long-term follow-up typically shows continuing disease relapse over many years. In contrast to the situation for other tumor types, cytoreductive surgery (debulking) for palliative purposes (decreasing the amount of hormone-producing tissue) should be considered for these tumors. Such surgery includes hepatic resection or resection of other intra-abdominal and thoracic metastases. Surgical palliation of bowel obstruction from tumor masses or mesenteric fibrosis associated with carcinoid tumors may substantially improve quality of life for patients. Hepatic surgery for liver metastasis may allow patients to remain disease-free for prolonged periods and may reduce hormone production.

Liver-directed therapy, such as (chemo-)embolization, high-frequency radioablation, or surgical resection, commonly is used for these tumor types.[347] These techniques are particularly useful for reducing symptoms caused by local growth of the tumor or by hormone production and should be regarded as nonsurgical debulking. These procedures also are associated with a greater likelihood of prolonged tumor regression.

Radiation therapy may offer relief for local recurrence or for symptomatic metastasis, such as bone metastases, which are relatively common for patients with advanced carcinoids. An emerging area of research involves the use of radiolabeled octreotide as treatment. The results of ongoing clinical trials may highlight substantial benefits from this approach; however, radioactive octreotide therapy is not yet approved by the FDA.[349]

Octreotide and its analogues have been used for some time to control the secretion of 5-hydroxyindoleacetic acid and other peptides.[350,351] More recently, the analogues have been assessed for their antitumor activity, despite their poor tumoricidal effect resulting in few regressions. There is substantial evidence from small phase II clinical studies that these agents have cytostatic effects and may prolong survival.[346] In a prospective, placebo-controlled, randomized trial in 85 patients with midgut neuroendocrine tumors (classic carcinoids), the use of long-acting octreotide (30 mg intramuscular monthly) was associated with significant delay in tumor progression and a trend toward improvement in overall survival.[352] Another biologic agent that may have benefit is interferon-alfa, which has been shown to decrease the tumor size for a few patients with metastatic disease.[353] Similar to octreotide, interferon appears to have a tumorstatic effect rather than a tumoricidal one. One trial demonstrated a survival advantage for interferon compared with the combination of streptozotocin and fluorouracil[353];

however, the role of interferon for the treatment of differentiated carcinoid tumors is still under debate.

Traditional chemotherapy has been tested extensively for the treatment of patients with carcinoid cancers. Agents commonly used include fluorouracil and its oral analogue capecitabine, streptozotocin, and anthracyclines, such as doxorubicin and liposomal doxorubicin. Unfortunately, response rates for chemotherapeutic agents in combination regimens have been poor (typically less than 20%).[346] Therefore, for most patients, the use of systemic chemotherapy either is reserved for end-of-life care or should not be considered at all. It is important to recognize that the slow-growing nature of carcinoid tumors may allow patients to be followed for a long period without any considerable intervention. Patients should be monitored closely to determine if the disease is slow growing. If so, simple observation often is sufficient.

The outcome with systemic chemotherapy may be better for patients with non-carcinoid pancreas neuroendocrine tumors. One trial, in which streptozotocin plus doxorubicin was compared with streptozotocin plus fluorouracil, demonstrated that the doxorubicin-containing regimen was superior (response rate: 69% vs. 45%, p = 0.05; overall survival: 2.2 vs. 1.4 years, p = 0.004).[354] A combination of capecitabine and temozolomide is currently being tested in prospective trials.

For patients who have poorly differentiated gut neuroendocrine tumors, the selection of chemotherapy is similar to that for small cell lung cancer, with the most consistent regression observed using combination etoposide and cisplatin. This distinction is important and emphasizes the need for pathologic evaluation to distinguish between the small cell variant and the more slow-growing pancreatic neuroendocrine/carcinoid tumors.

Novel biologics including VEGF inhibitors, such as sunitinib, and signal transduction inhibitors, such as mTOR inhibitors, have shown efficacy in pancreatic neuroendocrine tumors.[355,356] Data of a placebo-controlled phase III trial with sunitinib (37.5 mg/day) compared with best supportive care in 169 patients with advanced pancreatic neuroendocrine cancer, all of whom had progressed in the last 12 months, were released.[355] Progression-free survival increased from 5.5 months with placebo to 11.4 months in the sunitinib group (HR 0.42, 95% CI 0.26, 0.66; p < 0.001). Data on overall survival were not mature at the time of presentation, but a reduced death rate was noted in the sunitinib arm at the time of data cut-off (10% vs. 25%, p = 0.02). The most commonly reported grade 3/4 adverse events in the sunitinib group were neutropenia (12%), hypertension (9%), abdominal pain (7%), diarrhea (97%), hypoglycemia (7%), and hand-foot syndrome (7%). In a parallel placebo-controlled phase III trial in 410 patients with advanced low- to intermediate-grade pancreatic neuroendocrine tumors, the mTOR inhibitor everolimus (10 mg daily) likewise improved median progression-free survival from 4.6 months to 11.0 months (HR 0.35, 95% CI 0.27, 0.45; p < 0.001).[356] Overall survival data were still premature because of the indolent nature of these cancers. The most common side effects of everolimus were (all grades) stomatitis (64%), rash (49%), diarrhea (34%), fatigue (31%), and infections (23%). Based on these positive trial results, sunitinib and everolimus gained FDA approval for the treatment of pancreatic neuroendocrine tumors in 2011.

Although these positive results established a new medical standard of care in pancreatic neuroendocrine tumors, the same treatment appears to be less effective in carcinoids. Everolimus added to octreotide demonstrated only modest activity in patients with carcinoids, with only a borderline statistically significant improvement in progression-free survival.[357]

In summary, though, these results can be regarded as proof of principle for the role of multitargeted kinase inhibitors in neuroendocrine cancers. Ongoing studies are currently investigating the activity of combinations of targeted agents (e.g., VEGF plus mTOR inhibition) in neuroendocrine malignancies.[358]

References

1. Siegel R, Naishadham D, Jemal A. Cancer statistics, 2013. *CA Cancer J Clin.* 2013;63:11-30. PMID: 23335087.

2. Devesa SS, Blot WJ, Fraumeni JF Jr. Changing patterns in the incidence of esophageal and gastric carcinoma in the United States. *Cancer.* 1998; 83:2049-2053. PMID: 9827707.

3. Jemal A, Bray F, Center MM, et al. Global cancer statistics. *CA Cancer J Clin.* 2011;61:69-90. PMID: 21296855.

4. Vizcaino AP, Moreno V, Lambert R, et al. Time trends incidence of both major histologic types of esophageal carcinomas in selected countries, 1973-1995. *Int J Cancer.* 2002;99:860-868. PMID: 12115489.

5. Botterweck AA, Schouten LJ, Volovics A, et al. Trends in incidence of adenocarcinoma of the oesophagus and gastric cardia in ten European countries. *Int J Epidemiol.* 2000;29:645-654. PMID: 10922340.

6. Shaheen N, Ransohoff DF. Gastroesophageal reflux, barrett esophagus, and esophageal cancer: scientific review. *JAMA.* 2002;287:1972-1981. PMID: 11960540.

7. Schuchert MJ, Luketich JD. Management of Barrett's esophagus. *Oncology (Williston Park).* 2007;21:1382-1389, 1392; discussion 1392, 1394, 1396. PMID: 18080619.

8. Hvid-Jensen F, Pedersen L, Drewes AM, et al. Incidence of adenocarcinoma among patients with Barrett's esophagus. *N Engl J Med.* 2011;365:1375-1383. PMID: 21995385.

9. Ye W, Held M, Lagergren J, et al. Helicobacter pylori infection and gastric atrophy: risk of adenocarcinoma and squamous-cell carcinoma of the esophagus and adenocarcinoma of the gastric cardia. *J Natl Cancer Inst.* 2004;96:388-396. PMID: 14996860.

10. Gillison ML, Shah KV. Chapter 9: Role of mucosal human papillomavirus in nongenital cancers. *J Natl Cancer Inst Monogr.* 2003;31:57-65. PMID: 12807947.

11. van Vliet EP, Heijenbrok-Kal MH, Hunink MG, et al. Staging investigations for oesophageal cancer: a meta-analysis. *Br J Cancer.* 2008;98:547-557. PMID: 18212745.

12. Flamen P, Lerut A, Van Cutsem E, et al. Utility of positron emission tomography for the staging of patients with potentially operable esophageal carcinoma. *J Clin Oncol.* 2000;18:3202-3210. PMID: 10986052.

13. Juweid ME, Cheson BD. Positron-emission tomography and assessment of cancer therapy. *N Engl J Med.* 2006;354:496-507. PMID: 16452561.

14. Hulscher JB, Tijssen JG, Obertop H, et al. Transthoracic versus transhiatal resection for carcinoma of the esophagus: a meta-analysis. *Ann Thorac Surg.* 2001;72:306-313. PMID: 11465217.

15. Rindani R, Martin CJ, Cox MR. Transhiatal versus Ivor-Lewis oesophagectomy: is there a difference? *Aust N Z J Surg.* 1999;69:187-194. PMID: 10075357.

16. Veeramachaneni NK, Zoole JB, Decker PA, et al. Lymph node analysis in esophageal resection: American College of Surgeons Oncology Group Z0060 trial. *Ann Thorac Surg.* 2008;86:418-421; discussion 2008;421. PMID: 18640307.

17. Wolff CS, Castillo SF, Larson DR, et al. Ivor Lewis approach is superior to transhiatal approach in retrieval of lymph nodes at esophagectomy. *Dis Esophagus.* 2008;21:328-333. PMID: 18477255.

18. Herskovic A, Martz K, al-Sarraf M, et al. Combined chemotherapy and radiotherapy compared with radiotherapy alone in patients with cancer of the esophagus. *N Engl J Med.* 1992;326:1593-1598. PMID: 1584260.

19. Sun DR. Ten-year follow-up of esophageal cancer treated by radical radiation therapy: analysis of 869 patients. *Int J Radiat Oncol Biol Phys.* 1989;16:329-334. PMID: 2921133.

20. van Hagen P, Hulshof MC, van Lanschot JJ, et al. Preoperative chemoradiotherapy for esophageal or junctional cancer. *N Engl J Med.* 2012;366:2074-2084. PMID: 22646630.

21. al-Sarraf M, Martz K, Herskovic A, et al. Progress report of combined chemoradiotherapy versus radiotherapy alone in patients with esophageal cancer: an intergroup study. *J Clin Oncol.* 1997;15:277-284. PMID: 8996153.

22. Wong RK, Malthaner RA, Zuraw L, et al. Combined modality radiotherapy and chemotherapy in nonsurgical management of localized carcinoma of the esophagus: a practice guideline. *Int J Radiat Oncol Biol Phys.* 2003;55:930-942. PMID: 12605971.

23. Meluch AA, Greco FA, Gray JR, et al. Preoperative therapy with concurrent paclitaxel/carboplatin/infusional 5-FU and radiation therapy in locoregional esophageal cancer: final results of a Minnie Pearl Cancer Research Network phase II trial. *Cancer J.* 2003;9:251-260. PMID: 12967135.

24. Cooper JS, Guo MD, Herskovic A, et al. Chemoradiotherapy of locally advanced esophageal cancer: long-term follow-up of a prospective randomized trial (RTOG 85-01). Radiation Therapy Oncology Group. *JAMA.* 1999;281:1623-1627. PMID: 10235156.

25. Stahl M, Stuschke M, Lehmann N, et al. Chemoradiation with and without surgery in patients with locally advanced squamous cell carcinoma of the esophagus. *J Clin Oncol.* 2005;23:2310-2317. PMID: 15800321.

26. Cunningham D, Allum WH, Stenning SP, et al. Perioperative chemotherapy versus surgery alone for resectable gastroesophageal cancer. *N Engl J Med.* 2006;355:11-20. PMID: 16822992.

27. Gebski V, Burmeister B, Smithers BM, et al. Survival benefits from neoadjuvant chemoradiotherapy or chemotherapy in oesophageal carcinoma: a meta-analysis. *Lancet Oncol.* 2007;8:226-234. PMID: 17329193.

28. Urschel JD, Vasan H. A meta-analysis of randomized controlled trials that compared neoadjuvant chemoradiation and surgery to surgery alone for resectable esophageal cancer. *Am J Surg.* 2003;185:538-543. PMID: 12781882.

29. Tepper J, Krasna MJ, Niedzwiecki D, et al. Phase III trial of trimodality therapy with cisplatin, fluorouracil, radiotherapy, and surgery compared with surgery alone for esophageal cancer: CALGB 9781. *J Clin Oncol.* 2008;26:1086-1092. PMID: 18309943.

30. Armanios M, Xu R, Forastiere AA, et al. Adjuvant chemotherapy for resected adenocarcinoma of the esophagus, gastro-esophageal junction, and cardia: phase II trial (E8296) of the Eastern Cooperative Oncology Group. *J Clin Oncol.* 2004;22:4495-4499. PMID: 15542799.

31. Ku GY, Ilson DH. Esophageal cancer: adjuvant therapy. *Cancer J.* 2007;13:162-167. PMID: 17620765.

32. Hwang JJ. Role of chemotherapy in the treatment of gastroesophageal cancers. *Oncology (Williston Park).* 2007;21:579-586; discussion 587, 591-592. PMID: 17536343.

33. Aklilu M, Ilson DH. Targeted agents and esophageal cancer–the next step? *Semin Radiat Oncol.* 2007;17:62-69. PMID: 17185199.

34. Ohtsu A, Shah MA, Van Cutsem E, et al. Bevacizumab in combination with chemotherapy as first-line therapy in advanced gastric cancer: a randomized, double-blind, placebo-controlled phase III study. *J Clin Oncol.* 2011;29:3968-3976. PMID: 21844504.

35. Waddell T, Chau I, Cunningham D, et al. Epirubicin, oxaliplatin, and capecitabine with or without panitumumab for patients with previously untreated advanced oesophagogastric cancer (REAL3): a randomised, open-label phase 3 trial. *Lancet Oncol.* 2013;14:481-489. PMID: 23594787.

36. Fuchs CS, Tomasek J, Yong CJ, et al. Ramucirumab monotherapy for previously treated advanced gastric or gastro-oesophageal junction adenocarcinoma (REGARD): an international, randomised, multicentre, placebo-controlled, phase 3 trial. *Lancet.* 2014;383:31-39. PMID: 24094768.

37. Bang YJ, Van Cutsem E, Feyereislova A, et al. Trastuzumab in combination with chemotherapy versus chemotherapy alone for treatment of HER2-positive advanced gastric or gastro-oesophageal junction cancer (ToGA): a phase 3, open-label, randomised controlled trial. *Lancet.* 2010;376:687-697. PMID: 20728210.

38. Kamineni A, Williams MA, Schwartz SM, et al. The incidence of gastric carcinoma in Asian migrants to the United States and their descendants. *Cancer Causes Control.* 1999;10:77-83. PMID: 10334646.

39. Al-Refaie WB, Tseng JF, Gay G, et al. The impact of ethnicity on the presentation and prognosis of patients with gastric adenocarcinoma. Results from the National Cancer Data Base. *Cancer.* 2008;113:461-469. PMID: 18553367.

40. Kubo A, Corley DA. Body mass index and adenocarcinomas of the esophagus or gastric cardia: a systematic review and meta-analysis. *Cancer Epidemiol Biomarkers Prev.* 2006;15:872-878. PMID: 16702363.

41. Rothwell PM, Fowkes FG, Belch JF, et al. Effect of daily aspirin on long-term risk of death due to cancer: analysis of individual patient data from randomised trials. *Lancet*. 2011;377:31-41. PMID: 21144578.

42. Liu C, Russell RM. Nutrition and gastric cancer risk: an update. *Nutr Rev*. 2008;66:237-249. PMID: 18454810.

43. Eslick GD, Lim LL, Byles JE, et al. Association of Helicobacter pylori infection with gastric carcinoma: a meta-analysis. *Am J Gastroenterol*. 1999;94:2373-2379. PMID: 10483994.

44. Huang JQ, Sridhar S, Chen Y, et al. Meta-analysis of the relationship between Helicobacter pylori seropositivity and gastric cancer. *Gastroenterology*. 1998;114:1169-1179. PMID: 9609753.

45. Parsonnet J, Forman D. Helicobacter pylori infection and gastric cancer–for want of more outcomes. *JAMA*. 2004;291:244-245. PMID: 14722152.

46. Wong BC, Lam SK, Wong WM, et al. Helicobacter pylori eradication to prevent gastric cancer in a high-risk region of China: a randomized controlled trial. *JAMA*. 2004;291:187-194. PMID: 14722144.

47. Fuccio L, Zagari RM, Eusebi LH, et al. Meta-analysis: can Helicobacter pylori eradication treatment reduce the risk for gastric cancer? *Ann Intern Med*. 2009;151:121-128. PMID: 19620164.

48. Herrmann K, Ott K, Buck AK, et al. Imaging gastric cancer with PET and the radiotracers 18F-FLT and 18F-FDG: a comparative analysis. *J Nucl Med*. 2007;48:1945-1950. PMID: 18006614.

49. Bonenkamp JJ, Hermans J, Sasako M, et al. Extended lymph-node dissection for gastric cancer. *N Engl J Med*. 1999;340:908-914. PMID: 10089184.

50. Cuschieri A, Weeden S, Fielding J, et al. Patient survival after D1 and D2 resections for gastric cancer: long-term results of the MRC randomized surgical trial. Surgical Co-operative Group. *Br J Cancer*. 1999;79:1522-1530. PMID: 10188901.

51. Songun I, Putter H, Kranenbarg EM, et al. Surgical treatment of gastric cancer: 15-year follow-up results of the randomised nationwide Dutch D1D2 trial. *Lancet Oncol*. 2010;11:439-449. PMID: 20409751.

52. Earle CC, Maroun JA. Adjuvant chemotherapy after curative resection for gastric cancer in non-Asian patients: revisiting a meta-analysis of randomised trials. *Eur J Cancer*. 1999;35:1059-1064. PMID: 10533448.

53. Macdonald JS, Smalley SR, Benedetti J, et al. Chemoradiotherapy after surgery compared with surgery alone for adenocarcinoma of the stomach or gastroesophageal junction. *N Engl J Med*. 2001;345:725-730. PMID: 11547741.

54. Fuchs CS, Tepper JE, Niedzwiecki D, et al. Postoperative adjuvant chemoradiation for gastric or gastroesophageal junction (GEJ) adenocarcinoma using epirubicin, cisplatin, and infusional (CI) 5-FU (ECF) before and after CI 5-FU and radiotherapy (CRT) compared with bolus 5-FU/LV before and after CRT: Intergroup trial CALGB 80101. *J Clin Oncol*. 2011;29:15s (suppl; abstr 4003).

55. Cascinu S, Labianca R, Barone C, et al. Adjuvant treatment of high-risk, radically resected gastric cancer patients with 5-fluorouracil, leucovorin, cisplatin, and epidoxorubicin in a randomized controlled trial. *J Natl Cancer Inst*. 2007;99:601-607. PMID: 17440161.

56. Sakuramoto S, Sasako M, Yamaguchi T, et al. Adjuvant chemotherapy for gastric cancer with S-1, an oral fluoropyrimidine. *N Engl J Med*. 2007;357:1810-1820. PMID: 17978289.

57. Sasako M, Sakuramoto S, Katai H, et al. Five-year outcomes of a randomized phase III trial comparing adjuvant chemotherapy with S-1 versus surgery alone in stage II or III gastric cancer. *J Clin Oncol*. 2011;29:4387-4393. PMID: 22010012.

58. Bang YJ, Kim YW, Yang HK, et al. Adjuvant capecitabine and oxaliplatin for gastric cancer after D2 gastrectomy (CLASSIC): a phase 3 open-label, randomised controlled trial. *Lancet*. 2012;379:315-321. PMID: 22226517.

59. GASTRIC (Global Advanced/Adjuvant Stomach Tumor Research International Collaboration) Group, Paoletti X, Oba K, et al. Benefit of adjuvant chemotherapy for resectable gastric cancer: a meta-analysis. *JAMA*. 2010;303:1729-1737. PMID: 20442389.

60. Cascinu S, Scartozzi M, Labianca R, et al. High curative resection rate with weekly cisplatin, 5-fluorouracil, epidoxorubicin, 6S-leucovorin, glutathione, and filgastrim in patients with locally advanced, unresectable gastric cancer: a report from the Italian Group for the Study of Digestive Tract Cancer (GISCAD). *Br J Cancer*. 2004;90:1521-1525. PMID: 15083179.

61. Wagner AD, Grothe W, Haerting J, et al. Chemotherapy in advanced gastric cancer: a systematic review and meta-analysis based on aggregate data. *J Clin Oncol*. 2006;24:2903-2909. PMID: 16782930.

62. Webb A, Cunningham D, Scarffe JH, et al. Randomized trial comparing epirubicin, cisplatin, and fluorouracil versus fluorouracil, doxorubicin, and methotrexate in advanced esophagogastric cancer. *J Clin Oncol*. 1997;15:261-267. PMID: 8996151.

63. Van Cutsem E, Moiseyenko VM, Tjulandin S, et al. Phase III study of docetaxel and cisplatin plus fluorouracil compared with cisplatin and fluorouracil as first-line therapy for advanced gastric cancer: a report of the V325 Study Group. *J Clin Oncol*. 2006;24:4991-4997. PMID: 17075117.

64. Cunningham D, Starling N, Rao S, et al. Capecitabine and oxaliplatin for advanced esophagogastric cancer. *N Engl J Med*. 2008;358:36-46. PMID: 18172173.

65. Van Cutsem E, Dicato M, Geva R, et al. The diagnosis and management of gastric cancer: expert discussion and recommendations from the 12th ESMO/World Congress on Gastrointestinal Cancer, Barcelona, 2010. *Ann Oncol*. 2011;22 Suppl 5:v1-v9. PMID: 21633049.

66. Dank M, Zaluski J, Barone C, et al. Randomized phase III study comparing irinotecan combined with 5-fluorouracil and folinic acid to cisplatin combined with 5-fluorouracil in chemotherapy naive patients with advanced adenocarcinoma of the stomach or esophagogastric junction. *Ann Oncol*. 2008;19:1450-1457. PMID: 18558665.

67. Hofmann M, Stoss O, Shi D, et al. Assessment of a HER2 scoring system for gastric cancer: results from a validation study. *Histopathology*. 2008;52:797-805. PMID: 18422971.

68. Bang Y-J. A randomized, open-label, phase III study of lapatinib in combination with weekly paclitaxel versus weekly paclitaxel alone in the second-line treatment of HER2 amplified advanced gastric cancer (AGC) in Asian population: Tytan study. *J Clin Oncol*. 2013;31:4s (suppl; abstr 11).

69. Hecht JR, Bang Y-J, Qin S, et al. Lapatinib in combination with capecitabine plus oxaliplatin (CapeOx) in HER2-positive advanced or metastatic gastric, esophageal, or gastroesophageal adenocarcinoma (AC): The TRIO-013/LOGiC Trial. *J Clin Oncol*. 2013;31:4s (suppl; abstr LBA4001).

70. Lordick F, Kang YK, Chung HC, et al. Capecitabine and cisplatin with or without cetuximab for patients with previously untreated advanced gastric cancer (EXPAND): a randomised, open-label phase 3 trial. *Lancet Oncol*. 2013;14:490-499. PMID: 23594786.

71. Wilke H, Van Cutsem E, Oh SC, et al. RAINBOW: A global, phase III, randomized, double-blind study of ramucirumab plus paclitaxel versus placebo plus paclitaxel in the treatment of metastatic gastroesophageal junction (GEJ) and gastric adenocarcinoma following disease progression on first-line platinum- and fluoropyrimidine-containing combination therapy rainbow IMCL CP12-0922 (I4T-IE-JVBE). *J Clin Oncol*. 2014;32:15s (suppl; abstr LBA7).

72. Park SH, Lim DH, Park K, et al. A multicenter, randomized phase III trial comparing second-line chemotherapy (SLC) plus best supportive care (BSC) with BSC alone for pretreated advanced gastric cancer (AGC). *J Clin Oncol*. 2011;29:15s (suppl; abstr 4004).

73. Thuss-Patience PC, Kretzschmar A, Bichev D, et al. Survival advantage for irinotecan versus best supportive care as second-line chemotherapy in gastric cancer--a randomised phase III study of the Arbeitsgemeinschaft Internistische Onkologie (AIO). *Eur J Cancer*. 2011;47:2306-2314. PMID: 21742485.

74. Kang JH, Lee SI, Lim do H, et al. Salvage chemotherapy for pretreated gastric cancer: a randomized phase III trial comparing chemotherapy plus best supportive care with best supportive care alone. *J Clin Oncol*. 2012;30:1513-1518. PMID: 22412140.

75. Hironaka S, Ueda S, Yasui H, et al. Randomized, open-label, phase III study comparing irinotecan wth paclitaxel in patients with advanced gastric cancer without severe peritoneal metastasis after failure of prior combination chemotherapy using fluoropyrimidine plus platinum: WJOG 4007 Trial. *J Clin Oncol*. 2013;31:4438-4444. PMID: 24190112.

76. Popa EC, Shah MA. Met, IGF1R, and other new targets in upper GI malignancies. *Curr Treat Options Oncol*. 2013;14:321-336. PMID: 23873272.

77. Kleeff J, Michalski C, Friess H, et al. Pancreatic cancer: from bench to 5-year survival. *Pancreas*. 2006;33:111-118. PMID: 16868475.

78. Lowenfels AB, Maisonneuve P. Epidemiology and risk factors for pancreatic cancer. *Best Pract Res Clin Gastroenterol*. 2006;20:197-209. PMID: 16549324.

79. Iodice S, Gandini S, Maisonneuve P, et al. Tobacco and the risk of pancreatic cancer: a review and meta-analysis. *Langenbecks Arch Surg*. 2008;393:535-545. PMID: 18193270.

80. Everhart J, Wright D. Diabetes mellitus as a risk factor for pancreatic cancer. A meta-analysis. *JAMA*. 1995;273:1605-1609. PMID: 7745774.

81. Hruban RH, Petersen GM, Ha PK, et al. Genetics of pancreatic cancer. From genes to families. *Surg Oncol Clin N Am*. 1998;7:1-23. PMID: 9443984.

82. Delpu Y, Hanoun N, Lulka H, et al. Genetic and epigenetic alterations in pancreatic carcinogenesis. *Current Genomics* 2011;12:15-24. PMID: 21886451.

83. Jones S, Zhang X, Parsons DW, et al. Core signaling pathways in human pancreatic cancers revealed by global genomic analyses. *Science*. 2008;321:1801-1806. PMID: 18772397.

84. Hruban RH, Adsay NV, Albores-Saavedra J, et al. Pancreatic intraepithelial neoplasia: a new nomenclature and classification system for pancreatic duct lesions. *Am J Surg Pathol.* 2001;25:579-586. PMID: 11342768.

85. Pannala R, Leirness JB, Bamlet WR, et al. Prevalence and clinical profile of pancreatic cancer-associated diabetes mellitus. *Gastroenterology.* 2008;134:981-987. PMID: 18395079.

86. Beger HG, Rau B, Gansauge F, et al. Treatment of pancreatic cancer: challenge of the facts. *World J Surg.* 2003;27:1075-1084. PMID: 12925907.

87. Kalser MH, Ellenberg SS. Pancreatic cancer. Adjuvant combined radiation and chemotherapy following curative resection. *Arch Surg.* 1985;120:899-903. PMID: 4015380.

88. Klinkenbijl JH, Jeekel J, Sahmoud T, et al. Adjuvant radiotherapy and 5-fluorouracil after curative resection of cancer of the pancreas and peri-ampullary region: phase III trial of the EORTC gastrointestinal tract cancer cooperative group. *Ann Surg.* 1999;230:776-82; discussion 782-784. PMID: 10615932.

89. Neoptolemos JP, Dunn JA, Stocken DD, et al. Adjuvant chemoradiotherapy and chemotherapy in resectable pancreatic cancer: a randomised controlled trial. *Lancet.* 2001;358:1576-1585. PMID: 11716884.

90. Neoptolemos JP, Stocken DD, Friess H, et al. A randomized trial of chemoradiotherapy and chemotherapy after resection of pancreatic cancer. *N Engl J Med.* 2004;350:1200-1210. PMID: 15028824.

91. Neuhaus P, Riess H, Post S, et al. CONKO-001: Final results of the randomized, prospective, multicenter phase III trial of adjuvant chemotherapy with gemcitabine versus observation in patients with resected pancreatic cancer (PC). *J Clin Oncol.* 2008; 26:15s (suppl; abstr LBA4504).

92. Oettle H, Post S, Neuhaus P, et al. Adjuvant chemotherapy with gemcitabine vs observation in patients undergoing curative-intent resection of pancreatic cancer: a randomized controlled trial. *JAMA.* 2007;297:267-277. PMID: 17227978.

93. Oettle H, Neuhaus P, Hochhaus A, et al. Adjuvant chemotherapy with gemcitabine and long-term outcomes among patients with resected pancreatic cancer: the CONKO-001 randomized trial. *JAMA.* 2013;310:1473-1481. PMID: 24104372.

94. Neoptolemos JP, Stocken DD, Bassi C, et al. Adjuvant chemotherapy with fluorouracil plus folinic acid vs gemcitabine following pancreatic cancer resection: a randomized controlled trial. *JAMA.* 2010;304:1073-1081. PMID: 20823433.

95. Fukutomi A, Uesaka K, Boku N, et al. JASPAC 01: randomized phase III trial of adjuvant chemotherapy with gemcitabine versus S-1 for patients with resected pancreatic cancer. *J Clin Oncol.* 2013;31:15s (suppl; abstr 4008).

96. Ueno H, Ioka T, Ikeda M, et al. Randomized phase III study of gemcitabine plus S-1, S-1 alone, or gemcitabine alone in patients with locally advanced and metastatic pancreatic cancer in Japan and Taiwan: GEST study. *J Clin Oncol.* 2013;31:1640-1648. PMID: 23547081.

97. Regine WF, Winter KA, Abrams RA, et al. Fluorouracil vs gemcitabine chemotherapy before and after fluorouracil-based chemoradiation following resection of pancreatic adenocarcinoma: a randomized controlled trial. *JAMA.* 2008;299:1019-1026. PMID: 18319412.

98. Berlin JD. Adjuvant therapy for pancreatic cancer: to treat or not to treat? *Oncology (Williston Park).* 2007;21:712-718; discussion 720, 725-726, 730. PMID: 17564327.

99. Evans DB, Varadhachary GR, Crane CH, et al. Preoperative gemcitabine-based chemoradiation for patients with resectable adenocarcinoma of the pancreatic head. *J Clin Oncol.* 2008;26:3496-3502. PMID: 18640930.

100. Katz MH, Pisters PW, Evans DB, et al. Borderline resectable pancreatic cancer: the importance of this emerging stage of disease. *J Am Coll Surg.* 2008;206:833-846; discussion 846-848. PMID: 18471707.

101. Loehrer PJ, Sr., Feng Y, Cardenes H, et al. Gemcitabine alone versus gemcitabine plus radiotherapy in patients with locally advanced pancreatic cancer: an Eastern Cooperative Oncology Group trial. *J Clin Oncol.* 2011;29:4105-4112. PMID: 21969502.

102. Chauffert B, Mornex F, Bonnetain F, et al. Phase III trial comparing intensive induction chemoradiotherapy (60 Gy, infusional 5-FU and intermittent cisplatin) followed by maintenance gemcitabine with gemcitabine alone for locally advanced unresectable pancreatic cancer. Definitive results of the 2000-01 FFCD/SFRO study. *Ann Oncol.* 2008;19:1592-1599. PMID: 18467316.

103. Hammel P, Huguet F, Van Laethem J-L, et al. Comparison of chemoradiotherapy (CRT) and chemotherapy (CT) in patients with a locally advanced pancreatic cancer (LAPC) controlled after 4 months of gemcitabine with or without erlotinib: Final results of the international phase III LAP 07 study. *J Clin Oncol.* 2013;31:18s (suppl; abstr LBA4003).

104. Conroy T, Desseigne F, Ychou M, et al. FOLFIRINOX versus gemcitabine for metastatic pancreatic cancer. *N Engl J Med.* 2011;364:1817-1825. PMID: 21561347.

105. Kaw M, Singh S, Gagneja H, et al. Role of self-expandable metal stents in the palliation of malignant duodenal obstruction. *Surg Endosc.* 2003;17:646-650. PMID: 12404051.

106. van der Gaag NA, Rauws EA, van Eijck CH, et al. Preoperative biliary drainage for cancer of the head of the pancreas. *N Engl J Med.* 2010;362:129-137. PMID: 20071702.

107. Burris HA 3rd, Moore MJ, Andersen J, et al. Improvements in survival and clinical benefit with gemcitabine as first-line therapy for patients with advanced pancreas cancer: a randomized trial. *J Clin Oncol.* 1997;15:2403-2413. PMID: 9196156.

108. Nieto J, Grossbard ML, Kozuch P. Metastatic pancreatic cancer 2008: is the glass less empty? *Oncologist.* 2008;13:562-576. PMID: 18515741.

109. Moore MJ, Goldstein D, Hamm J, et al. Erlotinib plus gemcitabine compared with gemcitabine alone in patients with advanced pancreatic cancer: a phase III trial of the National Cancer Institute of Canada Clinical Trials Group. *J Clin Oncol.* 2007;25:1960-1966. PMID: 17452677.

110. Cunningham D, Chau I, Stocken DD, et al. Phase III randomized comparison of gemcitabine versus gemcitabine plus capecitabine in patients with advanced pancreatic cancer. *J Clin Oncol.* 2009;27:5513-5518. PMID: 19858379.

111. Heinemann V, Boeck S, Hinke A, et al. Meta-analysis of randomized trials: evaluation of benefit from gemcitabine-based combination chemotherapy applied in advanced pancreatic cancer. *BMC Cancer.* 2008;8:82. PMID: 18373843.

112. Von Hoff DD, Ervin T, Arena FP, et al. Increased survival in pancreatic cancer with nab-paclitaxel plus gemcitabine. *N Engl J Med.* 2013;369:1691-1703. PMID: 24131140.

113. Pelzer U, Schwaner I, Stieler J, et al. Best supportive care (BSC) versus oxaliplatin, folinic acid and 5-fluorouracil (OFF) plus BSC in patients for second-line advanced pancreatic cancer: a phase III-study from the German CONKO-study group. *Eur J Cancer.* 2011;47:1676-1681. PMID: 21565490.

114. Kindler HL, Niedzwiecki D, Hollis D, et al. Gemcitabine plus bevacizumab compared with gemcitabine plus placebo in patients with advanced pancreatic cancer: phase III trial of the Cancer and Leukemia Group B (CALGB 80303). *J Clin Oncol.* 2010;28:3617-3622. PMID: 20606091.

115. Philip PA, Benedetti J, Corless CL, et al. Phase III study comparing gemcitabine plus cetuximab versus gemcitabine in patients with advanced pancreatic adenocarcinoma: Southwest Oncology Group-directed intergroup trial S0205. *J Clin Oncol.* 2010;28:3605-3610. PMID: 20606093.

116. Van Cutsem E, Vervenne WL, Bennouna J, et al. Phase III trial of bevacizumab in combination with gemcitabine and erlotinib in patients with metastatic pancreatic cancer. *J Clin Oncol.* 2009;27:2231-2237. PMID: 19307500.

117. Parkin DM. The global health burden of infection-associated cancers in the year 2002. *Int J Cancer.* 2006;118:3030-3044. PMID: 16404738.

118. El-Serag HB. Epidemiology of hepatocellular carcinoma in USA. *Hepatol Res.* 2007;37 Suppl 2:S88-S94. PMID: 17877502.

119. Torbenson M. Review of the clinicopathologic features of fibrolamellar carcinoma. *Adv Anat Pathol.* 2007;14:217-223. PMID: 17452818.

120. Llovet JM, Burroughs A, Bruix J. Hepatocellular carcinoma. *Lancet.* 2003;362:1907-1917. PMID: 14667750.

121. Sterling RK, Jeffers L, Gordon F, et al. Clinical utility of AFP-L3% measurement in North American patients with HCV-related cirrhosis. *Am J Gastroenterol.* 2007;102:2196-2205. PMID: 17617202.

122. Llovet JM, Bruix J. Systematic review of randomized trials for unresectable hepatocellular carcinoma: chemoembolization improves survival. *Hepatology.* 2003;37:429-442. PMID: 12540704.

123. Sala M, Llovet JM, Vilana R, et al. Initial response to percutaneous ablation predicts survival in patients with hepatocellular carcinoma. *Hepatology.* 2004;40:1352-1360. PMID: 15565564.

124. Germani G, Pleguezuelo M, Gurusamy K, et al. Clinical outcomes of radiofrequency ablation, percutaneous alcohol and acetic acid injection for hepatocellular carcinoma: a meta-analysis. *J Hepatol.* 2010;52:380-388. PMID: 20149473.

125. Mazzaferro V, Llovet JM, Miceli R, et al. Predicting survival after liver transplantation in patients with hepatocellular carcinoma beyond the Milan criteria: a retrospective, exploratory analysis. *Lancet Oncol.* 2009;10:35-43. Epub 2008 Dec 4. PMID: 19058754.

126. Llovet JM, Bruix J. Novel advancements in the management of hepatocellular carcinoma in 2008. *J Hepatol.* 2008;48 Suppl 1:S20-S37. PMID: 18304676.

127. Qin S, Bai Y, Lim HY, et al. Randomized, multicenter, open-label study of oxaliplatin plus fluorouracil/leucovorin versus doxorubicin as palliative chemotherapy in patients with advanced hepatocellular carcinoma from Asia. *J Clin Oncol.* 2013;31:3501-3508. PMID: 23980077.

128. Llovet JM, Ricci S, Mazzaferro V, et al. Sorafenib in advanced hepatocellular carcinoma. *N Engl J Med.* 2008;359:378-390. PMID: 18650514.

129. Cheng AL, Kang YK, Lin DY, et al. Sunitinib versus sorafenib in advanced hepatocellular cancer: results of a randomized phase III trial. *J Clin Oncol.* 2013;31:4067-4075. PMID: 24081937.

130. Bartlett DL. Gallbladder cancer. *Semin Surg Oncol.* 2000;19:145-155. PMID: 11126379.

131. Duffy A, Capanu M, Abou-Alfa GK, et al. Gallbladder cancer (GBC): 10-year experience at Memorial Sloan-Kettering Cancer Centre (MSKCC). *J Surg Oncol.* 2008;98:485-489. PMID: 18802958.

132. Shaib Y, El-Serag HB. The epidemiology of cholangiocarcinoma. *Semin Liver Dis.* 2004;24:115-125. PMID: 15192785.

133. LaRusso NF, Shneider BL, Black D, et al. Primary sclerosing cholangitis: summary of a workshop. *Hepatology.* 2006;44:746-764. PMID: 16941705.

134. Eckel F, Schmid RM. Chemotherapy in advanced biliary tract carcinoma: a pooled analysis of clinical trials. *Br J Cancer.* 2007;96:896-902. PMID: 17325704.

135. Hezel AF, Zhu AX. Systemic therapy for biliary tract cancers. *Oncologist.* 2008;13:415-423. PMID: 18448556.

136. Nakeeb A, Pitt HA. Radiation therapy, chemotherapy and chemoradiation in hilar cholangiocarcinoma. *HPB (Oxford).* 2005;7:278-282. PMID: 18333207.

137. Nelson JW, Ghafoori AP, Willett CG, et al. Concurrent chemoradiotherapy in resected extrahepatic cholangiocarcinoma. *Int J Radiat Oncol Biol Phys.* 2009;73:148-153. PMID: 18805651.

138. Wang SJ, Lemieux A, Kalpathy-Cramer J, et al. Nomogram for predicting the benefit of adjuvant chemoradiotherapy for resected gallbladder cancer. *J Clin Oncol.* 2011;29:4627-4632. PMID: 22067404.

139. Valle J, Wasan H, Palmer DH, et al. Cisplatin plus gemcitabine versus gemcitabine for biliary tract cancer. *N Engl J Med.* 2010;362:1273-1281. PMID: 20375404.

140. Richter JA, Kahaleh M. Photodynamic therapy: palliation and endoscopic technique in cholangiocarcinoma. *World J Gastrointest Endosc.* 2010;2:357-361. PMID: 21173912.

141. Ibrahim SM, Mulcahy MF, Lewandowski RJ, et al. Treatment of unresectable cholangiocarcinoma using yttrium-90 microspheres: results from a pilot study. *Cancer.* 2008;113:2119-2128. PMID: 18759346.

142. Cole BF, Baron JA, Sandler RS, et al. Folic acid for the prevention of colorectal adenomas: a randomized clinical trial. *JAMA.* 2007;297:2351-2359. PMID: 17551129.

143. Park Y, Hunter DJ, Spiegelman D, et al. Dietary fiber intake and risk of colorectal cancer: a pooled analysis of prospective cohort studies. *JAMA.* 2005;294:2849-2857. PMID: 16352792.

144. Wactawski-Wende J, Kotchen JM, Anderson GL, et al. Calcium plus vitamin D supplementation and the risk of colorectal cancer. *N Engl J Med.* 2006;354:684-696. PMID: 16481636.

145. Meyerhardt JA, Giovannucci EL, Holmes MD, et al. Physical activity and survival after colorectal cancer diagnosis. *J Clin Oncol.* 2006;24:3527-3534. PMID: 16822844.

146. Meyerhardt JA, Heseltine D, Niedzwiecki D, et al. Impact of physical activity on cancer recurrence and survival in patients with stage III colon cancer: findings from CALGB 89803. *J Clin Oncol.* 2006;24:3535-3541. PMID: 16822843.

147. Meyerhardt JA, Niedzwiecki D, Hollis D, et al. Association of dietary patterns with cancer recurrence and survival in patients with stage III colon cancer. *JAMA.* 2007;298:754-764. PMID: 17699009.

148. Meyerhardt JA, Niedzwiecki D, Hollis D, et al. Impact of body mass index and weight change after treatment on cancer recurrence and survival in patients with stage III colon cancer: findings from Cancer and Leukemia Group B 89803. *J Clin Oncol.* 2008;26:4109-4115. PMID: 18757324.

149. Baron JA, Cole BF, Sandler RS, et al. A randomized trial of aspirin to prevent colorectal adenomas. *N Engl J Med.* 2003;348:891-899. PMID: 12621133.

150. Flossmann E, Rothwell PM, British Doctors Aspirin Trial and the UK-TIA Aspirin Trial. Effect of aspirin on long-term risk of colorectal cancer: consistent evidence from randomised and observational studies. *Lancet.* 2007;369:1603-1613. PMID: 17499602.

151. Koehne CH, Dubois RN. COX-2 inhibition and colorectal cancer. *Semin Oncol.* 2004;31:12-21. PMID: 15252926.

152. Sandler RS, Halabi S, Baron JA, et al. A randomized trial of aspirin to prevent colorectal adenomas in patients with previous colorectal cancer. *N Engl J Med.* 2003;348:883-890. PMID: 12621132.

153. Burn J, Bishop DT, Mecklin JP, et al. Effect of aspirin or resistant starch on colorectal neoplasia in the Lynch syndrome. *N Engl J Med.* 2008;359:2567-2578. PMID: 19073976.

154. Kinzler KW, Vogelstein B. Lessons from hereditary colorectal cancer. *Cell.* 1996;87:159-170. PMID: 8861899.

155. De Jong AE, Morreau H, Van Puijenbroek M, et al. The role of mismatch repair gene defects in the development of adenomas in patients with HNPCC. *Gastroenterology.* 2004;126:42-48. PMID: 14699485.

156. Goel A, Arnold CN, Niedzwiecki D, et al. Characterization of sporadic colon cancer by patterns of genomic instability. *Cancer Res.* 2003;63:1608-1614. PMID: 12670912.

157. Lindor NM, Burgart LJ, Leontovich O, et al. Immunohistochemistry versus microsatellite instability testing in phenotyping colorectal tumors. *J Clin Oncol.* 2002;20:1043-1048. PMID: 11844828.

158. Carethers JM, Chauhan DP, Fink D, et al. Mismatch repair proficiency and in vitro response to 5-fluorouracil. *Gastroenterology.* 1999;117:123-131. PMID: 10381918.

159. Jover R, Zapater P, Castells A, et al. The efficacy of adjuvant chemotherapy with 5-fluorouracil in colorectal cancer depends on the mismatch repair status. *Eur J Cancer.* 2009;45:365-373. Epub 2008 Aug 21. PMID: 18722765.

160. Meyers M, Wagner MW, Hwang HS, et al. Role of the hMLH1 DNA mismatch repair protein in fluoropyrimidine-mediated cell death and cell cycle responses. *Cancer Res.* 2001;61:5193-5201. PMID: 11431359.

161. Ribic CM, Sargent DJ, Moore MJ, et al. Tumor microsatellite-instability status as a predictor of benefit from fluorouracil-based adjuvant chemotherapy for colon cancer. *N Engl J Med.* 2003;349:247-257. PMID: 12867608.

162. Sargent DJ, Marsoni S, Monges G, et al. Defective mismatch repair as a predictive marker for lack of efficacy of fluorouracil-based adjuvant therapy in colon cancer. *J Clin Oncol.* 2010;28:3219-3226. PMID: 20498393.

163. Moreira L, Balaguer F, Lindor N, et al. Identification of Lynch syndrome among patients with colorectal cancer. *JAMA.* 2012;308:1555-1565. PMID: 23073952.

164. Munkholm P. Review article: the incidence and prevalence of colorectal cancer in inflammatory bowel disease. *Aliment Pharmacol Ther.* 2003;18 Suppl 2:1-5. PMID: 12950413.

165. Kim DH, Pickhardt PJ, Taylor AJ, et al. CT colonography versus colonoscopy for the detection of advanced neoplasia. *N Engl J Med.* 2007;357:1403-1412. PMID: 17914041.

166. Wilschut JA, Habbema JD, van Leerdam ME, et al. Fecal occult blood testing when colonoscopy capacity is limited. *J Natl Cancer Inst.* 2011;103:1741-1751. PMID: 22076285.

167. Levin B, Lieberman DA, McFarland B, et al. Screening and surveillance for the early detection of colorectal cancer and adenomatous polyps, 2008: a joint guideline from the American Cancer Society, the US Multi-Society Task Force on Colorectal Cancer, and the American College of Radiology. *CA Cancer J Clin.* 2008;58:130-160. PMID: 18322143.

168. Nishihara R, Wu K, Lochhead P, et al. Long-term colorectal-cancer incidence and mortality after lower endoscopy. *N Engl J Med.* 2013;369:1095-1105. PMID: 24047059.

169. Shaukat A, Mongin SJ, Geisser MS, et al. Long-term mortality after screening for colorectal cancer. *N Engl J Med.* 2013;369:1106-1114. PMID: 24047060.

170. Vasen HF, Möslein G, Alonso A, et al. Guidelines for the clinical management of Lynch syndrome (hereditary non-polyposis cancer). *J Med Genet.* 2007;44:353-362. PMID: 17327285.

171. Bernstein CN. Surveillance programmes for colorectal cancer in inflammatory bowel disease: have we got it right? *Gut.* 2008;57:1194-1196. PMID: 18719132.

172. Clinical Outcomes of Surgical Therapy Study Group. A comparison of laparoscopically assisted and open colectomy for colon cancer. *N Engl J Med.* 2004;350:2050-2059. PMID: 15141043.

173. van der Pas MH, Haglind E, Cuesta MA, et al. Laparoscopic versus open surgery for rectal cancer (COLOR II): short-term outcomes of a randomised, phase 3 trial. *Lancet Oncol.* 2013;14:210-218. PMID: 23395398.

174. Zlobec I, Lugli A. Prognostic and predictive factors in colorectal cancer. *J Clin Pathol.* 2008;61:561-569. PMID: 18326017.

175. Eschrich S, Yang I, Bloom G, et al. Molecular staging for survival prediction of colorectal cancer patients. *J Clin Oncol.* 2005;23:3526-3535. PMID: 15908663.

176. O'Connell MJ, Lavery I, Yothers G, et al. Relationship between tumor gene expression and recurrence in four independent studies of patients with stage II/III colon cancer treated with surgery alone or surgery plus adjuvant fluorouracil plus leucovorin. *J Clin Oncol.* 2010;28:3937-3944. PMID: 20679606.

177. Moertel CG, Fleming TR, Macdonald JS, et al. Levamisole and fluorouracil for adjuvant therapy of resected colon carcinoma. *N Engl J Med.* 1990;322:352-358. PMID: 2300087.

178. Haller DG, Catalano PJ, Macdonald JS, et al. Phase III study of fluorouracil, leucovorin, and levamisole in high-risk stage II and III colon cancer: final report of Intergroup 0089. *J Clin Oncol.* 2005;23:8671-8678. PMID: 16314627.

179. Sargent DJ, Wieand HS, Haller DG, et al. Disease-free survival versus overall survival as a primary end point for adjuvant colon cancer studies: individual patient data from 20,898 patients on 18 randomized trials. *J Clin Oncol.* 2005;23:8664-8670. PMID: 16260700.

180. Twelves C, Wong A, Nowacki MP, et al. Capecitabine as adjuvant treatment for stage III colon cancer. *N Engl J Med.* 2005;352:2696-2704. PMID: 15987918.

181. André T, Boni C, Mounedji-Boudiaf L, et al. Oxaliplatin, fluorouracil, and leucovorin as adjuvant treatment for colon cancer. *N Engl J Med.* 2004;350:2343-2351. PMID: 15175436.

182. Kuebler JP, Wieand HS, O'Connell MJ, et al. Oxaliplatin combined with weekly bolus fluorouracil and leucovorin as surgical adjuvant chemotherapy for stage II and III colon cancer: results from NSABP C-07. *J Clin Oncol.* 2007;25:2198-2204. PMID: 17470851.

183. André T, Boni C, Navarro M, et al. Improved overall survival with oxaliplatin, fluorouracil, and leucovorin as adjuvant treatment in stage II or III colon cancer in the MOSAIC trial. *J Clin Oncol.* 2009;27:3109-3116. PMID: 19451431.

184. Yothers G, O'Connell MJ, Allegra CJ, et al. Oxaliplatin as adjuvant therapy for colon cancer: updated results of NSABP C-07 trial, including survival and subset analyses. *J Clin Oncol.* 2011;29:3768-3774. PMID: 21859995.

185. Haller DG, Tabernero J, Maroun J, et al. Capecitabine plus oxaliplatin compared with fluorouracil and folinic acid as adjuvant therapy for stage III colon cancer. *J Clin Oncol.* 2011;29:1465-1471. PMID: 21383294.

186. Ychou M, Raoul JL, Douillard JY, et al. A phase III randomised trial of LV-5FU2 + irinotecan versus LV5FU2 alone in adjuvant high-risk colon cancer (FNCLCC Accord02/FFCD9802). *Ann Oncol.* 2009;20:674-680. PMID: 19179549.

187. Van Cutsem E, Labianca R, Bodoky G, et al. Randomized phase III trial comparing biweekly infusional fluorouracil/leucovorin alone or with irinotecan in the adjuvant treatment of stage III colon cancer: PETACC-3. *J Clin Oncol.* 2009;27:3117-3125. PMID: 19451425.

188. Saltz LB, Niedzwiecki D, Hollis D, et al. Irinotecan fluorouracil plus leucovorin is not superior to fluorouracil plus leucovorin alone as adjuvant treatment for stage III colon cancer: results of CALGB 89803. *J Clin Oncol.* 2007;25:3456-3461. PMID: 17687149.

189. André T, Iveson T, Labianca R, et al. The IDEA (International Duration Evaluation of Adjuvant Chemotherapy) Collaboration: prospective combined analysis of phase III trials investigating duration of adjuvant therapy with the FOLFOX (FOLFOX4 or modified FOLFOX6) or XELOX (3 versus 6 months) regimen for patients with stage III colon cancer: trial design and current status. *Curr Colorectal Cancer Rep.* 2013;9:261-269. PMID: 24032000.

190. Goldberg RM, Tabah-Fisch I, Bleiberg H, et al. Pooled analysis of safety and efficacy of oxaliplatin plus fluorouracil/leucovorin administered bimonthly in elderly patients with colorectal cancer. *J Clin Oncol.* 2006;24:4085-4091. PMID: 16943526.

191. Tournigand C, André T, Bonnetain F, et al. Adjuvant therapy with fluorouracil and oxaliplatin in stage II and elderly patients (between ages 70 and 75 years) with colon cancer: subgroup analyses of the Multicenter International Study of Oxaliplatin, Fluorouracil, and Leucovorin in the Adjuvant Treatment of Colon Cancer trial. *J Clin Oncol.* 2012;30:3353-3360. PMID: 22915656.

192. Jackson McCleary NA, Meyerhardt J, Green E, et al. Impact of older age on the efficacy of newer adjuvant therapies in >12,500 patients (pts) with stage II/III colon cancer: Findings from the ACCENT Database. *J Clin Oncol.* 2009;27:15s (suppl; abstr 4010).

193. Mamounas E, Wieand S, Wolmark N, et al. Comparative efficacy of adjuvant chemotherapy in patients with Dukes' B versus Dukes' C colon cancer: results from four National Surgical Adjuvant Breast and Bowel Project adjuvant studies (C-01, C-02, C-03, and C-04). *J Clin Oncol.* 1999;17:1349-1355. PMID: 10334518.

194. Efficacy of adjuvant fluorouracil and folinic acid in B2 colon cancer. International Multicentre Pooled Analysis of B2 Colon Cancer Trials (IMPACT B2) Investigators. *J Clin Oncol.* 1999;17:1356-1363. PMID: 10334519.

195. Schrag D, Rifas-Shiman S, Saltz L, et al. Adjuvant chemotherapy use for Medicare beneficiaries with stage II colon cancer. *J Clin Oncol.* 2002;20:3999-4005. PMID: 12351597.

196. Quasar Collaborative Group, Gray R, Barnwell J, et al. Adjuvant chemotherapy versus observation in patients with colorectal cancer: a randomised study. *Lancet.* 2007;370:2020-2029. PMID: 18083404.

197. Gray RG, Quirke P, Handley K, et al. Validation study of a quantitative multigene reverse transcriptase-polymerase chain reaction assay for assessment of recurrence risk in patients with stage II colon cancer. *J Clin Oncol.* 2011;29:4611-4619. PMID: 22067390.

198. Benson AB 3rd, Schrag D, Somerfield MR, et al. American Society of Clinical Oncology recommendations on adjuvant chemotherapy for stage II colon cancer. *J Clin Oncol.* 2004;22:3408-3419. PMID: 15199089.

199. Gill S, Loprinzi CL, Sargent DJ, et al. Pooled analysis of fluorouracil-based adjuvant therapy for stage II and III colon cancer: who benefits and by how much? *J Clin Oncol.* 2004;22:1797-1806. PMID: 15067028.

200. Mayo Clinic. Adjuvant Systemic Therapy for Melanoma. http://www.mayoclinic.com/calcs. Accessed January 7, 2012.

201. Bardia A, Loprinzi C, Grothey A. Adjuvant chemotherapy for resected stage II and III colon cancer: comparison of two widely used prognostic calculators. *Semin Oncol.* 2010;37:39-46. PMID: 20172363.

202. Gill S, Loprinzi C, Kennecke H, et al. Prognostic web-based models for stage II and III colon cancer: a population and clinical trials-based validation of numeracy and adjuvant! online. *Cancer.* 2011;117:4155-4165. PMID: 21365628.

203. Tejpar S, Bosman F, Delorenzi M, et al. Microsatellite instability (MSI) in stage II and III colon cancer treated with 5FU-LV or 5FU-LV and irinotecan (PETACC 3-EORTC 40993-SAKK 60/00 trial). *J Clin Oncol.* 2009;27:15s (suppl; abstr 4001).

204. Grothey A. Risk assessment in stage II colon cancer: to treat or not to treat? *Oncology.* 2010;24:1-2. PMID: 20225604.

205. Sargent DJ, Resnick MB, Meyers MO, et al. Evaluation of guanylyl cyclase C lymph node status for colon cancer staging and prognosis. *Ann Surg Oncol.* 2011;18:3261-3270. PMID: 21533822.

206. Salazar R, Roepman P, Capella G, et al. Gene expression signature to improve prognosis prediction of stage II and III colorectal cancer. *J Clin Oncol.* 2011;29:17-24. PMID: 21098318.

207. Allegra CJ, Yothers G, O'Connell MJ, et al. Phase III trial assessing bevacizumab in stages II and III carcinoma of the colon: results of NSABP protocol C-08. *J Clin Oncol.* 2011;29:11-16. PMID: 20940184.

208. de Gramont A, Van Cutsem E, Schmoll HJ, et al. Bevacizumab plus oxaliplatin-based chemotherapy as adjuvant treatment for colon cancer (AVANT): a phase 3 randomised controlled trial. *Lancet Oncol.* 2012;13:1225-1233. PMID: 23168362.

209. Alberts SR, Sargent DJ, Nair S, et al. Effect of oxaliplatin, fluorouracil, and leucovorin with or without cetuximab on survival among patients with resected stage III colon cancer: a randomized trial. *JAMA.* 2012;307:1383-1393. PMID: 22474202.

210. Blanke CD, Goldberg RM, Grothey A, et al. KRAS and colorectal cancer: ethical and pragmatic issues in effecting real-time change in oncology clinical trials and practice. *The Oncologist.* 2011;16:1061-1068. PMID: 21737577.

211. Taieb J, Tabernero J, Mini E, et al. Adjuvant FOLFOX4 with or without cetuximab (CTX) in patinets (pts) with resected stage III colon cancer (CC): DFS and OS results and subgroup analyses of the PETACC8 intergroup phase III trial. *Ann Oncol.* 2012;23:9s (suppl; abstr LBA4).

212. Meyerhardt JA. Beyond standard adjuvant therapy for colon cancer: role of nonstandard interventions. *Semin Oncol.* 2011;38:533-541. PMID: 21810512.

213. Liao X, Lochhead P, Nishihara R, et al. Aspirin use, tumor PIK3CA mutation, and colorectal-cancer survival. *N Engl J Med.* 2012;367:1596-1606. PMID: 23094721.

214. Domingo E, Church DN, Sieber O, et al. Evaluation of PIK3CA mutation as a predictor of benefit from nonsteroidal anti-inflammatory drug therapy in colorectal cancer. *J Clin Oncol.* 2013;31:4297-4305. PMID: 24062397.

215. Grothey A, Marshall JL. Optimizing palliative treatment of metastatic colorectal cancer in the era of biologic therapy. *Oncology (Williston Park).* 2007;21:553-64, 566; discussion 566-568, 577-578. PMID: 17536342.

216. Poon MA, O'Connell MJ, Moertel CG, et al. Biochemical modulation of fluorouracil: evidence of significant improvement of survival and quality of life in patients with advanced colorectal carcinoma. *J Clin Oncol.* 1989;7:1407-1418. PMID: 2476530.

217. Petrelli N, Douglass HO, Jr., Herrera L, et al. The modulation of fluorouracil with leucovorin in metastatic colorectal carcinoma: a prospective randomized phase III trial. Gastrointestinal Tumor Study Group. *J Clin Oncol.* 1989;7:1419-1426. PMID: 2674331.

218. de Gramont A, Bosset JF, Milan C, et al. Randomized trial comparing monthly low-dose leucovorin and fluorouracil bolus with bimonthly high-dose leucovorin and fluorouracil bolus plus continuous infusion for advanced colorectal cancer: a French intergroup study. *J Clin Oncol.* 1997;15:808-815. PMID: 9053508.

219. Köhne CH, Wils J, Lorenz M, et al. Randomized phase III study of high-dose fluorouracil given as a weekly 24-hour infusion with or without leucovorin

versus bolus fluorouracil plus leucovorin in advanced colorectal cancer: European organization of Research and Treatment of Cancer Gastrointestinal Group Study 40952. *J Clin Oncol.* 2003;21:3721-3728. PMID: 12963704.

220. Hoff PM, Ansari R, Batist G, et al. Comparison of oral capecitabine versus intravenous fluorouracil plus leucovorin as first-line treatment in 605 patients with metastatic colorectal cancer: results of a randomized phase III study. *J Clin Oncol.* 2001;19:2282-2292. PMID: 11304782.

221. Arkenau HT, Arnold D, Cassidy J, et al. Efficacy of oxaliplatin plus capecitabine or infusional fluorouracil/leucovorin in patients with metastatic colorectal cancer: a pooled analysis of randomized trials. *J Clin Oncol.* 2008;26:5910-5917. PMID: 19018087.

222. Cassidy J, Clarke S, Díaz-Rubio E, et al. Randomized phase III study of capecitabine plus oxaliplatin compared with fluorouracil/folinic acid plus oxaliplatin as first-line therapy for metastatic colorectal cancer. *J Clin Oncol.* 2008;26:2006-2012. PMID: 18421053.

223. Porschen R, Arkenau HT, Kubicka S, et al. Phase III study of capecitabine plus oxaliplatin compared with fluorouracil and leucovorin plus oxaliplatin in metastatic colorectal cancer: a final report of the AIO Colorectal Study Group. *J Clin Oncol.* 2007;25:4217-4223. PMID: 17548840.

224. Haller DG, Cassidy J, Clarke SJ, et al. Potential regional differences for the tolerability profiles of fluoropyrimidines. *J Clin Oncol.* 2008;26:2118-2123. PMID: 18445840.

225. Van Cutsem E, Findlay M, Osterwalder B, et al. Capecitabine, an oral fluoropyrimidine carbamate with substantial activity in advanced colorectal cancer: results of a randomized phase II study. *J Clin Oncol.* 2000;18:1337-1345. PMID: 10715306.

226. Hochster HS, Hart LL, Ramanathan RK, et al. Safety and efficacy of oxaliplatin and fluoropyrimidine regimens with or without bevacizumab as first-line treatment of metastatic colorectal cancer: results of the TREE Study. *J Clin Oncol.* 2008;26:3523-3529. PMID: 18640933.

227. Cunningham D, Pyrhönen S, James RD, et al. Randomised trial of irinotecan plus supportive care versus supportive care alone after fluorouracil failure for patients with metastatic colorectal cancer. *Lancet.* 1998;352:1413-1418. PMID: 9807987.

228. Douillard JY, Cunningham D, Roth AD, et al. Irinotecan combined with fluorouracil compared with fluorouracil alone as first-line treatment for metastatic colorectal cancer: a multicentre randomised trial. *Lancet.* 2000;355:1041-1047. PMID: 10744089.

229. Rougier P, Van Cutsem E, Bajetta E, et al. Randomised trial of irinotecan versus fluorouracil by continuous infusion after fluorouracil failure in patients with metastatic colorectal cancer. *Lancet.* 1998;352:1407-1412. PMID: 9807986.

230. Saltz LB, Cox JV, Blanke C, et al. Irinotecan plus fluorouracil and leucovorin for metastatic colorectal cancer. Irinotecan Study Group. *N Engl J Med.* 2000;343:905-914. PMID: 11006366.

231. Seymour MT, Maughan TS, Ledermann JA, et al. Different strategies of sequential and combination chemotherapy for patients with poor prognosis advanced colorectal cancer (MRC FOCUS): a randomised controlled trial. *Lancet.* 2007;370:143-152. PMID: 17630037.

232. Köhne CH, van Cutsem E, Wils J, et al. Phase III study of weekly high-dose infusional fluorouracil plus folinic acid with or without irinotecan in patients with metastatic colorectal cancer: European Organisation for Research and Treatment of Cancer Gastrointestinal Group Study 40986. *J Clin Oncol.* 2005;23:4856-4865. PMID: 15939923.

233. de Gramont A, Figer A, Seymour M, et al. Leucovorin and fluorouracil with or without oxaliplatin as first-line treatment in advanced colorectal cancer. *J Clin Oncol.* 2000;18:2938-2947. PMID: 10944126.

234. Giacchetti S, Perpoint B, Zidani R, et al. Phase III multicenter randomized trial of oxaliplatin added to chronomodulated fluorouracil-leucovorin as first-line treatment of metastatic colorectal cancer. *J Clin Oncol.* 2000;18:136-147. PMID: 10623704.

235. Grothey A, Deschler B, Kroening H, et al. Phase III study of bolus 5-fluorouracil (5-FU)/ folinic acid (FA) (Mayo) vs. weekly high-dose 24h 5-FU infusion/ FA + oxaliplatin (OXA) in advanced colorectal cancer (ACRC). *Proc Am Soc Clin Oncol.* 2002;21:129a (abstr 512).

236. Rothenberg ML, Oza AM, Bigelow RH, et al. Superiority of oxaliplatin and fluorouracil-leucovorin compared with either therapy alone in patients with progressive colorectal cancer after irinotecan and fluorouracil-leucovorin: interim results of a phase III trial. *J Clin Oncol.* 2003;21:2059-2069. PMID: 12775730.

237. Grothey A. Oxaliplatin-safety profile: neurotoxicity. *Semin Oncol.* 2003;30:5-13. PMID: 14523789.

238. Grothey A, Nikcevich DA, Sloan JA, et al. Intravenous calcium and magnesium for oxaliplatin-induced sensory neurotoxicity in adjuvant colon cancer: NCCTG N04C7. *J Clin Oncol.* 2011;29:421-427. PMID: 21189381.

239. Loprinzi CL, Qin R, Dakhil SR, et al. Phase III randomized, placebo-controlled, double-blind study of intravenous calcium and magnesium to prevent oxaliplatin-induced sensory neurotoxicity (N08CB/Alliance). *J Clin Oncol.* 2014;32:997-1005. PMID: 24297951.

240. Goldberg RM, Sargent DJ, Morton RF, et al. A randomized controlled trial of fluorouracil plus leucovorin, irinotecan, and oxaliplatin combinations in patients with previously untreated metastatic colorectal cancer. *J Clin Oncol.* 2004;22:23-30. PMID: 14665611.

241. Colucci G, Gebbia V, Paoletti G, et al. Phase III randomized trial of FOLFIRI versus FOLFOX4 in the treatment of advanced colorectal cancer: a multicenter study of the Gruppo Oncologico Dell'Italia Meridionale. *J Clin Oncol.* 2005;23:4866-4875. PMID: 15939922.

242. Tournigand C, André T, Achille E, et al. FOLFIRI followed by FOLFOX6 or the reverse sequence in advanced colorectal cancer: a randomized GERCOR study. *J Clin Oncol.* 2004;22:229-237. PMID: 14657227.

243. Grothey A, Sargent D, Goldberg RM, et al. Survival of patients with advanced colorectal cancer improves with the availability of fluorouracil-leucovorin, irinotecan, and oxaliplatin in the course of treatment. *J Clin Oncol.* 2004;22:1209-1214. PMID: 15051767.

244. Falcone A, Ricci S, Brunetti I, et al. Phase III trial of infusional fluorouracil, leucovorin, oxaliplatin, and irinotecan (FOLFOXIRI) compared with infusional fluorouracil, leucovorin, and irinotecan (FOLFIRI) as first-line treatment for metastatic colorectal cancer: the Gruppo Oncologico Nord Ovest. *J Clin Oncol.* 2007;25:1670-1676. PMID: 17470860.

245. Hicklin DJ, Ellis LM. Role of the vascular endothelial growth factor pathway in tumor growth and angiogenesis. *J Clin Oncol.* 2005;23:1011-1027. PMID: 15585754.

246. Hurwitz H, Fehrenbacher L, Novotny W, et al. Bevacizumab plus irinotecan, fluorouracil, and leucovorin for metastatic colorectal cancer. *N Engl J Med.* 2004;350:2335-2342. PMID: 15175435.

247. Giantonio BJ, Catalano PJ, Meropol NJ, et al. Bevacizumab in combination with oxaliplatin, fluorouracil, and leucovorin (FOLFOX4) for previously treated metastatic colorectal cancer: results from the Eastern Cooperative Oncology Group Study E3200. *J Clin Oncol.* 2007;25:1539-1544. PMID: 17442997.

248. Kabbinavar FF, Hambleton J, Mass RD, et al. Combined analysis of efficacy: the addition of bevacizumab to fluorouracil/leucovorin improves survival for patients with metastatic colorectal cancer. *J Clin Oncol.* 2005;23:3706-3712. PMID: 15867200.

249. Saltz LB, Clarke S, Díaz-Rubio E, et al. Bevacizumab in combination with oxaliplatin-based chemotherapy as first-line therapy in metastatic colorectal cancer: a randomized phase III study. *J Clin Oncol.* 2008;26:2013-2019. PMID: 18421054.

250. Fuchs CS, Marshall J, Mitchell E, et al. Randomized, controlled trial of irinotecan plus infusional, bolus, or oral fluoropyrimidines in first-line treatment of metastatic colorectal cancer: results from the BICC-C Study. *J Clin Oncol.* 2007;25:4779-4786. PMID: 17947725.

251. Grothey A. Recognizing and managing toxicities of molecular targeted therapies for colorectal cancer. *Oncology (Williston Park).* 2006;20:21-28. PMID: 17354514.

252. Nalluri SR, Chu D, Keresztes R, et al. Risk of venous thromboembolism with the angiogenesis inhibitor bevacizumab in cancer patients: a meta-analysis. *JAMA.* 2008;300:2277-2285. PMID: 19017914.

253. Hurwitz HI, Saltz LB, Van Cutsem E, et al. Venous thromboembolic events with chemotherapy plus bevacizumab: a pooled analysis of patients in randomized phase II and III studies. *J Clin Oncol.* 2011;29:1757-1764. PMID: 21422411.

254. Cunningham D, Lang I, Marcuello E, et al. Bevacizumab plus capecitabine versus capecitabine alone in elderly patients with previously untreated metastatic colorectal cancer (AVEX): an open-label, randomised phase 3 trial. *Lancet Oncol.* 2013;14:1077-1085. PMID: 24028813.

255. Saltz LB, Lenz HJ, Kindler HL, et al. Randomized phase II trial of cetuximab, bevacizumab, and irinotecan compared with cetuximab and bevacizumab alone in irinotecan-refractory colorectal cancer: the BOND-2 study. *J Clin Oncol.* 2007;25:4557-4561. PMID: 17876013.

256. Hecht JR, Mitchell E, Chidiac T, et al. A randomized phase IIIB trial of chemotherapy, bevacizumab, and panitumumab compared with chemotherapy and bevacizumab alone for metastatic colorectal cancer. *J Clin Oncol.* 2008;27:672-680. PMID: 19114685.

257. Tol J, Koopman M, Cats A, et al. Chemotherapy, bevacizumab, and cetuximab in metastatic colorectal cancer. *N Engl J Med.* 2009;360:563-572. PMID: 19196673.

258. Kuczynski EA, Sargent DJ, Grothey A, et al. Drug rechallenge and treatment beyond progression–implications for drug resistance. *Nat Rev Clin Oncol.* 2013;10:571-587. PMID: 23999218.

259. Koopman M, Simkens LH, Ten Tije AJ, et al. Maintenance treatment with capecitabine and bevacizumab versus observation after induction treatment with chemotherapy and bevacizumab in metastatic colorectal cancer (mCRC): The phase III CAIRO3 study of the Dutch Colorectal Cancer Group (DCCG). *J Clin Oncol.* 2013;31:15s (suppl; abstr 3502).

260. Bennouna J, Sastre J, Arnold D, et al. Continuation of bevacizumab after first progression in metastatic colorectal cancer (ML18147): a randomised phase 3 trial. *Lancet Oncol.* 2013;14:29-37. PMID: 23168366.

261. Saltz LB, Meropol NJ, Loehrer PJ Sr, et al. Phase II trial of cetuximab in patients with refractory colorectal cancer that expresses the epidermal growth factor receptor. *J Clin Oncol.* 2004;22:1201-1208. PMID: 14993230.

262. Cunningham D, Humblet Y, Siena S, et al. Cetuximab monotherapy and cetuximab plus irinotecan in irinotecan-refractory metastatic colorectal cancer. *N Engl J Med.* 2004;351:337-345. PMID: 15269313.

263. Van Cutsem E, Peeters M, Siena S, et al. Open-label phase III trial of panitumumab plus best supportive care compared with best supportive care alone in patients with chemotherapy-refractory metastatic colorectal cancer. *J Clin Oncol.* 2007;25:1658-1664. PMID: 17470858.

264. Jonker DJ, O'Callaghan CJ, Karapetis CS, et al. Cetuximab for the treatment of colorectal cancer. *N Engl J Med.* 2007;357:2040-2048. PMID: 18003960.

265. Bokemeyer C, Bondarenko I, Makhson A, et al. Fluorouracil, leucovorin, and oxaliplatin with and without cetuximab in the first-line treatment of metastatic colorectal cancer. *J Clin Oncol.* 2009;27:663-671. PMID: 19114683.

266. Douillard JY, Siena S, Cassidy J, et al. Randomized, phase III trial of panitumumab with infusional fluorouracil, leucovorin, and oxaliplatin (FOLFOX4) versus FOLFOX4 alone as first-line treatment in patients with previously untreated metastatic colorectal cancer: the PRIME study. *J Clin Oncol.* 2010;28:4697-4705. PMID: 20921465.

267. Van Cutsem E, Köhne CH, Láng I, et al. Cetuximab plus irinotecan, fluorouracil, and leucovorin as first-line treatment for metastatic colorectal cancer: updated analysis of overall survival according to tumor KRAS and BRAF mutation status. *J Clin Oncol.* 2011;29:2011-2019. PMID: 21502544.

268. Van Cutsem E, Köhne CH, Hitre E, et al. Cetuximab and chemotherapy as initial treatment for metastatic colorectal cancer. *N Engl J Med.* 2009;360:1408-1417. PMID: 19339720.

269. Price T, Peeters M, Kim T, et al. ASPECCT: a randomized, multicenter, open-label, phase 3 study of panitumumab (pmab) vs cetuximab (cmab) for previously treated wild-type (WT) KRAS metastatic colorectal cancer (mCRC). Paper presented at: the 38th Congress of the European Society for Medical Oncology (ESMO); September 27-October 1, 2013; Amsterdam, Netherlands.

270. Chung CH, Mirakhur B, Chan E, et al. Cetuximab-induced anaphylaxis and IgE specific for galactose-alpha-1,3-galactose. *N Engl J Med.* 2008;358:1109-1117. PMID: 18337601.

271. Amado RG, Wolf M, Peeters M, et al. Wild-type KRAS is required for panitumumab efficacy in patients with metastatic colorectal cancer. *J Clin Oncol.* 2008;26:1626-1634. PMID: 18316791.

272. Artale S, Sartore-Bianchi A, Veronese SM, et al. Mutations of KRAS and BRAF in primary and matched metastatic sites of colorectal cancer. *J Clin Oncol.* 2008;26:4217-4219. PMID: 18757324.

273. Bokemeyer C, Bondarenko I, Hartmann JT, et al. KRAS status and efficacy of first-line treatment of patients with metastatic colorectal cancer (mCRC) with FOLFOX with or without cetuximab: The OPUS experience. *J Clin Oncol.* 2008;26:15s (suppl; abstr 4000).

274. Karapetis CS, Khambata-Ford S, Jonker DJ, et al. K-ras mutations and benefit from cetuximab in advanced colorectal cancer. *N Engl J Med.* 2008;359:1757-1765. PMID: 18946061.

275. Lièvre A, Bachet JB, Le Corre D, et al. KRAS mutation status is predictive of response to cetuximab therapy in colorectal cancer. *Cancer Res.* 2006;66:3992-3995. PMID: 16618717.

276. Rajagopalan H, Bardelli A, Lengauer C, et al. Tumorigenesis: RAF/RAS oncogenes and mismatch-repair status. *Nature.* 2002;418:934. PMID: 12198537.

277. Malumbres M, Barbacid M. RAS oncogenes: the first 30 years. *Nat Rev Cancer.* 2003;3:459-465. PMID: 12778136.

278. Douillard JY, Oliner KS, Siena S, et al. Panitumumab-FOLFOX4 treatment and RAS mutations in colorectal cancer. *N Engl J Med.* 2013;369:1023-1034. PMID: 24024839.

279. Stinzing S, Jung A, Rossius L, et al. Analysis of KRAS/NRAS and BRAF mutations in FIRE-3: A randomized phase III study of FOLFIRI plus cetuximab or bevacizumab as first-line treatment for wild-type (WT) KRAS (exon 2) metastatic colorectal cancer (mCRC) patients. Paper presented at: the 38th Congress of the European Society for Medical Oncology (ESMO); September 27-October 1, 2013; Amsterdam, Netherlands.

280. De Roock W, Claes B, Bernasconi D, et al. Effects of KRAS, BRAF, NRAS, and PIK3CA mutations on the efficacy of cetuximab plus chemotherapy in chemotherapy-refractory metastatic colorectal cancer: a retrospective consortium analysis. *Lancet Oncol.* 2010;11:753-762. PMID: 20619739.

281. Frattini M, Saletti P, Romagnani E, et al. PTEN loss of expression predicts cetuximab efficacy in metastatic colorectal cancer patients. *Br J Cancer.* 2007;97:1139-1145. PMID: 17940504.

282. Khambata-Ford S, Garrett CR, Meropol NJ, et al. Expression of epiregulin and amphiregulin and K-ras mutation status predict disease control in metastatic colorectal cancer patients treated with cetuximab. *J Clin Oncol.* 2007;25:3230-3237. PMID: 17664471.

283. Loupakis F, Pollina L, Stasi I, et al. Evaluation of PTEN expression in colorectal cancer (CRC) metastases (mets) and in primary tumors as predictors of activity of cetuximab plus irinotecan treatment. *J Clin Oncol.* 2008;26:15s (suppl; abstr 4003).

284. Di Nicolantonio F, Martini M, Molinari F, et al. Wild-type BRAF is required for response to panitumumab or cetuximab in metastatic colorectal cancer. *J Clin Oncol.* 2008;26:5705-5712. PMID: 19001320.

285. Masi G, Loupakis F, Salvatore L, et al. Bevacizumab with FOLFOXIRI (irinotecan, oxaliplatin, fluorouracil, and folinate) as first-line treatment for metastatic colorectal cancer: a phase 2 trial. *Lancet Oncol.* 2010;11:845-852. PMID: 20702138.

286. Loupakis F, Cremolini C, Salvatore L, et al. FOLFOXIRI plus bevacizumab as first-line treatment in BRAF mutant metastatic colorectal cancer. *Eur J Cancer.* 2014;50:57-63. PMID: 24138831.

287. Heinemann V, Fischer von Weikersthal L, Decker T, et al. Randomized comparison of FOLFIRI plus cetuximab versus FOLFIRI plus bevacizumab as first-line treatment of KRAS wild-type metastatic colorectal cancer: German AIO study KRK-0306 (FIRE-3). *J Clin Oncol.* 2013;31:15s (suppl; abstr LBA3506).

288. Holash J, Davis S, Papadopoulos N, et al. VEGF-Trap: a VEGF blocker with potent antitumor effects. *Proc Natl Acad Sci U S A.* 2002;99:11393-11398. PMID: 12177445.

289. Van Cutsem E, Tabernero J, Lakomy R, et al. Addition of aflibercept to fluorouracil, leucovorin, and irinotecan improves survival in a phase III randomized trial in patients with metastatic colorectal cancer previously treated with an oxaliplatin-based regimen. *J Clin Oncol.* 2012;30:3499-3506. PMID: 22949147.

290. Wilhelm SM, Dumas J, Adnane L, et al. Regorafenib (BAY 73-4506): a new oral multikinase inhibitor of angiogenic, stromal and oncogenic receptor tyrosine kinases with potent preclinical antitumor activity. *Int J Cancer.* 2011;129:245-255. PMID: 21170960.

291. Grothey A, Van Cutsem E, Sobrero A, et al. Regorafenib monotherapy for previously treated metastatic colorectal cancer (CORRECT): an international, multicentre, randomised, placebo-controlled, phase 3 trial. *Lancet.* 2013;381:303-312. PMID: 23177514.

292. Poston GJ, Adam R, Alberts S, et al. OncoSurge: a strategy for improving resectability with curative intent in metastatic colorectal cancer. *J Clin Oncol.* 2005;23:7125-7134. PMID: 16192596.

293. Bismuth H, Adam R, Lévi F, et al. Resection of nonresectable liver metastases from colorectal cancer after neoadjuvant chemotherapy. *Ann Surg.* 1996;224:509-20; discussion 1996;520-522. PMID: 8857855.

294. Adam R, Chiche L, Aloia T, et al. Hepatic resection for noncolorectal nonendocrine liver metastases: analysis of 1,452 patients and development of a prognostic model. *Ann Surg.* 2006;244:524-535. PMID: 16998361.

295. Fong Y, Fortner J, Sun RL, et al. Clinical score for predicting recurrence after hepatic resection for metastatic colorectal cancer: analysis of 1001 consecutive cases. *Ann Surg.* 1999;230:309-318; discussion 318-321. PMID: 10493478.

296. Nordlinger B, Guiguet M, Vaillant JC, et al. Surgical resection of colorectal carcinoma metastases to the liver. A prognostic scoring system to improve case selection, based on 1568 patients. Association Française de Chirurgie. *Cancer.* 1996;77:1254-1262. PMID: 8608500.

297. Nordlinger B, Sorbye H, Glimelius B, et al. Perioperative chemotherapy with FOLFOX4 and surgery versus surgery alone for resectable liver metastases from colorectal cancer (EORTC Intergroup trial 40983): a randomised controlled trial. *Lancet.* 2008;371:1007-1016. PMID: 18358928.

298. Petrelli N. Update on surgical resection of liver metastases from colorectal cancer. *Clin Adv Hematol Oncol.* 2008;6:514-516. PMID: 18654118.

299. Folprecht G, Grothey A, Alberts S, et al. Neoadjuvant treatment of unresectable colorectal liver metastases: correlation between tumour response and resection rates. *Ann Oncol.* 2005;16:1311-1319. PMID: 15870084.

300. Kemeny N, Huang Y, Cohen AM, et al. Hepatic arterial infusion of chemotherapy after resection of hepatic metastases from colorectal cancer. *N Engl J Med.* 1999;341:2039-2048. PMID: 10615075.

301. Mitry E, Fields AL, Bleiberg H, et al. Adjuvant chemotherapy after potentially curative resection of metastases from colorectal cancer: a pooled

analysis of two randomized trials. *J Clin Oncol*. 2008;26:4906-4911. PMID: 18794541.

302. Folprecht G, Gruenberger T, Bechstein WO, et al. Tumour response and secondary resectability of colorectal liver metastases following neoadjuvant chemotherapy with cetuximab: the CELIM randomised phase 2 trial. *Lancet Oncol*. 2010;11:38-47. PMID: 19942479.

303. Primrose JN, Falk S, Finch-Jones M, et al. A randomized clinical trial of chemotherapy compared to chemotherapy in combination with cetuximab in k-RAS wild-type patients with operable metastases from colorectal cancer: The new EPOC study. *J Clin Oncol*. 2013;31:15s (suppl; abstr 3504).

304. Ellis LM, Curley SA, Grothey A. Surgical resection after downsizing of colorectal liver metastasis in the era of bevacizumab. *J Clin Oncol*. 2005;23:4853-4855. PMID: 16051943.

305. Cercek A, Saltz L. Factors dictating outcomes in patients with colorectal cancer and peritoneal carcinomatosis: selection, resection, or convection? *J Clin Oncol*. 2012;30:226-228. Epub 2011 Dec 12. PMID: 22162591.

306. Meyerhardt JA, Tepper JE, Niedzwiecki D, et al. Impact of hospital procedure volume on surgical operation and long-term outcomes in high-risk curatively resected rectal cancer: findings from the Intergroup 0114 Study. *J Clin Oncol*. 2004;22:166-174. PMID: 14701779.

307. Sebag-Montefiore D, Stephens RJ, Steele R, et al. Preoperative radiotherapy versus selective postoperative chemoradiotherapy in patients with rectal cancer (MRC CR07 and NCIC-CTG C016): a multicentre, randomised trial. *Lancet*. 2009;373:811-820. PMID: 19269519.

308. Nastro P, Beral D, Hartley J, et al. Local excision of rectal cancer: review of literature. *Dig Surg*. 2005;22:6-15. PMID: 15761225.

309. Heald RJ, Ryall RD. Recurrence and survival after total mesorectal excision for rectal cancer. *Lancet*. 1986;1:1479-1482. PMID: 2425199.

310. Kapiteijn E, Marijnen CA, Nagtegaal ID, et al. Preoperative radiotherapy combined with total mesorectal excision for resectable rectal cancer. *N Engl J Med*. 2001;345:638-646. PMID: 11547717.

311. Quirke P, Steele R, Monson J, et al. Effect of the plane of surgery achieved on local recurrence in patients with operable rectal cancer: a prospective study using data from the MRC CR07 and NCIC-CTG CO16 randomised clinical trial. *Lancet*. 2009;373:821-828. PMID: 19269520.

312. Sauer R, Becker H, Hohenberger W, et al. Preoperative versus postoperative chemoradiotherapy for rectal cancer. *N Engl J Med*. 2004;351:1731-1740. PMID: 15496622.

313. Improved survival with preoperative radiotherapy in resectable rectal cancer. Swedish Rectal Cancer Trial. *N Engl J Med*. 1997;336:980-987. PMID: 9091798.

314. Krook JE, Moertel CG, Gunderson LL, et al. Effective surgical adjuvant therapy for high-risk rectal carcinoma. *N Engl J Med*. 1991;324:709-715. PMID: 1997835.

315. Fisher B, Wolmark N, Rockette H, et al. Postoperative adjuvant chemotherapy or radiation therapy for rectal cancer: results from NSABP protocol R-01. *J Natl Cancer Inst*. 1988;80:21-29. PMID: 3276900.

316. O'Connell MJ, Martenson JA, Wieand HS, et al. Improving adjuvant therapy for rectal cancer by combining protracted-infusion fluorouracil with radiation therapy after curative surgery. *N Engl J Med*. 1994;331:502-507. PMID: 8041415.

317. Roh MS, Yothers GA, O'Connell MJ, et al. The impact of capecitabine and oxaliplatin in the preoperative multimodality treatment in patients with carcinoma of the rectum: NSABP R-04. *J Clin Oncol*. 2011;29:15s (suppl; abstr 3503).

318. Hofheinz RD, Wenz F, Post S, et al. Chemoradiotherapy with capecitabine versus fluorouracil for locally advanced rectal cancer: a randomised, multicentre, non-inferiority, phase 3 trial. *Lancet Oncol*. 2012;13:579-588. PMID: 22503032.

319. Bertolini F, Chiara S, Bengala C, et al. Neoadjuvant treatment with single-agent cetuximab followed by 5-FU, cetuximab, and pelvic radiotherapy: a phase II study in locally advanced rectal cancer. *Int J Radiat Oncol Biol Phys*. 2009;73:466-472. Epub 2008 Nov 10. PMID: 19004567.

320. Czito BG, Bendell JC, Willett CG, et al. Bevacizumab, oxaliplatin, and capecitabine with radiation therapy in rectal cancer: phase I trial results. *Int J Radiat Oncol Biol Phys*. 2007;68:472-478. PMID: 17498568.

321. Rodel C, Arnold D, Hipp M, et al. Phase I-II trial of cetuximab, capecitabine, oxaliplatin, and radiotherapy as preoperative treatment in rectal cancer. *Int J Radiat Oncol Biol Phys*. 2008;70:1081-1086. PMID: 17881150.

322. Willett CG, Duda DG, di Tomaso E, et al. Complete pathological response to bevacizumab and chemoradiation in advanced rectal cancer. *Nat Clin Pract Oncol*. 2007;4:316-321. PMID: 17464339.

323. Aschele C, Cionini L, Lonardi S, et al. Primary tumor response to preoperative chemoradiation with or without oxaliplatin in locally advanced rectal

324. Gérard JP, Azria D, Gourgou-Bourgade S, et al. Comparison of two neoadjuvant chemoradiotherapy regimens for locally advanced rectal cancer: results of the phase III trial ACCORD 12/0405-Prodige 2. *J Clin Oncol*. 2010;28:1638-1644. PMID: 20194850.

325. Rödel C, Liersch T, Becker H, et al. Preoperative chemoradiotherapy and postoperative chemotherapy with fluorouracil and oxaliplatin versus fluorouracil alone in locally advanced rectal cancer: initial results of the German CAO/ARO/AIO-04 randomised phase 3 trial. *Lancet Oncol*. 2012;13:679-687. PMID: 22627104.

326. Bujko K, Nowacki MP, Nasierowska-Guttmejer A, et al. Long-term results of a randomized trial comparing preoperative short-course radiotherapy with preoperative conventionally fractionated chemoradiation for rectal cancer. *Br J Surg*. 2006;93:1215-1223. PMID: 16983741.

327. Ngan S, Fisher R, Goldstein D, et al. A randomized trial comparing local recurrence (LR) rates between short-course (SC) and long-course (LC) preoperative radiotherapy (RT) for clinical T3 rectal cancer: An intergroup trial (TROG, AGITG, CSSANZ, RACS). *J Clin Oncol*. 2010;28:15s (suppl; abstr 3509).

328. Frisch M, Glimelius B, van den Brule AJ, et al. Sexually transmitted infection as a cause of anal cancer. *N Engl J Med*. 1997;337:1350-1358. PMID: 9358129.

329. Sischy B, Doggett RL, Krall JM, et al. Definitive irradiation and chemotherapy for radiosensitization in management of anal carcinoma: interim report on Radiation Therapy Oncology Group study no. 8314. *J Natl Cancer Inst*. 1989;81:850-856. PMID: 2724350.

330. Palefsky JM, Giuliano AR, Goldstone S, et al. HPV vaccine against anal HPV infection and anal intraepithelial neoplasia. *N Engl J Med*. 2011;365:1576-1585. PMID: 22029979.

331. Centers for Disease Control and Prevention. Recommendations on the use of quadrivalent human papillomavirus vaccine in males--Advisory Committee on Immunization Practices (ACIP), 2011. *MMWR Morb Mortal Wkly Rep*. 2011;60:1705-1708. PMID: 22189893.

332. Ajani JA, Winter KA, Gunderson LL, et al. Prognostic factors derived from a prospective database dictate clinical biology of anal cancer: the intergroup trial (RTOG 98-11). *Cancer*. 2010;116:4007-4013. PMID: 20564111.

333. Nigro ND, Seydel HG, Considine B, et al. Combined preoperative radiation and chemotherapy for squamous cell carcinoma of the anal canal. *Cancer*. 1983;51:1826-1829. PMID: 6831348.

334. Ajani JA, Winter KA, Gunderson LL, et al. Fluorouracil, mitomycin, and radiotherapy vs fluorouracil, cisplatin, and radiotherapy for carcinoma of the anal canal: a randomized controlled trial. *JAMA*. 2008;299:1914-1921. PMID: 18430910.

335. Gunderson LL, Winter KA, Ajani JA, et al. Long-term update of US GI intergroup RTOG 98-11 phase III trial for anal carcinoma: survival, relapse, and colostomy failure with concurrent chemoradiation involving fluorouracil/mitomycin versus fluorouracil/cisplatin. *J Clin Oncol*. 2012;30:4344-4351. PMID: 23150707.

336. James RD, Glynne-Jones R, Meadows HM, et al. Mitomycin or cisplatin chemoradiation with or without maintenance chemotherapy for treatment of squamous-cell carcinoma of the anus (ACT II): a randomised, phase 3, open-label, 2 x 2 factorial trial. *Lancet Oncol*. 2013;14:516-524. PMID: 23578724.

337. Das P, Crane CH, Ajani JA. Current treatment for localized anal carcinoma. *Curr Opin Oncol*. 2007;19:396-400. PMID: 17545807.

338. Van Damme N, Deron P, Van Roy N, et al. Epidermal growth factor receptor and K-RAS status in two cohorts of squamous cell carcinomas. *BMC Cancer*. 2010;10:189. PMID: 20459770.

339. Ryan DP, Compton CC, Mayer RJ. Carcinoma of the anal canal. *N Engl J Med*. 2000;342:792-800. PMID: 10717015.

340. Kauh J, Koshy M, Gunthel C, et al. Management of anal cancer in the HIV-positive population. *Oncology (Williston Park)*. 2005;19:1634-1638; discussion 1638-1640, 1645 passim. PMID: 16396154.

341. Kulke MH, Siu LL, Tepper JE, et al. Future directions in the treatment of neuroendocrine tumors: consensus report of the National Cancer Institute Neuroendocrine Tumor clinical trials planning meeting. *J Clin Oncol*. 2011;29:934-943. PMID: 21263089.

342. Tsukada T, Yamaguchi K, Kameya T. The MEN1 gene and associated diseases: an update. *Endocr Pathol*. 2001;12:259-273. PMID: 11740047.

343. Wermer P. Genetic aspects of adenomatosis of endocrine glands. *Am J Med*. 1954;16:363-371. PMID: 13138607.

344. Carney JA. Familial multiple endocrine neoplasia: the first 100 years. *Am J Surg Pathol*. 2005;29:254-274. PMID: 15644784.

345. Modlin IM, Lye KD, Kidd M. A 5-decade analysis of 13,715 carcinoid tumors. *Cancer*. 2003;97:934-959. PMID: 12569593.

346. Modlin IM, Kidd M, Drozdov I, et al. Pharmacotherapy of neuroendocrine cancers. *Expert Opin Pharmacother.* 2008;9:2617-2626. PMID: 18803449.

347. Kvols LK. Revisiting C.G. Moertel's land of small tumors. *J Clin Oncol.* 2008;26:5005-5007. PMID: 18838695.

348. Moertel CG, Weiland LH, Nagorney DM, et al. Carcinoid tumor of the appendix: treatment and prognosis. *N Engl J Med.* 1987;317:1699-1701. PMID: 3696178.

349. Kwekkeboom DJ, Mueller-Brand J, Paganelli G, et al. Overview of results of peptide receptor radionuclide therapy with 3 radiolabeled somatostatin analogs. *J Nucl Med.* 2005;46 Suppl 1:62S-66S. PMID: 15653653.

350. Kvols LK, Martin JK, Marsh HM, et al. Rapid reversal of carcinoid crisis with a somatostatin analogue. *N Engl J Med.* 1985;313:1229-1230. PMID: 2865675.

351. Kvols LK, Moertel CG, O'Connell MJ, et al. Treatment of the malignant carcinoid syndrome. Evaluation of a long-acting somatostatin analogue. *N Engl J Med.* 1986;315:663-666. PMID: 2427948.

352. Rinke A, Müller HH, Schade-Brittinger C, et al. Placebo-controlled, double-blind, prospective, randomized study on the effect of octreotide LAR in the control of tumor growth in patients with metastatic neuroendocrine midgut tumors: a report from the PROMID Study Group. *J Clin Oncol.* 2009;27:4656-4663. PMID: 19704057.

353. Oberg K, Eriksson B. The role of interferons in the management of carcinoid tumors. *Acta Oncol.* 1991;30:519-522. PMID: 1854509.

354. Moertel CG, Lefkopoulo M, Lipsitz S, et al. Streptozocin-doxorubicin, streptozocin-fluorouracil or chlorozotocin in the treatment of advanced islet-cell carcinoma. *N Engl J Med.* 1992;326:519-523. PMID: 1310159.

355. Raymond E, Dahan L, Raoul JL, et al. Sunitinib malate for the treatment of pancreatic neuroendocrine tumors. *N Engl J Med.* 2011;364:501-513. PMID: 21306237.

356. Yao JC, Shah MH, Ito T, et al. Everolimus for advanced pancreatic neuroendocrine tumors. *N Engl J Med.* 2011;364:514-523. PMID: 21306238.

357. Pavel ME, Hainsworth JD, Baudin E, et al. Everolimus plus octreotide long-acting repeatable for the treatment of advanced neuroendocrine tumours associated with carcinoid syndrome (RADIANT-2): a randomised, placebo-controlled, phase 3 study. *Lancet.* 2011;378:2005-2012. PMID: 22119496.

358. Yao JC, Hoff PM. Molecular targeted therapy for neuroendocrine tumors. *Hematol Oncol Clin North Am.* 2007;21:575-581; x. PMID: 17548041.

10

GENITOURINARY CANCERS

Matthew I. Milowsky, MD

Updates from 2012

Germ cell tumors

▶ Surveillance is now the preferred option for patients with stage I seminoma and stage IA non-seminoma. Based on the excellent outcome for the majority of patients with early-stage germ cell tumors, there is an important trend toward the use of less intense therapy for patients with stage I disease (Nichols CR, *J Clin Oncol* 2013).

Bladder cancer

▶ Next-generation genomic technology has defined molecular alterations in urothelial cancer that represent potential targets for novel therapeutics (Cancer Genome Atlas Research Network, *Nature* 2014).

Renal cancer

▶ In the first-line treatment of renal cell carcinoma, pazopanib is noninferior to sunitinib, with an improved safety profile and health-related quality of life (Motzer RJ, *N Engl J Med* 2013).

Prostate cancer

▶ Abiraterone acetate and enzalutamide improve the outcome of men with metastatic castrate-resistant prostate cancer not previously treated with chemotherapy (Ryan CJ, *N Engl J Med* 2013; Beer TM, *N Engl J Med* 2014).

▶ Radium-223 dichloride improves overall survival and has been approved by the U.S. Food and Drug Administration for the treatment of men with castrate-resistant prostate cancer and symptomatic bone metastases (Parker C, *N Engl J Med* 2013).

▶ For patients with metastatic prostate cancer, continuous androgen deprivation therapy (ADT) is superior to intermittent ADT, based on a noninferiority trial in which intermittent ADT was noninferior. This stands in contrast to patients with a rising prostate-specific antigen but no radiographic evidence of metastasis, for whom survival is similar with intermittent or continuous ADT (Hussain M, *N Eng J Med* 2013).

▶ Chemohormonal therapy with docetaxel in men with hormone-sensitive newly diagnosed metastatic prostate cancer is associated with a survival benefit compared to hormone therapy alone in patients with high-volume disease (Sweeney C, *J Clin Oncol* 2014).

I n the United States in 2013, genitourinary cancers accounted for 23% of new cancer cases and 10% of cancer-related deaths, with an estimated 390,000 cases and 60,000 deaths.[1] Aside from arising in genitourinary organs and requiring a multidisciplinary approach to management, each cancer type is unique with respect to its biology, natural history, and treatment options. The medical oncologist must understand the following: (1) the role for androgen deprivation therapy (ADT), chemotherapy, immunotherapy, and radiopharmaceuticals in the treatment of localized and advanced prostate cancer; (2) the use of a risk-adapted approach including surveillance, surgery, radiation therapy, and chemotherapy for patients with malignant germ cell tumors; (3) the integration of chemotherapy in the treatment of muscle-invasive and metastatic urothelial cancer; and (4) the use of targeted therapy and immunotherapy in advanced kidney cancer. The medical oncologist also plays a key role in the survivorship issues accompanying each disease, including management of the many side effects associated with ADT in men with prostate cancer; the potential for long-term toxicities related to radiation and chemotherapy in young men with germ cell tumors; the concerns related to chemotherapy effects on functional outcome in older patients with bladder cancer; and the treatment of a new spectrum of side effects and potential long-term toxicities associated with targeted agents for patients with advanced kidney cancer. Although many recent advances have led to novel treatment options with an associated improvement in outcome, a cure remains elusive for the majority of patients with advanced genitourinary cancers, and continued research is needed.

GERM CELL TUMORS

Germ cell tumors are the most common malignancies among men between ages 15 and 35. In 2013, 7,920 cases and 370 deaths were estimated to occur in the United States.[1] Germ cell tumors most frequently originate in the gonads (testis or ovary) and less commonly in the retroperitoneum and mediastinum. (For a discussion of germ cell tumors in women, see Chapter 11: Gynecologic Cancers.) Retroperitoneal tumors are often associated with an invasive tumor or carcinoma in situ within the testis, even in the absence of a palpable testicular mass. Primary mediastinal germ cell tumors are not associated with testicular involvement. Extragonadal germ cell neoplasms also rarely arise in the sacrum, pineal gland, paranasal sinuses, and liver. Regardless of the stage or extent of disease, the therapeutic objective is cure, which requires an integrated multidisciplinary approach.

EPIDEMIOLOGY

Germ cell tumors are primarily seen in white patients. Risk factors include both abdominal and inguinal cryptorchidism, spermatic or testicular dysgenesis, and a family history that confers a 4- to 10-fold increase in risk.[2] Orchiopexy or surgical correction of abdominal cryptorchidism results in improved ability to monitor the testis and reduces the risk of germ cell tumors—with those treated before puberty achieving the greatest benefit.[3] Factors associated with increased testicular cancer mortality include age older than 40, non-white race, and lower socioeconomic status.[4] Testicular seminoma occurs more frequently in men with HIV, and the treatment by stage is the same as for the HIV-negative population.[5] Klinefelter syndrome is a risk factor for the development of mediastinal germ cell tumors. Carcinoma in situ (intratubular germ cell neoplasia) is found in virtually all cases of testicular germ cell tumors. Men in whom in situ disease is identified during a testicular biopsy as part of an infertility evaluation have a 50% risk of an invasive tumor over a 5-year period. A metachronous or synchronous testicular primary germ cell tumor occurs in 2% of patients, with seminoma as the most common histology.[6] Regular self-examination of the remaining testis is recommended.

Table 10-1 **Histologic Classification of Germ Cell Neoplasms**[11]

Seminoma	▪ Classical (typical) ▪ Spermatocytic (present in elderly patients and associated with indolent course)

Nonseminoma	▪ Teratoma
	  □ Mature
	  □ Immature
	▪ With malignant transformation
	▪ Choriocarcinoma
	▪ Yolk sac tumor (endodermal sinus tumor)
	▪ Embryonal carcinoma

Adapted from Bosl GJ, Motzer RJ. Testicular germ-cell cancer. N Engl J Med. 1997;337(4):242-253.

BIOLOGY

Germ cell tumors are derived from the malignant transformation of premeiotic germ cells. To create a pluripotential tumor, these transformed germ cells must be able to differentiate in a manner similar to the totipotential zygote without the reciprocal genetic information that results from fertilization.[7] An isochromosome of the short arm of chromosome 12—i(12p)—is present in 80% of all histologic subtypes, including carcinoma in situ and extragonadal tumors. The remaining 20% of cases have excess 12p genetic material as an increase in copy number, tandem duplication, or transposition, which indicates that one or more genes on 12p are involved in malignant transformation. Although the 12p target genes have not been clearly defined, several candidate genes include *CCND2* at 12p13 and *SOX5*, *JAW1*, and *KRAS* mapped to an amplified region at 12p11.2-12.1.[8] Most germ cell tumors are hyperdiploid, and often triploid or tetraploid, implying that endoreduplication is important in the early steps of malignant transformation. A genome-wide analysis of genetic alterations in testicular primary seminoma identified copy number variations that correlated with progression, including deletions in chromosomes 4q, 5p, 13q, and 20p and amplifications in chromosomes 9q and 13q.[9] An integrated analysis of genome-wide messenger RNA and micro RNA expression profiles in testicular cancer demonstrated alterations in gene sets implicated in processes related to male reproductive function.[10]

DIAGNOSIS

A painless testicular mass is highly suggestive of a testicular tumor; however, the majority of patients present with diffuse testicular swelling, hardness, pain, or some combination of these findings. For patients who present with pain, the initial therapy often is antibiotics for presumed infectious epididymitis or orchitis. If symptoms do not resolve within 2 weeks, an ultrasound of the testis is indicated. If the ultrasound is abnormal and a testicular tumor is suspected, a radical inguinal orchiectomy with removal of the testis and ligation of the spermatic cord at the level of the internal ring is performed. Because the testes originate in the genital ridge and migrate through the abdomen

Table 10-2 Staging of Testicular Germ Cell Tumors[12]

Primary Tumor (T)

pTX	Primary tumor cannot be assessed (if no radical orchiectomy has been performed)
pT0	No evidence of primary tumor (e.g., histologic scar in testis)
pTis	Intratubular germ cell neoplasia (carcinoma in situ)
pT1	Tumor limited to testis and epididymis; no vascular or lymphatic invasion; tumor may invade into the tunica albuginea but not the tunica vaginalis
pT2	Tumor limited to testis and epididymis with vascular or lymphatic invasion, or tumor extending through the tunica albuginea with involvement of tunica vaginalis
pT3	Tumor invades the spermatic cord with or without vascular or lymphatic invasion
pT4	Tumor invades the scrotum with or without vascular or lymphatic invasion

Regional Lymph Nodes (N) Clinical

NX	Regional lymph nodes cannot be assessed
N0	No regional lymph node metastasis
N1	Metastasis with a lymph node mass 2 cm or less in greatest dimension; or multiple lymph nodes, none more than 2 cm in greatest dimension
N2	Metastasis with a lymph node mass more than 2 cm but not more than 5 cm in greatest dimension; or multiple lymph nodes, any one mass more than 2 cm but not more than 5 cm in greatest dimension
N3	Metastasis with a lymph node mass more than 5 cm in greatest dimension

Pathologic (pN)

pNX	Regional lymph nodes cannot be assessed
pN0	No regional lymph node metastasis
pN1	Metastasis with a lymph node mass 2 cm or less in greatest dimension and less than or equal to five nodes positive, none more than 2 cm in greatest dimension
pN2	Metastasis with a lymph node mass more than 2 cm but not more than 5 cm in greatest dimension; or more than five nodes positive, none more than 5 cm in greatest dimension; or evidence of extranodal extension of tumor
pN3	Metastasis with a lymph node mass more than 5 cm in greatest dimension

Distant Metastases (M)

M0	No distant metastasis
M1	Distant metastasis
M1a	Nonregional nodal or pulmonary metastasis
M1b	Distant metastasis other than to nonregional lymph nodes and lung

Table 10-2 continued

Serum Tumor Markers (S)

SX	Marker studies not available or not performed
S0	Marker study levels within normal limits
S1	LDH is < 1.5 times the upper limit of normal (ULN) **and** HCG (mIU/mL) is < 5,000 **and** AFP (ng/mL) level is < 1,000
S2	LDH is 1.5 to 10 times ULN **or** HCG is 5,000 to 50,000 **or** AFP is 1,000 to 10,000
S3	LDH is > 10 times ULN **or** HCG is > 50,000 **or** AFP is > 10,000

Anatomic Stage/Prognostic Groupings

Stage 0	pTis N0 M0 S0
Stage I	pT1-4 N0 M0 SX
Stage IA	pT1 N0 M0 S0
Stage IB	pT2 N0 M0 S0 pT3 N0 M0 S0 pT4 N0 M0 S0
Stage IS	Any pT/TX N0 M0 S1-3
Stage II	Any pT/TX N1-3 M0 SX
Stage IIA	Any pT/TX N1 M0 S0 Any pT/TX N1 M0 S1
Stage IIB	Any pT/TX N2 M0 S0 Any pT/TX N2 M0 S1
Stage IIC	Any pT/TX N3 M0 S0 Any pT/TX N3 M0 S1
Stage III	Any pT/TX Any N M1 SX
Stage IIIA	Any pT/TX Any N M1a S0 Any pT/TX Any N M1a S1
Stage IIIB	Any pT/TX N1-3 M0 S2 Any pT/TX Any N M1a S2
Stage IIIC	Any pT/TX N1-3 M0 S3 Any pT/TX Any N M1a S3 Any pT/TX Any N M1b Any S

Abbreviations: LDH, lactate dehydrogenase; HCG, human chorionic gonadotropin; AFP, alpha-fetoprotein.
The original source for this material is the AJCC Cancer Staging Manual, 7th Edition *(2010) published by Springer Science and Business Media LLC, www.springerlink.com.*

and inguinal canal into the scrotum, the vascular and lymphatic drainage of the testes is to the renal or great vessels and the retroperitoneal nodes, respectively. A testicular biopsy or transscrotal orchiectomy is contraindicated because the normal vascular and lymphatic drainage is disturbed. Levels of alphafetoprotein (AFP), human chorionic gonadotropin (HCG), and lactate dehydrogenase (LDH) also should be determined. Less common presentations include gynecomastia (as a result of elevated levels of HCG), back pain related to retroperitoneal nodal disease, superior vena cava syndrome from primary mediastinal tumors, and hemoptysis from extensive pulmonary metastases.

Table 10-3 Risk Stratification According to the International Germ Cell Consensus Classification[13]

Seminoma	**Good risk** Any primary and any markers and no nonpulmonary visceral metastases
	Intermediate risk Any primary and any markers and nonpulmonary visceral metastases
Nonseminoma	**Good risk** Testis or retroperitoneal primary and good-risk markers and no nonpulmonary visceral metastases
	Intermediate risk Testis/retroperitoneal primary and intermediate-risk markers and no nonpulmonary visceral metastases
	Poor risk Mediastinal primary site or testis or retroperitoneal primary with either nonpulmonary visceral metastases or poor-risk markers

Reprinted with permission from International Germ Cell Consensus classification: A prognostic factor-based staging system for metastatic germ cell cancers. J Clin Oncol. 1997;15:594-603. PMID: 9053482.

PATHOLOGY

Germ cell tumors are classified histologically into seminomas and nonseminomas. Seminomas, which account for approximately one-half of testicular germ cell tumors, retain totipotentiality and are exquisitely sensitive to radiation and chemotherapy. Nonseminomas are composed of the following cell types: embryonal carcinoma, teratoma, choriocarcinoma, and yolk sac or endodermal-sinus tumors (Table 10-1).[11] Embryonal carcinoma is the most undifferentiated, with totipotential capacity to differentiate into extraembryonic malignant cell types, such as yolk sac tumors and choriocarcinoma, and somatic cell types, such as teratoma. Teratoma is composed of somatic cells from two or more germ cell layers (i.e., ectoderm, mesoderm, or endoderm) and thus can differentiate into tissue types such as cartilage, muscle, mucinous glandular epithelium, and others. The presence of any component of nonseminoma with seminoma is treated as a nonseminomatous germ cell tumor. In addition, an abnormal serum AFP level is not seen in seminoma and indicates a nonseminomatous germ cell tumor. Most nonseminomas show mixed histologies, including embryonal carcinoma, yolk sac tumors, teratoma, and choriocarcinoma. When reporting histology, all subtypes present must be noted, starting with the most prevalent and ending with the least common component.

Seminomas are positive for placental alkaline phosphatase (PLAP), CD117 (c-kit), OCT-4, and SALL-4. They are negative for cytokeratins and CD30. However, embryonal carcinoma almost universally expresses cytokeratins, epithelial membrane antigen, CD30, OCT-4, and SALL-4; approximately 50% express PLAP. Yolk sac tumors are positive for cytokeratins, AFP, and SALL-4, but negative for CD117 and CD30. Immunohistochemical analysis may be useful in the evaluation of patients with midline tumors of uncertain histiogenesis.

PATTERNS OF SPREAD

The primary lymphatic drainage for testicular germ cell tumors is to the retroperitoneal lymph nodes (primary landing zones). The right testicular artery originates from the aorta, and the right testicular vein drains into the inferior vena cava. The left testicular artery originates near the left renal artery, and the left testicular vein terminates in the left renal vein. Right-sided tumors spread to the interaortocaval lymph nodes immediately below the renal blood vessels, and left-sided tumors spread to the para-aortic lymph nodes immediately below the left renal artery and vein. Cross-metastases are more commonly seen from right to left. Invasion of the epididymis or spermatic cord may be associated with iliac nodal involvement, and inguinal metastases may be seen with scrotal invasion or if there has been disturbance of the normal lymphatic drainage related to prior surgery. Additional metastatic sites include retrocrural, mediastinal, and supraclavicular lymph nodes; the lungs; and, less commonly, the liver, central nervous system, and bone.

STAGING

Pretreatment Evaluation

The extent of disease evaluation for patients with newly diagnosed germ cell tumors includes a chest x-ray, computed tomography (CT) of the abdomen and pelvis, and tumor markers. Indications for a CT scan of the chest include an abnormal chest x-ray, known mediastinal disease, and risk for pulmonary metastases. A bone scan and magnetic resonance imaging (MRI) of the brain are indicated only if related symptoms are present. Measurement of tumor markers, including AFP, HCG, and LDH, is used to establish the diagnosis and may assist in determining histologic subtype. Sperm banking should be performed before treatment is pursued.

Stage Groupings

A tumor, node, metastasis (TNM) staging classification system was developed by the American Joint Committee on Cancer (AJCC) and incorporates serum tumor markers, including AFP, HCG, and LDH (Table 10-2).[12] Adverse factors include mediastinal primary site; degree of elevation of AFP, HCG, and LDH; and presence of nonpulmonary visceral metastases. Based on these findings, advanced germ cell tumors are risk-stratified as follows: good risk (60% of germ cell tumors and resulting in a 5-year survival rate of 91%); intermediate risk (26% of germ cell tumors and a 5-year survival rate of 79%); and poor risk (14% of germ cell tumors and a 5-year survival rate of 48%). All seminomas are either good or intermediate risk (Table 10-3).[13]

TUMOR MARKERS

Tumor markers are measured before, during, and after treatment. An initial rise in tumor markers may occur with chemotherapy, particularly in the setting of bulky advanced disease.

The serum half-lives of AFP and HCG are 5 to 7 days and 30 hours, respectively, and a slow marker decline after orchiectomy or during chemotherapy implies residual active disease. Elevated or rising AFP and/or HCG levels that occur without radiologic or clinical findings imply active disease and must be managed accordingly. Other conditions associated with elevated AFP levels include hepatocellular carcinoma, liver damage, and other gastrointestinal malignancies. HCG elevations may occur as a result of treatment-related hypogonadism or cross-reactivity with pituitary hormones, including luteinizing hormone. This cross-reactivity is typically less of an issue with current assays specific for the beta subunit of HCG. Hyperthyroidism may be associated with elevated levels of HCG related to cross-reactivity of HCG with the thyroid-stimulating receptor. A spurious elevation in HCG also has been associated with marijuana use.[14] With these exceptions, increased levels of AFP are pathognomonic of a nonseminoma and not seen in seminoma, whereas elevated levels of HCG may be seen in both seminoma and nonseminoma. LDH levels can increase for patients with advanced seminoma or nonseminoma and are used for staging and assessment of outcome. Elevations in any one marker or combination are found in approximately 20% of patients with stage I disease, 40% of patients with stage II disease, and 60% or more of patients with stage III disease.

SEMINOMA

Approximately 70% of patients with seminoma have stage I disease. After radical inguinal orchiectomy, standard treatment options include surveillance, adjuvant infradiaphragmatic radiotherapy to include the para-aortic nodes, and single-agent carboplatin, recognizing that approximately 80% of these patients will not have required treatment. Findings from observational studies of patients with clinical stage I seminoma indicate a 15% to 20% likelihood of disease relapse, mostly in the retroperitoneum; however, the median time to relapse exceeds 15 months, which is twice as long as for clinical stage I nonseminomatous tumors and may occur as late as 8 to 10 years. Based on the excellent outcome for patients with stage I seminoma and the potential for long-term radiation-related toxicity, including secondary malignancies, surveillance represents a preferred strategy for the treatment of patients with clinical stage I disease.[15-18] Radiation therapy is contraindicated in the setting of inflammatory bowel disease or a horseshoe kidney. Radiotherapy using a para-aortic field compared with a dogleg field is associated with reduced toxicity and a low rate of recurrence.[19] A randomized trial comparing radiotherapy with single-dose carboplatin in the adjuvant treatment of stage I seminoma has shown a noninferior relapse-free rate for single-dose carboplatin, with a reduced risk of a second primary germ cell tumor in the carboplatin arm.[20,21] Although chemotherapy represents a potential strategy for the management of clinical stage I disease, concerns have been raised based on the relatively short follow-up period (median follow-up, 6.5 years) to evaluate for late relapse and late toxicity.[22,23]

Patients with stage IIA disease are treated with radiotherapy to the retroperitoneal and ipsilateral pelvic lymph nodes with doses of up to 25 Gy, with a boost to gross disease of up to 30 to 35 Gy. Chemotherapy or radiotherapy may be considered for patients with clinical stage IIB seminoma. Chemotherapy will cure more than 90% of the patients who experience disease relapse after radiotherapy; approximately 99% of patients with early-stage seminoma are cured.

Advanced Seminoma

Approximately 10% of patients with seminoma require chemotherapy; 15% to 20% of patients with advanced seminoma present with an elevated HCG. An elevated AFP indicates a nonseminomatous tumor, and the patient should be treated accordingly. Patients with retroperitoneal masses larger than 5 cm (stage IIC), supradiaphragmatic lymphadenopathy, visceral disease, bulky retroperitoneal tumors, tumor-related back pain, and mediastinal extragonadal presentations are treated with primary chemotherapy. Approximately 90% of patients with advanced seminoma will be classified as good prognosis and receive treatment with good-risk chemotherapy, with an 86% 5-year survival (see Management of Advanced Germ Cell Tumors by Risk Classification section below).[12] Prophylactic radiation therapy to sites of initial bulky disease after chemotherapy is not indicated because it does not alter the probability of relapse or survival.

Surgery after chemotherapy is technically more difficult for patients with seminomas than for patients with nonseminomas. A classical retroperitoneal lymph node dissection is typically not carried out in this setting because of fibrosis and an increased likelihood of damage to the great vessels; however, surgery after chemotherapy typically is not necessary. Postchemotherapy residual masses usually represent fibrosis rather than persistent seminoma. Options have included surgery for postchemotherapy masses larger than 3 cm or close observation with CT imaging and intervention if there is evidence of disease progression. 18-fluorodeoxyglucose positron emission tomography (FDG-PET) has been shown to be a reliable predictor for viable tumors in postchemotherapy seminoma.[24] The specificity, sensitivity, and negative predictive value of FDG-PET are improved if performed 6 weeks after the end of the last chemotherapy cycle compared with before 6 weeks.[25] In summary, FDG-PET should be performed for patients with a residual mass larger than 3 cm and normal tumor markers. A positive FDG-PET scan indicates viable seminoma and surgery is indicated.

NONSEMINOMATUOUS GERM CELL TUMORS
Stage I Disease
Most patients with clinical stage I disease have normal findings on imaging and normalization of serum tumor markers after radical inguinal orchiectomy. Approximately 30% to 40% of patients with nonseminomatous germ cell tumors present with stage I disease. The management options include surveillance, retroperitoneal lymph node dissection, or primary chemotherapy.

Surveillance is a preferred option for compliant patients with stage IA (pT1 tumors; i.e., those with no vascular/lymphatic invasion or with invasion into the tunica vaginalis, spermatic cord, or scrotum) who have a low risk for recurrence. Absence of a predominant embryonal carcinoma component in the primary tumor is also favorable. Approximately 20% of patients will experience a recurrence of the disease (most commonly in the retroperitoneum) and will need chemotherapy. Most recurrences of germ cell tumors will occur in the first 2 years after therapy, and these patients must have meticulous follow-up that includes a history, physical examination, chest x-ray, and measurement of serum tumor markers every 1 to 2 months, as well as an abdominal CT scan every 3 to 4 months during the first year.[26] During the second year, the history, physical examination, tumor markers, and chest x-ray are performed at 2-month intervals, and CT scan occurs every 4 to 6 months. Although the intervals for follow-up increase during subsequent years, it is important to remember that late recurrences can occur.[27] Compliance with this surveillance schedule, and with salvage therapy as indicated, produces cure rates of 98% to 99% and spares 75% to 80% of patients without micrometastatic disease from additional therapy. The potential long-term risk of secondary cancers associated with exposure to low-dose ionizing radiation with medical imaging procedures has generated particular concern for young patients with germ cell tumors.[28] Although one report suggested that the risk of secondary cancers was not associated with the amount of diagnostic radiation, the observation period was relatively short at only 11 years.[16,29]

Patients with stage I disease with more than 50% risk of recurrence based on pathologic features—including embryonal carcinoma predominant (greater than 50%) and/or the presence of lymphatic, vascular, scrotal, or spermatic-cord invasion (stage IB)—may be considered for a nerve-sparing retroperitoneal lymph node dissection by a surgeon experienced in the procedure. Surveillance in a compliant patient with stage IB is an accepted option and preferred by some experts in the field. Low recurrence rates were seen in two studies evaluating the use of short-course adjuvant chemotherapy with one or two cycles of combination bleomycin/etoposide/cisplatin (BEP) for patients with clinical stage I nonseminomatous germ cell tumors; however, concerns remain regarding the many men exposed to unnecessary chemotherapy with the potential for long-term adverse effects.[30,31] The decision to recommend adjuvant chemotherapy after a retroperitoneal lymph node dissection is made on the basis of pathologic findings, as described for patients with pathologic stage II disease. Patients without evidence of clinical disease and persistently elevated tumor markers, including HCG, AFP, or both after orchiectomy (stage IS), should receive standard chemotherapy rather than surgery.

Stage II Disease

The standard treatment for a patient with stage IIA disease (nodes 2 cm or smaller in diameter) is a modified, bilateral retroperitoneal lymph node dissection. In this procedure, the dissection becomes unilateral at the level of the inferior mesenteric artery. Experience with the technique is essential because, depending on the location of the tumor, a nerve-sparing procedure can be performed.

Approximately 20% to 25% of patients will have pathologic N1 (metastases with node diameter of 2 cm or smaller

or five or fewer involved nodes) with an approximate 20% risk of relapse such that surveillance is preferred in a compliant patient. The likelihood of micrometastatic disease is 50% or more for patients with an involved node diameter of more than 2 cm, more than five involved nodes, or any extranodal extension (pathologic N2). Assuming that serum tumor marker levels return to normal after surgery, these patients should receive two cycles of adjuvant chemotherapy, which results in a 98% to 99% likelihood of cure.[32] For patients with pathologic N3 (node diameter of more than 5 cm), three to four cycles of chemotherapy are administered. In circumstances wherein disease relapses or serum tumor markers do not normalize, indicating residual active disease, then three to four cycles of chemotherapy and subsequent surgical excision of residual macroscopically documented disease, if present, are indicated—as is required for any patient with disseminated disease.

The majority of patients with clinical stage IIB disease (nodes more than 2 cm but not more than 5 cm in diameter) are typically advised to receive primary chemotherapy. In addition, patients with back pain related to psoas invasion, bilateral retroperitoneal involvement, suprahilar or retrocrural adenopathy, or other signs that the disease may be unresectable should undergo primary chemotherapy. Clinical stage IIC disease (nodes more than 5 cm in diameter) also are treated with initial chemotherapy.

Stage III Disease

Approximately 70% to 80% of patients with metastatic disease will be cured with cisplatin-based chemotherapy combined with surgery to resect residual disease as an integral part of management. The therapeutic objective is cure, with distinct approaches for disease deemed good risk (i.e., high probability of cure) and poor risk (i.e., lower probability of cure).[33] For patients with good-risk disease, the goal is to minimize toxicity without compromising cure, whereas management of poor-risk disease focuses less on minimizing toxicity and more on increasing the probability of cure.

MANAGEMENT OF ADVANCED GERM CELL TUMORS BY RISK CLASSIFICATION

The treatment of germ cell tumors is based on the International Germ Cell Consensus Classification, developed in 1996 (Table 10-3).[13]

Good Risk

Approximately 60% of patients with nonseminomatous germ cell tumors present with good-risk disease. Patients with good risk include those with stage II or III disease with testis/retroperitoneal primary tumors, no nonpulmonary visceral metastases, and good-risk tumor markers. The majority of patients with advanced seminoma have good-risk disease. Based on the results of clinical trials, more than 90% of these patients will be cured with the use of combination chemotherapy, including cisplatin and etoposide with or without bleomycin.[34-38] Summaries of the trials are as follows:

- Four cycles of etoposide plus cisplatin and three cycles of BEP achieve a durable complete response in approximately 90% of patients with good-risk disease.
- The elimination of bleomycin can compromise cure if only three cycles of therapy with etoposide and cisplatin are given or adequate doses of etoposide are not administered.[39,40]
- Although carboplatin has less toxicity, it cannot be substituted for cisplatin because it is less effective.[41,42]

A trial from the Genito-Urinary Group of the French Federation of Cancer Centers randomly assigned patients with good-risk nonseminomatous germ cell tumors to three cycles of BEP or to four cycles of etoposide plus cisplatin.[38] In 257 assessable patients, there was no significant difference, respectively, in response (94.7% vs. 96.8%; p = 0.34), 4-year event-free survival (91% vs. 86%; p = 0.135) and 4-year overall survival (OS; 96% vs. 92%; p = 0.096). One additional cycle of treatment is required with the regimen of etoposide plus cisplatin, but the nine bleomycin treatments are avoided. Bleomycin is associated with Raynaud phenomenon and pulmonary toxicity, although clinically significant pulmonary toxicity is rare.[43] Three cycles of BEP or four cycles of etoposide plus cisplatin are the standard regimens for the treatment of patients with good-risk germ cell tumors.

The lower limit of dose for bleomycin and etoposide was addressed in a trial comparing three cycles of standard BEP (20 mg/m^2 of cisplatin on days 1 to 5; 100 mg/m^2 of etoposide on days 1 to 5; and 30 kU of bleomycin on days 1, 8, and 15 repeated every 21 days) with four cycles of the same combination at different dosages (100 mg/m^2 of cisplatin on day 1; 120 mg/m^2 of etoposide on days 1 to 3; and 30 kU of bleomycin on day 1, repeated every 21 days). The trial was stopped when an interim analysis attributed a higher cancer death rate with the alternative regimen, which was felt to be related to the lower total dose and dose intensity of bleomycin and to the lower-dose intensity of etoposide.[44]

In an attempt to decrease toxicity, the substitution of carboplatin for cisplatin was addressed in a randomized trial in which etoposide plus cisplatin was compared with etoposide plus carboplatin (500 mg/m^2 on day 1 of each cycle) for four cycles.[41] There were significantly inferior event-free and relapse-free survival rates for patients who received etoposide plus carboplatin. Therefore, carboplatin should not be substituted for cisplatin in the treatment of patients with germ cell tumors.

Intermediate Risk
The intermediate-risk group includes patients with nonseminomatous tumors with intermediate-risk tumor markers, as well as patients with seminoma who have nonpulmonary visceral metastases or primary mediastinal seminoma. These patients comprise 20% to 30% of germ cell tumors and have a 5-year survival rate of approximately 80%. A regimen that includes four cycles of BEP is the standard treatment.

Poor Risk
Patients with poor-risk disease include nonseminomatous germ cell tumors with nonpulmonary visceral metastases, poor-risk

tumor markers, or a primary mediastinal site. These patients comprise 10% to 20% of nonseminomas and have a 5-year survival of approximately 50%. For patients with poor-risk disease, the standard of care remains four cycles of conventional-dose BEP. A randomized trial showed that the substitution of ifosfamide for bleomycin has similar efficacy but significantly greater toxicity.[45] Additionally, the use of high-dose cisplatin (200 mg/m^2) is not superior to standard-dose cisplatin (100 mg/m^2) when administered in combination with etoposide and bleomycin.[46] A randomized phase III trial in 219 patients with intermediate- or poor-risk germ cell tumors compared two cycles of standard BEP followed by two cycles of high-dose chemotherapy (cyclophosphamide/etoposide/carboplatin) plus stem cell rescue to four cycles of conventional-dose BEP.[47] The primary endpoint was the percentage of patients with complete response at 1 year. Final analysis showed that there was not a significant difference, with a complete response at 1 year of 52% for BEP plus high-dose chemotherapy and 48% for BEP alone (p = 0.53). A second randomized phase III study comparing standard-dose BEP with sequential high-dose cisplatin/etoposide/ifosfamide plus stem cell support for patients with poor-prognosis germ cell cancer did not demonstrate a benefit for high-dose chemotherapy given as part of first-line therapy.[48] In a population-based study of treatment guided by tumor marker decline in patients with metastatic nonseminomatous germ cell tumors, intensification of therapy based on prolonged marker decline was associated with improved outcome such that the survival rate for patients with intermediate-risk disease approached that of patients with good-risk disease.[49] A recently reported phase III trial in poor-prognosis germ cell tumors of personalized chemotherapy based on serum tumor marker decline demonstrated that treatment intensification determined by the rate of early marker decline reduces the risk of progression or death; but the dose-dense intensification used in the study is not a standard regimen.[50]

SALVAGE THERAPY FOR GERM CELL TUMORS
For 20% to 30% of patients with advanced germ cell tumors, their disease will fail to achieve a durable response to chemotherapy regimens, including cisplatin and etoposide with or without bleomycin. Approximately 25% of these patients will experience a durable complete response using vinblastine/ifosfamide/cisplatin as salvage therapy.[51] Patients whose disease does not achieve a durable complete response to induction chemotherapy have a particularly poor prognosis. In addition, patients with a mediastinal primary tumor site rarely experience a durable complete response to cisplatin plus ifosfamide-based salvage chemotherapy. The timing of relapse also is important, with late relapse beyond 2 years associated with a high degree of resistance to standard salvage chemotherapy and with an overall poor prognosis.[27] The combination of paclitaxel, ifosfamide, and cisplatin (TIP) was evaluated as second-line therapy for patients with favorable prognostic features for response, including testis primary tumor site and a prior complete response to a first-line chemotherapy program.[52] Four cycles of TIP as second-line therapy resulted in a

70% complete response rate to treatment, with a 63% durable complete response rate and a 2-year progression-free survival (PFS) rate of 65%. The high level of activity with TIP as salvage therapy is, in part, related to the patient selection criteria used to identify patients more likely to benefit from conventional-dose second-line therapy. A retrospective study demonstrated that the TIP regimen followed by surgery may be effective for patients with late-relapse germ cell tumors who are not candidates for primary surgery.[53] Ifosfamide-based therapy has been associated with significant hematologic, renal, and neurologic toxicities, and the use of hematopoietic growth factors is considered standard. A phase II study of cisplatin plus epirubicin also has demonstrated activity in the salvage setting.[54] Additional regimens—such as those incorporating gemcitabine and oxaliplatin—have demonstrated antitumor activity in patients who have been heavily pretreated.[55] Clinical trials should be considered in the salvage setting. For patients experiencing treatment failure with cisplatin-based first-line chemotherapy, prognostic variables including histology, primary tumor location, response, progression-free interval after first-line treatment, AFP, and HCG, as well as the presence of liver, bone, or brain metastases, have been used to develop a prognostic model to guide salvage therapies.[56]

HIGH-DOSE CHEMOTHERAPY WITH PERIPHERAL STEM CELL RESCUE FOR GERM CELL TUMORS

The use of high-dose chemotherapy with peripheral stem cell rescue should be considered for patients who do not have an initial complete response to induction chemotherapy or who experience relapse after first-line salvage therapy. The use of high-dose carboplatin and etoposide followed by peripheral blood stem cell transplantation or autologous bone marrow transplantation rescue with a repeat course of therapy given after hematopoietic reconstitution was evaluated as initial salvage therapy in 65 patients with testicular cancer.[57] Postchemotherapy resection of residual disease was performed in selected patients. At a median follow-up of 39 months, 37 (57%) of the 65 patients were continuously disease-free, and three additional patients were rendered disease-free with surgery. The use of sequential, dose-intensive combination paclitaxel, ifosfamide, carboplatin, and etoposide with stem cell rescue was evaluated in 107 patients with germ cell tumors whose disease was resistant to cisplatin and who had unfavorable prognostic features for response to conventional-dose salvage therapy, including extragonadal primary site, incomplete response to first-line therapy, or relapse/incomplete response to ifosfamide/cisplatin-based conventional-dose salvage therapy.[58] Fifty-four patients (50%) achieved a complete response, and eight patients (8%) achieved a partial response with negative tumor markers. With a median follow-up of 61 months, the 5-year disease-free survival (DFS) was 47%; OS was 52% with no relapses occurring after 2 years. In a retrospective review of 184 consecutive patients with metastatic testicular cancer who had disease progression after receiving cisplatin-containing combination chemotherapy and who were treated with high-dose chemotherapy and stem cell rescue, 116 had a complete remission of disease without relapse with a median

follow-up of 48 months (range, 14 months to 118 months).[59] Durable remissions were seen in patients receiving high-dose chemotherapy plus stem cell rescue as second-line therapy, as third-line (or later) therapy, and in patients with platinum-refractory disease. Results for patients with primary mediastinal germ cell tumors treated with high-dose chemotherapy and with stem cell rescue demonstrate a worse outcome, and these patients should be enrolled in clinical trials at specialized centers.[60] Treatment-related morbidity following high-dose therapy can be significant, and all patients should be referred to major treatment centers specializing in this approach.[61]

SURGERY AFTER CHEMOTHERAPY FOR NONSEMINOMATOUS TUMORS

Surgery after chemotherapy is an integral part of the treatment of patients with germ cell tumors and should be considered for individuals with residual radiographic abnormalities but with normal serum tumor markers after treatment. A retroperitoneal lymph node dissection is the standard surgery for patients with evidence of disease in the retroperitoneum. All residual masses at all sites should be excised, as the histology at one site does not adequately predict the histology at other sites. Approximately 45% of residual masses will consist of necrotic debris or fibrosis, 40% will consist of mature teratoma, and 15% will harbor a viable germ cell tumor. If the viable germ cell tumor has been completely resected, two additional cycles of chemotherapy are administered. Although histologically benign, teratoma arises from malignant germ cells and may grow over time; surgical removal is needed. Additionally, a minority of resected teratomas will have malignant transformation to cell types including rhabdomyosarcoma, adenocarcinoma, and others. Surgical resection is the mainstay of treatment; however, chemotherapy for metastases of a particular cell type may result in major responses and long-term survival in select patients.[62]

The role for surgery in all patients who initially present with visible disease on imaging and have normalization or minimal residual disease on repeat imaging after chemotherapy is controversial. CT scans of the chest can identify small residual masses in the pulmonary parenchyma. The sensitivity of this technique in the retroperitoneum remains uncertain, leading to controversy over the definition of residual retroperitoneal masses. In 87 patients with minimal residual tumor masses (largest diameter of the residual mass on transaxial plane was 20 mm or less) after chemotherapy, 58 patients (67%) had complete fibrosis or necrosis, 23 patients (26%) had teratoma, and six patients (7%) had viable malignant germ cell tumor. Thus, approximately one-third of patients had vital tumor tissue with teratoma at risk for growth and/or malignant transformation and viable germ cell tumor at risk for progression.[63] Additional concerns include the poor outcome associated with late relapses and the finding that a lack of prior retroperitoneal surgery is a major predisposing factor.[27,64] Patients with a late relapse who are symptomatic at presentation, as well as those with multifocal disease, have a significantly decreased survival.[65] With nonseminomatous germ cell tumors, FDG-PET scans are unable to distinguish fibrosis from teratoma, thereby limiting the utility of PET imaging in determining the histology of residual masses after chemotherapy.

An exception to the requirement for normal tumor markers is the patient with elevated serum tumor markers whose disease did not respond to salvage chemotherapy. This clinical scenario is rare because less than 5% of patients who do not have normal marker status are candidates for surgical excision of a solitary residual mass. Surgery in the setting of elevated markers should only be considered by specialists with experience in the management of these cases.

ASSOCIATED MALIGNANT DISEASE

Malignant transformation of a somatic teratomatous component of a nonseminoma to somatic malignancies, including rhabdomyosarcoma, adenocarcinoma, primitive neuroectodermal tumor, and leukemia, as well as others, has been well described.[62] The presence of i(12p) or excess 12p copy number in these tumors establishes the clonal germ cell tumor origin. The finding of i(12p) or excess 12p genetic material by either molecular or cytogenetic studies correlates with response to cisplatin therapy.[66] Mediastinal nonseminomatous germ cell tumors also are associated with the presence of myeloproliferative disorders, including acute nonlymphocytic leukemia and acute megakaryocytic leukemia. A minority of patients with poorly differentiated carcinomas of unknown primary origin have a complete response to cisplatin-based chemotherapy. The presence of additional clinical features, including male sex, predominant midline tumor, relatively young age, and elevated serum tumor markers, has suggested that the minority of patients with poorly differentiated carcinomas of unknown primary origin may have germ cell tumors. Clinical features as well as molecular and cytogenetic studies are important in the management of carcinomas of unknown primary or midline tumors of uncertain histiogenesis.

SURVIVORSHIP AND LATE EFFECTS

An evaluation of the long-term risk of cardiovascular disease in survivors of testicular cancer demonstrated a moderately increased myocardial infarction risk at young ages for patients with nonseminomatous germ cell tumors.[67] Increased risk was associated with prior chemotherapy regimens including cisplatin, vinblastine, and bleomycin, as well as BEP, and with previous mediastinal irradiation and recent tobacco use. In a 20-year follow-up study of 990 men treated for unilateral testicular cancer, treatment with infradiaphragmatic radiation therapy and/or cisplatin-based chemotherapy increased the long-term risk for cardiovascular disease.[68] Patients who were treated with BEP alone had a 5.7-fold higher risk (95% CI 1.9-fold, 17.1-fold) for coronary artery disease compared with surgery only and a 3.1-fold higher risk (95% CI 1.2-fold, 7.7-fold) for myocardial infarction compared with age-matched controls from the general population. Acute chemotherapy-induced cardiovascular changes have been observed in patients treated with cisplatin-based chemotherapy, including an increase in plasma von Willebrand factor levels and an increased intima-media thickness of the carotid artery.[69] In addition to chemotherapy-induced endothelial damage, cardiovascular toxicity also is likely related to the metabolic syndrome and gonadal dysfunction.[70]

Patients with testicular cancer are at an increased risk of secondary malignancies that is related to prior radiotherapy or chemotherapy for at least 35 years after treatment.[18] Increased risks have been seen for cancers of the stomach, gallbladder, bile ducts, pancreas, bladder, kidney, and thyroid, as well as for soft tissue sarcoma, nonmelanoma skin cancer, and myeloid leukemia.[71] The long-term risks of second malignant neoplasms and cardiovascular disease were evaluated in a cohort of 2,707 5-year testicular cancer survivors from the Netherlands.[72] Radiotherapy and chemotherapy increased the risk of second malignant neoplasms or cardiovascular disease to a similar extent as smoking. Subdiaphragmatic radiation strongly increased the risk of secondary malignancies but not of cardiac disease, whereas chemotherapy increased the risks for both. Median survival was 1.4 years after a secondary malignancy and 4.7 years after cardiovascular disease. In a recently reported population-based study evaluating the risk for solid tumors after chemotherapy or surgery for testicular nonseminoma, a significantly increased risk for solid tumors was seen among patients treated in the modern era of cisplatin-based chemotherapy with no increase in risk following surgery (standardized incidence ratio, 1.43 [95% CI 1.18, 1.73] for chemotherapy versus 0.93 [95% CI 0.76, 1.14] for surgery alone).[73]

Newly diagnosed patients with testicular cancer are at risk for decreased sperm counts or impaired sperm motility. With treatment, infertility can result from retrograde ejaculation after retroperitoneal lymph node dissection or as a result of radiation or chemotherapy. Although some patients will have long-standing chemotherapy-induced oligospermia or azoospermia, normal or near-normal spermatogenesis resumes in most patients. In a survey study of patients treated with two to four cycles of standard cisplatin-based chemotherapy without

KEY POINTS

- Germ cell tumor staging includes serum tumor markers, and management of advanced disease requires the use of a risk-adapted classification system.
- The different main histologic subtypes of germ cell tumors (i.e., seminoma and nonseminoma) have biologic significance and require different treatment strategies.
- Surveillance represents an important management option for patients with early-stage germ cell tumors.
- Combined-modality treatment approaches are used to achieve the highest probability of cure with the least morbidity.
- Survivorship issues are an important component of the treatment of patients with germ cell tumors.

additional treatment after surgery, the 15-year actuarial paternity rate was 85%, with decreased success with an increasing number of cycles.[74] Patients who are scheduled to have a retroperitoneal lymph node dissection, radiation therapy, or chemotherapy are advised to bank sperm. Other late effects of treatment include ototoxicity, chronic neurotoxicity, renal impairment, pulmonary toxicity, and anxiety disorder. In light of a young age at diagnosis and high cure rates, patients with testicular cancer require specialized follow-up care with close attention to monitoring for late effects of cancer and cancer therapy.[75]

BLADDER CANCER
EPIDEMIOLOGY

Approximately 72,570 (54,610 men and 17,960 women) new cases of bladder cancer and 15,210 (10,820 men and 4,390 women) related deaths were estimated to occur in the United States in 2013.[1] The incidence of bladder cancer is 3 to 4 times higher in men than in women, and the median age at diagnosis is 73. The approximate 5:1 ratio of incidence to mortality reflects the frequency of noninvasive tumors compared with muscle-invasive tumors and metastatic disease. In the United States, white individuals have a 2-fold higher incidence of bladder cancer, but black individuals have a higher mortality rate, with a higher incidence of high-grade and muscle-invasive tumors.[76] The difference in mortality does not appear to be related to the intensity and quality of care received.[77] Risk factors for bladder cancer include tobacco use, occupational exposures, urinary tract diseases, and pharmaceutical drug use. Cigarette smoking is strongly associated with an increased risk of bladder cancer among men and women. In the United States, the risk of bladder cancer in former smokers (hazard ratio [HR] 2.22, 95% CI 2.03, 2.44) and current smokers (HR 4.06, 95% CI 3.66, 4.50) compared with the risk in never-smokers has increased over time.[78] Although smoking cessation is associated with a reduced risk of bladder cancer, the risk compared with that in never-smokers remains elevated for those who have quit, even after 10 years or more. This risk increases in proportion to the amount and duration of cigarette exposure with heavy smokers (more than 20 cigarettes per day and/or more than 40 years), resulting in up to a 5-fold higher relative risk [RR] than for nonsmokers. Occupational exposure to aromatic amines (particularly 2-naphthylamine, benzidine, and polycyclic aromatic hydrocarbons) is associated with an increased incidence of bladder cancer (e.g., workers in dyestuff manufacturing and rubber and aluminum industries). Infection with the trematode schistosoma haematobium leads to chronic irritation of the urothelium and an increased risk of both squamous and urothelial carcinomas. Other chronic urinary tract infections, including stones and cystitis, also may lead to chronic inflammation and an increased risk of bladder cancer. Heavy use of phenacetin-containing analgesics is associated with tumors of the renal pelvis and ureter, and cyclophosphamide also has been associated with an increased risk of urothelial carcinoma. These myriad risk factors lead to field changes within the urothelium that predispose individuals to the development of recurrent tumors,

as well as to the involvement of new locations in the urothelial tract (polychronotropism). Hereditary nonpolyposis colon cancer or Lynch syndrome is associated with an increased risk for the development of bladder and other urothelial cancers.[79]

The three general categories of disease—non–muscle-invasive, muscle-invasive, and metastatic—differ in tumor biology, clinical phenotype, management, and prognosis. For non–muscle-invasive tumors, the goal is to prevent recurrence and progression to an incurable state. For muscle-invasive disease, the goal is to maximize the chance for cure using a multimodality approach incorporating chemotherapy with surgery or radiation therapy. The management of metastatic disease requires the use of established prognostic and predictive factors to determine the therapeutic objectives and potential for treatment-related toxicity. The main goals are prolongation of survival and palliation of symptoms.

PATHOLOGY

Urothelial carcinoma may occur throughout the urinary tract (i.e., in any structure lined by the urothelium), with more than 90% of tumors originating in the bladder. Upper urinary tract tumors, including the renal pelvis and ureter, account for 5% to 7% of urothelial carcinomas, with renal pelvis tumors composing the majority. In the United States, 92% of lower urinary tract tumors are urothelial carcinomas, 5% are squamous cell cancers, 2% are adenocarcinomas, and 1% are small cell carcinomas. Lesions of mixed histology typically are variants of urothelial carcinoma. Adenocarcinomas may be of urachal origin, occurring at the junction of the urachal ligament and bladder dome. In Northern Africa and other parts of the world where there is a high prevalence of infection with schistosoma haematobium, up to 75% of tumors are pure squamous cell carcinomas.

BIOLOGY

Molecular profiling has demonstrated that urothelial tumors evolve through divergent pathways corresponding to the clinical phenotypes of nonlethal, recurrent non–muscle-invasive lesions and lethal, muscle-invasive, and metastatic disease.[80] Deletions of both arms of chromosome 9 are seen during the earliest stages of urothelial tumorigenesis. Overexpression of HRAS—the first human oncogene identified in urothelial carcinoma—is seen in the majority of human urothelial cancers. The RAS signaling pathway appears to have a major role in the development of low-grade noninvasive lesions; 30% to 40% are characterized by activating mutations in the HRAS gene, and 70% have mutations in FGFR3, an upstream tyrosine kinase receptor involved in cellular proliferation and angiogenesis. Although approximately 70% of these low-grade lesions will recur, only 10% to 15% will progress to invasive lesions. Progression of low-grade lesions to invasive disease is characterized by structural and functional alterations in the tumor suppressors p53 and Rb, in addition to chromosome aberrations, including deletions in chromosome 8p, 11p, 13q, and 14q. Approximately 20% to 30% of patients will present with high-grade muscle-invasive tumors, with more than 50% of these tumors containing alterations in *p53* and *Rb.* Despite radical cystectomy and the use of perioperative chemotherapy, up to 50% of invasive tumors will progress to local and distant metastases. This ability to invade and metastasize not only is a function of alterations in the tumor cells but also involves the interactions of the tumor cells with the local microenvironment. The following are seen in urothelial carcinoma: defects in cell–cell adhesion, with loss or reduced expression of E-cadherin; increased levels of matrix metalloproteinases, such as MMP9 and MMP2, which lead to degradation of the extracellular matrix; and increased angiogenic factors, such as vascular endothelial growth factor (VEGF).

Retrospective studies have suggested that p53 nuclear overexpression is an independent predictor of progression and decreased survival. Immunohistochemical staining for p53, p21, pRB, and p16 in a series of patients with bladder cancer who underwent radical cystectomy and bilateral pelvic lymphadenectomy demonstrated that altered expression of each of the four cell cycle regulators was associated with bladder cancer outcome, with p53 as the strongest predictor.[81] A phase III study of molecularly targeted adjuvant therapy in locally advanced bladder cancer based on p53 status failed to confirm both the prognostic value of p53 and the benefit of chemotherapy in p53-positive tumors.[82] Using oligonucleotide microarrays, a genetic profile consisting of 174 probes has identified patients with lymph node metastases and poor survival.[83]

In an attempt to identify actionable genomic alterations in high-grade bladder cancer, an integrative genomic analysis including mutational profiling and DNA copy number alterations was performed on 97 high-grade tumors.[84] Core pathway alterations included the RTK/RAS/RAF pathway (e.g., *ERBB2* amplification and *FGFR3* mutation), TP53 (e.g., *TP53* mutation and *MDM2* amplification), RB1/E2F3 (e.g., *RB1* mutation and *E2F3* amplification) and phosphoinositide 3-kinase (PI3K)/AKT (e.g., *PIK3CA* mutation and *TSC1* mutation). Overall, 61% of the tumors harbored genetic alterations representing potential drug targets. The recently published Cancer Genome Atlas Research Network "Comprehensive Molecular Characterization of Urothelial Bladder Carcinoma" revealed recurrent mutations in genes involved in cell-cycle regulation, chromatin regulation, and kinase signaling with potential therapeutic targets identified in 69% of tumors, including targets in the PI3K/AKT/mammalian target of rapamycin (mTOR) pathway and the RTK/MAPK pathway.[85]

DIAGNOSIS AND STAGING

The most common presenting symptom is hematuria, and patients may also present with irritative urinary symptoms. Less frequently, patients present with symptoms related to distant metastases. The diagnosis is established by cystoscopy and biopsy. The TNM staging system for bladder cancer is listed below:

- Ta tumors are noninvasive papillary lesions that tend to recur but not invade.

- Tis, or carcinoma in situ, is the precursor of a more aggressive and invasive variant.
- T1 tumors invade the subepithelial connective tissue, including lamina propria or muscularis mucosa.
- T2 tumors invade the muscle.
- pT2a tumors invade superficial muscle.
- pT2b tumors invade deep muscle.
- T3 tumors invade perivesical tissue.
- pT3a are evident microscopically.
- pT3b are evident macroscopically (extravesical mass).
- T4 tumors invade the prostate, uterus, vagina, pelvic, and/or abdominal wall.

The major problem with staging is that the correlation of depth of invasion determined by cystoscopy and biopsy with the results of cystectomy is only 50% to 60%. Noninvasive imaging with CT or MRI can identify extravesical or nodal disease and is more reliable if done prior to the transurethral resection with a distended bladder. FDG-PET/CT may have a role in the staging of muscle-invasive disease and in the detection of metastatic bladder cancer.[86,87] The histologic grading system of low grade and high grade is more relevant for noninvasive tumors, because virtually all invasive neoplasms are high grade.

THERAPY FOR BLADDER CANCER BY DISEASE STAGE

Non–Muscle-Invasive Disease

Seventy percent of patients with newly diagnosed bladder cancer will present with non–muscle-invasive disease, with 70% confined to the mucosa (Ta or Tis) and 30% involving the submucosa (T1). The treatment involves complete removal of the lesion by transurethral resection followed by rigorous surveillance with cystoscopy and urine cytology at 3-month intervals for recurrence and/or progression to a more advanced stage. The sensitivity of urine cytology ranges from 13% to 75%, and the limitations of cystoscopy include impaired visualization related to bleeding and difficulty distinguishing flat carcinoma in situ from benign lesions; however, urine markers under investigation—such as nuclear matrix protein, NMP22, and fluorescence in situ hybridization—to detect chromosomal alterations might complement cystoscopy and urine cytology in the detection of recurrence.[88,89] Approximately 70% of patients with non–muscle-invasive bladder cancer will have a recurrence or a new occurrence within 5 years, and approximately 15% will progress to a more advanced stage. When urine cytology is positive but cystoscopy reveals no visible lesions in the bladder or urethra, selective catheterization and visualization of the upper urinary tract is warranted. The management of non–muscle-invasive bladder cancer involves a complete transurethral resection with or without intravesical therapy.[90] Intravesical therapy has two uses: as prophylaxis—to prevent or delay tumor recurrence and/or progression—and as therapy for carcinoma in situ. Although the indications for prophylaxis vary, intravesical therapy typically is recommended for multifocal or recurrent Ta lesions, carcinoma in situ, and T1 disease. Randomized trials have established bacille Calmette-Guérin (BCG) with six weekly installations as the intravesical treatment of choice to limit recurrence and reduce the incidence of progression.[91] There is data to suggest a benefit from maintenance therapy with BCG. Salvage intravesical therapy with BCG and interferon (IFN)-alpha-2b may be effective for patients whose disease does not respond to BCG alone. Alternative intravesical agents including mitomycin C, gemcitabine, doxorubicin, and valrubicin have been shown to prevent recurrence with minimal effect on progression. For disease that does not respond to BCG, these alternative agents may be considered. In some cases, cystectomy is indicated, with a delay in cystectomy leading to a worse outcome.[92,93]

Muscle-Invasive Disease

Although the majority of patients present with non–muscle-invasive disease, approximately 20% to 40% of patients either present with more advanced disease or experience disease progression after therapy for non–muscle-invasive disease. Staging for patients with muscle-invasive disease includes a CT scan of the abdomen and pelvis, chest x-ray or CT scan of the chest, and, if clinically indicated, a bone scan. The standard treatment for a muscle-invasive tumor is a radical cystectomy with bilateral pelvic lymphadenectomy that includes removal of the bladder, prostate, seminal vesicles, and proximal urethra for men, and removal of the bladder, urethra, and uterus (including bilateral salpingo-oophorectomy) and excision of a portion of the anterior vaginal wall for women. The pelvic lymph node dissection is a necessary part of the radical cystectomy surgery, with a more extended lymph node dissection associated with an improvement in outcome.[94,95] The three main types of urinary diversions include an ileal conduit that drains to an appliance on the anterior abdominal wall, a continent cutaneous reservoir constructed from detubularized bowel segments, and an orthotopic neobladder. More men are candidates for continent urethral reservoirs than women because of anatomic considerations. It is not clear that continent reconstruction after radical cystectomy is associated with an improvement in quality of life (QOL) compared with conduit diversion.[96] In fact, most patients report a favorable QOL regardless of the type of diversion used.

Prognosis varies inversely with higher T stage, lymphatic or vascular invasion in the primary tumor, and lymph node involvement. In addition, extracapsular extension of lymph node metastases is associated with a worse outcome.[97] In a series of 1,054 patients undergoing radical cystectomy and pelvic lymphadenectomy, the overall recurrence-free survival rates at 5 and 10 years were 68% and 66%, respectively.[98] Patients with non–organ-confined, lymph node–negative tumors had a significantly higher (p < 0.001) probability of recurrence compared with patients who had organ-confined bladder cancers (Table 10-4). The 5- and 10-year recurrence-free survival rates for the 246 patients with lymph node involvement were 35% and 34%, respectively. Patients with organ-confined tumors and fewer than five involved lymph nodes had improved survival rates. The median time to recurrence among the 311 patients in whom the cancer recurred was 12 months (range, approximately 5 months to 11 years).

Table 10-4 **Survival Rates for Bladder Cancer According to Stage[98]**

	5-Year Survival (%)	**10-Year Survival (%)**
Node-Negative Disease		
P2	77	57
P3a	64	44
P3b	49	29
P4	44	23
Lymph Node Involvement	31	23

Reprinted with permission from Stein JP, Lieskovsky G, Cote R, et al. Radical cystectomy in the treatment of invasive bladder cancer: long-term results in 1,054 patients. J Clin Oncol. 2001;19:666-675. PMID: 11157016.

Multivariate nomograms have been developed to predict outcome after radical cystectomy.[99,100] A partial cystectomy can provide adequate local control of invasive bladder cancer in select patients.[101] Less invasive surgical techniques, including laparoscopic and robotic radical cystectomy, are being evaluated.[102] The use of bladder-sparing protocols as alternatives to surgery in the management of invasive bladder cancer will be reviewed in the Bladder Preservation section.

Metastatic Disease

Urothelial tumors are sensitive to several chemotherapy agents with different mechanisms of action, including methotrexate, vinblastine, doxorubicin, cisplatin, the taxanes, ifosfamide, pemetrexed, and gemcitabine. Two-, three-, and four-drug combinations have been used, with the combination of methotrexate, vinblastine, doxorubicin, and cisplatin (MVAC) and gemcitabine plus cisplatin (GC) representing the standard regimens.[103-105] Randomized trials comparing MVAC with single-agent cisplatin and with the three-drug combination of doxorubicin, cyclophosphamide, and cisplatin demonstrated superior response rates, prolongation of time to progression, and improved OS for patients treated with MVAC. Increasing the dose intensity of MVAC in a 2-week schedule with growth factor support compared with classic MVAC on a 4-week schedule led to a borderline statistically significant relative reduction in the risk of progression and death compared with MVAC.[106]

MVAC was compared with GC in patients with locally advanced or metastatic urothelial carcinoma.[104] Although this trial was not designed as a noninferiority study, the results demonstrated a similar response rate (GC, 49%; MVAC, 46%; p = 0.51), PFS (GC, 7.7 months; MVAC, 8.3 months; p = 0.63), and median survival (GC, 14 months; MVAC, 15.2 months; p = 0.66), as well as less toxicity for GC than for MVAC. Specifically, treatment with GC produced less neutropenia, neutropenic fever, sepsis, and mucositis but more anemia and thrombocytopenia than MVAC. The combination of docetaxel and cisplatin plus granulocyte colony-stimulating factor (G-CSF) has been compared with MVAC plus G-CSF in advanced urothelial carcinoma.[107] Treatment with MVAC resulted in a superior response rate (54.2% vs. 37.4%; p = 0.17), median time to progression (9.4 months vs. 6.1 months; p = 0.003), and median survival (14.2 months vs. 9.3 months; p = 0.026).

Several trials using taxanes have demonstrated promising results with ifosfamide/paclitaxel/cisplatin, gemcitabine/paclitaxel/cisplatin, and gemcitabine/paclitaxel/carboplatin.

The superiority of triplet regimens has not been established, with a randomized, international trial of patients with advanced urothelial cancer without prior systemic therapy comparing GC with combination paclitaxel, cisplatin, and gemcitabine (PCG) demonstrating a higher overall response rate for PCG that did not translate into a higher PFS or median survival for the PCG triplet.[108] A sequential regimen using gemcitabine and doxorubicin followed by the combination of ifosfamide, paclitaxel, and cisplatin demonstrated a high overall response rate; but the regimen was associated with toxicity without a clear benefit compared with other nonsequential, cisplatin-based regimens.[109]

As a disease of older individuals with coexisting medical problems, including impaired performance status and renal insufficiency, approximately 40% to 50% of patients with advanced bladder cancer are not eligible for cisplatin-based chemotherapy. Recently proposed criteria to determine ineligibility for cisplatin-based chemotherapy include at least one of the following: Eastern Cooperative Oncology Group (ECOG) performance status of 2, creatinine clearance less than 60 mL/min, grade 2 or greater hearing loss, grade 2 or greater neuropathy, and/or New York Heart Association Class III heart failure.[110] For patients with renal insufficiency who are not candidates for cisplatin, alternative regimens such as gemcitabine or paclitaxel with carboplatin have been used. Multiple phase II trials have suggested an improvement in outcome with cisplatin- versus carboplatin-based chemotherapy.[111] A phase II/III trial of gemcitabine and carboplatin compared with methotrexate and vinblastine plus carboplatin (M-CAVI) in patients with metastatic urothelial cancer ineligible for cisplatin-based chemotherapy (World Health Organization performance status of 2 and/or creatinine clearance of 30 mL/min to 60 mL/min) demonstrated no difference in outcome and improved tolerability for gemcitabine and carboplatin compared with M-CAVI.[112]

The prognostic factors predicting long-term survival of patients with metastatic urothelial carcinoma receiving MVAC chemotherapy include Karnofsky performance status (less than or greater than 80%) and presence or absence of visceral metastases (lung, liver, or bone).[113] Median survival times for patients who had zero, one, or two risk factors were 33 months, 13.4 months, and 9.3 months, respectively. Two nomograms for predicting survival of patients with metastatic urothelial cancer have recently been published.[114,115] The pretreatment variables used to predict OS in the models include the presence and number of visceral metastases, albumin, performance status, hemoglobin, site of the primary tumor, lymph node metastases and leukocyte count. Toxicity varies as a function of risk group. For patients with poor-risk disease, treatment-related mortality has been reported in 3% to 4% of cases. Although the frequency of these events may be reduced with the use of hematopoietic growth factors, MVAC is typically avoided for patients with poor-risk disease.

There is no accepted standard of care for second-line chemotherapy in advanced bladder cancer.[116] Evaluations of single agents—such as ifosfamide, docetaxel, gemcitabine, paclitaxel, and pemetrexed—have demonstrated response rates between 9% and 27%, with a PFS in the range of 2 months to 3 months and no documented improvement in OS. In a randomized phase III trial of vinflunine (a microtubule inhibitor) plus best supportive care compared with best supportive care alone as second-line therapy after a platinum-containing regimen, vinflunine did not demonstrate a significant survival benefit.[117] Although multidrug regimens have been associated with higher response rates, this does not appear to translate into an improvement in survival. For patients with metastatic disease who experience treatment failure after a platinum-based regimen, three adverse risk factors, including ECOG performance status greater than 0, hemoglobin level less than 10 g/dL, and the presence of liver metastasis, have been shown to predict for OS.[118] The median OS times for patients with zero, one, two, or three risk factors are 14.2, 7.3, 3.8, and 1.7 months, respectively. A nomogram including baseline prognostic factors has been developed to estimate the activity of second-line therapy.[119]

Metastasectomy is routinely performed in the management of advanced testicular germ cell tumors and may be considered in the management of other advanced urologic malignancies. In highly select patients with metastatic urothelial carcinoma, resection of metastatic disease can result in long-term disease control.[120,121]

PERIOPERATIVE CHEMOTHERAPY FOR MUSCLE-INVASIVE AND LOCALLY ADVANCED BLADDER CANCER

The use of perioperative chemotherapy in the management of invasive and locally advanced bladder cancer has been studied in the neoadjuvant (preoperative) and adjuvant (postoperative) settings. The potential advantages for neoadjuvant chemotherapy include (1) evaluation of response to therapy in vivo with continuation of effective chemotherapy, (2) discontinuation of chemotherapy and early cystectomy in the setting of no response or progression, (3) tumor downstaging to allow for a less complicated surgery, and (3) delivery of full-dose chemotherapy without the problems associated with postoperative recovery. The major advantages for the use of adjuvant chemotherapy include treatment based on pathologic criteria with the ability to select those patients at high risk who are most likely to benefit from chemotherapy and to avoid the unnecessary treatment of patients with lower-risk disease.

Neoadjuvant Chemotherapy for Bladder Cancer

Several of the initial prospective randomized trials of neoadjuvant chemotherapy using single agents and combination chemotherapy failed to demonstrate a benefit. The largest phase III neoadjuvant chemotherapy trial performed to date randomly assigned 976 patients with T2 G3, T3, T4a, N0 to NX, or M0 bladder cancer undergoing cystectomy or radiotherapy or both to three cycles of neoadjuvant chemotherapy with cisplatin, methotrexate, and vinblastine or to no chemotherapy. Chemotherapy-associated mortality was 1%, and cystectomy-associated mortality was 3.7%. At a median follow-up of 8 years, a statistically significant 16% reduction in the risk of death (HR 0.84; 95% CI 0.72, 0.99; p = 0.037) corresponding to an increase in 10-year survival from 30% to 36% was seen in the chemotherapy arm.[122] The chemotherapy regimen was associated with a higher pathologic complete response rate. A U.S. phase III Intergroup trial randomly assigned patients with T2-4aN0M0 bladder cancer to neoadjuvant MVAC plus cystectomy (153 patients) or to cystectomy alone (154 patients).[123] At a median follow-up of 8.7 years, the estimated risk of death was reduced by 25% for the patients who received MVAC and cystectomy. Median survival of patients assigned to surgery alone was 46 months, compared with 77 months among patients assigned to MVAC plus cystectomy. The survival benefit of neoadjuvant MVAC was associated with tumor downstaging to pT0 (38% in those patients who received MVAC compared with 15% of those who received cystectomy), with an 85% 5-year survival for patients who experienced a pathologic complete response to neoadjuvant chemotherapy. A meta-analysis of neoadjuvant chemotherapy in invasive bladder cancer performed with data from 3,005 patients enrolled in 11 randomized trials showed a significant OS benefit for platinum-based combination chemotherapy, with a 14% reduction in the risk of death and 5% absolute survival benefit at 5 years, with OS increasing from 45% to 50%.[124] This effect did not vary between subgroups of patients or type of local treatment. Based on these data, neoadjuvant cisplatin combination chemotherapy represents a standard of care in the management of muscle-invasive bladder cancer (Table 10-5). Although not formally evaluated in a randomized trial in the neoadjuvant setting, the

most widely used regimen is the combination of gemcitabine and cisplatin.[125] Two recently reported trials suggest that dose-dense or accelerated MVAC with growth factor support is safe and effective in the neoadjuvant setting.[125a,125b] Despite the evidence supporting neoadjuvant chemotherapy, it remains grossly underutilized.[126] There are insufficient data to support the use of non-cisplatin chemotherapy regimens in the neoadjuvant setting. Thus, renal insufficiency or coexisting medical problems may limit the ability to use perioperative chemotherapy.

Adjuvant Chemotherapy for Bladder Cancer

Although many physicians favor the use of adjuvant chemotherapy for patients with nodal involvement and extravesical tumor extension, definitive trials are lacking. Unfortunately, the adjuvant studies that have been performed have major limitations, including flawed statistical methodology with underpowered trials and early termination, as well as the use of suboptimal chemotherapy with non–cisplatin-containing regimens. For example, in one study, 91 patients with P3, P4, or node-positive disease were randomly assigned to receive either four cycles of adjuvant cisplatin, cyclophosphamide, and doxorubicin or to observation. Although the trial demonstrated a significant delay in time to disease progression in patients who received chemotherapy—with 70% of patients disease-free at 3 years compared with 46% of untreated patients—the 5-year OS was not significantly different.[127] Several methodologic problems with this trial include the small sample size, premature closure, and the fact that 25% of patients assigned to chemotherapy never received it. A German study randomly assigned patients with pT3b, pT4a, and/or lymph node involvement to observation after cystectomy or to three cycles of adjuvant MVAC or combination methotrexate, vinblastine, epirubicin, and cisplatin.[128] The trial was terminated early when an interim analysis indicated an inferior DFS rate and a significantly

Table 10-5 **Randomized Trials of Neoadjuvant Cisplatin-Based Combination Chemotherapy for Muscle-Invasive Bladder Cancer**[122,123]

Clinical Trial	Eligible Disease	Comparison	Median Survival (years)	pT0 Rate (%)	Survival Rates (%)
Grossman et al.	T2-4a, N0, M0	Three cycles of MVAC plus cystectomy	6.4	38	57 (5 years)*
		Cystectomy alone	3.8	15	42 (5 years)*
Hall et al.	T2(G3), T3-T4a, N0/NX, M0	Three cycles of CMV plus cystectomy or radiotherapy or both	NA	33	56, 49, 36** (3, 5, 10 years)
		Cystectomy or radiotherapy or both	NA	12	50, 43, 30** (3, 5, 10 years)

*p = 0.06 by a stratified log-rank test
**p = 0.037; HR 0.84, 95% CI (0.72, 0.99)

Abbreviations: MVAC, methotrexate, vinblastine, doxorubicin, and cisplatin; NA, not available; CMV, cisplatin, methotrexate, and vinblastine.

Adapted from Hall RR et al. The Intl Collaboration of Trialists of the MRC Advanced Bladder Cancer Group, MRC Clinical Trials Unit. ASCO Annual Meeting. Proc Am Soc Clin Oncol. 2002:21:Abstract 710, No. 18S; Adapted from Grossman HB, Natale RB, Tangen CM, et al. Neoadjuvant chemotherapy plus cystectomy compared with cystectomy alone for locally advanced bladder cancer. N Engl J Med. 2003;349(9): 859-866; and adapted from International Collaboration of Trialists, Medical Research Council Advanced Bladder Cancer Working Party (now the National Cancer Research Institute Bladder Cancer Clinical Studies Group), European Organisation for Research and Treatment of Cancer Genito-Urinary Tract Cancer Group, et al. International phase III trial assessing neoadjuvant cisplatin, methotrexate, and vinblastine chemotherapy for muscle-invasive bladder cancer: long-term results of the BA06 30894 trial. J Clin Oncol. 2011;29:2171-2177.

higher relapse rate (18 of 22 patients, 82%) among untreated patients compared with patients who received chemotherapy (three of 18 patients, 17%; p = 0.0012). For patients with nodal involvement, disease progressed for 92% of patients on observation compared with 73% of patients who received adjuvant chemotherapy (p < 0.002). A survival difference was subsequently shown; however, patients did not receive chemotherapy at the time of relapse.[129] An Italian multicenter randomized phase III trial comparing adjuvant GC chemotherapy with chemotherapy at relapse for patients with muscle-invasive bladder cancer after radical cystectomy did not demonstrate a significant difference in DFS and OS between the groups; however, the study was underpowered, having not met its accrual goal.[130] Another recent randomized phase III trial comparing adjuvant paclitaxel/ gemcitabine/cisplatin (PGC) to observation in patients with resected high-risk bladder cancer (pT3-4 and/or pN+) by the Spanish Oncology Genitourinary Group demonstrated an improvement in DFS and OS; however, this trial also was prematurely closed and underpowered, limiting the conclusion.[131] The final results of the EORTC randomized phase III trial comparing immediate versus deferred chemotherapy after radical cystectomy in patients with pT3, T4 and/or N+ M0 bladder cancer was recently presented. With only 284 of a planned 660 patients ultimately enrolled, immediate chemotherapy led to a statistically significant improvement in the secondary endpoint of PFS (median and 5-year PFS are 2.9 years and 46.8% on the immediate and 0.9 years and 29.5% on the deferred arm [p < 0.0001]) and a nonsignificant decrease of 22% in the risk of death after radical cystectomy, the primary endpoint.[131a] A systemic review and meta-analysis based on 491 patients with bladder cancer treated on six randomized controlled trials comparing local treatment plus adjuvant chemotherapy with local treatment alone revealed an overall HR for survival of 0.75 (95% CI 0.60, 0.96; p = 0.019) suggesting a 25% relative reduction in the risk of death associated with adjuvant chemotherapy.[132] The power of the meta-analysis is clearly limited by the sample size and the flawed trials from which the analysis was derived.

BLADDER PRESERVATION

A bladder-sparing approach is only justified when the treatment can completely eradicate the tumor in the bladder, the risk of recurrence is low, and bladder function is not substantially compromised.[133] It is estimated that this approach is applicable to 15% to 20% of patients who present with invasive disease, but select series suggest that this rate may be higher.

Although neoadjuvant chemotherapy in combination with local therapy has been shown to improve OS, the role of chemotherapy alone in bladder preservation is problematic because of the inability to definitively determine which bladders are truly without residual tumor. In addition, pathologic complete response rates after neoadjuvant chemotherapy at the time of cystectomy are only 20% to 40%. At a minimum, chemotherapy alone cannot replace definitive treatment of the bladder by surgery or radiation.

In randomized trials, radiation therapy alone has been shown to be inferior to cystectomy with respect to survival, particularly for patients with T3 or T4 disease. Although radical cystectomy has not been formally compared with a multimodality bladder-sparing approach, multiple studies have evaluated trimodality treatment consisting of transurethral resection (as complete as safely possible) together with chemotherapy plus radiation therapy for select patients resulting in long-term DFS and OS rates approaching those seen in radical cystectomy series. An analysis of long-term outcomes of selective bladder preservation in 348 patients at Massachusetts General Hospital demonstrated 5-year disease-specific survival and OS rates of 64% and 52%, respectively, with preservation of the native bladder in more than 70% of patients.[134] The majority of trimodality protocols have used cisplatin-based chemotherapy; however, other agents such as paclitaxel and gemcitabine have been used as well. In the largest randomized study to compare chemoradiotherapy using fluorouracil and mitomycin with radiotherapy alone in muscle-invasive bladder cancer, the chemoradiotherapy arm was associated with a 32% reduction in the risk of locoregional recurrence (HR 0.68, 95% CI 0.48, 0.96; p = 0.03) at a median follow-up of 69.9 months.[135] An important component of bladder-sparing protocols is an evaluation of early response of the primary tumor to treatment, with less than a complete response requiring cystectomy. Approximately one-third of patients initiated on a bladder-sparing protocol will ultimately require cystectomy for a less-than-complete response or for recurrent muscle-invasive tumors. QOL is another important consideration. Radiation therapy can induce disturbances in the function of the bladder, anal sphincter, and large bowel. The morbidity of radiation therapy has decreased with the availability of better imaging, allowing for a boost to the primary tumor and a reduction in fraction size. An evaluation of late pelvic toxicity after bladder-sparing therapy in patients with invasive bladder cancer treated on four prospective Radiation Therapy Oncology Group (RTOG) protocols showed low rates of significant late pelvic toxicity (7% of patients with late grade 3 or greater pelvic toxicity: 5.7% genitourinary and 1.9% gastrointestinal) at a median follow-up of 5.4 years.[136] The main disadvantage for bladder preservation is the requirement for lifelong surveillance because of the risk of recurrence or development of a new bladder cancer. However, many of these new or recurrent tumors are noninvasive and can be managed endoscopically. In a series of 121 patients treated with sequential chemotherapy followed by concurrent chemotherapy and radiation therapy, 48 patients had a recurrence, of which 32 (66%) were noninvasive, occurring 2 years after treatment. Of these, 21 patients were treated conservatively. Thus, even when a complete remission is accomplished, continued endoscopic monitoring is essential.[137]

OTHER UROTHELIAL TRACT CANCERS

Cancers of the renal pelvis, ureter, and proximal urethra also are of urothelial origin and should be treated on the basis of primary histology. Because approximately 20% to 50% of patients with urothelial carcinomas of the upper urinary tract will develop bladder cancer, surveillance cystoscopy is necessary. The two theories for the multifocal nature of urothelial carcinoma include the field cancerization effect and monoclonality (i.e., tumor cells spreading from their origin to multiple sites). Thus, simultaneous or metachronous primary tumors of the urothelium at multiple sites may occur, and monitoring is required, including follow-up cystoscopies and CT or MRI scans of the upper tracts.

Regarding the management of noninvasive bladder cancer with intravesical BCG, it is not uncommon for relapse to occur at the ureteral orifices, ureter, or urethra—areas that are less accessible to intravesical treatment. As such, monitoring must include periodic evaluations of the remaining urothelium with cytology and imaging to ensure relapses or new primary tumors are identified and treated early.

The chemotherapy used for urothelial carcinoma has been considered to be less effective in nonurothelial histology tumors; however, a secondary analysis of the U.S. phase III Intergroup trial of neoadjuvant MVAC in patients with nonurothelial components in the tumor, including squamous and glandular differentiation, demonstrated a survival benefit from chemotherapy in these mixed histology tumors.[138] For patients with pure small cell carcinoma or adenocarcinoma, the use of chemotherapy regimens demonstrating activity in other sites with similar histology is typically used (e.g., etoposide and cisplatin for small cell carcinoma of the lung may be used for the management of small cell carcinoma of the bladder). Micropapillary bladder cancer, a rare variant of urothelial carcinoma, has been associated with a poor prognosis.[139] Intravesical therapy may be less effective, and early radical cystectomy is often recommended.

KEY POINTS

- Urothelial tumorigenesis results in three general categories of urothelial tract tumors—non–muscle-invasive, muscle-invasive, and metastatic—that differ with respect to tumor biology, clinical phenotype, prognosis, and management.
- The staging of localized urothelial tract tumors requires a transurethral resection specimen that includes muscle to ensure that a muscle-invasive tumor is not missed.
- Level 1 evidence supports the use of neoadjuvant cisplatin-based combination chemotherapy for patients with muscle-invasive bladder cancer. Although the data for adjuvant chemotherapy are less compelling, it may be considered for patients with high-risk features after radical cystectomy.
- Bladder preservation may be considered in select patients using a trimodality approach: a maximal transurethral resection followed by concurrent chemotherapy and radiation therapy.

RENAL CANCER

Renal cell carcinoma (RCC) accounts for 90% of all malignant neoplasms of the kidney, with an estimated 65,150 newly diagnosed cases of kidney and renal pelvis tumors (40,430 men and

Table 10-6 Staging of Kidney Cancer[12]

Primary Tumor (T)	
TX	Primary tumor cannot be assessed
T0	No evidence of primary tumor
T1	Tumor 7 cm or less in greatest dimension, limited to the kidney
T1a	Tumor 4 cm or less in greatest dimension, limited to the kidney
T1b	Tumor more than 4 cm but not more than 7 cm in greatest dimension, limited to the kidney
T2	Tumor more than 7 cm in greatest dimension, limited to the kidney
T2a	Tumor more than 7 cm but less than or equal to 10 cm in greatest dimension, limited to the kidney
T2b	Tumor more than 10 cm, limited to the kidney
T3	Tumor extends into major veins or perinephric tissues but not into the ipsilateral adrenal gland and not beyond Gerota fascia
T3a	Tumor grossly extends into the renal vein or its segmental (muscle-containing) branches, or tumor invades perirenal and/or renal sinus fat but not beyond Gerota fascia
T3b	Tumor grossly extends into the vena cava below the diaphragm
T3c	Tumor grossly extends into the vena cava above the diaphragm or invades the wall of the vena cava
T4	Tumor invades beyond Gerota fascia (including contiguous extension into the ipsilateral adrenal gland)
Regional Lymph Nodes (N)	
NX	Regional lymph nodes cannot be assessed
N0	No regional lymph node metastasis
N1	Metastasis in regional lymph node(s)
Distant Metastasis (M)	
M0	No distant metastasis
M1	Distant metastasis
Anatomic Stage/Prognostic Groups	
Stage I	T1 N0 M0
Stage II	T2 N0 M0
Stage III	T1 or T2 N1 M0 T3 N0 or N1 M0
Stage IV	T4 Any N M0 Any T Any N M1

The original source for this material is the AJCC Cancer Staging Manual, 7th Edition (2010) published by Springer Science and Business Media LLC, www.springerlink.com.

24,720 women) and 13,680 deaths (8,780 men and 4,900 women) in 2013.[1] Between 1975 and 2008, the annual incidence of kidney tumors increased by 1.8% and 3.3% in white men and women, respectively, and by 2.9% in black men and women. Based on rates from 2005 to 2007, 1.49% of individuals (1 in 67)

Table 10-7 Molecular Classification of Renal Epithelial Neoplasms

Type of Cancer	Cytogenetics	Molecular Alteration	Familial Syndrome
Clear cell (conventional)	3p–	VHL inactivating mutation or hypermethylation, PBRM1, SETD2, BAP1, and TORC1 pathway mutations	von Hippel-Lindau
Papillary	+7, +17, –Y	c-met activating mutation; fumarate hydratase inactivating mutation	Hereditary papillary renal cell carcinoma; hereditary leiomyomatosis renal cell carcinoma
Chromophobe	–1, –Y hypodiploid	FLCN mutation	Birt-Hogg-Dubé syndrome
Oncocytoma	–1, –Y		Birt-Hogg-Dubé syndrome
Collecting-duct carcinoma	Not defined		

will be diagnosed with cancer of the kidney or renal pelvis during their lifetime. Renal cancers were historically called the "internist's tumor" because of the variable clinical presentations, including fatigue, weight loss, and anemia. Today, less than 10% of cases present with the classic triad of hematuria, abdominal pain, and a palpable mass. Between 1993 and 2004, the proportion of patients diagnosed with stage I RCC increased from 43.0% to 57.1%, whereas the proportion of patients diagnosed with stage IV disease decreased from 27.4% to 18.7%, likely resulting from the increased use of radiographic testing done for other diagnostic purposes.[140] Risk factors for RCC include smoking, obesity, hypertension, and acquired cystic kidney disease, which is associated with end-stage renal disease.[141,142] Tobacco use (longer duration and exposure) is associated with an increased risk of advanced RCC.[143] Approximately 2% of cases are associated with inherited syndromes.

CT scan with contrast media is used for detecting and staging renal cancers. MRI is useful when renal function is poor, for evaluating local invasion, or for assessing the renal vein and inferior vena cava for thrombus. Although negative FDG-PET imaging does not reliably exclude renal cancer, it may be useful in evaluating for local recurrence and distant metastases.[144] Staging is performed using the AJCC staging classification (Table 10-6).[12]

Surgical excision by open or laparoscopic nephrectomy is the primary treatment for patients with localized disease, either by radical nephrectomy or nephron-sparing partial nephrectomy for small tumors. In one prospective randomized trial, a lymph node dissection did not prolong OS,[145] although the role for lymphadenectomy remains controversial.[146] Cryoablation or radiofrequency ablation is a reasonable alternative for incidentally detected small renal masses in select patients.[147,148] Tumor extension into the renal vein or inferior vena cava—indicating stage III disease—does not preclude resection, and cardiopulmonary bypass may be required; approximately 50% of such patients have prolonged survival with a successful resection. There is no benefit to postoperative radiation therapy for patients with locally advanced disease. Signs and symptoms of hepatic dysfunction may occur in patients with localized renal cancer (i.e., without evidence of metastatic disease). This is a rare paraneoplastic syndrome referred to as Stauffer syndrome. Patients with this syndrome should undergo resection, which leads to reversal of the hepatopathy.

Cytoreductive nephrectomy should be considered as an initial treatment for patients with metastatic disease or to relieve symptoms or control bleeding. Two prospective randomized studies demonstrated improved survival for patients subsequently treated with IFN, with a combined analysis showing a median survival of 13.6 months for patients undergoing nephrectomy plus IFN compared with 7.8 months for patients receiving IFN alone, despite similar low response rates to IFN.[149] The role for cytoreductive nephrectomy is less well defined in the new era of novel agents targeting angiogenesis. A retrospective study of cytoreductive nephrectomy in patients with metastatic RCC receiving VEGF-targeted therapy revealed a prolonged survival with nephrectomy.[150] The use of an antiangiogenic agent preoperatively for patients with metastases or for those with a large primary tumor to reduce tumor size prior to nephrectomy is under investigation.[151] Use of embolization is often recommended preoperatively for large primary tumors and metastases because of the highly vascular nature of RCC. Surgical excision of oligometastatic disease at presentation or following prolonged disease-free intervals may be appropriate.

PATHOLOGY AND MOLECULAR PATHOGENESIS

The Heidelberg classification of renal tumors introduced in 1997 correlated histopathologic features with genetic abnormalities.[152] The classification of adult epithelial kidney tumors has significantly expanded to include less common histologies that are associated with distinct clinical outcomes.[153,154] The most common histopathologic subtypes of renal cancer in adults, based on tumor morphology, immunohistochemistry, cytogenetics, and other molecular studies, are clear cell, papillary, chromophobe, and collecting-duct or Bellini duct tumors, with 4% to 6% of tumors remaining unclassified. Sarcomatoid differentiation, which is associated with a worse prognosis, can occur in any major histologic subtype. Specific cytogenetic and molecular abnormalities that frequently result in dysregulation of metabolic pathways are associated with each major histologic subtype (Table 10-7).[155,156]

Von Hippel-Lindau (VHL) disease is an autosomal-dominant, familial cancer syndrome that predisposes individuals to renal clear cell cancers, retinal angiomas, hemangioblastomas of the spinal cord and cerebellum, pheochromocytomas, and other rare

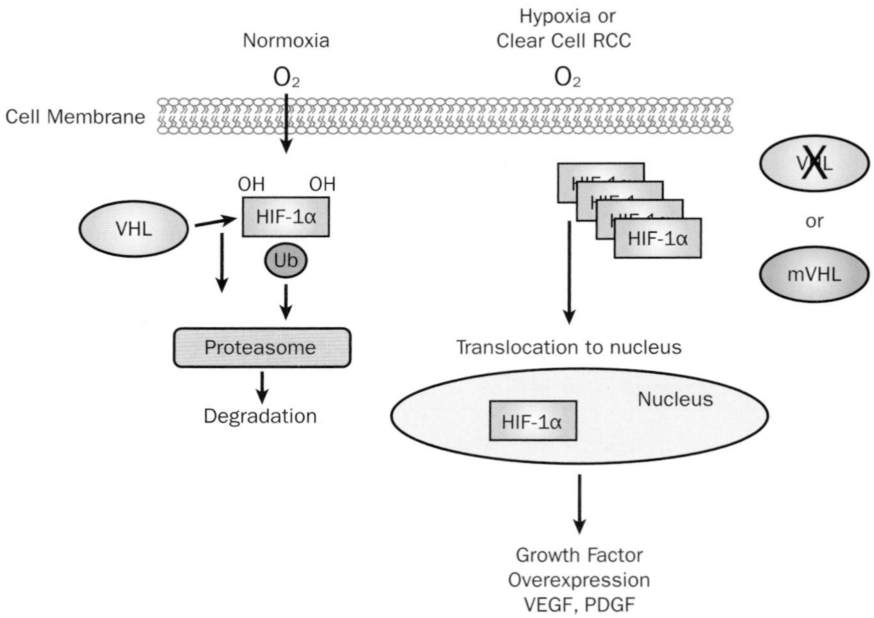

Fig. 10-1 Von Hippel-Lindau (VHL) pathway in clear cell renal cancer.

Under normoxic conditions, HIF-1 alpha is hydroxylated, allowing VHL to bind and target hypoxia inducible factor (HIF)-1 alpha for ubiquitination (Ub) and degradation via the 26S proteasome pathway. Under hypoxic conditions, HIF-1 alpha is not hydroxylated or marked by VHL for degradation, resulting in HIF-1 alpha accumulation which translocates to the nucleus to form a complex with HIF-1 beta. It then functions to induce transcription of growth stimulatory genes such as VEGF, PDGF, and TGF-alpha, as well as erythropoietin. Similarly, in clear cell carcinomas where VHL is lost or mutated (mVHL), HIF-1 alpha accumulates, tranlocates to the nucleus, and stimulates growth factor expression that promotes angiogenesis and tumor cell growth.

Abbreviations: RCC, renal cell carcinoma; TGF, transforming growth factor; VEGF, vascular endothelial growth factor; PDGF, platelet-derived growth factor.

neoplasms. Frequent loss of at least one allele on chromosome 3p in renal tumors of patients with VHL disease led to the identification of the *VHL* tumor-suppressor gene. This gene encodes a protein that promotes the ubiquitination and destruction of hypoxia-inducible factor (HIF-alpha; Fig. 10-1).[157] Several proteins encoded by HIF-alpha are involved in angiogenesis, such as VEGF and platelet-derived growth factor B chain (PDGF-B). When the VHL protein is lost in renal cancers, VEGF, PDGF-B, and other proteins are overexpressed, promoting angiogenesis and tumor cell growth. Defects in the *VHL* gene, including mutation or gene silencing through methylation, also occur in the majority of tumors from patients with sporadic clear cell carcinomas. Tumor angiogenesis also is stimulated by other growth factors that activate AKT and mTOR signaling, which also increases HIF-alpha expression.[158] Therapies that target VHL-regulated and AKT signaling pathways have demonstrated significant antitumor activity. Several new mutations in genes involved in histone modification have recently been identified in clear cell RCCs,[159,159a] including the SWI/SNF chromatin remodeling complex gene *PBRM1*, which was mutated in 41% of sporadic clear cell carcinomas,[160] suggesting new potential targets for therapy.

Activating mutations in the MET receptor tyrosine kinase located on chromosome 7 occur in hereditary papillary renal carcinoma and in occasional sporadic papillary tumors.[161] Germline mutations in tricarboxylic acid cycle enzymes that are part of mitochondrial oxidative phosphorylation result in an increased risk of renal tumors. The syndrome of hereditary leiomyomatosis and renal cell cancer is associated with loss-of-function mutations in the Krebs cycle enzyme fumarate hydratase leading to a risk for cutaneous and uterine leiomyomas and solitary papillary renal carcinomas.[162] Early-onset renal tumors also occur in patients with germ-line mutations of the succinate dehydrogenase gene *SDHB*.[155,156] Sporadic cases of papillary (or clear cell) renal carcinomas containing chromosomal translocations involving the *TFE3* gene at chromosome Xp11.2 are rare, more commonly occurring in children and young adults.[163] The Birt-Hogg-Dubé syndrome is another rare autosomal-dominant disorder characterized by hair-follicle hamartomas of the face and neck, renal and pulmonary cysts, and, for some patients, multiple chromophobe or mixed chromophobe-oncocytoma renal tumors.[164] Collecting-duct carcinomas are more similar to transitional cell carcinomas.[165] Medullary carcinoma, a variant of the collecting-duct subtype, is associated with sickle cell trait or disease.

BIOLOGY

RCC can have a variable natural history that reflects the biology of the histologic tumor type. Oncocytomas are considered benign. Chromophobe carcinomas also are typically indolent and uncommonly result in metastases and cancer-related death,[166] while tumor necrosis and sarcomatoid differentiation predict a more aggressive phenotype.[167] The clinical course of clear cell carcinomas, which compromise the majority of renal tumors, is typically aggressive; although some patients can have an indolent course with stable metastases for years, or metastases occurring decades after complete resection of a primary tumor. Molecular studies are attempting to identify markers that may predict prognosis. The prognosis for papillary renal cancers typically is more favorable than for clear cell tumors.[168] Papillary tumors are divided into type 1 and type 2 lesions according to architectural, cytologic, and genetic features. Type 2 papillary RCC is associated with more aggressive clinicopathologic features and a worse outcome.[169] Collecting-duct carcinomas have a very aggressive clinical course, with over one-half of patients presenting with metastases, and a median survival of only a few months for patients with metastatic disease.[170]

SYSTEMIC THERAPIES

Patients with metastatic RCC may have a varied, unpredictable, and, in some cases, protracted clinical course. Thus, an important consideration for initiating systemic therapy is the documentation of clinical progression. One nomogram used to predict survival based on patients treated in the cytokine era includes the following as poor prognostic variables: no prior nephrectomy, low Karnofsky performance status (< 80%), low hemoglobin level, high "corrected" serum calcium, and high serum LDH. The median survival was 24 months (good risk), 12 months (intermediate risk), and 5 months (poor risk) for patients with 0, 1 to 2, or 3 or more risk factors, respectively.[171] Newer prognostic models for patients with metastatic RCC treated with contemporary targeted therapies have typically included these prognostic factors in addition to others, such as platelet count, alkaline phosphatase, and number and sites of metastases. Although the International Metastatic Renal Cell Carcinoma Database Consortium model (risk factors: anemia, thrombocytosis, neutrophilia, hypercalcemia, Karnofsky performance status less than 80%, and less than 1 year from diagnosis to treatment) has been externally validated in patients treated with first-line VEGF-targeted treatment; prospective validation has not yet been performed.[172-174]

Increased expression of VEGF in clear cell renal carcinomas led to a phase II randomized trial of bevacizumab, a humanized VEGF-neutralizing antibody, in patients with cytokine-refractory disease demonstrating a 10% response proportion and a prolonged PFS of 4.8 months compared with 2.5 months for patients receiving placebo.[175] Hypertension and asymptomatic proteinuria were the most common adverse events. Two subsequent multicenter phase III studies compared bevacizumab plus IFN-alpha to IFN-alpha alone as first-line treatment in patients with metastatic RCC.[176,177] In the AVOREN study, the addition of bevacizumab significantly increased PFS (10.2 months vs. 5.4 months, HR 0.63; p < 0.001) and objective tumor response rate (30.6% vs. 12.4%; p < 0.0001). In the Cancer and Leukemia Group B (CALGB) 90206 trial, the median PFS was 8.5 months for patients receiving bevacizumab plus IFN (95% CI 7.5, 9.7 months) compared with 5.2 months (95% CI 3.1, 5.6 months) for patients receiving IFN monotherapy (HR 0.71; p < 0.0001), with a significant increase in objective tumor response rate (25.5% vs. 13.1%; p < 0.0001). Although the contribution of IFN to bevacizumab therapy is uncertain, the combination and not bevacizumab monotherapy must be considered the standard.

Sunitinib malate is an oral broad-spectrum receptor tyrosine kinase inhibitor that targets VEGF receptor, PDGF receptor, the Fms-like tyrosine kinase (FLT3), and the c-KIT receptor tyrosine kinase. Two phase II trials in patients with cytokine-refractory disease demonstrating a response proportion of 41% and PFS of 8.2 months[178,179] led to U. S. Food and Drug Administration (FDA) approval of sunitinib for second-line therapy in 2006. A randomized phase III trial of sunitinib compared with IFN in previously untreated patients with clear cell carcinoma demonstrated a 47% objective response rate and a median PFS and OS of 11 months and 26.4 months, respectively, in patients treated with sunitinib compared with a 12% objective response rate, 5-month median PFS, and 21.8-month median OS for patients treated with IFN.[180,181] In this study, 90% of patients had undergone nephrectomy and 93% of patients had good- or intermediate-risk disease. The recommended dosing schedule for sunitinib is 50 mg daily, 4 weeks on and 2 weeks off. A randomized phase II study comparing the intermittent schedule to lower-dose (37.5 mg) continuous dosing did not demonstrate a benefit for continuous dosing in terms of QOL or PFS, with a nonstatistically significant trend toward inferior time to progression and PFS with the continuous dosing regimen.[182]

Pazopanib is another oral broad-spectrum receptor tyrosine kinase inhibitor with similar targets to sunitinib. In a phase III 2:1 randomized clinical trial comparing pazopanib with placebo, PFS was significantly improved both in patients who had not been previously treated (11.1 months vs. 2.8 months; HR 0.40, 95% CI 0.27, 0.60; p < 0.0001) and in patients pretreated with cytokines (7.4 months vs. 4.2 months; HR 0.54, 95% CI 0.35, 0.84; p < 0.001) with an overall response rate of 30% in patients receiving pazopanib.[183] This study led to FDA approval of pazopanib for metastatic RCC. A recently reported randomized phase III noninferiority trial compared the efficacy and safety of pazopanib and sunitinib as first-line therapy.[184] The PFS for patients treated with pazopanib was noninferior to patients treated with sunitinib (HR 1.05, 95% CI 0.90, 1.22), and the OS was similar (HR 0.91, 95% CI 0.76, 1.08). The safety profile favored pazopanib with less fatigue (63% vs. 55%), hand-foot syndrome (50% vs. 29%), and thrombocytopenia (78% vs. 41%). A higher incidence of increased alanine aminotransferase was seen with pazopanib (60% vs. 43%). Health-related QOL (HRQOL) measures favored pazopanib with less fatigue and soreness of the mouth, hands, and feet.

Sorafenib tosylate is another multikinase inhibitor designed as a c-RAF and BRAF kinase inhibitor, but it also inhibits VEGF receptor, PDGF receptor, FLT3, and c-KIT. Encouraging results from a phase II randomized discontinuation trial of sorafenib in patients with renal cancer[185] led to a phase III randomized Treatment Approaches in RCC Global Evaluation Trial (TARGET) of sorafenib compared with placebo for second-line therapy in patients with cytokine-refractory disease. Based on the results of this study—which showed that patients who received sorafenib had a significantly prolonged median PFS compared with placebo (24 weeks vs. 12 weeks)—sorafenib was FDA-approved for second-line therapy.[186] Similar to studies with sunitinib, patients had clear cell histology with the majority undergoing nephrectomy, an excellent performance status, and good- or intermediate-risk disease. A randomized phase II trial of first-line treatment with sorafenib (400 mg twice daily) compared with IFN for patients with previously untreated clear cell RCC demonstrated a median PFS of 5.7 months and 5.6 months for sorafenib compared with IFN, respectively (HR 0.88; p = 0.504).[187] Major response rates were less than 10% in both treatment arms. Of note, patients whose treatment was dose-escalated to 600 mg twice daily after progression had disease stabilization for a further 3.6 months, suggesting a dose response.

Toxicity from this class of drugs includes fatigue, hypertension, diarrhea, rash, hand-foot syndrome, myelosuppression including thrombocytopenia, hypothyroidism, and congestive heart failure.[188] Pazopanib therapy may also be associated with serious hepatotoxicity. Sunitinib-associated hypertension defined as a maximum or mean systolic blood pressure of greater

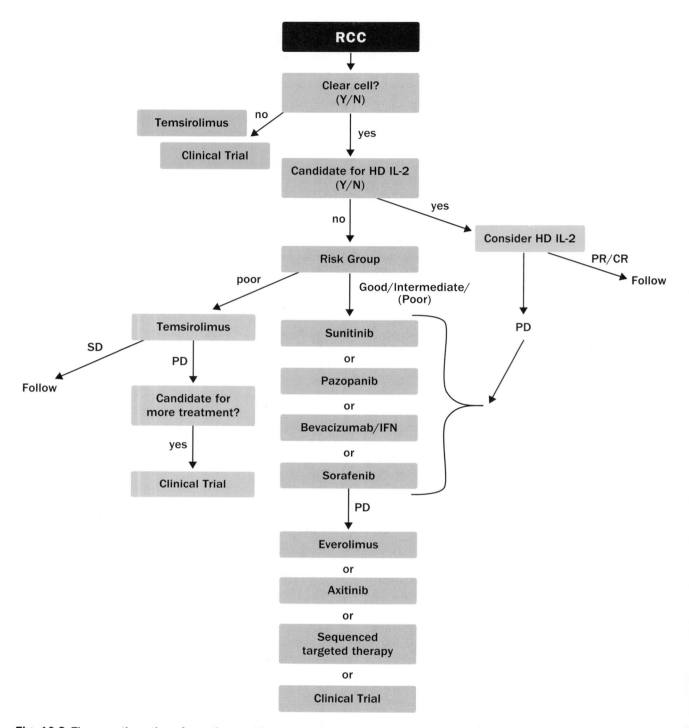

Fig. 10-2 Therapeutic options for patients with metastatic renal cell carcinoma.

Abbreviations: CR, complete response; HD IL-2, high-dose interleukin-2; IFN, interferon; PD, progressive disease; PR, partial response; RCC, renal cell carcinoma; SD, stable disease.

than 140 mm/Hg was associated with an improvement in clinical outcome, suggesting that the development of hypertension on therapy may be a biomarker of response to sunitinib.[189]

The mTOR protein is frequently activated in RCC, which can result in increased production of HIF-1-alpha and HIF-2-alpha. Consequently, agents that inhibit mTOR have been studied in patients with metastatic RCC. The mTOR inhibitor temsirolimus

demonstrated evidence of an improvement in survival in a phase II study of patients with cytokine-refractory RCC,[190] resulting in a phase III, multicenter study in patients with previously untreated advanced RCC. Patients with three or more of six poor prognostic factors (a serum LDH greater than 1.5 times the upper limit of normal, a hemoglobin level below the lower limit of the normal range, a corrected serum calcium level of more than 10 mg/dL

[2.5 mmoL/L], a time from initial diagnosis of RCC to random assignment of less than 1 year, a Karnofsky performance score of 60 or 70, or metastases in multiple organs) were randomly assigned to 25 mg of temsirolimus weekly, IFN alone, or the combination of 15 mg of temsirolimus weekly plus IFN.[191] Single-agent temsirolimus was associated with an improvement in OS compared with IFN (HR 0.73, 95% CI 0.58, 0.92; p = 0.0078), with a median OS of 10.9 months compared with 7.3 months for patients receiving IFN alone. PFS was 5.5 months on the temsirolimus arm and 3.1 months on the IFN arm (HR 0.66, 95% CI 0.53, 0.81). The combination arm did not increase survival. This led to FDA approval of single-agent temsirolimus in 2007.

Everolimus is an orally administered mTOR inhibitor. A phase III, 2:1 randomized, double-blind trial compared everolimus with placebo for patients whose disease had progressed on sunitinib (46%), sorafenib (28%), or both agents (26%).[192] Median PFS for patients receiving everolimus was 4.0 months compared with 1.9 months for patients receiving placebo (HR 0.3; p < 0.0001). The probability of being progression-free at 6 months was 26% for the treatment arm compared with 2% for the placebo arm. Adverse reactions from mTOR inhibitors include rash, asthenia, mucositis, nausea, edema, myelosuppression, hyperlipidemia, hyperglycemia, and drug-induced pneumonitis. This study was the first phase III randomized trial to demonstrate efficacy of second-line therapy for patients whose disease progressed on a VEGF inhibitor.

Previous phase II studies had shown that patients whose disease progresses on a VEGF-targeted therapy may experience a response to another VEGF-targeted therapy.[193] A prospective randomized trial compared the VEGF selective receptor tyrosine kinase inhibitor axitinib to sorafenib in patients whose disease had progressed on first-line therapy (AXIS trial). The overall median PFS was 6.7 months for patients receiving axitinib compared with 4.7 months for patients treated with sorafenib (HR 0.665, 95% CI 0.544, 0.812; p < 0.0001).[194] Subgroup analysis showed that PFS was 12 months compared with 6.5 months (HR 0.46; p < 0.0001) after prior cytokine therapy and 4.8 months compared with 3.4 months (HR 0.74; p = 0.011) after prior sunitinib therapy for patients treated with axitinib and sorafenib, respectively.

The combination of two targeted therapy agents may improve response proportions but results in increased toxicity.[195,196] Combination studies have failed to demonstrate an improvement in PFS,[197,198] whereas sequential use of targeted agents does appear to improve both PFS and OS in patients with metastatic RCC.[199] Ongoing randomized studies will determine which sequence or combination therapy will result in the greatest benefit.

Sunitinib and sorafenib also have shown activity in patients with non–clear cell RCC, including patients with metastatic papillary RCC and chromophobe carcinoma.[200-203] In a subset analysis of the randomized phase III trial that compared temsirolimus, IFN, or the combination,[191] patients with non–clear cell histology receiving temsirolimus had a significant improvement in PFS (7 months vs. 1.8 months) and OS (11.6 months vs. 4.3 months) compared with patients receiving IFN, suggesting temsirolimus has activity in non–clear cell RCC.[204]

Until 2006, immunotherapy had represented the primary treatment for patients with advanced renal cancer. The most extensively studied agents were IFN-alpha and aldesleukin (IL-2). IFN-alpha demonstrated low but reproducible response rates of 10% to 20% with occasional durable responses. Response rates of higher than 30% have been reported for patients with small-volume disease that is primarily limited to the lung. Two randomized trials showed that patients treated with IFN-alpha compared with vinblastine or medroxyprogesterone achieved a small survival advantage,[205,206] although other studies have not demonstrated a survival benefit.[207] A dose response to IFN-alpha is suggested, as few responses are associated with a dose of less than 3 million units per day, with maximum benefit seen in the dose range of 5 to 20 million units daily. In randomized trials, no consistent survival benefit has been demonstrated with the addition of vinblastine, IL-2, 13-cis retinoic acid, or floxuridine to IFN therapy.

Therapy with IL-2 results in major responses in 10% to 15% of patients with clear cell histology, with durable responses in 4% to 5% of cases. High-dose regimens appear to be more effective than low-dose regimens.[208] Prolonged and durable responses occur more commonly in patients with a good performance status and young age. One study demonstrated a higher response proportion with IL-2 compared with prior studies but failed to confirm carbonic anhydrase IX expression as a predictor of response.[209] Toxicity associated with high-dose bolus IL-2 is related to increased vascular permeability and often necessitates treating patients in an intensive-care setting. IL-2 has been associated with a 4% incidence of treatment-related death. IL-2 in combination with autologous lymphokine-activated killer cells obtained by leukapheresis did not result in any added benefit.[210] IL-2 remains the only therapy that is associated with durable complete responses and may be most appropriate for young, good-risk patients.

Variability in trial design and eligibility criteria for the multiple studies makes it difficult to compare results and to determine if one agent is superior as first- or second-line therapy. Figure 10-2 provides therapeutic options for metastatic RCC. These recommendations will most certainly be revised as additional studies are completed and results reported.

RCC is, in general, highly resistant to single-agent and combination chemotherapy, except for patients with sarcomatoid or collecting-duct carcinomas, for whom chemotherapy may be beneficial.[211] The combination of weekly gemcitabine with continuous infusional 5-fluorouracil or oral capecitabine showed modest activity in clear cell renal cancers.[212] A phase II trial investigated doxorubicin and gemcitabine in patients with sarcomatoid features (ECOG 8802).[213] The objective response rate (complete plus partial response) was 16% (one complete and five partial responses), and 10 patients (26%) had stable disease. The median PFS was 3.5 months and the median OS was 8.8 months. Similarly, a prospective phase II trial of patients with metastatic collecting-duct carcinoma treated with gemcitabine and cisplatin or carboplatin demonstrated antitumor activity.[214] VEGF-targeted agents have also shown activity in clear cell RCC with varying degrees of sarcomatoid differentiation, with a PFS in most studies of 4 months to 5 months.[188,215]

Activation of the c-met signaling pathway in papillary RCCs has led to early-phase trials with agents that target the c-met tyrosine kinase receptor or its ligand hepatocyte growth factor in patients with metastatic papillary RCC.[216-218] In a single-arm uncontrolled multicenter phase II trial from the Southwest Oncology Group (SWOG; S0317), 45 patients with advanced papillary RCC were treated with the oral EGFR kinase inhibitor erlotinib.[219] An overall partial response rate of 11% and a disease control rate of 64%, with five partial responses and 24 patients with stable disease, was seen. The 6-month PFS was 29%, and the median OS was 27 months.

There is no proven role for adjuvant cytokine therapy for patients who undergo nephrectomy and who are at high risk for recurrence. Studies examining the potential benefit of multi-kinase inhibitors as adjuvant therapy have been completed and results are pending. Renal cancer that metastasizes to the bone is typically osteolytic. Treatment with bone-targeting agents, such as zoledronic acid or denosumab, has been shown to decrease the risk of skeletal-related events in patients with bone metastases.[220,221] Brain metastases are a frequent complication in patients with metastatic clear cell renal cancer. Surgical resection or stereotactic radiosurgery are feasible alternatives to whole-brain radiation and may result in long-term survival.[222] Patients with treated brain metastases may safely receive systemic therapy with a multikinase inhibitor.[223] Limited studies also suggest that patients with severe renal impairment or end-stage renal disease on hemodialysis may safely be treated with targeted therapies.[224]

PROSTATE CANCER

Prostate cancer represents 28% of all newly diagnosed cancers in males and 10% of cancer-related deaths. In 2013, there were an estimated 238,590 new cases of prostate cancer and 29,720 deaths.[1] The 8:1 ratio of incidence to mortality demonstrates that although the disease is lethal for some men, the majority of men with prostate cancer die of other causes. Autopsy series show that nearly 70% of men older than 80 have occult prostate cancer. These facts highlight the variable biology and clinical course of prostate cancer. Although some prostate cancers do not require immediate intervention as the risk of death from non-cancer-related causes exceeds that of the cancer, other prostate cancers require combined modality approaches, both to eradicate the tumor locally and to eliminate micrometastases.

A risk-adapted approach for prostate cancer was first proposed in 2000 to categorize prostate cancer into a series of clinical states for which the therapeutic objectives are distinct (Fig. 10-3). Each state represents a clinically important milestone for which an intervention may or may not be needed. For example, for patients with a prostate cancer diagnosis, a treatment decision must incorporate an understanding of the individual's risk of developing metastases or death from prostate cancer in a given time frame. Using this model, it is clear that some patients may not be at risk for the development of metastases or symptoms for years (such that the risk of death from non-cancer-related causes exceeds that of prostate cancer), whereas other patients may require a more immediate intervention. Until a patient has progressive castrate-resistant prostate cancer (CRPC; previously referred to as hormone-refractory or androgen-independent prostate cancer), he is unlikely to die of his illness. The following are examples of the distinct therapeutic objectives for each disease state:

- For men who do not have a diagnosis but who may be at high risk for the disease, prevention is the objective (e.g., black males or those with a family history of prostate cancer).
- In the setting of localized disease, the objectives are to identify patients who can be cured by local modalities directed at the prostate only, patients who have indolent tumors that can be safely observed, and patients who have aggressive disease that will require combined-modality approaches aimed at eradicating the tumor locally and eliminating micrometastases.
- For patients with CRPC, the goal is to prevent or eliminate symptoms of disease and prolong life.

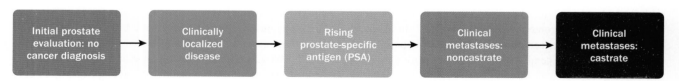

Fig. 10-3 Clinical states of prostate cancer.

Reprinted from Urology, Volume 55(3). Scher HI, Heller G. Clinical states in prostate cancer: toward a dynamic model of disease progression. Pages 323-327, copyright 2000. With permission from Elsevier.

ANATOMY

The prostate is composed of branching tubuloalveolar glands that are arranged in lobules and surrounded by stroma. Prostatic fluid is secreted through ducts to the urethra and comprises the bulk of seminal emissions. Associated structures are the dorsal vein complex responsible for passive urinary control and the pelvic plexus that provides innervation to the pelvic organs and corpora cavernosa through the neurovascular bundle and is responsible for erectile function. Protection of these fibers is essential to preserve potency. The peripheral zone is palpable by digital rectal examination (DRE) and is the site of origin of 70% of cancers. The transition zone surrounds the urethra and cannot be assessed by DRE. Up to 20% of all cancers develop in the transition zone; however, benign prostatic hypertrophy is more common than prostate cancer in the transition zone.

EPIDEMIOLOGY

In the United States, approximately one in six men will develop prostate cancer. Individuals with one first-degree relative diagnosed with prostate cancer have a 2-fold increased lifetime risk, which increases to 4-fold if two or more relatives are affected before age 70. Current estimates suggest that 5% to 10% of all cases of prostate cancer are hereditary and follow a Mendelian inheritance pattern. Identification of genes that result in hereditary prostate cancer have led to the elucidation of more than 30 single-nucleotide polymorphisms (SNPs) that are consistently associated with prostate cancer, yet the magnitude of risk elevation attributed to an individual SNP is low. A rare but recurrent mutation (G84E) in *HOXB13* (rs138213197), a homeobox transcription factor, was strongly associated with early-onset, familial prostate cancer, suggesting that rare genetic variants exist that contribute to familial clustering of prostate cancer.[225]

Although the frequency of histologic cancers at autopsy is similar throughout the world, the clinical incidence is significantly higher in Western countries, suggesting a role for environmental factors. High consumption of dietary fats, in particular the fatty acid alpha-linoleic acid, is believed to increase risk by 2- to 3-fold. Several potential protective dietary factors for prostate cancer incidence have been proposed, including tomatoes (lycopenes), cruciferous vegetables, carotenoids, fish, long-chain marine omega-3 fatty acids, soy, and polyphenols.[226] The biology of prostate cancer appears to differ in certain racial groups. For example, matched for age, black men have both a greater number of precursor prostatic intraepithelial neoplasia lesions and larger tumors compared with white men.

PATHOLOGY AND MOLECULAR PATHOGENESIS

Prostatic intraepithelial neoplasia (PIN) is an epithelial cellular proliferation within benign-appearing glands and acini. Approximately 50% of men with PIN as demonstrated on prostate biopsy will have prostate cancer in 5 years.[227] More than 99% of prostate cancers are adenocarcinomas; less than 1% are pure ductal and mucinous variants. In atypical prostatic lesions, expression of alpha-methylacyl-coenzyme-A racemase is useful to confirm adenocarcinoma. Other histologic subtypes include small cell carcinoma and rare mesenchymal tumors (rhabdomyosarcomas in younger patients and leiomyosarcomas in older patients). Urothelial carcinomas of the prostate are confined to the periurethral ducts and are more common among patients who have been successfully treated for noninvasive bladder cancer. Lymphomas and leukemias may also occur in the prostate gland.

The Gleason grading system is most commonly used to describe the morphology of adenocarcinomas of the prostate. Using the original system, the morphology was described using a score of 1 to 5 for the primary and secondary growth patterns within the tumor. Pattern 1 tumors were the most differentiated, with discrete glandular formation, whereas pattern 5 lesions were the most undifferentiated, with virtually complete loss of the glandular architecture. In 2005, a consensus conference modified Gleason grading to include the use of immunohistochemistry.[228] This resulted in a more narrow definition of Gleason 3 pattern (discrete glandular units) and widened the scope of Gleason 4 pattern. The Gleason score is determined by adding the Gleason grade of the two most predominant histologies. A higher Gleason score is associated with more aggressive disease and a greater probability of extracapsular extension, nodal involvement, and the subsequent development of metastases.

Androgens are the primary regulators of prostate cancer cell growth and proliferation. Prostate cancer rarely develops in castrated men or in those who become hypopituitary before age 40. The androgen receptor, located on chromosome Xq11-13, is a member of a super-family of ligand-dependent transcription factors that have a similar structure with different functional domains. The development of prostate cancer involves a multistep process in which androgen receptor signaling plays a key role. Specific genetic changes have been identified in tumors representing different clinical states. In early-stage cancers, loss of function of genes that detoxify carcinogens may contribute to hypermethylation, leading to loss of function of multiple genes including the PI-class glutathione S-transferase.[229] Gene fusions in prostate cancer, including the androgen-regulated gene *TMPRSS2* (21q22.3) and an ETS transcription factor family member, either *ERG* (21q22.2), *ETV1* (7p21.2), or *ETV4* (17q21), were first described in 2005.[230] Among these, the *TMPRSS2-ERG* fusion is the most prevalent, occurring in up to 40% to 70% of clinically localized prostate cancers. Subsequently, gene fusions have been identified involving additional ETS family members, *RAF* kinases and *SPINK-1*. Some studies suggest that patients with *TMPRSS2-ERG* fusions have an inferior prognosis, but the clinical and therapeutic implications of this and other molecular abnormalities are unclear and require further study.

Gene expression profiling has identified numerous molecular abnormalities that may differ between primary, metastatic, and CRPCs. As such, the targets relevant for the treatment of early-stage disease may not be the same as those for late-stage tumors. For example, the frequency of expression of *HER2* and *BCL-2* is higher in castrate-metastatic lesions than untreated localized tumors.[231,232] In contrast, the frequency of expression

Table 10-8 Staging of Prostate Cancer[12]

Primary Tumor (T)

Clinical

TX	Primary tumor cannot be assessed
T0	No evidence of primary tumor
T1	Clinically inapparent tumor neither palpable nor visible by imaging
T1a	Tumor incidental histologic finding in 5% or less of tissue resected
T1b	Tumor incidental histologic finding in more than 5% of tissue resected
T1c	Tumor identified by needle biopsy (e.g., because of elevated PSA)
T2	Tumor confined within prostate*
T2a	Tumor involves one-half of one lobe or less
T2b	Tumor involves more than one-half of one lobe but not both lobes
T2c	Tumor involves both lobes
T3	Tumor extends through the prostate capsule**
T3a	Extracapsular extension (unilateral or bilateral)
T3b	Tumor invades seminal vesicle(s)
T4	Tumor is fixed or invades adjacent structures other than seminal vesicles, such as external sphincter, rectum, bladder, levator muscles, and/or pelvic wall

*Tumor found in one or both lobes by needle biopsy, but not palpable or reliably visible by imaging, is classified as T1c.

**Invasion into the prostatic apex or into (but not beyond) the prostatic capsule is classified not as T3 but as T2.

Pathologic (pT)[†]

pT2[†]	Organ-confined
pT2a	Unilateral, involving one-half of one side or less
pT2b	Unilateral, involving more than one-half of one side but not both sides
pT2c	Bilateral disease
pT3	Extraprostatic extension
pT3a	Extraprostatic extension or microscopic invasion of bladder neck[‡]
pT3b	Seminal vesicle invasion
pT4	Invasion of rectum, levator muscles, and/or pelvic wall

[†]There is no pathologic T1 classification.

[‡]Positive surgical margin should be indicated by an R1 descriptor (residual microscopic disease).

Table 10-8 continued

Regional Lymph Nodes (N)

Clinical

NX	Regional lymph nodes were not assessed
N0	No regional lymph node metastasis
N1	Metastasis in regional lymph node(s)

Pathologic

pNX	Regional nodes not sampled
pN0	No positive regional nodes
pN1	Metastases in regional node(s)

Distant Metastasis (M)[§]

M0	No distant metastasis
M1	Distant metastasis
M1a	Nonregional lymph node(s)
M1b	Bone(s)
M1c	Other site(s) with or without bone disease

[§]When more than one site of metastasis is present, the most advanced category is used; pM1c is most advanced.

Prognostic State Groupings[◊]

Group	TNM	PSA	Gleason
I	T1a-c N0 M0	< 10	≤ 6
	T2a N0 M0	< 10	≤ 6
	T1-2a N0 M0	Not available	Not available
IIA	T1a-c N0 M0	< 20	7
	T1a-c N0 M0	≥ 10 < 20	≤ 6
	T2a N0 M0	≥ 10 < 20	≤ 6
	T2a N0 M0	< 20	7
	T2b N0 M0	< 20	≤ 7
	T2b N0 M0	Not available	Not available
IIB	T2c N0 M0	Any PSA	Any Gleason
	T1-2 N0 M0	≥ 20	Any Gleason
	T1-2 N0 M0	Any PSA	≥ 8
III	T3a-b N0 M0	Any PSA	Any Gleason
IV	T4 N0 M0	Any PSA	Any Gleason
	Any T N1 M0	Any PSA	Any Gleason
	Any T Any N M1	Any PSA	Any Gleason

[◊]When either PSA or Gleason is not available, grouping should be determined by T stage and/or either PSA or Gleason as available.

Abbreviations: TNM, tumor-node-metastasis; PSA, prostate-specific antigen.
The original source for this material is the AJCC Cancer Staging Manual, 7th Edition (2010) published by Springer Science and Business Media LLC, www.springerlink.com.

of prostate-specific membrane antigen is relatively constant across all clinical states, although the intensity of staining is higher in castrate-metastatic tumors.[233] Potential molecular targets that have undergone clinical investigation include *HER2*, *BCL-2*, VEGF, *Src*, the endothelin receptor, interleukin-6, and prostate-specific membrane antigen. The recent demonstration that neuroendocrine prostate cancer is associated with

amplification of the genes aurora kinase A (*AURKA*) and N-myc (*MYCN*) provides a rationale for exploring the use of aurora kinase inhibitor therapy.[234]

TUMOR STAGING

The TNM system describes the extent of the primary tumor (T), status of the regional nodes (N), and presence or absence of distant metastases (M; Table 10-8).[12] Tumors detected by biopsy on the basis of an elevated prostate-specific antigen (PSA) level and no palpable disease detected by DRE are designated T1c. Staging for T2 tumors includes (1) T2a, a tumor involving one-half of one lobe or less; (2) T2b, a tumor involving more than one-half of one lobe but not both lobes; and (3) T2c, a tumor involving both lobes. In T3 disease, a tumor extends through the prostate capsule (T3a) or invades the seminal vesicles (T3b), whereas a tumor is considered T4 if it invades adjacent structures or organs. With the widespread use of PSA testing, T1c is the most frequent classification at the time of diagnosis. T1c disease should be reclassified in the appropriate T category for nonpalpable disease if a tumor is reliably visible on an imaging study. Margin positivity, which is influenced by surgical technique and anatomic extent of disease, should be specified in the pathology report by an R1 descriptor (residual microscopic disease). Positive surgical margin status is not classified specifically in the pathologic T stage because the data were inconclusive regarding effect on disease outcomes when the TNM system was last revised.[235]

The clinical studies used to assess the primary tumor, including DRE, transrectal ultrasound (TRUS), CT, and MRI, have limitations in determining whether a tumor is organ-confined. To improve diagnostic precision and to guide treatment selection, nomograms based on the findings of the DRE, PSA level, and Gleason score are frequently used to predict the probability of capsular penetration, seminal vesicle, and lymph node involvement.[236]

PREVENTION

A number of chemoprevention strategies have been studied in prostate cancer. The Prostate Cancer Prevention Trial (PCPT) was a randomized, double-blind, multicenter study designed to investigate the use of finasteride, a 5-alpha reductase inhibitor, to prevent prostate cancer in men 55 and older. Over 18,000 men were enrolled, of whom one-half received 5 mg of finasteride daily for 7 years and one-half received placebo. The results initially demonstrated a 24.8% reduction in prostate cancer risk among men treated with finasteride, with a higher frequency of high-grade lesions for this same group[237]; although the clinical significance of the high-grade disease was uncertain.[238] In a recently reported trial update, prostate cancer was diagnosed in 989 of 9,423 (10.5%; 3.5% high grade) in the finasteride group and 1,412 of 9,457 (14.9%; 3.0% high grade) in the placebo group (RR 0.70, 95% CI 0.65, 0.76; p < 0.001; and for high-grade cancer [Gleason score, 7 to 10] RR 1.17, 95% CI 1.00, 1.37; p = 0.05).[239] A complementary study of another 5-alpha reductase inhibitor, the Reduction by Dutasteride of Prostate Cancer Events (REDUCE) trial in high-risk men had PSA-based entry criteria: baseline values of 2.5 ng/mL to 10 ng/mL for men younger than 60, and of 3.0 ng/mL to 10 ng/mL for older men.[240] Participants had a negative prostate biopsy in the 6 months prior to enrollment and no evidence of prostate cancer, PIN, or atypical small acinar proliferation. Men were randomly assigned to 0.5 mg/day of dutasteride or to placebo for 4 years, with prostate biopsies performed after 2 years

and at the end of the study. Eight hundred fifty-seven cases of prostate cancer were diagnosed in the patients who received placebo compared with 659 in those who received dutasteride, representing a 23% risk reduction (p < 0.0001). Subgroup analysis consistently favored dutasteride regardless of patient age, family history of prostate cancer, or baseline prostate symptom score, prostate volume, or PSA level. As in the PCPT trial, there was a small increase in the number of high-grade cancers. In 2011, an FDA advisory committee analysis of both trials confirmed a relative reduction of approximately 25% in the overall incidence of prostate cancer. The analysis noted, however, that this was limited to tumors with a modified Gleason score of 6 or lower and that many of the detected cancers were diagnosed by prostate biopsy in response to an elevated PSA level or to an abnormal DRE.[241] The reassessment of the PCPT and REDUCE trials confirmed a significantly increased incidence of high-grade prostate cancers, and the committee estimated that use of a 5-alpha reductase inhibitor for prevention of prostate cancer would result in one additional high-grade cancer to avert three to four potentially clinically relevant lower-grade cancers. The advisory committee concluded that finasteride and dutasteride do not have a favorable risk–benefit profile for chemoprevention of prostate cancer in healthy men. In the recently reported update of the PCPT with up to 18 years of follow-up, there was no significant difference in OS or survival after the diagnosis of prostate cancer between the finasteride and the placebo groups (10-year survival rates were 83.0% in the finasteride group and 80.9% in the placebo group for men with low-grade prostate cancer and 73.0% and 73.6% for patients with high-grade prostate cancer).[239]

The Physicians' Health Study II randomized, double-blind, placebo-controlled trial of vitamins E and C supplementation in 14,641 male physicians in the United States initially 50 or older did not reduce the risk of prostate cancer.[242] The Selenium and Vitamin E Cancer Prevention Trial (SELECT) evaluated 35,553 men in a double-blind, 2×2 factorial study of selenium and vitamin E alone and in combination for black men 50 or older or all other men 55 or older, a serum PSA of 4 ng/mL or less, and a normal DRE.[243] The endpoint was clinical incidence of prostate cancer. With a median follow-up of 5.46 years, there were no significant differences in the development of prostate cancer in any cohort (p > 0.15). At a median follow-up of 7 years, there was a 17% increased risk of prostate cancer in the vitamin E group (p = 0.008) but not in the selenium plus vitamin E group (p = 0.46), suggesting that vitamin E supplementation at 400 IU daily significantly increases the risk of prostate cancer.[244] Of note, the recommended daily dietary allowance for vitamin E is 22.4 IU.

EARLY DECTECTION AND SCREENING

The rationale for prostate cancer screening is that early detection and treatment of early-stage, asymptomatic cancers compared with diagnosis and treatment at the time of clinical diagnosis (e.g., a palpable mass on DRE) may result in an improvement in survival. Although case-controlled studies suggest an association between PSA screening and a decrease in

Table 10-9 **Prostate Cancer Screening Guidelines**[245]

Recommendation		American Urological Association[248]	American Cancer Society[248a]	U.S. Preventive Services Task Force[247]
Shared decision-making between patient and clinician		Yes, for men age 55 to 69	Yes (consider use of decision aid)	Yes (when patients request screening)
Average age to begin offering screening	Average-risk patients	55	50	Not applicable
	High-risk patients (black patients and patients with a first-degree relative with prostate cancer)	Not applicable	40 to 45	Not applicable
Discontinuation of screening		In men age 70+ or any man with less than a 10- to 15-year life expectancy	Life expectancy < 10 years	Not applicable
Screening tests		PSA, DRE	PSA, optional DRE	Not applicable
Frequency of screening		To reduce the harms of screening, a routine screening interval of 2 years or more may be preferred over annual screening in those men who have participated in shared decision-making and decided on screening.	Annually (every other year when PSA < 2.5 ng/mL)	Not applicable
Criteria for biopsy referral		At this point, the use of DRE, PSA derivatives (PSA density and age-specific reference ranges) and PSA kinetics (velocity and doubling time), PSA molecular forms (percent free PSA and proPSA), novel urinary markers (PCA3), and prostate imaging should be considered secondary tests (not primary screening tests) with potential utility for determining the need for a prostate biopsy, but with unproven benefit as primary screening tests.	PSA ≥ 4.0 ng/mL, abnormal DRE, individualized risk assessment if PSA is 2.5 ng/mL to 4.0 ng/mL	Not applicable

Abbreviations: DRE, digital rectal examination; PCA, prostate cancer antigen; PSA, prostate-specific antigen.
Adapted from N Engl J Med, Hoffman RM, Screening for Prostate Cancer. 2011; 365;21:2013-2019 Copyright © (2011) Massachusetts Medical Society. Reprinted with permission from Massachusetts Medical Society.

mortality, prospective randomized trials have not convincingly proven that PSA screening decreases mortality.[245] Consequently, there is significant controversy regarding PSA screening for prostate cancer.[246] In 2012, the U.S. Preventive Services Task Force updated its 2008 recommendation statement on screening for prostate cancer and recommended against PSA-based screening for prostate cancer for men in the general U.S. population, regardless of age (grade D recommendation).[247] This recommendation has generated significant controversy, with some other organizations concluding that PSA screening is warranted and should not be dismissed as nonbeneficial.

The risk of prostate cancer overdetection and overtreatment with screening are substantial, and a significant proportion of men are diagnosed with prostate cancer that would otherwise not progress to clinically significant disease during their lifetime. Serial PSA screening has at best a modest effect on prostate cancer mortality during the first decade of follow-up. With the recognition that no randomized trial has convincingly indicated a benefit for screening in terms of reducing mortality from prostate cancer, several national groups—including the American College of Physicians and the American Academy of

Family Physicians—modified their positions on screening and recommend that a patient be informed of the implications related to PSA screening prior to a PSA measurement. The American Urological Association now recommends shared decision-making for PSA-based screening for men age 55 to 69; however, outside this age range, routine PSA-based screening is not recommended.[248] Recommendations for prostate cancer screening are summarized in Table 10-9.[245]

PSA is a single-chain glycoprotein with a molecular weight of 34 kD that functions as a kallikrein-like serine protease causing liquefaction of seminal coagulum. It is prostate-specific but not prostate cancer–specific, and an elevated PSA may occur as a result of prostatitis, nonmalignant enlargement of the gland, biopsy of the prostate, ejaculation, and prostate cancer. A DRE does not alter PSA levels appreciably. The half-life of PSA is estimated to be 2 to 3 days, and levels should remain undetectable if the prostate has been removed. A PSA level greater than 4 ng/mL has predictive value for the diagnosis of prostate cancer; however, lower PSA values may also be associated with prostate cancer, as well as high-grade cancers, as demonstrated in an analysis of the prevalence of prostate cancer among men with a PSA level less than 4 ng/mL in the placebo group of the PCPT.[249] The prevalence of prostate cancer was 6.6% with a PSA up to 0.5 ng/mL, 10.1% with a PSA between 0.6 ng/mL to 1.0 ng/mL, 17% with values of 1.1 ng/mL to 2.0 ng/mL, 23.9% with values of 2.1 ng/mL to 3.0 ng/mL, and 26.9% with values of 3.1 ng/mL to 4.0 ng/mL. Of the prostate cancers diagnosed with a PSA less than 4.0 ng/mL, approximately 15% had a Gleason score of 7 or higher. This highlights the limitations of using a PSA cutoff value in the diagnosis of prostate cancer and specifically in detecting high-grade disease. For men with a PSA value between 4 ng/mL and 10 ng/mL, a PSA velocity of at least 0.75 ng/mL per year is suspicious for cancer. PSA measurement should be made on at least three consecutive occasions over at least 12 to 18 months because of variability. Because 5-alpha reductase inhibitors, including finasteride and dutasteride, are associated with a lowering of the PSA level, failure to have a substantial decrease in PSA (approximately 50%) or an increase in PSA while receiving these agents can be associated with an increased risk of prostate cancer.

An abnormal DRE necessitates a referral to a urologist for additional diagnostic testing. The sensitivity, specificity, and positive predictive value have been determined for DRE and PSA (using a cutoff of 4 ng/mL).[250] The positive predictive value of an abnormal DRE is 21%, whereas 25% of men with an elevated PSA level and abnormal DRE have cancer. Conditions that mimic prostate cancer on DRE include acute and granulomatous prostatitis and a prostatic calculus. When establishing a diagnosis, a TRUS is used to ensure that biopsy specimens encompass all portions of the gland. A TRUS has no role in screening. The diagnosis of prostate cancer is established with a TRUS-guided needle biopsy using a biopsy gun. An extended-pattern 12-core biopsy is recommended, and additional biopsies may be performed if clinically indicated.

PSA testing has produced a shift in the frequency and proportion of men with early-stage disease. It remains controversial whether prostate cancer screening of the general population decreases prostate cancer mortality. Two large randomized trials of PSA screening for prostate cancer—the Prostate, Lung, Colorectal, and Ovarian (PLCO) Cancer Screening Trial of the National Cancer Institute and the European Randomized Study for Screening for Prostate Cancer (ERSPC) Trial, both with the common endpoint of prostate cancer–specific mortality—were begun in the 1990s to assess the effectiveness of PSA screening.[251,252] In the ERSPC study, the initial mortality results were presented for 162,243 men between age 55 and 69 randomly assigned to PSA screening every 4 years or to a control group with no PSA screening. During a median follow-up of 9 years, the cumulative incidence of prostate cancer was 8.2% in the screened group and 4.8% in the control group (71% increase in diagnosis). The rate ratio for death from prostate cancer in the screening group, compared with the control group, was 0.80 (95% CI 0.65, 0.98; adjusted p = 0.04)—a 20% lower mortality from prostate cancer in the screened group. The absolute risk difference was 0.71 deaths per 1,000 men, indicating that 1,410 men would need to be screened and 48 additional cases of prostate cancer would need to be treated to prevent one death. A recent update after 11 years of follow-up indicated that 1,055 men would need to be invited for screening and 37 cancers would need to be detected to prevent one death from prostate cancer.[253] In the PLCO study, 76,693 men were assigned to either annual screening for 6 years and DRE for 4 years or to no screening with no reduction in mortality with screening. After 7 years of follow-up, the incidence of prostate cancer per 10,000 person-years was 116 (2,820 cancers) in the screening group and 95 (2,322 cancers) in the control group (rate ratio, 1.22; 95% CI 1.16, 1.29). The incidence of death per 10,000 person-years was 2.0 (50 deaths) in the screening group and 1.7 (44 deaths) in the control group (rate ratio, 1.13; 95% CI 0.75, 1.70). There are numerous criticisms of both of these studies, including a significant proportion of men having undergone PSA screening prior to enrollment, contamination with PSA screening in the control group, and the relatively short follow-up.[254,255] Subsequent analyses suggest a greater benefit to screening.[256] In a third screening trial from Sweden, which included ERSPC subjects and had a 14-year median follow-up, only 293 men needed to be screened and 12 diagnosed with prostate cancer to prevent one death from prostate cancer.[257]

Improving Specificity and Sensitivity of PSA Testing

PSA testing should be considered as a continuum, particularly as more men are diagnosed on the basis of a change in the measurement over time. A number of modifications to PSA testing have been proposed to increase its sensitivity, including PSA doubling time, PSA density (determined by dividing the serum PSA concentration by the volume of the prostate gland measured by TRUS), and PSA velocity (the change in serum PSA level over time)[258]; however, the utility of these modifications is disputed.[259] PSA exists in serum in a complexed form bound to either alpha l-antichymotrypsin or beta-2 macroglobulin, two extracellular protease inhibitors. When bound to these elements, the enzyme is inactive but still detectable using conventional immunoassays. For men with total PSA levels of 4 ng/mL to 10 ng/mL, cancer is more likely if the percent free (the fraction not protein bound in the serum) is less than 25%.[260] Free PSA is not typically recommended to determine whether to perform a prostate biopsy. Elevation of prostate cancer antigen 3 (PCA3) in the urine following a DRE may suggest the presence of prostate cancer and may assist in determining whether a prostate biopsy is indicated in a patient with an elevated PSA.[261]

MANAGEMENT OF PROSTATE CANCER BY DISEASE STAGE

Localized Disease

Localized prostate cancers are those confined to the prostate gland without nodal involvement or metastases. Treatment selection considers whether the disease can be eradicated by a treatment directed solely at the prostate, whether a combined local and systemic approach is necessary for cure, or whether therapy can be deferred because of a low risk of progression. In general, therapy is aimed at complete local control to decrease the potential for recurrence while preserving optimal bowel, bladder, and sexual function.

Within each T category are tumors with a range of prognoses—especially for men with T1c disease—mandating the consideration of other factors to assess outcomes and select treatment. Many groups have developed prognostic models based on the combination of the initial T stage, Gleason score, and baseline PSA level. Some prognostic models use discrete cut points, and others are nomograms that use PSA level and Gleason score as continuous variables. These algorithms are used to predict disease extent (i.e., organ-confined versus non-organ-confined), node status (negative or positive), and the probability of success using a PSA-based definition of failure specific to the local therapy under consideration. Specific nomograms have been developed for radical prostatectomy, external beam radiation therapy, and brachytherapy (radioactive seed implantation). The seventh edition of the AJCC Cancer Staging System includes prognostic groupings that incorporate anatomic stage and PSA (Table 10-8).[12]

Pelvic Lymph Node Involvement

Pelvic CT or MRI scans are recommended if the tumor is T3, T4, or T1 to T2 and the nomogram indicates the probability of lymph node involvement is greater than 20%. The FDA has approved the radioimmunoconjugate capromab pendetide that recognizes prostate-specific membrane antigen for the detection of prostate cancer nodal metastases.[262,263]

Distant Metastases

Prostate cancers spread by local extension through the capsule and seminal vesicles, through the lymphatic system to regional nodes, or hematogenously to bone and visceral sites. Bone metastases are predominantly osteoblastic rather than osteolytic, although both types likely coexist. Radionuclide bone scans are used to detect metastases to the skeleton. The yield of a bone scan is low for patients with tumors that are T2 or less, with a Gleason score of less than 7, and a PSA level of less than 10 ng/mL. Bone scans are recommended if the following criteria are met: tumor is T1 to T2, and the PSA level is greater than 20 ng/mL; the Gleason score is 8; the tumor is T3 or T4; or the patient has symptoms of bone metastases. CT scans are also useful for evaluating focal areas of the skeleton and for identifying healing fractures, arthritis, Paget's disease, bone infections, and other inflammatory bone conditions that may mimic prostate cancer on a bone scan.

RISING PSA

The disease state of a rising PSA refers to men who have no detectable metastases on a scan and in whom the PSA level increases after radical prostatectomy, radiation therapy, or both. It does not refer to an increase in PSA level for patients in whom disease is managed by watchful waiting. Issues in management include whether the rising PSA value represents a local recurrence that could be eliminated with additional treatment to the prostate or prostate bed, whether it represents metastatic disease, or both.

In most cases, a rising PSA level represents micrometastatic disease that is not detectable on conventional imaging studies. The time to development of metastases is highly variable. In one series of patients experiencing a PSA recurrence following radical prostatectomy, the median time to the detection of metastatic disease was 8 years, and 63% of the patients with a rising PSA level remained free of metastases at 5 years.[264] Time to biochemical progression, Gleason score, and PSA doubling time were predictive of the probability and time to development of metastatic disease. In a follow-up report, significant risk factors for time to prostate cancer–specific mortality included PSA doubling time (< 3.0 vs. 3.0-8.9 vs. 9.0-14.9 vs. ≥ 15.0 months), Gleason score (≤ 7 vs. 8-10), and time from surgery to PSA recurrence (≤ 3 vs. > 3 years).[265] PSA velocity at recurrence is significantly associated with an increased risk of all-cause mortality among men treated with radiation therapy with or without ADT.[266] A major issue for patients with a rising PSA level is the use of early versus deferred ADT. Although guidelines for evaluating and treating men in this state were updated in 2013, there is no gold standard.[267]

If the decision is made to begin ADT in a patient with a rising PSA value but no evidence of metastases, data suggest that intermittent androgen suppression is a reasonable alternative to continuous androgen suppression without adversely affecting survival. In a phase III noninferiority trial that enrolled 1,386 men with nonmetastatic prostate cancer who had a rising PSA level of greater than 3.0 ng/mL 1 year after the completion of radiotherapy, men were randomly assigned to either ADT with a luteinizing hormone-releasing hormone (LHRH) continuously until their cancer became castrate-resistant or intermittently (for 8 months in each cycle with restart when the PSA reached greater than 10 ng/mL) until progression, at which time they were switched to continuous ADT. Median OS was 9.1 years for patients on continuous therapy compared with 8.8 years for the intermittent group (HR 1.02; 95% CI 0.86, 1.21; p for noninferiority [HR intermittent vs. continuous ≥ 1.25] = 0.009). The majority of patients (59%) died of causes unrelated to prostate cancer, with more prostate cancer–related deaths in the intermittent arm (120 of 690) compared to the continuous arm (94 of 696; 7-year cumulative rates of disease-related deaths were 18% and 15%, respectively [p = 0.24]). Time to the development of castration resistance was statistically significantly improved on the intermittent arm (HR 0.80, 95% CI 0.67, 0.98; p = 0.024). Patients who received intermittent androgen suppression had reduced hot flashes, but otherwise there was no evidence of differences in toxicity, including myocardial events or osteoporotic fractures.[268]

A rising PSA can also occur in patients who have received ADT but have no sign of metastases (nonmetastatic CRPC). In these patients, radiographic imaging should be performed in an attempt to document metastases. In an analysis of the placebo group of a randomized controlled trial of men with a rising PSA level—despite ADT and no radiographic evidence of metastases—46% of men developed bone metastases at 2 years, and the median metastasis-free survival was 25 months.[269] Higher baseline PSA (≥ 13.2 ng/mL) was significantly associated with shorter time to first bone metastasis, OS, and bone metastasis–free survival. A higher PSA velocity was also associated with shorter overall and bone metastasis–free survival.

THERAPY FOR TUMORS CONFINED TO THE PROSTATE

Tumors that are confined to the prostate are typically managed by radical surgery, radiation therapy, or, in some cases, active surveillance. All are considered options by the American Urological Association Prostate Cancer Clinical Guidelines Update Panel.[270] An assessment of the patient's life expectancy, overall health status, and tumor characteristics should be undertaken before a treatment decision is made. For patients with low-risk localized prostate cancer, active surveillance, interstitial prostate brachytherapy, external beam radiation therapy, and radical prostatectomy are appropriate monotherapy treatment options. For patients with intermediate-risk or high-risk localized prostate cancer, combined-modality therapy may be indicated (see Hormone Therapy for Systemic Relapse section below). With few randomized trials, comparisons among treatments have been limited by selection bias and differences in outcomes reporting, both with respect to cancer control and QOL. Nomograms and other prognostic models have been developed to assist in decision-making, while QOL assessments have become more standardized.

Reported complication rates for each modality vary widely in the literature. For radical prostatectomy, impotence rates range from 25% to 89%, and incontinence ranges from 2% to 47%. The differences are related to the different definitions used, whether the patient or physician is reporting, and the time from the treatment to the assessment of symptoms. Recent HRQOL studies are more accurately defining the patient's satisfaction with the different treatments for localized prostate cancer. For example, in one study, adjuvant hormone therapy was associated with worse QOL outcomes among patients receiving brachytherapy or radiotherapy, whereas urinary incontinence was observed after prostatectomy but urinary irritation and obstruction improved, particularly in patients with large prostates.[271] In one large study of erectile function at 2 years in men after prostatectomy, external radiotherapy, or brachytherapy for prostate cancer, the estimated 2-year function probabilities ranged from as low as 10% or less to as high as 70% or greater depending on the individual's pretreatment patient characteristics and treatment details (i.e., pretreatment sexual HRQOL score, age, serum PSA level, race/ethnicity, body mass index, and intended treatment details).[272] These analyses have led to the development of HRQOL nomograms that may help guide treatment choice in an individual patient with localized prostate cancer.

Radical Retropubic Prostatectomy

The goal of radical retropubic prostatectomy is to completely excise the cancer while maintaining urinary control and preserving potency. After the prostate has been removed, PSA levels should decline to undetectable. Cancer control is assessed by PSA relapse-free survival, time to objective progression (local or systemic), cancer-specific survival, and OS. The procedure continues to evolve as clinicians use biopsy algorithms that include more extensive sampling and imaging to determine both the extent and location of the tumor within the prostate. This approach has resulted in refined selection of cases and surgical planning, which, in turn, has led to more rapid recovery, higher rates of continence, and improved potency. In a large series, continence returned in 2 months, predicted by younger age and preservation of both neurovascular bundles. Overall, 6% of patients had mild stress urinary incontinence (requiring one pad daily), 2% had moderate incontinence (more than one pad daily), and 0.3% had severe incontinence that required an artificial urinary sphincter, with 92% having complete continence at 1 year. With preservation of both neurovascular bundles, erectile function returns in a median of 4 to 6 months. Sacrificing one nerve bundle decreases recovery by 50%. Minimally invasive surgery, including both conventional and robotic laparoscopic radical prostatectomy, has emerged as an alternative to open surgery for patients with clinically localized prostate cancer.[273]

Radiation Therapy

Radiation can be administered using external beam techniques, an implant or radioactive seeds, or a combination of both. ADT may or may not be administered. As is the case with surgery, the reported outcomes vary, but most trials measure the proportion of patients who have a decline in PSA level to less than 0.5 ng/mL or 1 ng/mL, the proportion with nonrising PSA, and/or the proportion with negative findings on biopsy of the prostate 2 years after the completion of treatment. The standard Phoenix definition for a biochemical failure after external beam radiation therapy with or without hormone therapy is PSA nadir plus 2 ng/ml.[274] Contemporary external beam radiation therapy incorporates three-dimensional conformal treatment planning with intensity modulation to maximize the administered dose to the tumor while minimizing the exposure of surrounding normal structures. These techniques allow for the safe administration of higher doses, which in turn have resulted in improved outcomes. Compared with surgery, radiation therapy is associated with a higher frequency of bowel complications, mainly loose stools and diarrhea, and lower rates of urinary incontinence and sexual dysfunction.

The use of interstitial radiation or implantation of radioactive seeds is based on the principle that deposition of radiation energy in tissues decreases exponentially as a square function of the distance from the radiation source. Older techniques relied on digital placement of the seeds, whereas modern techniques use computer-generated templates to place the seeds more accurately under direct visualization. The result is better cancer control and reduced toxicity. An acute toxicity associated with implantation is irritative urinary symptoms including urinary frequency. Incontinence is rare, and potency may be better than that observed with radical surgery.[272,275-279]

Four prospective randomized trials have demonstrated that radiotherapy doses less than 70 Gy are inadequate for the curative treatment of clinically localized prostate cancer.[280] It is not clear if doses exceeding 78 Gy to 79 Gy render additional benefit. The role for hypofractionated external beam radiotherapy for prostate cancer is still being defined.[281,282] The relative efficacy of external beam radiation therapy compared with permanent prostate implants remains controversial; however, implant alone is unable to treat disease outside of the prostate, which is increasingly likely in patients with intermediate- and high-risk disease.

Cryosurgical Ablation and High-Intensity Focused Ultrasound

Cryosurgery and high-intensity focused ultrasound are minimally invasive procedures aimed at local control with low complication rates and favorable functional outcomes. These approaches often are considered for patients who are not suitable for radical surgery or who have local recurrences. Sufficient long-term follow-up is lacking to estimate efficacy in terms of prostate cancer–specific mortality.

Neoadjuvant and Adjuvant ADT

Although neoadjuvant ADT before surgery leads to a reduction in the rate of positive surgical margins, it has not had an effect on overall outcome and is not recommended. The benefit of immediate adjuvant ADT following surgery in men with localized disease at high risk for relapse is not proven. Limited studies suggest that perioperative chemotherapy with or without ADT may improve outcomes, but this approach should be considered investigational. A prospective randomized trial (CALGB 90203) of men with high-risk localized prostate cancer is randomly assigning patients to radical prostatectomy alone or to six cycles of docetaxel chemotherapy followed by radical prostatectomy to assess the potential benefit of neoadjuvant chemotherapy.

In contrast to surgery, the role of neoadjuvant and concurrent ADT for patients receiving radiation is well established. Results of numerous randomized trials suggest that neoadjuvant and concurrent androgen deprivation is beneficial for patients with intermediate-risk disease receiving external beam radiation therapy with an optimal duration of 3 to 6 months.[280,283-286] Six months of ADT was associated with a longer time to PSA recurrence and decreased mortality for men with a pretreatment PSA velocity more than 2 ng/mL per year.[287] Patients with high-risk disease should receive long-term adjuvant ADT for at least 2 years.[288,289] Pelvic nodal radiation with concurrent androgen deprivation for patients at intermediate and high risk for nodal involvement remains controversial.[290]

The role for immediate long-term androgen suppression in patients with pathologically documented lymph node involvement is supported by subset analysis of patients with lymph node–positive disease in RTOG 85-31. Patients randomly assigned to immediate androgen suppression in conjunction with standard external beam radiation therapy had significantly improved outcomes compared with patients receiving radiation alone.[291] In a study of patients undergoing radical prostatectomy, patients with lymph node–positive disease at surgery were randomly assigned to undergo castration (surgically or medically) or observation. PSA testing was not in wide use during this study, so objective progression was defined as

the development of metastases on imaging tests. At a median follow-up of 11.9 years, men assigned to immediate androgen suppression had a significant improvement in PFS, prostate cancer–specific survival, and OS.[292] Although there is evidence that early (adjuvant) androgen deprivation may benefit patients with node-positive disease after radical prostatectomy, it is based on only 98 men and a control arm with a lower than predicted cancer-specific survival.

Watchful Waiting and Active Surveillance

Watchful waiting or deferred therapy is a policy of no therapeutic intervention after a diagnosis has been established until disease progression is evidenced by changes in the PSA level, local tumor growth, or the development of metastases. The approach evolved from studies of predominantly older men with well-differentiated tumors in whom tumor progression was found to occur over a protracted period of time, and studies in which, during the follow-up interval, a substantial proportion of men died of intercurrent disease. In a structured literature review of patients treated with a deferred approach, radical prostatectomy, or external beam radiation, the 10-year mean weighted survivals were 93% for patients who received radical prostatectomy, 84% for patients treated with a deferred approach, and 74% for patients who received external beam radiation.[293] A retrospective, population-based cohort study using the Connecticut Tumor Registry indicated that the 20-year prostate cancer–specific survival for men with a Gleason score of 6 or less treated with watchful waiting was 80% to 90%.[294]

Randomized trials to establish the utility of watchful waiting are lacking. A retrospective study of 44,630 men age 65 to 80 who were diagnosed between 1991 and 1999 with organ-confined, well- or moderately differentiated prostate cancer stratified as having received treatment or observation found a statistically significant survival advantage associated with treatment (HR 0.69, 95% CI 0.66, 0.72).[295] A benefit associated with treatment was seen in all subgroups examined, including older men (age 75 to 80 at diagnosis), black men, and men with low-risk disease. In a prospective trial of 695 men randomly assigned to watchful waiting or radical prostatectomy, death from prostate cancer after over 13 years of follow-up occurred in 20.7% of men assigned to watchful waiting compared with 14.6% of patients who had radical surgery (relative hazard, 0.62, 95% CI 0.44, 0.97; p = 0.01).[296] At 15 years, 21.7% of men in the surgery group and 33.4% of men in the watchful waiting group had been diagnosed with distant metastases (difference = 11.7%; 95% CI 4.8%, 18.6%), for a RR of 0.59 (95% CI 0.45, 0.79; p = 0.001). Of note, the mean PSA value was 12.3 ng/mL, and 74% of patients had T2 disease in the observation arm, making it unlikely that these results are applicable to the current U.S. population, where nearly one-half of newly diagnosed patients are diagnosed with T1c prostate cancer.

As a consequence of PSA screening resulting in overdiagnosis and overtreatment of men with indolent tumors, active surveillance or close monitoring of patients with good-risk disease (defined as a Gleason score of 6 or less, PSA less than 10 ng/mL, and T1c-2a disease) for delayed intervention has gained increased acceptance as an initial strategy for men diagnosed with prostate cancer. Men are actively monitored by serial PSA, DRE, and periodic prostate rebiopsies every 1 to 2 years. Therapy is offered based on various risk progression criteria that may include biochemical (change in PSA), histologic (increase in Gleason score or number of positive biopsies), and stage (by DRE or imaging) measures.[297] This approach may also be considered in select men with intermediate-risk prostate cancer.[298]

Adjuvant Compared with Salvage Radiation Therapy for Local Failure

For men treated with radical prostatectomy, salvage radiation therapy to the prostatic bed is administered in selected patients who develop a biochemical recurrence following surgery. A local recurrence is more likely if the PSA first became detectable more than 1 year after surgery, the PSA doubling time is greater than 10 months, the radical prostatectomy specimen contained a cancer of low Gleason score (less than 7), and there was no seminal vesicle invasion or lymph node metastases in the pathologic specimen.[264] In a retrospective review of 1,540 patients who received salvage radiotherapy, the 6-year progression-free probability was 32% (95% CI 31%, 51%).[299] Forty-eight percent of patients (95% CI 40%, 56%) treated with salvage radiotherapy alone at PSA levels of 0.50 ng/mL or lower were disease-free at 6 years, including 41% (95% CI 31%, 51%) who also had a PSA doubling time of 10 months or less or poorly differentiated cancer (Gleason grade 8 to 10). Furthermore, another retrospective study demonstrated that salvage radiotherapy alone was associated with a significant 3-fold increase in prostate cancer–specific survival relative to those who received no salvage treatment (HR 0.32, 95% CI 0.19, 0.54; p < 0.001).[300] The increase in prostate cancer–specific survival associated with salvage radiotherapy was limited to men with a PSA doubling time of less than 6 months and remained after adjustment for pathologic stage and other established prognostic factors. Other studies suggest that PSA kinetics—specifically a pretreatment PSA velocity greater than 2 ng/mL per year, an interval to PSA failure of less than 3 years, and a post-treatment PSA doubling time of less than 3 months—increase the risk for metastases and subsequent prostate cancer–specific mortality, making these men poor candidates for salvage radiation therapy.[301]

Three prospective randomized trials suggested that immediate postoperative radiotherapy in men with advanced pathologic features (stage pT3a or pT3b) and/or positive surgical margins improves biochemical PFS.[302] In each of these studies, there was an improvement in biochemical PFS for patients receiving immediate postoperative radiotherapy but no improvement in OS. At nearly 13 years of follow-up in the SWOG 8794 trial, in which men with pT3N0M0 or margin-positive disease were randomly assigned to immediate radiation to the prostatic fossa or to usual care, the metastasis-free survival rate was 43% in the radiation-treated group and 54% in the untreated group (p = 0.016).[303] Moreover, OS was significantly improved for men treated with adjuvant radiotherapy (52% vs. 41% for men initially observed; p = 0.023). Of note, there was also a significant benefit of radiotherapy in those men with a detectable PSA after surgery. In this study, 9.1 men with pathologic T3 disease needed to receive adjuvant radiotherapy to prevent one death at a median follow-up of 12.6 years.

Patients treated initially with radiation therapy may be considered for salvage prostatectomy if they were surgical candidates at the time of diagnosis, have a life expectancy of more than 10 years, and have no metastatic disease. Biopsy confirmation of persistent disease in the gland and no evidence of spread are essential before surgery is considered. Despite refinements in case selection, incontinence rates remain high and virtually all patients are impotent after the procedure.

ANDROGEN DEPRIVATION THERAPY FOR SYSTEMIC RELAPSE

ADT that negates androgen effects is the standard approach for relapsed prostate cancer. More than 90% of male hormones originate in the testes, with the remaining hormones synthesized in the adrenal gland. Surgical orchiectomy was the gold standard treatment but is the least preferred by patients. ADT options can be divided into those that lower serum testosterone levels (such as gonadotropin-releasing hormone [GnRH] agonists or antagonists, and estrogens) and antiandrogens that do not lower testosterone but block androgen action at the level of the androgen receptor. Medical or surgical castration is associated with gynecomastia, impotence, loss of libido, weakness, fatigue, hot flashes, loss of muscle mass, changes in personality, anemia, depression, and loss of bone over time. Resistance and aerobic exercise can improve muscle mass, strength, and physical function.[304]

Prolonged time on ADT that lowers testosterone can result in osteoporosis. Dual-energy x-ray absorptiometry scans may be used at baseline and to screen for the development of osteopenia and/or osteoporosis. Bisphosphonates, denosumab (a fully humanized anti-RANKL monoclonal antibody), and selective estrogen receptor modulators (SERMS) have been shown to increase bone mineral density in men on ADT.[305]

Prolonged ADT is frequently used in men without metastases, as in men receiving radiation therapy as definitive therapy for high-risk prostate cancer (see Therapy for Tumors Confined to the Prostate section above). The Denosumab Hormone Ablation Bone Loss Trial (HALT) examined the role of denosumab at a dose of 60 mg subcutaneously every 6 months in men receiving ADT for nonmetastatic prostate cancer. Fifteen hundred sixty-eight men were randomly assigned to either denosumab or to placebo.[306] Bone mineral density of the lumbar spine increased by 5.6% in the denosumab group compared with a loss of 1.0% in the placebo group (p < 0.001) at 24 months, and there was also a decreased incidence of new vertebral fractures at 36 months (1.5% vs. 3.9% with placebo; RR 0.38, 95% CI 0.19, 0.78; p = 0.006). In 2011, the FDA approved denosumab (60 mg every 6 months) to increase bone mass in men at high risk for fracture who are receiving ADT for nonmetastatic prostate cancer.

ADT for Metastatic Prostate Cancer

Non-castrate-resistant metastatic prostate cancer is defined by metastases on an imaging study (either at the time of diagnosis or following local therapy) in patients who have non-castrate levels of testosterone. At this point, the risk of death from prostate cancer exceeds that of non-cancer-related mortality. Response to ADT can be measured by a decline in PSA values, decrease in the size of nodal or visceral metastases, or improvement in cancer-related symptoms. Overall, 60% to 70% of patients with abnormal PSA levels will have normalization of the value to below 4 ng/mL after castration, 30% to 50% of measurable tumor masses will regress by 50% or more, and approximately 60% of patients will have palliation of symptoms (either urinary or osseous symptoms). Serial bone scans will show improvement in only 30% to 40% of patients, and a scintigraphic flare on bone scans can occur following ADT between 3 and 6 months after initiation of therapy; this should not be confused with progression of skeletal metastases. In an analysis of survival in more than 1,000 patients treated with ADT, the PSA value measured at 7 months after initiating therapy was predictive of outcomes, with a median survival of 13 months for patients with a PSA nadir of greater than 4 ng/mL, 44 months for patients with PSA nadir of greater than 0.2 ng/mL to less than 4 ng/mL, and 75 months for patients with PSA nadir of less than 0.2 ng/mL.[307]

The initial rise in testosterone after treatment with a GnRH agonist can result in a clinical flare of the disease. These agents should be cautiously used as monotherapy for patients with severe pain, urinary symptoms, or spinal cord compromise. Under such circumstances, antiandrogens to block the flare response in combination with a GnRH agonist or a GnRH antagonist that suppresses testosterone without a testosterone surge are preferred. The combination of an antiandrogen and a GnRH analog also has the additional potential to block the effects of adrenal androgens, which can contribute anywhere from 5% to 45% of the residual androgens present in tumors following surgical castration alone. Whether the antitumor effects of a combined or maximum androgen-blockade approach were superior to castration alone or to GnRH monotherapy was in question for many years. In 2000, the Prostate Cancer Trialists' Collaborative Group (PCTCG) published a meta-analysis of combined androgen blockade, showing that nonsteroidal antiandrogens conferred a small but statistically significant improvement in 5-year survival over castration therapy alone (72.4% vs. 75.3%; HR 0.92; p < 0.005).[308] In a recent update after a median of 5.2 years follow-up of a phase III randomized trial comparing combined androgen blockade using LHRH agonist plus 80 mg of bicalutamide compared with LHRH agonist alone in patients with advanced prostate cancer, there was a significant improvement in OS for patients receiving combined androgen blockade (HR 0.78, 95% CI 0.60, 0.99; p = 0.0498), although there was no significant difference in cause-specific survival between the two groups.[309] Thus, several thousand patients have been enrolled in trials, with the results showing that antiandrogens do not add to the antitumor effects of surgical castration but may provide a very modest improvement in survival for patients treated in combination with GnRH agonists or antagonists.

Nonsteroidal antiandrogens, such as flutamide, bicalutamide, and nilutamide, block the binding of androgens to the androgen receptor. They have been evaluated for several purposes:

- To block the flare secondary to the initial rise in testosterone that results following administration of GnRH agonists
- To simultaneously inhibit testicular and adrenal androgens as part of a combined androgen-blockade approach

Other approaches that have been investigated include high-dose bicalutamide (150 mg), which is associated with fewer hot flashes, less effect on libido, less muscle wasting, fewer personality changes, and less bone loss. Gynecomastia remains a substantial problem but may be alleviated, in part, with prophylactic breast irradiation. Whether this approach is equivalent to more traditional therapies that lower testosterone levels is questionable because the results of clinical trials have been conflicting. For patients with established metastatic disease, however, antiandrogen monotherapy was inferior to testosterone-lowering therapy.[310]

Early versus Delayed ADT

Recommendations for the initial treatment of patients with androgen-sensitive, metastatic, recurrent, or progressive prostate cancer were updated in 2007.[311] A continuing controversy is the question of early versus delayed ADT. Data in support of early ADT date back to the findings from early randomized studies in which diethylstilbestrol or orchiectomy was found to delay the development of metastases for patients with T3 disease. In a study conducted by the Medical Research Council, 938 patients with locally advanced or asymptomatic metastatic prostate cancer were randomly assigned to either immediate treatment (orchiectomy or medical castration) or to the same treatment deferred until an indication occurred. Treatment was commenced for local progression almost as frequently as for metastatic disease. Compared with patients treated with deferred therapy, patients treated with early therapy were less likely to have progression from M0 to M1 disease (p < 0.001), have pain (p < 0.001), and die of prostate cancer.[312]

Several randomized trials provide support for early ADT in conjunction with local therapy in patients with high-risk disease. In one study conducted by Bolla et al,[313] patients with localized disease were randomly assigned to receive radiotherapy alone or radiation therapy and 3 years of androgen ablation. Although the results showed a survival benefit, the trial was criticized for the poor outcomes in the control group. Ten-year follow-up of RTOG 8531—which tested whether the use of lifelong ADT after radiation therapy improved outcomes—showed that patients treated with early ADT had superior local, biochemical, and distant disease control rates (all p < 0.0001), as well as improved disease-specific survival (83% vs. 78%; p = 0.0053) and OS (47% vs. 38%; p = 0.0043) compared with patients treated at relapse.[314,315] Use of early ADT also is supported by the trials previously described in which patients with pathologically confirmed lymph node involvement receiving immediate ADT had improved survival.[291,294] In SWOG 9921, 983 men with high-risk prostate cancer were randomly assigned postprostatectomy to adjuvant therapy with ADT alone (GnRH agonist plus bicalutamide for 2 years) or ADT with mitoxantrone chemotherapy. An early analysis of the 481 men treated on the ADT-alone arm at a median follow-up of 4.4 years found a 5-year biochemical-free survival of 92.5% and an OS of 95.9%.[316] However, this trial was not designed specifically to address the role of adjuvant androgen ablation after prostatectomy and has many inherent problems (e.g., selection bias and PSA-driven stage migration).

In the Early Prostate Cancer Program, patients with localized disease were randomly assigned to receive 150 mg of bicalutamide or placebo. The primary endpoint was objective clinical progression that included detectable disease in soft tissue or the documentation of bone metastases at 2 years. Early combined results of three trials showed that the proportion of patients in whom osseous metastases developed within 2 years was 9% for patients who received bicalutamide and 14% for patients who received placebo. This finding represented a HR reduction of 0.58 (95% CI 0.51, 0.66; p < 0.001).[317] No effect on survival was demonstrated. Subgroup analysis showed the greatest benefit in patients with nodal disease.[318] A recent update, however, showed no benefit for early bicalutamide therapy for patients with localized disease at low risk for recurrence.[319] No prospective randomized study has demonstrated the utility of initiating ADT to patients with biochemical-only (PSA) progression after definitive local therapy.

Continuous versus Intermittent ADT in Metastatic Prostate Cancer

The use of continuous (long-term) ADT in patients with metastatic prostate cancer is associated with many adverse effects including hot flashes, loss of libido, bone loss, and muscle atrophy. Androgen-dependent animal models have suggested that intermittent androgen deprivation increases the time to castrate-resistant disease. A trial of intermittent versus continuous ADT in men with metastatic prostate cancer randomly assigned 3,040 patients to intermittent or continuous ADT after an initial 7 months of treatment with a luteinizing hormone-releasing hormone analogue and an antiandrogen if PSA fell to ≤ 4 ng/mL.[320] The co-primary endpoints were to determine whether intermittent therapy was noninferior to continuous therapy for survival (upper boundary of HR 1.20) and whether QOL differed at 3 months. At a median follow-up of 9.8 years, the median survival for continuous and intermittent ADT was 5.8 and 5.1 years, respectively (HR for death with intermittent therapy, 1.10, 90% CI 0.99, 1.23). Although intermittent therapy was associated with improved erectile function and mental health at 3 months, there was no difference thereafter. Since the confidence interval for survival exceeded the upper boundary for noninferiority, the findings were statistically inconclusive (i.e., could not rule out a 20% greater risk of death with intermittent ADT). A systemic review of randomized clinical trials of intermittent versus continuous ADT including nine studies with 5,508 patients demonstrated no significant differences in OS or PFS, with more prostate cancer–related deaths with intermittent ADT balanced by more non-prostate cancer–related deaths with continuous therapy. Intermittent ADT was associated with improvement in general well-being, sexual function, and physical activity in some studies as well as a median cost saving of 48%.[321]

CHEMOTHERAPY FOR METASTATIC NON-CASTRATE PROSTATE CANCER

At the 2014 ASCO Annual Meeting, the results of an ECOG-led phase III randomized trial of chemohormonal therapy versus hormone therapy for hormone-sensitive newly metastatic prostate cancer were presented. Seven hundred ninety men were randomly assigned to ADT alone or ADT plus docetaxel every 3 weeks for six cycles within 4 months of starting ADT with a primary endpoint of OS. At a median follow-up of 29 months, the median OS was 42.3 months versus 52.7 months for the ADT and ADT plus docetaxel arms, respectively (HR 0.63, 95% CI 0.48, 0.82; p = 0.0006). The benefit was seen in patients with high-volume disease (visceral metastases and/or four or more bone metastases) with a median survival of 32.2 months for ADT alone and 49.2 months for ADT plus docetaxel (HR 0.62, 95% CI 0.46, 0.83, p = 0.0012). There was no significant benefit seen in patients with low-volume disease, although longer follow-up is needed. This is the first trial to demonstrate a survival benefit for chemotherapy in the setting of newly diagnosed castration-sensitive metastatic disease.[321a]

TREATMENT FOR CASTRATE-RESISTANT PROSTATE CANCER

The treatment of patients with disease that progresses during ADT requires documentation that the patient is medically castrated (serum testosterone level less than 50 ng/mL) and a determination of the extent of disease. Some patients will experience disease progression with a rising PSA level alone (non-metastatic CRPC), and others will experience disease progression with the development of or progression in bone, soft tissue, or visceral metastases (metastatic CRPC). The terminology "hormone refractory" is no longer accurate because progression of disease during ADT is not necessarily refractory to additional treatment targeting androgen signaling. Despite the development of CRPC, androgen receptor signaling continues to play a major role in many prostate cancers. Mechanisms leading to androgen receptor activation include androgen receptor overexpression, ligand-independent activation, de novo synthesis of intratumoral androgens, and alterations in the androgen receptor, including splice variants and circulating subcastrate levels of androgens.[322,323] Patients who are taking an antiandrogen are first given a trial of antiandrogen withdrawal based on the observation that these agents, although initially providing benefit, can later contribute to prostate cancer progression. Thereafter, a second agent, such as another nonsteroidal antiandrogen, or ketoconazole with hydrocortisone, may be considered. Responses, when they occur, are frequently of short duration (2- to 4-month median), although there are patients who achieve a prolonged response. The recent development of new classes of agents including novel nonsteroidal antiandrogens, CYP 17 inhibitors, and androgen receptor–targeted compounds has already led to substantial improvements in outcome for patients with CRPC. Abiraterone acetate and enzalutamide (formerly MDV3100) have been approved, and other androgen receptor pathway–targeted agents (see Targeted Therapies section) are under investigation in patients whose disease progressed on primary

ADT and may represent effective second-line hormone therapy prior to chemotherapy.

For patients with overt symptomatic metastatic disease at the time of initiating ADT, disease typically relapses first with rising PSA levels, followed by progression on a radionuclide bone scan evaluation, then by symptoms. The presence of back pain should raise concern for possible spinal cord or cauda equina syndrome, and, if clinically indicated, an MRI should be performed. In approximately 10% to 15% of patients, disease will relapse with aggressive local or distant metastases, where the level of PSA appears to be disproportionately low for the tumor burden present. The results on repeat biopsy may indicate a neuroendocrine phenotype. With the use of novel highly potent androgen receptor–targeted therapies (e.g., abiraterone acetate and enzalutamide), it has been hypothesized that treatment-related neuroendocrine prostate cancer may arise.[324]

TREATMENT EVALUATION CRITERIA

A major issue in the development of effective therapies for patients with castrate-resistant disease has been designing endpoints for phase II clinical trials in prostate cancer. In 2008, the Prostate Cancer Clinical Trials Working Group (PCWG2) published recommendations to define eligibility and outcome measures in clinical trials that evaluate systemic treatment for patients with progressive prostate cancer and castrate levels of testosterone.[325] It was suggested that outcomes be reported independently for PSA, imaging, and clinical measures and that grouped categorizations be avoided, such as complete or partial response. In most trials, early changes in PSA and/or pain should not be acted on without other evidence of disease progression, and treatment should be continued for at least 12 weeks to ensure adequate drug exposure. Bone scans should be assessed as "new lesions" or "no new lesions," changes in soft-tissue disease assessed by Response Evaluation Criteria in Solid Tumor (RECIST), and pain measured using validated scales. PCWG2 recommended an increased emphasis on time-to-event endpoints (i.e., failure to progress) as decision aids in assessing the activity of new agents and in proceeding from phase II to phase III studies.

In addition to clinical assessments, measurement of circulating prostate cancer tumor cells has been studied in patients with metastatic CRPC as a prognostic marker[326] and to assess response to systemic chemotherapy.[327] This has led to FDA approval of an assay to count circulating tumor cells in patients with metastatic CRPC. A recently reported study validated the prognostic utility of circulating tumor cell counts in a large docetaxel-based prospective cohort.[328]

IMMUNOTHERAPY

A variety of studies using various immune-based therapies suggested a benefit in survival for men with metastatic CRPC. Sipuleucel-T is an autologous cellular vaccine composed of prostatic acid phosphatase and G-CSF. It is administered intravenously every 2 weeks for a total of three infusions designed to elicit an immune response to prostatic acid phosphatase. In a randomized 2:1, phase III, placebo-controlled trial of men

with minimally symptomatic metastatic CRPC, patients who received sipuleucel-T had a median OS of 25.8 months compared with 21.7 months in patients who received placebo (HR 0.78, 95% CI 0.61, 0.98; p = 0.03).[329] No significant effect on PSA values or PFS was observed. The proportion of patients receiving sipuleucel-T who were alive was 50% higher than in the control group at 3 years (31.7% versus 21.7%, respectively). Based on the 4.1-month improvement in OS, sipuleucel-T was FDA approved in 2010. Another immunotherapy, ipilimumab—the fully humanized antibody that binds to CTLA-4—failed to improve survival in postdocetaxel metastatic CRPC[330] with an ongoing prechemotherapy study.

CHEMOTHERAPY

Patients with metastatic CRPC who experience disease progression on ADT should be considered for systemic chemotherapy. Prior to 2004, chemotherapeutic regimens demonstrated antitumor activity determined by changes in measurable disease, a greater than 50% decline in the PSA level, and objective improvements in bone scan, but did not demonstrate an effect on OS. In 2004, two randomized trials (SWOG 9916 and TAX 327) were reported that compared docetaxel-based therapy to mitoxantrone and prednisone in patients with metastatic CRPC. A significant improvement in OS was demonstrated for patients who received docetaxel, with a median survival of more than 18 months.[331-333] Docetaxel was also superior to mitoxantrone with respect to pain response rate, PSA response rate, and QOL indicies.[334] Based on these studies, the FDA approved the use of docetaxel (75 mg/m^2 every 21 days) together with prednisone as front-line therapy for men with metastatic CRPC. CALGB 90401 tested if the addition of bevacizumab to docetaxel and prednisone prolonged survival. There was no improvement in OS (22.6 months vs. 21.5 months; p = 0.181), although there was an improvement in PFS (9.9 months) in patients receiving bevacizumab compared with patients receiving placebo (7.5 months; p < 0.0001).[335] Similarly, the addition of lenalidomide to docetaxel and prednisone in the discontinued MAINSAIL trial did not result in an improved survival. Three recently completed randomized phase III trials evaluating the addition of dasatinib, aflibercept, or zibotentan to docetaxel did not lead to an improvement in survival.[336-338] The benefit of chemotherapy for patients with nonmetastatic CRPC has not been established.

A number of agents have been studied in patients with metastatic CRPC whose disease progresses on first-line chemotherapy. A phase III study of prednisone plus either the oral platinum analog satraplatin or placebo for patients with CRPC who had received prior chemotherapy showed that the addition of satraplatin did not improve OS.[339] Similarly, sunitinib plus prednisone did not improve OS compared with placebo plus prednisone in men with CRPC who had progressed after treatment with docetaxel-based chemotherapy. Cabazitaxel is a microtubule stabilizing taxane that was FDA-approved as second-line chemotherapy after docetaxel, based on the results of a phase III trial of men with CRPC who previously received docetaxel and who were randomly assigned to either 25 mg/m^2 of cabazitaxel or to 12 mg/m^2 of mitoxantrone every 3 weeks in combination with 10 mg/day of prednisone.[340] Median survival was 15.1 months and 12.7 months for patients treated with cabazitaxel and mitoxantrone, respectively (HR 0.70, 95% CI 0.59, 0.83; p < 0.0001). Grade 3 to 4 neutropenia was the major serious toxicity in patients who received cabazitaxel, suggesting primary prophylaxis with G-CSF should be considered. Mitoxantrone and other regimens that have demonstrated activity in CRPC may be beneficial as third-line therapy for patients with a good performance status.[341-343] In patients with neuroendocrine or small cell histologies, the use of platinum-containing chemotherapy regimens such as etoposide and cisplatin may be beneficial.[344,345]

TARGETED THERAPIES

Numerous studies indicate that androgen signaling via biosynthesis of extragonadal or intratumoral androgens or an activated androgen receptor, despite low levels of circulating dihydrotestosterone, may contribute to CRPC progression. Phase I and II trials demonstrated that therapy with drugs that inhibit the androgen receptor axis can result in significant and prolonged declines in PSA levels in patients with CRPC both before (chemotherapy naive) and after docetaxel therapy.[346] Two similarly designed, phase III, randomized 2:1, double-blind, placebo-controlled trials in patients with CRPC postdocetaxel therapy, with a primary endpoint of OS, have been completed. Abiraterone acetate is an oral CYP17 inhibitor that inhibits androgen biosynthesis. In the first phase III trial, patients received abiraterone (1,000 mg daily) or placebo plus prednisone (5 mg twice daily). OS was significantly longer in patients treated with abiraterone compared with placebo (14.8 months vs. 10.9 months; HR 0.65, 95% CI 0.54, 0.77; p < 0.001), as were all secondary endpoints: time to PSA progression (10.2 months vs. 6.6 months; p < 0.001), PFS (5.6 months vs. 3.6 months; p < 0.001), and PSA response rate (29% vs. 6%; p < 0.001).[347] Mineralocorticoid-related toxicities in patients receiving abiraterone included fluid retention, hypertension, and hypokalemia. Abiraterone acetate was FDA-approved in 2011 for postdocetaxel therapy. It was subsequently FDA-approved in 2012 for the treatment of metastatic prostate cancer without previous chemotherapy based on a phase III randomized trial of abiraterone acetate (1,000 mg) plus prednisone (5 mg twice daily) versus placebo plus prednisone in patients with CRPC who had not been previously treated with chemotherapy.[348] Abiraterone acetate plus prednisone improved radiographic PFS (rPFS) compared to placebo plus prednisone (16.5 months vs. 8.3 months; HR 0.53, 95% CI 0.45, 0.62; p < 0.001) with a trend toward improvement in survival (median not reached vs. 27.2 months for prednisone alone; HR 0.75, 95% CI 0.61, 0.93; p = 0.01) as well as a significant delay in clinical decline and initiation of chemotherapy. Enzalutamide is a highly potent oral androgen receptor antagonist that blocks androgens from binding to the androgen receptor.[349] A phase III trial in patients with postdocetaxel CRPC compared enzalutamide with placebo.[350] An interim analysis performed in 2011 reported a median OS of 18.4 months in the enzalutamide arm compared with 13.6 months in patients receiving placebo (p < 0.0001), with an overall 37% risk reduction in death (HR 0.63, 95% CI 0.53, 0.75). Enzalutamide

was superior to placebo with respect to all secondary endpoints (50% reduction in PSA, soft-tissue response rate, QOL response rate, time to PSA progression, and the time to the first skeletal-related event). A randomized phase III trial comparing enzalutamide to placebo in asymptomatic or mildly symptomatic chemotherapy-naive men with CRPC demonstrated a significant benefit of enzalutamide over placebo with a 29% reduction in risk of death (OS: HR 0.71, 95% CI 0.60, 0.84; p < 0.001), 81% reduction in risk of radiographic progression or death (rPFS: HR 0.19, 95% CI 0.15, 0.23; p < 0.001) and a delay in the median time to chemotherapy initiation of 17 months when compared to placebo (28 months vs. 10.8 months; HR 0.35, 95% CI 0.30, 0.40; p < 0.001).[351] Finally, early studies with the dual met-VEGF receptor tyrosine kinase inhibitor cabozantinib have resulted in significant pain relief and clinical, soft tissue, and bone scan responses in patients with CRPC who were heavily pretreated.[352] Phase III studies are ongoing.

BONE-TARGETED THERAPY

The alpha-emitter radium-223 is a bone-seeking radionuclide that demonstrated an improvement in time to progression in a randomized phase II study, which led to a phase III trial in which 921 men with metastatic CRPC with symptomatic bone metastases who had received, were not eligible for, or declined docetaxel were randomly assigned 2:1 to radium-223 dichloride or to placebo every 4 weeks for six treatments.[353] At the updated analysis involving 921 patients, OS was significantly improved with radium-223 dichloride with a median survival of 14.9 months versus 11.3 months for men treated with placebo (HR 0.70, 95% CI 0.58, 0.83; p < 0.001). Time to first symptomatic skeletal event and all main secondary endpoints were improved with radium-223 dichloride. Toxicity was mild, with low myelosuppression rates. This study led to the FDA approval of radium-223 dichloride for the treatment of patients with CRPC and symptomatic bone metastases with no known visceral metastatic disease in 2013.

Zoledronate has been shown to palliate symptoms and reduce the frequency of skeletal-related events, such as new pain, need for radiation therapy, and microfractures.[354] Renal insufficiency has been reported with zoledronate and other bisphosphonate use, and serum creatinine should be monitored and the dose adjusted accordingly. An uncommon (2% to 4%) complication of bisphosphonate therapy is osteonecrosis of the jaw, the incidence of which increases with treatment duration and is associated with dental procedures.[355]

A phase III noninferiority trial compared denosumab with zoledronate administered every 4 weeks for the prevention of skeletal-related events in men with CRPC and bone metastases.[356] The median time to first on-study skeletal-related event was 20.7 months (95% CI 18.8, 24.9) with denosumab compared with 17.1 months (95% CI 15.0, 19.4) with zoledronic acid (HR 0.82, 95% CI 0.71, 0.95; p = 0.0002 for noninferiority; p = 0.008 for superiority). Hypocalcemia was more common in patients treated with denosumab, and osteonecrosis of the jaw occurred infrequently in both arms. Either therapy is recommended for men with CRPC

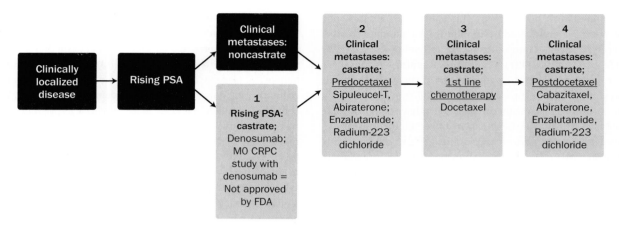

Fig. 10-4 Prostate cancer clinical states model; framework for castrate-resistant prostate cancer (CRPC) management.

Adapted from Scher HI, Morris MJ, Basch E, et al. End points and outcomes in castration-resistant prostate cancer: from clinical trials to clinical practice. J Clin Oncol. 2011;29:3695-704. PMID: 21859988.

and bone metastases together with calcium and vitamin D supplementation.

The FDA approval of multiple agents for the treatment of CRPC has resulted in numerous therapeutic choices. This has led to reformulation of the prostate cancer clinical-states model to provide a framework for patient treatment to guide clinicians (Fig. 10-4).[357]

PALLIATION

An important aspect of patient care is the palliation of pain. Durable relief in selected sites can be achieved with external beam radiation therapy delivered in a focal or hemibody technique. Systemic therapies can also provide palliation. The combination of mitoxantrone and prednisone is FDA-approved for the palliation of pain of osseous metastases.[358] Two bone-seeking radiopharmaceutical agents, strontium-89 and samarium-153, have been shown to reduce the pain of skeletal metastases despite the lack of a survival benefit.

SURVIVORSHIP

With early detection and treatment, significant numbers of men will be cured of prostate cancer by radiation or surgery. These patients may have a variety of adverse effects related to therapy, including urinary incontinence, erectile dysfunction, and post-treatment psychosocial issues. Men undergoing ADT suffer from numerous adverse effects, including decreased libido, impotence, decreased lean body mass and muscle strength, increased fat mass, decreased QOL, and osteoporosis.[359] It also has been recognized that patients receiving long-term ADT (12 months or longer) may develop metabolic complications such as insulin resistance, hyperglycemia, and metabolic syndrome, which may be responsible for an increased risk of cardiovascular mortality.[360] Men receiving long-term ADT should be monitored for the development of diabetes, and those who develop an adverse lipid profile should be treated according to the established guidelines for hyperlipidemia. One study reported that the SERM toremifene significantly decreased fasting serum lipid levels in men with prostate cancer on ADT.[361] It has been

suggested that men who receive as little as 6 months of ADT with radiation therapy may have an increased risk of cardiovascular-related mortality,[362] but this observation was not confirmed in other retrospective analyses[363-365] or in a recent meta-analysis.[366] Other studies suggest that men with previous cardiovascular disease may be at increased risk of cardiovascular morbidity while receiving ADT.[367]

KEY POINTS

- Prostate cancer may be classified into clinical states from clinically localized disease to clinical metastases: castrate disease for which the prognosis and therapeutic objectives are distinct.
- Prostate-specific antigen (PSA) has a role in the diagnosis and management of prostate cancer; however, limitations in PSA sensitivity, specificity, and positive and negative predictive values have led to differing opinions regarding screening recommendations.
- The risks and benefits associated with different treatment modalities must be carefully considered when choosing the best therapeutic option for a particular patient and disease state.
- Chemotherapy and novel hormone agents improve survival in men with metastatic castrate-resistant prostate cancer (previously referred to as hormone-refractory prostate cancer).

MALIGNANT ADRENAL TUMORS

Malignant adrenal tumors are extremely rare cancers with only limited information to make specific treatment recommendations. Malignant adrenal cortical carcinoma is derived from the adrenal cortex, with approximately 60% of cases associated with hormone secretion leading to symptoms and signs of hypercortisolism, virilization, and mineralocorticoid excess. Localized disease is managed with surgery. The overall prognosis is poor—particularly in patients with larger tumors (more than 5 cm) and/or evidence of local invasion. The adrenocorticolytic agent mitotane is commonly used for patients with metastatic disease; however, response rates are low with no clear survival benefit.[368] Although several studies suggest higher response rates with chemotherapy plus mitotane, it is not at all clear that this translates into an improvement in outcome. A retrospective analysis suggested a potential benefit for mitotane in the adjuvant setting, and it is commonly used in patients at high risk of recurrence following surgery.[369] The FIRM-ACT study compared mitotane plus either a combination of etoposide, doxorubicin, and cisplatin (EDP) every 4 weeks or streptozotocin every 3 weeks in patients with advanced adrenocortical carcinoma and demonstrated significant improvements in response and PFS with EDP plus mitotane but no difference in OS.[370] Malignant pheochromocytomas arise from chromaffin tissue of the adrenal medulla and are extremely rare—accounting for approximately 10% of all pheochromocytomas. Functional pheochromocytomas secrete catecholamines, leading to an array of clinical symptoms, including the classic triad of headache, diaphoresis, and tachycardia. There is no curative therapy for malignant pheochromocytoma, and the mainstay of management includes surgical resection of the tumor. Based on limited data, no definitive recommendations regarding systemic therapy can be made; however, the association of pheochromocytomas with VHL has led to the use of VEGF receptor–targeted agents in this disease.

References

1. Siegel R, Naishadham D, Jemal A. Cancer statistics, 2013. *CA Cancer J Clin.* 2013;63:11-30. PMID: 23335087.

2. Lutke Holzik MF, Rapley EA, Hoekstra HJ, et al. Genetic predisposition to testicular germ-cell tumours. *Lancet Oncol.* 2004;5:363-371. PMID: 15172357.

3. Pettersson A, Richiardi L, Nordenskjold A, et al. Age at surgery for undescended testis and risk of testicular cancer. *N Engl J Med.* 2007;356:1835-1841. PMID: 17476009.

4. Fosså SD, Cvancarova M, Chen L, et al. Adverse prognostic factors for testicular cancer-specific survival: a population-based study of 27,948 patients. *J Clin Oncol.* 2011;29:963-970. Epub 2011 Feb 7. PMID: 21300926.

5. Powles T, Bower M, Daugaard G, et al. Multicenter study of human immunodeficiency virus-related germ cell tumors. *J Clin Oncol.* 2003;21:1922-1927. PMID: 12743144.

6. Holzbeierlein JM, Sogani PC, Sheinfeld J. Histology and clinical outcomes in patients with bilateral testicular germ cell tumors: the Memorial Sloan Kettering Cancer Center experience 1950 to 2001. *J Urol.* 2003;169:2122-2125. PMID: 12771732.

7. Chaganti RS, Houldsworth J. Genetics and biology of adult human male germ cell tumors. *Cancer Res.* 2000;60:1475-1482. PMID: 10749107.

8. Reuter VE. Origins and molecular biology of testicular germ cell tumors. *Mod Path.* 2005;18 Suppl 2:S51-S60. PMID: 15761466.

9. LeBron C, Pal P, Brait M, et al. Genome-wide analysis of genetic alterations in testicular primary seminoma using high resolution single nucleotide polymorphism arrays. *Genomics.* 2011;97:341-349. Epub 2011 Mar 2. PMID: 21376111.

10. Li X, Chen J, Hu X, et al. Comparative mRNA and microRNA expression profiling of three genitourinary cancers reveals common hallmarks and cancer-specific molecular events. *PLoS One.* 2011;6:e22570. Epub 2011 Jul 25. PMID: 21799901.

11. Bosl GJ, Motzer RJ. Testicular germ-cell cancer. *N Engl J Med.* 1997;337:242-253. PMID: 9227931.

12. Edge SB, Byrd DR, Compton CC, et al (eds). *AJCC Cancer Staging Manual, 7th ed.* New York: Springer Science and Business Media LLC; 2010.

13. International Germ Cell Consensus Classification: a prognostic factor-based staging system for metastatic germ cell cancers. International Germ Cell Cancer Collaborative Group. *J Clin Oncol.* 1997;15:594-603. PMID: 9053482.

14. Garnick MB. Spurious rise in human chorionic gonadotropin induced by marihuana in patients with testicular cancer. *N Engl J Med.* 1980;303:1177. PMID: 7421935.

15. Warde P, Huddart R, Bolton D, et al. Management of localized seminoma, stage I-II: SIU/ICUD Consensus Meeting on Germ Cell Tumors (GCT), Shanghai 2009. *Urology.* 2011;78:S435-S443. PMID: 21986223.

16. van Walraven C, Fergusson D, Earle C, et al. Association of diagnostic radiation exposure and second abdominal-pelvic malignancies after testicular cancer. *J Clin Oncol.* 2011;29:2883-2888. Epub 2011 Jun 20. PMID: 21690479.

17. Lewinshtein D, Gulati R, Nelson PS, et al. Incidence of second malignancies after external beam radiotherapy for clinical stage I testicular seminoma. *BJU Int.* 2012;109:706-712. Epub 2011 Aug 22. PMID: 21883828.

18. Travis LB, Fosså SD, Schonfeld SJ, et al. Second cancers among 40,576 testicular cancer patients: focus on long-term survivors. *J Natl Cancer Inst.* 2005;97:1354-1365. PMID: 16174857.

19. Fosså SD, Horwich A, Russell JM, et al. Optimal planning target volume for stage I testicular seminoima: a Medical Research Council randomized trial. Medical Research Council Testicular Tumor Working Group. *J Clin Oncol.* 1999;17:1146-1154. PMID: 10561173.

20. Oliver RT, Mason MD, Mead GM, et al. Radiotherapy versus single-dose carboplatin in adjuvant treatment of stage I seminoma: a randomised trial. *Lancet.* 2005;366:293-300. PMID: 16039331.

21. Oliver RT, Mead GM, Rustin GJ, et al. Randomized trial of carboplatin versus radiotherapy for stage I seminoma: mature results on relapse and contralateral testis cancer rates in MRC TE19/EORTC 30982 study (ISRCTN27163214). *J Clin Oncol.* 2011;29:957-962. Epub 2011 Jan 31. PMID: 21282539.

22. Loehrer PJ, Bosl GJ. Carboplatin for stage I seminoma and the sword of Damocles. *J Clin Oncol.* 2005;23:8566-8569. Epub 2005 Oct 31. PMID: 16260692.

23. Bosl GJ, Patil S. Carboplatin in clinical stage I seminoma: too much and too little at the same time. *J Clin Oncol.* 2011;29:949-952. Epub 2011 Jan 31. PMID: 21282532.

24. De Santis M, Becherer A, Bokemeyer C, et al. 2-18fluoro-deoxy-D-glucose positron emission tomography is a reliable predictor for viable tumor in postchemotherapy seminoma: an update of the prospective multicentric SEMPET trial. *J Clin Oncol.* 2004;22:1034-1039. PMID: 15020605.

25. Bachner M, Loriot Y, Gross-Goupil M, et al. 2-18fluoro-deoxy-D-glucose positron emission tomography (FDG-PET) for postchemotherapy seminoma residual lesions: a retrospective validation of the SEMPET trial. *Ann Oncol.* 2012;23:59-64. Epub 2011 Apr 2. PMID: 21460378.

26. NCCN Clinical Practice Guidelines in Oncology. Testicular Cancer. Version 2.2011. www.nccn.org/professionals/physician_gls/pdf/testicular.pdf. Accessed October 10, 2012.

27. Carver BS, Motzer RJ, Kondagunta GV, et al. Late relapse of testicular germ cell tumors. *Urol Oncol.* 2005;23:441-445. PMID: 16301125.

28. Fazel R, Krumholz HM, Wang Y, et al. Exposure to low-dose ionizing radiation from medical imaging procedures. *N Engl J Med.* 2009;361:849-857. PMID: 19710483.

29. Brenner DJ, Shuryak I. Ten years of follow-up is not long enough to assess lifetime cancer risks caused by computed tomography scans in a young population. *J Clin Oncol.* 2011;29:4062. Epub 2011 Sep 19. PMID: 21931034.

30. Albers P, Siener R, Krege S, et al. Randomized phase III trial comparing retroperitoneal lymph node dissection with one course of bleomycin and etoposide plus cisplatin chemotherapy in the adjuvant treatment of clinical stage I Nonseminomatous testicular germ cell tumors: AUO trial AH 01/94 by the German Testicular Cancer Study Group. *J Clin Oncol.* 2008;26:2966-2972. Epub 2008 May 5. Erratum in: *J Clin Oncol.* 2010;28:1439. Dosage error in article text. PMID: 18458040.

31. Cullen MH, Stenning SP, Parkinson MC, et al. Short-course adjuvant chemotherapy in high-risk stage I nonseminomatous germ cell tumors of the testis: a Medical Research Council report. *J Clin Oncol.* 1996;14:1106-1113. PMID: 8648364.

32. Motzer RJ, Sheinfeld J, Mazumdar M, et al. Etoposide and cisplatin adjuvant therapy for patients with pathologic stage II germ cell tumors. *J Clin Oncol.* 1995;13:2700-2704. PMID: 7595727.

33. Feldman DR, Bosl GJ, Sheinfeld J, et al. Medical treatment of advanced testicular cancer. *JAMA*. 2008;299:672-684. PMID: 18270356.

34. Bosl GJ, Gluckman R, Geller NL, et al. VAB-6: an effective chemotherapy regimen for patients with germ-cell tumors. *J Clin Oncol*. 1986;4:1493-1499. PMID: 2428948.

35. Williams SD, Birch R, Einhorn LH, et al. Treatment of disseminated germ-cell tumors with cisplatin, bleomycin, and either vinblastine or etoposide. *N Engl J Med*. 1987;316:1435-1440. PMID: 2437455.

36. Bosl GJ, Geller NL, Bajorin D, et al. A randomized trial of etoposide + cisplatin versus vinblastine + bleomycin + cisplatin + cyclophosphamide + dactinomycin in patients with good-prognosis germ cell tumors. *J Clin Oncol*. 1988;6:1231-1238. PMID: 2457657.

37. Kondagunta GV, Bacik J, Bajorin D, et al. Etoposide and cisplatin chemotherapy for metastatic good-risk germ cell tumors. *J Clin Oncol*. 2005;23:9290-9294. PMID: 16361627.

38. Culine S, Kerbrat P, Kramar A, et al. Refining the optimal chemotherapy regimen for good-risk metastatic nonseminomatous germ-cell tumors: a randomized trial of the Genito-Urinary Group of the French Federation of Cancer Centers (GETUG T93BP). *Ann Oncol*. 2007;18:917-924. Epub 2007 Mar 9. PMID: 17351252.

39. Loehrer PJ Sr, Johnson D, Elson P, et al. Importance of bleomycin in favorable-prognosis disseminated germ cell tumors: an Eastern Cooperative Oncology Group Trial. *J Clin Oncol*. 1995;13:470-476. PMID: 7531223.

40. de Wit R, Stoter G, Kaye SB, et al. Importance of bleomycin in combination chemotherapy for good-prognosis testicular nonseminoma: a randomized study of the European Organization for Research and Treatment of Cancer Genitourinary Tract Cancer Cooperative Group. *J Clin Oncol*. 1997;15:1837-1843. PMID: 9164193.

41. Bajorin DF, Sarosdy MF, Pfister DG, et al. Randomized trial of etoposide and cisplatin versus etoposide and carboplatin in patients with good-risk germ cell tumors: a multiinstitutional study. *J Clin Oncol*. 1993;11:598-606. PMID: 8386751.

42. Horwich A, Sleijfer DT, Fosså SD, et al. Randomized trial of bleomycin, etoposide, and cisplatin compared with bleomycin, etoposide, and carboplatin in good-prognosis metastatic nonseminomatous germ cell cancer: a Multiinstitutional Medical Research Council/European Organization for Research and Treatment of Cancer Trial. *J Clin Oncol*. 1997;15:1844-1852. PMID: 9164194.

43. Einhorn LH, Foster RS. Bleomycin, etoposide, and cisplatin for three cycles compared with etoposide and cisplatin for four cycles in good-risk germ cell tumors: is there a preferred regimen? *J Clin Oncol*. 2006;24:2597-2598, author reply 2598-2599. PMID: 16735718.

44. Toner GC, Stockler MR, Boyer MJ, et al. Comparison of two standard chemotherapy regimens for good-prognosis germ-cell tumours: a randomised trial. Australian and New Zealand Germ Cell Trial Group. *Lancet*. 2001;357:739-745. PMID: 11253966.

45. Nichols CR, Catalano PJ, Crawford ED, et al. Randomized comparison of cisplatin and etoposide and either bleomycin or ifosfamide in treatment of advanced disseminated germ cell tumors: an Eastern Cooperative Oncology Group, Southwest Oncology Group, and Cancer and Leukemia Group B Study. *J Clin Oncol*. 1998;16:1287-1293. PMID: 9552027.

46. Ozols RF, Ihde DC, Linehan WM, et al. A randomized trial of standard chemotherapy v a high-dose chemotherapy regimen in the treatment of poor prognosis nonseminomatous germ-cell tumors. *J Clin Oncol*. 1988;6:1031-1040. PMID: 2453619.

47. Motzer RJ, Nichols CJ, Margolin KA, et al. Phase III randomized trial of conventional-dose chemotherapy with or without high-dose chemotherapy and autologous hematopoietic stem-cell rescue as first-line treatment for patients with poor-prognosis metastatic germ cell tumors. *J Clin Oncol*. 2007;25:247-256. PMID: 17235042.

48. Daugaard G, Skoneczna I, Aass N, et al. A randomized phase III study comparing standard dose BEP with sequential high-dose cisplatin, etoposide, and ifosfamide (VIP) plus stem-cell support in males with poor-prognosis germ-cell cancer. An intergroup study of EORTC, GTCSG, and Grupo Germinal (EORTC 30974). *Ann Oncol*. 2011;22:1054-1061. Epub 2010 Nov 8. PMID: 21059637.

49. Olofsson SE, Tandstad T, Jerkeman M, et al. Population-based study of treatment guided by tumor marker decline in patients with metastatic nonseminomatous germ cell tumor: a report from the Swedish-Norwegian Testicular Cancer Group. *J Clin Oncol*. 2011;29:2032-2039. Epub 2011 Apr 11. PMID: 21482994.

50. Fizazi K, Pagliaro LC, Flechon A, et al. A phase III trial of personalized chemotherapy based on serum tumor marker decline in poor-prognosis germ-cell tumors: Results of GETUG 13. *J Clin Oncol*. 2013;31 (suppl; abstr LBA4500).

51. Loehrer PJ Sr, Gonin R, Nichols CR, et al. Vinblastine plus ifosfamide plus cisplatin as initial salvage therapy in recurrent germ cell tumor. *J Clin Oncol*. 1998;15:2500-2504. PMID: 9667270.

52. Kondagunta GV, Bacik J, Donadio A, et al. Combination of paclitaxel, ifosfamide, and cisplatin is an effective second-line therapy for patients with relapsed testicular germ cell tumors. *J Clin Oncol*. 2005;23:6549-6555. PMID: 16170162.

53. Ronnen EA, Kondagunta GV, Bacik J, et al. Incidence of late-relapse germ cell tumor and outcome to salvage chemotherapy. *J Clin Oncol*. 2005;23:6999-7004. PMID: 16192587.

54. Bedano PM, Brames MJ, Williams SD, et al. Phase II study of cisplatin plus epirubicin salvage chemotherapy in refractory germ cell tumors. *J Clin Oncol*. 2006;24:5403-5407. PMID: 17135640.

55. Kollmannsberger C, Beyer J, Liersch R, et al. Combination chemotherapy with gemcitabine plus oxaliplatin in patients with intensively pretreated or refractory germ cell cancer: a study of the German Testicular Cancer Study Group. *J Clin Oncol*. 2004;22:108-114. PMID: 14701772.

56. Lorch A, Beyer J, Bascoul-Mollevi C, et al. Prognostic factors in patients with metastatic germ cell tumors who experienced treatment failure with cisplatin-based first-line chemotherapy. *J Clin Oncol*. 2010;28:4906-4911. Epub 2010 Oct 18. PMID: 20956623.

57. Bhatia S, Abonour R, Porcu P, et al. High-dose chemotherapy as initial salvage chemotherapy in patients with relapsed testicular cancer. *J Clin Oncol*. 2000;18:3346-3351. PMID: 11013274.

58. Feldman DR, Sheinfeld J, Bajorin DF, et al. TI-CE high-dose chemotherapy for patients with previously treated germ cell tumors: results and prognostic factor analysis. *J Clin Oncol*. 2010;28:1706-1713. Epub 2010 Mar 1. PMID: 20194867.

59. Einhorn LH, Williams SD, Chamness A, et al. High-dose chemotherapy and stem-cell rescue for metastatic germ-cell tumors. *N Engl J Med*. 2007;357:340-348. PMID: 17652649.

60. Vaena DA, Abonour R, Einhorn LH. Long-term survival after high-dose salvage chemotherapy for germ cell malignancies with adverse prognostic variables. *J Clin Oncol*. 2003;21:4100-4104. PMID: 14615439.

61. Collette L, Sylvester RJ, Stenning SP, et al. Impact of the treating institution on survival of patients with "poor-prognosis" metastatic nonseminoma. European Organization for Research and Treatment of Cancer Genito-Urinary Tract Cancer Collaborative Group and the Medical Research Council Testicular Cancer Working Party. *J Natl Cancer Inst*. 1999;91:839-846. PMID: 10340903.

62. Donadio AC, Motzer RJ, Bajorin DF, et al. Chemotherapy for teratoma with malignant transformation. *J Clin Oncol*. 2003;21:4285-4291. PMID: 14645417.

63. Oldenburg J, Alfsen GC, Lien HH, et al. Postchemotherapy retroperitoneal surgery remains necessary in patients with nonseminomatous testicular cancer and minimal residual tumor masses. *J Clin Oncol*. 2003;21:3310-3317. PMID: 12947067.

64. Oldenburg J, Alfsen GC, Waehre H, et al. Late recurrences of germ cell malignancies: a population-based experience over three decades. *Br J Cancer*. 2006;94:820-827. PMID: 16508636.

65. Sharp DS, Carver BS, Eggener SE, et al. Clinical outcome and predictors of survival in late relapse of germ cell tumor. *J Clin Oncol*. 2008;26:5524-5529. Epub 2008 Oct 20. PMID: 18936477.

66. Motzer RJ, Rodriguez E, Reuter VE, et al. Molecular and cytogenetic studies in the diagnosis of patients with poorly differentiated carcinomas of unknown primary site. *J Clin Oncol*. 1995;13:274-282. PMID: 7799031.

67. van den Belt-Dusebout AW, Nuver J, de Wit R, et al. Long-term risk of cardiovascular disease in 5-year survivors of testicular cancer. *J Clin Oncol*. 2006;24:467-475. PMID: 16421423.

68. Haugnes HS, Wethal T, Aass N, et al. Cardiovascular risk factors and morbidity in long-term survivors of testicular cancer: a 20-year follow-up study. *J Clin Oncol*. 2010;28:4649-4657. Epub 2010 Sep 20. PMID: 20855830.

69. Nuver J, Smit AJ, van der Meer J, et al. Acute chemotherapy-induced cardiovascular changes in patients with testicular cancer. *J Clin Oncol*. 2005;23:9130-9137. Epub 2005 Nov 21. PMID: 16301596.

70. Nuver J, Smit AJ, Wolffenbuttel BH, et al. The metabolic syndrome and disturbances in hormone levels in long-term survivors of disseminated testicular cancer. *J Clin Oncol*. 2005;23:3718-3725. Epub 2005 Feb 28. PMID: 15738540.

71. Richiardi L, Scélo G, Boffetta P, et al. Second malignancies among survivors of germ-cell testicular cancer: a pooled analysis between 13 cancer registries. *Int J Cancer*. 2007;120:623-631. PMID: 17096341.

72. van den Belt-Dusebout AW, de Wit R, Gietema JA, et al. Treatment-specific risks of second malignancies and cardiovascular disease in 5-year survivors of testicular cancer. *J Clin Oncol*. 2007;25:4370-4378. PMID: 17906202.

73. Fung C, Fossa SD, Milano MT et al. Solid tumors after chemotherapy or surgery for testicular nonseminoma: a population-based study. *J Clin Oncol.* 2013;31:3807-3814. PMID: 24043737.

74. Brydoy M, Fossa SD, Klepp O, et al. Paternity and testicular function among testicular cancer survivors treated with two to four cycles of cisplatin-based chemotherapy. *Eur Urol.* 2010;58:134-140. Epub 2010 Apr 2. PMID: 20395037.

75. Travis LB, Beard C, Allan JM, et al. Testicular cancer survivorship: research strategies and recommendations. *J Natl Cancer Inst.* 2010;102:1114-1130. Epub 2010 Jun 28. PMID: 20585105.

76. Mallin K, David KA, Carroll PR, et al. Transitional cell carcinoma of the bladder: racial and gender disparities in survival (1993 to 2002), stage and grade (1993 to 2007). *J Urol.* 2011;185:1631-1636. Epub 2011 Mar 21. PMID: 21419456.

77. Hollenbeck BK, Dunn RL, Ye Z, et al. Racial differences in treatment and outcomes among patients with early stage bladder cancer. *Cancer.* 2010;116:50-56. PMID: 19877112.

78. Freedman ND, Silverman DT, Hollenbeck AR, et al. Association between smoking and risk of bladder cancer among men and women. *JAMA.* 2011;306:737-745. PMID: 21846855.

79. Engel C, Loeffler M, Steinke V, et al. Risks of less common cancers in proven mutation carriers with lynch syndrome. *J Clin Oncol.* 2012;30:4409-4415. PMID: 23091106.

80. Wu XR. Urothelial tumorigenesis: a tale of divergent pathways. *Nat Rev Cancer.* 2005;5:713-725. PMID: 16110317.

81. Shariat SF, Tokunaga H, Zhou J, et al. p53, p21, pRB, and p16 expression predict clinical outcome in cystectomy with bladder cancer. *J Clin Oncol.* 2004;22:1014-1024. Epub 2004 Feb 23. PMID: 14981102.

82. Stadler WM, Lerner SP, Groshen S, et al. Phase III study of molecularly targeted adjuvant therapy in locally advanced urothelial cancer of the bladder based on p53 status. *J Clin Oncol.* 2011;29:3443-3449. Epub 2011 Aug 1. PMID: 21810677.

83. Sanchez-Carbayo M, Socci ND, Lozano J, et al. Defining molecular profiles of poor outcome in patients with invasive bladder cancer using oligonucleotide microarrays. *J Clin Oncol.* 2006;24:778-789. Epub 2006 Jan 23. PMID: 16432078.

84. Iyer G, Al-Ahmadie H, Schultz N, et al. Prevalence and co-occurrence of actionable genomic alterations in high-grade bladder cancer. *J Clin Oncol.* 2013;31:3133-3140. PMID: 23897969.

85. Cancer Genome Atlas Research Network. Comprehensive molecular characterization of urothelial bladder carcinoma. *Nature.* 2014;507:315-322. PMID: 24476821.

86. Kibel AS, Dehdashti F, Katz MD, et al. Prospective study of [18F]fluoro-deoxyglucose positron emission tomography/computed tomography for staging of muscle-invasive bladder carcinoma. *J Clin Oncol.* 2009;27:4314-4320. PMID: 19652070.

87. Apolo AB, Riches J, Schöder H, et al. Clinical value of fluorine-18 2-fluoro-2-deoxy-D-glucose positron emission tomography/computed tomography in bladder cancer. *J Clin Oncol.* 2010;28:3973-3978. PMID: 20679618.

88. Grossman HB, Soloway M, Messing E, et al. Surveillance for recurrent bladder cancer using a point-of-care proteomic assay. *JAMA.* 2006;295:299-305. PMID: 16418465.

89. Gudjónsson S, Isfoss BL, Hansson K, et al. The value of the UroVysion assay for surveillance of non-muscle-invasive bladder cancer. *Eur Urol.* 2008;54:402-408. Epub 2007 Dec 7. PMID: 18082934.

90. Brausi M, Witjes JA, Lamm D, et al. A review of current guidelines and best practice recommendations for the management of nonmuscle invasive bladder cancer by the International Bladder Cancer Group. *J Urol.* 2011;186:2158-2167. Epub 2011 Oct 19. PMID: 22014799.

91. Clark PE, Agarwal N, Biagioli MC, et al. Bladder cancer. *J Natl Compr Canc Netw.* 2013;11:446-475. PMID: 23584347.

92. Jager W, Thomas C, Haag S, et al. Early vs delayed radical cystectomy for 'high-risk' carcinoma not invading bladder muscle: delay of cystectomy reduces cancer-specific survival. *BJU Int.* 2011;108:E284-E288. Epub 2011 Jan 18. PMID: 21244611.

93. Segal R, Yafi FA, Brimo F, et al. Prognostic factors and outcome in patients with T1 high-grade bladder cancer: can we identify patients for early cystectomy? *BJU Int.* 2012;109:1026-1030. Epub 2011 Aug 24. PMID: 21883838.

94. Herr HW, Bochner BH, Dalbagni G, et al. Impact of the number of lymph nodes retrieved on outcome in patients with muscle invasive bladder cancer. *J Urol.* 2002;167:1295-1298. PMID: 11832716.

95. Kassouf W, Leibovici D, Munsell MF, et al. Evaluation of the relevance of lymph node density in a contemporary series of patients undergoing radical cystectomy. *J Urol.* 2006;176:53-57. PMID: 16753366.

96. Gerharz EW, Månsson A, Hunt S, et al. Quality of life after cystectomy and urinary diversion: an evidence based analysis. *J Urol.* 2005;174:1729-1736. PMID: 16217273.

97. Fleischmann A, Thalmann GN, Markwalder R, et al. Extracapsular extension of pelvic lymph node metastases from urothelial carcinoma of the bladder is an independent prognostic factor. *J Clin Oncol.* 2005;23:2358-2365. PMID: 15800327.

98. Stein JP, Lieskovsky G, Cote R, et al. Radical cystectomy in the treatment of invasive bladder cancer: long-term results in 1,054 patients. *J Clin Oncol.* 2001;19:666-675. PMID: 11157016.

99. International Bladder Cancer Nomogram Consortium, Bochner BH, Kattan MW, et al. Postoperative nomogram predicting risk of recurrence after radical cystectomy for bladder cancer. *J Clin Oncol.* 2006;24:3967-3972. Epub 2006 Jul 24. PMID: 16864855.

100. Shariat SF, Karakiewicz PI, Palapattu GS, et al. Nomograms provide improved accuracy for predicting survival after radical cystectomy. *Clin Cancer Res.* 2006;12:6663-6676. PMID: 17121885.

101. Kassouf W, Swanson D, Kamat AM, et al. Partial cystectomy for muscle invasive urothelial carcinoma of the bladder: a contemporary review of the M. D. Anderson Cancer Center experience. *J Urol.* 2006;175:2058-2062. PMID: 16697803.

102. Pruthi RS, Nielsen ME, Nix J, et al. Robotic radical cystectomy for bladder cancer: surgical and pathological outcomes in 100 consecutive cases. *J Urol.* 2010;183:510-514. Epub 2009 Dec 14. PMID: 20006884.

103. Sternberg CN, Yagoda A, Scher HI, et al. M-VAC (methotrexate, vinblastine, doxorubicin, and cisplatin) for advanced transitional cell carcinoma of the urothelium. *J Urol.* 1988;139:461-469. PMID: 3343727.

104. von der Maase H, Hansen SW, Roberts JT, et al. Gemcitabine and cisplatin versus methotrexate, vinblastine, doxorubicin, and cisplatin in advanced or metastatic bladder cancer: results of a large, randomized, multinational, multicenter, phase III study. *J Clin Oncol.* 2000;18:3068-3077. PMID: 11001674.

105. von der Maase H, Sengelov L, Roberts JT, et al. Long-term survival results of a randomized trial comparing gemcitabine plus cisplatin, with methotrexate, vinblastine, doxorubicin, plus cisplatin in patients with bladder cancer. *J Clin Oncol.* 2005;23:4602-4608. PMID: 16034041.

106. Sternberg CN, de Mulder P, Schornagel JH, et al. Seven year update of an EORTC phase III trial of high-dose intensity M-VAC chemotherapy and G-CSF versus classic M-VAC in advanced urothelial tract tumours. *Eur J Cancer.* 2006;42:50-54. Epub 2005 Dec 5. PMID: 16330205.

107. Bamias A, Aravantinos G, Deliveliotis C, et al. Docetaxel and cisplatin with granulocyte colony-stimulating factor (G-CSF) versus MVAC with G-CSF in advanced urothelial carcinoma: a multicenter, randomized, phase III study from the Hellenic Cooperative Oncology Group. *J Clin Oncol.* 2004;22:220-228. Epub 2003 Dec 9. PMID: 14665607.

108. Bellmunt J, von der Maase H, Mead GM, et al. Randomized phase III study comparing paclitaxel/cisplatin/gemcitabine and gemcitabine/cisplatin in patients with locally advanced or metastatic urothelial cancer without prior systemic therapy: EORTC Intergroup Study 30987. *J Clin Oncol.* 2012;30:1107-1113. Epub 2012 Feb 27. PMID: 22370319.

109. Milowsky MI, Nanus DM, Maluf FC, et al. Final results of sequential doxorubicin plus gemcitabine and ifosfamide, paclitaxel, and cisplatin chemotherapy in patients with metastatic or locally advanced transitional cell carcinoma of the urothelium. *J Clin Oncol.* 2009;27:4062-4067. Epub 2009 Jul 27. PMID: 19636012.

110. Galsky MD, Hahn NM, Rosenberg J, et al. Treatment of patients with metastatic urothelial cancer "unfit" for Cisplatin-based chemotherapy. *J Clin Oncol.* 2011;29:2432-2438. Epub 2011 May 9. PMID: 21555688.

111. Galsky MD, Chen GJ, Oh WK, et al. Comparative effectiveness of cisplatin-based and carboplatin-based chemotherapy for treatment of advanced urothelial carcinoma. *Ann Oncol.* 2012;23:406-410. Epub 2011 May 4. PMID: 21543626.

112. De Santis M, Bellmunt J, Mead G, et al. Randomized phase II/III trial assessing gemcitabine/carboplatin and methotrexate/carboplatin/vinblastine in patients with advanced urothelial cancer who are unfit for cisplatin-based chemotherapy: EORTC study 30986. *J Clin Oncol.* 2012;30:191-199. PMID: 22162575.

113. Bajorin DF, Dodd PM, Mazumdar M, et al. Long-term survival in metastatic transitional-cell carcinoma and prognostic factors predicting outcome of chemotherapy. *J Clin Oncol.* 1999;17:3173-3181. PMID: 10506615.

114. Galsky MD, Moshier E, Krege S, et al. Nomogram for predicting survival in patients with unresectable and/or metastatic urothelial cancer who are treated with cisplatin-based chemotherapy. *Cancer.* 2013;119:3012-3019. PMID: 23720216.

115. Apolo AB, Ostrovnaya I, Halabi S, et al. Prognostic model for predicting survival of patients with metastatic urothelial cancer treated with cisplatin-based chemotherapy. *J Natl Cancer Inst.* 2013;105:499-503. PMID: 23411591.

116. Gallagher DJ, Milowsky MI, Bajorin DF. Advanced bladder cancer: status of first-line chemotherapy and the search for active agents in the second-line setting. *Cancer.* 2008;113:1284-1293. PMID: 18629841.

117. Bellmunt J, Théodore C, Demkov T, et al. Phase III trial of vinflunine plus best supportive care compared with best supportive care alone after a platinum-containing regimen in patients with advanced transitional cell carcinoma of the urothelial tract. *J Clin Oncol.* 2009;27:4454-4461. Epub 2009 Aug 17. PMID: 19687335.

118. Bellmunt J, Choueiri TK, Fougeray R, et al. Prognostic factors in patients with advanced transitional cell carcinoma of the urothelial tract experiencing treatment failure with platinum-containing regimens. *J Clin Oncol.* 2010;28:1850-1855. Epub 2010 Mar 15. PMID: 20231682.

119. Pond GR, Agarwal N, Bellmunt J, et al. A nomogram including baseline prognostic factors to estimate the activity of second-line therapy for advanced urothelial carcinoma. *BJU Int.* 2014;113:E137-E143 PMID: 24219029.

120. Siefker-Radtke AO, Walsh GL, Pisters LL, et al. Is there a role for surgery in the management of metastatic urothelial cancer? The M. D. Anderson experience. *J Urol.* 2004;171:145-148. PMID: 14665863.

121. Herr HW, Donat SM, Bajorin DF. Post-chemotherapy surgery in patients with unresectable or regionally metastatic bladder cancer. *J Urol.* 2001;165:811-814. PMID: 11176475.

122. International Collaboration of Trialists, Medical Research Council Advanced Bladder Cancer Working Party (now the National Cancer Research Institute Bladder Cancer Clinical Studies Group), European Organisation for Research and Treatment of Cancer Genito-Urinary Tract Cancer Group, et al. International phase III trial assessing neoadjuvant cisplatin, methotrexate, and vinblastine chemotherapy for muscle-invasive bladder cancer: long-term results of the BA06 30894 trial. *J Clin Oncol.* 2011;29:2171-2177. Epub 2011 Apr 18. PMID: 21502557.

123. Grossman HB, Natale RB, Tangen CM, et al. Neoadjuvant chemotherapy plus cystectomy compared with cystectomy alone for locally advanced bladder cancer. *N Engl J Med.* 2003;349:859-866. PMID: 12944571.

124. Advanced Bladder Cancer (ABC) Meta-analysis Collaboration. Neoadjuvant chemotherapy in invasive bladder cancer. update of a systematic review and meta-analysis of individual patient data advanced bladder cancer (ABC) meta-analysis collaboration. *Eur Urol.* 2005;48:202-205. Epub 2005 Apr 21. PMID: 15939524.

125. Dash A, Pettus JA 4th, Herr HW, et al. A role for neoadjuvant gemcitabine plus cisplatin in muscle-invasive urothelial carcinoma of the bladder: a retrospective experience. *Cancer.* 2008;113:2471-2477. PMID: 18823036.

125a. Choueiri TK, Jacobus S, Bellmunt J, et al. Neoadjuvant dose-dense methotrexate, vinblastine, doxorubicin, and cisplatin with pegfilgrastim support in muscle-invasive urothelial cancer: pathologic, radiologic, and biomarker correlates. *J Clin Oncol.* 2014;32:1889-1894. PMID: 24821883.

125b. Plimack ER, Hoffman-Censits JH, Viterbo R, et al. Accelerated methotrexate, vinblastine, doxorubicin, and cisplatin is safe, effective, and efficient neoadjuvant treatment for muscle-invasive bladder cancer: results of a multicenter phase II study with molecular correlates of response and toxicity. *J Clin Oncol.* 2014;32:1895-1901. PMID: 24821881.

126. Fedeli U, Fedewa SA, Ward EM. Treatment of muscle invasive bladder cancer: evidence from the National Cancer Database, 2003 to 2007. *J Urol.* 2011;185:72-78. PMID: 21074192.

127. Skinner DG, Daniels JR, Russell CA, et al. The role of adjuvant chemotherapy following cystectomy for invasive bladder cancer: a prospective comparative trial. *J Urol.* 1991;145:459-464. PMID: 1997689.

128. Stöckle M, Meyenburg W, Wellek S, et al. Advanced bladder cancer (stages pT3b, pT4a, pN1 and pN2): improved survival after radical cystectomy and 3 adjuvant cycles of chemotherapy. Results of a controlled prospective study. *J Urol.* 1992;148:302-306. PMID: 1635123.

129. Stöckle M, Meyenburg W, Wellek S, et al. Adjuvant polychemotherapy of nonorgan-confined bladder cancer after radical cystectomy revisited: long-term results of a controlled prospective study and further clinical experience. *J Urol.* 1995;153:47-52. PMID: 7966789.

130. Cognetti F, Ruggeri EM, Felici A, et al. Adjuvant chemotherapy with cisplatin and gemcitabine versus chemotherapy at relapse in patients with muscle-invasive bladder cancer submitted to radical cystectomy: an Italian, multicenter, randomized phase III trial. *Ann Oncol.* 2012;23:695-700. Epub 2011 Aug 22. PMID: 21859900.

131. Paz-Ares LG, Solsona E, Esteban E, et al. Randomized phase III trial comparing adjuvant paclitaxel/gemcitabine/cisplatin (PGC) to observation in patients with resected invasive bladder cancer: Results of the Spanish Oncology Genitourinary Group (SOGUG) 99/01 study. *J Clin Oncol.* 2010;28:18s (suppl; abstr LBA4518).

131a. Sternberg CN, Skoneczna IA, Kerst JM, et al. Final results of EORTC intergroup randomized phase III trial comparing immediate versus deferred chemotherapy after radical cystectomy in patients with pT3T4 and/or N+ M0 transitional cell carcinoma (TCC) of the bladder. *J Clin Oncol.* 2014;32;5s (suppl; abstr 4500).

132. Advanced Bladder Cancer (ABC) Meta-analysis Collaboration. Adjuvant chemotherapy in invasive bladder cancer. a systematic review and meta-analysis of individual patient data Advanced Bladder Cancer (ABC) Meta-analysis Collaboration. *Eur Urol.* 2005;48:189-199. Epub 2005 Apr 25. PMID: 15939530.

133. Balar A, Bajorin DF, Milowsky MI. Management of invasive bladder cancer in patients who are not candidates for or decline cystectomy. *Ther Adv Oncol.* 2011;3:107-117. PMID: 21904567.

134. Efstathiou JA, Spiegel DY, Shipley WU, et al. Long-term outcomes of selective bladder preservation by combined-modality therapy for invasive bladder cancer: the MGH experience. *Eur Urol.* 2012;61:705-711. PMID: 22101114.

135. James ND, Hussain SA, Hall E, et al. Radiotherapy with or without chemotherapy in muscle-invasive bladder cancer. *N Engl J Med.* 2012;366:1477-1488. PMID: 22512481.

136. Efstathiou JA, Bae K, Shipley WU, et al. Late pelvic toxicity after bladder-sparing therapy in patients with invasive bladder cancer: RTOG 89-03, 95-06, 97-06, 99-06. *J Clin Oncol.* 2009;27:4055-4061. Epub 2009 Jul 27. PMID: 19636019.

137. Shipley WU, Winter KA, Kaufman DS, et al. Phase III trial of neoadjuvant chemotherapy in patients with invasive bladder cancer treated with selective bladder preservation by combined radiation therapy and chemotherapy: initial results of Radiation Therapy Oncology Group 89-03. *J Clin Oncol.* 1998;16:3576-3583. PMID: 9817278.

138. Scosyrev E, Ely BW, Messing EM, et al. Do mixed histological features affect survival benefit from neoadjuvant platinum-based combination chemotherapy in patients with locally advanced bladder cancer? A secondary analysis of Southwest Oncology Group-Directed Intergroup Study (S8710). *BJU Int.* 2011;108:693-699. Epub 2010 Nov 24. PMID: 21105991.

139. Kamat AM, Dinney CP, Gee JR, et al. Micropapillary bladder cancer: a review of the University of Texas M. D. Anderson Cancer Center experience with 100 consecutive patients. *Cancer.* 2007;110:62-67. PMID: 17542024.

140. Kane CJ, Mallin K, Ritchey J, et al. Renal cell cancer stage migration: analysis of the National Cancer Data Base. *Cancer.* 2008;113:78-83. PMID: 18491376.

141. Chow WH, Gridley G, Fraumeni JF Jr, et al. Obesity, hypertension, and the risk of kidney cancer in men. *N Engl J Med.* 2000;343:1305-1311. PMID: 11058675.

142. Setiawan VW, Stram DO, Nomura AM, et al. Risk factors for renal cell cancer: the multiethnic cohort. *Am J Epidemiol.* 2007;166:932-940. Epub 2007 Jul 26. PMID: 17656615.

143. Tsivian M, Moreira DM, Caso JR, et al. Cigarette smoking is associated with advanced renal cell carcinoma. *J Clin Oncol.* 2011;20;29:2027-2031. Epub 2011 Apr 18. PMID: 21502558.

144. Mueller-Lisse UG, Mueller-Lisse UL. Imaging of advanced renal cell carcinoma. *World J Urol.* 2010;28:253-261. Epub 2010 May 11. PMID: 20458484.

145. Blom JH, van Poppel H, Maréchal JM, et al. Radical nephrectomy with and without lymph-node dissection: final results of European Organization for Research and Treatment of Cancer (EORTC) randomized phase 3 trial 30881. *Eur Urol.* 2008;55:28-34. PMID: 18848382.

146. Whitson JM, Harris CR, Reese AC, et al. Lymphadenectomy improves survival of patients with renal cell carcinoma and nodal metastases. *J Urol.* 2011;185:1615-1620. Epub 2011 Mar 21. PMID: 21419453.

147. Kunkle DA, Uzzo RG. Cryoablation or radiofrequency ablation of the small renal mass: a meta-analysis. *Cancer.* 2008;113:2671-2680. PMID: 18816624.

148. Choueiri TK, Schutz FA, Hevelone ND, et al. Thermal ablation vs surgery for localized kidney cancer: a Surveillance, Epidemiology, and End Results

(SEER) database analysis. *Urology*. 2011;78:93-98. Epub 2011 May 7. PMID: 21550636.

149. Flanigan RC, Mickisch G, Sylvester R, et al. Cytoreductive nephrectomy in patients with metastatic renal cancer: a combined analysis. *J Urol*. 2004;171:1071-1076. PMID: 14767273.

150. Choueiri TK, Xie W, Kollmannsberger C, et al. The impact of cytoreductive nephrectomy on survival of patients with metastatic renal cell carcinoma receiving vascular endothelial growth factor targeted therapy. *J Urol*. 2011;185:60-66. PMID: 21074201.

151. Chapin BF, Delacroix SE Jr, Culp SH, et al. Safety of presurgical targeted therapy in the setting of metastatic renal cell carcinoma. *Eur Urol*. 2011;60:964-971. Epub 2011 May 25. PMID: 21621907.

152. Kovacs G, Akhtar M, Beckwith BJ, et al. The Heidelberg classification of renal cell tumours. *J Pathol*. 1997;183:131-133. PMID: 9390023.

153. Lopez-Beltran A, Carrasco JC, Cheng L, et al. 2009 update on the classification of renal epithelial tumors in adults. *Int J Urol*. 2009;16:432-443. Epub 2009 Apr 20. PMID: 19453547.

154. Reuter VE, Tickoo SK. Differential diagnosis of renal tumours with clear cell histology. *Pathology*. 2010;42:374-383. PMID: 20438412.

155. Linehan WM, Grubb RL, Coleman JA, et al. The genetic basis of cancer of kidney cancer: implications for gene-specific clinical management. *BJU Int*. 2005;95:2-7. PMID: 15720328.

156. Linehan WM, Srinivasan R, Schmidt LS. The genetic basis of kidney cancer: a metabolic disease. *Nat Rev Urol*. 2010;7:277-285. PMID: 20448661.

157. Kim WY, Kaelin WG. Role of VHL gene mutation in human cancer. *J Clin Oncol*. 2004;22:4991-5004. PMID: 15611513.

158. Hudson CC, Liu M, Chiang GG, et al. Regulation of hypoxia-inducible factor 1alpha expression and function by the mammalian target of rapamycin. *Mol Cell Biol*. 2002;22:7004-7014. PMID: 12242281.

159. Dalgliesh GL, Furge K, Greenman C, et al. Systematic sequencing of renal carcinoma reveals inactivation of histone modifying genes. *Nature*. 2010;463:360-363. Epub 2010 Jan 6. PMID: 20054297.

159a. Brugarolas J. Molecular genetics of clear-cell renal cell carcinoma. *J Clin Oncol*. 2014;32:1968-1976. PMID: 24821879.

160. Varela I, Tarpey P, Raine K, et al. Exome sequencing identifies frequent mutation of the SWI/SNF complex gene PBRM1 in renal carcinoma. *Nature*. 2011;469:539-542. Epub 2011 Jan 19. PMID: 21248752.

161. Schmidt L, Duh FM, Chen F, et al. Germline and somatic mutations in the tyrosine kinase domain of the MET proto-oncogene in papillary renal carcinomas. *Nat Genet*. 1997;16:68-73. PMID: 9140397.

162. Wei MH, Toure O, Glenn GM, et al. Novel mutations in FH and expansion of the spectrum of phenotypes expressed in families with hereditary leiomyomatosis and renal cell cancer. *J Med Genet*. 2006;43:18-27. Epub 2005 Jun 3. PMID: 15937070.

163. Wu A, Kunju LP, Cheng L, et al. Renal cell carcinoma in children and young adults: analysis of clinicopathological, immunohistochemical and molecular characteristics with an emphasis on the spectrum of Xp11.2 translocation-associated and unusual clear cell subtypes. *Histopathology*. 2008;53:533-544. PMID: 18983462.

164. Nickerson ML, Warren MB, Toro JR, et al. Mutations in a novel gene lead to kidney tumors, lung wall defects, and benign tumors of the hair follicle in patients with the Birt-Hogg-Dubé syndrome. *Cancer Cell*. 2002;2:157-164. PMID: 12204536.

165. Milowsky MI, Rosmarin A, Tickoo SK, et al. Active chemotherapy for collecting duct carcinoma of the kidney: a case report and review of the literature. *Cancer*. 2002;94:111-116. PMID: 11815966.

166. Cindolo L, de la Taille A, Schips L, et al. Chromophobe renal cell carcinoma: comprehensive analysis of 104 cases from multicenter European database. *Urology*. 2005;65:681-686. PMID: 15833508.

167. Amin MB, Paner GP, Alvarado-Cabrero I, et al. Chromophobe renal cell carcinoma: histomorphologic characteristics and evaluation of conventional pathologic prognostic parameters in 145 cases. *Am J Surg Pathol*. 2008;32:1822-1834. PMID: 18813125.

168. Beck SD, Patel MI, Snyder ME, et al. Effect of papillary and chromophobe cell type on disease-free survival after nephrectomy for renal cell carcinoma. *Ann Surg Oncol*. 2004;11:71-77. PMID: 14699037.

169. Pignot G, Elie C, Conquy S, et al. Survival analysis of 130 patients with papillary renal cell carcinoma: prognostic utility of type 1 and type 2 subclassification. *Urology*. 2007;69:230-235. Epub 2007 Jan 31. PMID: 17275070.

170. Motzer RJ, Bacik J, Mariani T, et al. Treatment outcome and survival associated with metastatic renal cell carcinoma of non-clear-cell histology. *J Clin Oncol*. 2002;20:2376-2381. PMID: 11981011.

171. Motzer RJ, Mazumdar M, Bacik J, et al. Survival and prognostic stratification of 670 patients with advanced renal cell carcinoma. *J Clin Oncol*. 1999;17:2530-2540. PMID: 10561319.

172. Heng DY, Xie W, Regan MM, et al. Prognostic factors for overall survival in patients with metastatic renal cell carcinoma treated with vascular endothelial growth factor-targeted agents: results from a large, multicenter study. *J Clin Oncol*. 2009;27:5794-5799. Epub 2009 Oct 13. PMID: 19826129.

173. Manola J, Royston P, Elson P, et al. Prognostic model for survival in patients with metastatic renal cell carcinoma: results from the international kidney cancer working group. *Clin Cancer Res*. 2011;17:5443-5450. Epub 2011 Aug 9. PMID: 21828239.

174. Heng DY, Xie W, Regan MM, et al. External validation and comparison with other models of the International Metastatic Renal-Cell Carcinoma Database Consortium prognostic model: a population-based study. *Lancet Oncol*. 2013;14:141-148. PMID: 23312463.

175. Yang JC, Haworth L, Sherry RM, et al. A randomized trial of bevacizumab, an anti-vascular endothelial growth factor antibody, for metastatic renal cancer. *N Engl J Med*. 2003;349:427-434. PMID: 12890841.

176. Escudier B, Bellmunt J, Négrier S, et al. Phase III trial of bevacizumab plus interferon alfa-2a in patients with metastatic renal cell carcinoma (AVOREN): final analysis of overall survival. *J Clin Oncol*. 2010;28:2144-2150. Epub 2010 Apr 5. PMID: 20368553.

177. Rini BI, Halabi S, Rosenberg JE, et al. Phase III trial of bevacizumab plus interferon alfa versus interferon alfa monotherapy in patients with metastatic renal cell carcinoma: final results of CALGB 90206. *J Clin Oncol*. 2010;28:2137-2143. Epub 2010 Apr 5. PMID: 20368558.

178. Motzer RJ, Michaelson MD, Redman BG, et al. Activity of SU11248, a multitargeted inhibitor of vascular endothelial growth factor receptor and platelet-derived growth factor receptor, in patients with metastatic renal cell carcinoma. *J Clin Oncol*. 2006;24:16-24. Epub 2005 Dec 5. PMID: 16330672.

179. Motzer RJ, Rini BI, Bukowski RM, et al. Sunitinib in patients with metastatic renal cell carcinoma. *JAMA*. 2006;295:2516-2524. PMID: 16757724.

180. Motzer RJ, Hutson TE, Tomczak P, et al. Sunitinib versus interferon alfa in metastatic renal-cell carcinoma. *N Engl J Med*. 2007;356:115-124. PMID: 17215529.

181. Motzer RJ, Hutson TE, Tomczak P, et al. Overall survival and updated results for sunitinib compared with interferon alfa in patients with metastatic renal cell carcinoma. *J Clin Oncol*. 2009;27:3584-3590. Epub 2009 Jun 1. PMID: 19487381.

182. Motzer RJ, Hutson TE, Olsen MR, et al. Randomized phase II trial of sunitinib on an intermittent versus continuous dosing schedule as first-line therapy for advanced renal cell carcinoma. *J Clin Oncol*. 2011;29: Epub 2012 Mar 19. PMID: 22430274.

183. Sternberg CN, Davis ID, Mardiak J, et al. Pazopanib in locally advanced or metastatic renal cell carcinoma: results of a randomized phase III trial. *J Clin Oncol*. 2010;20;28:1061-1068. Epub 2010 Jan 25. PMID: 20100962.

184. Motzer RJ, Hutson TE, Cella D, et al. Pazopanib versus sunitinib in metastatic renal-cell carcinoma. *N Engl J Med*. 2013;369:722-731. PMID: 23964934.

185. Ratain MJ, Eisen T, Stadler WM, et al. Phase II placebo-controlled randomized discontinuation trial of sorafenib in patients with metastatic renal cell carcinoma. *J Clin Oncol*. 2006;24:2505-2512. Epub 2006 Apr 24. PMID: 16636341.

186. Escudier B, Eisen T, Stadler WM, et al. Sorafenib for treatment of renal cell carcinoma: Final efficacy and safety results of the phase III treatment approaches in renal cancer global evaluation trial. *J Clin Oncol*. 2009;27:3312-3318. Epub 2009 May 18. PMID: 19451442.

187. Escudier B, Szczylik C, Hutson TE, et al. Randomized phase II trial of first-line treatment with sorafenib versus interferon Alfa-2a in patients with metastatic renal cell carcinoma. *J Clin Oncol*. 2009;27:1280-1289. Epub 2009 Jan 26. PMID: 19171708.

188. Beck J, Procopio G, Bajetta E, et al. Final results of the European Advanced Renal Cell Carcinoma Sorafenib (EU-ARCCS) expanded-access study: a large open-label study in diverse community settings. *Ann Oncol*. 2011;22:1812-2183. Epub 2011 Feb 15. PMID: 21324953.

189. Rini BI, Cohen DP, Lu DR, et al. Hypertension as a biomarker of efficacy in patients with metastatic renal cell carcinoma treated with sunitinib. *J Natl Cancer Inst*. 2011;103:763-773. Epub 2011 Apr 28. PMID: 21527770.

190. Atkins MB, Hidalgo M, Stadler WM, et al. Randomized phase II study of multiple dose levels of CCI-779, a novel mammalian target of rapamycin kinase inhibitor, in patients with advanced refractory renal cell carcinoma. *J Clin Oncol*. 2004;22:909-918. PMID: 14990647.

191. Hudes G, Carducci M, Tomczak P, et al. Temsirolimus, interferon alfa, or both for advanced renal-cell carcinoma. *N Engl J Med.* 2007;356:2271-2281. PMID: 17538086.

192. Motzer RJ, Escudier B, Oudard S, et al. Efficacy of everolimus in advanced renal cell carcinoma: a double-blind, randomised, placebo-controlled phase III trial. *Lancet.* 2008;372:449-456. Epub 2008 Jul 22. PMID: 18653228.

193. Rini BI, Michaelson MD, Rosenberg JE, et al. Antitumor activity and biomarker analysis of sunitinib in patients with bevacizumab-refractory metastatic renal cell carcinoma. *J Clin Oncol.* 2008;26:3743-3748. PMID: 18669461.

194. Rini BI, Escudier B, Tomczak P, et al. Comparative effectiveness of axitinib versus sorafenib in advanced renal cell carcinoma (AXIS): a randomised phase 3 trial. *Lancet.* 2011;378:1931-1939. PMID: 22056247.

195. Azad NS, Posadas EM, Kwitkowski VE, et al. Combination targeted therapy with sorafenib and bevacizumab results in enhanced toxicity and antitumor activity. *J Clin Oncol.* 2008;26:3709-3714. PMID: 18669456.

196. Molina AM, Feldman DR, Voss MH, et al. Phase 1 trial of everolimus plus sunitinib in patients with metastatic renal cell carcinoma. *Cancer.* 2012;118:1868-1876. Epub 2011 Sep 6. PMID: 21898375.

197. Hainsworth JD, Spigel DR, Burris HA 3rd, et al. Phase II trial of bevacizumab and everolimus in patients with advanced renal cell carcinoma. *J Clin Oncol.* 2010;28:2131-2136. Epub 2010 Apr 5. PMID: 20368560.

198. Négrier S, Gravis G, Pérol D, et al. Temsirolimus and bevacizumab, or sunitinib, or interferon alfa and bevacizumab for patients with advanced renal cell carcinoma (TORAVA): a randomised phase 2 trial. *Lancet Oncol.* 2011;12:673-680. Epub 2011 Jun 12. PMID: 21664867.

199. Escudier B, Goupil MG, Massard C, et al. Sequential therapy in renal cell carcinoma. *Cancer.* 2009;115:2321-2326. PMID: 19402067.

200. Strumberg D. Efficacy of sunitinib and sorafenib in non-clear cell renal cell carcinoma: results from expanded access studies. *J Clin Oncol.* 2008;26:3469-3471; author reply 2471. PMID: 18612169.

201. Choueiri TK, Plantade A, Elson P, et al. Efficacy of sunitinib and sorafenib in metastatic papillary and chromophobe renal cell carcinoma. *J Clin Oncol.* 2008;26:127-131. PMID: 18165647.

202. Gore ME, Szczylik C, Porta C, et al. Safety and efficacy of sunitinib for metastatic renal-cell carcinoma: an expanded-access trial. *Lancet Oncol.* 2009;10:757-763. Epub 2009 Jul 15. PMID: 19615940.

203. Stadler WM, Figlin RA, McDermott DF, et al. Safety and efficacy results of the advanced renal cell carcinoma sorafenib expanded access program in North America. *Cancer.* 2010;116:1272-1280. PMID: 20082451.

204. Dutcher JP, de Souza P, McDermott D, et al. Effect of temsirolimus versus interferon-alpha on outcome of patients with advanced renal cell carcinoma of different tumor histologies. *Med Oncol.* 2009;26:202-209. Epub 2009 Feb 20. PMID: 19229667.

205. Pyrhönen S, Salminen E, Ruutu M, et al. Prospective randomized trial of interferon alfa-2a plus vinblastine versus vinblastine alone in patients with advanced renal cell cancer. *J Clin Oncol.* 1999;17:2859-2867. PMID: 10561363.

206. Interferon-alpha and survival in metastatic renal carcinoma: early results of a randomised controlled trial. Medical Research Council Renal Cancer Collaborators. *Lancet.* 1999;353:14-17. PMID: 10023944.

207. Negrier S, Perol D, Ravaud A, et al. Medroxyprogesterone, interferon alfa-2a, interleukin 2, or combination of both cytokines in patients with metastatic renal carcinoma of intermediate prognosis: results of a randomized controlled trial. *Cancer.* 2007;110:2468-2477. PMID: 17932908.

208. McDermott DF, Regan MM, Clark JI, et al. Randomized phase III trial of high-dose interleukin-2 versus subcutaneous interleukin-2 and interferon in patients with metastatic renal cell carcinoma. *J Clin Oncol.* 2005;23:133-141. PMID: 15625368.

209. McDermott DF, Ghebremichael MS, Signoretti S, et al. The high-dose aldesleukin (HD IL-2) "SELECT" trial in patients with metastatic renal cell carcinoma (mRCC)_. *J Clin Oncol.* 2010;28:15s. (suppl; abstr 4514).

210. Atkins MB, Dutcher J, Weiss G, et al. Kidney cancer: the Cytokine Working Group experience (1986-2001): part I. IL-2-based clinical trials. *Med Oncol.* 2001;18:197-207. PMID: 11917944.

211. Nanus DM, Garino A, Milowsky MI, et al. Active chemotherapy for sarcomatoid and rapidly progressing renal cell carcinoma. *Cancer.* 2004;101:1545-1551. PMID: 15378501.

212. Stadler WM, Halabi S, Rini B, et al. A phase II study of gemcitabine and capecitabine in metastatic renal cancer: a report of Cancer and Leukemia Group B protocol 90008. *Cancer.* 2006;107:1273-1279. PMID: 16909426.

213. Haas NB, Lin X, Manola J, et al. A phase II trial of doxorubicin and gemcitabine in renal cell carcinoma with sarcomatoid features: ECOG 8802. *Med Oncol.* 2012;29:761-767. Epub 2011 Feb 6. PMID: 21298497.

214. Oudard S, Banu E, Vieillefond A, et al. Prospective multicenter phase II study of gemcitabine plus platinum salt for metastatic collecting duct carcinoma: results of a GETUG (Groupe d'Etudes des Tumeurs Uro-Génitales) study. *J Urol.* 2007;177:1698-1702. PMID: 17437788.

215. Molina AM, Tickoo SK, Ishill N, et al. Sarcomatoid-variant renal cell carcinoma: treatment outcome and survival in advanced disease. *Am J Clin Oncol.* 2011;34:454-459. PMID: 21127411.

216. Giubellino A, Linehan WM, Bottaro DP. Targeting the Met signaling pathway in renal cancer. *Expert Rev Anticancer Ther.* 2009;9:785-793. PMID: 19496715.

217. Schöffski P, Garcia JA, Stadler WM, et al. A phase II study of the efficacy and safety of AMG 102 in patients with metastatic renal cell carcinoma. *BJU Int.* 2011;108:679-686. Epub 2010 Dec 13. PMID: 21156020.

218. Eder JP, Shapiro GI, Appleman LJ, et al. A phase I study of foretinib, a multi-targeted inhibitor of c-Met and vascular endothelial growth factor receptor 2. *Clin Cancer Res.* 2010;16:3507-3516. Epub 2010 May 14. PMID: 20472683.

219. Gordon MS, Hussey M, Nagle RB, et al. Phase II study of erlotinib in patients with locally advanced or metastatic papillary histology renal cell cancer: SWOG S0317. *J Clin Oncol.* 2009;27:5788-5793. Epub 2009 Nov 2. PMID: 19884559.

220. Lipton A, Zheng M, Seaman J. Zoledronic acid delays the onset of skeletal-related events and progression of skeletal disease in patients with advanced renal cell carcinoma. *Cancer.* 2003;98:962-969. PMID: 12942563.

221. Henry DH, Costa L, Goldwasser F, et al. Randomized, double-blind study of denosumab versus zoledronic acid in the treatment of bone metastases in patients with advanced cancer (excluding breast and prostate cancer) or multiple myeloma. *J Clin Oncol.* 2011;29:1125-1132. Epub 2011 Feb 22. PMID: 21343556.

222. Samlowski WE, Majer M, Boucher KM, et al. Multidisciplinary treatment of brain metastases derived from clear cell renal cancer incorporating stereotactic radiosurgery. *Cancer.* 2008;113:2539-2548. PMID: 18780316.

223. Gore ME, Hariharan S, Porta C, et al. Sunitinib in metastatic renal cell carcinoma patients with brain metastases. *Cancer.* 2011;117:501-509. Epub 2010 Sep 22. PMID: 20862748.

224. Josephs D, Hutson TE, Cowey CL, et al. Efficacy and toxicity of sunitinib in patients with metastatic renal cell carcinoma with severe renal impairment or on haemodialysis. *BJU Int.* 2011;108:1279-1283. Epub 2011 Jan 18. PMID: 21244613.

225. Ewing CM, Ray AM, Lange EM, et al. Germline mutations in HOXB13 and prostate-cancer risk. *N Engl J Med.* 2012;366:141-149. PMID: 22236224.

226. Chan JM, Gann PH, Giovannucci EL. Role of diet in prostate cancer development and progression. *J Clin Oncol.* 2005;23:8152-8160. PMID: 16278466.

227. DeMarzo AM, Nelson WG, Isaacs WB, et al. Pathological and molecular aspects of prostate cancer. *Lancet.* 2003;361:955-964. PMID: 12648986.

228. Epstein JI. An update of the Gleason grading system. *J Urol.* 2010;183:433-440. Epub 2009 Dec 14. PMID: 20006878.

229. Bastian PJ, Yegnasubramanian S, Palapattu GS, et al. Molecular biomarker in prostate cancer: the role of CpG island hypermethylation. *Eur Urol.* 2004;46:698-708. PMID: 15548435.

230. Rubin MA, Maher CA, Chinnaiyan AM. Common gene rearrangements in prostate cancer. *J Clin Oncol.* 2011;29:3659-3668. Epub 2011 Aug 22. PMID: 21859993.

231. McDonnell TJ, Troncoso P, Brisbay SM, et al. Expression of the protooncogene bcl-2 in the prostate and its association with emergence of androgen-independent prostate cancer. *Cancer Res.* 1992;52:6940-6944. PMID: 1458483.

232. Morris MJ, Reuter VE, Kelly WK, et al. HER-2 profiling and targeting in prostate carcinoma. *Cancer.* 2002;94:980-986. PMID: 11920466.

233. Ross JS, Gray KE, Webb IJ, et al. Antibody-based therapeutics: focus on prostate cancer. *Cancer Metastasis Rev.* 2005;24:521-537. PMID: 16408160.

234. Beltran H, Rickman DS, Park K, et al. Molecular characterization of neuroendocrine prostate cancer and identification of new drug targets. *Cancer Discov.* 2011;1:487-495. PMID: 22389870.

235. Kawachi MH, Bahnson RR, Barry M, et al. Prostate cancer early detection. Clinical practice guidelines in oncology. *J Natl Compr Canc Netw.* 2007;5:714-736. PMID: 17692177.

236. Lughezzani G, Briganti A, Karakiewicz PI, et al. Predictive and prognostic models in radical prostatectomy candidates: a critical analysis of the literature. *Eur Urol.* 2010;58:687-700. Epub 2010 Aug 6. PMID: 20727668.

237. Thompson IM, Goodman PJ, Tangen CM, et al. The influence of finasteride on the development of prostate cancer. *N Engl J Med.* 2003;349:215-224. Epub 2003 Jun 24. PMID: 12824459.

238. Lucia MS, Epstein JI, Goodman PJ, et al. Finasteride and high-grade prostate cancer in the Prostate Cancer Prevention Trial. *J Natl Cancer Inst.* 2007;99:1375-1383. Epub 2007 Sep 11. PMID: 17848673.

239. Thompson IM Jr, Goodman PJ, Tangen CM, et al. Long-term survival of participants in the prostate cancer prevention trial. *N Engl J Med.* 2013;369:603-610. PMID: 23944298.

240. Andriole GL, Bostwick DG, Brawley OW, et al. Effect of dutasteride on the risk of prostate cancer. *N Engl J Med.* 2010;362:1192-1202. PMID: 20357281.

241. Theoret MR, Ning YM, Zhang JJ, et al. The risks and benefits of 5alpha-reductase inhibitors for prostate-cancer prevention. *N Engl J Med.* 2011;365:97-99. Epub 2011 Jun 15. PMID: 21675880.

242. Gaziano JM, Glynn RJ, Christen WG, et al. Vitamins E and C in the prevention of prostate and total cancer in men: the Physicians' Health Study II randomized controlled trial. *JAMA.* 2009;301:52-62. Epub 2008 Dec 9. PMID: 19066368.

243. Lippman SM, Klein EA, Goodman PJ, et al. Effect of selenium and vitamin E on risk of prostate cancer and other cancers: the Selenium and Vitamin E Cancer Prevention Trial (SELECT). *JAMA.* 2009;301:39-51. Epub 2008 Dec 9. PMID: 19066370.

244. Klein EA, Thompson IM Jr., Tangen CM, et al. Vitamin E and the risk of prostate cancer: the Selenium and Vitamin E Cancer Prevention Trial (SELECT). *JAMA.* 2011;306:1549-1556. PMID: 21990298.

245. Hoffman RM. Clinical Practice. Screening for prostate cancer. *N Engl J Med.* 2011;365:2013-2019. Epub 2011 Oct 26. PMID: 22029754.

246. McNaughton-Collins MF, Barry MJ. One man at a time--resolving the PSA controversy. *N Engl J Med.* 2011;365:1951-1953. Epub 2011 Oct 26. PMID: 22029758.

247. Moyer VA, U.S. Preventive Services Task Force. Screening for prostate cancer: U.S. Preventive Services Task Force recommendation statement. *Ann Intern Med.* 2012;157:120-134. PMID: 22801674.

248. Carter HB, Albertsen PC, Barry MJ, et al. Early detection of prostate cancer: AUA Guideline. *J Urol.* 2013;190:419-426. PMID: 23659877.

248a. American Cancer Society Recommendations for Prostate Cancer Early Detection. http://www.cancer.org/cancer/prostatecancer/moreinformation/prostatecancerearlydetection/prostate-cancer-early-detection-acsrecommendations. Accessed May 30, 2014.

249. Thompson IM, Pauler DK, Goodman PJ, et al. Prevalence of prostate cancer among men with a prostate-specific antigen level < or =4.0 ng per milliliter. *N Engl J Med.* 2004;350:2239-2246. PMID: 15163773.

250. Cupp MR, Oesterling JE. Prostate-specific antigen, digital rectal examination, and transrectal ultrasonography: their roles in diagnosing early prostate cancer. *Mayo Clin Proc.* 1993;68:297-306. PMID: 7682639.

251. Schroder FH, Hugosson J, Roobol MJ, et al. Screening and prostate-cancer mortality in a randomized European study. *N Engl J Med.* 2009;360:1320-1328. Epub 2009 Mar 18. PMID: 19297566.

252. Andriole GL, Crawford ED, Grubb RL 3rd, et al. Mortality results from a randomized prostate-cancer screening trial. *N Engl J Med.* 2009;360:1310-1319. Epub 2009 Mar 18. PMID: 19297565.

253. Schröder FH, Hugosson J, Roobol MJ, et al. Prostate-cancer mortality at 11 years of follow-up. *N Engl J Med.* 2012;366:981-990. PMID: 22417251.

254. Barry MJ. Screening for prostate cancer–the controversy that refuses to die. *N Engl J Med.* 2009;360:1351-1354. Epub 2009 Mar 18. PMID: 19297564.

255. Canfield SE. ACP Journal Club. Periodic screening with prostate-specific antigen testing reduced mortality from prostate cancer. *Ann Intern Med.* 2009;150:JC6-5, JC6-4. PMID: 19528550.

256. Carroll PR, Whitson JM, Cooperberg MR. Serum prostate-specific antigen for the early detection of prostate cancer: always, never, or only sometimes? *J Clin Oncol.* 2011;29:345-347. PMID: 21189396.

257. Hugosson J, Carlsson S, Aus G, et al. Mortality results from the Goteborg randomised population-based prostate-cancer screening trial. *Lancet Oncol.* 2010;11:725-732. Epub 2010 Jul 2. PMID: 20598634.

258. Loeb S, Catalona WJ. Prostate-specific antigen in clinical practice. *Cancer Lett.* 2007;249:30-39. Epub 2007 Jan 26. PMID: 17258389.

259. Vickers AJ, Savage C, O'Brien MF, et al. Systematic review of pretreatment prostate-specific antigen velocity and doubling time as predictors for prostate cancer. *J Clin Oncol.* 2009;20;27:398-403. Epub 2008 Dec 8. PMID: 19064972.

260. Catalona WJ, Partin AW, Slawin KM, et al. Use of the percentage of free prostate-specific antigen to enhance differentiation of prostate cancer from benign prostatic disease: a prospective multicenter clinical trial. *JAMA.* 1998;279:1542-1547. PMID: 9605898.

261. Auprich M, Bjartell A, Chun FK, et al. Contemporary role of prostate cancer antigen 3 in the management of prostate cancer. *Eur Urol.* 2011;60:1045-1054. Epub 2011 Aug 25. PMID: 21871709.

262. Freeman LM, Krynyckyi BR, Li Y, et al. The role of (111)In Capromab Pendetide (Prosta-ScintR) immunoscintigraphy in the management of prostate cancer. *Q J Nucl Med.* 2002;46:131-137. PMID: 12114876.

263. Keane TE, Rosner IL, Wingo MS, et al. The emergence of radioimmunoscintigraphy for prostate cancer. *Rev Urol.* 2006;8 Suppl 1:S20-S28. PMID: 17021623.

264. Pound CR, Partin AW, Eisenberger MA, et al. Natural history of progression after PSA elevation following radical prostatectomy. *JAMA.* 1999;281:1591-1597. PMID: 10235151.

265. Freedland SJ, Humphreys EB, Mangold LA, et al. Risk of prostate cancer-specific mortality following biochemical recurrence after radical prostatectomy. *JAMA.* 2005;294:433-439. PMID: 16046649.

266. Wo JY, Chen MH, Nguyen PL, et al. Evaluating the combined effect of comorbidity and prostate-specific antigen kinetics on the risk of death in men after prostate-specific antigen recurrence. *J Clin Oncol.* 2009;27:6000-6005. PMID: 19858385.

267. Mohler JL, Kantoff PW, Armstrong AJ, et al. Prostate cancer, version 1.2014. *J Natl Compr Canc Netw.* 2013;11:1471-1479. PMID: 24335682.

268. Crook JM, O'Callaghan CJ, Duncan G, et al. Intermittent androgen suppression for rising PSA level after radiotherapy. *N Engl J Med.* 2012;367:895-903. PMID: 22931259.

269. Smith MR, Cook R, Lee KA, et al. Disease and host characteristics as predictors of time to first bone metastasis and death in men with progressive castration-resistant nonmetastatic prostate cancer. *Cancer.* 2011;117:2077-2085. Epub 2010 Nov 16. PMID: 21523719.

270. Thompson I, Thrasher JB, Aus G, et al. Guideline for the management of clinically localized prostate cancer: 2007 update. *J Urol.* 2007;177:2106-2131. PMID: 17509297.

271. Sanda MG, Dunn RL, Michalski J, et al. Quality of life and satisfaction with outcome among prostate-cancer survivors. *N Engl J Med.* 2008;358:1250-1261. PMID: 18354103.

272. Alemozaffar M, Regan MM, Cooperberg MR, et al. Prediction of erectile function following treatment for prostate cancer. *JAMA.* 2011;306:1205-1214. PMID: 21934053.

273. Coelho RF, Rocco B, Patel MB, et al. Retropubic, laparoscopic, and robot-assisted radical prostatectomy: a critical review of outcomes reported by high-volume centers. *J Endourol.* 2010;24:2003-2015. Epub 2010 Oct 13. PMID: 20942686.

274. Roach M 3rd, Hanks G, Thames H Jr, et al. Defining biochemical failure following radiotherapy with or without hormonal therapy in men with clinically localized prostate cancer: recommendations of the RTOG-ASTRO Phoenix Consensus Conference. *Intl J Radiat Oncol Biol Phys.* 2006;65:965-974. PMID: 16798415.

275. Gore JL, Kwan L, Lee SP, et al. Survivorship beyond convalescence: 48-month quality-of-life outcomes after treatment for localized prostate cancer. *J Natl Cancer Inst.* 2009;101:888-892. Epub 2009 Jun 9. PMID: 19509365.

276. Sanda MG, Dunn RL, Michalski J, et al. Quality of life and satisfaction with outcome among prostate-cancer survivors. *N Engl J Med.* 2008;358:1250-1261. PMID: 18354103.

277. Alemozaffar M, Regan MM, Cooperberg MR, et al. Prediction of erectile function following treatment for prostate cancer. *JAMA.* 2011;306:1205-1214. PMID: 21934053.

278. Chen RC, Clark JA, Talcott JA. Individualizing quality-of-life outcomes reporting: how localized prostate cancer treatments affect patients with different levels of baseline urinary, bowel, and sexual function. *J Clin Oncol.* 2009;27:3916-3922. PMID: 19620493.

279. Pardo Y, Guedea F, Aguiló F, et al. Quality-of-life impact of primary treatments for localized prostate cancer in patients without hormonal treatment. *J Clin Oncol.* 2010;28:4687-4696. PMID: 20921463.

280. Speight JL, Roach M 3rd. Radiotherapy in the management of clinically localized prostate cancer: evolving standards, consensus, controversies and new directions. *J Clin Oncol.* 2005;23:8176-8185. PMID: 16278470.

281. Lee WR. Prostate cancer and the hypofractionation hypothesis. *J Clin Oncol.* 2013;31:3849-3851. PMID: 24101055.

282. Pollack A, Walker G, Horwitz EM, et al. Randomized trial of hypofractionated external-beam radiotherapy for prostate cancer. *J Clin Oncol.* 2013;31:3860-3868. PMID: 24101042.

283. Horwitz EM, Bae K, Hanks GE, et al. Ten-year follow-up of radiation therapy oncology group protocol 92-02: a phase III trial of the duration of elective

androgen deprivation in locally advanced prostate cancer. *J Clin Oncol.* 2008;26:2497-2504. Epub 2008 Apr 14. PMID: 18413638.

284. Roach M 3rd, Bae K, Speight J, et al. Short-term neoadjuvant androgen deprivation therapy and external-beam radiotherapy for locally advanced prostate cancer: long-term results of RTOG 8610. *J Clin Oncol.* 2008;26:585-591. Epub 2008 Jan 2. PMID: 18172188.

285. Jones CU, Hunt D, McGowan DG, et al. Radiotherapy and short-term androgen deprivation for localized prostate cancer. *N Engl J Med.* 2011;365:107-118. PMID: 21751904.

286. D'Amico AV, Chen MH, Renshaw AA, et al. Androgen suppression and radiation vs radiation alone for prostate cancer: a randomized trial. *JAMA.* 2008;299:289-295. PMID: 18212313.

287. D'Amico AV, Loffredo M, Renshaw AA, et al. Six-month androgen suppression plus radiation therapy compared with radiation therapy alone for men with prostate cancer and a rapidly increasing pretreatment prostate-specific antigen level. *J Clin Oncol.* 2006;24:4190-4195. PMID: 16943536.

288. Bolla M, de Reijke TM, Van Tienhoven G, et al. Duration of androgen suppression in the treatment of prostate cancer. *N Engl J Med.* 2009;360:2516-2527. PMID: 19516032.

289. Hanks GE, Pajak TF, Porter A, et al. Phase III trial of long-term adjuvant androgen deprivation after neoadjuvant hormonal cytoreduction and radiotherapy in locally advanced carcinoma of the prostate: the Radiation Therapy Oncology Group Protocol 92-02. *J Clin Oncol.* 2003;21:3972-3978. PMID: 14581419.

290. Morikawa LK, Roach M 3rd. Pelvic nodal radiotherapy in patients with unfavorable intermediate and high-risk prostate cancer: evidence, rationale, and future directions. *Int J Radiat Oncol Biol Phys.* 2011;80:6-16. PMID: 21481721.

291. Lawton CA, Winter K, Grignon D, et al. Androgen suppression plus radiation versus radiation alone for patients with stage D1/pathologic node-positive adenocarcinoma of the prostate: updated results based on national prospective randomized trial Radiation Therapy Oncology Group 85-31. *J Clin Oncol.* 2005;23:800-807. PMID: 15681524.

292. Messing EM, Manola J, Yao J, et al. Immediate versus deferred androgen deprivation treatment in patients with node-positive prostate cancer after radical prostatectomy and pelvic lymphadenectomy. *Lancet Oncol.* 2006;7:472-479. PMID: 16750497.

293. Chodak GW, Thisted RA, Gerber GS, et al. Results of conservative management of clinically localized prostate cancer. *N Engl J Med.* 1994;330:242-248. PMID: 8272085.

294. Albertsen PC, Hanley JA, Fine J. 20-year outcomes following conservative management of clinically localized prostate cancer. *JAMA.* 2005;293:2095-2101. PMID: 15870412.

295. Wong YN, Mitra N, Hudes G, et al. Survival associated with treatment vs observation of localized prostate cancer in elderly men. *JAMA.* 2006;296:2683-2693. PMID: 17164454.

296. Bill-Axelson A, Holmberg L, Ruutu M, et al. Radical prostatectomy versus watchful waiting in early prostate cancer. *N Engl J Med.* 2011;364:1708-1717. PMID: 21542742.

297. Cooperberg MR, Carroll PR, Klotz L. Active surveillance for prostate cancer: progress and promise. *J Clin Oncol.* 2011;29:3669-3676. Epub 2011 Aug 8. PMID: 21825257.

298. Cooperberg MR, Cowan JE, Hilton JF, et al. Outcomes of active surveillance for men with intermediate-risk prostate cancer. *J Clin Oncol.* 2011;29:228-234. Epub 2010 Nov 29. PMID: 21115873.

299. Stephenson AJ, Scardino PT, Kattan MW, et al. Predicting the outcome of salvage radiation therapy for recurrent prostate cancer after radical prostatectomy. *J Clin Oncol.* 2007;25:2035-2041. PMID: 17513807.

300. Trock BJ, Han M, Freedland SJ, et al. Prostate cancer-specific survival following salvage radiotherapy vs observation in men with biochemical recurrence after radical prostatectomy. *JAMA.* 2008;299:2760-2769. PMID: 18560003.

301. Lee AK, D'Amico AV. Utility of prostate-specific antigen kinetics in addition to clinical factors in the selection of patients for salvage local therapy. *J Clin Oncol.* 2005;23:8192-8197. PMID: 16278472.

302. Pasquier D, Ballereau C. Adjuvant and salvage radiotherapy after prostatectomy for prostate cancer: a literature review. *Int J Radiat Oncol Biol Phys.* 2008;72:972-979. PMID: 18954710.

303. Thompson IM, Tangen CM, Paradelo J, et al. Adjuvant radiotherapy for pathological T3N0M0 prostate cancer significantly reduces risk of metastases and improves survival: long-term followup of a randomized clinical trial. *J Urol.* 2009;181:956-962. Epub 2009 Jan 23. PMID: 19167731.

304. Galvão DA, Taaffe DR, Spry N, et al. Combined resistance and aerobic exercise program reverses muscle loss in men undergoing androgen suppression therapy for prostate cancer without bone metastases: a randomized controlled trial. *J Clin Oncol.* 2010;28:340-347. Epub 2009 Nov 30. PMID: 19949016.

305. Saylor PJ, Lee RJ, Smith MR. Emerging therapies to prevent skeletal morbidity in men with prostate cancer. *J Clin Oncol.* 2011;29:3705-3714. Epub 2011 Aug 22. PMID: 21860001.

306. Smith MR, Egerdie B, Hernández Toriz N, et al. Denosumab in men receiving androgen-deprivation therapy for prostate cancer. *N Engl J Med.* 2009;361:745-755. Epub 2009 Aug 11. PMID: 19671656.

307. Hussain M, Tangen CM, Higano C, et al. Absolute prostate-specific antigen value after androgen deprivation is a strong independent predictor of survival in new metastatic prostate cancer: data from Southwest Oncology Group Trial 9346 (INT-0162). *J Clin Oncol.* 2006;24:3984-3990. PMID: 16921051.

308. Maximum androgen blockade in advanced prostate cancer: an overview of the randomised trials. Prostate Cancer Trialists' Collaborative Group. *Lancet.* 2000;355:1491-1498. PMID: 10801170.

309. Akaza H, Hinotsu S, Usami M, et al. Combined androgen blockade with bicalutamide for advanced prostate cancer: long-term follow-up of a phase 3, double-blind, randomized study for survival. *Cancer.* 2009;115:3437-3445. PMID: 19536889.

310. Tyrrell CJ, Kaisary AV, Iversen P, et al. A randomised comparison of 'Casodex' (bicalutamide) 150 mg monotherapy versus castration in the treatment of metastatic and locally advanced prostate cancer. *Eur Urol.* 1998;33:447-456. PMID: 9643663.

311. Loblaw DA, Virgo KS, Nam R, et al. Initial hormonal management of androgen-sensitive metastatic, recurrent, or progressive prostate cancer: 2006 update of an American Society of Clinical Oncology practice guideline. *J Clin Oncol.* 2007;25:1596-1605. Epub 2007 Apr 2. PMID: 17404365.

312. Immediate versus deferred treatment for advanced prostatic cancer: initial results of the Medical Research Council Trial. The Medical Research Council Prostate Cancer Working Party Investigators Group. *Br J Urol.* 1997;79:235-246. PMID: 9052476.

313. Bolla M, Collette L, Blank L, et al. Long-term results with immediate androgen suppression and external irradiation in patients with locally advanced prostate cancer (an EORTC study): a phase III randomised trial. *Lancet.* 2002;360:103-106. PMID: 12126818.

314. Lawton CA, Winter K, Grignon D, et al. Androgen suppression plus radiation versus radiation alone for patients with stage D1/pathologic node-positive adenocarcinoma of the prostate: updated results based on national prospective randomized trial Radiation Therapy Oncology Group 85-31. *J Clin Oncol.* 2005;23:800-807. PMID: 15681524.

315. Ryan CJ, Small EJ. Early versus delayed androgen deprivation for prostate cancer: new fuel for an old debate. *J Clin Oncol.* 2005;23:8225-8231. PMID: 16278477.

316. Dorff TB, Flaig TW, Tangen CM, et al. Adjuvant androgen deprivation for high-risk prostate cancer after radical prostatectomy: SWOG S9921 study. *J Clin Oncol.* 2011;29:2040-2045. Epub 2011 Apr 18. PMID: 21502546.

317. See WA, Wirth MP, McLeod DG, et al. Bicalutamide as immediate therapy either alone or as adjuvant to standard care of patients with localized or locally advanced prostate cancer: first analysis of the early prostate cancer program. *J Urol.* 2002;168:429-435. PMID: 12131282.

318. Iversen P, Wirth MP, See WA, et al. Is the efficacy of hormonal therapy affected by lymph node status? data from the bicalutamide (Casodex) Early Prostate Cancer program. *Urology.* 2004;63:928-933. PMID: 15134983.

319. McLeod DG, See WA, Klimberg I, et al. The bicalutamide 150 mg early prostate cancer program: findings of the North American trial at 7.7-year median followup. *J Urol.* 2006;176:75-80. PMID: 16753373.

320. Hussain M, Tangen CM, Berry DL, et al. Intermittent versus continuous androgen deprivation in prostate cancer. *N Engl J Med.* 2013;368:1314-1325. PMID: 23550669.

321. Niraula S, Le LW, Tannock IF. Treatment of prostate cancer with intermittent versus continuous androgen deprivation: a systematic review of randomized trials. *J Clin Oncol.* 2013;31:2029-2036. PMID: 23630216.

321a. Sweeney C, Chen Y, Carducci MA, et al. Impact on overall survival (OS) with chemohormonal therapy versus hormonal therapy for hormone-sensitive newly diagnosed metastatic prostate cancer (mPRCa): An ECOG-led phase III randomized trial. *J Clin Oncol.* 2014;32:5s (suppl; abstr LBA2).

322. Sridhar SS, Freedland SJ, Gleave ME, et al. Castration-resistant prostate cancer: from new pathophysiology to new treatment. *Eur Urol.* 2014;65:289-299. PMID: 23957948.

323. Azzouni F, Mohler J. Biology of castration-recurrent prostate cancer. *Urol Clin North Am.* 2012;39:435-452. PMID: 23084522.

324. Beltran H, Tagawa ST, Park K, et al. Challenges in recognizing treatment-related neuroendocrine prostate cancer. *J Clin Oncol.* 2012;30:e386-e389. PMID: 23169519.

325. Scher HI, Halabi S, Tannock I, et al. Design and end points of clinical trials for patients with progressive prostate cancer and castrate levels of testosterone: recommendations of the Prostate Cancer Clinical Trials Working Group. *J Clin Oncol.* 2008;26:1148-1159. PMID: 18309951.

326. Danila DC, Heller G, Gignac GA, et al. Circulating tumor cell number and prognosis in progressive castration-resistant prostate cancer. *Clin Cancer Res.* 2007;13:7053-7058. PMID: 18056182.

327. de Bono JS, Scher HI, Montgomery RB, et al. Circulating tumor cells predict survival benefit from treatment in metastatic castration-resistant prostate cancer. *Clin Cancer Res.* 2008;14:6302-6309. PMID: 18829513.

328. Goldkorn A, Ely B, Quinn DI, et al. Circulating tumor cell counts are prognostic of overall survival in SWOG S0421: a phase III trial of docetaxel with or without atrasentan for metastatic castration-resistant prostate cancer. *J Clin Oncol.* 2014;32:1136-1142. PMID: 24616308.

329. Beer TM, Bernstein GT, Corman JM, et al. Randomized trial of autologous cellular immunotherapy with sipuleucel-T in androgen-dependent prostate cancer. *Clin Cancer Res.* 2011;17:4558-4567. Epub 2011 May 10. PMID: 21558406.

330. Gerritsen W, Kwon ED, Fizazi K, et al. CA184-043: A randomized, multicenter, double-blind phase 3 trial comparing overall survival (OS) in patients (pts) with post-docetaxel castration-resistant prostate cancer (CRPC) and bone metastases treated with ipilimumab (ipi) vs placebo (pbo), each following single-dose radiotherapy (RT). *European Cancer Congress.* 2013 (abstr 2850).

331. Petrylak DP, Tangen CM, Hussain MH, et al. Docetaxel and estramustine compared with mitoxantrone and prednisone for advanced refractory prostate cancer. *N Engl J Med.* 2004;351:1513-1520. PMID: 15470214.

332. Tannock IF, de Wit R, Berry WR, et al. Docetaxel plus prednisone or mitoxantrone plus prednisone for advanced prostate cancer. *N Engl J Med.* 2004;351:1502-1512. PMID: 15470213.

333. Berthold DR, Pond GR, Soban F, et al. Docetaxel plus prednisone or mitoxantrone plus prednisone for advanced prostate cancer: updated survival in the TAX 327 study. *J Clin Oncol.* 2008;26:242-245. PMID: 18182665.

334. Southwest Oncology Group, Berry DL, Moinpour CM, et al. Quality of life and pain in advanced stage prostate cancer: results of a Southwest Oncology Group randomized trial comparing docetaxel and estramustine to mitoxantrone and prednisone. *J Clin Oncol.* 2006;20;24:2828-2835. PMID: 16782921.

335. Kelly WK, Halabi S, Carducci M, et al. Randomized, double-blind, placebo-controlled phase III trial comparing docetaxel and prednisone with or without bevacizumab in men with metastatic castration-resistant prostate cancer: CALGB 90401. *J Clin Oncol.* 2012;30:1534-1540. Epub 2012 Mar 26. PMID: 22454414.

336. Araujo JC, Trudel GC, Saad F, et al. Docetaxel and dasatinib or placebo in men with metastatic castration-resistant prostate cancer (READY): a randomised, double-blind phase 3 trial. *Lancet Oncol.* 2013;14:1307-1316. PMID: 24211163.

337. Tannock IF, Fizazi K, Ivanov S, et al. Aflibercept versus placebo in combination with docetaxel and prednisone for treatment of men with metastatic castration-resistant prostate cancer (VENICE): a phase 3, double-blind randomised trial. *Lancet Oncol.* 2013;14:760-768. PMID: 23742877.

338. Fizazi KS, Higano CS, Nelson JB, et al. Phase III, randomized, placebo-controlled study of docetaxel in combination with zibotentan in patients with metastatic castration-resistant prostate cancer. *J Clin Oncol.* 2013;31:1740-1747. PMID: 23569308.

339. Sternberg CN, Petrylak DP, Sartor O, et al. Multinational, double-blind, phase III study of prednisone and either satraplatin or placebo in patients with castrate-refractory prostate cancer progressing after prior chemotherapy: the SPARC trial. *J Clin Oncol.* 2009;27:5431-5438. Epub 2009 Oct 5. PMID: 19805692.

340. de Bono JS, Oudard S, Ozguroglu M, et al. Prednisone plus cabazitaxel or mitoxantrone for metastatic castration-resistant prostate cancer progressing after docetaxel treatment: a randomised open-label trial. *Lancet.* 2010;376:1147-1154. PMID: 20888992.

341. Berthold DR, Sternberg CN, Tannock IF. Management of advanced prostate cancer after first-line chemotherapy. *J Clin Oncol.* 2005;23:8247-8252. PMID: 16278480.

342. Nakabayashi M, Ling J, Xie W, et al. Response to vinorelbine with or without estramustine as second-line chemotherapy in patients with hormone-refractory prostate cancer. *Cancer J.* 2007;13:125-129. PMID: 17476141.

343. Oh WK, Tay MH, Huang J. Is there a role for platinum chemotherapy in the treatment of patients with hormone-refractory prostate cancer? *Cancer.* 2007;109:477-486. PMID: 17186531.

344. Papandreou CN, Daliani DD, Thall PF, et al. Results of a phase II study with doxorubicin, etoposide, and cisplatin in patients with fully characterized small-cell carcinoma of the prostate. *J Clin Oncol.* 2002;20:3072-3080. PMID: 12118020.

345. Steineck G, Reuter V, Kelly WK, et al. Cytotoxic treatment of aggressive prostate tumors with or without neuroendocrine elements. *Acta Oncol.* 2002;41:668-674. PMID: 14651212.

346. Ryan CJ, Tindall DJ. Androgen receptor rediscovered: the new biology and targeting the androgen receptor therapeutically. *J Clin Oncol.* 2011;29:3651-3658. Epub 2011 Aug 22. PMID: 21859989.

347. de Bono JS, Logothetis CJ, Molina A, et al. Abiraterone and increased survival in metastatic prostate cancer. *N Engl J Med.* 2011;364:1995-2005. PMID: 21612468.

348. Ryan CJ, Smith MR, de Bono JS, et al. Abiraterone in metastatic prostate cancer without previous chemotherapy. *N Engl J Med.* 2013;368:138-148. PMID: 23228172.

349. Scher HI, Beer TM, Higano CS, et al. Antitumour activity of MDV3100 in castration-resistant prostate cancer: a phase 1-2 study. *Lancet.* 2010;375:1437-1446. Epub 2010 Apr 14. PMID: 20398925.

350. Scher HI, Fizazi K, Saad F, et al. Increased survival with enzalutamide in prostate cancer after chemotherapy. *N Engl J Med.* 2012;367:1187-1197. PMID: 22894553.

351. Beer TM, Armstrong AJ, Rathkopf DE, et al. Enzalutamide in metastatic prostate cancer before chemotherapy. *N Engl J Med.* Epub 2014 Jun 1. PMID: 24881730.

352. Smith DC, Smith MR, Sweeney C, et al. Cabozantinib in patients with advanced prostate cancer: results of a phase II randomized discontinuation trial. *J Clin Oncol.* 2013;31:412-419. PMID: 23169517.

353. Parker C, Nilsson S, Heinrich D, et al. Alpha emitter radium-223 and survival in metastatic prostate cancer. *N Engl J Med.* 2013;369:213-223. PMID: 23863050.

354. Saad F, Gleason DM, Murray R, et al. Long-term efficacy of zoledronic acid for the prevention of skeletal complications in patients with metastatic hormone-refractory prostate cancer. *J Natl Cancer Inst.* 2004;96:879-882. PMID: 15173273.

355. Bamias A, Kastritis E, Bamia C, et al. Osteonecrosis of the jaw in cancer after treatment with bisphosphonates: incidence and risk factors. *J Clin Oncol.* 2005;23:8580-8587. PMID: 16314620.

356. Fizazi K, Carducci M, Smith M, et al. Denosumab versus zoledronic acid for treatment of bone metastases in men with castration-resistant prostate cancer: a randomised, double-blind study. *Lancet.* 2011;377:813-822. Epub 2011 Feb 25. PMID: 21353695.

357. Scher HI, Morris MJ, Basch E, et al. End points and outcomes in castration-resistant prostate cancer: from clinical trials to clinical practice. *J Clin Oncol.* 2011;29:3695-3704. Epub 2011 Aug 22. PMID: 21859988.

358. Tannock IF, Osoba D, Stockler MR, et al. Chemotherapy with mitoxantrone plus prednisone or prednisone alone for symptomatic hormone-resistant prostate cancer: a Canadian randomized trial with palliative end points. *J Clin Oncol.* 1996;14:1756-1764. PMID: 8656243.

359. Basaria S, Lieb J 2nd, Tang AM, et al. Long-term effects of androgen deprivation therapy in prostate cancer patients. *Clin Endocrinol (Oxf).* 2002;56:779-786. PMID: 12072048.

360. Braga-Basaria M, Dobs AS, Muller DC, et al. Metabolic syndrome in men with prostate cancer undergoing long-term androgen-deprivation therapy. *J Clin Oncol.* 2006;24:3979-3983. PMID: 16921050.

361. Smith MR, Malkowicz SB, Chu F, et al. Toremifene improves lipid profiles in men receiving androgen-deprivation therapy for prostate cancer: interim analysis of a multicenter phase III study. *J Clin Oncol.* 2008;26:1824-1829. PMID: 18398147.

362. D'Amico AV, Denham JW, Crook J, et al. Influence of androgen suppression therapy for prostate cancer on the frequency and timing of fatal myocardial infarctions. *J Clin Oncol.* 2007;25:2420-2425. PMID: 17557956.

363. Efstathiou JA, Bae K, Shipley WU, et al. Cardiovascular mortality after androgen deprivation therapy for locally advanced prostate cancer: RTOG 85-31. *J Clin Oncol.* 2009;27:92-99. Epub 2008 Dec 1. PMID: 19047297.

364. Punnen S, Cooperberg MR, Sadetsky N, et al. Androgen deprivation therapy and cardiovascular risk. *J Clin Oncol.* 2011;29:3510-3516. Epub 2011 Aug 15. PMID: 21844498.

365. Smith MR, Klotz L, van der Meulen E, et al. Gonadotropin-releasing hormone blockers and cardiovascular disease risk: analysis of prospective

clinical trials of degarelix. *J Urol.* 2011;186:1835-1842. Epub 2011 Sep 25. PMID: 21944083.

366. Nguyen PL, Je Y, Schutz FA, et al. Association of androgen deprivation therapy with cardiovascular death in patients with prostate cancer: a meta-analysis of randomized trials. *JAMA.* 2011;306:2359-2366. PMID: 22147380.

367. Hedlund PO, Johansson R, Damber JE, et al. Significance of pretreatment cardiovascular morbidity as a risk factor during treatment with parenteral oestrogen or combined androgen deprivation of 915 patients with metastasized prostate cancer: evaluation of cardiovascular events in a randomized trial. *Scand J Urol Nephrol.* 2011;45:346-353. Epub 2011 May 31. PMID: 21627403.

368. Veytsman I, Nieman L, Fojo T. Management of endocrine manifestations and the use of mitotane as a chemotherapeutic agent for adrenocortical carcinoma. *J Clin Oncol.* 2009;20;27:4619-4629. Epub 2009 Aug 10. PMID: 19667279.

369. Dickstein G, Shechner C, Nativ O. Adjuvant mitotane in adrenocortical carcinoma. *N Engl J Med.* 2007;20;357:1257-1258. PMID: 17891838.

370. Fassnacht M, Terzolo M, Allolio B, et al. Combination chemotherapy in advanced adrenocortical carcinoma. *N Engl J Med.* 2012;366:2189-2197. PMID: 22551107.

11

GYNECOLOGIC CANCERS

Martee L. Hensley, MD, MSc

Updates from 2012

Cervix cancer

▶ In a prospective phase III trial, the addition of bevacizumab to dual-agent chemotherapy for patients with recurrent and metastatic cervix cancer improved overall survival by nearly 4 months (Tewari KS, *N Engl J Med* 2014).

Endometrial cancer

▶ Genomic characterization of endometrial carcinoma may lead to reclassification of endometrial cancer types, which may lead to changes in post-surgical adjuvant therapy decisions (Cancer Genome Atlas Research Network, *Nature* 2013).

▶ Long-term follow-up of patients with stage I endometrial carcinoma treated on a phase III trial comparing pelvic radiation plus vaginal brachytherapy versus vaginal brachytherapy alone showed no improvement in overall survival with pelvic radiation; in the subset of patients younger than age 60, pelvic radiation was associated with poorer overall survival and increased risk for second cancers (Onsrud M, *J Clin Oncol* 2013).

Ovarian cancer

▶ The addition of bevacizumab to weekly paclitaxel, liposomal doxorubicin, or topotecan improved response rates and progression-free survival compared with chemotherapy alone among patients with platinum-resistant, recurrent ovarian cancer (Pujade-Lauraine E, *J Clin Oncol* 2014).

Uterine sarcoma

▶ Pazopanib is approved by the U.S. Food and Drug Administration for the treatment of metastatic sarcoma based on a randomized phase III trial of pazopanib versus placebo. Progression-free survival was 4.6 months among patients assigned to pazopanib versus 1.6 months among patients assigned to placebo. Objective response was observed in 6% of patients on pazopanib. There was no difference in overall survival (van der Graaf WT, *Lancet* 2012).

Approximately 92,000 women in the United States were expected to be diagnosed with a gynecologic malignancy in 2013, of whom more than 28,000 women were expected to die.[1] Figure 11-1 illustrates the estimated number of new gynecologic cancers that will be diagnosed in the United States in 2014. Figure 11-2 illustrates the estimated number of deaths from gynecologic cancers for 2014.[2] The management of most gynecologic malignancies is multidisciplinary. Important roles for the medical oncologist include the decision-making for and clinical management of adjuvant chemotherapy for epithelial and nonepithelial ovarian cancer, adjuvant treatment decisions for high-risk endometrial cancers, concurrent chemotherapy with

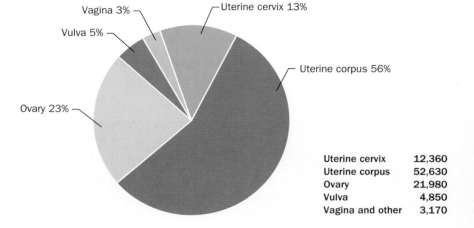

Fig. 11-1 Estimated frequency of new gynecologic cancer diagnoses in the United States for 2014.

Adapted from Siegel R, et al. CA Cancer J Clin. 2014;64:9-29.

Uterine cervix	12,360
Uterine corpus	52,630
Ovary	21,980
Vulva	4,850
Vagina and other	3,170

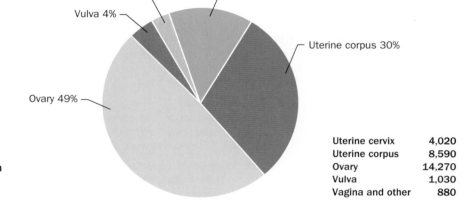

Fig. 11-2 Estimated number of deaths from gynecologic cancers in the United States in 2014.

Adapted from Siegel R, et al. CA Cancer J Clin. 2014;64:9-29.

Uterine cervix	4,020
Uterine corpus	8,590
Ovary	14,270
Vulva	1,030
Vagina and other	880

radiation for cervix cancer, appropriate use of chemotherapy for recurrent and metastatic gynecologic cancers, and appropriate supportive care. The medical oncologist also plays a vital role in identifying women who are potential carriers of a heritable predisposition to gynecologic (and other) cancers and in making appropriate referrals for genetic counseling and testing. For survivors of gynecologic malignancies, the medical oncologist can help women cope with issues related to premature, treatment-related menopause and may recommend appropriate screening for other cancers.

CERVIX CANCER

Cervix cancer is the most common cause of death resulting from gynecologic cancers worldwide. While it is estimated that more than 500,000 new cases of invasive cervix cancer are diagnosed globally each year, the burden of the disease is greatest in developing countries, where more than 85% of the worldwide cases are found. In the United States, an estimated 12,000 cases are diagnosed annually, and there are approximately 4,000 cervix cancer deaths.[2] Pap smear screening in the United States has led to a decline in the number of cases of invasive cervix cancer in recent decades. The mean age at the

time of diagnosis of cervix cancer is approximately 47 years. The relatively slow growth rate of most cervix cancers means that preinvasive changes in the cells of the surface of the cervix can be detected by Pap smear screening, yielding an opportunity for intervention to prevent the development of invasive cancer.

Cervix cancers may be squamous cell carcinomas, adenocarcinomas, or mixed histology tumors (Table 11-1). Neuroendocrine cancers of the cervix and small cell carcinomas of the cervix are rare histologies that carry a high risk for metastases and death, even when apparently localized at the time of diagnosis. These rare histologic types require a specialized therapeutic approach.

RISK FACTORS

The major contributor to the development of invasive cervix cancer is the presence of persistent infection with one of the high-risk types of human papillomavirus (HPV). HPV is transmitted by sexual contact. Certain HPV types specifically infect mucosal surfaces.[3] HPV infection prevalence rates as high as 45% have been observed among women age 25 to 29 in the United States.[4] With increased use of routine HPV vaccination,

Table 11-1 **Histologic Subtypes of Cervix Cancer, Endometrial Cancer, Uterine Sarcomas, and Epithelial Ovarian Cancer**

Cervix Cancer	Endometrial Cancer	Uterine Sarcomas	Epithelial Ovarian Cancer
Squamous cell carcinoma	Endometrioid adenocarcinoma	Carcinosarcoma (mixed Mullerian tumors)	Serous or papillary serous carcinomas
Adenocarcinoma	Papillary serous carcinoma	Leiomyosarcoma	Endometrioid carcinomas
Mixed squamous and adenocarcinoma	Adenosquamous cell carcinoma	Endometrial stromal sarcoma	Clear cell carcinomas
Neuroendocrine carcinoma	Clear cell carcinoma	High-grade undifferentiated sarcoma	Transitional cell carcinomas
Small cell carcinoma		Adenosarcoma	Mucinous carcinomas

these rates should decrease in coming decades. Although the majority of women infected with HPV clear the virus without specific intervention, in a minority of patients, the virus persists.[5] With persistent infection, HPV genes *E6* and *E7* are incorporated into cervix cells, and viral proteins capable of binding to and inactivating tumor suppressor proteins (RB1 and TP53) are produced, initiating carcinogenesis.[6] Other risk factors for the development of cervix cancer include smoking (which increases risk of persistent cervical dysplastic changes) and immunocompromise (such as HIV infection). Behavioral factors such as early age at coitarche, short interval between menarche and coitarche, having multiple sexual partners, and having partners who have had multiple partners—all of which increase the risk of exposure to HPV—are associated with an increased risk of cervix cancer. Use of an intrauterine device has been associated with a lower risk of cervix cancer, independent of HPV status.[7]

Of the more than 100 types of HPV, approximately 15 are considered high risk for causing cervix cancer; among these 15 high-risk types, HPV subtypes 16 and 18 are by far the most prevalent. In one study, HPV subtypes 16 and 18 were associated with approximately 70% of cervix cancer cases, with other high-risk subtypes (31, 33, 35, 39, 45, 51, 52, 56, 58, 59, 68, 73, and 82) accounting for the rest.[8]

SCREENING AND PREINVASIVE DISEASE

Pap smears are effective for detecting preinvasive cervical changes. Cytologists generally report Pap smear results through the Bethesda system, which accounts for specimen adequacy as well as for cytologic interpretation. The advent of liquid-based cytology has resulted in fewer inadequate samples. The incorporation of HPV DNA testing into the screening process helps guide treatment choices, considering that patients who test positive for high-risk HPV serotypes should be followed much more closely for the development of cancer. HPV testing is more sensitive for the detection of grade II or III cervical intraepithelial neoplasia (CIN) than is Pap smear liquid cytology testing.[9] Stand-alone HPV testing as screening for cervix cancer (replacing liquid cytology testing) is not currently recommended in the United States but may be a reasonable option in other countries.[10] So-called co-testing with both

cytologic evaluation and HPV testing continues to be recommended for women over age 30 in the United States.[11] After an abnormal Pap smear or a positive test for high-risk HPV, a patient is referred for colposcopy for directed biopsies to determine whether there is evidence of CIN or invasive cancer. CIN is characterized by dysplastic changes in the epithelium. The more severe the morphologic changes, which are labeled CIN I, CIN II, and CIN III, the greater the risk for transformation into invasive cervix cancer. If a colposcopy shows low-grade changes (CIN I), the patient usually is observed, because these changes will resolve without intervention for approximately 60% of patients. For patients with negative colposcopy, HPV testing is helpful for determining which women are at risk for development of CIN II or greater. In one study, among women with abnormal Pap smear and negative colposcopy, the risk for developing CIN II or worse was 0.44% among the HPV-negative patients and 41.8% among the HPV-positive patients.[12] A diagnosis of CIN II or III requires an excisional procedure, usually a loop electrosurgical excision procedure or a cone biopsy, to rule out invasive carcinoma.

PREVENTION

Large randomized controlled phase III trials of HPV vaccination have shown that vaccination dramatically reduces the incidence of premalignant lesion development in the cervix, vagina, and vulva.[13,14] Ideally, vaccination occurs prior to exposure to HPV. Unfortunately, data suggest that uptake and completion of HPV vaccination among younger women is low, particularly among poor and uninsured women.[15] In older women age 24 to 45 who have not been infected with HPV, vaccination with the quadrivalent vaccine (which includes HPV serotypes 6, 11, 16, and 18) may be effective at preventing premalignant disease.[16] However, HPV vaccination given after age 18 or when cervical dysplasia is already present is less effective.[17] Several national and international health organizations have strongly endorsed routine immunization of all girls and young women as an effective approach to reduce the worldwide burden associated with cervix cancer. HPV vaccination of boys and young men with the quadrivalent vaccine has been shown to decrease the risk of development of external genital lesions related to HPV (i.e., genital warts, anal cancer).[18] Consistent use of condoms has also been associated with lower rates of HPV infection. Routine vaccination against HPV is expected to reduce the burden of HPV-related malignancies in the coming decades.

INVASIVE CERVIX CANCER

The most common presenting symptom of invasive cervix cancer is abnormal vaginal bleeding (i.e., postmenopausal, intermenstrual, or postcoital). Bleeding accompanied by other symptoms, such as pelvic pain and vaginal discharge, usually indicates more advanced disease. Because the rate of false-negative Pap smear findings may be as high as 50% for women with invasive cancer, negative findings should not preclude further diagnostic evaluation of a woman with signs and symptoms consistent with cervix cancer.

Staging of cervix cancer is performed by clinical examination. Table 11-2 details cervix cancer stages, provides an overview of treatment, and lists estimates of 5-year overall survival.

Patients with very early-stage disease (IA1 without lymphovascular space invasion) can be treated with a simple hysterectomy because the risk of lymph node involvement is low. The rate of long-term survival for patients with early-stage disease is greater than 95%. If a patient with such low-risk, early-stage disease wishes to maintain fertility, observation following conization may be considered if the cone margins are negative.

Patients with stage IA1 with lymphovascular space invasion, IA2, and IB1 disease are candidates for radical hysterectomy and lymph node dissection. The role of postsurgical adjuvant radiation treatment for early-stage cervix cancer was investigated in a Gynecologic Oncology Group trial (GOG 92).[19] Patients with stage IB cervix cancer who had undergone radical hysterectomy and lymph node dissection, and who met specified criteria for being at intermediate risk for relapse (lymph nodes negative but with a tumor having two of the following three pathologic features: large tumor diameter, deep stromal invasion, capillary-lymphatic space invasion), were randomly assigned to receive adjuvant whole-pelvis radiation or no further treatment. Five-year overall survival was 88% for the group assigned to receive radiation compared with 79% for the group assigned to undergo observation. This study established postresection radiation as a standard intervention for early-stage cervix cancer. A subsequent study showed that administering concurrent cisplatin-based chemotherapy with radiation was superior to pelvic radiation alone for patients with certain high-risk pathologic features.[20] Thus, currently, patients with clinically early-stage, resectable cervix cancer undergo radical hysterectomy and lymph node dissection. Pathologic factors from the surgery are used to determine which patients require adjuvant therapy; patients with positive lymph nodes, positive margins, or positive parametria benefit from adjuvant cisplatin-based chemoradiation.

The optimal treatment for patients with IB2 disease is controversial. Patients with larger tumors are likely to have pathologic features found at the time of radical hysterectomy that require adjuvant radiation, and thus may be better served with platinum-based chemoradiation rather than radical surgery. If surgery is elected as the initial treatment, the likelihood of finding high-risk features that necessitate postsurgery treatment with chemoradiation is high, and thus morbidity may be higher.[21,22] It has not been determined whether hysterectomy following initial chemoradiation improves outcomes. The long-term survival rates range from approximately 60% to 80%.

With extensive locally advanced disease (stage IIB to IVA) there is no role for primary surgery, and standard treatment includes the simultaneous delivery of external beam radiation with concurrent cisplatin-based chemotherapy, followed by brachytherapy. Several phase III randomized trials have demonstrated that concurrent cisplatin-based chemoradiation yields superior progression-free and overall survival rates compared with radiation alone.[23,24]

METASTATIC AND RECURRENT CERVIX CANCER

The prognosis is poor for patients with metastatic cervix cancer or for those who have recurrence after primary treatment of localized disease. For carefully selected patients who have an isolated pelvic recurrence within a previously irradiated field, aggressive resection (i.e., pelvic exenteration) can be considered because it offers the potential to provide long-term disease-free survival for approximately 25% of patients. Patients who have not previously undergone pelvic radiation therapy may undergo salvage radiation.

A number of cytotoxic agents have been evaluated for activity against cervix cancer. Cisplatin, which is associated with a 20% objective response rate, is the most widely used. Other drugs with demonstrated activity include carboplatin, paclitaxel, topotecan, vinorelbine, gemcitabine, and ifosfamide. Although palliation of symptoms may be achieved with these drugs, the duration of response generally is less than 4 months.

Stage (FIGO 2009)	Definition	Treatment Overview	5-Year Overall Survival (%)
0*	Carcinoma in situ	Observation (CIN I); LEEP or conization (CIN II, III)	100
I	Carcinoma limited to the uterus		80-95
IA	Invasive carcinoma diagnosed only by microscopy		
IA1	Lesions ≤ 3 mm depth of stromal invasion and < 7 mm horizontal spread	If no lymphovascular invasion, simple hysterectomy, or observation if cone margins negative and fertility desired; if lymphovascular invasion, radical hysterectomy with lymph node dissection†	
IA2	> 3 mm and < 5 mm depth of invasion and ≤ 7 mm horizontal spread	Radical hysterectomy with lymph node dissection†	
IB	Lesions greater than IA2, or clinically visible lesions		85-90
IB1	Lesion ≤ 4 cm in greatest dimension	Radical hysterectomy with lymph node dissection†	
IB2	Lesions > 4 cm in greatest dimension	Cisplatin-based chemoradiation	60-80
II	Tumor extends beyond the cervix but not to the pelvic side wall or to lower one-third of vagina		60-80
IIA1	No parametrial invasion and clinically visible lesion is < 4 cm in size	Cisplatin-based chemoradiation	
IIA2	Clinically visible lesion is > 4 cm in size	Cisplatin-based chemoradiation	
IIB	Lesion extends to the parametria	Cisplatin-based chemoradiation	
III	Tumor extends to the pelvic side wall or to lower one-third of the vagina, or causes hydronephrosis	Cisplatin-based chemoradiation	35-45
IV	Tumor extends beyond the true pelvis; and/or invades the mucosa of the bladder or rectum; or distant metastases		5
IVA	Tumor extends beyond the true pelvis; and/or invades the mucosa of the bladder or rectum	Cisplatin-based chemoradiation	
IVB	Distant metastases	Palliative cisplatin-based chemotherapy	

*FIGO no longer includes stage 0 in cervix cancer staging.

†Patients with high-risk pathologic features (positive lymph nodes, positive tumor margins, or positive parametria) require adjuvant cisplatin-based chemoradiation.

Abbreviations: FIGO, International Federation of Gynecology and Obstetrics; CIN, cervical intraepithelial neoplasia; LEEP, loop electrosurgical excision procedure.

An objective response is more likely to be noted in a non-irradiated area and for patients who have never received chemotherapy. For patients with metastatic and recurrent cervix cancer, cisplatin plus topotecan has produced a significantly higher objective response rate, as well as superior progression-free and overall survival rates, compared with single-agent cisplatin.[25] The combination of cisplatin plus paclitaxel also is associated with a higher response rate and better progression-free survival compared with single-agent cisplatin, but this regimen was not shown to improve overall survival.[26] A recent randomized trial (GOG 240) investigated whether a nonplatinum doublet (topotecan plus paclitaxel) may be as efficacious as a platinum doublet (paclitaxel plus cisplatin), and whether the addition of bevacizumab to cytotoxic therapy improves outcomes. Although the data for the topotecan/paclitaxel versus paclitaxel/cisplatin research question are not yet reported, the results from the bevacizumab portion of this study showed that the addition of bevacizumab to chemotherapy increased overall survival by nearly 4 months.[27]

HIGH-RISK HISTOLOGY CERVIX CANCERS

Small cell carcinoma of the cervix and neuroendocrine tumors of the cervix are high-risk histologies. The rarity of these histologic subtypes precludes the conduct of large, prospective trials. Treatment has been informed by experience with treating small cell histology lung cancers. Patients frequently receive treatment with regimens including platinum and etoposide. Many patients are treated with concurrent radiation in conjunction with chemotherapy.[28]

ENDOMETRIAL CANCER

It is estimated that in 2013, approximately 49,000 women in the United States would be diagnosed with endometrial cancer, and more than 8,000 would die as a result of this disease. Seventy-five percent of women diagnosed with endometrial cancer are postmenopausal, with an average age of 60. Approximately 80% of patients present with early-stage, uterine-confined disease. Although the risk of endometrial cancer is 40% lower for black women than for white women in the United States, the mortality rate for black women is approximately 50% higher. Black women present with more advanced-stage disease and have a higher incidence of aggressive histology tumors. The cause of this mortality discrepancy between black and white women is likely complex, involving environmental, socioeconomic, and biologic factors.

Endometrial cancers have been classified as either type I or type II cancers. These types differ in histologic appearance, epidemiologic risk factors, and molecular characteristics. Type I cancers compose approximately 85% of endometrial cancer and show endometrioid histology. Type II cancers have non-endometrioid histology, most commonly papillary serous or clear cell histology. The pathogenesis of type I endometrial cancer appears to be related to the effect of unopposed estrogen on the glandular cells of the endometrial lining of the uterus. Estrogen stimulation leads to endometrial hyperplasia and atypical adenomatosis hyperplasia, which may be regarded as in situ carcinoma of the endometrium. Women with simple endometrial hyperplasia have a low risk of developing invasive adenocarcinoma; however, approximately 25% of women with complex endometrial hyperplasia with atypia will develop invasive cancer.[29] The pathogenesis of type II endometrial cancer is less clear. The median age of women with type II endometrial cancers is older than that of women with type I cancers.[30] In general, women with type II cancers have not been considered to have conditions associated with excess estrogen exposure. However, a recent large epidemiologic study showed that women with type I and type II cancers did not differ in terms of parity, oral contraceptive use, smoking, age at menarche, or diabetes. High body mass index (and thus excess endogenous estrogen) was more likely to be associated with type I tumors than with type II tumors.[31] The risk for death is higher for type II cancers compared to type I cancers.[32] It is likely that genomic characterization will augment our understanding of endometrial cancer pathogenesis and improve classification of these cancers.[33]

RISK FACTORS AND DISEASE PRESENTATION

The major risk factors for endometrial carcinoma are unopposed estrogen (for example, estrogen replacement therapy after menopause without concomitant use of progestins), obesity, nulliparity, late menopause, complex atypical endometrial hyperplasia, and tamoxifen use.[34] Combined oral contraceptive use may decrease the risk of endometrial cancer. Smoking is associated with a lower risk, likely through an antiestrogenic effect.

The risk of endometrial cancer is 3- to 7-fold higher for women receiving tamoxifen than for women who do not take the drug.[35] Tamoxifen-associated endometrial cancers are usually well differentiated and present at an early stage. However, not all studies have supported the generally favorable treatment outcome for tamoxifen-associated endometrial cancer. Oncologists caring for women taking tamoxifen should ask these patients about abnormal vaginal bleeding. Any abnormal bleeding requires evaluation; however, no clinical data justify routine screening for endometrial cancer among all women taking tamoxifen.[36] In the STAR trial, a randomized clinical trial comparing these drugs for breast cancer risk reduction, there was no significant difference in the incidence of endometrial cancer between individuals receiving tamoxifen or raloxifene.[37]

Women with hereditary nonpolyposis colon cancer (HNPCC) syndrome carry a 20% to 60% lifetime risk of developing endometrial cancer.[38] HNPCC-related endometrial cancers occur at a younger age than do sporadic endometrial cancers. These women require special surveillance for endometrial cancer, such as annual transvaginal sonography and consideration of endometrial biopsy, even in the absence of symptoms or abnormal uterine bleeding.[39]

The most common symptom associated with endometrial cancer is postmenopausal bleeding. Approximately 15% of patients with postmenopausal bleeding will have endometrial cancer; thus, all postmenopausal women with abnormal uterine bleeding require evaluation with endometrial sampling. Most endometrial cancers are localized to the uterus at the time of diagnosis, have a well-differentiated histologic appearance, carry a lower propensity to spread, and are curable. Type II endometrial cancers are high-grade cancers that include the

Table 11-3 Endometrial Cancer Staging, Treatment Overview, and Estimates of Overall Survival

Stage (FIGO 2009)	Definition	Treatment Overview*	5-Year Overall Survival (%)
I	Tumor confined to the uterine corpus	Hysterectomy and complete surgical staging	83
IA	Tumor confined to the endometrium or tumor invades to < 50% of the myometrium	No adjuvant therapy for grade 1 and 2 cancers	
IB	Tumor invades to > 50% of the myometrium	May consider postsurgical pelvic + intravaginal radiation or only intravaginal radiation; may consider adjuvant chemotherapy for high-grade or high-risk histologies and for patients meeting high-intermediate risk criteria	
II	Tumor invades the cervical stroma but does not invade beyond the uterus	May consider postsurgical pelvic and intravaginal radiation; may consider adjuvant chemotherapy for high-grade or high-risk histologies and for patients meeting high-intermediate risk criteria	73
III	Local and/or regional spread of tumor	Hysterectomy and complete surgical staging; adjuvant chemotherapy; or combined radiation and chemotherapy	52
IIIA	Tumor invades the uterine serosa and/or adnexae		
IIIB	Vaginal and/or parametrial involvement		
IIIC	Metastatic involvement of pelvic and/or para-aortic lymph nodes		30
IIIC1	Positive pelvic lymph nodes		
IIIC2	Positive para-aortic lymph nodes with or without positive pelvic lymph nodes		
IV	Tumor involves bowel or bladder mucosa or distant metastatic disease	If patient underwent surgery and has no residual disease in peritoneal cavity > 2 cm, consider adjuvant chemotherapy	27
IVA	Tumor involves bowel mucosa and/or bladder mucosa		
IVB	Distant metastases, including intra-abdominal and/or inguinal lymph nodes	If disease is not potentially completely resectable, treatment is with palliative systemic therapy; consider hormone treatments for lower-grade cancers; combination chemotherapy for advanced, higher-grade, disseminated disease	

*Standards for postsurgical treatment of stage I, II, and III endometrial cancer are still evolving. Clinical trial participation should be encouraged.
Abbreviation: FIGO, International Federation of Gynecology and Obstetrics.

histologic subtypes called papillary serous and clear cell carcinomas. These endometrial cancers are more likely to demonstrate high-risk features such as deep myometrial invasion, lymph node involvement, and metastatic spread at the time of diagnosis.

STAGING AND TREATMENT

Endometrial cancer is surgically staged. Postsurgical treatment recommendations are based on the surgical stage and the specifics of the endometrial cancer grade and histologic subtype. Histologic subtypes of endometrial cancer include endometrioid adenocarcinoma, papillary serous carcinomas, adenosquamous carcinomas, and clear cell carcinomas (Table 11-1). The standard surgical staging procedure includes hysterectomy,

bilateral salpingo-oophorectomy, washings, and examination of the entire abdominal cavity. Whether routine pelvic and para-aortic lymph node dissection is necessary for all patients is highly controversial.[40] The use of sentinel lymph node dissection as a way to spare some patients full lymph node dissection is under investigation.[41]

Patients who are not candidates for surgery as a result of comorbidities and/or poor performance status can be treated with radiation, but outcomes will not be as favorable as with surgery. Table 11-3 summarizes endometrial cancer staging, treatment, and survival rates.

Endometrial carcinomas are staged using the International Federation of Gynecology and Obstetrics (FIGO) system. The staging system was revised in 2009; older literature should be interpreted in light of the changes of certain stage definitions.[42] Approximately 80% of patients with endometrial cancer have stage I disease at initial diagnosis. Stages II, III, and IV are found in 11%, 6%, and 2% of patients, respectively. Survival is substantially influenced by stage. Five-year survival is 83% for patients with stage I disease, 73% for those with stage II disease, 52% for those with stage III disease, and 27% for those with stage IV disease. In addition to stage, features associated with a poorer prognosis include older age, higher tumor grade, vascular invasion, and high-risk histologic subtypes (papillary serous and clear cell carcinomas). Lower-grade tumors are more likely to be estrogen and/or progesterone receptor–positive than high-grade cancers.

Postsurgical adjuvant treatment strategies for endometrial cancer continue to evolve. The role of postresection adjuvant pelvic radiation has been investigated in randomized trials. In the GOG99 study, all patients underwent total abdominal hysterectomy, bilateral salpingo-oophorectomy, peritoneal cytology, and lymph node dissection. Patients with FIGO 1988 stage IB or IC, or stage II (occult), endometrial cancer were randomly assigned to receive adjuvant radiation or to no additional treatment. Although there was no significant difference in overall survival in this relatively good-risk population, the risk of pelvic and/or vaginal recurrence was significantly lower in the pelvic-radiation group compared with the no-additional-treatment group (12% vs. 3%). Data from GOG99 have been used to define "low-risk" and "high-intermediate" risk subgroups of early-stage endometrial cancers. Low-risk patients are those with FIGO 1988 stage IA or IB (these patients would all be FIGO 2009 stage IA), grade 1 or 2 cancers. These patients have an approximately 6% risk of recurrence. Surgery alone is generally considered adequate treatment for grade 1 or 2 endometrial cancers with less than 50% muscle invasion (FIGO 2009 stage IA).[43,44] Patients in the GOG99 high-intermediate risk group were defined using patient age and the following histologic features: grade 2 or 3, outer-third invasion of the myometrium, and lymphovascular invasion. Patients older than age 70 with one feature, older than age 50 with two features, or any age with all three features were considered high-intermediate risk. The risk of recurrence in this subgroup was 13% among patients assigned to pelvic radiation compared with 27% among patients assigned to no additional treatment. Thus, adjuvant pelvic radiation has been recommended for patients meeting these criteria.

More recently, results from a study of adjuvant pelvic radiation compared with intravaginal brachytherapy for high-intermediate risk endometrial cancer suggested that outcomes are equivalent (pelvic recurrence rates, 5.1% with vaginal brachytherapy vs. 2.1% with pelvic radiation; no difference in metastatic disease, relapse-free survival, or overall survival), with less toxicity and superior quality of life, among patients assigned to adjuvant intravaginal brachytherapy.[45,46] Long-term follow-up (median follow-up, 20.5 years) of 568 patients with early-stage endometrial cancer treated with either whole-pelvis radiation plus vaginal brachytherapy or with vaginal brachytherapy alone showed no survival benefit to whole-pelvis

radiation and, among women younger than age 60, pelvic radiation was associated with decreased survival and increased risk for second malignancies.[47] A GOG study comparing chemotherapy plus intravaginal brachytherapy to pelvic radiation for patients at high-intermediate risk will report results in 2014. Patients with FIGO 2009 stage II disease generally receive treatment that is similar to that for higher-risk stage I cancers. Clinical trial participation is encouraged for all patients with early-stage endometrial cancer since optimal treatment standards are not yet defined.

Patients with stage III endometrial cancer are at risk for both local and distant treatment failure. Optimal adjuvant treatment approaches have not yet been defined. In a phase III trial conducted by GOG, patients with stage III and stage IV disease with no residual disease greater than 2 cm in the peritoneal cavity were randomly assigned to receive adjuvant whole-abdomen radiation therapy or to receive chemotherapy (cisplatin plus doxorubicin). Superior 5-year survival rates and overall survival were seen in the chemotherapy arm (55% vs. 42%).[48] These data support a role for systemic chemotherapy in the adjuvant treatment of stage III disease. Whether or how to incorporate radiation into the adjuvant strategy remains to be defined. Among the chemotherapy agents with demonstrated activity in endometrial cancer are doxorubicin, cisplatin, carboplatin, and paclitaxel; however, the optimal adjuvant chemotherapy regimen remains under investigation. In a phase III trial (GOG184) for patients with completely resected stage III or IV disease, all patients received adjuvant radiation followed by doxorubicin/cisplatin with or without paclitaxel. Three-year progression-free survival was about 60% for both treatment arms.[49] A current phase III trial is comparing a chemotherapy-only strategy (paclitaxel/carboplatin) with a combined chemotherapy/radiation strategy.

Patients with the rare, high-risk histologies—papillary serous and clear cell carcinoma—are at higher risk for recurrent disease than are patients with lower-grade, endometrioid cancers, even when these high-risk histologies present at an early stage. Data showing that combination chemotherapy improves survival for stage III disease suggest that adjuvant chemotherapy may be appropriate for these early-stage, high-risk histology tumors; however, prospective data are lacking to define the optimal adjuvant treatment for these patients.

KEY POINTS

- Patients with early-stage, low-risk (stage IA, grade 1 or 2) endometrial cancer have a high chance of being cured with surgery alone. Patients with "high-intermediate" risk for recurrence may be offered adjuvant treatment, although optimal strategies are under investigation.
- Chemotherapy has an important role in adjuvant therapy of completely resected stage III and IV endometrial cancer.

METASTATIC OR RECURRENT DISEASE

Endometrial cancer, particularly type I, lower-grade endometrial cancer, is a hormonally sensitive malignant disease. Responses of up to 38% have been reported in studies of hormonal agents for endometrial carcinoma. Responses are more likely among patients with grade 1 and 2 tumors.[50] Grade 3 or undifferentiated and serous histology endometrial cancers rarely respond to hormone therapy, thus chemotherapy should be the primary treatment for most patients with metastatic, high-grade disease. Clinical features that are predictors of response to a progestational agent include grade 1 or 2 histology, a long disease-free interval from diagnosis, and the presence of estrogen or progesterone receptors on the tumor cells.

Chemotherapy agents that have demonstrated activity in metastatic endometrial cancer include the platinum drugs (cisplatin and carboplatin), paclitaxel, and doxorubicin. The overall response rates to these single agents range from 25% to 35%. In metastatic or recurrent endometrial cancer, the combination of cisplatin plus doxorubicin produced a higher objective response rate and a slight improvement in progression-free survival but no difference in overall survival compared with doxorubicin alone.[51] Subsequently, a phase III randomized trial conducted by GOG showed that the combination of cisplatin, doxorubicin, and paclitaxel yielded a small but significant improvement in overall survival compared with cisplatin plus doxorubicin (15.3 months vs. 12.3 months); however, this was at the expense of a greater risk of toxicity.[52] Results of a phase III trial comparison of combination cisplatin, doxorubicin, and paclitaxel with paclitaxel and carboplatin showed that these two regimens are equivalent in terms of progression-free and overall survival rates.[53]

Targeted therapies are under active investigation in endometrial cancer. Endometrioid endometrial cancers frequently have mutations in the tumor suppressor gene phosphatase and tensin homolog (PTEN).[54] PTEN mutations are much less common in nonendometrioid-histology endometrial cancers. PTEN is a negative regulator of the phosphatidylinositol-3 kinase/serine-threonine kinase (PI3K/AKT) pathway. Inhibitors of the mammalian target of rapamycin (mTOR), which is downstream of Akt, may have activity in endometrial cancer.[55] The vascular endothelial growth factor inhibitor bevacizumab achieved objective response in 13.5% of previously treated patients, and 40% of patients remained progression-free at 6 months.[56]

UTERINE CARCINOSARCOMAS AND SARCOMAS

Uterine carcinosarcomas, leiomyosarcomas, endometrial stromal sarcomas, and adenosarcomas compose approximately 4% of uterine cancers. These cancers differ from endometrial cancer in their prognosis and management. Among the uterine sarcomas, carcinosarcomas (sometimes still referred to as uterine mixed Mullerian tumors) make up approximately 50%, leiomyosarcomas approximately 40%, and adenosarcomas and endometrial stromal sarcomas the remaining 10%.

Carcinosarcomas are high-risk tumors that show both carcinoma- and sarcoma-like histologic features due to bidifferentiation from a single malignant precursor. They are associated with high rates of recurrence, even among patients with early-stage disease at diagnosis. Results of a phase III trial established the role of adjuvant chemotherapy for completely resected stage I, II, III, or IV uterine carcinosarcoma. In this trial, women with minimal residual disease after surgical resection were randomly assigned to receive adjuvant whole-abdomen radiation or chemotherapy (cisplatin plus ifosfamide). Recurrence rates at 5 years were lower for patients in the chemotherapy arm (52% with chemotherapy vs. 58% with radiation) for all patients and for subgroups of patients by stage.[57] For patients with advanced, recurrent carcinosarcoma, the combination of paclitaxel plus ifosfamide yielded higher response rates (45% vs. 29%) and longer overall survival (13.5 months vs. 8.4 months) than did ifosfamide alone.[58] The combination of paclitaxel plus carboplatin achieved objective response in 54% of patients with measurable disease in a phase II trial.[59] Paclitaxel/carboplatin is being compared to paclitaxel/ifosfamide in a randomized phase III trial for patients with any stage carcinosarcoma. It is standard to consider two-agent adjuvant chemotherapy (for example, paclitaxel/carboplatin, ifosfamide/paclitaxel, or ifosfamide/cisplatin) for all patients with completely resected uterine carcinosarcoma. However, the optimal chemotherapy regimens for adjuvant treatment and for advanced disease have not been defined.

Leiomyosarcoma is a high-risk cancer of the uterine smooth muscle with a propensity for early hematogenous dissemination. Patients with uterus-limited disease have a 50% to 70% risk of recurrence. A randomized trial comparing adjuvant pelvic radiation with observation for stage I or II uterine leiomyosarcoma did not show a benefit to adjuvant pelvic radiation.[60] One very small randomized trial of adjuvant doxorubicin compared with observation did not show a survival benefit to chemotherapy.[61] The current standard of care after resection of uterus-limited leiomyosarcoma is observation. Whether adjuvant chemotherapy can improve overall survival is being investigated in a prospective phase III trial, with observation as the standard control arm. Active agents for the treatment of advanced, metastatic disease include the combination of gemcitabine plus docetaxel,[62,63] doxorubicin, ifosfamide,[64] single-agent gemcitabine, and dacarbazine. A prospective phase III trial showed that the addition of bevacizumab to gemcitabine/docetaxel did not improve response rates, nor progression-free survival.[65] The multi-kinase inhibitor pazopanib was approved for treatment of soft tissue sarcomas that have progressed after prior cytotoxic therapy based on results of a phase III trial of pazopanib versus placebo. Progression-free survival was 4.6 months among patients assigned to pazopanib compared with 1.6 months among patients assigned to placebo. Objective response was observed in 6% of patients on pazopanib. There was no difference in overall survival.[66] Although trabectedin is approved for treatment of soft tissue sarcomas in Europe, in a prospective phase II study for patients with uterine leiomyosarcoma who had received no prior treatment, trabectedin achieved response in only 10% of patients.[67]

True endometrial stromal sarcomas are low-grade tumors that generally express estrogen and progesterone receptors. Treatment with hormone blockade approaches may be effective for patients with recurrent disease. High-grade endometrial stromal sarcomas are now called high-grade undifferentiated sarcomas. These tumors do not generally express estrogen or progesterone receptors. They are very high-risk cancers. Because of their rarity, there are no prospective studies addressing active agents for these tumors. A characteristic fusion gene has been identified in these cancers that may help with histologic diagnosis.[68] It is recommended to enroll these patients onto soft tissue sarcoma trials.

KEY POINTS

- Patients with completely resected stage I, II, III, or IV uterine carcinosarcoma are generally treated with adjuvant two-agent chemotherapy.
- Observation is the standard management for patients with completely resected, uterus-limited leiomyosarcoma.
- Careful histologic review is recommended for patients with a diagnosis of a uterine sarcoma because these rare cancers differ greatly in their clinical behavior and management.

EPITHELIAL OVARIAN CANCER, FALLOPIAN TUBE CANCER, AND PRIMARY PERITONEAL CANCER

Ovarian cancer is the leading cause of gynecologic cancer death. Ovarian cancer accounts for about 3% of cancers among women in the United States but is the fifth most common cause of cancer-related death. It was estimated that approximately 22,240 women would be diagnosed with ovarian cancer in the United States in 2013, and that approximately 14,030 women would die as a result of ovarian cancer in 2013. Epithelial ovarian cancer accounts for 90% of all cases of malignant tumors of the ovaries. Fallopian tube cancer and primary peritoneal cancer are much rarer but share histologic, prognostic, and treatment response features with epithelial ovarian cancer. Fallopian tube and primary peritoneal cancers are rarely studied prospectively as separate cancers; rather, patients with these cancers are generally eligible for clinical trials for epithelial ovarian cancer, and treatment strategies used for epithelial ovarian cancer are applied to patients with fallopian tube and primary peritoneal cancer. Epithelial ovarian cancers are adenocarcinomas, and they can be subclassified as serous, endometrioid, transitional cell, mucinous, and clear cell carcinomas.

RISK FACTORS AND DISEASE PRESENTATION

Patients with early-stage ovarian cancer often have nonspecific discomfort, including irregular menses (for a premenopausal woman), urinary frequency, persistent bloating, and constipation. With advanced disease, patients may note abdominal pain, bloating, dyspnea, emesis, early satiety, anorexia, and constipation. In early-stage disease, the major physical finding is a pelvic mass; patients with advanced disease may have large-volume ascites on examination. Because symptoms referable to the upper abdomen often are predominant at the time of presentation for patients with advanced ovarian cancer, this clinical feature may delay the time before a definitive diagnosis is established, unless the possibility of gynecologic pathology is considered.

Overall, approximately one woman in 70 will develop ovarian cancer. The mean age at diagnosis of ovarian cancer is 59. Increasing age is one of the strongest risk factors for developing ovarian cancer. The age-specific risk of the disease steadily increases from age 20 to 80 and then declines.

Family history is the next strongest risk factor after age. A woman with a single first-degree relative with ovarian cancer has a relative risk of 3.6 for developing ovarian cancer, meaning her lifetime risk for developing ovarian cancer is approximately 5%. Women from families with multiple cases of breast and/or ovarian cancer should consider genetic testing to determine whether they carry a genetic predisposition to breast and ovarian cancer as a result of a mutation in the *BRCA1* or *BRCA2* genes. Deleterious *BRCA1* or *BRCA2* mutation carriers have a lifetime risk of ovarian cancer estimated at 16% to 60%, with the higher risk among *BRCA1* mutation heterozygous women with strong family histories of the disease.[69] Women with genetic mutations that are part of the HNPCC syndrome also have an increased risk of ovarian cancer. The lifetime risk likely varies depending on the specific mismatch repair enzyme mutation. For example, in one study, women with *MLH1* mutations had an estimated 20% lifetime risk, *MSH2* a 24% risk, and *MSH6* a 1% risk.[70]

Other risk factors for ovarian cancer include white race and diets high in animal fat. Nulliparity or first birth after age 35, involuntary infertility, late menopause, and early menarche increase the risk of ovarian cancer, perhaps because each of these factors is associated with prolonged, uninterrupted periods of ovulation, which might increase the probability of genetic errors occurring during repair of the ovary surface epithelium, which, in turn, may increase the risk for malignant transformation. Oral contraceptive use is associated with a decreased risk of ovarian cancer: the relative risk is approximately 0.5 for women who used oral contraceptives for 5 years or more, compared with never-users. Smoking does not appear to increase risk.

SCREENING FOR OVARIAN CANCER

There are no data to support the routine use of ovarian cancer screening of any type in the general population. Transvaginal sonography and serum cancer antigen 125 (CA-125) testing have been proposed as noninvasive tests. Some reports place the sensitivity of these tests at 90% to 96%, and specificity at 98% to 99%. However, because of the relative rarity of ovarian cancer in the general population, even these high screening test performance estimates would yield a positive predictive value for only 7% of patients. Unlike breast cancer, where biopsy of a mammogram-detected abnormality carriers a very minimal risk, false-positive test results from ovarian cancer screening require laparotomy or laparoscopy to rule out cancer. Although screening strategies with high sensitivity and specificity for the general-risk population are actively being sought, currently, screening by sonogram or CA-125 for the general population is not recommended.[71] A randomized trial of screening with CA-125 and transvaginal sonogram compared with usual care enrolled 78,216 women age 55 to 74. Screening did not decrease mortality, and there was evidence of harm from interventions required for women with false-positive screening results.[72] For women with strong family histories of breast/ovarian cancer and for women with *BRCA1, BRCA2,* or HNPCC genetic mutations, screening may be recommended for the years until childbearing has been completed, after which risk-reducing surgery may be recommended (discussed further in the following subsection). Although there are no prospective data to demonstrate longer survival with screening of women at high risk for developing ovarian cancer, the prevalence of the disease in these populations makes screening a reasonable choice for women who wish to preserve fertility.[73] High-risk women who elect to undergo screening should recognize that false-positive results are very common, particularly with serial screening taking place across several years. False-positive results can cause significant emotional distress in this population,[74] and studies to date have not suggested that screening achieves diagnosis at an earlier stage or improves survival.[75,76]

RISK-REDUCING SALPINGO-OOPHORECTOMY

Several studies indicate that performing a bilateral prophylactic salpingo-oophorectomy may substantially reduce the risk of ovarian cancer for women who are carriers of deleterious *BRCA1* or *BRCA2* mutations (approximately 80% lower risk of ovarian and fallopian tube cancers with follow-up of less than 10 years from surgical procedure).[77,78] A meta-analysis of 10 studies confirmed this level of risk reduction across a large population of high-risk women.[79] Longer follow-up of these patient cohorts will yield information about the consequences of estrogen deprivation, which can include bone loss and cardiac effects. Hormone-replacement therapy may not be considered an appropriate option for all patients because of the heightened risk of breast cancer for this patient population.[80,81] Data show that outcomes of risk-reducing salpingo-oophorectomy may differ by the type of genetic mutation. Patients at higher lifetime risk *(BRCA1* mutation carriers) derive greater ovarian cancer risk reduction than do *BRCA2* mutation carriers, whose lifetime risk is lower.[82]

DIAGNOSIS AND SURGICAL STAGING

For premenopausal women, the majority of ovarian masses are functional cysts that usually decrease in size after several

menstrual cycles. Performing a transvaginal ultrasound can assist in the differential diagnosis of cysts that do not spontaneously regress. For postmenopausal women, a palpable pelvic mass is of greater concern as an indicator of the presence of malignant disease. A computed tomography (CT) scan of the chest, abdomen, and pelvis can help determine the extent of tumor involvement, but it cannot confirm that advanced disease is from an ovarian cancer primary. For a patient with ascites, a paracentesis may be performed to enable cytologic analysis of the fluid. CA-125 level is elevated in more than 80% of patients with advanced ovarian cancer; however, only approximately 50% of patients with early-stage ovarian cancer have elevated CA-125 levels. Normal CA-125 levels should not deter the treating physician from further evaluating a suspicious pelvic mass.

The definitive diagnosis of ovarian, fallopian tube, or primary peritoneal cancer is made by surgical exploration. Prognosis is linked to the amount of residual tumor after surgical cytoreduction (debulking surgery). Optimal cytoreduction is defined as no residual tumor measuring more than 1 cm at the end of the surgical procedure. A standard approach in the United States has been for all patients with suspected ovarian cancer to be considered for surgical cytoreduction, followed by chemotherapy according to the surgical stage and amount of residual disease. However, a number of studies have provided support for offering initial chemotherapy (neoadjuvant chemotherapy) followed by surgery to patients with clinically advanced ovarian cancer. One randomized trial showed equivalent outcomes for patients with stage III or IV ovarian cancer whether treated with neoadjuvant chemotherapy followed by surgery or with cytoreductive surgery followed by chemotherapy.[83] A subset analysis of this trial suggested that initial cytoreductive surgery achieved better outcomes among patients with stage III, lower-volume disease, while initial neoadjuvant chemotherapy achieved better outcomes among patients with stage IV, bulky disease.[84] Most patients in the United States who are considered to have a high likelihood of achieving optimally debulked disease receive initial treatment with initial cytoreductive surgery.[85] In patients for whom there is clear evidence that optimal cytoreduction will not be possible (e.g., multiple large, unresectable, parenchymal liver metastases; parenchymal lung involvement) or for patients not medically fit for major surgery, a biopsy of accessible tissue (such as a large omental mass) may be performed to confirm a diagnosis prior to chemotherapy treatment. Patients who are treated with neoadjuvant chemotherapy and who have evidence of disease response are offered subsequent cytoreductive surgery. Whether treated with initial debulking surgery or with neoadjuvant chemotherapy followed by cytoreductive surgery, patients who have a complete resection of all macroscopic disease have superior survival outcomes compared with patients in whom the disease cannot be completely resected.

Cytoreduction surgery for ovarian cancer includes total abdominal hysterectomy, bilateral salpingo-oophorectomy, pelvic and para-aortic lymph node sampling, infracolic omentectomy, pelvic and peritoneal biopsies, and pelvic and peritoneal washings. The importance of appropriate surgical staging in ovarian cancer—particularly in cases of apparent early-stage disease—cannot be overemphasized. Failure to perform complete surgical staging may result in the need for chemotherapy when it may be unnecessary, or it may lead to an inappropriate decision to withhold adjuvant chemotherapy when disease in the abdominal cavity or regional lymph nodes has gone undetected. In the United States, national surveys indicate that an appropriate and complete staging procedure is carried out in less than 15% of women with suspected early-stage ovarian cancer.[86] An initial appropriate staging procedure is much more likely if the surgeon is a gynecologic oncologist.

Considerable retrospective data have documented that survival is better for women who begin receiving chemotherapy after surgery in the presence of low-volume intraperitoneal disease than it is for women who do not have surgery or for whom surgery did not result in optimal cytoreduction. These data strongly support the conclusion that a reasonable attempt at maximal cytoreduction is an important component in treating patients with ovarian cancer. However, for patients in whom it is possible to carry out optimal cytoreduction, it remains uncertain whether survival outcomes are better because of the surgery itself or because the same tumor biologic factors that permit a successful surgery (such as the local growth pattern of the tumor) are also responsible for overall chemosensitivity, risk of inherent or acquired resistance to chemotherapy, and the rate of disease progression.

PROGNOSTIC FACTORS

The most important prognostic factor is tumor stage. Approximately 25% of women present with stage I disease, 15% with stage II, 42% with stage III, and 17% with stage IV. Table 11-4 gives an overview of ovarian cancer staging, treatment, and 5-year survival estimates. Other important prognostic factors include extent of residual disease at completion of cytoreductive surgery, tumor grade, patient age, and performance status. Histologic subtype may affect prognosis. For example, all clear cell carcinomas are considered to be grade 3, and mucinous carcinomas carry a less-favorable prognosis for patients with advanced-stage disease. Some ovarian serous carcinomas may be classified as "low-grade serous" carcinomas. These low-grade cancers differ from high-grade serous cancers in their molecular signatures (for example, *p53* mutations are rare, but *KRAS* and *BRAF* mutations, and mitogen-activated protein kinase pathway alterations, are more common), exhibit a more indolent disease course, and may be more resistant to platinum/taxane chemotherapy.[87] Advances in our understanding of the molecular differences among ovarian cancers may lead to treatment changes involving therapies that are specifically directed to identifiable driver abnormalities.

Some studies have shown that ovarian cancer prognosis is more favorable among women with a *BRCA1* mutation, but results of other studies have not found improved survival among *BRCA1* mutation–related ovarian cancers.[88,89] Tumor grade is particularly important in stage I ovarian cancers, guiding both prognosis and treatment decisions.

CHEMOTHERAPY FOR EARLY-STAGE OVARIAN CANCER

Patients with early-stage ovarian cancer can be classified into favorable and less-favorable prognostic groups. Patients with stage IA or IB, grade 1 or 2 cancers have 5-year disease-free survival rates of more than 90%. Two randomized trials for

KEY POINTS

- Surgery for staging and tumor cytoreduction plays a key role in the management of epithelial ovarian cancer.
- Neoadjuvant chemotherapy followed by surgical cytoreduction yields equivalent outcomes to those for surgical cytoreduction followed by adjuvant chemotherapy for patients with clinically advanced epithelial ovarian cancer.
- Important prognostic factors include stage, optimal compared with suboptimal cytoreduction, tumor grade (particularly for stage I cancers), poor-risk histology such as clear cell or mucinous cancers, patient age, and performance status.
- Patients with favorable-risk, early-stage ovarian cancer (stage IA or IB, grade 1 or 2 cancers) do not require adjuvant chemotherapy after complete surgical staging.
- Patients with less-favorable risk, early-stage ovarian cancer (stage IA or IB, grade 3, all stage IC, all clear cell carcinomas, and stage II cancers) should receive adjuvant platinum-based chemotherapy after complete surgical staging.

Table 11-4 **Epithelial Ovarian Cancer Staging, Treatment Overview, and Estimates of Overall Survival**

Stage	Definition	Treatment Overview	5-Year Overall Survival (%)
I	Tumor confined to the ovaries	Hysterectomy, bilateral salpingo-oophorectomy, lymph node sampling, washings, and complete surgical staging*	85-90
IA	Tumor limited to one ovary; capsule intact, no tumor on ovarian surface, no malignant cells in ascites or peritoneal washings	No adjuvant chemotherapy for grade 1 or 2 tumors; adjuvant platinum-based chemotherapy for grade 3 and clear cell tumors	
IB	Tumor limited to both ovaries; capsule intact, no tumor on ovarian surface, no malignant cells in ascites or peritoneal washings	No adjuvant chemotherapy for grade 1 or 2 tumors; adjuvant platinum-based chemotherapy for grade 3 and clear cell tumors	
IC	Tumor limited to one or both ovaries; capsule rupture or tumor on the ovarian surface or malignant cells in ascites or peritoneal washings	Adjuvant platinum-based chemotherapy	
II	Tumor involves one or both ovaries with pelvic extension		80
IIA	Extension and/or implants on uterus and/or fallopian tubes; no malignant cells in ascites or peritoneal washings	Adjuvant platinum-based chemotherapy	
IIB	Extension to other pelvic tissues; no malignant cells in ascites or peritoneal washings	Adjuvant platinum-based chemotherapy	
IIC	Pelvic extension with malignant cells in ascites or peritoneal washings	Adjuvant platinum-based chemotherapy	
III	Tumor involves one or both ovaries with peritoneal metastasis outside the pelvis and/or retroperitoneal or inguinal lymph node metastasis		15-50[†]
IIIA	Microscopic peritoneal metastasis beyond the pelvis		
IIIB	Macroscopic peritoneal metastasis beyond the pelvis, measuring ≤ 2 cm in greatest dimension		
IIIC-optimally debulked	Macroscopic peritoneal metastasis beyond the pelvis measuring > 2 cm and/or regional lymph node metastases; no residual disease > 1 cm at completion of cytoreductive surgery	Intraperitoneal platinum- and taxane-based chemotherapy, or dose-dense weekly taxane plus platinum intravenous chemotherapy (see text for details)	30-50
IIIC-suboptimally debulked	Macroscopic peritoneal metastasis beyond the pelvis measuring > 2 cm and/or regional lymph node metastases; residual disease > 1 cm at completion of cytoreductive surgery	Intravenous platinum plus taxane combination chemotherapy	10-20
IV	Distant metastases (excluding peritoneal metastases) to liver parenchyma or malignant pleural effusion	Intravenous platinum plus taxane combination chemotherapy	5-10

*Fertility-sparing surgery (unilateral salpingo-oophorectomy, lymph node sampling, washings, and biopsies) may be appropriate for selected young patients with stage IA disease who have not completed childbearing.

[†]Survival is longer among patients who undergo optimal cytoreduction at time of initial surgery.

this favorable prognostic group failed to show a disease-free or overall survival benefit from chemotherapy.[90] Women with stage IA or IB, grade 1 or 2 ovarian cancer do not require adjuvant chemotherapy if complete surgical staging was performed.

Patients with stage IA or IB, grade 3 cancer, all patients with stage IC disease, all patients with clear cell carcinomas, and patients with stage II disease have a less favorable prognosis, with 5-year survival rates of 80% to 90%. A number of randomized trials have demonstrated that adjuvant chemotherapy can prolong the time to progression for women with high-risk, early-stage ovarian cancer. An analysis of data from more than 900 patients with high-risk, early-stage disease showed that adjuvant platinum-based chemotherapy administered postoperatively led to an 11% improvement in 5-year progression-free survival and an 8% improvement in 5-year overall survival, compared with a strategy of observation until evidence of recurrent disease.[91,92] These data strongly support the recommendation for treating women with less-favorable prognosis, early-stage ovarian cancer (stage IA or IB, grade 3, all stage IC, all clear cell carcinomas, and stage II) with adjuvant platinum-based chemotherapy after complete surgical staging. The optimal duration of therapy for early-stage disease has not been defined. A large phase III trial showed that adding 24 weeks of maintenance paclitaxel after three cycles of intravenous paclitaxel plus carboplatin did not improve progression-free or overall survival (85.4% with maintenance vs. 86.2% without, at 5 years).[93]

CHEMOTHERAPY FOR ADVANCED OVARIAN CANCER

A series of randomized phase III trials have been conducted in advanced ovarian cancer, the results of which have established combination platinum (cisplatin or carboplatin) and taxane (paclitaxel or docetaxel) chemotherapy as the standard of care for first-line treatment.[94,95] Results generally have shown a significant improvement in overall survival with combination platinum/taxane regimens. One large randomized trial failed to demonstrate a survival advantage for platinum/paclitaxel compared with single-agent carboplatin,[96] but this discrepancy may be explained by trial design differences and the eventual use of paclitaxel in one-third of patients in the single-agent carboplatin arm.

Carboplatin and cisplatin are equally efficacious for ovarian cancer, but their adverse effect profiles differ. Carboplatin is more myelosuppressive, but cisplatin has a greater risk for nausea, vomiting, neurotoxicity, and nephrotoxicity. Carboplatin is chosen more frequently for use in combination with paclitaxel because it can be administered safely with a 3-hour paclitaxel infusion, whereas cisplatin needs to be administered with a 24-hour paclitaxel infusion to minimize the risk of combined neurotoxicity.[97]

Approximately 60% to 80% of patients with advanced ovarian cancer experience objective response to platinum/taxane treatment with improvement of disease-related symptoms. Median progression-free survival is approximately 26 months, and overall survival approximately 60 months, for women with advanced ovarian cancer who had optimal cytoreduction at initial surgery. For patients with suboptimal cytoreduction or stage IV disease, median progression-free survival is 18 months and median overall survival is 38 months.

Newer agents and alternative treatment schedules that have shown activity in recurrent disease are being investigated in the first-line setting for advanced ovarian cancer. The angiogenesis inhibitor bevacizumab, which achieved objective responses in patients with recurrent ovarian cancer,[98,99] was tested in a phase III trial for first-line treatment of stage III and IV ovarian cancer. In this randomized, placebo-controlled study, patients who were assigned to treatment with paclitaxel plus carboplatin with bevacizumab followed by bevacizumab maintenance had a progression-free survival of 14.1 months compared with 10.3 months for the patients assigned to chemotherapy without bevacizumab and without bevacizumab maintenance. Overall survival was not improved.[100] A progression-free survival advantage of similar magnitude was observed in a similarly designed European study (ICON7), which employed a lower dose and shorter duration of bevacizumab treatment.[101] Weekly paclitaxel plus every-3-weeks carboplatin was compared with standard every-3-weeks paclitaxel plus carboplatin in a phase III trial. The weekly paclitaxel/every-3-weeks carboplatin schedule was associated with an overall survival advantage of 72% compared with 65% at 3 years.[102] However, subsequent studies do not appear to corroborate this advantage for the weekly paclitaxel schedule. Liposomal doxorubicin plus carboplatin was not superior to paclitaxel plus carboplatin as first-line treatment for patients with stage IC to IV disease in terms of survival outcomes; quality-of-life outcomes were also similar in the two treatment arms.[103]

In terms of surveillance for relapse in patients who experience a complete clinical remission (normal serum CA-125 level and no evidence of disease by CT scan) with first-line treatment for ovarian cancer, a randomized trial showed that there was no advantage to routine monitoring of CA-125 for detection of relapse because early treatment on the basis of rising CA-125 levels did not improve survival.[104] However, in the United States, post-treatment surveillance by CA-125 levels is commonly utilized.

INTRAPERITONEAL CHEMOTHERAPY FOR STAGE III DISEASE WITH OPTIMAL CYTOREDUCTION

Managing ovarian cancer by delivering drugs directly into the peritoneal cavity has particular appeal for treating a disease that is largely confined to the peritoneum. Phase I and II clinical trials have demonstrated the biologic activity and safety of intraperitoneal delivery of chemotherapy. Because drug delivery is by diffusion, intraperitoneal therapy is limited to patients with small-volume residual disease.

Several randomized phase III clinical trials have been completed, suggesting an advantage to intraperitoneal cisplatin-based therapy compared with intravenous treatment.[105,106] In a large phase III trial, patients with optimally cytoreduced stage III ovarian cancer were randomly assigned to receive intravenous cisplatin plus paclitaxel or intraperitoneal cisplatin plus intravenous and intraperitoneal paclitaxel.[107] Patients assigned to the intraperitoneal treatment arm had significantly longer progression-free survival (23.8 months vs. 18.3 months) and overall survival (65.6 months vs. 49.7 months) compared with patients

KEY POINTS

- Standard first-line therapy for patients with stage III and stage IV ovarian cancer is platinum plus taxane combination chemotherapy.
- Patients with optimally cytoreduced, stage III ovarian cancer have a significant survival advantage when receiving a combination of intraperitoneal cisplatin plus intraperitoneal and intravenous paclitaxel.
- Carboplatin and cisplatin are equally efficacious when delivered intravenously for advanced ovarian cancer but have important differences in adverse effect profiles.

assigned to intravenous-only therapy. Toxicity was greater in the intraperitoneal arm, with an initial decrease in quality of life; however, at 1 year, there were no quality-of-life differences between the two treatment arms.[108] The use of intraperitoneal chemotherapy varies among different academic medical centers. Areas of active investigation include whether and how to incorporate bevacizumab, poly (adenosine diphosphate-ribose) polymerase (PARP) inhibitors (see Treatment of Recurrent or Resistant Disease below), and weekly taxane schedules into first-line treatment of optimally debulked ovarian cancer.

SECONDARY SURGICAL PROCEDURES

In addition to its importance in staging and primary cytoreduction for ovarian cancer, surgery has additional roles in the management of ovarian cancer. Patients for whom primary surgical cytoreduction was not recommended but whose disease exhibited a response to neoadjuvant chemotherapy may be candidates for surgical resection of residual macroscopic disease. For such patients, a residual mass may not be an area of resistant disease; rather, it may be a necrotic or poorly vascularized region where potentially chemosensitive cancer cells have not been exposed to cytotoxic drugs. Thus, removal of bulky residual tumors may improve the clinical outcome for inherently chemosensitive cancers. A European randomized trial has provided limited confirmation of this theory by demonstrating a survival advantage with interval surgical cytoreduction— performed after three cycles of cytotoxic drugs—for women with advanced ovarian cancer who have evidence of an initial response to chemotherapy and who have not had an initial attempt at complete surgical cytoreduction.[109] In contrast, GOG conducted a randomized trial to determine whether secondary surgery was beneficial for patients whose residual tumor was larger than 1 cm after primary cytoreduction surgery. Patients whose disease was stable or improved with cisplatin plus paclitaxel were randomly assigned to continue with chemotherapy or to have a second attempt at cytoreduction followed by additional chemotherapy. This study indicated that such patients do not benefit from a second attempt at cytoreduction surgery; rather, treatment with chemotherapy should continue.[110]

Although patients with recurrent ovarian cancer are sometimes offered secondary cytoreduction surgery after a relatively long disease-free interval, there are no prospective data from randomized trials to determine whether such surgery improves outcomes. The GOG is currently conducting a study in which patients with recurrent ovarian cancer who are potential candidates for surgery are randomly assigned to secondary cytoreduction surgery followed by chemotherapy or to chemotherapy without surgery.

In the past, some patients underwent a second surgery after the completion of chemotherapy to determine whether there had been complete pathologic response to treatment. This procedure was termed second-look laparotomy. A negative second look was defined as patients with no visible disease and no microscopic evidence of disease on multiple biopsies from the abdominal cavity. Although second-look laparotomy may provide prognostic information (patients with no microscopic evidence of disease on biopsy have longer overall survival than patients with microscopic or visible residual disease after chemotherapy),[111] it does not improve survival outcomes.[112]

CONSOLIDATION AND MAINTENANCE THERAPY

Disease will recur in approximately 70% of women with advanced ovarian cancer who have a clinically defined complete response to standard chemotherapy with a platinum agent and a taxane. A number of studies have been conducted to determine whether consolidation or maintenance chemotherapy can improve overall survival. In the largest prospective randomized trial, women who had a complete clinical response to platinum/taxane first-line treatment were randomly assigned to receive three additional cycles of monthly paclitaxel or 12 additional monthly cycles.[113] Patients assigned to receive 12 cycles of consolidation paclitaxel had a median progression-free survival of 28 months compared with a median of 21 months for patients assigned to receive three cycles. Data were premature for any demonstrable overall survival benefit, and early closure of this study means that survival data are unlikely to be meaningful. Patients who continue with prolonged paclitaxel treatment continue to have alopecia and are at increased risk for developing worsening peripheral neuropathy. It is reasonable to discuss these data with patients for individuals to consider the potential for a 7-month improvement in progression-free survival. As detailed above, GOG218 and ICON7 showed that maintenance bevacizumab after treatment with paclitaxel plus carboplatin plus bevacizumab provided an approximately 3.5-month improvement in progression-free survival compared with the no-bevacizumab treatment arm. In contrast, consolidation with the epidermal growth factor receptor (EGFR)-targeted agent erlotinib did not improve survival outcomes following first-line platinum-based chemotherapy for patients with stage I, II, III, or IV ovarian cancer. No subgroup (EGFR status by immunohistochemistry, *EGFR* mutation, erlotinib rash) was found to

---

KEY POINTS

- Second-look laparotomy at completion of first-line chemotherapy is not a standard approach. Although it may provide prognostic information, the procedure does not improve survival outcomes.
- Consolidation treatment with paclitaxel provides a moderate prolongation of progression-free survival at the cost of continued alopecia and increased risk for neuropathy.
- The addition of bevacizumab to paclitaxel/carboplatin followed by bevacizumab maintenance provides a modest prolongation in progression-free survival but no overall survival advantage.
- Consolidation with other chemotherapy agents for patients in first clinical remission at completion of first-line platinum/taxane treatment has not been shown to be beneficial.

benefit from erlotinib.[114] To date, consolidation with other chemotherapy agents has not been shown to be beneficial. In one study, patients who received consolidation therapy with topotecan had a shorter progression-free survival than patients who received no consolidation.[115]

TREATMENT OF RECURRENT OR RESISTANT DISEASE

Patients with recurrent ovarian cancer are often classified according to whether their recurrent disease is platinum-refractory (defined as progressing during treatment with platinum-based therapy), platinum-resistant (defined as progressing within 6 months of completing first-line platinum-based therapy), potentially/intermediate platinum-sensitive (defined as progression more than 6 but fewer than 12 months from completing first-line platinum-based therapy), or platinum-sensitive (defined as recurrence 12 months or more from the completion of first-line platinum-based therapy). Approximately 20% of women with advanced ovarian cancer do not have a disease response to first-line treatment with platinum/taxane combination chemotherapy. These patients with platinum-refractory disease have a very poor prognosis and a very low likelihood of achieving objective response to second-line therapy; they are excellent candidates for clinical trials of novel agents. Patients who experience disease response to first-line treatment followed by progression/recurrence have a somewhat better prognosis. Treatment options and prognosis are linked to the duration of disease control achieved with first-line treatment. Patients with platinum-sensitive disease have a high likelihood of response to retreatment with platinum-based therapy. Two randomized trials have shown that platinum-based combination therapy (carboplatin/gemcitabine or carboplatin/paclitaxel) is superior to single-agent platinum for this patient population.[116,117] Liposomal doxorubicin plus carboplatin was superior to paclitaxel plus carboplatin in terms of progression-free survival (11.3 months vs. 9.4 months) and toxicity profile.[118] In a phase III trial comparing gemcitabine plus carboplatin with or without bevacizumab for platinum-sensitive recurrent ovarian cancer, progression-free survival was superior in the group assigned to receive bevacizumab (12.4 months with bevacizumab vs. 8.4 months with placebo).[119] Similarly, in a blinded, placebo-controlled trial for patients with platinum-sensitive recurrent disease that responded to platinum-based therapy, maintenance treatment with the PARP inhibitor olaparib was superior to placebo for progression-free survival (8.4 months with olaparib vs. 4.8 months with placebo), but there was no difference in overall survival.[120]

Patients retreated with carboplatin should be cautioned about the risk of acquired platinum allergy.[121] Carboplatin is associated with an acquired allergy, generally seen in patients who have had multiple prior cycles of this drug. Reactions can range from minor itching and rash to respiratory distress, hypotension, and anaphylactic shock.[122] Clinical trials are investigating potential methods for mitigating risk of developing hypersensitivity such as use of pre-medications and prolonged, desensitizing infusion times.[123]

A number of chemotherapy agents can achieve objective responses for a minority of patients with platinum-resistant disease (generally 10% to 20%).[124] Chemotherapy agents with demonstrated activity as second-line therapy for ovarian cancer include liposomal doxorubicin, topotecan, gemcitabine, docetaxel, weekly paclitaxel, oral etoposide, pemetrexed, irinotecan, vinorelbine, and bevacizumab. Patients with low-volume recurrent disease may experience disease control with the use of hormone agents such as tamoxifen. Bevacizumab in combination with either weekly paclitaxel or liposomal doxorubicin or topotecan has also been shown to improve response and progression-free survival among patients with platinum-resistant ovarian cancer.[125]

For patients with an intermediate interval of time from completion of first-line platinum-based treatment (more than 6 months, less than 12 months), the response rate to platinum-based therapy is higher than 20%. Treatment with platinum or nonplatinum single agents is appropriate for this group. Second-line treatment options differ in dosing schedules and adverse effect profiles. Choices among the agents can be individualized according to prior treatments received, existing toxicities, patient convenience, and patient preferences. All patients with refractory or recurrent ovarian cancer are appropriate candidates for clinical trial participation because no current strategy is known to result in long-term disease control or cure.

BRCA mutation–associated ovarian cancers (like breast cancers) harbor DNA repair defects that render them more dependent on PARP for DNA repair.[126] Inhibition of PARP may lead to improved tumor cell kill. Some data suggest that inhibition of PARP may also be successful in non–*BRCA*-mutated cancers. In a prospective phase II trial, 63 assessable patients with high-grade serous or poorly differentiated ovarian cancer received the PARP inhibitor olaparib. Among the 17 patients with *BRCA1* or *BRCA2* mutations, seven (41%) experienced objective responses; among the 46 without mutations, 11 (24%) experienced objective responses.[127] PARP inhibitors are under active investigation in combination with chemotherapy for first-line treatment, for recurrent disease, and as maintenance therapy. In a randomized phase II study, maintenance treatment with olaparib following a response to platinum-based chemotherapy improved progression-free survival in platinum-sensitive recurrent disease compared to placebo.[128]

Low-grade serous ovarian cancers commonly have *KRAS* or *BRAF* mutations, which has led to interest in testing MAP kinase inhibitors in patients with these cancers, which are often resistant to taxane-platinum therapy.[129] Most patients with recurrent ovarian cancer will receive a series of chemotherapy regimens over time. The median time for disease control with any given agent is approximately 4 months. Patients who develop organ dysfunction from progressive ovarian cancer may receive palliative care with selected interventions such as paracentesis for relief of large-volume ascites, thoracentesis/pleurodesis for symptomatic pleural effusion, ureteral stent placement for hydronephrosis, bowel surgery/diversion for small or large bowel obstruction, or decompressing gastrostomy for persistent, symptomatic small bowel obstruction.

LOW MALIGNANT POTENTIAL TUMORS OF THE OVARY

For some patients, the histologic diagnosis is low malignant potential (LMP) tumor of the ovary. Patients with LMP tumors who wish to preserve fertility can undergo fertility-sparing surgery.[130] All areas of visible tumor involvement should be removed at time of surgery and carefully reviewed by the pathologist to confirm that there is no evidence of invasive disease. Patients who do not desire preservation of fertility may undergo standard surgical staging for ovarian cancer. Patients who have no evidence of invasive carcinoma and no evidence of extra-ovarian tumor may be considered for fertility-sparing surgery. Most women with LMP tumors have early-stage disease at diagnosis, and the 5-year overall survival rates for such patients exceed 95%; progression-free survival exceeds 80%. There is no evidence that adjuvant therapy (chemotherapy or radiation) is beneficial for patients with LMP tumors of any stage if pathology review confirms there is no evidence of invasive implants. Five-year overall survival rates for patients with stage III or IV LMP tumors are approximately 90%, and progression-free survival rates are more than 65%.[131] Patients who are found to have histologic evidence of invasive cancer may be considered for adjuvant chemotherapy, as would be offered to patients with invasive epithelial ovarian cancer; however, data are limited for this rare situation.

NONEPITHELIAL CANCERS OF THE OVARY

About 10% of cancers of the ovary are nonepithelial cancers. These tumors are classified as either sex-cord stromal cell tumors of the ovary or germ cell tumors. Each of these groups is further subclassified by histology. It is important to identify the stromal tumors and germ cell tumors because they differ markedly from epithelial ovarian cancer in prognosis and treatment.

SEX-CORD STROMAL CELL TUMORS OF THE OVARY

Sex-cord stromal tumors are subclassified as granulosa cell tumors and androgen-producing tumors such as Sertoli-Leydig cell tumors. Adult-type granulosa cell tumors are generally stage I at diagnosis and are diagnosed in women age 40 to 70. Granulosa cell tumors frequently produce estrogen. The excess estrogen production may cause abnormal uterine bleeding, endometrial hyperplasia, and even endometrial cancer. Endometrial cancers that are found concurrently with granulosa cell tumors are typically early stage and low grade. The treatment for granulosa cell tumors is surgical resection.[132] Patients with early-stage disease who desire fertility preservation may undergo fertility-sparing surgery. If the uterus is not removed, an endometrial biopsy should be done to rule out a concurrent endometrial cancer. Patients who have completed childbearing should undergo hysterectomy and bilateral salpingo-oophorectomy. Occult lymph node metastases are rare, and routine lymphadenectomy is not routinely recommended.[133] Adjuvant chemotherapy is not generally administered after complete resection of newly diagnosed disease. Granulosa cell tumors may recur, and it is typical for recurrences to be years or even decades later. There are some data supporting the use of combination platinum-based chemotherapy for patients with recurrent, unresectable disease.[134,135]

Sertoli-Leydig tumors commonly present before age 40. More than 90% are stage I at diagnosis. Androgen production can lead to virilization. Five-year survival rates are 70% to 90%, with prognosis related to stage and degree of tumor differentiation. Patients with advanced-stage disease have an unfavorable prognosis. Platinum-based chemotherapy may be considered for patients with poorly differentiated tumors and for patients with advanced or recurrent disease.

GERM CELL TUMORS OF THE OVARY

Germ cell tumors of the ovary usually affect adolescent girls and young women. Fertility-sparing surgery is appropriate for most patients. Fifty percent of germ cell tumors are dysgerminomas; other histologies include yolk sac tumors, immature teratomas, embryonal cell carcinoma, nongestational choriocarcinomas, and mixed tumors. Dysgerminomas are more likely to be confined to one ovary at diagnosis (stage I) and carry a favorable prognosis. Patients with stage I dysgerminomas who have had complete staging surgery (with or without fertility preservation) do not require chemotherapy. Similarly, patients with stage I, grade 1 immature teratomas can be treated with surgery only. All other nondysgerminomas and higher-stage dysgerminomas should be treated with chemotherapy after surgical resection. Standard treatment is combination platinum/etoposide-based therapy, with most data supporting three to four cycles of bleomycin, etoposide, and cisplatin. Patient outcomes are excellent with chemotherapy for these higher-risk germ cell tumors. In a GOG study, 93 patients with completely resected nondysgerminoma received three cycles of bleomycin, etoposide, and cisplatin; 91 of 93 patients (96%) remained disease-free with follow-up ranging from 4 to 90 months.[136]

Serum levels of human chorionic gonadotropin (hCG) and alpha-fetoprotein may be elevated in some germ cell tumors at diagnosis and can be used in follow-up monitoring. Most patients who have had fertility-sparing surgery either continue to menstruate during chemotherapy or resume normal menstrual cycles after completion of chemotherapy.[137,138] The majority of women remain fertile, and pregnancy outcomes are favorable.[139]

GESTATIONAL TROPHOBLASTIC DISEASE

Gestational trophoblastic diseases are diseases of the human placenta that occur in women of childbearing age. There is a spectrum of malignant potential, from lesions with very low malignant potential (complete and partial hydatidiform moles) to invasive tumors with metastatic potential (invasive moles and placental site trophoblastic tumors) to tumors with exceedingly high risk for systemic metastases (gestational choriocarcinoma). Despite the risk for metastatic disease, nearly all women with gestational trophoblastic disease can be cured with the appropriate use of chemotherapy, careful monitoring for treatment response, and surveillance for evidence of relapse using sensitive beta-hCG assays. A major role of the medical oncologist is to consider the possibility of gestational trophoblastic disease in women of childbearing age who present with a diagnosis of metastatic cancer.

Malignant gestational trophoblastic disease is classified as either nonmetastatic (disease is limited to the uterus) or metastatic. Patients with metastatic disease are further classified as low risk (good prognosis) or high risk (poorer prognosis). Risk assessment incorporates such variables as patient age, type of antecedent pregnancy, interval of time from the antecedent pregnancy, hCG level, largest tumor size, metastatic sites, number of metastases, and prior chemotherapy.[140,141] Treatment recommendations are based on risk assessment. Patients with low-risk disease may be treated with single-agent methotrexate.[142] Other chemotherapy agents with activity include dactinomycin[143] and etoposide.[144] For high-risk patients, combination chemotherapy is administered, usually incorporating etoposide, methotrexate, and dactinomycin, alternating with cyclophosphamide and vincristine.[145] Response to chemotherapy is assessed by following the quantitative level of the serum hCG.

VULVAR CANCER

Most vulvar carcinomas are squamous cell carcinomas. There are about 4,000 cases annually in the United States and occur most often in postmenopausal, older women. Risk factors include smoking, vulvar dystrophy, HPV infection, and a prior history of cervix cancer and immunodeficiency syndromes. Most vulvar cancers are localized at time of diagnosis and managed with complete surgical resection of the primary tumor. Assessment of lymph node involvement is considered standard for nearly all lesions; sentinel lymph node biopsies are increasingly incorporated in the surgical approach to vulvar cancer in order to decrease the morbidity associated with inguinofemoral lymphadenectomy. Patients with completely resected disease whose lymph nodes are negative may be observed. Five-year survival rates are estimated to be 70% to 93%. Patients with lymph node involvement are at much greater risk for recurrence and death (5-year survival rate, 25% to 41%)[146] and are recommended to receive adjuvant chemoradiation. Similarly, patients with locally advanced disease that cannot be completely resected are treated with primary chemoradiation. Patients who have an excellent clinical response to chemoradiation may subsequently be considered for resection of residual disease if such resection is feasible and the patient is medically fit for surgery. The efficacy of chemoradiation for locally advanced disease was shown in a prospective study of 52 patients with one or more clinically involved lymph nodes. Patients received radiation to the primary tumor and the lymph nodes with concurrent cisplatin plus 5-fluorouracil. Patients who experienced a clinical response underwent subsequent surgical resection. Among the 46 eligible patients, four did not complete chemoradiation (three died, one refused treatment), and four did not have surgery (two died of noncancer-related causes, two experienced an inadequate disease response). Thirty-eight patients had surgery; 37 had lymph node dissections. The lymph nodes were histologically negative in 15 of the 37, providing good evidence for the efficacy of chemoradiation, although it is noted that two patients died of treatment-related complications.[147]

Whether patients with initially resectable disease benefit from adjuvant chemoradiation has not been prospectively studied. Based on retrospective data that showed improved survival for patients with positive lymph nodes who received adjuvant radiation,[148] some physicians recommend adjuvant chemoradiation for patients with large tumors, lymph node involvement, extensive lymphovascular invasion, or positive margins.

Patients with locally recurrent disease should be considered for re-excision. Radiation may be considered if the recurrence is not resectable and the patient has not had prior radiation. Patients with multisite, unresectable metastatic disease may be offered palliative chemotherapy, although there are no prospective data evaluating the efficacy of systemic chemotherapy for metastatic vulvar cancer. Agents such as platinum and taxanes that have demonstrated efficacy in cervix cancer are reasonable options for patients who are fit for chemotherapy.

VAGINAL CANCER

Like vulvar cancer, most vaginal carcinomas are squamous cell carcinomas and associated with HPV infection.[149] Other risk factors include tobacco use, early age at first intercourse, multiple lifetime sexual partners, and a history of prior cervix cancer. Other histologies of vaginal cancer are rarer and include clear cell carcinoma (in utero diethylstilbestrol [DES] exposure increases the risk for vaginal-cervix clear cell cancers), melanoma, sarcoma, and adenocarcinoma. It is important to consider metastatic or recurrent disease from other sites (cervix, vulva, ovary, breast, endometrium, uterine sarcoma) in the evaluation of a new vaginal lesion since metastatic disease is more common than primary vaginal carcinoma.

Most women with vaginal cancer present with abnormal bleeding. Diagnosis is established by biopsy. Colposcopy may be required to visualize the lesion. There are no prospective studies upon which to base treatment recommendations for vaginal carcinomas. Both surgery and radiation can be difficult due to proximity of the bladder, urethra, and rectum. Small, upper vaginal lesions may be treated with surgery or radiation. For vaginal cancers that invade the paravaginal tissues but do not extend to the pelvic side wall, treatment with radiation can be considered, or treatment with platinum-based chemotherapy may achieve sufficient response to permit resection.[150]

For patients with more extensive, locally advanced disease, radiation or platinum-based chemoradiation is reasonable. While there are no prospective comparison data showing chemoradiation to be superior to radiation alone, many extrapolate the data from randomized trials in cervix cancer, and interpret data from retrospective studies in vaginal cancer, to support the recommendation of chemoradiation.[151]

As with cervix cancer, patients with a central recurrence may be considered for pelvic exenteration surgery. Patients with unresectable, metastatic disease may be offered palliative cytotoxic chemotherapy, but there are no prospective data to establish which agents are active.

References

1. American Cancer Society. Cancer Facts & Figures 2013. http://www.cancer.org/acs/groups/content/@epidemiologysurveilance/documents/document/acspc-036845.pdf. Accessed February 8, 2014.

2. Siegel R, Ma J, Zou Z, et al. Cancer statistics, 2014. *CA Cancer J Clin.* 2014;64:9-29. PMID: 24399786.

3. de Villiers EM, Fauquet C, Broker TR, et al. Classification of papillomaviruses. *Virology.* 2004;324:17-27. PMID: 15183049.

4. Dunne EF, Unger ER, Sternberg M, et al. Prevalence of HPV infection among females in the United States. *JAMA.* 2007;297:813-819. PMID: 17327523.

5. Plummer M, Schiffman M, Castle PE, et al. A 2-year prospective study of human papillomavirus persistence among women with a cytological diagnosis of atypical squamous cells of undetermined significance or low-grade squamous intraepithelial lesion. *J Infect Dis.* 2007;195:1582-1589. PMID: 17471427.

6. Phelps WC, Yee CL, Munger K, et al. The human papillomavirus type 16 E7 gene encodes transactivation and transforming functions similar to those of adenovirus E1A. *Cell.* 1988;58:539-547. PMID: 2836062.

7. Castellsagué X, Díaz M, Vaccarella S, et al. Intrauterine device use, cervical infection with human papillomavirus, and risk of cervical cancer: a pooled analysis of 26 epidemiological studies. *Lancet Oncol.* 2011;12:1023-1031. PMID: 21917519.

8. Muñoz N, Bosch FX, de Sanjosé S, et al. Epidemiologic classification of human papillomavirus types associated with cervical cancer. *N Engl J Med.* 2003;348:518-527. PMID: 12571259.

9. Mayrand MH, Duarte-Franco E, Rodrigues I, et al. Human papillomavirus DNA versus Papanicolaou screening tests for cervical cancer. *N Engl J Med.* 2007;357:1579-1588. PMID: 17942871.

10. Rijkaart DC, Berkhof J, van Kemenade FJ, et al. HPV DNA testing in population-based cervical screening (VUSA-Screen study): results and implications. *Br J Cancer.* 2012;106:975-981. PMID: 22251922.

11. Moyer VA, U.S. Preventive Services Task Force. Screening for cervical cancer: U.S. Preventive Services Task Force recommendation statement. *Ann Intern Med.* 2012;156:880-891, W312. PMID: 22711081.

12. Carozzi F, Visioli CB, Confortini M, et al. hr-HPV testing in the follow-up of women with cytological abnormalities and negative colposcopy. *Br J Cancer.* 2013;109:1766-1774. PMID: 24008667.

13. Ault KA, FUTURE II Study Group. Effect of prophylactic human papillomavirus L1 virus-like-particle vaccine on risk of cervical intraepithelial neoplasia grade 2, grade 3, and adenocarcinoma in situ: a combined analysis of four randomised clinical trials. *Lancet.* 2007;369:1861-1868. PMID: 17544766.

14. Muñoz N, Kjaer SK, Sigurdsson K, et al. Impact of human papillomavirus (HPV)-6/11/16/18 vaccine on all HPV-associated genital diseases in young women. *J Natl Cancer Inst.* 2010;102:325-339. PMID: 20139221.

15. Laz TH, Rahman M, Berenson AB. Human papillomavirus vaccine uptake among 18- to 26-year-old women in the United States: National Health Interview Survey, 2010. *Cancer.* 2013;119:1386-1392. PMID: 23508594.

16. Muñoz N, Manalastas R Jr, Pitisuttithum P, et al. Safety, immunogenicity, and efficacy of quadrivalent human papillomavirus (types 6, 11, 16, 18) recombinant vaccine in women aged 24-45 years: a randomised, double-blind trial. *Lancet.* 2009;373:1949-1957. PMID: 19493565.

17. Mahmud SM, Kliewer EV, Lambert P, et al. Effectiveness of the quadrivalent human papillomavirus vaccine against cervical dysplasia in Manitoba, Canada. *J Clin Oncol.* 2014;32:438-443. PMID: 24395857.

18. Giuliano AR, Palefsky JM, Goldstone S, et al. Efficacy of quadrivalent HPV vaccine against HPV infection and disease in males. *N Engl J Med.* 2011;364:401-411. PMID: 21288094.

19. Sedlis A, Bundy BN, Rotman MZ, et al. A randomized trial of pelvic radiation therapy versus no further therapy in selected patients of stage IB carcinoma of the cervix after radical hysterectomy and pelvic lymphadenectomy: A Gynecologic Oncology Group Study. *Gyn Oncol.* 1999;73:177-183. PMID: 10329031.

20. Peters WA 3rd, Liu PY, Barrett RJ 2nd, et al. Concurrent chemotherapy and pelvic radiation therapy compared with pelvic radiation therapy alone as adjuvant therapy after radical surgery in high-risk early-stage cancer of the cervix. *J Clin Oncol.* 2000;18:1606-1613. PMID: 10764420.

21. Zivanovic O, Alektiar KM, Sonoda Y, et al. Treatment patterns of FIGO Stage IB2 cervical cancer: a single-institution experience of radical hysterectomy

with individualized postoperative therapy and definitive radiation therapy. *Gynecol Oncol.* 2008;111:265-270. PMID: 18774596.

22. Keys HM, Bundy BN, Stehman FB, et al. Cisplatin, radiation, and adjuvant hysterectomy compared with radiation and adjuvant hysterectomy for bulky stage IB cervical carcinoma. *N Engl J Med.* 1999;340:1154-1161. PMID: 10202166.

23. Green JA, Kirwan JM, Tierney JF, et al. Survival and recurrence after concomitant chemotherapy and radiotherapy for cancer of the uterine cervix: a systematic review and meta-analysis. *Lancet.* 2001;358:781-786. PMID: 11564482.

24. Whitney CW, Sause W, Bundy BN, et al. Randomized comparison of fluorouracil plus cisplatin versus hydroxyurea as an adjunct to radiation therapy in stage IIB-IVA carcinoma of the cervix with negative para-aortic lymph nodes: a Gynecologic Oncology Group and Southwest Oncology Group study. *J Clin Oncol.* 1999;17:1339-1348. PMID: 10334517.

25. Long HJ 3rd, Bundy BN, Grendys EC Jr, et al. Randomized phase III trial of cisplatin with or without topotecan in carcinoma of the uterine cervix: a Gynecologic Oncology Group Study. *J Clin Oncol.* 2005;23:4626-4633. PMID: 15911865.

26. Moore DH, Blessing JA, McQuellon RP, et al. Phase III study of cisplatin with or without paclitaxel in stage IVB, recurrent, or persistent squamous cell carcinoma of the cervix: a gynecologic oncology group study. *J Clin Oncol.* 2004;22:3113-3119. PMID: 15284262.

27. Tewari KS, Sill MW, Long HJ 3rd, et al. Improved survival with bevacizumab in advanced cervical cancer. *N Engl J Med.* 2014;370:734-743. PMID: 24552320.

28. Siva M, Mahmood R, Kakumanu S, et al. Small cell neuroendocrine carcinoma of uterine cervix: The Scottish experience. *J Clin Oncol.* 2006;24:18s (suppl; abstr 15026).

29. Kurman RJ, Kaminski PF, Norris HJ. The behavior of endometrial hyperplasia. A long-term study of "untreated" hyperplasia in 170 patients. *Cancer.* 1985;56:403-412. PMID: 4005805.

30. Madison T, Schottenfeld D, James SA, et al. Endometrial cancer: socioeconomic status and racial/ethnic differences in stage at diagnosis, treatment, and survival. *Am J Public Health.* 2004;94:2104-2111. PMID: 15569961.

31. Setiawan VW, Yang HP, Pike MC, et al. Type I and II endometrial cancers: have they different risk factors? *J Clin Oncol.* 2013;31:2607-2618. PMID: 23733771.

32. Moore KN, Fader AN. Uterine papillary serous carcinoma. *Clin Obstet Gynecol.* 2011;54:278-291. PMID: 21508697.

33. Cancer Genome Atlas Research Network, Kandoth C, Schultz N, et al. Integrated genomic characterization of endometrial carcinoma. *Nature.* 2013;497:67-73. PMID: 23636398.

34. Bergman L, Beelen ML, Gallee MP, et al. Risk and prognosis of endometrial cancer after tamoxifen for breast cancer. Comprehensive Cancer Centres' ALERT Group. Assessment of Liver and Endometrial cancer Risk following Tamoxifen. *Lancet.* 2000;356:881-887. PMID: 11036892.

35. Fisher B, Costantino JP, Redmond CK, et al. Endometrial cancer in tamoxifen-treated breast cancer patients: findings from the National Surgical Adjuvant Breast and Bowel Project (NSABP) B-14. *J Natl Cancer Inst.* 1994;86:527-537. PMID: 8133536.

36. Barakat RR. Screening for endometrial cancer in the patient receiving tamoxifen for breast cancer. *J Clin Oncol.* 1999;17:1967-1968. PMID: 10561245.

37. Vogel VG, Costantino JP, Wickerham DL, et al. Effects of tamoxifen vs raloxifene on the risk of developing invasive breast cancer and other disease outcomes: the NSABP Study of Tamoxifen and Raloxifene (STAR) P-2 trial. *JAMA.* 2006;295:2727-2741. PMID: 16754727.

38. Aarnio M, Mecklin JP, Aaltonen LA, et al. Life-time risk of different cancers in hereditary non-polyposis colorectal cancer (HNPCC) syndrome. *Int J Cancer.* 1995;64:430-433. PMID: 8550246.

39. Helder-Woolderink JM, De Bock GH, Sijmons RH, et al. The additional value of endometrial sampling in the early detection of endometrial cancer in women with Lynch syndrome. *Gynecol Oncol.* 2013;131:304-308. PMID: 23769810.

40. Colombo N, Preti E, Landoni F, et al. Endometrial cancer: ESMO Clinical Practice Guidelines for diagnosis, treatment and follow-up. *Ann Oncol.* 2011; 22 (suppl 6):vi35–vi39. PMID: 21908501.

41. Leitao MM Jr, Khoury-Collado F, Gardner G, et al. Impact of incorporating an algorithm that utilizes sentinel lymph node mapping during minimally invasive procedures on the detection of stage IIIC endometrial cancer. *Gynecol Oncol.* 2013;129:38-41. PMID: 23321065.

42. Pecorelli S. Revised FIGO staging for carcinoma of the vulva, cervix, and endometrium. *Int J Gynaecol Obstet.* 2009;105:103-104. PMID: 19367689.

43. Keys HM, Roberts JA, Brunetto VL, et al. A phase III trial of surgery with or without adjunctive external pelvic radiation therapy in intermediate risk endometrial adenocarcinoma: a Gynecologic Oncology Group study. *Gyn Oncol.* 2004;92:744-751. PMID: 14984936.

44. Creutzberg CL, van Putten WL, Koper PC, et al. Surgery and postoperative radiotherapy versus surgery alone for patients with stage-1 endometrial carcinoma: multicentre randomised trial. PORTEC Study Group. Post Operative Radiation Therapy in Endometrial Carcinoma. *Lancet.* 2000;355:1404-1411. PMID: 10791524.

45. Nout RA, Smit VT, Putter H, et al. Vaginal brachytherapy versus pelvic external beam radiotherapy for patients with endometrial cancer of high-intermediate risk (PORTEC-2): an open-label, non-inferiority, randomised trial. *Lancet.* 2010;375:816-823. PMID: 20206777.

46. Nout RA, Putter H, Jürgenliemk-Schulz IM, et al. Five-year quality of life of endometrial cancer patients treated in the randomised Post Operative Radiation Therapy in Endometrial Cancer (PORTEC-2) trial and comparison with norm data. *Eur J Cancer.* 2012;48:1638-48. PMID: 22176868.

47. Onsrud M, Cvancarova M, Hellebust TP, et al. Long-term outcomes after pelvic radiation for early-stage endometrial cancer. *J Clin Oncol.* 2013;31:3951-3956. PMID: 24019546.

48. Randall ME, Filiaci VL, Muss H, et al. Randomized phase III trial of whole-abdominal irradiation versus doxorubicin and cisplatin chemotherapy in advanced endometrial carcinoma: a Gynecologic Oncology Group Study. *J Clin Oncol.* 2006;24:36-44. PMID: 16330675.

49. Homesley HD, Filiaci V, Gibbons SK, et al. A randomized phase III trial in advanced endometrial carcinoma of surgery and volume directed radiation followed by cisplatin and doxorubicin with or without paclitaxel: A Gynecologic Oncology Group study. *Gyn Oncol.* 2009;112:543-552. PMID: 19108877.

50. Fiorica JV, Brunetto VL, Hanjani P, et al. Phase II trial of alternating courses of megestrol acetate and tamoxifen in advanced endometrial carcinoma: a Gynecologic Oncology Group study. *Gyn Oncol.* 2004;92:10-14. PMID: 14751131.

51. Thigpen JT, Brady MF, Homesley HD, et al. Phase III trial of doxorubicin with or without cisplatin in advanced endometrial carcinoma: a Gynecologic Oncology Group study. *J Clin Oncol.* 2004;22:3902-3908. PMID: 15459211.

52. Fleming GF, Brunetto VL, Cella D, et al. Phase III trial of doxorubicin plus cisplatin with or without paclitaxel plus filgrastim in advanced endometrial carcinoma: a Gynecologic Oncology Group Study. *J Clin Oncol.* 2004;22:2159-2166. PMID: 15169803.

53. Miller D, Filiaci V, Fleming G, et al. Late-Breaking Abstract 1: Randomized phase III noninferiority trial of first-line chemotherapy for metastatic or recurrent endometrial carcinoma: A Gynecologic Oncology Group study. *Gynecol Oncol.* 2012;125:771.

54. Kanamori Y, Kigawa J, Itamochi H, et al. Correlation between loss of PTEN expression and Akt phosphorylation in endometrial carcinoma. *Clin Cancer Res.* 2001;7:892-895. PMID: 11309338.

55. Oza AM, Elit L, Tsao MS, et al. Phase II study of temsirolimus in women with recurrent or metastatic endometrial cancer: a trial of the NCIC Clinical Trials Group. *J Clin Oncol.* 2011;29:3278-3285. PMID: 21788564.

56. Aghajanian C, Sill MW, Darcy KM, et al. Phase II trial of bevacizumab in recurrent or persistent endometrial cancer: a Gynecologic Oncology Group study. *J Clin Oncol.* 2011;29:2259-2265. PMID: 21537039.

57. Wolfson AH, Brady MF, Rocereto T, et al. A Gynecologic Oncology Group randomized phase III trial of whole abdominal irradiation (WAI) vs. cisplatin-ifosfamide and mesna (CIM) as post-surgical therapy in stage I-IV carcinosarcoma (CS) of the uterus. *Gyn Oncol.* 2007;107:177-185. PMID: 17822748.

58. Homesley HD, Filiaci V, Markman M, et al. Phase III trial of ifosfamide with or without paclitaxel in advanced uterine carcinosarcoma: a Gynecologic Oncology Group Study. *J Clin Oncol.* 2007;25:526-531. PMID: 17290061.

59. Powell MA, Filiaci VL, Rose PG, et al. Phase II evaluation of paclitaxel and carboplatin in the treatment of carcinosarcoma of the uterus: a Gynecologic Oncology Group study. *J Clin Oncol.* 2010;28:2727-2731. PMID: 20421537.

60. Reed NS, Mangioni C, Malmström H, et al. Phase III randomised study to evaluate the role of adjuvant pelvic radiotherapy in the treatment of uterine sarcomas stages I and II: an European Organisation for Research and Treatment of Cancer Gynaecological Cancer Group Study (protocol 55874). *Eur J Cancer.* 2008;44:808-818. PMID: 18378136.

61. Omura GA, Blessing JA, Major F, et al. A randomized clinical trial of adjuvant adriamycin in uterine sarcomas: a Gynecologic Oncology Group Study. *J Clin Oncol.* 1985;3:1240-1245. PMID: 3897471.

62. Hensley ML, Blessing JA, Mannel R, et al. Fixed-dose rate gemcitabine plus docetaxel as first-line therapy for metastatic uterine leiomyosarcoma: a Gynecologic Oncology Group phase II trial. *Gynecol Oncol.* 2008;109:329-334. PMID: 18534250.

63. Hensley ML, Blessing JA, Degeest K, et al. Fixed-dose rate gemcitabine plus docetaxel as second-line therapy for metastatic uterine leiomyosarcoma: a Gynecologic Oncology Group phase II study. *Gyn Oncol.* 2008;109:323-328. PMID: 18394689.

64. Sutton G, Blessing JA, Malfetano JH. Ifosfamide and doxorubicin in the treatment of advanced leiomyosarcomas of the uterus: a Gynecologic Oncology Group study. *Gyn Oncol.* 1996;62:226-229. PMID: 8751554.

65. Hensley ML, Miller A, O'Malley DM, et al. A randomized phase III trial of gemcitabine + docetaxel + bevacizumab or placebo as first-line treatment for metastatic uterine leiomyosarcoma (uLMS): a Gynecologic Oncology Group study (Abstract 1239). Presented at: Society of Gynecologic Oncology 45th Annual Meeting on Women's Cancer; March 2014; Tampa, FL.

66. van der Graaf WT, Blay JY, Chawla SP, et al. Pazopanib for metastatic soft-tissue sarcoma (PALETTE): a randomised, double-blind, placebo-controlled phase 3 trial. *Lancet.* 2012;379:1879-1886. PMID: 22595799.

67. Monk BJ, Blessing JA, Street DG, et al. A phase II evaluation of trabectedin in the treatment of advanced, persistent, or recurrent uterine leiomyosarcoma: a gynecologic oncology group study. *Gynecol Oncol.* 2012;124:48-52. PMID: 21996263.

68. Croce S, Hostein I, Ribeiro A, et al. YWHAE rearrangement identified by FISH and RT-PCR in endometrial stromal sarcomas: genetic and pathological correlations. *Mod Pathol.* 2013;26:1390-1400. PMID: 23599159.

69. Satagopan JM, Boyd J, Kauff ND, et al. Ovarian cancer risk in Ashkenazi Jewish carriers of BRCA1 and BRCA2 mutations. *Clin Cancer Res.* 2002;8:3776-3781. PMID: 12473589.

70. Bonadona V, Bonaïti B, Olschwang S, et al. Cancer risks associated with germline mutations in MLH1, MSH2, and MSH6 genes in Lynch syndrome. *JAMA.* 2011;305:2304-2310. PMID: 21642682.

71. U.S. Preventive Services Task Force. Screening for ovarian cancer: recommendation statement. *Ann Fam Med.* 2004;2:260-262. PMID: 15209204.

72. Buys SS, Partridge E, Black A, et al. Effect of screening on ovarian cancer mortality: the Prostate, Lung, Colorectal and Ovarian (PLCO) Cancer Screening Randomized Controlled Trial. *JAMA.* 2011;305:2295-2303. PMID: 21642681.

73. Burke W, Daly M, Garber J, et al. Recommendations for follow-up care of individuals with inherited predisposition to cancer. II. BRCA1 and BRCA2. Cancer Genetics Studies Consortium. *JAMA.* 1997;277:997-1003. PMID: 9091675.

74. Hensley ML, Robson ME, Kauff ND, et al. Pre- and postmenopausal high-risk women undergoing screening for ovarian cancer: anxiety, risk perceptions, and quality of life. *Gyn Oncol.* 2003;89:440-446. PMID: 12798709.

75. van der Velde NM, Mourits MJ, Arts HJ, et al. Time to stop ovarian cancer screening in BRCA1/2 mutation carriers? *Int J Cancer.* 2009;124:919-923. PMID: 19035463.

76. Meeuwissen PA, Seynaeve C, Brekelmans CT. Outcome of surveillance and prophylactic salpingo-oophorectomy in asymptomatic women at high risk for ovarian cancer. *Gyn Oncol.* 2005;97:476-482. PMID: 15863147.

77. Rebbeck TR, Lynch HT, Neuhausen SL, et al. Prophylactic oophorectomy in carriers of BRCA1 or BRCA2 mutations. *N Engl J Med.* 2002;346:1616-1622. PMID: 12023993.

78. Finch A, Beiner M, Lubinski J, et al. Salpingo-oophorectomy and the risk of ovarian, fallopian tube, and peritoneal cancers in women with a BRCA1 or BRCA2 mutation. *JAMA.* 2006;296:185-192. PMID: 16835424.

79. Rebbeck TR, Kauff ND, Domchek SM. Meta-analsis of risk reduction estimates associated with risk-reducing salpingo-oophorectomy in BRCA1 and BRCA2 mutation carriers. *J Natl Cancer Inst.* 2009;101:80-87. PMID: 19141781.

80. Eisen A, Rebbeck TR, Wood WC, et al. Prophylactic surgery in women with a hereditary predisposition to breast and ovarian cancer. *J Clin Oncol.* 2000;18:1980-1995. PMID: 10784640.

81. Rocca WA, Grossardt BR, de Andrade M, et al. Survival patterns after oophorectomy in premenopausal women: a population-based cohort study. *Lancet Oncol.* 2006;7:821-828. PMID: 17012044.

82. Kauff ND, Domchek SM, Friebel TM, et al. Risk-reducing salpingo-oophorectomy for the prevention of BRCA1- and BRCA2-associated breast and gynecologic cancer: a multicenter, prospective study. *J Clin Oncol.* 2008;26:1331-1337. PMID: 18268356.

83. Vergote I, Tropé CG, Amant F, et al. Neoadjuvant chemotherapy or primary surgery in stage IIIC or IV ovarian cancer. *N Engl J Med.* 2010;363:943-953. PMID: 20818904.

84. van Meurs HS, Tajik P, Hof MH, et al. Which patients benefit most from primary surgery or neoadjuvant chemotherapy in stage IIIC or IV ovarian cancer? An exploratory analysis of the European Organisation for Research and Treatment of Cancer 55971 randomised trial. *Eur J Cancer.* 2013;49:3191-3201. PMID: 23850170.

85. Chi DS, Musa F, Dao F, et al. An analysis of patients with bulky advanced stage ovarian, tubal, and peritoneal carcinoma treated with primary debulking surgery (PDS) during an identical time period as the randomized EORTC-NCIC trial of PDS vs neoadjuvant chemotherapy (NACT). *Gyn Oncol.* 2012;124:10-14. PMID: 21917306.

86. Muñoz KA, Harlan LC, Trimble EL. Patterns of care for women with ovarian cancer in the United States. *J Clin Oncol.* 1997;15:3408-3415. PMID: 9363873.

87. Vang R, Shih IeM, Kurman RJ. Ovarian low-grade and high-grade serous carcinoma: pathogenesis, clinicopathologic and molecular biologic features, and diagnostic problems. *Adv Anat Pathol.* 2009;16:267-282. PMID: 19700937.

88. Boyd J, Sonoda Y, Federici MG, et al. Clinicopathologic features of BRCA-linked and sporadic ovarian cancer. *JAMA.* 2000;283:2260-2265. PMID: 10807385.

89. Buller RE, Shahin MS, Geisler JP, et al. Failure of BRCA1 dysfunction to alter ovarian cancer survival. *Clin Cancer Res.* 2002;8:1196-1202. PMID: 12006538.

90. Young RC, Walton LA, Ellenberg SS, et al. Adjuvant therapy in stage I and II epithelial ovarian cancer. Results of two prospective randomized trials. *N Engl J Med.* 1990;322:1021-1027. PMID: 2181310.

91. Trimbos JB, Parmar M, Vergote I, et al. International Collaborative Ovarian Neoplasm trial 1 and Adjuvant ChemoTherapy in Ovarian Neoplasm trial: two parallel randomized phase III trials of adjuvant chemotherapy in patients with early-stage ovarian carcinoma. *J Natl Cancer Inst.* 2003;95:105-112. PMID: 12529343.

92. Colombo N, Guthrie D, Chiari S, et al. International Collaborative Ovarian Neoplasm trial 1: a randomized trial of adjuvant chemotherapy in women with early-stage ovarian cancer. *J Natl Cancer Inst.* 2003;95:125-132. PMID: 12529345.

93. Mannel RS, Brady MF, Kohn EC, et al. A randomized phase III trial of IV carboplatin and paclitaxel × 3 courses followed by observation versus weekly maintenance low-dose paclitaxel in patients with early-stage ovarian carcinoma: a Gynecologic Oncology Group Study. *Gyn Oncol.* 2011;122:89-94. PMID: 21529904.

94. Covens A, Carey M, Bryson P, et al. Systematic review of first-line chemotherapy for newly diagnosed postoperative patients with stage II, III, or IV epithelial ovarian cancer. *Gyn Oncol.* 2002;85:71-80. PMID: 11925123.

95. Muggia FM, Braly PS, Brady MF, et al. Phase III randomized study of cisplatin versus paclitaxel versus cisplatin and paclitaxel in patients with suboptimal stage III or IV ovarian cancer: a Gynecologic Oncology Group study. *J Clin Oncol.* 2000;18:106-115. PMID: 10623700.

96. International Collaborative Ovarian Neoplasm Group. Paclitaxel plus carboplatin versus standard chemotherapy with single-agent carboplatin or cyclophosphamide, doxorubicin, and cisplatin in women with ovarian cancer: the ICON3 randomised trial. *Lancet.* 2002;360:505-515. PMID: 12241653.

97. Piccart MJ, Bertelsen K, James K, et al. Randomized intergroup trial of cisplatin-paclitaxel versus cisplatin-cyclophosphamide in women with advanced epithelial ovarian cancer: three-year results. *J Natl Cancer Inst.* 2000;92:699-708. PMID: 10793106.

98. Cannistra SA, Matulonis UA, Penson RT, et al. Phase II study of bevacizumab in patients with platinum-resistant ovarian cancer or peritoneal serous cancer. *J Clin Oncol.* 2007;25:5180-5186. PMID: 18024865.

99. Burger RA, Sill MW, Monk BJ, et al. Phase II trial of bevacizumab in persistent or recurrent epithelial ovarian cancer or primary peritoneal cancer: a Gynecologic Oncology Group Study. *J Clin Oncol.* 2007;25:5165-5171. PMID: 18024863.

100. Burger RA, Brady MF, Bookman MA, et al. Phase III trial of bevacizumab (BEV) in the primary treatment of advanced epithelial ovarian cancer (EOC), primary peritoneal cancer (PPC), or fallopian tube cancer (FTC): a Gynecologic Oncology Group study. *J Clin Oncol.* 2010;28:18s (suppl; abstr LBA1).

101. Stark D, Nankivell M, Pujade-Lauraine E, et al. Standard chemotherapy with or without bevacizumab in advanced ovarian cancer: quality-of-life outcomes from the International Collaboration on Ovarian Neoplasms (ICON7) phase 3 randomised trial. *Lancet Oncol.* 2013;14:236-243. PMID: 23333117.

102. Katsumata N, Yasuda M, Takahashi F, et al. Dose-dense paclitaxel once a week in combination with carboplatin every 3 weeks for advanced ovarian cancer: a phase 3, open-label, randomised controlled trial. *Lancet.* 2009;374:1331-1338. PMID: 19767092.

103. Pignata S, Scambia G, Ferrandina G, et al. Carboplatin plus paclitaxel versus carboplatin plus pegylated liposomal doxorubicin as first-line treatment for patients with ovarian cancer: the MITO-2 randomized phase III trial. *J Clin Oncol.* 2011;29:3628-3635. PMID: 21844495.

104. Rustin GJ, van der Burg ME, Griffin CL, et al. Early versus delayed treatment of relapsed ovarian cancer (MRC OV05/EORTC 55955): a randomized trial. *Lancet.* 2010;376:1155-1163. PMID: 20888993.

105. Alberts DS, Liu PY, Hannigan EV, et al. Intraperitoneal cisplatin plus intravenous cyclophosphamide versus intravenous cisplatin plus intravenous cyclophosphamide for stage III ovarian cancer. *N Engl J Med.* 1996;335:1950-1955. PMID: 8960474.

106. Markman M, Bundy BN, Alberts DS, et al. Phase III trial of standard-dose intravenous cisplatin plus paclitaxel versus moderately high-dose carboplatin followed by intravenous paclitaxel and intraperitoneal cisplatin in small-volume stage III ovarian carcinoma: an intergroup study of the Gynecologic Oncology Group, Southwestern Oncology Group, and Eastern Cooperative Oncology Group. *J Clin Oncol.* 2001;19:1001-1007. PMID: 11181662.

107. Armstrong DK, Bundy B, Wenzel L, et al. Intraperitoneal cisplatin and paclitaxel in ovarian cancer. *N Engl J Med.* 2006;354:34-43. PMID: 16394300.

108. Wenzel LB, Huang HQ, Armstrong DK. Health-related quality of life during and after intraperitoneal versus intravenous chemotherapy for optimally debulked ovarian cancer: a Gynecologic Oncology Group Study. *J Clin Oncol.* 2007;25:437-443. PMID: 17264340.

109. van der Burg ME, van Lent M, Buyse M, et al. The effect of debulking surgery after induction chemotherapy on the prognosis in advanced epithelial ovarian cancer. Gynecological Cancer Cooperative Group of the European Organization for Research and Treatment of Cancer. *N Engl J Med.* 1995;332:629-634. PMID: 7845426.

110. Rose PG, Nerenstone S, Brady MF, et al. Secondary surgical cytoreduction for advanced ovarian carcinoma. *N Engl J Med.* 2004;351:2489-2497. PMID: 15590951.

111. Barakat RR, Sabbatini P, Bhaskaran D, et al. Intraperitoneal chemotherapy for ovarian carcinoma: results of long-term follow-up. *J Clin Oncol.* 2002;20:694-698. PMID: 11821450.

112. Rubin SC, Hoskins WJ, Hakes TB, et al. Recurrence after negative second-look laparotomy for ovarian cancer: analysis of risk factors. *Am J Obstet Gynecol.* 1988;159:1094-1098. PMID: 3189442.

113. Markman M, Liu PY, Wilczynski S, et al. Phase III randomized trial of 12 versus 3 months of maintenance paclitaxel in patients with advanced ovarian cancer after complete response to platinum and paclitaxel-based chemotherapy: a Southwest Oncology Group and Gynecologic Oncology Group trial. *J Clin Oncol.* 2003;2:2460-2465. PMID: 12829663.

114. Vergote IB, Jimeno A, Joly F, et al. Randomized phase III study of erlotinib versus observation in patients with no evidence of disease progression after first-line platin-based chemotherapy for ovarian carcinoma: a European Organisation for Research and Treatment of Cancer-Gynaecological Cancer Group, and Gynecologic Cancer Intergroup study. *J Clin Oncol.* 2014;32:320-326. PMID: 24366937.

115. De Placido S, Scambia G, Di Vagno G, et al. Topotecan compared with no therapy after response to surgery and carboplatin/paclitaxel in patients with ovarian cancer: Multicenter Italian Trials in Ovarian Cancer (MITO-1) randomized study. *J Clin Oncol.* 2004;22:2635-2642. PMID: 15226331.

116. Parmar MK, Ledermann JA, Colombo N, et al. Paclitaxel plus platinum-based chemotherapy versus conventional platinum-based chemotherapy in women with relapsed ovarian cancer: the OCON4/AGO-OVAR-2.2 trial. *Lancet.* 2003;361:2099-2106. PMID: 12826431.

117. Pfisterer J, Plante M, Vergote I, et al. Gemcitabine plus carboplatin compared with carboplatin in patients with platinum-sensitive recurrent ovarian cancer: an intergroup trial of the AGO-OVAR, the NCIC CTG, and the EORTC GCG. *J Clin Oncol.* 2006;24:4699-4707. PMID: 16966687.

118. Pujade-Lauraine E, Wagner U, Aavall-Lundqvist E, et al. Pegylated liposomal doxorubicin and carboplatin compared with paclitaxel and carboplatin for patients with platinum-sensitive ovarian cancer in late relapse. *J Clin Oncol.* 2010;28:3323-3329. PMID: 20498395.

119. Aghajanian C, Blank SV, Goff BA, et al. OCEANS: a randomized, double-blind, placebo-controlled phase III trial of chemotherapy with or without bevacizumab in patients with platinum-sensitive recurrent epithelial ovarian, primary peritoneal, or fallopian tube cancer. *J Clin Oncol.* 2012;30:2039-2045. PMID: 22529265.

120. Ledermann J, Harter P, Gourley C, et al. Olaparib maintenance therapy in platinum-sensitive relapsed ovarian cancer. *N Engl J Med.* 2012;366:1382-1392. PMID: 22452356.

121. Markman M. The dilemma of carboplatin-associated hypersensitivity reactions in ovarian cancer management. *Gyn Oncol.* 2007;107:163-165. PMID: 17675141.

122. Sood AK, Gelder MS, Huang SW, et al. Anaphylaxis to carboplatin following multiple previous uncomplicated courses. *Gyn Oncol.* 1995;57:131-132. PMID: 7705695.

123. O'Cearbhaill R, Zhou Q, Iasonos A, et al. The prophylactic conversion to an extended infusion schedule and use of premedication to prevent hypersensitivity reactions in ovarian cancer patients during carboplatin retreatment. *Gynecol Oncol.* 2010;116:326-331. PMID: 19944454.

124. Markman M, Bookman MA. Second-line treatment of ovarian cancer. *Oncologist.* 2000;5:26-35. PMID: 10706647.

125. Pujade-Lauraine E, Hilpert F, Weber B, et al. AURELIA: A randomized phase III trial evaluating bevacizumab (BEV) plus chemotherapy (CT) for platinum (PT)-resistant recurrent ovarian cancer (OC). *J Clin Oncol.* 2012;30:18s (suppl; abstr LBA5002).

126. Fong PC, Boss DS, Yap TA, et al. Inhibition of poly(ADP-ribose) polymerase in tumors from BRCA mutation carriers. *N Engl J Med.* 2009;361:123-134. PMID: 19553641.

127. Gelmon KA, Tischkowitz M, Mackay H, et al. Olaparib in patients with recurrent high-grade serous or poorly differentiated ovarian carcinoma or triple-negative breast cancer: a phase 2, multicentre, open-label, non-randomised study. *Lancet Oncol.* 2011;12:852-861. PMID: 21862407.

128. Ledermann J, Harter P, Gourley C, et al. Olaparib maintenance therapy in platinum-sensitive relapsed ovarian cancer. *N Engl J Med.* 2012;366:1382-1392. PMID: 22452356.

129. Farley J , Brady WE, Vathipadiekal V, et al. Selumetinib in women with recurrent low-grade serous carcinoma of the ovary or peritoneum: an open-label, single-arm, phase 2 study. *Lancet Oncol.* 2013;14:134-140. PMID: 23261356.

130. Kennedy AW, Hart WR. Ovarian papillary serous tumors of low malignant potential (serous borderline tumors). A long-term follow-up study, including patients with microinvasion, lymph node metastasis, and transformation to invasive serous carcinoma. *Cancer.* 1996;78:278-286. PMID: 8674004.

131. Longacre TA, McKenney JK, Tazelaar HD, et al. Ovarian serous tumors of low malignant potential (borderline tumors): outcome-based study of 276 patients with long-term (> or =5-year) follow-up. *Am J Surg Pathol.* 2005;29:707-723. PMID: 15897738.

132. Schumer ST, Cannistra SA. Granulosa cell tumor of the ovary. *J Clin Oncol.* 2003;21:1180-1189. PMID: 12637488.

133. Thrall MM, Paley P, Pizer E, et al. Patterns of spread and recurrence of sex cord-stromal tumors of the ovary. *Gyn Oncol.* 2011;122:242-245. PMID: 21481441.

134. Colombo N, Parma G, Zanagnolo V, et al. Management of ovarian stromal cell tumors. *J Clin Oncol.* 2007;25:2944-2951. PMID: 17617526.

135. Homesley, HD, Bundy BN, Hurteau JA et al. Bleomycin, etoposide, and cis-platin combination therapy of ovarian granulosa cell tumors and other stromal malignancies: A Gynecologic Oncology Group study. *Gyn Oncol.* 1999;72:131-137. PMID: 10021290.

136. Williams S, Blessing JA, Liao SY, et al. Adjuvant therapy of ovarian germ cell tumors with cisplatin, etoposide, and bleomycin: a trial of the Gynecologic Oncology Group. *J Clin Oncol.* 1994;12:701-706. PMID: 7512129.

137. Gershenson DM. Menstrual and reproductive function after treatment with combination chemotherapy for malignant ovarian germ cell tumors. *J Clin Oncol.* 1988;6:270-275. PMID: 2828558.

138. Brewer M, Gershenson DM, Herzog CE, et al. Outcome and reproductive function after chemotherapy for ovarian dysgerminoma. *J Clin Oncol.* 1999;17:2670-2675. PMID: 10561340.

139. Tangir J, Zelterman D, Ma W, et al. Reproductive function after conservative surgery and chemotherapy for malignant germ cell tumors of the ovary. *Obstet Gynecol.* 2003;101:251-257. PMID: 12576247.

140. World Health Organization. *Gestational Trophoblastic Diseases. Report of a WHO Scientific Group.* Technical Report Series No. 692. Geneva: World Health Organization; 1983.

141. Lurain JR, Casanova LA, Miller DS, et al. Prognostic factors in gestational trophoblastic tumors: a proposed new scoring system based on multivariate analysis. *Am J Obstet Gynecol.* 1991;164:611. PMID: 1847005.

142. Homesley HD, Blessing JA, Schlaerth J, et al. Rapid escalation of weekly intramuscular methotrexate for nonmetastatic gestational trophoblastic disease: a Gynecologic Oncology Group study. *Gyn Oncol.* 1990;39:305-308. PMID: 2175286.

143. Petrilli ES, Twiggs LB, Blessing JA, et al. Single-dose actinomycin-D treatment for nonmetastatic gestational trophoblastic disease. A prospective phase II trial of the Gynecologic Oncology Group. *Cancer.* 1990;60:2173-2176. PMID: 2449942.

144. Wong LC, Choo YC, Ma HK. Primary oral etoposide therapy in gestational trophoblastic disease. An update. *Cancer.* 1986;58:14-17. PMID: 3011237.

145. Newlands ES, Bagshawe KD, Begent RH, et al. Results with the EMA/CO (etoposide, methotrexate, actinomycin D, cyclophosphamide, vincristine) regimen in high risk gestational trophoblastic tumours, 1979 to 1989. *Br J Obstet Gynaecol.* 1991;98:550-557. PMID: 1651757.

146. Gadducci A, Cionini L, Romanini A, et al. Old and new perspectives in the management of high-risk, locally advanced or recurrent, and metastatic vulvar cancer. *Crit Rev Oncol Hematol.* 2006;60:227-241. PMID: 16945551.

147. Montana GS, Thomas GM, Moore DH, et al. Preoperative chemo-radiation for carcinoma of the vulva with N2/N3 nodes: a gynecologic oncology group study. *Int J Radiat Oncol Biol Phys.* 2000;48:1007-1013. PMID: 11072157.

148. Mahner S, Jueckstock JK, Hilpert F, et al. Impact of adjuvant therapy in lymph-node positive vulvar cancer. The AGO CARE 1 study. *J Clin Oncol.* 2012;30s: (suppl; abstr 5007).

149. Daling JR, Madeleine MM, Schwartz SM, et al. A population-based study of squamous cell vaginal cancer: HPV and cofactors. *Gynecol Oncol.* 2002;84:263-270. PMID: 11812085.

150. Benedetti Panici P, Bellati F, Plotti F, et al. Neoadjuvant chemotherapy followed by radical surgery in patients with vaginal carcinoma. *Gynecol Oncol.* 2008;111:307-311. PMID: 18708243.

151. Dalrymple JL, Russell AH, Lee SW, et al. Chemoradiation for primary invasive squamous carcinoma of the vagina. *Int J Gynecol Cancer.* 2004;14:110-117. PMID: 14764038.

12

MALIGNANT MELANOMA

Lynn M. Schuchter, MD

Updates from 2012

▶ Dabrafenib, a highly selective and effective BRAF inhibitor, was approved by the U.S. Food and Drug Administration (FDA) for the treatment of unresectable stage III and stage IV melanoma with *BRAF V600* mutation in 2013 (Ascierto P, *J Clin Oncol* 2013; Hauschild A, *Lancet* 2012).

▶ Trametinib, a MEK inhibitor, was approved by the FDA for the treatment of advanced *BRAF V600E-* or *V600K*-mutant melanoma in 2013 (Flaherty KT, *N Engl J Med* 2012).

▶ Combination therapy with dabrafenib and trametinib for *BRAF*-mutant melanoma was approved by the FDA for patients with metastatic melanoma (Flaherty KT, *N Engl J Med* 2012).

▶ Encouraging results with anti-programmed cell death (PD)-1 and anti-programmed death-ligand (PD-L)-1 antibodies have been reported for patients with metastatic melanoma (Brahmer JR, *N Engl J Med* 2012; Hamid O, *N Engl J Med* 2013).

Current estimates indicate that one out of every 37 men and one out of every 56 women will be diagnosed with melanoma in their lifetime. In the United States in 2013, approximately 76,690 new cases of invasive melanoma were diagnosed, and 9,480 patients died from melanoma.[1] The incidence of melanoma continues to increase, with a tripling in the incidence during the past 20 years.[2] Melanoma is the leading cause of death from cutaneous malignancies and accounts for 1% to 2% of all cancer deaths in the United States. Melanoma affects all age groups; the median age at diagnosis is 50.

RISK FACTORS AND GENETICS OF MELANOMA

Risk factors for developing melanoma are both environmental and genetic. Exposure to sunlight (ultraviolet [UV] radiation) has been strongly implicated as a causative factor in the development of melanoma. Ultraviolet B (UVB) radiation appears to be more closely associated with the development of melanoma than ultraviolet A (UVA) radiation. The rates of melanoma are higher for patients with a tendency to burn rather than tan when exposed to sunlight. The pattern of sun exposure may also be important. Intermittent intense exposure and sunburns in areas exposed to the sun only sporadically (e.g., the back for men and the legs for women), rather than chronic exposure, may carry more risk for melanoma. Blistering sunburns, particularly in childhood, are associated with an increased risk for melanoma. However, melanoma can occur in any ethnic group and without significant sun exposure. There is growing evidence that the use of tanning beds increases the risk for melanoma. In 2009, the World Health Organization International Agency for Research on Cancer classified UV light emitted from tanning beds as a human carcinogen based on evidence from multiple studies.

High nevus counts and atypical nevi (dysplastic nevi) are also strongly associated with melanoma.[3] The proportion of melanomas that develop from melanocytic nevi ranges from 18% to 85%. Dysplastic nevi are important precursor lesions of melanoma and also serve as markers for increasing risk. The presence of dysplastic nevi is associated with a 6% lifetime chance of melanoma. This risk is as high as 80% for patients who have dysplastic nevi and a family history of melanoma. Phenotypic traits associated with melanoma risk include skin pigmentation, hair color (red or blond), freckles, and light eye color (blue, green, or hazel). Other risk factors for melanoma include a personal history of the disease, nonmelanoma skin cancers, immunosuppression, and xeroderma pigmentosum.

HEREDITARY BASIS OF MELANOMA: GENES INVOLVED IN MELANOMA SUSCEPTIBILITY

Approximately 10% of cutaneous melanoma is hereditary and known to involve germ-line mutations in highly penetrant autosomal-dominant genes. Several genetic loci determine susceptibility to melanoma, the most important of these being *p16/CDKN2A*, a gene located on chromosome 9p21. *CDKN2A* gene encodes two proteins, p16 and p14ARF, which are cell-cycle inhibitors. Of the members of melanoma-prone families, 25% to 40% have mutations in this gene. A few rare kindreds have mutations in *CDK4*. The risk for developing cutaneous melanoma in an individual who is a *CDKN2A* carrier is between 30% and 90% by age 80 and varies by geographic location.[4] Some familial melanoma occurs in the setting of the familial atypical multiple mole and melanoma syndrome, also called the dysplastic nevus syndrome. A family history of melanoma in multiple first-degree relatives and younger age at diagnosis are important features of this syndrome. As many as 10% of patients with multiple primary melanomas have been found to have a *CDKN2A* mutation. Pancreas cancer is also seen in melanoma-prone families with *CDKN2A* germ-line mutations. Testing for mutations in the *p16/CDKN2A* locus is available on a commercial basis. However, the clinical utility of genetic testing for melanoma susceptibility is limited at this time. Other genes that predispose to melanoma include xeroderma pigmentosum, a rare inherited disorder in which DNA repair mechanisms are compromised. In addition, carriers of the *BRCA2* gene have an increased risk for cutaneous melanoma. Melanocortin-1 receptor *(MC1R)* is one of the primary genes that regulate skin color; patients with *MC1R* variants are at increased risk for developing melanoma.[5] At this time, diligent skin exams by trained physicians, as well as educating patients in skin self-exam, remains the standard of care for patients, even in high-risk families. Recently, germ-line mutations in *BAP1* have been described in several kindreds of familial uveal melanoma.[6]

GENES INVOLVED IN SPORADIC MELANOMA

A number of somatic genetic changes have been described in primary melanomas, which are summarized in Table 12-1.[7,8] The *BRAF* oncogene is the most common somatic mutation in melanoma, present in approximately 50% to 60% of tumors.[9] Although more than 60 mutations have been mapped in *BRAF*,

Table 12-1 Molecular Alterations in Melanoma

Oncogene	Frequency
BRAF	50%; Some association with superficial spreading melanoma
NRAS	15% to 20%
c-KIT	10%; Acral, mucosal, lentigo maligna melanoma
GNAQ/GNA11	50%; Uveal melanoma

a valine to glutamic acid change at codon 600 (*V600E* mutation) occurs in more than 80% of cases, locking the kinase into an active conformation. Immediately upstream of *BRAF* is *NRAS*, which is mutated and activated in 15% to 20% of melanomas. Mutations of both *NRAS* and *BRAF* rarely occur together. Melanomas with somatic mutations of either *NRAS* or *BRAF* may be associated with poorer prognosis. Molecular alterations in melanoma have been linked with subtypes of melanoma, anatomic location, and sun exposure. For example, activating mutations in *BRAF* are more common in melanomas occurring in skin that has little chronic sun-induced damage and are less frequent in melanomas associated with severe chronic solar damage. *BRAF* mutation is also associated with younger age of onset of melanoma. Studies found that melanomas on mucosal membranes, acral skin (i.e., soles, palms, and nail beds), and skin with chronic sun-induced damage (i.e., lentigo maligna melanoma) have frequent mutations in *KIT*,[10] and these types of melanoma lack mutation in *BRAF* or *NRAS* (although *BRAF* and *NRAS* mutations can be found rarely in these subtypes, supporting the need for genotyping). Microphthalmia-associated transcription factor *(MITF)*, the master regulator of melanocyte differentiation, has also been identified as an oncogene in melanoma. Activation of the phosphoinositide 3-kinase (PI3K) pathway in melanoma is common; one of its main mechanisms is loss of PTEN through inactivating missense mutations or allele deletion. Recent studies have shown that uveal melanoma is associated with mutations in *GNAQ/GNA11*. Monosomy of chromosome 3 has been associated with the development of metastatic disease and poor overall survival (OS) in patients with uveal melanoma.[11] In addition, somatic mutations in the gene encoding BRCA1-associated protein (BAP) on chromosome 3 have been associated with worse

KEY POINTS

- Risk factors for melanoma include dysplastic (atypical) nevi, an increased number of benign nevi, family history of melanoma, and fair skin that burns.
- Germ-line mutation in the *p16* gene is the most common cause of familial or inherited melanoma.
- Approximately 50% of melanomas have a somatic *BRAF* mutation.

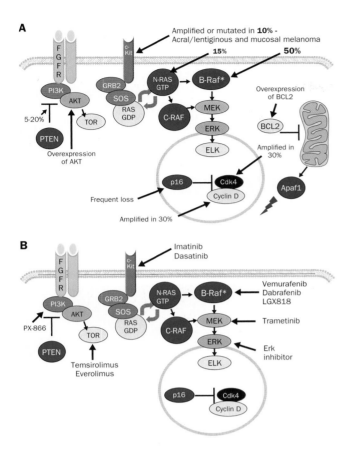

Fig. 12-1 Molecular alterations (A) and examples of targeted therapies (B) in melanoma.

outcome.[12] The discovery of somatic genetic mutations and underlying aberrant signal transduction has provided leads for the development of molecularly targeted therapy for patients with advanced melanoma.[13,14] Figure 12-1 summarizes the signaling pathways and examples of targeted therapies in melanoma.

PREVENTION AND SCREENING

The most important melanoma preventive measures are to reduce excessive sun exposure and avoid sunburns. Strategies to reduce exposure include avoiding the midday sun, using sunscreen products with a sun protection factor (SPF) higher than 15 on a regular basis, and wearing protective clothing. Although data show that sunscreens may prevent nonmelanoma skin cancer, it has been difficult to prove that regular use of sunscreen protects against melanoma. There is recent evidence from an Australian community-based clinical trial that the regular use of sunscreen may prevent the development of melanoma.[15] Tools for ascertaining risk for melanoma have been developed. The Melanoma Risk Assessment Tool is available online through the National Cancer Institute (NCI; www.cancer.gov/melanomarisktool). This tool helps clinicians identify individuals at increased risk for melanoma in order to plan appropriate screening interventions.

Screening for skin cancer, whether by self-examination or by a health care provider, is a controversial area. No randomized

trials have established the efficacy of clinician screening for melanoma. However, patients with clinically atypical nevi or an increased number of nevi, particularly if they have a family history of melanoma, require a regular surveillance program by a clinician who has had appropriate training to identify melanoma. Regular skin examinations should be performed every 6 to 12 months and can be supplemented with photographs of the atypical nevi.

CLINICAL PRESENTATION AND DIAGNOSIS

Early detection and recognition of melanoma is important to improving OS of patients with melanoma. The signs of early melanoma are based on the clinical appearance of the pigmented lesion in addition to a history of change in an existing mole, including change in shape, color, or surface. More than 70% of melanomas are associated with an increase in size and a change in color of a pigmented lesion. Most patients report having a pre-existing mole at the site of the melanoma. Itching, burning, or pain in a pigmented lesion should increase suspicion, although melanomas often are not associated with local discomfort. Bleeding and ulceration are signs of a more advanced melanoma. Most melanomas are varying shades of brown, but they also may be black, blue, or pink. The "ABCDEs" for the recognition of melanoma are asymmetry, border, color, diameter, and evolution. The "ugly duckling" sign is recognizing a pigmented lesion that looks different from other surrounding lesions and, therefore, suspicious. Handheld instruments for skin-surface microscopy (dermoscopy) or epiluminescence microscopy are now available, and may aid clinicians in more reliably differentiating between benign and malignant skin lesions.

A biopsy should be performed on any skin lesion suspicious for melanoma. The proper biopsy is essential not only to establish a diagnosis, but also to allow precise histologic interpretation that will determine the prognosis and plan of therapy. For most clinically suspicious skin lesions, complete excision with a 1-mm to 2-mm margin of normal skin is best. Shallow shave biopsy or curettage is contraindicated for lesions suspicious for melanoma.

Cutaneous melanoma has been divided into four subtypes based on distinct clinical and histologic features. In descending order of frequency, these are superficial spreading melanoma, nodular melanoma, lentigo maligna melanoma, and acral lentiginous melanoma (Table 12-2 and Figs. 12-2 to 12-6). Histologic subtype does not directly correlate with clinical behavior; however, data suggest that histologic subtype may correlate with specific genetic abnormalities. For example, lentigo maligna melanoma may be more commonly associated with a mutation in *cKIT*.[10] Primary melanomas also can occur from mucosal epithelial cells lining the respiratory, alimentary, and genitourinary tracts, although such melanomas are rare. Ocular melanomas arise from the pigmented layer of the eye that includes the iris, ciliary body, and choroid; these lesions are referred to as uveal melanomas. Uveal melanoma is the most common primary intraocular malignancy in adults.

During the past decade, critical molecular alterations have been identified (Table 12-1) and these oncogenic mutations

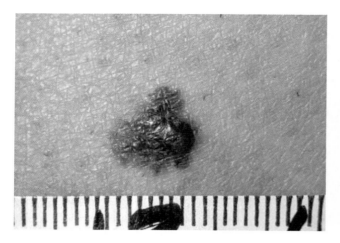

Fig. 12-2 Superficial spreading melanoma.

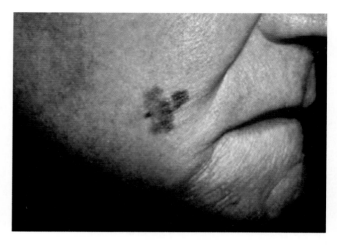

Fig. 12-3 Lentigo malignant melanoma.

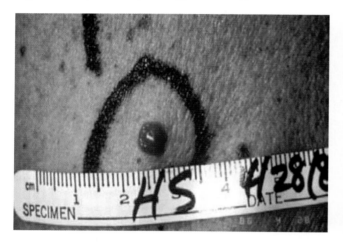

Fig. 12-4 Nodular melanoma.

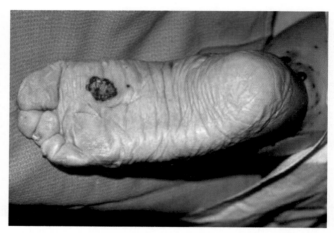

Fig. 12-5 Acral lentiginous melanoma with in-transit metastases.

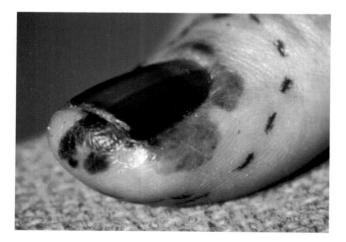

Fig. 12-6 Acral lentiginous melanoma.

in melanoma are now being exploited as therapeutic targets. Going forward, it will be necessary to modify the traditional clinicopathologic classification for melanoma by incorporating the new understanding of the molecular pathogenesis of melanoma.[16,17]

KEY POINTS

- A history of recent change in a pigmented lesion or a new pigmented lesion should alert the clinician that a biopsy is needed. Changes in size, color, and border are important clues to the diagnosis of melanoma.
- "Ugly duckling" sign is a pigmented lesion that looks different from other lesions.

PROGNOSTIC FACTORS

A number of clinical and pathologic factors have been identified that influence the probability of survival of a patient with melanoma. The most important prognostic factors for patients with localized melanoma are tumor thickness, mitotic rate, and presence or absence of ulceration. These factors have been incorporated in the seventh (2010) edition of the American Joint Committee on Cancer (AJCC) staging system.[18] The single most predictive factor is the depth of invasion (Breslow thickness) of the original lesion, measured in millimeters from the uppermost

| Table 12-2 | **Four Histologic Subtypes of Cutaneous Melanoma** |

Superficial Spreading Melanoma (Fig. 12-2)

- Incidence: Accounts for 70% of all melanomas, tends to occur in young patients (median age, 50)
- Anatomic site: Any, predominantly trunk and extremities, anatomic sites associated with intermittent sun exposure
- Clinical appearance: Change in the appearance of a large mole, asymmetry, irregular border, variegated color (brown, black, pink, white, gray, and blue), often arising in a precursor mole
- Can be associated with *BRAF* mutation

Lentigo Maligna Melanoma (Fig. 12-3)

- Incidence: Accounts for 4% to 10% of all melanoma; tends to occur more commonly in older patients
- Anatomic site: Areas with chronic exposure to the sun, head and neck regions, and distal extremities
- Clinical appearance: Macular (flat) lesion, arising in a lentigo maligna, which often appears as a flat, light brown skin lesion
- Can be associated with mutation in *c-KIT*

Nodular Melanoma (Fig. 12-4)

- Incidence: Accounts for 15% of melanomas
- Anatomic site: Any
- Clinical appearance: Rapidly enlarging, elevated, or polypoid lesion, often arising in normal skin, often blue, black, or pink as can be amelanotic (The A-B-C-D-E rule does not apply*)

Acral Lentiginous Melanoma (Figs. 12-5 and 12-6)

- Incidence: 5% to 10%
- Anatomic site: Most commonly on the palms, soles, or subungual (under the nail bed)
- Clinical appearance: Darkly pigmented, flat to nodular lesion, highly irregular borders
- Can be associated with *c-KIT* mutation

*The A-B-C-D-E rule is defined as the following: A, asymmetry; B, border (irregular); C, color (heterogeneous, variegated); D, diameter greater than 5 mm; and E, evolution.

Adapted with permission from Balch CM, Buzaid AC, Soong S-J, et al. Final version of the American Joint Committee on Cancer staging system for cutaneous melanoma. J Clin Oncol. 2001;19:3635–3648. PMID: 11504745.

layer of the epidermis to the deepest melanoma cell in the underlying dermis. Increasing thickness is associated with a higher risk for recurrence of melanoma and, therefore, death (Table 12-3). In addition, the thicker the primary melanoma, the more likely there is microscopic involvement of regional lymph nodes. Ulcerated melanomas are associated with a poorer prognosis.

Mitotic count has been identified as an independent predictor of survival for primary melanoma. In multivariate analysis, the mitotic count was the second most important prognostic factor after thickness of the primary tumor.[19,20] The mitotic count should be assessed in all primary melanomas. The recommended approach to determining the mitotic count is to identify the area of the dermis containing the most mitoses and then count the number of mitoses within 1 mm². Other poor prognostic factors include increasing level of invasion (Clark

level), lack of tumor-infiltrating lymphocytes (TILs), and presence of microscopic satellites. Primary tumor location, patient age, and sex are clinical variables associated with prognosis. In general, patients with primary melanoma of the extremities have a significantly better clinical prognosis than those with primary lesions of the trunk and head. Increased patient age and male sex is associated with a worse outcome. The involvement of regional lymph nodes is a poor prognostic sign, regardless of the primary tumor thickness. In addition, the number of involved lymph nodes correlates with the risk for distant metastatic disease and, therefore, survival. Patients with one regional lymph node involved have an approximately 40% to 50% risk for systemic recurrence. Patients with multiple lymph nodes involved have a 75% risk for systemic recurrence. Ongoing studies are exploring the effect of somatic mutation status of the primary melanoma (*BRAF*, *NRAS*, etc.) on outcome or OS.

STAGING SYSTEM

The tumor/node/metastasis (TNM) staging system for melanoma, which was developed by the AJCC and updated in 2010, now more accurately classifies patients into groups with similar survival (Table 12-3).[18] Stages I and II melanoma indicate clinically localized primary melanoma to the skin, and stage III melanoma indicates regional involvement (lymph nodes or in-transit metastases). Stage IV is metastatic disease beyond regional lymph nodes (i.e., lung, liver, and brain). The T categories (primary tumor) are subdivided into "a" or "b" based upon the presence or absence of ulceration and the mitotic count. The 5-year survival rates associated with each of the four stages are noted in the staging system in Table 12-3. About 80% of patients with melanoma present with localized disease (stage I or II); 15% present with regional lymph node disease (stage III); and 5% present with distant metastatic disease.

PATIENT EVALUATION

The initial evaluation of a patient with melanoma includes taking personal and family histories and conducting an appropriate physical examination, including a total skin examination and palpation of regional (draining) lymph nodes. The focus of this evaluation is to identify risk factors, signs or symptoms of metastases, dysplastic nevi, and additional primary melanomas. The extent of the work-up for patients with the initial diagnosis of melanoma is based on the risk for recurrence associated with the primary melanoma. In general, for low-risk melanomas (i.e., less than 1.0 mm thick, low mitotic count, and no ulceration) no further search for occult metastatic disease is indicated. In patients with higher-risk primary melanomas, a chest x-ray, liver function tests, and measurement of lactate dehydrogenase often are performed; however, there are no data to support this common practice. A more extensive staging evaluation with computed tomography (CT) alone or in combination with positron emission tomography (PET) scans of the chest, abdomen, or pelvis can be considered for patients with thick primary melanomas (larger than 4 mm, high-risk stage II melanoma) or node-positive disease (stage III melanoma) for whom the risk for distant metastatic disease is greater. Again, there are no data to support this

Table 12-3 **American Joint Committee on Cancer Staging System for Cutaneous Melanoma**

Stage	TNM Classification	Definition	5-Year Survival Rate, % ± SE
IA	T1a N0 M0	≤ 1 mm; no ulceration and mitotic rate < 1 mitosis/mm^2	95.3 ± 0.4
IB	T1b N0 M0	≤ 1 mm with ulceration or mitotic rate > 1 mitosis/mm^2	90.9 ± 1.0
	T2a N0 M0	1.01 to 2 mm; no ulceration	89.0 ± 0.7
IIA	T2b N0 M0	1.01 to 2 mm with ulceration	77.4 ± 1.7
	T3a N0 M0	2.01 to 4 mm; no ulceration	78.7 ± 1.2
IIB	T3b N0 M0	2.01 to 4 mm with ulceration	63.0 ± 1.5
	T4a N0 M0	> 4 mm; no ulceration	67.4 ± 2.4
IIC	T4b N0 M0	> 4 mm with ulceration	45.1 ± 1.9
IIIA	T1-4a N1a M0	Single nodal micrometastasis; no ulceration	69.5 ± 3.7
	T1-4a N2a M0	2 to 3 nodal micrometastases; no ulceration	63.3 ± 5.6
IIIB	T1-4a N1b-2c M0	1 to 3 nodal macrometastases or in-transit metastases; no ulceration	40 – 60
	T1-4b N1a-2a M0	1 to 3 nodal micrometastases; ulceration	40 – 55
IIIC	T1-4b N1b-2b M0	1 to 3 nodal macrometastases; ulceration	20 – 35
	Any T N3 M0	≥ 4 nodes, matted, or nodes plus in-transit metastasis	26.7 ± 2.5
IV	Any T Any N M1a-1b	Distant skin, SC, nodal, or lung metastasis	5 – 20
	Any T Any N M1c	All visceral metastases or elevated LDH with metastases	9.5 ± 1.1

Abbreviations: TNM, tumor, node, metastases; SE, standard error; SC, subcutaneous; LDH, lactate dehydrogenase.
Adapted with permission from Balch CM, Gershenwald JE, Soong SJ, et al. Final version of the 2009 American Joint Committee on Cancer staging system and classification for cutaneous melanoma. J Clin Oncol. 2009;27:6199-6206. PMID: 19917835.

approach, and there is considerable variation in clinical practice. CT or PET imaging is not indicated for patients with stage I melanoma nor for most patients with stage II melanoma. Currently, no tumor markers are sensitive and specific for melanoma. Assays to detect molecular markers of melanoma cells in the blood and sentinel lymph nodes are being investigated. *BRAF* mutation status should be determined for most patients with stage III and all patients with stage IV melanoma.

TREATMENT

Once melanoma has been diagnosed, the standard treatment is surgical excision of the primary lesion (Fig. 12-7). The extent of surgery depends on the thickness of the primary melanoma. Large surgical excisions are no longer necessary, and most wide excisions can be performed with primary closure. Findings from randomized clinical studies of optimal surgical margins have demonstrated that less radical surgery results in excellent local control with no adverse effect on survival.[21,22] Current recommendations for the optimal width of surgical margins are summarized in Table 12-4.

The wide excision should include underlying subcutaneous tissue down to fascia. In cosmetically sensitive areas, such as

the face, or anatomically difficult areas, such as the ears and hands, it may be difficult to achieve the desired margin. In those situations, obtain at least a 1-cm margin.

KEY POINTS

- Surgery is the mainstay of treatment for early melanoma. The extent of surgical margins depends on the thickness of the primary melanoma, but the overall trend is for narrower surgical margins.
- The goal of wide excision is to minimize the risk for local recurrence with optimal functional and cosmetic outcome.
- Extensive imaging is not indicated for patients with stage I and stage II melanoma.

MANAGEMENT OF REGIONAL LYMPH NODES
Clinically Normal (Negative) Regional Lymph Nodes
The surgical management of clinically normal lymph nodes is determined by the characteristics of the primary melanoma.

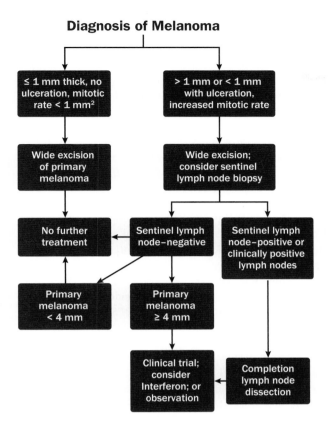

Diagnosis of Melanoma

- ≤ 1 mm thick, no ulceration, mitotic rate < 1 mm²
  - Wide excision of primary melanoma
    - No further treatment

- > 1 mm or < 1 mm with ulceration, increased mitotic rate
  - Wide excision; consider sentinel lymph node biopsy
    - Sentinel lymph node–negative
      - Primary melanoma < 4 mm
      - Primary melanoma ≥ 4 mm
        - Clinical trial; consider Interferon; or observation
    - Sentinel lymph node–positive or clinically positive lymph nodes
      - Completion lymph node dissection

Fig. 12-7 Treatment algorithm for patients with newly diagnosed melanoma.

There is a direct relationship between thickness of the primary melanoma and risk for regional lymph node involvement. Sentinel lymph node biopsy (SLNB) is the primary method for regional nodal staging. Sentinel lymph node mapping is generally considered for patients with primary melanomas that are at least 1 mm thick. For melanomas that are less than 1 mm thick, the likelihood of regional lymph node involvement is decreased (less than 10%); thus, sentinel node mapping is generally not indicated unless there are worrisome histologic features such as ulceration of the primary melanoma or high mitotic count (greater than 1 mitosis/mm²) or Clark level IV or V. The false-negative rate for sentinel lymph node mapping is approximately 4%. Lymphoscintigraphy is performed preoperatively to identified regional nodal basin and facilitates intraoperative identification of the sentinel nodes. SLNB is typically performed on an outpatient basis, with excision of the sentinel nodes, followed by wide local excision of the primary tumor. [23] If the sentinel lymph node is negative for melanoma, no further lymph node surgery is required. If melanoma is detected in the sentinel lymph node, a complete lymph node dissection of the involved nodal basin is currently recommended, although no randomized trial has demonstrated therapeutic value of completion node dissection.

The Multicenter Selective Lymphadenectomy Trial (MSLT-I) is the largest trial to date to address the role of lymphatic

Table 12-4 Recommended Surgical Margins for Primary Melanoma

Tumor Thickness	Surgical Margin
≤ 1.0 mm	1.0 cm
1.0 mm to 2.0 mm	1.0 cm to 2.0 cm
2.01 mm to 4.0 mm	2.0 cm
> 4.0 mm	At least 2.0 cm

mapping with SLNB in determining prognosis and effect on survival.[24] This trial evaluated the role of sentinel lymph node mapping compared with observation in patients with intermediate-thickness melanoma. Patients were randomly assigned to wide excision followed by observation of regional lymph nodes with lymphadenectomy if nodal relapse occurred, or to wide excision and SLNB with immediate lymphadenectomy if nodal micrometastases were detected on biopsy. The 5-year melanoma-specific survival rates were similar for the two groups. However, even in the absence of a proven survival benefit, the staging advantages of SLNB are sufficiently compelling to justify its routine use for patients with melanoma. A follow-up study, MSLT-II, is currently being conducted to determine the role of complete lymph node dissection compared with close surveillance in patients with sentinel lymph node–positive melanoma.

KEY POINTS

- Sentinel lymph node mapping is a useful staging procedure for melanoma and provides important prognostic information.
- Sentinel lymph node biopsy should be performed if the primary melanoma is greater than 1 mm in thickness. Sentinel lymph node biopsy may be considered for melanomas that are less than 1 mm thick, but have high-risk features (i.e., ulceration, mitotic rate higher than 1 mitosis/mm², lymphovascular invasion, or Clark level IV or V).
- At this time, complete lymph node dissection is recommended for patients with a positive sentinel lymph node.

Clinically Enlarged (Positive) Regional Lymph Nodes

For patients who present with palpable regional lymph node metastases, a therapeutic lymph node dissection should be performed. The goal of nodal dissection is to provide long-term, disease-free survival and, possibly, to cure or provide optimum local-regional control of disease. Satellite metastases and in-transit metastases are usually surgically resected. Negative margins are generally sufficient without large, wide excisions.

ADJUVANT THERAPY FOLLOWING SURGERY

The primary treatment for most patients with stage I and II melanoma is surgical resection. Postoperative adjuvant therapy can be considered for patients at high risk for recurrence. High risk is generally defined as melanomas that are larger than 4 mm thick or node-positive (stage III) disease. Adjuvant therapy options include high-dose interferon alpha-2b (IFN-α-2b), a clinical trial, or observation. Similar treatment options are considered for patients with resected in-transit melanoma or for those patients with stage IV melanoma who are free of disease after surgical resection of metastases, although there are no data yet to support any particular adjuvant therapy approach for patients with stage IV melanoma who are free of disease.

Adjuvant IFN Therapy

On the basis of the potent immunologic effects of IFN and its modest activity in patients with metastatic melanoma, numerous studies with this drug have been conducted in the postoperative adjuvant setting. The U.S. Food and Drug Administration (FDA) recommended approval for IFN-α-2b in 1995 based on study E1684 conducted by the Eastern Cooperative Oncology Group (ECOG).[25] In that study, 280 patients with thick primary melanoma (larger than 4 mm thick) and node-negative disease (T4, stage IIB) or with node-positive disease (stage III) were randomly assigned to receive either dose-intensive IFN-α-2b for 1 year or to observation. The patients were treated with an intravenous induction phase of 20 million IU/m² given 5 days per week for 1 month followed by an 11-month course of 10 million IU/m² given subcutaneously 3 days per week. For patients who were assigned to treatment with IFN, there was a 9-month prolongation in median relapse-free survival (RFS; 1.7 vs. 1.0 years; p = 0.002) and there was a 1-year prolongation in median OS (3.8 vs. 2.8 years; p = 0.02), with a 9% absolute increase in survival at 5 years (47% vs. 36%). However, with longer follow-up, the benefit in terms of OS was no longer significant. Several subsequent studies of adjuvant IFN therapy were conducted addressing dose and schedule. In the Intergroup adjuvant trial E1690 high-dose IFN therapy was compared with a lower-dose regimen (3 million IU/m² 3 days per week for 2 years) and with observation after complete resection of all known disease. The results of the trial confirmed the disease-free survival advantage of high-dose IFN seen in study E1684, but not the OS advantage.[26] This discrepancy may be the result of differences in eligibility criteria for the two studies and the subsequent availability of cross-over treatment with IFN after relapse in the E1690 trial. A third trial, E1694, evaluated a 1-year course of high-dose IFN compared with a 2-year course of treatment with a ganglioside GM2 vaccine.[27] The trial was closed prematurely when the interim analysis showed a significantly worse RFS and OS for patients treated with the GM2-KLH vaccine compared with the high-dose IFN (hazard ratio [HR] 1.47 and 1.52, respectively).

Intermediate-dose regimens of IFN have also been evaluated in several clinical trials. European Organisation for Research and Treatment of Cancer (EORTC) 18991 is a randomized clinical trial of adjuvant pegylated IFN-α-2b compared with observation for patients with stage III melanoma.[28] In this study, 1,256 patients were randomly assigned to observation or weekly adjuvant pegylated IFN-α at a dose of 6 μg/kg per week for 8 weeks (induction), then 3 μg/kg per week (maintenance) for an intended duration of 5 years. There was no difference in OS or distant metastasis-free survival (DMFS) between the groups (DMFS and OS: HR 0.88, 95% CI 0.75, 1.03; p = 0.107). There was a significant reduction in hazard for relapse for the patients treated with IFN, with risk reduction in RFS (HR 0.82, 95% CI 0.71, 0.96; p = 0.011) at 4 years of median follow-up. Based on these data, pegylated IFN was approved by the FDA for treatment of patients with stage III melanoma. The favorable pharmacokinetic properties of pegylated IFN allow its administration on a weekly basis. Available data suggest that the schedule is more convenient than a high-dose regimen, but it is unclear if acute and chronic side effects differ significantly.

Thus, the results from a series of randomized clinical trials show that high-dose IFN improves RFS but not OS. These results come with substantial cost regarding toxicity, which has limited the acceptance of high-dose IFN therapy by patients and physicians. Toxicities of high-dose IFN include flu-like symptoms, fatigue, fever, chills, myalgia, anorexia, nausea, vomiting, headache, depression, and suicidal ideation. Significant laboratory abnormalities include elevated levels of hepatic transaminases, neutropenia, thyroid dysfunction, and anemia. Patients who are treated with high-dose IFN must be monitored closely and the dose of IFN must be modified appropriately for toxicity.

In addition, low-dose IFN regimens have been evaluated. A randomized controlled trial evaluated low-dose adjuvant pegylated IFN-α-2a compared with observation, and there was no improvement in RFS or OS.[29] Ongoing studies are exploring alternative schedules and doses of IFN (in particular, 1 month of high-dose induction intravenous IFN). Gogas et al reported the results of a small randomized trial that compared 1 month of induction IFN-alpha with 1 year of induction IFN-alpha followed by maintenance with a modified dosage.[30] This trial enrolled 364 patients with high-risk melanoma (stage IIB, IIC, or III). At a median follow-up of 63 months, there was no significant difference in median RFS (24 vs. 28 months) or OS (64 vs. 65 months) for the induction alone compared with induction with maintenance IFN. The use of a brief induction course of IFN-alpha without maintenance was formally studied in ECOG 1697, in which patients with stage IIA melanoma were randomly assigned to high-dose IFN-alpha for 4 weeks or to observation. This study showed no benefit for the 1-month induction regimen.[31]

Approximately 15% to 30% of patients treated with IFN-alpha develop signs and symptoms of autoimmunity, including development of auto-antibodies (e.g., antinuclear antibodies, antithyroglobulin, and anticardiolipin antibodies) and/or the clinical manifestations of autoimmunity (e.g., vitiligo, autoimmune thrombocytopenia, and retinopathy). At this time, there are conflicting reports on whether the development of autoimmunity is associated with an improved outcome in terms of RFS and OS, with some studies suggesting a relationship between the development of autoimmunity and improvement in both disease-free survival and OS and other studies not showing this association.[32,33] Because autoimmunity may not be observed for months after the initiation of IFN therapy, this cannot be used as a selection criterion for identifying which patients may derive benefit from IFN therapy.

In summary, all the trials with high-dose IFN have shown a significant improvement in RFS but no improvement in OS. A meta-analysis compared the outcomes of patients treated with IFN with patients who were observed.[34,35] Disease-free survival was significantly better in patients treated with IFN-alpha (HR 0.82, 95% CI 0.77, 0.87), as well as OS (HR 0.89, 95% CI 0.83, 0.96). Overall, the decision regarding the use of adjuvant IFN should be made carefully, and it involves a thorough conversation between the patient and physician that includes review of risks and benefits, as well as potential contraindications to treatment with IFN.

KEY POINTS

- Interferon therapy may be considered as adjuvant therapy after surgery for patients with high-risk primary melanomas (greater than 4 mm thick) or for patients with stage III, node-positive disease, based on results from phase III trials showing a modest improvement in relapse-free survival.
- Interferon therapy requires close monitoring for side effects with appropriate dose modification for toxicity.
- Observation or participation in a clinical trial are additional options for patients with stage III or high-risk stage II melanoma.

Other Adjuvant Approaches

A variety of experimental approaches are being evaluated to improve on the outcomes seen with high-dose IFN in the adjuvant setting, including melanoma vaccine clinical trials. Two approaches are under clinical investigation: whole-cell vaccines (autologous or allogeneic) and peptide-based, or defined, antigens. Peptides have been selected from two classes: melanocyte differentiation antigens and cancer-testis antigens. The most widely studied peptides are derived from glycoprotein (gp) 100, tyrosinase, melan-A (all melanocyte-specific), and NY-ESO-1 and melanoma antigen encoding gene proteins. Results from melanoma vaccine clinical trials either have shown no benefit or demonstrated worse survival compared with observation. EORTC 18961, a randomized postoperative adjuvant clinical trial for patients with stage II melanoma, tested a ganglioside GM2-KLH21 vaccine compared with observation. Preliminary results show that the vaccine was ineffective and could possibly be detrimental.[36]

Ipilimumab, a monoclonal antibody targeting cytotoxic T-lymphocyte antigen (CTLA)-4, has been to shown to prolong survival in patients with metastatic melanoma. Currently, ipilimumab is being studied in multiple phase III trials as an adjuvant therapy in patients with high-risk melanoma. Similarly, given overall high response rates (RRs) and improvement in OS for patients with stage IV melanoma, adjuvant studies with BRAF and MEK inhibitors are now open and enrolling patients with stage III melanoma. Other studies have evaluated the role of biochemotherapy in the adjuvant setting. Results from S-0008 were presented at the 2012 ASCO Annual Meeting. In this study, 402 patients with high-risk stage III melanoma were randomly assigned to high-dose IFN for 1 year compared with cisplatin, vincristine, dacarbazine, interleukin (IL)-2, and IFN for 9 weeks. At 5 years, median RFS for the chemotherapy/IL-2 arm was 4.31 years compared with 1.90 years for the IFN arm (HR 0.76; p = 0.034). However, there was no difference in OS (5-year OS, 56% for both arms of the study [HR 1.02]).[37] Combination chemotherapy, IL-2, and IFN treatments are associated with substantial toxicity, although therapy is completed in 9 weeks.

SURVEILLANCE AFTER PRIMARY THERAPY

Patients with a history of melanoma should be followed regularly for evidence of local-regional recurrence, distant metastatic disease, and a second primary melanoma. The most important components of surveillance are the patient's history and physical examination. The physical examination should include a thorough skin examination, because the risk for a second primary melanoma is increased for patients who have a history of melanoma. An annual skin examination is recommended for life, or more frequently, based on patient risk factors. Regional lymph nodes should be thoroughly examined, especially in patients who have not had surgical resection of nodes. The remainder of the examination should be comprehensive, with awareness of frequent metastases to the lung, liver, and brain. Patient education is an integral part of the treatment of patients with melanoma, and they should receive instruction on how to perform monthly self-examinations of the skin for detection of new primary melanomas and recurrent disease. Patients should be taught about the clinical characteristics of melanoma and the importance of safe sun strategies. Educating family members about melanoma risk factors and changes in behavior related to sun exposure also is important.

The optimal follow-up and surveillance program for patients with melanoma has not been defined. To date, there are no data to show that regular screening with radiologic studies affects OS for patients with melanoma. The follow-up schedule and the extent of the evaluation (i.e., blood test or radiographic evaluation) is influenced by the risk for recurrence. For patients with thin melanomas, no specific radiologic or laboratory investigations to detect occult disease are recommended. For patients with melanomas larger than 1 mm in thickness, follow-up studies generally include a complete blood count, serum chemistry analyses with liver function tests, and a serum lactate dehydrogenase level. An elevated level of lactate dehydrogenase is suggestive of metastatic melanoma. Because the lungs are the most frequent sites of distant disease, periodic chest x-rays may be considered. The routine use of screening CT, magnetic resonance imaging, PET (with or without CT), or bone scans is not viewed as necessary but may be performed as clinically indicated. The National Comprehensive Cancer Network has proposed surveillance guidelines. In general, for patients with stage I or stage II melanoma, regular physical examination and annual skin exam are recommended. Chest x-ray and blood tests for lactate dehydrogenase levels are optional. In addition to these tests, CT or PET scanning (or a combination of both) can be considered for patients with stage III melanoma. There is significant variability in clinical practice so these guidelines allow for flexibility in follow-up. The clinician should choose a follow-up schedule and selection of tests based on the patient's risk for recurrence, symptoms, and the physician's experience.

TREATMENT OF METASTATIC MELANOMA

Metastatic melanoma can affect virtually any organ of the body, with the most common sites being lung, skin, liver, and brain. Until recently, the OS for patients with metastatic melanoma ranged from 5 to 11 months, with a median survival of 9 months. However, as described in subsequent sections, new treatments are now available for patients with metastatic melanoma, with much improved outcomes for patients with this historically treatment-refractory disease.

The treatment of patients with metastatic melanoma depends on multiple factors, including the overall condition and performance status, the sites and number of metastases, the pace of the disease, and the patient's preferences for treatment. New approaches in immunotherapy and molecularly targeted therapy have led to several recent FDA approvals of new agents that have redefined the standard of care for patients with metastatic melanoma. Treatment options for metastatic melanoma

include molecularly targeted therapy based on somatic mutation status, immunotherapy, chemotherapy, surgical resection of isolated metastases, and participation in a clinical trial. There are no randomized trials that compare these different approaches and there are no data on the appropriate sequencing of these therapies. Therefore, the selection of treatment needs to be individualized, taking into account the overall condition of the patient, a molecular analysis for the presence of mutated *BRAF* gene, and the extent of metastatic disease. Patients with metastatic melanoma have a particularly high incidence of brain metastases. Surgery or radiation therapy (whole-brain or stereotactic radiosurgery) may be considered based on symptoms, number of lesions present, and location of lesions.

MOLECULARLY TARGETED THERAPY

The identification of activating mutations in *BRAF* in approximately 50% of melanomas in 2002 was the beginning for the investigation of molecularly targeted therapy in melanoma.[9] The MAPK (i.e., Ras-Raf-Erk) pathway and oncogenic *BRAF* are attractive targets for the development of new therapies for patients with melanoma (Fig. 12-1B) that have focused on the inhibition of BRAF, MEK, NRAS, and KIT. BRAF is a key protein kinase component of the RAS-RAF pathway.[8] This critical intracellular signaling pathway relays extracellular signals to the nucleus in order to regulate gene expression (Fig. 12-1A). The most commonly identified mutation in the *BRAF* gene occurs in the region that encodes the kinase domain of the protein at position V600 and results in constitutive activation of the kinase. Almost 80% of *BRAF* mutations are *V600E* with most of the remainder consisting of *V600K*. All patients with advanced cutaneous melanoma should have their tumors assessed for presence or absence of *BRAF* mutation.

The first RAF inhibitor to be tested in patients with advanced melanoma was the multikinase inhibitor sorafenib. It is a broad RAF kinase inhibitor, which suppresses BRAF as well as CRAF. Phase II and phase III clinical trials with sorafenib, either as a single agent or combined with chemotherapy, failed to show meaningful clinical activity in patients with advanced disease.[38,39] Subsequently, more potent and selective BRAF inhibitors were developed that specifically inhibit mutant *BRAF* over other RAF kinases. These include the FDA-approved vemurafenib and dabrafenib (BRAF inhibitors), and trametinib (MEK inhibitor).

Vemurafenib is a potent inhibitor of the mutated *BRAF V600E* kinase. The clinical efficacy of vemurafenib in patients with *BRAF V600E*-mutated melanoma has been firmly established in three clinical trials.[40] In the phase II study of vemurafenib (BRIM2), 132 patients with metastatic melanoma harboring a *BRAF V600E* mutation were enrolled. The overall RR was 53%, the median progression-free survival (PFS) was 6.2 months, and the median duration of response was 6.8 months.[41] The median OS was 15.9 months (95% CI 11.6, 18.3). The pivotal phase III study (BRIM3) enrolled 675 patients with previously untreated metastatic melanoma with *BRAF V600E* mutation. Patients were randomly assigned to oral vemurafenib (960 mg twice daily) or intravenous dacarbazine (1,000 mg/m²

KEY POINTS

- New treatment options are available for patients with metastatic melanoma, including immunotherapy such as ipilimumab and molecularly targeted therapy. *BRAF*-targeted therapies should only be used for patients with *BRAF V600*-mutant melanoma.
- All patients with advanced cutaneous melanoma should have their tumors evaluated for the presence of *BRAF* mutation. Patients with acral or mucosal primary melanoma tumors that do not contain a *BRAF* mutation should have their tumors assessed for *KIT* mutation.
- Other treatment options for metastatic melanoma include interleukin-2 in carefully selected patients, resection of solitary metastasis, and dacarbazine- or temozolomide-based therapy. Participation in clinical trials is highly recommended.

every 3 weeks).[42] The overall RR was 48% in the vemurafenib arm compared with 5% in the dacarbazine arm. At the 6-month evaluation, OS was 84% in the vemurafenib arm and 64% in the dacarbazine arm (HR 0.37; p < 0.001). The estimated median PFS was 5.3 months in the vemurafenib arm and 1.6 months in the dacarbazine arm. Based on these results, the FDA approved vemurafenib for patients with *BRAF V600E*-mutant unresectable stage III or stage IV melanoma. These results were recently updated with 12.5 months median follow-up. Vemurafenib is still associated with an OS benefit compared with dacarbazine (median OS, 13.6 months; HR 0.70).[43]

The most frequent adverse events associated with vemurafenib treatment are arthralgias, rash, nausea, photosensitivity, pruritus, and hand-foot syndrome. Cutaneous squamous cell carcinomas (SCC) or keratoacanthoma can occur in approximately 25% of patients treated with vemurafenib. Mutations in *RAS,* particularly *HRAS*, are frequent in SCC that develops in patients treated with vemurafenib.[44] Based upon the frequent skin-associated adverse events, patients undergoing treatment with vemurafenib (and other *BRAF*-targeted therapies) should be counseled to perform regular self-examination of their skin and report any new or changing skin lesions to their physicians. Additionally, patients starting therapy should be advised of sun-protective measures. Dermatologic skin exams should be performed prior to initiation of therapy and every 2 months while on therapy. Surveillance for other sites of SCC is also a topic of consideration, although to date no other secondary malignancies have been associated. Electrocardiography should be performed before treatment and regularly thereafter because of the risk for QT prolongation.

Dabrafenib is a potent, ATP-competitive inhibitor of RAF kinases, including BRAF, which is highly active in melanoma, both as monotherapy and in combination with MEK inhibitors. In a multicenter phase II study (BREAK-2), 92 patients with stage IV *BRAF*-mutant (*V600E* and *V600K*) melanoma received 150 mg of dabrafenib twice daily until disease progression or unacceptable adverse events. The overall RR was 51% and was higher in the *V600E* cohort compared with *V600K*. Median PFS was 6.3 months and median OS was 13.1 months for the *BRAF V600E* group. Therapy was well tolerated. The most common adverse events were arthralgias, hyperkeratosis, and pyrexia. Ten percent of patients developed SCC.[45] A phase III trial randomly assigned 250 patients with *BRAF*-mutant melanoma to dabrafenib or dacarbazine. Median PFS was 5.1 months for dabrafenib and 2.7 months for dacarbazine.[46] Based on these results, the FDA approved dabrafenib for the treatment of unresectable or metastatic *BRAF*-mutant melanoma (*V600E*). The FDA-approved dose is 150 mg orally twice daily. Overall, dabrafenib is well tolerated. Side effects include fever, skin rash, skin cancer, and uveitis/iritis. Cardiomyopathy has been reported in 9% of patients and baseline echocardiogram is recommended followed by monitoring for patients receiving dabrafenib. Ophthalmologic evaluation should be performed for any visual disturbances.

An alternative strategy to targeting BRAF is inhibition of MEK (MAPK/extracellular signal-regulated kinase), the immediate downstream signaling component in the MAPK pathway.

Ongoing studies are exploring MEK inhibitors in patients with *BRAF*-mutant metastatic melanoma with encouraging results. In a recent randomized phase III trial comparing trametinib (MEK inhibitor) with dacarbazine chemotherapy for patients with *BRAF V600E*- or *V600K*-mutant advanced melanoma, results showed improvement in PFS and OS in favor of trametinib.[47] The RR to trametinib was 22%. On the basis of these results, the FDA approved trametinib in 2013 for patients with unresectable or metastatic melanoma with *BRAF V600E* or *V600K*. The toxicities of the MEK inhibitor include rash, diarrhea, transient mild and reversible cardiac dysfunction, and ocular toxicities. Baseline and ongoing monitoring with echocardiogram is recommended.

Ongoing studies are combining BRAF and MEK inhibitors in patients with mutated *BRAF*. The rationale behind this approach is to prolong PFS by delaying or preventing the development of MAPK-dependent resistance mechanisms and to reduce BRAF inhibitor–related toxicities as a result of paradoxical activation of the MAPK pathway in nonmelanoma *BRAF* wild-type cells. Dabrafenib (a BRAF inhibitor) plus trametinib (MEK inhibitor) was first evaluated in a large phase I/II clinical trial (CombiDT) for patients with advanced *BRAF*-mutant melanoma. Recent results showed that the RR was higher with combination dabrafenib and trametinib than for those previously reported with single-agent dabrafenib. The RR was greater than 70% with an acceptable safety profile. The median PFS in the combination arm (dabrafenib 150 mg twice daily and trametinib 2 mg once daily) was 9.4 months compared with 5.8 months in the monotherapy arm of dabrafenib alone (HR for progression or death 0.39, 95% CI 0.025 to 0.62, p < 0.001). The combination was associated with a lower incidence of treatment-associated rash and hyperproliferative lesions compared with single-agent treatment.[48] The rate of cutaneous SCC with combination therapy was one-third that of dabrafenib monotherapy (7% vs. 19%). Fever was the most common toxicity with combination therapy and occurred in approximately 70% of patients. Fever can be an early side effect and is often managed with brief dose interruption, or in the case of persistent fever, with corticosteroids. Two phase III trials are ongoing to evaluate combination BRAF and MEK inhibitors compared with BRAF inhibitors alone.

In summary, two BRAF inhibitors (vemurafenib and dabrafenib) and one MEK inhibitor (trametinib) have been approved by the FDA as monotherapy for *BRAF*-mutant melanoma. These drugs should not be used in BRAF wild-type tumors because of the risks for potential tumor promotion. Vemurafenib and dabrafenib have similar efficacy with a RR of greater than 50%, and a median PFS of approximately 7 months. Both drugs have activity against *V600E* and *V600K*, and both are active in patients with brain metastases. Vemurafenib is FDA approved for *BRAF V600E*-mutant melanoma and dabrafenib is FDA-approved for *V600E*- and *V600K*-mutant melanoma. The side effect profiles appear somewhat different. There is higher rate of SCC, elevated liver enzymes, photosensitivity, and arthralgias in vemurafenib compared with dabrafenib and more fever associated with dabrafenib. Vemurafenib has been associated with prolonged QT interval and echocardiogram monitoring is recommended. Cardiomyopathy has been reported on the clinical trials of dabrafenib and monitoring with echocardiogram is recommended. For both drugs, side effects are manageable and rarely require discontinuation of medications. Although trametinib, the first MEK inhibitor approved by the FDA, has activity in patients with melanoma, BRAF inhibitors have consistently shown greater single-agent activity. Preliminary results suggest increased RRs, longer PFS, and less toxicity in terms of cutaneous side effects with combinations of BRAF and MEK inhibitors. Combination treatment with dabrafenib and trametinib was recently FDA approved. Results of ongoing phase III clinical trials will determine whether combination therapy is superior to monotherapy.

Although clinical activity of the selective BRAF inhibitors is quite impressive, complete responses are uncommon and approximately 80% of patients develop progressive disease as a result of de novo or acquired drug resistance. Understanding the molecular basis for primary-resistance and secondary-resistance mechanisms to BRAF inhibitors is a major focus of investigation. Early evidence from direct sequencing of BRAF exons suggests that new point mutations in BRAF V600E are not present. Preliminary results from different labs have described several different potential mechanisms of resistance, activating NRAS mutations, mutated BRAF splice variants, and overexpression of mutated BRAF.[49]

This remains an intense area of investigation. A recent analysis of patients receiving dabrafenib showed that patients with BRAF-mutant melanoma having concurrent PTEN dysfunction exhibited lower response rates than those patients whose tumors retained PTEN function.[50]

Alterations in the PI3K/AKT pathway also occur frequently in patients with melanoma. Therefore, approaches to simultaneously inhibit both the MAPK and PI3K/AKT pathways are currently undergoing clinical development. In addition, angiogenesis inhibitors are currently undergoing evaluation in combination with chemotherapy in randomized clinical trials. Patients with cKIT-mutant metastatic melanoma have also been treated with cKIT inhibitors such as imatinib, with some clinical responses reported.[51]

IMMUNOTHERAPY

Immunotherapy is another important treatment strategy for patients with metastatic melanoma, and recent breakthroughs in understanding T-cell activation and anergy have led to new therapeutic approaches. The use of targeted immunotherapy such as the CTLA-4-blocking antibody ipilimumab has shown clinical activity in patients with advanced melanoma. Evidence from numerous studies indicates that CTLA-4 provides a braking mechanism on T-cell activation and serves a critical role in controlling the immune response. CTLA-4 blockade results in enhanced antitumor immunity, most likely through direct activation of T cells as well as inhibition of regulatory (suppressor) T cells.

Ipilimumab is a monoclonal antibody directed against CTLA-4 that has been shown to increase survival in patients with metastatic melanoma, leading to its regulatory approval in the United States in 2011. Two large phase III trials have been conducted with ipilimumab. In the first study, 676 previously treated patients with metastatic melanoma were randomly assigned to one of three arms in a 3:1:1 ratio: ipilimumab plus peptide vaccine (gp100), ipilimumab alone, or peptide vaccine alone. Ipilimumab (3 mg/kg) and/or peptide vaccine were given every 3 weeks for four doses.[52] Patients with confirmed partial or complete response were allowed to receive reinduction with their original therapy provided they had not experienced significant toxicity. Results showed that the median OS was 10.0 months and 10.1 months in the ipilimumab-containing arms compared with 6.4 months in the peptide-alone arm (HR 0.68; p < 0.003). The objective RR was significantly improved in the groups of patients who received ipilimumab compared with those who received the peptide vaccine alone (5.7% and 10.9% vs. 1.5%, respectively). In a second phase III clinical trial, 502 patients with previously untreated metastatic melanoma were randomly assigned to ipilimumab (10 mg/kg) plus intravenous dacarbazine (850 mg/m^2) or dacarbazine plus placebo with maintenance ipilimumab or placebo for patients with responding disease and no dose-limiting toxicity. Results of this study showed that OS was longer in the group receiving ipilimumab plus dacarbazine compared with dacarbazine alone (11.2 vs. 9.1 months), with higher survival rates in the ipilimumab/dacarbazine group at 1 year (47.3% vs. 36.3%) and at 3 years (20.8% vs. 12.2%; HR for death, 0.72; p < 0.001).[53] Overall incidence of grade 3 and 4 toxicity was significantly higher in the ipilimumab and chemotherapy arm, especially hepatic toxicity. Objective responses were low (15.2% vs. 10.3%), but the response duration was long—19.3 months for ipilimumab plus dacarbazine compared with 8.1 months for dacarbazine alone. Based on clinical activity results, the FDA approved ipilimumab for the treatment of unresectable stage III or stage IV melanoma. Although different schedules and doses have been explored, the FDA-approved dose and schedule is 3 mg/kg intravenously every 3 weeks for four treatments without maintenance. Preliminary results from phase II studies show that ipilimumab has activity in patients with brain metastases and is safe to administer in this clinical situation.

There are two important features of ipilimumab that are unique compared with other standard cancer therapies. First, some patients receiving therapy with ipilimumab have radiographic evidence of disease progression during treatment before disease stabilizes or regresses. Therefore, caution should be taken in stopping therapy early. Further, responses generally take much longer, with disease regression at times occurring well after completion of induction therapy. Second, treatment with ipilimumab results in immune-mediated adverse reactions because of T-cell activation and proliferation. These immune-mediated reactions may involve any organ system; however, the most common immune-adverse reactions are colitis, hepatitis, dermatitis, neuropathy, and endocrinopathy. Endocrinopathies include hypopituitarism and hypothyroidism. The majority of these immune-mediated reactions occur during treatment; however, a minority occurs weeks to months after discontinuation of ipilimumab. Treatment of immune-mediated toxicity requires interruption of ipilimumab and use of corticosteroids, depending upon severity of symptoms. Patients receiving ipilimumab require close monitoring with blood tests, including liver and thyroid function, before and during treatment. Meticulous attention to gastrointestinal symptoms and other immune-related adverse events is required in order to safely prescribe this treatment. The FDA has created a Risk Evaluation and Mitigation Strategy to provide additional information regarding side effects and management of ipilimumab-associated adverse events. Ongoing studies will further define the activity of these agents in the treatment of metastatic melanoma and in the adjuvant setting. The addition of other immune modulators is also an active area of clinical investigation. The addition of granulocyte-macrophage colony stimulating factor to ipilimumab is currently being studied in an ECOG clinical trial.

A second investigational approach to inhibit negative regulation of T-cell activation and thereby activate the immune response against melanoma is to block the PD-1/PD-L1 pathway. PD-1 protein, a T-cell co-inhibitory receptor, and one of its ligands, PD-L1, play an important role in the ability of tumor cells to evade the host's immune system. Monoclonal antibodies targeting both PD-1 and PD-L1 are being developed to augment the antitumor T-cell response against melanoma. The first-in-class PD-1 antibody nivolumab, a fully human IgG4 monoclonal PD-1 antibody, was evaluated in a phase I/II study which included a large cohort of patients with melanoma. Preliminary results show substantial clinical activity with a 28% RR and a favorable side effect profile.[54] Another PD-1 inhibitor in clinical development is lambrolizumab, a humanized monoclonal antibody. In a study investigating lambrolizumab, 135 patients with advanced melanoma were treated on one of three dose schedules. The overall RR was 37% with a higher RR at the highest dose tested.[55] Treatment was well tolerated. Treatment with PD-1 inhibitors is associated with immune-related adverse events, although these adverse events may be less frequent compared with ipilimumab. However, pulmonary toxicity has been reported with PD-1 inhibitors and requires careful monitoring. Clinical trials with anti-PD-L1 monoclonal antibodies are also ongoing, with clear activity in patients with advanced melanoma.[56] Ongoing randomized clinical trials are in progress or planned comparing PD-1 and PD-L1 with chemotherapy. Tumor expression of PD-L1 may be a potential biomarker of response to this new class of treatment. Combining anti-CTLA-4 and anti-PD-1 immunotherapy is currently being explored in several clinical trials. The combination of ipilimumab (anti-CTLA-4) plus nivolumab (anti-PD-1 antibody) was evaluated in a phase I study for patients with advanced melanoma.[57] Remarkably, evidence of clinical activity was observed in 65% of patients. At the maximum tolerated dose, 53% of patients had an objective response, all with tumor reduction of more than 80%. Grade 3 or 4 adverse events occurred in one-half of the patients, which were mostly immune-related adverse events and reversible.

Building upon the success of targeted therapies and immunotherapies, ongoing studies are combining BRAF inhibitors with new immunotherapies. However, in the first phase I study that combined vemurafenib (BRAF inhibitor) with ipilimumab, unexpected hepatotoxicity lead to early closure of the clinical trial, reinforcing the need for carefully conducted clinical trials of new combination treatments.[58]

IL-2 is a potent T-cell activator. IL-2 is a well-established therapy that can cause durable complete responses. The overall RR in patients with melanoma is 16%, with a 6% complete RR.[59] The current FDA-approved regimen consists of two 5-day courses of IL-2 separated by a rest period of 7 to 10 days. Two high-dose regimens have been used: 600,000 IU/kg or 720,000 IU/kg, administered every 8 hours. Repeat courses can be given at 8 to 12 weeks if the disease responds to treatment. Typically, two or three courses are given when there is a good response, with a maximum of five courses. The toxicity of IL-2 is clearly dose-related. The most common side effects include hypotension, diarrhea, renal dysfunction with oliguria, respiratory failure, fever, chills, and vomiting. Many of the adverse effects of this treatment result from a capillary-leak syndrome caused by the drug. Most of the side effects are self-limiting and resolve after discontinuation. Because of low RRs and the substantial toxicity of high-dose IL-2, its use should be restricted to carefully selected patients and should be administered by experienced clinicians at established cancer treatment centers. Careful assessment of cardiac and pulmonary function is mandatory prior to initiation of high-dose IL-2 therapy.

Other dosing regimens include continuous intravenous infusion or subcutaneous administration with lower doses of IL-2. Less serious side effects with these alternative doses and methods of delivery have been reported in some studies, but it remains unclear whether efficacy is comparable. In a recent randomized phase III clinical trial, the gp100 vaccine was tested in combination with high-dose IL-2 and compared with the same dose of IL-2 alone. RRs were significantly higher in the IL-2 and gp100 vaccine combination arm (16% vs. 6%; p = 0.03); longer PFS was seen in favor of the combination.[60]

Ongoing clinical trials are investigating the role of adoptive immunotherapy—activated T cells and autologous TILs. In patients treated at the NCI Surgery Branch, use of TILs with prior lymphodepletion results in significant responses.[61] Current studies are focused on optimizing this type of treatment and applying it at other cancer centers to assess feasibility.

CHEMOTHERAPY

Numerous chemotherapy agents have demonstrated modest activity in the treatment of metastatic melanoma. However, neither single-agent nor combination chemotherapy has been shown to consistently improve OS. Dacarbazine remains the only chemotherapy agent approved by the FDA for the treatment of metastatic melanoma. Results from clinical trials have demonstrated overall RRs of approximately 10% to 20%. Responses are not durable, lasting a median of 3 to 4 months, and long-term complete responses are seen in only 1% to 2% of patients. Doses and schedules of dacarbazine vary widely, with no data to suggest that RRs are influenced by these variables. The most commonly used regimen is intravenous dacarbazine at a dose of 800 mg/m^2 to 1,000 mg/m^2 repeated every 3 to 4 weeks or 200 mg/m^2 for 5 days every 3 to 4 weeks.

Dacarbazine is generally well tolerated. The most frequent side effects are nausea and vomiting, which can be severe. Mild to moderate myelosuppression is a common dose-related side effect.

Temozolomide is a second-generation oral alkylating agent with a mechanism of action similar to that of dacarbazine, through the active metabolite 5-(3-methyl triazen-1-yl)-imidazole-4-carboxamide. The results from several phase II studies suggest that temozolomide is at least as effective as dacarbazine in metastatic disease. Temozolomide, which crosses the blood–brain barrier, was approved by the FDA in 1999 for the treatment of primary brain cancer. Although not FDA-approved for melanoma, temozolomide is used to treat patients with advanced melanoma based upon its ease of administration and favorable toxicity profile. Two different schedules have been evaluated. The first regimen is a 5-day regimen with a daily dose of 150 mg/m^2 to 200 mg/m^2 on days 1 to 5. Courses are repeated every 3 to 4 weeks. The major side effect is mild to moderate myelosuppression. Mild nausea and vomiting also are common but can be readily controlled with standard antiemetic therapy. This schedule of temozolomide was compared with dacarbazine in a phase III clinical trial of 305 patients with stage IV melanoma.[62] Temozolomide was associated with a nonsignificant improvement in median survival (7.7 vs. 6.4 months with dacarbazine). RRs were 13.5% and 12.1%, respectively. A second regimen, known as extended dosing of temozolomide, has been investigated, which comprises a lower daily dose for prolonged periods (75 mg/m^2 daily for 6 weeks on, 2 weeks off). This dosing regimen of temozolomide is associated with more lymphopenia and opportunistic infections; specifically, pneumocystis pneumonia has been reported. Newer approaches combine temozolomide and other agents, including antiangiogenesis and immunotherapeutic agents. Other chemotherapy drugs with single-agent activity include cisplatin, the taxanes, carmustine, fotemustine, lomustine, and vinblastine.

Several combination chemotherapy regimens have been evaluated in patients with metastatic melanoma with limited benefit. More recently, paclitaxel/carboplatin combination therapies have been evaluated, with modest activity in patients with metastatic melanoma. In one study, carboplatin/paclitaxel was associated with a 20% RR and median PFS of 4.2 months.[39]

BIOCHEMOTHERAPY

Biochemotherapy, the combination of immunotherapy and cytotoxic chemotherapy, has been studied in patients with metastatic melanoma and is currently being evaluated in the adjuvant setting by ECOG. Biochemotherapy is associated with considerable toxicity, including myelosuppression, nausea, vomiting, rash, hypotension, and fluid retention. Given the lack of survival benefit, which was evaluated in a randomized clinical trial,[63] along with the toxicity, biochemotherapy is not the standard of care for patients with stage IV melanoma. However, biochemotherapy continues to be evaluated in the adjuvant[37] and neoadjuvant settings in clinical trials.

In summary, there have been tremendous advances in the treatment of patients with metastatic melanoma, both in targeted therapy and immunotherapy. All patients with metastatic disease should have their tumors assessed for the presence of the *V600* mutation in the *BRAF* gene. *KIT* mutation testing should be performed in patients with *BRAF*-mutation–negative melanoma when primary melanoma is mucosal or acral. The presence of *V600E* or *V600K* predicts responsiveness of the BRAF inhibitors (vemurafenib, dabrafenib) or MEK inhibitors (trametinib). The optimal treatment and sequence of treatments has not been defined. For patients with *BRAF V600* mutation with minimal symptoms and good performance, it is reasonable to begin initial systemic treatment with immunotherapy (i.e., ipilimumab). For patients with metastatic melanoma with *BRAF V600* mutation, and high disease burden and symptoms related to melanoma, beginning systemic treatment with targeted therapy is most appropriate. For patients with *BRAF V600*-mutation melanoma who were initially treated with immunotherapy and who have disease progression, beginning treatment with a targeted therapy is appropriate. For patients with *KIT* mutation, *KIT* inhibitors may be useful. For the 50% of patients without *BRAF* mutation, immunotherapy is the preferred initial treatment. Chemotherapy is now considered second- or third-line therapy for patients with advanced melanoma. Participation in a clinical trial should always be considered.

RADIATION THERAPY

The main indication for radiation therapy for patients with metastatic disease is the palliative treatment of symptomatic lesions, including painful bone, skin, or subcutaneous metastases. Whole-brain radiation therapy or stereotactic radiosurgery may be helpful for palliating the symptoms of brain metastases in patients. However, durable local control of brain metastases is rarely achieved, with the occasional exception of some patients with oligometastatic disease who are treated with stereotactic radiosurgery. Radiation therapy also is indicated for spinal cord compression.

SURGICAL RESECTION

Surgical resection is a very effective palliative treatment for isolated metastases, offering quick palliation and, in some patients, long-lasting survival. Surgical excision of solitary metastases in visceral organs can lead to survival of longer than 5 years in 5% to 20% of patients.

ISOLATED LIMB PERFUSION/INFUSION

Isolated limb perfusion or infusion is used to treat patients with melanoma that is confined to a limb, such as unresectable local recurrence and in-transit metastases. The most commonly used chemotherapy agent is melphalan, which is used in conjunction with hyperthermia. RRs have ranged from 40% to 80%. Alternative approaches to the management of in-transit metastases include surgery when feasible, as well as systemic treatment approaches as described above.

References

1. Siegel R, Naishadham D, Jemal A. Cancer statistics, 2013. *CA Cancer J Clin.* 2013;63:11-30. PMID: 23335087.

2. Purdue MP, Freeman LE, Anderson WF, et al. Recent trends in incidence of cutaneous melanoma among US Caucasian young adults. *J Invest Dermat.* 2008;128;2905-2908. PMID: 18615112.

3. Fears TR, Guerry D 4th, Pfeiffer RM, et al. Identifying individuals at high risk of melanoma: a practice predictor of absolute risk. *J Clin Oncol.* 2006;24:3590-3596. PMID: 16728488.

4. Orlow I, Begg CB, Cotignola J, et al. CDKN2A germline mutations in individuals with cutaneous malignant melanoma. *J Invest Dermatol.* 2007;127:1234-1243. PMID: 17218939.

5. Kanetsky PA, Rebbeck TR, Hummer AJ, et al. Population-based study of natural variation in the melanocortin-1 receptor gene and melanoma. *Cancer Res.* 2006;66:9330-9337. PMID: 16982779.

6. Abdel-Rahman MH, Pilarski R, Cebulla CM, et al. Germline BAP1 mutation predisposes to uveal melanoma, lung adenocarcinoma, meningioma, and other cancers. *J Med Genet* 2011;48:856-859. PMID:21941004.

7. Fecher LA, Cummings SD, Keefe MJ, et al. Toward a molecular classification of melanoma. *J Clin Oncol.* 2007;25:1606-1620. PMID: 17443002.

8. Curtin JA, Fridlyand J, Kageshita T, et al. Distinct sets of genetic alterations in melanoma. *N Engl J Med.* 2005;353:2135-2147. PMID: 16291983.

9. Davies H, Bignell GR, Cox C, et al. Mutations of the BRAF gene in human cancer. *Nature.* 2002;417:949-954. PMID: 12068308.

10. Curtin JA, Busam K, Pinkel D, et al. Somatic activation of KIT in distinct subtypes of melanoma. *J Clin Oncol.* 2006;24:4340-4346. PMID: 16908931.

11. Van Raamsdonk CD, Griewank KG, Crosby MB, et al. Mutations in GNA11 in uveal melanoma. *N Engl J Med.* 2010;363:2191-2199. PMID: 21083380.

12. Shields CL, Ganguly A, Bianciotto CG, et al. Prognosis of uveal melanoma in 500 cases using genetic testing of fine-needle aspiration biopsy specimens. *Opthalmology.* 2011;118:396-401. PMID: 20869116.

13. Smalley KS, McArthur GA. The current state of targeted therapy in melanoma: this time it's personal. *Semin Oncol.* 2012;39:204-214. PMID: 22484192.

14. Romano E, Schwartz GK, Chapman PB, et al. Treatment implications of the emerging molecular classification system for melanoma. *Lancet Oncol.* 2011;9:913-922. PMID: 21349766.

15. Green AC, Williams GM, Logan V, et al. Reduced melanoma after regular sunscreen use: randomized trial follow-up. *J Clin Oncol.* 2011;29:257-263. PMID: 21135266.

16. Scolyer RA, Long GV, Thompson JF. Evolving concepts in melanoma classification and their relevance to multidisciplinary melanoma patient care. *Mol Oncol.* 2011;5:124-136. PMID: 21482206.

17. Long GV, Menzies AM, Nagrial AM, et al. Prognostic and clinicopathologic associations of oncogenic BRAF in metastatic melanoma. *J Clin Oncol.* 2011;29:1239-1246. PMID: 21343559.

18. Balch CM, Gershenwald JE, Soong SJ, et al. Final version of 2009 AJCC melanoma staging and classification. *J Clin Oncol.* 2009;27:6199-6206. PMID: 19917835.

19. Thompson JF, Soong SJ, Balch CM, et al. Prognostic significance of mitotic rate in localized primary cutaneous melanoma: an analysis of patients in the multi-institutional American Joint Committee on Cancer melanoma staging database. *J Clin Oncol.* 2011;29:2199-2205. PMID: 21519009.

20. Gimotty PA, Elder DE, Fraker DL, et al. Identification of high-risk patients among those diagnosed with thin cutaneous melanomas. *J Clin Oncol.* 2007;25:1129-1134. PMID: 17369575.

21. Balch CM, Soong SJ, Smith T, et al. Long-term results of a prospective surgical trial comparing 2 cm vs. 4 cm excision margins for 740 patients with 1-4 mm melanomas. *Ann Surg Oncol.* 2001;8:101-108. PMID: 11258773.

22. Thomas JM, Newton-Bishop J, A'Hern R, et al. Excision margins in high-risk malignant melanoma. *N Engl J Med.* 2004;350:757-766. PMID: 14973217.

23. Gershenwald JE, Ross MI. Sentinel-lymph-node biopsy for cutaneous melanoma. *N Engl J Med.* 2011;364:1738-1745. PMID: 21542744.

24. Morton DL, Thompson JF, Cochran AJ, et al. Final trial report of sentinel-node biopsy versus observation in melanoma. *N Engl J Med.* 2014;370:599-609. PMID: 24521106.

25. Kirkwood JM, Strawderman MH, Ernstoff MS, et al. Interferon alfa-2b adjuvant therapy of high-risk resected cutaneous melanoma: the Eastern Cooperative Oncology Group Trial EST 1684. *J Clin Oncol.* 1996;14:7-17. PMID: 8558223.

26. Kirkwood JM, Ibrahim JG, Sondak VK, et al. High- and low-dose interferon alfa-2b in high-risk melanoma: first analysis of intergroup trial E1690/S9111/C9190. *J Clin Oncol.* 2000;18:2444-2458. PMID: 10856105.

27. Kirkwood JM, Ibrahim JG, Sosman JA, et al. High-dose interferon alfa-2b significantly prolongs relapse-free and overall survival compared with the GM2-KLH/QS-21 vaccine in patients with resected stage IIB-III melanoma: results of intergroup trial E1694/S9512/C509801. *J Clin Oncol.* 2001;19:2370-2380. PMID: 11331315.

28. Eggermont AM, Suciu S, Santinami M, et al. Adjuvant therapy with pegylated interferon alfa-2b versus observation alone in resected stage III melanoma: final results of EORTC 18991, a randomised phase III trial. *Lancet.* 2008;372:117-126. PMID: 18620949.

29. Hancock BW, Wheatley K, Harris S, et al. Adjuvant interferon in high-risk melanoma: the AIM HIGH Study--United Kingdom Coordinating Committee on Cancer Research randomized study of adjuvant low-dose extended-duration interferon Alfa-2a in high-risk resected malignant melanoma. *J Clin Oncol.* 2004;22:53-61. PMID: 14665609.

30. Pectasides D, Dafni U, Bafaloukos D, et al. Randomized phase III study of 1 month versus 1 year of adjuvant high-dose interferon alfa-2b in patients with resected high-risk melanoma. *J Clin Oncol.* 2009;27:939-944. PMID: 19139440.

31. Agarwala SS, Lee SJ, Flaherty LE, et al. Randomized phase III trial of high-dose interferon alfa-2b (HDI) for 4 weeks induction only in patients with intermediate- and high-risk melanoma (Intergroup trial E1697). *J Clin Oncol.* 2011;29:15s (suppl; abstr 8505).

32. Gogas H, Ioannovich J, Dafni U, et al. Prognostic significance of autoimmunity during treatment of melanoma with interferon. *N Engl J Med.* 2006;354:709-718. PMID: 16481638.

33. Bouwhuis MG, Suciu S, Collette S, et al. Autoimmune antibodies and recurrence-free interval in melanoma patients treated with adjuvant interferon. *J Natl Cancer Inst.* 2009;101:869-877. PMID: 19509353.

34. Mocellin S, Pasquali S, Rossi CR, et al. Interferon alpha adjuvant therapy in patients with high-risk melanoma: a systematic review and meta-analysis. *J Natl Cancer Inst.* 2010;102:493-501. PMID: 20179267.

35. Wheatley K, Ives N, Hancock B, et al. Does adjuvant interferon-alpha for high-risk melanoma provide a worthwhile benefit? A meta-analysis of the randomised trials. *Cancer Treat Rev.* 2003;29:241-252. PMID: 12927565.

36. Eggermont AS, Suciu S, Ruka W, et al. EORTC 18961: Post-operative adjuvant ganglioside GM2-KLH21 vaccination treatment vs observation in stage II (T3-T4N0M0) melanoma: 2nd interim analysis led to an early disclosure of the results. *J Clin Oncol.* 2008;26:15s (May 20 suppl; abstr 9004).

37. Flaherty L, Moon J, Atkins M, et al. Phase III trial of high-dose interferon alpha-2b versus cisplatin, vinblastine, DTIC plus IL-2 and interferon in patients with high-risk melanoma (SWOG S0008): An intergroup study of CALGB, COG, ECOG, and SWOG. *J Clin Oncol.* 2012;30:15s (suppl; abstr 8504).

38. Amaravadi RK, Schuchter LM, McDermott DF, et al. Phase II trial of temozolomide and sorafenib in advanced melanoma patients with or without brain metastases. *Clin Cancer Res.* 2009;15:771-7718. PMID: 19996224.

39. Flaherty KT, Lee SJ, Zhao F, et al. Phase III trial of carboplatin and paclitaxel with or without sorafenib in metastatic melanoma. *J Clin Onc.* 2013;31:373-379. PMID: 23248256.

40. Flaherty KT, Puzanov I, Kim KB, et al. Inhibition of mutated, activated BRAF in metastatic melanoma. *N Engl J Med.* 2010;363:809-819. PMID: 20818844.

41. Sosman JA, Kim KB, Schuchter L, et al. Survival in BRAF V600-mutant advanced melanoma treated with vemurafenib. *N Engl J Med.* 2012;366:707-714. PMID: 22356324.

42. Chapman PB, Hauschild A, Robert C, et al. Improved survival with vemurafenib in melanoma with BRAF V600E mutation. *N Engl J Med.* 2011;364:2507-2516. PMID: 21639808.

43. Chapman PB, Hauschild A, Robert C, et al. Updated overall survival (OS) results for BRIM-3, a phase III randomized, open-label, multicenter trial comparing BRAF inhibitor vemurafenib (vem) with dacarbazine (DTIC) in previously untreated patients with *BRAF V600E*-mutated melanoma. *J Clin Oncol.* 2012;30:15s (suppl; abstr 8502).

44. Su F, Viros A, Milagre C, et al. RAS mutations in cutaneous squamous-cell carcinomas in patients treated with BRAF inhibitors. *N Engl J Med.* 2012;366:207-215. PMID: 22256804.

45. Ascierto PA, Minor D, Ribas A, et al. Phase II trial (BREAK-2) of the BRAF inhibitor dabrafenib (GSK2118436) in patients with metastatic melanoma. *J Clin Oncol.* 2013;31:3205-3211. PMID: 23918947.

46. Hauschild A, Grob JJ, Demidov LV, et al. Dabrafenib in BRAF-mutated metastatic melanoma: a muticentre, open-label, phase 3 randomised controlled trial. *Lancet.* 2012; 380:358-365. PMID: 22735384.

47. Flaherty KT, Robert C, Hersey P, et al. Improved survival with MEK inhibition in BRAF-mutated melanoma. *N Engl J Med.* 2012;367:107-114. PMID: 22663011.

48. Flaherty KT, Infante JR, Daud A et al. Combined BRAF and MEK inhibition in melanoma with BRAF V 600 mutations. *N Engl J Med.* 2012;367:1694-703. PMID: 23020132.

49. Villanueva J, Vultur A, Herlyn M. Resistance to BRAF inhibitors: unraveling mechanisms and future treatment options. *Cancer Res.* 2011;71:7137-7140. PMID: 22131348.

50. Nathanson KL, Martin AM, Wubbenhorst B, et al. Tumor genetic analyses of patients with metastatic melanoma treated with the BRAF inhibitor dabrafenib (GSK2118436). *Clin Cancer Res.* 2013;19:4868-4878. PMID: 23833299.

51. Carvajal RD, Antonescu CR, Wolchok JD, et al. KIT as a therapeutic target in metastatic melanoma. *JAMA.* 2011;305:2327-2334. PMID: 21642685.

52. Hodi FS, O'Day SJ, McDermott DF, et al. Improved survival with ipilimumab in patients with metastatic melanoma. *N Engl J Med.* 2010;363:711-723. PMID: 20525992.

53. Robert C, Thomas L, Bondarenko I, et al. Ipilimumab plus dacarbazine for previously untreated metastatic melanoma. *N Engl J Med.* 2011;364:2517-2526. PMID: 21639810.

54. Topalian SL, Hodi FS, Brahmer JR, et al. Safety, activity, and immune correlates of anti-PD-1 antibody in cancer. *N Engl J Med.* 2012;366:2443-2454. PMID: 22658127.

55. Hamid O, Robert C, Daud A, et al. Safety and tumor responses with lambrolizumab (anti-PD-1) in melanoma. *N Engl J Med.* 2013;369:133-144. PMID: 23724846.

56. Brahmer JR, Tykodi SS, Chow LQ, et al. Safety and activity of anti-PD-L1 antibody in patients with advanced cancer. *N Engl J Med.* 2012;366:2455-2465. PMID: 22658128.

57. Wolchok JD, Kluger H, Callahan MK, et al. Nivolumab plus ipilimumab in advanced melanoma. *N Engl J Med.* 2013;369:122-133. PMID: 23724867.

58. Ribas A, Hodi FS, Callahan M, et al. Hepatotoxicity with combination of vemurafenib and ipilimumab. *N Engl J Med.* 2013;368:1365-6. PMID: 23550685.

59. Atkins MB, Lotze MT, Dutcher JP, et al. High-dose recombinant interleukin 2 therapy for patients with metastatic melanoma: analysis of 270 patients treated between 1985 and 1993. *J Clin Oncol.* 1999;17:2105-2116. PMID: 10561265.

60. Schwartzentruber DJ, Lawson DH, Richards JM, et al. gp100 peptide vaccine and interleukin-2 in patients with advanced melanoma. *N Engl J Med.* 2011;364:2119-2127. PMID: 21631324.

61. Parkhurst MR, Riley JP, Dudley ME, et al. Adoptive transfer of autologous natural killer cells leads to high levels of circulating natural killer cells but does not mediate tumor regression. *Clin Cancer Res.* 2011;17:6287-6297 PMID: 21844012.

62. Middleton MR, Grob JJ, Aaronson N, et al. Randomized phase III study of temozolomide versus dacarbazine in the treatment of patients with advanced metastatic malignant melanoma. *J Clin Oncol.* 2000;18:158-166. PMID: 10623706.

63. Atkins MB, Hsu J, Lee S, et al. Phase III trial comparing concurrent biochemotherapy with cisplatin, vinblastine, dacarbazine, interleukin-2, and interferon alfa-2b with cisplatin, vinblastine, and dacarbazine alone in patients with metastatic melanoma (E3695): a trial coordinated by the Eastern Cooperative Oncology Group. *J Clin Oncol.* 2008;26:5748-5754. PMID: 19001327.

13

SARCOMA

Scott M. Schuetze, MD, PhD

Updates from 2012

Drugs approved for treatment of specific connective tissue tumors

▶ Regorafenib is approved by the U.S. Food and Drug Administration (FDA) for treatment of metastatic *KIT*-positive gastrointestinal stromal tumor (GIST) after failure of imatinib and sunitinib. In a randomized, placebo-controlled trial of regorafenib (160 mg daily for 3 out of every 4 weeks) versus placebo in patients with advanced GIST previously treated with imatinib and sunitinib, the median progression-free survival (PFS) was 4.8 and 0.9 months, respectively, and 6-month PFS rate was 38% and 0%, respectively (Demetri GD, *Lancet* 2013).

▶ Everolimus is approved by the FDA for treatment of angiomyolipoma of the kidney associated with tuberous sclerosis complex that does not require immediate surgery. In a randomized trial the objective tumor response rate was 42% and 6-month PFS rate was 98% for patients receiving 10 mg of everolimus daily versus 0% and 83%, respectively, for patients receiving placebo (Bissler JJ, *Lancet* 2013).

▶ Denosumab is approved by the FDA for treatment of unresectable giant cell tumor of bone or in situations in which complete resection would result in severe morbidity in adults and skeletally mature adolescents based on a high rate of tumor control and low rate of serious toxicity in a proof-of-concept phase II study and interim analysis of a larger confirmatory phase II trial (Thomas D, *Lancet Oncol* 2010; Chawla S, *Lancet Oncol* 2013).

Ewing sarcoma

▶ Administration of standard chemotherapy cycles every 2 weeks versus every 3 weeks using myeloid growth factor support reduces Ewing sarcoma relapse in patients younger than age 50 with localized sarcoma. In a randomized Children's Oncology Group trial, the 5-year event-free survival rate was improved from 65% in the standard arm to 73% in the dose-dense arm with no significant difference in rate of severe toxicity (Womer RB, *J Clin Oncol* 2012).

Non-GIST soft tissue sarcoma

▶ Doxorubicin (75 mg/m^2/cycle) is a good standard treatment for patients with unresectable locally advanced or metastatic soft tissue sarcoma (excluding subtypes not responsive to conventional chemotherapy). In patients with bulky or symptomatic advanced soft tissue sarcoma, who would benefit from tumor regression or prolongation of time to tumor progression for palliation, combination therapy with doxorubicin (75 mg/m^2/cycle) and ifosfamide (10 g/m^2/cycle) should be considered. A randomized phase III trial demonstrated improved sarcoma response rate (26% vs. 14%), longer median PFS (7.4 vs. 4.6 months), and lower rate of primary tumor progression on treatment (13% vs. 32%), with similar median and 2-year overall survival and rate of toxic death from doxorubicin and ifosfamide compared with doxorubicin alone, respectively (Judson I, *Lancet Oncol* 2014).

Sarcoma is the term used for cancers of connective tissue. Most sarcomas arise from mesoderm-derived cells. Sarcomas of soft tissue and bone are uncommon, constituting less than 1% of cancers occurring in adults, but about 15% of cancers in children. Sarcomas are remarkably heterogeneous, with more than 50 subtypes recognized by the World Health Organization classification of tumors of soft tissue and bone.[1] In adults, soft tissue sarcomas are about four times more common than sarcomas of bone (11,400 compared with 3,000 cases, respectively, in 2013).[2] Approximately 40% of patients diagnosed with sarcoma will die from the disease, with the majority dying from metastatic disease.[2] Complete surgical removal of the primary tumor is required for cure in most cases and is often an essential component in the management of oligometastases; appropriate multidisciplinary treatment is essential for patients presenting with sarcoma. Radiation is also important in many sarcoma subtypes to provide optimal local control in the site of the primary tumor or palliation of tumor-related symptoms. With appropriate multidisciplinary management, the rates of long-term survivors of localized osteosarcoma and Ewing sarcoma have improved from less than 20% to more than 70%.[3] Similar gains in cure rates have occurred in patients with pediatric rhabdomyosarcoma but have been less impressive in other soft tissue sarcoma subtypes. Dramatic improvement in the long-term survival rate of patients with metastatic gastrointestinal stromal tumor (GIST) has occurred following the introduction of tyrosine kinase inhibitor therapy, with 20% to 30% of patients surviving 9 to 10 years after initiation of treatment, and kinase inhibitor therapy is being integrated into management of other selected sarcoma subtypes.[4]

EPIDEMIOLOGY AND ETIOLOGY

The more common subtypes of sarcoma include GIST, leiomyosarcoma, liposarcoma, and undifferentiated pleomorphic sarcoma (previously called malignant fibrous histiocytoma). Approximately 10% to 15% of soft tissue sarcomas cannot be characterized beyond noting that they are sarcomas (sarcoma, not otherwise specified). Other relatively common subtypes include synovial sarcoma, fibrosarcoma, malignant peripheral nerve sheath tumor, and angiosarcoma. Osteosarcomas and chondrosarcomas are the two most common sarcomas arising from bone in adults. Ewing sarcoma can arise in either bone or soft tissue. Figure 13-1 indicates the relative frequency of some of these sarcoma subtypes.

Most sarcomas arise in the absence of a genetic cancer-predisposition syndrome or exposure to known environmental factors including toxins, radiation, or virus associated with development of sarcoma. The incidence of sarcomas increases with age, although specific subtypes, such as Ewing sarcoma, rhabdomyosarcoma (embryonal and alveolar subtypes), and osteosarcoma, occur much more frequently in children and young adults. Adults younger than age 35 are at a greater risk of synovial sarcoma and desmoplastic small round cell tumors; individuals older than age 60 are at a greater risk of myxofibrosarcoma, undifferentiated pleomorphic sarcoma, and sarcoma, not otherwise specified.

There are many genetic syndromes associated with sarcoma, including Li-Fraumeni syndrome (TP53 mutation); retinoblastoma (RB1 gene deletion); neurofibromatosis type-1 (NF1 mutation); Gardner syndrome (APC mutation); McCune-Albright syndrome (GNAS1 mutation); Bloom, Rothmund-Thomson, and Werner syndromes (associated with loss of helicase function); Costello syndrome (HRAS mutation); and Nijmegen breakage syndrome (NBN mutation), among others.[1] Individuals with Li-Fraumeni syndrome are at significant risk of developing osteosarcoma or soft tissue sarcoma. In one large study of patients with sarcoma, germ-line TP53 mutations were present in about 3% of cases.[5] The most common secondary cancers in

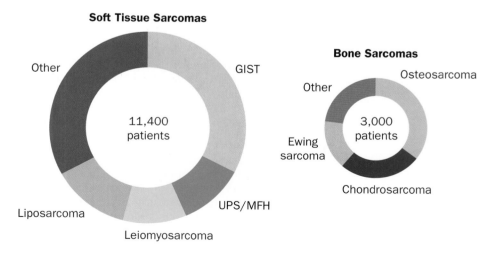

Fig. 13-1 Soft tissue and bone sarcomas: relative frequency.

The number of estimated cases and breakdown of subtypes for soft tissue and bone sarcomas is indicated. The area of each circle is proportional to the frequency of such tumors.

Abbreviations: GIST, gastrointestinal stromal tumor; UPS, undifferentiated pleomorphic sarcoma; MFH, malignant fibrous histiocytoma.

Table 13-1 Representative Genetic Alterations in Sarcomas[1,14]

Class of Alteration	Sarcoma Subtype	Genetic Change	Frequency
Activating mutation	Gastrointestinal stromal tumor	*KIT* or *PDGFRA* mutation	> 90%
Ligand expression	Dermatofibrosarcoma protuberans	PDGF expression	~ 100%
	Giant cell tumor of the bone	RANK ligand	~ 100%
Inactivation/deletion	Myxofibrosarcoma	*NF1* mutation	~ 10% to 20%
	Malignant peripheral nerve sheath	*NF1* deletion	> 90%
Gene amplification	Well-differentiated and dedifferentiated liposarcoma	*CDK4, MDM2* amplification	> 90%
Translocation	Synovial sarcoma	t(X;18) *SYT-SSX1* or *SYT-SSX2*	> 90%
	Ewing sarcoma	t(11;22) *EWSR1-FLI1*	> 85%
		t(21;22) *EWSR1-ERG*	5% to 10%
	Alveolar rhabdomyosarcoma	t(2;13) *PAX3-FOXO1*	~ 70%
		t(1;13) *PAX7-FOXO1*	~ 15%

patients with retinoblastoma syndrome are leiomyosarcoma and osteosarcoma. Individuals with neurofibromatosis type-1 have a 5% to 10% risk of developing a soft tissue sarcoma (malignant peripheral nerve sheath tumor or GIST) in their lifetime. Desmoid tumors (aggressive fibromatosis) are associated with Gardner syndrome.

There is epidemiologic evidence that associates occupational exposure to vinyl chloride or exposure to the imaging agent thorotrast with development of hepatic angiosarcoma, but few other environmental exposures are linked to sarcoma.[6] Some studies have suggested exposure to dioxins or phenoxyacetic acid herbicides, such as Agent Orange, increases the risk of sarcoma, but others have not; meta-analyses of such data remain inconclusive.[7-10]

There is a small but measurable long-term risk of soft tissue or bone sarcoma after exposure to therapeutic radiation.[11] The mean latency time is 16 years (range, 4 to 30 or more years). Angiosarcoma tends to have a shorter latency than other radiation-associated sarcomas. Recent analysis of sarcoma incidence in survivors of atomic bomb blasts suggests moderate levels of ionizing radiation, lower than typically administered for therapy, also increase the risk of developing bone and soft tissue sarcoma.[12,13] Although one-half of such sarcomas are high-grade, their prognoses do not appear to be worse than that of sporadic soft tissue sarcomas of the same stage. Local control can be challenging because of long-term effects of radiation on tissue planes and wound healing and the inability to deliver additional cytotoxic doses of radiation.

Other risk factors for the development of soft tissue sarcoma include lymphedema (angiosarcoma) and human herpesvirus-8 (HHV-8) infection (Kaposi sarcoma [KS]). KS is associated with concurrent HHV-8 and HIV infections but may also arise in elderly patients in the absence of HIV. Trauma does not appear to cause sarcomas; rather, it may unmask the presence of a sarcoma.

GENETIC CHARACTERISTICS

Sarcomas exhibit a wide range of genetic abnormalities, including complex chromosomal aberrations (e.g., leiomyosarcoma and undifferentiated pleomorphic sarcoma), chromosomal translocations involving transcription factors (e.g., Ewing sarcoma and synovial sarcomas), overexpression of ligands to receptor kinases (e.g., dermatofibrosarcoma protuberans and giant cell tumor of bone), gene mutations resulting in activated cellular kinases (e.g., GIST), gene amplification (e.g., well-differentiated liposarcoma), and regulatory protein inactivation (e.g., malignant peripheral nerve sheath tumor), among others (Table 13-1).[1,14] Approximately 30% to 40% of sarcomas have defined recurring specific genetic alterations such as chromosome translocation, gene amplification, or mutation that contributes to pathogenesis. Given the broad differential diagnosis for many sarcomas, molecular analysis has proven extremely useful in the definitive diagnosis of specific sarcoma subtypes. Modern analysis of chromosome translocations using fluorescence in situ hybridization or polymerase chain reaction can be performed on paraffin-embedded, fixed tissue. Tumor genome sequencing and protein arrays may add to diagnosis and

KEY POINTS

- Individuals with certain cancer susceptibility syndromes have an increased risk for sarcoma.
- Therapeutic radiation confers a small but definite risk for the development of sarcoma.
- Human herpesvirus-8 infection is associated with Kaposi sarcoma.
- Approximately 30% to 40% of sarcomas have defined recurring specific genetic alterations such as chromosome translocation, gene amplification, or mutation that contributes to pathogenesis.

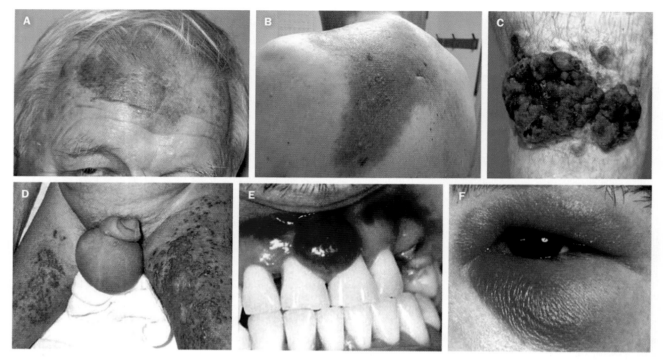

Fig. 13-2 Selected manifestations of angiosarcoma and Kaposi sarcoma.

(**A**) Angiosarcoma involving the scalp. (**B**) Angiosarcoma arising in prior radiation field. (**C**) Angiosarcoma associated with chronic lymphedema. (**D**) Kaposi sarcoma involving thighs causing lymphedema and scrotal edema. (**E**) Kaposi sarcoma of gingiva. (**F**) Kaposi sarcoma of head causing periorbital erythema and edema.

prognostication for sarcomas in the near future as genes characteristic of each subtype of sarcoma are recognized and validated.

CLINICAL PRESENTATION AND DIAGNOSIS

Soft tissue sarcomas generally present as painless, growing masses. They are generally differentiated from benign tumors, such as lipomas, by either their texture (generally firmer) or their location (typically deep to subcutaneous fat). Lipomas remain at least 100 times more common than their neoplastic counterpart. For many masses, a diagnosis of sarcoma can be rendered with a core needle biopsy, although this procedure may not yield adequate tissue to classify tumor subtype or grade. When diagnostic material cannot be obtained by core needle biopsy, incisional biopsy is performed, with the understanding that the subsequent oncologic procedure will likely need to encompass the prior biopsy site and scar. Fine-needle aspiration generally is inadequate to confirm the diagnosis of sarcoma, and its use usually is limited to confirming recurrence of sarcomas. Similarly, attention must be paid to the biopsy technique when attempting to diagnose a sarcoma of bone because it has implications for the extent of definitive surgery to follow.

Dermal vascular neoplasms such as angiosarcoma and KS often appear as indistinct red, purple, blue, or brown discoloration in the skin (Fig. 13-2). A mass-like lesion is often not present. Angiosarcoma arising in the dermis in elderly patients and KS arising in the setting of HIV/AIDS frequently involve the

head/neck and often are multicentric. KS arising in absence of HIV infection (typically referred to as classic KS) frequently involves the legs and feet. Advanced KS (usually in setting of AIDS) may involve lymph nodes, resulting in severe edema; oropharynx; gastrointestinal tract; or respiratory tract. Approximately 30% of patients with HIV and cutaneous KS will have involvement of the gastrointestinal tract, which may result in dysphagia, blood loss/anemia, or obstipation. Diagnosis of cutaneous vascular sarcoma is usually made by skin biopsy and appropriate immunohistochemistry (e.g., CD31, CD34, and ERG for angiosarcoma, ERG and HHV-8 for KS).

PATHOLOGIC FEATURES AND PROGNOSTIC FACTORS

Because of the diversity of sarcoma subtypes and their differential diagnoses, such as sarcomatoid carcinoma (which is treated as a carcinoma, not a sarcoma), uterine carcinosarcoma, melanoma, or lymphoma, the pathologist is a critical contributor to patient care. Important considerations for sarcoma staging include an evaluation of sarcoma grade and histologic subtype. It is important to recognize that pathologists may use different grading systems, with two grades (low and high), three grades (low, intermediate, and high), or four grades (grades 1 to 4). Evaluation of the extent of sarcoma is generally accomplished by magnetic resonance imaging or computed tomography (CT) of the site of the primary tumor and imaging of the chest. For patients with high-grade sarcoma, a chest CT is usually performed to evaluate for the

Stage	Three-Grade System	T*	N†	M‡
IA	Grade 1	T1a, T1b,	N0	M0
IB	Grade 1	T2a, T2b	N0	M0
IIA	Grades 2 and 3	T1a, T1b	N0	M0
IIB	Grade 2	T2a, T2b	N0	M0
III	Grade 3	T2a, T2b	N0	M0
	Any grade	Any	N1	M0
IV	Any grade	Any	Any	M1

*T1, tumor of no more than 5 cm in greatest dimension; T2, tumor of more than 5 cm in greatest dimension; a, superficial to investing fascia; b, deep to investing fascia.
†N0, no lymph node metastasis; N1, lymph node metastasis.
‡M0, no distant metastasis; M1, distant metastasis.

The original source for this material is the AJCC Cancer Staging Manual, 7th Edition (2010) published by Springer Science and Business Media LLC, www.springerlink.com.

presence of lung metastasis and to serve as a baseline for future comparison. CT of the abdomen/pelvis is performed for sarcomas originating in the abdomen, pelvis, or retroperitoneum and for myxoid/round cell liposarcoma of the extremity, which has an unusual propensity to spread to this body region. Additionally, for high-grade bone sarcomas, radionuclide bone scan or positron emission tomography (PET) is recommended to evaluate presence of metastasis to bone. In the absence of symptoms, the yield from routine imaging of the brain in patients with tumors originating outside the head/neck region is low. PET has relatively low accuracy in staging soft tissue sarcomas because of false-negative and false-positive findings.

The American Joint Committee on Cancer (AJCC) staging system for soft tissue sarcoma includes the tumor grade, size, and location (superficial or deep to any overlying investing fascia), as well as presence of nodal disease or overt metastatic disease (Table 13-2).[15] The preferred histopathologic grading system in the seventh edition of the *AJCC Cancer Staging Manual* is a three-tier (low, intermediate, and high) classification.[16] Nodal metastatic disease is an unfavorable prognostic feature but is associated with better overall survival compared to patients with blood-borne metastases, and the seventh edition of the *AJCC Cancer Staging Manual* has reclassified the presence of nodal metastasis from stage IV to stage III disease to reflect the better prognosis. Nodal metastatic disease is observed in less than 10% of patients with soft tissue sarcomas, however, certain subtypes of sarcoma including angiosarcoma, clear cell sarcoma, epithelioid sarcoma, extraskeletal Ewing sarcoma, pediatric rhabdomyosarcoma, and synovial sarcoma have a relatively higher propensity for spread through lymphatics. Sentinel node biopsy evaluations have been studied in the management of localized clear cell, epithelioid, and synovial sarcomas, but yield of a positive node is low.[17]

Table 13-3 **5-Year Disease-Free Survival Rates According to Size of High-Grade Soft Tissue Sarcoma**

Size of Tumor (cm)	5-Year Disease-Free Survival Rate (%)
2.6 to 4.9	77
5.0 to 9.9	62
10.0 to 14.9	51
15.0 to 20.0	42
> 20.0	17

Tumors 5 cm or smaller were generally treated with surgery; tumors larger than 5 cm were typically treated with surgery and radiation.

Histology, grade, and completeness of resection are the most important factors in determining risk of relapse. Of primary importance in determining overall survival is tumor grade; overall survival is also dependent on the initial size and location of the tumor. For example, as the size of the primary tumor increases, the risk of relapse increases, even within a given stage (Table 13-3).[18,19] It is important to recognize that sarcomas of different primary sites (and typically different histologic subtypes) are associated with different patterns of distant and local failure (Table 13-4). A nomogram using tumor histology, grade, size, depth, and patient age is available to help estimate the risk of death from soft tissue sarcoma after definitive local therapy.[20]

The AJCC staging system for bone cancers is shown in Table 13-5. Primary malignant lymphoma of bone and multiple myeloma are not included in the bone cancer system. Metastases of osteosarcomas to lymph nodes are extremely unusual and constitute stage IV disease. Patients with osteosarcoma with metastases only to the lungs have lower-stage disease and are treated differently than patients with metastasis to non-lung sites, because surgical resection of lung metastases can be curative.

TREATMENT OF NON-GIST SOFT TISSUE SARCOMAS
GENERAL PRINCIPLES

The primary curative treatment for most sarcomas of soft tissue is surgery. A planned oncologic resection to remove the tumor intact with a rim of normal tissue at the surgical margin (R0 resection) results in a lower risk of local relapse and better long-term survival than removal in which sarcoma touches the surgical margin (R1 resection).[21]

Adjuvant radiation to the site of the primary tumor is a standard of care for all soft tissue sarcomas of the extremities or body wall that are larger than 5 cm, independent of the grade. One exception to this rule is well-differentiated liposarcoma/atypical lipomatous tumor arising in a location amenable to additional non-mutilating surgery in case of local recurrence. This subtype of sarcoma has a very indolent clinical course and negligible risk of metastasizing. Patients with soft tissue sarcoma smaller than 5 cm arising in an extremity or body wall do not uniformly require

Table 13-4 Site of Recurrence According to Primary Site of Soft Tissue Sarcoma

Primary Site	Local	Lung	Other	Multiple Sites
Extremity (%)	10	70	15	5
Trunk (%)	41	29	12	18
Retroperitoneum (%)	30	17	6	47

Table 13-5 American Joint Committee on Cancer Staging System for Bone[15]

Stage	Grade (four tiers)	T*	N†	M‡
IA	1 to 2 (low)	T1	N0	M0
IB	1 to 2 (low)	T2, T3	N0	M0
IIA	3 to 4 (high)	T1	N0	M0
IIB	3 to 4 (high)	T2	N0	M0
III	3 to 4 (high)	T3	N0	M0
IVA	Any	Any	N0	M1a
IVB	Any	Any	N1	Any
	Any	Any	Any	M1b

*T1, tumor of no more than 8 cm in dimension; T2, tumor of more than 8 cm in greatest dimension; T3, discontinuous tumor in primary bone site.

†N0, no lymph node metastasis; N1, lymph node metastasis.

‡M0, no distant metastasis; M1a, lung metastasis; M1b, other distant metastasis.

The original source for this material is the AJCC Cancer Staging Manual, 7th Edition *(2010) published by Springer Science and Business Media LLC,* www.springerlink.com.

adjuvant radiation following an R0 resection.[22] Radiation therapy using external beam radiation[23] or brachytherapy[24] has been effective as an adjuvant to surgery for soft tissue sarcomas of the extremity in randomized studies. A randomized study performed in Canada of preoperative versus postoperative radiation as an

KEY POINTS

- Tumor grade is a key factor in sarcoma staging, treatment, and patient prognosis. Patients with low-grade sarcoma have a low risk of metastases and excellent prognosis. Patients with high-grade (grade 3) sarcoma have a high risk of metastases.
- Lung is the most common location for sarcoma metastases. For most patients, abdominal/pelvic imaging and lymph node dissection are not required for tumor staging.
- Ten percent to 20% of patients with sarcoma metastatic only to lung survive more than 5 to 10 years with appropriate multimodality treatment.

adjunct to complete resection of extremity soft tissue sarcoma demonstrated similar rates of local disease control. The risk of wound complications (delayed healing, infection, or need for re-operation) is increased (most significantly in the leg) with preoperative radiation, but the treatment field is smaller and radiation dose is lower than with postoperative radiation.[25] The risk of late complications, including fibrosis and lymphedema, appears greater with the larger fields treated and higher dose used in postoperative radiation.[26] The timing of radiation should be decided in conjunction with the orthopedic or surgical oncologist performing the definitive procedure, because of the effect on the postoperative course and longer-term complications.

In contrast to the benefit of radiation for soft tissue sarcomas of the extremities or body wall, there is no clear role for radiation for retroperitoneal or visceral sarcomas; the doses that can be administered postoperatively for abdominal sarcomas generally are not tumoricidal because of normal organ dose limits for radiation. However, for high-grade or large abdominal or retroperitoneal sarcomas, preoperative radiation may be considered because the tumor serves as its own tissue expander, pushing normal abdominal components, such as bowel, out of the radiation field. This anatomic feature increases the likelihood that a tumoricidal dose of radiation can be delivered to the abdomen. Intraoperative radiation and preoperative intensity-modulated radiation therapy remain largely investigational. New techniques such as image-guided, proton, or carbon ion radiation therapy are useful for treatment of sarcoma in anatomic areas where there is little tolerance for radiation scatter, such as the spine, sacrum, or base of the skull, but are not widely available.

ADJUVANT CHEMOTHERAPY

The role of chemotherapy in the adjuvant setting for adult soft tissue sarcoma remains controversial. Adjuvant chemotherapy is generally not used in management of soft tissue sarcoma smaller than 5 cm in size, regardless of tumor grade, or disease confined to a superficial location because of the low risk of metastases. Many of the trials of adjuvant chemotherapy have enrolled patients with AJCC stage IIB or III disease because of a high risk of metastases. In 1997, the Sarcoma Meta-analysis Collaboration (SMAC) published the finding of significant benefit from adjuvant doxorubicin-based chemotherapy in time to local and distant recurrence and recurrence-free survival in patients with localized soft tissue sarcoma.[27] However, there was only a trend for improved overall survival in patients receiving chemotherapy with an absolute benefit of 4% (7% for patients with extremity sarcoma) at 10 years, representing improvement in survival rate from 50% to 54%. A newer meta-analysis that included more contemporary trials not included in the original SMAC analysis showed a statistically significant survival benefit for adjuvant chemotherapy, with an odds ratio of 0.56 (95% CI 0.36, 0.85; p = 0.01) and absolute average overall survival risk reduction of 10% for anthracycline/ifosfamide combination therapy.[28] A randomized multisite study performed in Italy of epirubicin/ifosfamide given for five cycles compared with no adjuvant chemotherapy after resection of high-grade, 5-cm or larger (median diameter,

- Surgical resection remains the standard of care for most sarcomas.
- Adjuvant or neoadjuvant external beam radiation is used for larger soft tissue sarcomas (more than 5 cm in greatest dimension) in areas where tumoricidal doses can be delivered.
- Adjuvant radiation may be used for smaller soft tissue sarcoma in areas in which local recurrence would be difficult to manage using surgery.
- Adjuvant radiation is usually avoided in the initial treatment of atypical lipomatous tumors of the extremity or body wall.

10 cm) soft tissue sarcomas of the extremities or the pelvic girdle observed an overall survival benefit for patients who received adjuvant chemotherapy.[29] With longer follow-up, the 5-year overall survival remained superior for the study arm employing adjuvant chemotherapy (66% vs. 46%; p = 0.04).[30] Analysis of a prospective database of patients treated in France for localized soft tissue sarcoma found a significant improvement in metastasis-free survival and overall survival rates in the patients with grade 3, but not grade 2, sarcomas who received chemotherapy.[31] However, the analysis was limited to patients treated during 1980 to 1999, and the adjuvant chemotherapy was neither standardized nor randomized. Additionally, retrospective nonrandomized data support the contention that patients with synovial sarcoma or high-grade myxoid/round cell liposarcoma may benefit from adjuvant chemotherapy.[32] Any potential benefit from adjuvant chemotherapy, as well as the expected and possible severe toxicity, should be discussed with the patient on an individual basis.

Other studies have refuted the role of adjuvant chemotherapy in treatment of localized adult soft tissue sarcoma. Two small randomized studies did not show a significant benefit in overall survival after chemotherapy but were underpowered to detect a small difference in survival.[33,34] A large randomized study performed in Europe demonstrated no benefit in overall survival when comparing patients with completely resected soft tissue sarcoma treated with five cycles of adjuvant doxorubicin and ifosfamide with patients who underwent observation only.[35] The study included sarcomas arising at any site, but the majority had sarcoma of the extremity or proximal limb girdle. It was designed to enroll only patients with grade 2 or 3 tumors; however, 6% of the patients had grade 1 sarcoma. Less than 75% of the patients randomly assigned to adjuvant chemotherapy completed five cycles of treatment, and the dose of ifosfamide used (5 g/m^2/cycle) was lower than doses used in treatment of pediatric or advanced/metastatic sarcoma. Adding to the controversy, a retrospective analysis of the dataset from this trial and a preceding European Organisation for Research and Treatment of Cancer (EORTC) randomized adjuvant chemotherapy trial reported a significant improvement in relapse-free

survival for patients age 30 or older receiving chemotherapy, but not for younger patients.[36]

There are patients for whom adjuvant therapy is not indicated. A survival benefit from adjuvant chemotherapy for soft tissue sarcomas that arise from visceral or abdominal sites has not been demonstrated, and surgery remains a standard of care. In addition, there are a number of sarcoma subtypes (e.g., alveolar soft part sarcoma, epithelioid sarcoma, clear cell sarcoma, extraskeletal myxoid chondrosarcomas, and hemangiopericytomas) that are known to be poorly sensitive to doxorubicin/ifosfamide chemotherapy and for which the risks of adjuvant chemotherapy outweigh the potential benefit.

In contrast to adjuvant therapy for adult-type soft tissue sarcoma, adjuvant or neoadjuvant chemotherapy and radiation have dramatically improved overall survival for patients with pediatric rhabdomyosarcoma (e.g., embryonal and alveolar rhabdomyosarcoma) and extraskeletal Ewing sarcoma regardless of the age of the patient at the time of diagnosis. Although these sarcomas are typically seen in the pediatric population and occur less frequently in adults, treatment of adults follows the schedules of therapy administered to pediatric patients when feasible. Neoadjuvant/adjuvant chemotherapy should be administered to all patients with embryonal or alveolar rhabdomyosarcoma or extraskeletal Ewing sarcoma who have a good clinical performance status, adequate organ function, and sufficient bone marrow reserve to tolerate such therapy. Extraskeletal Ewing sarcoma is treated similarly to Ewing sarcoma arising in bone (see Ewing Sarcoma section). Based on phase III data, combination vincristine, dactinomycin, and cyclophosphamide form the backbone of adjuvant chemotherapy for most patients with primary pediatric-type rhabdomyosarcomas,[37] although for adult patients, doxorubicin is often incorporated. In contrast to embryonal and alveolar rhabdomyosarcoma for which chemotherapy is recommended, pleomorphic rhabdomyosarcoma is an "adult-type" high-grade soft tissue sarcoma, and thus the role of adjuvant chemotherapy is less clearly defined.

METASTATIC NON-GIST SOFT TISSUE SARCOMA

As single drugs or in combination, anthracyclines (such as doxorubicin) and the alkylating agent ifosfamide yield the best response rates for metastatic non-GIST sarcoma (rates of 10% to 25% for each drug in various studies).[38] Single-agent therapy may be as useful as combination therapy because doxorubicin and ifosfamide are not synergistic, although combinations generally are used when patients are symptomatic and rapid reduction in tumor burden is desired for palliation. Standard doses of doxorubicin are 75 mg/m^2 per cycle, usually administered in split daily doses or by continuous intravenous infusion to minimize cardiac toxicity. Ifosfamide is administered in a variety of schedules, from 5 g/m^2 over 24 hours once every 3 weeks, to 2 g/m^2 to 4 g/m^2 per day, to a total dose per cycle of 6 g/m^2 to 16 g/m^2, every 3 to 4 weeks, with support of mesna and usually growth factors as well.[39,40] A randomized EORTC trial of doxorubicin (75 mg/m^2/cycle) combined with ifosfamide (10 g/m^2/cycle) compared with the same dose of doxorubicin alone for up to six cycles in patients with locally advanced or metastatic high-grade soft tissue sarcoma demonstrated an improved objective response rate (26% vs. 14%, respectively) but similar overall survival rates.[41] The median progression-free survival was significantly higher and rate of primary progression was lower for the combination arm (7.4 months and 13%, respectively) than the single-agent arm (4.6 months and 32%, respectively). Study enrollment was limited to patients with good performance status and age younger than 60; however, 18% of patients receiving the combination discontinued treatment because of toxicity prior to completing six cycles, compared with 3% of patients receiving doxorubicin alone. The rate of toxic death was low (2% or lower) and similar in the two treatment arms. A recommendation by the study authors based on the available data is for the use of sequential single-agent therapy in the palliative setting when there are minimal symptoms from sarcoma and consideration of combination therapy if sarcoma regression would relieve acute symptoms or improve likelihood of tumor control from surgery or radiation.

At least three studies have confirmed the activity of the combination of gemcitabine/docetaxel in leiomyosarcoma[42-44]; the combination also has activity against undifferentiated pleomorphic sarcoma. Progression-free and overall survival rates were improved for patients who received gemcitabine/docetaxel compared with gemcitabine alone, even at a higher gemcitabine dose.[42] However, as borne out by toxicity data, the docetaxel dose from this study (100 mg/m² per cycle) is too high for routine use, and many physicians recommend a docetaxel dose of 75 mg/m² per cycle.[42] There is no consensus as to the duration of therapy for metastatic disease. Some physicians treat until progression or toxicity, whereas others administer a defined number of cycles or to maximum clinical or tumor response and then closely follow patients off therapy for symptoms or signs of tumor progression.

Pazopanib was approved by the U.S. Food and Drug Administration (FDA) in 2012 for treatment of patients with locally advanced or metastatic soft tissue sarcoma after treatment with standard chemotherapy based on results of a phase III randomized, placebo-controlled trial which demonstrated significant improvement in median progression-free survival in patients receiving pazopanib compared with placebo (20 vs. 7 weeks, respectively).[45] Objective sarcoma responses were infrequent at 6% in the group receiving pazopanib. Median overall survival was not significantly different between the groups taking pazopanib versus placebo (12.5 vs. 10.7 months, respectively). Patients with liposarcoma or GIST were not included in the trial. Notable severe toxicities experienced by more patients taking pazopanib compared with placebo included fatigue, anorexia, nausea, mucositis, hypertension, diarrhea, rash/desquamation, hypopigmentation, and decline in cardiac ejection fraction. The recommended starting dose is 800 mg daily.

Because sarcomas are a biologically heterogeneous group of diseases, it is not surprising that specific sarcoma subtypes have distinct sensitivity patterns to chemotherapy. Ifosfamide is particularly active for synovial sarcoma and myxoid/round cell liposarcoma and appears to be less active for leiomyosarcomas.

Dacarbazine has modest activity against leiomyosarcoma, and paclitaxel is active against angiosarcomas. Studies have demonstrated activity of sorafenib against angiosarcomas and desmoid tumors, and sunitinib against alveolar soft part sarcoma.[46-48]

Recently, improved understanding of the biology of certain connective tissue tumors has led to clinical introduction of serine/threonine and tyrosine kinase inhibitors in the management of disease. Angiomyolipomas are benign tumors often arising in patients with tuberous sclerosis and lead to serious morbidity or death. Loss of tuberous sclerosis complex results in constitutive activation of the mammalian target of rapamycin complex 1 (mTORC1), which is thought to be responsible for tumor growth. Everolimus is an inhibitor of mTORC1, and treatment of patients with angiomyolipomas resulted in an objective tumor response rate of 42% using 10 mg daily of everolimus compared with 0% using placebo in a double-blind, randomized trial.[49] The estimated tumor progression-free rates at 6 months were 98% for patients treated with everolimus and 83% for placebo. Adverse effects attributed to everolimus in more than 20% of patients were stomatitis, nasopharyngitis, acne-like skin reaction, headache, cough, and hypercholesterolemia. Everolimus was approved by the FDA in 2012 for treatment of angiomyolipoma associated with tuberous sclerosis and not requiring immediate surgery. Other examples of rare connective tissue tumors significantly affected by inhibitors of kinases include dermatofibrosarcoma protuberans, with overexpression of platelet-derived growth factor, and tenosynovial giant cell tumor/pigmented villonodular synovitis, with overexpression of colony stimulating factor-1, which may be effectively controlled using imatinib.[50,51] Clinical activity of the anaplastic lymphoma kinase (ALK) inhibitor crizotinib in a patient with inflammatory myofibroblastic tumor (IMT) aberrantly expressing ALK as a result of translocation (which occurs in about 50% of IMT) has also been reported.[52]

KEY POINTS

- Doxorubicin and ifosfamide are the most effective drugs for metastatic non-GIST soft tissue sarcomas. The benefit of such drugs appears additive, not synergistic.
- Gemcitabine/docetaxel is active in advanced/metastatic soft tissue sarcoma.
- Pazopanib (800 mg daily) is approved for the treatment of advanced or metastatic non-GIST soft tissue sarcoma after treatment with chemotherapy based on improvement in progression-free survival compared with placebo. Effectiveness has not been established in liposarcoma.

KAPOSI SARCOMA

Treatment of KS varies by extent of the disease. Asymptomatic lesions may be observed without direct therapy. In patients with AIDS and KS, introduction of highly active antiretroviral therapy (HAART) resulting in decline in viral load and increase in CD4 cell count frequently leads to regression in KS lesions with durable clinical response rates of more than 60%.[53] However, a substantial minority of patients with AIDS-associated KS may have undetectable HIV viral loads and CD4+ cell counts above the threshold typically associated with opportunistic infections or malignancies and require treatment for the sarcoma.[54-56] Occasionally—and sometimes dramatically—patients with KS who subsequently receive HAART experience a sudden flare or burst in KS lesion growth. This phenomenon, known as immune reconstitution inflammatory syndrome (IRIS) resulting from immune response against pathogens, may occur within weeks to a few months after initiation of HAART despite control of virologic and immunologic parameters. In a cohort study of 150 patients with HIV-associated KS who began HAART as the sole treatment for KS, 10 (6.6%) developed progressive IRIS-associated KS.[57] In such instances, HAART usually can be successfully continued, although for a time, chemotherapy also may be required to control KS growth.[58,59]

The decision to provide local or systemic treatment for KS should be based on several factors, including assessment of disease abundance, site of the disease, rate of disease progression, patient-specific psychologic factors, and presence of organ dysfunction.[60,61] Patients should be educated about treatment options for the various stages of the disease. Local treatment may be possible for patients who have limited, nonbulky, and accessible lesions. Alitretinoin gel (0.1%) is the only topical patient-administered therapy approved by the FDA for the treatment of KS.[62] Other local treatments for KS include intralesional chemotherapy, radiation therapy, laser therapy, and cryotherapy, all of which can be effective at controlling local tumor growth.[63-66] Radiation therapy has a role in the treatment of KS, particularly when the disease is bulky, symptomatic, and when rapid tumor shrinkage is required.[67] In a series of 36 patients with KS of the feet, a fractionation schedule of three fractions per week at 3.5 Gy/fraction (up to a total dose of 21.0 Gy) yielded an overall RR of 91% (complete responses, 80%).[68] Although discomfort from radiation therapy was frequent, it usually resolved without intervention within 2 weeks of completion of therapy.

Patients with KS-associated edema, extensive mucocutaneous disease, or symptomatic pulmonary or gastrointestinal involvement need a rapid response that is best achieved with systemic chemotherapy. Many cytotoxic chemotherapy agents have moderate activity in KS including bleomycin, vinca alkaloids, etoposide, taxanes, and anthracyclines.[60] Most of the reports of drug activity in classic or HIV-associated KS are from small retrospective series, case reports, or relatively small phase II trials. Few larger randomized studies of chemotherapy have been conducted in KS. Because many anticancer agents are also metabolized by CYP450, the potential for drug reactions with HAART is high. Liposomal formulations of doxorubicin and daunorubicin are the gold standard of clinical treatment for patients with extensive or advanced disease or who require rapid tumor shrinkage. In randomized multicenter trials, each of the two available liposomal anthracyclines proved superior to conventional chemotherapy (bleomycin and vincristine, with or without non-liposomal doxorubicin) in terms of response rates and toxicity profiles.[69-71] Liposomal doxorubicin also has significant activity in classic KS and is usually given at a dose of 20 mg/m^2 every 3 weeks.[72] Patients with KS whose tumors initially respond well to this treatment may require further therapy. Among 98 patients who received pegylated liposomal doxorubicin, after a median follow-up of 50 months, 13% had experienced a relapse, most within the first year of stopping chemotherapy.[73] Paclitaxel is an established second-line therapy for KS treatment and has shown efficacy even for patients with AIDS-associated KS and anthracycline-resistant disease. For patients in whom one previous systemic chemotherapy regimen had failed, the response rates in two trials were 59% and 71%, respectively, and the median duration of response in these studies was 8.9 months and 10.4 months, respectively.[74,75] Drug-related adverse events occurring in the majority of patients were severe neutropenia and alopecia. Oral etoposide, vinorelbine, gemcitabine, and bevacizumab have also been evaluated individually in patients with anthracycline-treated KS and demonstrated objective responses, but randomized comparison between agents has not been reported.

GASTROINTESTINAL STROMAL TUMORS
BIOLOGY AND PRESENTATION

During the past decade, it became clear that a group of sarcomas of the gastrointestinal tract is very distinct from gastrointestinal leiomyosarcomas. Now called GIST, these sarcomas are characterized by the presence of the CD117 (KIT) and/or DOG-1 (discovered on GIST) immunohistochemical markers, and most are positive for stem-cell marker CD34. Most GISTs have activating mutations in the *KIT* or platelet-derived growth factor receptor alpha *(PDGFRA)* gene, and approximately 10% to 15% have alternate mechanisms of activation.[76]

With increasing recognition, GISTs are the most common form of sarcoma (incidence, 5 to 10 cases per 1 million persons in the United States). These tumors arise from the interstitial cells of Cajal, the pacemaker cells of the gastrointestinal

---

KEY POINTS

- Kaposi sarcoma (KS) may be followed without antineoplastic therapy when the disease burden is limited and asymptomatic.
- Immune reconstitution following introduction of HAART in patients with AIDS-associated KS often leads to regression of KS but may result in tumor flare in 5% to 10% of cases.
- Liposomal anthracycline is a standard first-line chemotherapy for patients requiring treatment of KS because of tumor growth, tumor symptoms, or involvement of visceral organs.
- Paclitaxel is active in anthracycline-resistant KS.

tract. Approximately 65% of GISTs arise in the stomach, 25% in the small bowel, and the remainder in other sites along the gastrointestinal tract or in the abdomen. Surgery is the primary treatment for these tumors when localized, but many will recur in the peritoneum, liver, or both. Nodal, bone, and pulmonary metastasis from GIST have been described but are rare. GISTs are included in the AJCC staging system as a separate category.[15] Tumors are staged based on tumor size, number of mitoses, and presence of metastasis (to lymph nodes or other sites). Small tumors (smaller than 5 cm) with few mitoses (fewer than 5 per 50 high-power microscopic fields [HPF]) have a low risk of recurrence, whereas large tumors (larger than 10 cm), tumors with many mitoses (more than 5 per 50 HPF), and ruptured tumors have a high risk of recurrence after complete resection. GISTs larger than 2 cm in size that arise in the small bowel have a higher risk of recurrence after complete resection compared to those that originate in the stomach.

ADJUVANT THERAPY

The role of imatinib in the adjuvant setting has been the subject of a number of studies. A large randomized, prospective, placebo-controlled trial of imatinib after surgery for patients with GIST larger than 3 cm was stopped early because of a beneficial effect of imatinib on delaying disease recurrence, and led to the approval of imatinib in the adjuvant setting in the United States and Europe (the latter only for those patients at substantial risk of relapse).[77] Only 3% of patients who received imatinib experienced disease progression at 1 year (the end of the mandated treatment), compared with 17% of patients who were assigned to the placebo arm. However, there was no demonstrable overall survival benefit, owing to the high response rate in patients receiving imatinib after recurrence was detected and the short follow-up of the study, a median of 15 months. A large randomized, open-label trial of imatinib taken for 1 year compared with 3 years following complete resection of high-risk GIST (higher than 50% risk of tumor recurrence) detected an approximate 20% improvement in relapse-free survival at 5 years for the cohort receiving 3 years of adjuvant imatinib (65% vs. 48%).[78] Importantly, overall survival was significantly better at 5 years (92% vs. 82%) in the group receiving adjuvant therapy for 3 years compared with 1 year. Imatinib therapy can be associated with intolerable side effects, and one-quarter of the patients assigned to take imatinib for 3 years discontinued treatment early for reasons other than disease recurrence. Based on information currently available, it is reasonable to discuss adjuvant imatinib therapy for at least 3 years with patients who are at high risk of tumor relapse (a GIST that is larger than 5 cm in maximum dimension and has more than 5 mitoses per 50 HPF, GISTs that are either larger than 10 cm in greatest dimension or with more than 10 mitoses per 50 HPF, or ruptured tumors). However, the optimal duration of adjuvant therapy in patients with high-risk GIST continues to be the subject of ongoing clinical trials.

ADVANCED DISEASE

Cytotoxic chemotherapy (including intraperitoneal chemotherapy) is ineffective for most cases of GIST; however, imatinib, a small molecule inhibitor of KIT and PDGFRA kinase activity, has remarkable activity against GIST. In early-phase studies of imatinib therapy for metastatic GIST, the Response Evaluation Criteria in Solid Tumors (RECIST) response rates were approximately 60%, at least 10-fold greater than rates associated with previously available therapy.[79] In randomized phase II and phase III studies, a once-daily dose of 400 mg was as effective as 600 mg or 800 mg of imatinib daily.[80,81] As a result, 400 mg daily of oral imatinib is the standard treatment for metastatic GIST. The KIT genotype of a GIST predicts for the responsiveness of the tumor to imatinib. Patients with mutations in exon 11 of KIT have a greater chance of response to imatinib than patients with exon 9 KIT mutations or wild-type KIT.[76] Tumors that harbor the PDGFR mutation D842V are particularly insensitive to imatinib, although other mutations in PDGFR are imatinib-sensitive. The mutation in KIT (or in PDGFRA), and not mere expression of the protein, appears to correlate with sensitivity to imatinib and other tyrosine kinase inhibitors in GIST.

Patients with GIST harboring an activating mutation in exon 9 of KIT may benefit from a higher starting dose of imatinib (400 mg twice daily) based on a small, but statistically significant, improvement in median progression-free survival compared to patients receiving 400 mg of imatinib daily.[82] A meta-analysis of two large, randomized trials comparing 400 mg daily to 400 mg twice daily of imatinib for treatment of advanced or metastatic GIST confirmed a small progression-free survival advantage and detected a higher objective response rate from the higher dose in patients with the exon 9 KIT mutations.[83] However, with a median follow-up of more than 40 months, documented GIST progression or death in patients with exon 9 mutations occurred in 40 of 42 and 42 of 49 patients randomly assigned to 400 mg daily compared with 400 mg twice daily, respectively. There was a trend toward improved survival in the patients receiving the higher dose but it did not reach statistical significance. There was no difference in outcome between the standard- and high-dose groups among patients with the more-common exon 11 KIT mutations. Dose-limiting side effects of imatinib include nausea and vomiting, diarrhea, rash, mucositis, and/or diuretic-resistant peripheral edema. At imatinib doses higher than 800 mg daily, dose-limiting toxicities are frequently encountered.

In contending with advanced disease progressing on first-line therapy (i.e., imatinib at an oral dose of 400 mg daily), a conventional approach is to increase the dose to a total daily dose of 800 mg (or 600 mg if the higher dose is not tolerated).[80,81] Approximately one-third of patients may have some degree of tumor control after escalation of imatinib dose. For patients with imatinib-refractory disease or in patients intolerant of imatinib, sunitinib is the standard second-line therapy, as this agent was shown to be superior to placebo in a randomized phase III study in this setting.[84] The median progression-free survival duration in the arm receiving sunitinib was 24 weeks compared to 6 weeks in patients treated with placebo; however, objective tumor responses were infrequent (less than 10%). Overall survival was also better in the sunitinib-treated arm compared with the placebo-treated arm. Patients less likely to benefit from sunitinib had a primary mutation in exon 11 of *KIT* and likely had developed secondary mutations, rendering GIST resistant to both imatinib and sunitinib. The most frequently reported side effects of sunitinib were fatigue, diarrhea, skin discoloration, and nausea, each occurring in more than 20% of patients. Hypertension and hypothyroidism are also known toxicities of sunitinib, which are readily treated when identified. Rare cases of liver or cardiac fatal events have been reported and patients should be monitored closely on therapy.

Recently, regorafenib, at a dose of 160 mg daily for 3 out of every 4 weeks, was approved for treatment of GIST after development of resistance to imatinib and sunitinib based on results of a randomized, blinded, placebo-controlled trial.[85] Median progression-free survivals were 5 months compared with 1 month for patients receiving regorafenib or placebo, respectively. The most common severe adverse regorafenib-related events were hypertension and hand-foot skin reaction, which occurred in 24% and 20%, respectively, of patients.

Surgery can play a role in the treatment of metastatic disease. In some patients, the tumor progresses in a limited number of disease sites (e.g., one or two deposits of progression in the background of responding disease). Patients with this pattern of limited progression on imatinib (isolated secondary resistance to imatinib) may have a long period before future progression with resection of the resistant clone and continuation of imatinib therapy. All such patients should receive postoperative maintenance imatinib, owing to rapid progression off of systemic treatment. For patients with multiple sites of disease progression (generalized resistance to imatinib), a change in systemic therapy is warranted, because patients with resection of disease almost universally experience further progression within a few months of surgery.[86]

BONE SARCOMAS
OSTEOSARCOMA

Osteosarcomas are the most common tumors of bone, with two peaks of incidence: one between age 10 and 20 and a smaller peak between age 60 and 80. Disease in the latter age group often is associated with Paget disease of bone. Osteosarcomas generally arise in the metaphysis of the bone (between the bone end [epiphysis] and the shaft [diaphysis]). They are characterized by lytic and blastic features in admixed bone. If the tumors extend to soft tissue, they can cause both a periosteal reaction (Codman triangle) and ossification in a pattern perpendicular to the surface of the bone (sunburst pattern; Fig. 13-3).

Adjuvant and/or neoadjuvant chemotherapy is the standard of care for most patients with osteosarcomas. The exception is superficial low-grade osteosarcomas, for which adjuvant chemotherapy is not indicated.[87] For conventional osteosarcomas, the combination of neoadjuvant and adjuvant cisplatin and doxorubicin was found to be as effective as a more complex methotrexate-containing regimen in one randomized multicenter study.[88]

Data regarding the use of methotrexate remain somewhat controversial in adult patients; however, in the U.S. pediatric oncology community, doxorubicin/cisplatin/high-dose methotrexate is the standard of care. In practice, methotrexate most frequently is used in younger patients, owing to delayed clearance and risk of nephrotoxicity and acute lung injury in older adults. Ifosfamide is effective for osteosarcomas, but its role in standard neoadjuvant and adjuvant therapy remains under investigation. Muramyl tripeptide, a nonspecific immune stimulator, was shown to improve overall survival when used in the adjuvant setting in one large cooperative group study; however, the compound is unavailable for use in the United States, although it was approved for adjuvant use in patients younger than age 30 in Europe.[89,90]

The response of osteosarcomas to neoadjuvant chemotherapy can be assessed by pathologic examination at the time of operation, which provides prognostic information. However, there

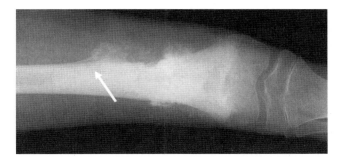

Fig. 13-3 Plain radiograph of osteogenic sarcoma of the distal part of the femur.

Note the Codman triangle (arrow) and the blastic changes in the bone and soft tissue.

is no evidence that changing therapy improves overall survival in patients with osteosarcoma that had a poor response to preoperative chemotherapy. This strategy was the subject of an international randomized study that completed accrual in 2011; results are forthcoming. Because patients with poorly responding osteosarcoma treated with chemotherapy have higher survival rates than patients who do not receive chemotherapy, all patients should be offered a full course of chemotherapy for treatment of primary osteosarcoma regardless of histologic response. Osteosarcomas typically metastasize to the lung. Resection of pulmonary metastases (stage IVA disease) is one of the few examples in nonhematologic cancer of possible cure in a significant minority of patients with metastatic disease.[91] Patients with fewer than three pulmonary metastases who are more than 2 years from diagnosis to the development of lung metastases have the best survival rates after metastasectomy. Ifosfamide plus etoposide with or without methotrexate has activity in relapsed osteosarcoma.[92,93]

CHONDROSARCOMA

Chondrosarcomas are the second most common tumor of the bone and usually affect patients older than age 60. There is no role for chemotherapy in the management of most chondrosarcomas, which are typically low- to intermediate-grade tumors that resemble cartilage both macroscopically and microscopically and are highly chemotherapy-resistant. On radiographs, chondrosarcomas generally appear as a radiolucent area with obvious bony destruction and a moderate number of discrete calcified areas and often involve the medullary cavity. They often have scalloped edges consistent with a multinodular growth pattern. Metastases from conventional chondrosarcoma often involve lung, follow an indolent growth rate, and may be managed by surgery if limited in number. Dedifferentiated chondrosarcoma occasionally responds to chemotherapy used for osteosarcoma. Patients with mesenchymal chondrosarcoma, another high-grade variant that resembles Ewing sarcoma on routine staining, may benefit from chemotherapy, often using a Ewing regimen. Extraskeletal mesenchymal chondrosarcoma is not a cartilaginous tumor but is a soft tissue malignancy that often arises in deep soft tissues, has a relatively indolent growth rate and a high risk of dissemination, and is relatively chemotherapy-resistant.[1]

EWING SARCOMA

Ewing sarcoma typically arises in the bones of children and less commonly in adults. Extracranial (peripheral) primitive neuroectodermal tumor arises in soft tissues and is more common than skeletal Ewing in adults. Askin tumor is an Ewing-like neoplasm typically arising in the soft tissues of the chest or pleura of young adults. These tumors are part of a spectrum of diseases referred to as Ewing sarcoma family of tumors (ESFT), characterized by a varying degree of differentiation and always considered high-grade. On microscopy, Ewing sarcoma appears as monotonous sheets of small round blue cells that express high levels of a cell surface glycoprotein (CD99) and the nuclear factor FLI-1, which can be detected using immunohistochemistry.

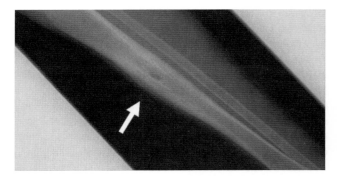

Fig. 13-4 Plain radiograph of Ewing sarcoma of the tibia. Note the diffuse infiltrative changes, or "onion-skinning" characteristic of Ewing sarcoma, in the middle part of the shaft (arrow).

However, expression of CD99 and FLI-1 are not specific for Ewing sarcoma, and molecular studies may be performed to detect the characteristic chromosome translocations present in the disease. Skeletal Ewing sarcoma usually affects the shaft of the bone in an infiltrative pattern called "onion-skinning," which is easily visible on CT scans (less so on plain x-rays; Fig. 13-4). Multimodality therapy with surgery, chemotherapy, and radiation is the standard of care for ESFT and results in rates of cure of higher than 50% for patients presenting with localized disease. Approximately 20% to 30% of patients presenting with metastasis may be long-term survivors after multimodality therapy.[94,95] Local treatment of the primary site of disease is usually performed after an initial 12 weeks of chemotherapy. Complete resection of the tumor is preferred, which reduces risk of local recurrence and secondary radiation-associated malignancy. Radiation is administered adjuvantly for treatment of microscopic residual tumor or if surgery cannot be performed with acceptable morbidity. Radiation-induced sarcomas develop in approximately 1% to 2% of long-term Ewing sarcoma survivors treated with radiation for local tumor control.[94,96,97]

The addition of ifosfamide and etoposide to the combination of vincristine, doxorubicin, and cyclophosphamide is the standard chemotherapy for this malignancy, and this regimen yielded improvement in relapse-free and overall survival compared to vincristine, doxorubicin, dactinomycin, and cyclophosphamide in patients with nonmetastatic Ewing sarcoma.[94] A randomized trial of cyclophosphamide, vincristine, and doxorubicin given in cycles alternating with ifosfamide and etoposide administered every 2 versus every 3 weeks for a total of 14 cycles in patients younger than age 50 with localized Ewing sarcoma demonstrated improvement in recurrence-free survival, with an absolute difference of 8% at 5 years for the arm receiving dose-dense treatment, which resulted in fewer distant relapses.[96] The toxicity profile and frequency did not differ between arms. The development of secondary malignancies including acute leukemia, osteosarcoma, and lymphoma occurred in approximately 3% of patients.

For metastatic Ewing sarcomas, the simpler combination of vincristine/doxorubicin/cyclophosphamide was shown to be as efficacious as the five-drug combination used for primary disease, probably because patients who had disease progression on the three-drug regimen could cross over to ifosfamide and etoposide at time of progression.[94] Assuming patients have received the standard multidrug regimen for Ewing sarcoma, options for therapy are limited, and these patients are good candidates for clinical trials. Relapsed or refractory ESFT may respond to treatment with cyclophosphamide plus topotecan or irinotecan plus temozolomide.[98,99]

GIANT CELL TUMOR OF BONE

Giant cell tumor of bone (GCT) is considered a benign disease, which often causes severe morbidity from destruction of bone. In a small number of cases, GCT has the potential to metastasize (primarily to the lungs). The tumor is composed of malignant stromal cells that secrete receptor activator of nuclear factor kappa-B (RANK) ligand and recruit multinucleated osteoclast-like cells that result in bone lysis. Patients usually present with lytic bone destruction, pain, and restricted mobility of the joint adjacent to the lesion. Current primary management involves complete curettage of the lesion, often followed by intralesional adjuvant therapy with heat, freezing, or chemicals (e.g., phenol). About 10% to 20% of tumors will recur locally, often necessitating joint resection and replacement; metastasis occurs in approximately 1% of cases. Denosumab, an inhibitory monoclonal antibody to RANK ligand, administered monthly resulted in evidence of GCT response in more than 80% of the patients treated in a phase II trial.[100] Reports from an interim analysis of a larger trial of denosumab in patients with GCT discussed occurrence of osteonecrosis of the jaw in 1%, hypocalcemia in 5%, and hypophosphatemia in 3% of patients, attributed to the drug.[101] Based on the high rate of tumor control and relatively low rate of adverse effects from denosumab treatment of GCT, in 2013 the FDA approved denosumab (120 mg administered subcutaneously monthly) for the treatment of patients with unresectable GCT or in situations in which complete resection would result in severe morbidity (e.g., GCT involving pelvis or sacrum or requiring joint replacement) in adults and skeletally mature adolescents.

SURVIVORSHIP

Survivors of childhood cancer are at risk for the development of secondary cancers, including sarcomas. The Childhood Cancer Survivor Study identified a 9-fold higher risk of developing a secondary sarcoma among survivors of childhood cancer compared to the general population.[102] Moreover, the significant improvement in long-term survival rates of children and adults with sarcoma, especially Ewing sarcoma, osteosarcoma, and rhabdomyosarcoma, from multimodality treatment comes at a heavy cost for a minority of patients. Serious late effects of treatment include secondary malignancy, infertility, cardiomyopathy, nephropathy, neuropathy, hearing impairment, and limb dysfunction. The cumulative incidence of secondary malignancy in children treated for sarcoma is approximately 1% to 3% at 10 to 20 years, with the highest risk in patients who received chemotherapy and radiation. There is a 3- to 6-fold higher risk of secondary cancer in children treated for sarcoma than in an age-matched general population.[103,104] Adults treated for sarcoma with chemotherapy and/or radiation also are at risk for long-term complications, including secondary malignancies. Approximately 1% to 2% of patients treated for sarcoma with doxorubicin and ifosfamide develop symptomatic cardiomyopathy, and 5% to 10% develop renal tubular and/or glomerular dysfunction, with risk related to cumulative dose received. Infertility is most often related to alkylating agent exposure and affects postpubescent males more often than females.

KEY POINTS

- Chemotherapy is used in the neoadjuvant/adjuvant setting to treat osteosarcoma. Doxorubicin/cisplatin is commonly used as standard therapy, and high-dose methotrexate is usually included in the treatment of children and young adults with normal renal function.
- Neoadjuvant/adjuvant chemotherapy using five drugs is the standard treatment for Ewing sarcoma of bone or soft tissue. Radiation may be used in the case of positive tumor margin during surgery or for unresectable disease.
- Patients with metastatic bone sarcomas may be cured by appropriate multidisciplinary management. Resection of osteosarcoma metastases to the lung should be considered, especially for patients with fewer than three metastases and a long disease-free interval after treatment of the primary sarcoma.
- Giant cell tumor of bone (GCT) causes osteoclast activation resulting in lysis of bone and carries a small risk of metastasis. Denosumab blocks differentiation and activation of osteoclasts in GCT and halts further bone destruction in the majority of cases.

References

1. Fletcher CDM (ed). WHO classification of tumours of soft tissue and bone. *World Health Organization Classification of Tumours, 4th ed.* Lyon: IARC Press, 2013;468.
2. Siegel R, Naishadham D, Jemal A. Cancer statistics, 2013. *CA Cancer J Clin.* 2013;63:11-30. PMID: 23335087.
3. Arndt CA, Crist WM. Common musculoskeletal tumors of childhood and adolescence. *N Engl J Med.* 1999;341:342-352. PMID: 10423470.
4. Patel S. Long-term efficacy of imatinib for treatment of metastatic GIST. *Cancer Chemother Pharmacol.* 2013;72:277-286. PMID: 23503753.
5. Mitchell G, Ballinger ML, Wong S, et al. High frequency of germline TP53 mutations in a prospective adult-onset sarcoma cohort. *PLoS One.* 2013;8:e69026. PMID: 23894400.
6. Falk H, Herbert J, Crowley S, et al. Epidemiology of hepatic angiosarcoma in the United States: 1964-1974. *Environ Health Perspect.* 1981;41:107-113. PMID: 7199426.
7. Bertazzi PA, Zocchetti C, Guercilena S, et al. Dioxin exposure and cancer risk: a 15-year mortality study after the "Seveso accident". *Epidemiology.* 1997;8:646-652. PMID: 9345664.
8. Collins JJ, Bodner K, Aylward LL, et al. Mortality rates among trichlorophenol workers with exposure to 2,3,7,8-tetrachlorodibenzo-p-dioxin. *Am J Epidemiol.* 2009;170:501-506. PMID: 19561065.
9. Ruder AM, Yiin JH. Mortality of US pentachlorophenol production workers through 2005. *Chemosphere.* 2011;83:851-861. PMID: 21440286.
10. Zambon P, Ricci P, Bovo E, et al. Sarcoma risk and dioxin emissions from incinerators and industrial plants: a population-based case-control study (Italy). *Environ Health.* 2007;6:19. PMID: 17634118.

11. Dores GM, Metayer C, Curtis RE, et al. Second malignant neoplasms among long-term survivors of Hodgkin's disease: a population-based evaluation over 25 years. *J Clin Oncol.* 2002;20:3484-3494. PMID: 12177110.

12. Samartzis D, Nishi N, Hayashi M, et al. Exposure to ionizing radiation and development of bone sarcoma: new insights based on atomic-bomb survivors of Hiroshima and Nagasaki. *J Bone Joint Surg Am.* 2011;93:1008-1015. PMID: 21984980.

13. Samartzis D, Nishi N, Cologne J, et al. Ionizing radiation exposure and the development of soft tissue sarcomas in atomic-bomb survivors. *J Bone Joint Surg Am.* 2013;95:222-229. PMID: 23389785.

14. Nielsen TO, West RB. Translating gene expression into clinical care: sarcomas as a paradigm. *J Clin Oncol.* 2010;28:1796-1805. PMID: 20194847.

15. Edge SB, Byrd DR, Compton CC, et al (eds). *AJCC Cancer Staging Manual, 7th ed.* New York: Springer; 2010.

16. Guillou L, Coindre JM, Bonichon F, et al. Comparative study of the National Cancer Institute and French Federation of Cancer Centers Sarcoma Group grading systems in a population of 410 adult patients with soft tissue sarcoma. *J Clin Oncol.* 1997;15:350-362. PMID: 8996162.

17. Maduekwe UN, Hornicek FJ, Springfield DS, et al. Role of sentinel lymph node biopsy in the staging of synovial, epithelioid, and clear cell sarcomas. *Ann Surg Oncol.* 2009;16:1356-1363. PMID: 19259743.

18. Brennan MF. Staging of soft tissue sarcomas. *Ann Surg Oncol.* 1999;6:8-9. PMID: 10030406.

19. Pisters PW, Leung DH, Woodruff J, et al. Analysis of prognostic factors in 1,041 patients with localized soft tissue sarcomas of the extremities. *J Clin Oncol.* 1996;14:1679-1689. PMID: 8622088.

20. Kattan MW, Leung DH, Brennan MF. Postoperative nomogram for 12-year sarcoma-specific death. *J Clin Oncol.* 2002;20:791-796. PMID: 11821462.

21. Gronchi A, Lo Vullo S, Colombo C, et al. Extremity soft tissue sarcoma in a series of patients treated at a single institution: local control directly impacts survival. *Ann Surg.* 2010;251:506-511. PMID: 20130465.

22. Pisters PW, Pollock RE, Lewis VO, et al. Long-term results of prospective trial of surgery alone with selective use of radiation for patients with T1 extremity and trunk soft tissue sarcomas. *Ann Surg.* 2007;246:675-681; discussion 681-682. PMID: 17893504.

23. Yang JC, Chang AE, Baker AR, et al. Randomized prospective study of the benefit of adjuvant radiation therapy in the treatment of soft tissue sarcomas of the extremity. *J Clin Oncol.* 1998;16:197-203. PMID: 9440743.

24. Pisters PW, Harrison LB, Leung DH, et al. Long-term results of a prospective randomized trial of adjuvant brachytherapy in soft tissue sarcoma. *J Clin Oncol.* 1996;14:859-868. PMID: 8622034.

25. O'Sullivan B, Davis AM, Turcotte R, et al. Preoperative versus postoperative radiotherapy in soft-tissue sarcoma of the limbs: a randomised trial. *Lancet.* 2002;359:2235-2241. PMID: 12103287.

26. Davis AM, O'Sullivan B, Turcotte R, et al. Late radiation morbidity following randomization to preoperative versus postoperative radiotherapy in extremity soft tissue sarcoma. *Radiother Oncol.* 2005;75:48-53. PMID: 15948265.

27. Adjuvant chemotherapy for localised resectable soft-tissue sarcoma of adults: meta-analysis of individual data. Sarcoma Meta-analysis Collaboration. *Lancet.* 1997;350:1647-1654. PMID: 9400508.

28. Pervaiz N, Colterjohn N, Farrokhyar F, et al. A systematic meta-analysis of randomized controlled trials of adjuvant chemotherapy for localized resectable soft-tissue sarcoma. *Cancer.* 2008;113:573-581. PMID: 18521899.

29. Frustaci S, Gherlinzoni F, De Paoli A, et al. Adjuvant chemotherapy for adult soft tissue sarcomas of the extremities and girdles: results of the Italian randomized cooperative trial. *J Clin Oncol.* 2001;19:1238-1247. PMID: 11230464.

30. Frustaci S, De Paoli A, Bidoli E, et al. Ifosfamide in the adjuvant therapy of soft tissue sarcomas. *Oncology.* 2003;65 Suppl 2:80-84. PMID: 14586155.

31. Italiano A, Delva F, Mathoulin-Pelissier S, et al. Effect of adjuvant chemotherapy on survival in FNCLCC grade 3 soft tissue sarcomas: a multivariate analysis of the French Sarcoma Group Database. *Ann Oncol.* 2010;21:2436-2441. PMID: 20439343.

32. Eilber FC, Eilber FR, Eckardt J, et al. The impact of chemotherapy on the survival of patients with high-grade primary extremity liposarcoma. *Ann Surg.* 2004;240:686-695; discussion 695-697. PMID: 15383796.

33. Gortzak E, Azzarelli A, Buesa J, et al. A randomised phase II study on neo-adjuvant chemotherapy for 'high-risk' adult soft-tissue sarcoma. *Eur J Cancer.* 2001;37:1096-1103. PMID: 11378339.

34. Brodowicz T, Schwameis E, Widder J, et al. Intensified adjuvant IFADIC chemotherapy for adult soft tissue sarcoma: a prospective randomized feasibility trial. *Sarcoma.* 2000;4:151-160. PMID: 18521295.

35. Woll PJ, Reichardt P, Le Cesne A, et al. Adjuvant chemotherapy with doxorubicin, ifosfamide, and lenograstim for resected soft-tissue sarcoma (EORTC 62931): a multicentre randomised controlled trial. *Lancet Oncol.* 2012;13:1045-1054. PMID: 22954508.

36. Kasper B, Ouali M, van Glabbeke M, et al. Prognostic factors in adolescents and young adults (AYA) with high risk soft tissue sarcoma (STS) treated by adjuvant chemotherapy: a study based on pooled European Organisation for Research and Treatment of Cancer (EORTC) clinical trials 62771 and 62931. *Eur J Cancer.* 2013;49:449-456. PMID: 22975215.

37. Crist WM, Anderson JR, Meza JL, et al. Intergroup rhabdomyosarcoma study-IV: results for patients with nonmetastatic disease. *J Clin Oncol.* 2001;19:3091-3102. PMID: 11408506.

38. Santoro A. Advanced soft tissue sarcoma: how many more trials with anthracyclines and ifosfamide? *Ann Oncol.* 1999;10:151-154. PMID: 10093682.

39. Patel SR, Vadhan-Raj S, Papadopolous N, et al. High-dose ifosfamide in bone and soft tissue sarcomas: results of phase II and pilot studies--dose-response and schedule dependence. *J Clin Oncol.* 1997;15:2378-2384. PMID: 9196153.

40. Edmonson JH, Ryan LM, Blum RH, et al. Randomized comparison of doxorubicin alone versus ifosfamide plus doxorubicin or mitomycin, doxorubicin, and cisplatin against advanced soft tissue sarcomas. *J Clin Oncol.* 1993;11:1269-1275. PMID: 8315424.

41. Judson I, Verweij J, Gelderblom H, et al. Doxorubicin alone versus intensified doxorubicin plus ifosfamide for first-line treatment of advanced or metastatic soft-tissue sarcoma: a randomised controlled phase 3 trial. *Lancet Oncol.* 2014;15:415-423. PMID: 24618336.

42. Maki RG, Wathen JK, Patel SR, et al. Randomized phase II study of gemcitabine and docetaxel compared with gemcitabine alone in patients with metastatic soft tissue sarcomas: results of sarcoma alliance for research through collaboration study 002 [corrected]. *J Clin Oncol.* 2007;25:2755-2763. PMID: 17602081.

43. Hensley ML, Blessing JA, Mannel R, et al. Fixed-dose rate gemcitabine plus docetaxel as first-line therapy for metastatic uterine leiomyosarcoma: a Gynecologic Oncology Group phase II trial. *Gyn Oncol.* 2008;109:329-334. PMID: 18534250.

44. Bay JO, Ray-Coquard I, Fayette J, et al. Docetaxel and gemcitabine combination in 133 advanced soft-tissue sarcomas: a retrospective analysis. *Int J Cancer.* 2006;119:706-711. PMID: 16496406.

45. van der Graaf WT, Blay JY, Chawla SP, et al. Pazopanib for metastatic soft-tissue sarcoma (PALETTE): a randomised, double-blind, placebo-controlled phase 3 trial. *Lancet.* 2012;379:1879-1886. PMID: 22595799.

46. Maki RG, D'Adamo DR, Keohan ML, et al. Phase II study of sorafenib in patients with metastatic or recurrent sarcomas. *J Clin Oncol.* 2009;27:3133-3140. PMID: 19451436.

47. Gounder MM, Lefkowitz RA, Keohan ML, et al. Activity of sorafenib against desmoid tumor/deep fibromatosis. *Clin Cancer Res.* 2011;17:4082-4090. PMID: 21447727.

48. Stacchiotti S, Negri T, Zaffaroni N, et al. Sunitinib in advanced alveolar soft part sarcoma: evidence of a direct antitumor effect. *Ann Oncol.* 2011;22:1682-1690. PMID: 21242589.

49. Bissler JJ, Kingswood JC, Radzikowska E, et al. Everolimus for angiomyolipoma associated with tuberous sclerosis complex or sporadic lymphangioleiomyomatosis (EXIST-2): a multicentre, randomised, double-blind, placebo-controlled trial. *Lancet.* 2013;381:817-824. PMID: 23312829.

50. Rutkowski P, Van Glabbeke M, Rankin CJ, et al. Imatinib mesylate in advanced dermatofibrosarcoma protuberans: pooled analysis of two phase II clinical trials. *J Clin Oncol.* 2010;28:1772-1779. PMID: 20194851.

51. Cassier PA, Gelderblom H, Stacchiotti S, et al. Efficacy of imatinib mesylate for the treatment of locally advanced and/or metastatic tenosynovial giant cell tumor/pigmented villonodular synovitis. *Cancer.* 2012;118:1649-1655. PMID: 21823110.

52. Butrynski JE, D'Adamo DR, Hornick JL, et al. Crizotinib in ALK-rearranged inflammatory myofibroblastic tumor. *N Engl J Med.* 2010;363:1727-1733. PMID: 20979472.

53. Aversa SM, Cattelan AM, Salvagno L, et al. Treatments of AIDS-related Kaposi's sarcoma. *Crit Rev Oncol Hematol.* 2005;53:253-265. PMID: 15718150.

54. Krown SE, Lee JY, Dittmer DP. More on HIV-associated Kaposi's sarcoma. *N Engl J Med.* 2008;358:535-536; author reply 536. PMID: 18234764.

55. Stebbing J, Powles T, Bower M. AIDS-associated Kaposi's sarcoma associated with a low viral load and a high CD4 cell count. *AIDS.* 2008;22:551-552. PMID: 18301078.

56. Mani D, Neil N, Israel R, et al. A retrospective analysis of HIV-associated Kaposi's sarcoma in patients with undetectable HIV viral loads and CD4 counts greater than 300 cells/mm(3). *J Int Assoc Physicians AIDS Care (Chic)*. 2009;8:279-285. PMID: 19721098.

57. Bower M, Nelson M, Young AM, et al. Immune reconstitution inflammatory syndrome associated with Kaposi's sarcoma. *J Clin Oncol*. 2005;23:5224-5228. PMID: 16051964.

58. Jaffe HW, De Stavola BL, Carpenter LM, et al. Immune reconstitution and risk of Kaposi sarcoma and non-Hodgkin lymphoma in HIV-infected adults. *AIDS*. 2011;25:1395-1403. PMID: 21572307.

59. Leidner RS, Aboulafia DM. Recrudescent Kaposi's sarcoma after initiation of HAART: a manifestation of immune reconstitution syndrome. *AIDS Patient Care and STDs*. 2005;19:635-644. PMID: 16232048.

60. Di Lorenzo G, Kostantinopolous PA, Pantanowitz L, et al. Management of AIDS-related Kaposi's sarcoma. *Lancet Oncol*. 2007;8:167-176. PMID: 17267331.

61. Nguyen HQ, Magaret AS, Kitahata MM, et al. Persistent Kaposi sarcoma in the era of highly active antiretroviral therapy: characterizing the predictors of clinical response. *AIDS*. 2008;22:937-945. PMID: 18453853.

62. Walmsley S, Northfelt DW, Melosky B, et al. Treatment of AIDS-related cutaneous Kapossi's sarcoma with topical alitretinoin (9-cis-retinoic acid) gel. Panretin Gel North American Study Group. *J Acquir Immune Defic Syndr*. 1999;22:235-246. PMID: 10770343.

63. Boudreaux AA, Smith LL, Cosby CD, et al. Intralesional vinblastine for cutaneous Kaposi's sarcoma associated with acquired immunodeficiency syndrome. A clinical trial to evaluate efficacy and discomfort associated with infection. *J Am Acad Dermatol*. 1993;28:61-65. PMID: 8381146.

64. Dupuy J, Price M, Lynch G, et al. Intralesional interferon-alpha and zidovudine in epidemic Kaposi sarcoma. *J Am Acad Dermatol*. 1993;28:966-972. PMID: 8496462.

65. Boente P, Sampaio G, Brandão MA, et al. Localized peri-lesional therapy with rhGM-CSF for Kaposi's sarcoma. *Lancet*. 1993;341:1154. PMID: 8097837.

66. Zouboulis CC. Cryosurgery in dermatology. *Eur J Dermatol*. 1998;8:466-474. PMID: 9854156.

67. Swift PS. The role of radiation therapy in the management of HIV-related Kaposi's sarcoma. *Hematol Oncol* Clin North Am. 1996;10:1069-1080. PMID: 8880197.

68. Gressen EL, Rosenstock JG, Xie Y, et al. Palliative treatment of epidemic Kaposi sarcoma of the feet. Am *J Clin Oncol*. 1999;22:286-290. PMID: 10362338.

69. Gill PS, Wernz J, Scadden DT, et al. Randomized phase III trial of liposomal daunorubicin versus doxorubicin, bleomycin, and vincristine in AIDS-related Kaposi's sarcoma. *J Clin Oncol*. 1996;14:2353-2364. PMID: 8708728.

70. Northfelt DW, Dezube BJ, Thommes JA, et al. Pegylated-liposomal doxorubicin versus doxorubicin, bleomycin, and vincristine in the treatment of AIDS-related Kaposi's sarcoma: results of a randomized phase III clinical trial. *J Clin Oncol*. 1998;16:2445-2451. PMID: 9667262.

71. Stewart S, Jablonowski H, Goebel FD, et al. Randomized comparative trial of pegylated liposomal doxorubicin versus bleomycin and vincristine in the treatment of AIDS-related Kaposi's sarcoma. International Pegylated Liposomal Doxorubicin Study Group. *J Clin Oncol*. 1998;16:683-691. PMID: 9469358.

72. Di Lorenzo G, Kreuter A, Di Trolio R, et al. Activity and safety of pegylated liposomal doxorubicin as first-line therapy in the treatment of non-visceral classic Kaposi's sarcoma: a multicenter study. *J Invest Dermatol*. 2008;128:1578-1580. PMID: 18185536.

73. Martín-Carbonero L, Palacios R, Valencia E, et al. Long-term prognosis of HIV-infected patients with Kaposi sarcoma treated with pegylated liposomal doxorubicin. *Clin Infect Dis*. 2008;47:410-417. PMID: 18582203.

74. Gill PS, Tulpule A, Espina BM, et al. Paclitaxel is safe and effective in the treatment of advanced AIDS-related Kaposi's sarcoma. *J Clin Oncol*. 1999;17:1876-1883. PMID: 10561228.

75. Welles L, Saville MW, Lietzau J, et al. Phase II trial with dose titration of paclitaxel for the therapy of human immunodeficiency virus-associated Kaposi's sarcoma. *J Clin Oncol*. 1998;16:1112-1121. PMID: 9508198.

76. Heinrich MC, Corless CL, Demetri GD, et al. Kinase mutations and imatinib response in patients with metastatic gastrointestinal stromal tumor. *J Clin Oncol*. 2003;21:4342-4349. PMID: 14645423.

77. Dematteo RP, Ballman KV, Antonescu CR, et al. Adjuvant imatinib mesylate after resection of localised, primary gastrointestinal stromal tumour: a randomised, double-blind, placebo-controlled trial. *Lancet*. 2009;373:1097-1104. PMID: 19303137.

78. Joensuu H, Eriksson M, Sundby Hall K, et al. One vs three years of adjuvant imatinib for operable gastrointestinal stromal tumor: a randomized trial. *JAMA*. 2012;307:1265-1272. PMID: 22453568.

79. Demetri GD, von Mehren M, Blanke CD, et al. Efficacy and safety of imatinib mesylate in advanced gastrointestinal stromal tumors. *N Engl J Med*. 2002;347:472-480. PMID: 12181401.

80. Verweij J, Casali PG, Zalcberg J, et al. Progression-free survival in gastrointestinal stromal tumours with high-dose imatinib: randomised trial. *Lancet*. 2004;364:1127-1134. PMID: 15451219.

81. Blanke CD, Rankin C, Demetri GD, et al. Phase III randomized, intergroup trial assessing imatinib mesylate at two dose levels in patients with unresectable or metastatic gastrointestinal stromal tumors expressing the kit receptor tyrosine kinase: S0033. *J Clin Oncol*. 2008;26:626-632. PMID: 18235122.

82. Debiec-Rychter M, Sciot R, Le Cesne A, et al. KIT mutations and dose selection for imatinib in patients with advanced gastrointestinal stromal tumours. *Eur J Cancer*. 2006;42:1093-1103. PMID: 16624552.

83. Gastrointestinal Stromal Tumor Meta-Analysis Group (MetaGIST). Comparison of two doses of imatinib for the treatment of unresectable or metastatic gastrointestinal stromal tumors: a meta-analysis of 1,640 patients. *J Clin Oncol*. 2010;28:1247-1253. PMID: 20124181.

84. Demetri GD, van Oosterom AT, Garrett CR, et al. Efficacy and safety of sunitinib in patients with advanced gastrointestinal stromal tumour after failure of imatinib: a randomised controlled trial. *Lancet*. 2006;368:1329-1338. PMID: 17046465.

85. Demetri GD, Reichardt P, Kang YK, et al. Efficacy and safety of regorafenib for advanced gastrointestinal stromal tumours after failure of imatinib and sunitinib (GRID): an international, multicentre, randomised, placebo-controlled, phase 3 trial. *Lancet*. 2013;381:295-302. PMID: 23177515.

86. DeMatteo RP, Maki RG, Singer S, et al. Results of tyrosine kinase inhibitor therapy followed by surgical resection for metastatic gastrointestinal stromal tumor. *Ann Surg*. 2007;245:347-352. PMID: 17435539.

87. Okada K, Frassica FJ, Sim FH, et al. Parosteal osteosarcoma. A clinicopathological study. *J Bone Joint Surg Am*. 1994;76:366-378. PMID: 8126042.

88. Souhami RL, Craft AW, Van der Eijken JW, et al. Randomised trial of two regimens of chemotherapy in operable osteosarcoma: a study of the European Osteosarcoma Intergroup. *Lancet*. 1997;350:911-917. PMID: 9314869.

89. Meyers PA, Schwartz CL, Krailo M, et al. Osteosarcoma: a randomized, prospective trial of the addition of ifosfamide and/or muramyl tripeptide to cisplatin, doxorubicin, and high-dose methotrexate. *J Clin Oncol*. 2005;23:2004-2011. PMID: 15774791.

90. Meyers PA, Schwartz CL, Krailo MD, et al. Osteosarcoma: the addition of muramyl tripeptide to chemotherapy improves overall survival--a report from the Children's Oncology Group. *J Clin Oncol*. 2008;26:633-638. PMID: 18235123.

91. Pastorino U, Gasparini M, Tavecchio L, et al. The contribution of salvage surgery to the management of childhood osteosarcoma. *J Clin Oncol*. 1991;9:1357-1362. PMID: 2072139.

92. Gentet JC, Brunat-Mentigny M, Demaille MC, et al. Ifosfamide and etoposide in childhood osteosarcoma. A phase II study of the French Society of Paediatric Oncology. *Eur J Cancer*. 1997;33:232-237. PMID: 9135494.

93. Michelagnoli MP, Lewis IJ, Gattamaneni HR, et al. Ifosfamide/etoposide alternating with high-dose methotrexate: evaluation of a chemotherapy regimen for poor-risk osteosarcoma. *Br J Cancer*. 1999;79:1174-1178. PMID: 10098754.

94. Grier HE, Krailo MD, Tarbell NJ, et al. Addition of ifosfamide and etoposide to standard chemotherapy for Ewing's sarcoma and primitive neuroectodermal tumor of bone. *N Engl J Med*. 2003;348:694-701. PMID: 12594313.

95. Paulussen M, Ahrens S, Craft AW, et al. Ewing's tumors with primary lung metastases: survival analysis of 114 (European Intergroup) Cooperative Ewing's Sarcoma Studies patients. *J Clin Oncol*. 1998;16:3044-3052. PMID: 9738574.

96. Womer RB, West DC, Krailo MD, et al. Randomized controlled trial of interval-compressed chemotherapy for treatment of localized Ewing sarcoma: a report from the Children's Oncology Group. *J Clin Oncol*. 2012;30:4148-4154. PMID: 23091096.

97. Bacci G, Forni C, Longhi A, et al. Long-term outcome for patients with nonmetastatic Ewing's sarcoma treated with adjuvant and neoadjuvant chemotherapy. 402 patients treated at Rizzoli between 1972 and 1992. *Eur J Cancer*. 2004;40:73-83. PMID: 14687792.

98. Hunold A, Weddeling N, Paulussen M, et al. Topotecan and cyclophosphamide in patients with refractory or relapsed Ewing tumors. *Pediatr Blood Cancer*. 2006;47:795-800. PMID: 16411206.

99. Wagner LM, McAllister N, Goldsby RE, et al. Temozolomide and intravenous irinotecan for treatment of advanced Ewing sarcoma. *Pediatr Blood Cancer*. 2007;48:132-139. PMID: 16317751.

100. Thomas D, Henshaw R, Skubitz K, et al. Denosumab in patients with giant-cell tumour of bone: an open-label, phase 2 study. *Lancet Oncol*. 2010;11:275-280. PMID: 20149736.

101. Chawla S, Henshaw R, Seeger L, et al. Safety and efficacy of denosumab for adults and skeletally mature adolescents with giant cell tumour of bone: interim analysis of an open-label, parallel-group, phase 2 study. *Lancet Oncol*. 2013;14:901-908. PMID: 23867211.

102. Henderson TO, Whitton J, Stovall M, et al. Secondary sarcomas in childhood cancer survivors: a report from the Childhood Cancer Survivor Study. *J Natl Cancer Inst*. 2007;99:300-308. PMID: 17312307.

103. Cohen RJ, Curtis RE, Inskip PD, et al. The risk of developing second cancers among survivors of childhood soft tissue sarcoma. *Cancer*. 2005;103:2391-2396. PMID: 15852362.

104. Goldsby R, Burke C, Nagarajan R, et al. Second solid malignancies among children, adolescents, and young adults diagnosed with malignant bone tumors after 1976: follow-up of a Children's Oncology Group cohort. *Cancer*. 2008;113:2597-2604. PMID: 18823030.

14

CENTRAL NERVOUS SYSTEM TUMORS

Sani Kizilbash, MBBS, and Jan Buckner, MD

Updates from 2012

Molecular pathogenesis of diffuse gliomas

▶ Molecular aberrations such as *IDH* mutation, 1p/19q codeletion, and *ATRX* mutation are challenging the understanding and classification of diffuse gliomas (Jiao Y, *Oncotarget* 2012).

Glioblastoma

▶ The addition of bevacizumab to standard chemoradiation with temozolomide in patients with newly diagnosed glioblastoma does not improve overall survival (Chinot OL, *N Engl J Med* 2014; Gilbert MR, *N Engl J Med* 2014).

▶ Temozolomide may be noninferior to radiation as initial therapy in elderly patients with newly diagnosed glioblastoma (Wick W, *Lancet Oncol* 2012).

Anaplastic oligodendroglioma and anaplastic oligoastrocytoma

▶ The addition of chemotherapy with procarbazine, lomustine, and vincristine (PCV) after radiation improves overall survival in patients with anaplastic oligodendroglioma and oligoastrocytoma with either 1p/19q codeletion or *IDH* mutation (Cairncross JG, *J Clin Oncol* 2014).

▶ Patients with neither 1p/19q codeletion nor *IDH* mutations do not benefit from adjuvant PCV chemotherapy (Cairncross JG, *J Clin Oncol* 2014).

Grade II astrocytoma, oligodendroglioma, and oligoastrocytoma

▶ PCV chemotherapy after radiation improves overall survival in high-risk, progressive, or symptomatic low-grade gliomas compared with radiation alone (Buckner JC, presented at 2014 ASCO Annual Meeting).

Medulloblastoma

▶ Vismodegib, a small molecule inhibitor of the hedgehog (SHH) pathway, has recently demonstrated activity in patients with recurrent SHH-type medulloblastoma (Gajjar AJ, presented at 2013 ASCO Annual Meeting).

Meningioma

▶ Genomic analyses suggest that meningiomas with *NF2* mutations and/or chromosome 22 losses are more likely to be atypical and follow a more aggressive course than meningiomas without these genetic aberrations (Clark VE, *Science* 2013).

Brain metastases

▶ Patients with *BRAF*-mutated melanoma metastatic to the brain benefit from treatment with dabrafenib (Long GV, *Lancet Oncol* 2012).

Primary central nervous system (CNS) tumors consist of a diverse range of pathologic entities, each with a distinct natural history. In 2007 the World Health Organization (WHO) defined the current classification for CNS tumors[1] and broadly categorized them into several groups. Tumors of neuroepithelial tissue comprise most of the malignant primary CNS tumors such as astrocytic tumors (e.g., glioblastoma), oligodendroglial tumors, oligoastrocytic tumors, and embryonal tumors (e.g., medulloblastoma). Tumors of the meninges (e.g., meningioma) represent the most common benign primary CNS tumors. Other less common primary CNS tumor categories include tumors of the cranial and paraspinal nerves (e.g., vestibular schwannoma), tumors of the sellar region (e.g., craniopharyngioma), hematopoietic neoplasms (e.g., primary CNS lymphoma), and germ cell tumors. Metastatic tumors are also included in the classification, as these represent the overwhelming majority of intracranial masses in adults.

CLASSIFICATION

GRADING

Unlike most other malignancies, primary CNS tumors rarely metastasize and hence staging is usually irrelevant (with some exceptions such as medulloblastoma and ependymoma).

Alternatively, histologic grading plays a much more significant role in determining prognosis and therapeutic interventions. The use of different grading systems for brain tumors has resulted in considerable confusion in the past. Since 1993, the WHO classification system has been the internationally accepted four-tier grading system. This includes a general grading scheme to describe a scale of malignancy across the various subtypes of primary CNS tumors[1] (Table 14-1):

- Grade I tumors include well-circumscribed tumors with low proliferative potential that may be excised with curative intent.
- Grade II tumors are more infiltrative and cellular. Although relatively slow-growing, these tumors often recur and tend to progress to higher grades of malignancy.
- Grade III tumors demonstrate histologic evidence for malignancy such as cytologic atypia and increased mitotic activity.
- Grade IV tumors are more cytologically malignant, mitotically active, and prone to necrosis. Endothelial proliferation may also be seen. These tumors are usually rapidly fatal.

This system extrapolates from the grading of astrocytoma, as that has been more extensively evaluated and systematically defined. Astrocytoma grading is based on four key histologic

Table 14-1 World Health Organization Classification and Grading of Selected Primary CNS Tumors

	I	II	III	IV		I	II	III	IV
Astrocytic tumors					**Ependymal tumors**				
Subependymal giant cell astrocytoma	X				Subependymoma	X			
Pilocytic astrocytoma	X				Myxopapillary ependymoma	X			
Pilomyxoid astrocytoma		X			Ependymoma		X		
Diffuse astrocytoma		X			Anaplastic ependymoma			X	
Pleomorphic xanthoastrocytoma		X			**Embryonal tumors**				
Anaplastic astrocytoma			X		Medulloblastoma				X
Glioblastoma				X	Supratentorial primitive neuroectodermal tumor				X
Giant cell glioblastoma				X	**Tumors of the cranial and paraspinal nerves**				
Gliosarcoma				X	Schwannoma	X			
Oligodendroglial tumors					**Meningeal tumors**				
Oligodendroglioma		X			Meningioma	X			
Anaplastic oligodendroglioma			X		Atypical meningioma		X		
Oligoastrocytic tumors					Anaplastic/malignant meningioma			X	
Oligoastrocytoma		X			**Tumors of the sellar region**				
Anaplastic oligoastrocytoma			X		Craniopharyngioma	X			

Modified from Louis DN, Ohgaki H, Wiestler OD, et al (eds). WHO Classification of Tumours of the Central Nervous System, 4th ed. Lyon, France: IARC Press; 2007.

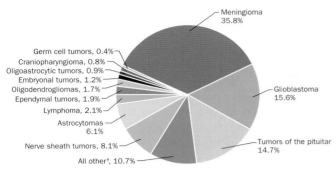

Gliomas (†ICD-O-3: 9380-9384,9391-9460,9480) account for
28% of all tumors and 80% of malignant tumors

Fig. 14-1 Distribution of primary brain and CNS tumors by histology (326,711 patients).

Abbreviation: NOS, not otherwise specified.

Reprinted from Ostrom QT, Gittleman H, Farah P, et al. CBTRUS Statistical Report: Primary Brain and Central Nervous System Tumors Diagnosed in the United States 2006-2010. Neuro-Oncol 2013 Nov; 15(sup 2): ii1 – ii56.

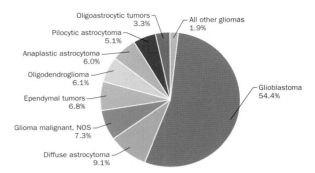

Astrocytomas and glioblastomas account for 75% of all gliomas

Fig. 14-2 Distribution of primary brain and CNS gliomas by histology subtypes (92,504 patients).

features: increased cellularity (in grade II astrocytomas), mitotic activity (in grade III astrocytomas), and endothelial proliferation and necrosis (in grade IV astrocytomas). Grade I astrocytomas have none of the above described characteristics. Of note, molecular markers in primary CNS tumors are increasingly being used to better define groups of patients with significantly different prognoses irrespective of the tumor grade (e.g., isocitrate dehydrogenase [*IDH*] mutation in high-grade glioma[2]). Molecular markers will be discussed in more detail in later sections.

EPIDEMIOLOGY

Primary malignant CNS tumors represent approximately 2% of all cancers but account for a disproportionate share of morbidity and mortality. They are the most common solid tumor in children and are the second leading cause of death from cancer in children, with leukemia being the first. CNS tumors are the third leading cause of cancer-related death for adolescents and young adults (ages 15 to 34). Malignant brain tumors occur more frequently in men, while meningiomas are more common in women. The median age-adjusted incidence for primary brain tumors is 21.0 cases per 100,000 individuals per year, varying from 5.3 in children and adolescents to 27.4 in adults. Of all primary brain tumors, approximately one-third are meningiomas, one-third are gliomas, and the remainder are a variety of other benign and malignant tumors (Fig. 14-1). Of all primary gliomas, 54% are glioblastomas (Fig. 14-2).[3]

It has been difficult to identify environmental factors associated with primary brain tumors. Although there is limited evidence that long-term use of cell phones may increase the risk of brain tumors, reports are conflicting and convincing evidence is lacking.[4] A large national study of 358,403 cell phone subscribers in Denmark followed from 1990 to 2007 (3.8 million person-years) revealed no evidence of increased risk in primary brain tumors in general or in gliomas in particular.[5] The one environmental risk factor identified is exposure to ionizing radiation. For example, radiation treatment for

children with tinea capitis, acute lymphocytic leukemia, craniopharyngioma, or non-Hodgkin lymphoma has been associated with an increased risk of subsequent brain tumors, especially gliomas. The risk of primary CNS lymphoma, but not other types of primary brain tumors, is increased for patients with immunodeficient conditions such as HIV.[6]

MOLECULAR EPIDEMIOLOGY

Genetic predisposition to primary CNS tumors is relatively uncommon, although they may be associated with several familial cancer syndromes (Table 14-2).[7,8] For example, astrocytomas are associated with Li-Fraumeni syndrome, neurofibromatosis 1, tuberous sclerosis, and Lynch syndrome. Medulloblastoma is associated with Li-Fraumeni syndrome, basal cell nevus syndrome, and familial adenomatous polyposis.

Germ-line polymorphisms in the *CDKN2B* and *RTEL1* genes have been associated with a greater risk of developing primary glioblastoma, while germ-line polymorphisms in *CCDC26* are associated with lower-grade tumors, 1p/19q codeletion, and *IDH* mutations.[9-11] In fact, one particular single nucleotide polymorphism near the *CCDC26* gene, rs55705857, is present in nearly 40% of patients with oligodendroglial tumors and gliomas with *IDH* mutations, compared with approximately 8% of the normal population.[12]

CLINICAL FEATURES AND DIAGNOSTIC EVALUATION

SYMPTOMATOLOGY

The presenting symptoms of a brain tumor are related to mass effect, parenchymal infiltration, hydrocephalus, and tissue destruction. Headaches are a common presenting symptom and occur in approximately 35% of patients. The sudden onset of headaches in a patient who has not previously had headaches is most characteristic, especially if the headaches are more severe in the morning and are associated with nausea, vomiting, or focal neurologic deficits. Seizures occur in approximately one-third of patients with gliomas, especially in patients with low-grade tumors. However, seizures may be associated with any CNS tumor. Focal neurologic deficits are related to the location of the tumor. Altered mental status may develop in 15% to 20% of patients with gliomas. Posterior fossa masses, and occasionally supratentorial masses, may obstruct the third or fourth ventricle, resulting in hydrocephalus associated with headache, nausea, vomiting, somnolence, lethargy, or coma.

DIAGNOSTIC IMAGING

Computed tomography (CT) of the brain typically shows a mass that may or may not be enhanced with use of contrast medium. Low-grade gliomas may be isodense with normal brain parenchyma and may not enhance with contrast medium. Consequently, findings on CT may not indicate the diagnosis. Lesions in the posterior fossa may not be identifiable on CT scans.

Magnetic resonance imaging (MRI) is more sensitive than CT for confirming the presence of a brain tumor. On T1-weighted MRI scans, a brain tumor appears as a mass lesion that may or may not be enhanced with contrast; there also may be signal abnormality on T2-weighted scans, especially visible on fluid attenuation and inversion recovery (FLAIR) images. The amount of contrast enhancement usually increases with higher grades of malignant disease. Ring enhancement is characteristic of glioblastoma and is a consequence of central tumor necrosis. However, some low-grade (benign) tumors, such as pilocytic astrocytoma, may also demonstrate contrast enhancement. In addition, some high-grade tumors may not demonstrate contrast enhancement. Furthermore, contrast enhancement does not reflect the true extent of disease as the blood-brain barrier may remain intact at the infiltrating tumor rim.[13,14]

MRI perfusion imaging may demonstrate increased blood flow in high-grade tumors, whereas MRI diffusion imaging may show reduced water movement, presumably secondary to increased cellularity and increased interstitial pressure. Although not definitive, MRI perfusion/diffusion imaging may assist clinical decision-making regarding tumor progression, pseudoprogression, and radiation necrosis. Both MRI spectroscopy and positron emission tomography (PET) imaging provide physiologic information about the tumor and may provide supplemental information in special clinical scenarios. However, the sensitivity and specificity of MRI spectroscopy and PET imaging for particular tumor histology or radiation necrosis are currently too low to recommend their routine use in the clinic.

DIAGNOSTIC PATHOLOGY

Definitive diagnosis of a CNS tumor requires a surgical biopsy or resection with histologic examination of the tissue for nearly

Table 14-2 Genetic Syndromes Associated with Primary CNS Tumors

Genetic Syndrome	Gene Alteration(s)	Associated Primary CNS Tumors
Basal cell nevus (Gorlin) syndrome	PTCH1	Medulloblastoma
Cowden syndrome	PTEN	Gangliocytoma
Li-Fraumeni syndrome	TP53	High-grade glioma Medulloblastoma
Neurofibromatosis 1	NF1	Malignant peripheral nerve sheath tumor Low-grade astrocytoma (usually pilocytic astrocytoma)
Neurofibromatosis 2	NF2	Vestibular schwannoma (frequently bilateral) Meningioma
Tuberous sclerosis	TSC1, TSC2	Subependymal giant cell astrocytoma
Familial adenomatous polyposis	APC	Medulloblastoma
Lynch syndrome (hereditary nonpolyposis colorectal cancer)	MSH2, MLH1, MSH6, PMS2	Glioblastoma
Von Hippel-Lindau syndrome	VHL	Hemangioblastoma

all patients. However, patients with brainstem gliomas may not be candidates for biopsy, both because of the associated risk to the patient and because of the characteristic imaging findings. Patients with CNS germ cell tumors may have elevated serum or cerebrospinal fluid human chorionic gonadotropin levels, or alpha-fetoprotein levels, which confirm the diagnosis for germ cell tumors.

Accurate pathologic diagnosis requires the review of an experienced tumor neuropathologist, as the rate of discordance between general pathologists and neuropathologists is very high. The diagnosis may change substantially for at least one-third of patients when pathologic review is performed by an experienced neuropathologist.

Certain CNS tumors have characteristic histologic features (e.g., "fried egg" appearance of oligodendroglioma). Nevertheless, the key role of immunohistochemistry and molecular markers in diagnosis and prognosis is undisputed. Markers of good prognosis in gliomas include 1p/19q codeletion,[15] O6-methylguanine-DNA-methyltransferase (*MGMT*) promoter hypermethylation,[16] and *IDH* mutation.[17] Furthermore, 1p/19q codeletion and *IDH* mutation independently predict response to chemotherapy in anaplastic oligodendrogliomas and anaplastic oligoastrocytomas,[18] while *MGMT* promoter hypermethylation is associated with a greater likelihood of benefit from temozolomide in glioblastoma.[19] Current clinical trials are using these biomarkers for either stratification or patient inclusion.

STAGING

Most primary brain tumors remain localized so extensive staging procedures are not necessary. Primitive neuroectodermal tumors, such as medulloblastoma, CNS germ cell tumors, ependymoma, and primary CNS lymphoma are exceptions as they frequently spread by way of the subarachnoid space to the leptomeninges. Consequently, MRI of the spine and/or cytologic examination of cerebrospinal fluid (CSF) are necessary for patients with these diagnoses.

KEY POINTS

- The best imaging tool for CNS tumors is magnetic resonance imaging (MRI). Contrast enhancement on MRI scans is the primary imaging hallmark of high-grade tumors. Physiologic imaging methods such as position emission tomography (PET) and MRI spectroscopy may be useful in special clinical scenarios.
- Experienced neuropathology review of brain tumor tissue is essential to establish an accurate diagnosis.
- Patients with medulloblastoma, CNS germ cell tumors, ependymoma, and primary CNS lymphoma may require MRI of the entire spine, as well as cerebrospinal fluid examination.

GENERAL TREATMENT STRATEGIES

SURGERY

The goals of surgery are to obtain sufficient representative tissue to assure accurate histologic diagnosis, to reduce mass effect while preserving neurologic function, to cytoreduce the tumor, and to treat hydrocephalus, if present. Surgery remains the initial therapy for nearly all patients with brain tumors and can be curative for most benign tumors, including meningiomas and some low-grade gliomas (e.g., pilocytic astrocytoma). Unfortunately, most gliomas are characterized by diffuse infiltration of brain parenchyma, making curative surgical extirpation impossible. In these cases, relief of mass effect and debulking results in symptomatic improvement and permits time for safe administration of subsequent treatment. Postoperative MRI is usually performed prior to the development of post-surgical contrast enhancement to assess the adequacy of resection.

Current stereotactic techniques allow for biopsy specimens to be obtained from nearly any part of the brain, including the brainstem. Biopsy alone is generally reserved for patients with tumors in critical functional portions of the brain, where resection would result in unacceptable neurologic deficit. In addition, patients with primary CNS lymphoma or CNS germ cell tumors may only need a biopsy because primary treatment usually involves radiation therapy, chemotherapy, or both.

Meningiomas may be incidentally discovered on imaging. In the presence of benign radiographic features, meningiomas may undergo surveillance alone without resection.

RADIATION THERAPY

External beam radiation therapy is an essential component of treatment for many patients with brain tumors. It can be curative for some patients, and it prolongs survival for others. Radiation often is also the primary treatment modality for patients with metastatic brain tumors, epidural spinal cord compression, and leptomeningeal metastases. Whereas whole-brain radiation may be administered for certain tumors, such as medulloblastoma or primary CNS lymphoma, involved field radiation using multiple field techniques has become the standard treatment for most patients with glioma. Involved field radiation has been as effective as whole-brain radiation and reduces the dose and volume of radiation to normal brain tissue, potentially reducing late neurotoxic effects.

Radiation therapy, especially when used concurrently with temozolomide, commonly causes an increase in the size of contrast-enhancing lesions or new areas of contrast enhancement soon after treatment, with spontaneous improvement without any further treatment.[20] This phenomenon has been labelled pseudoprogression and is crucial to recognize, as it mimics tumor progression.

Side effects and late effects of therapeutic radiation include radionecrosis and leukoencephalopathy. Radionecrosis presents as a focal mass lesion with contrast enhancement and mass effect. The clinical scenario is difficult to distinguish from recurrent tumor and may require surgical resection to relieve mass effect, as well as to establish a histologic diagnosis. Radiation-induced leukoencephalopathy often occurs months to years after treatment, and usually appears as a more diffuse increased T2/FLAIR signal abnormality on MRI with associated atrophy. Patients with characteristic MRI changes may be asymptomatic or may be severely compromised with dementia, gait instability, and urinary incontinence. The frequency of radiation injury is related to total radiation dose, fraction size, volume of brain radiated, treatment technique, and age. In general, morbidity is reduced by using smaller fraction size, lower total dose, and smaller treatment volumes.

Stereotactic radiotherapy techniques have demonstrated efficacy for well-circumscribed lesions such as meningioma and limited brain metastases. However, for the infiltrative malignant tumors, the clinical efficacy of stereotactic radiotherapy has not been proven. In two phase III trials, investigators found no survival advantage for patients with glioblastoma who received radiation with a stereotactic boost or brachytherapy compared with patients receiving standard whole-brain radiation.[21,22] The clinical benefits of other focal radiation therapy techniques, such as the use of nonspecific or targeted radioactive isotopes, are being investigated and are not recommended for routine clinical use. Evidence is emerging that external beam radiation, especially fractionated stereotactic radiation, may be beneficial in patients with high-grade gliomas whose tumors have recurred despite initial radiation and optimal chemotherapy.[23,24] The magnitude of efficacy in relationship to potential harm, and in comparison with other treatment approaches, remains to be determined.

CHEMOTHERAPY

Although chemotherapy provides only modest benefit for most patients with primary brain tumors, chemotherapy has a role in palliation and in adjuvant treatment. Alkylating agents remain the mainstay of treatment in gliomas. Temozolomide, the most commonly used agent, penetrates the intact blood-brain barrier and provides survival benefit for patients with glioblastoma,[19,25] however, the effect is usually not durable. Lomustine, a nitrosourea, in combination with procarbazine and vincristine (PCV) has antitumor activity in patients with low-grade gliomas[26] and anaplastic oligodendroglioma.[27] Platinum drugs have antitumor efficacy for medulloblastoma[28] and germ cell tumors. High-dose methotrexate regimens result in clear clinical benefit for patients with primary CNS lymphomas.[29] Bevacizumab, a vascular endothelial growth factor (VEGF) pathway inhibitor, has been approved by the U.S. Food and Drug Administration (FDA) for use in patients with recurrent or progressing glioblastoma following radiation therapy and temozolomide,[30] however, it does not prolong survival in patients with newly diagnosed glioblastoma.[31,32] Multiple other agents that target aberrant signaling pathways are under investigation.

There have been efforts to improve the efficacy of chemotherapy by improving the delivery of antineoplastic agents by bypassing the blood-tumor barrier. These techniques have included intra-arterial chemotherapy with or without blood-brain barrier disruption, intratumoral administration of agents by convection-enhanced delivery, and placement of intratumoral biodegradable polymers. The efficacy of local administration of various agents directly into brain tumors has generally been modest. However, the FDA has approved the use of carmustine-impregnated degradable polymers for the treatment of newly diagnosed high-grade gliomas and recurrent glioblastoma based on a significant survival benefit in clinical trials.[33,34]

IMPORTANT SUPPORTIVE CARE AGENTS

Corticosteroids, antiepileptic drugs, and anticoagulant drugs are important ancillary agents for the treatment of patients with brain tumors. Corticosteroids are indispensable for controlling edema. Unfortunately, the long-term use of corticosteroids can result in substantial toxic effects. Notably, bevacizumab may also be considered to control severe edema secondary to radiation necrosis.[35]

Antiepileptic drugs are administered for the treatment of seizure disorders. Clinical trials have also demonstrated that some antiepileptic agents, including phenytoin, phenobarbital, and carbamazepine, induce common hepatic enzyme systems, such as cytochrome P450 (especially CYP3A4/5) and glucuronidation enzymes. Induction of these enzymes results in decreased exposure to chemotherapy agents and other drugs metabolized by the same enzyme systems, such as warfarin and small molecule inhibitors. The use of antiepileptic drugs clearly reduces the blood concentration of camptothecins (topotecan and irinotecan), as well as taxanes (paclitaxel). At this point, it is not known if the reduced drug concentration affects chemotherapy efficacy. In contrast, valproate inhibits cytochrome P450 and may reduce chemotherapy metabolism with a consequent increase in toxicity. Newer antiepileptic drugs, such as levetiracetam, zonisamide, lacosamide, lamotrigine, topiramate, and pregabalin do not result in drug interactions with current treatment regimens. These agents may simplify other pharmaceutical interventions, and are preferred when feasible.

Clinical trials have not yet demonstrated a discernible benefit for the use of routine prophylactic antiepileptic therapy for patients in whom seizures have not occurred,[36] however, an ongoing phase III clinical trial is currently examining this question with a newer antiepileptic agent.[37] Similarly, there is no clear evidence supporting the efficacy or lack of efficacy of antiepileptic therapy in the post-craniotomy setting.[38] Prospective randomized trials have demonstrated a lack of efficacy of perioperative seizure prophylaxis,[39] however, the heterogeneity of included patients and the use of older antiepileptic agents in these trials has led to limited acceptance of these results. Hence, antiepileptics are frequently administered following surgical resection. If antiepileptics are initiated perioperatively, current practice recommendations are to taper and discontinue use after the first postoperative week.[40]

Clinically apparent deep vein thrombosis or pulmonary emboli that require treatment with anticoagulation drugs may occur in 20% to 30% of patients with primary brain tumors. Presumably, injury to brain parenchyma results in the release of tissue thromboplastins and increases the risk for clotting. Spontaneous bleeding while on anticoagulation only occurs in 2% of patients with malignant glioma and does not appear to be more frequent than for patients who do not need anticoagulant drugs.[41,42] Low molecular weight heparin is generally considered to be more effective than warfarin in patients with an active malignancy.[43] Clinical trials evaluating newer oral anticoagulants, including factor Xa inhibitors (e.g., rivaroxaban) and direct thrombin inhibitors (e.g., dabigatran), have not assessed the safety of these drugs in patients with brain tumors. Further clinical evaluation is necessary before these drugs can be recommended for routine use in this population.

MOLECULAR PATHOGENESIS IN DIFFUSE GLIOMAS

The current understanding of the pathobiology of diffuse gliomas has rapidly increased over the past decade. Several molecular abnormalities have been discovered which seem to play key roles in glioma development. Precise molecular characterization of diffuse gliomas is still subject to discussion and extensive research, however, diffuse gliomas may be considered to fall under three broad categories (Fig. 14-3)[3,44]:

1. Gliomas arising from mutations in *IDH* with 1p/19q codeletion—These gliomas predominantly consist of the oligodendroglial tumors. The 5-year survival of these tumors typically ranges from 50% to 80%.
2. Gliomas arising from mutations in *IDH* and *ATRX*—These gliomas predominantly consist of grade II and grade III astrocytomas along with secondary glioblastomas (glioblastoma that has arisen from a lower-grade glioma). The 5-year survival of these tumors typically ranges from 25% to 50%.
3. Gliomas arising from mutations other than *IDH/ATRX* and without 1p/19q codeletion—These gliomas predominantly consist of primary glioblastoma (de novo glioblastoma). The 5-year survival of these tumors is less than 5%.

The above classification does not account for many other recent discoveries (e.g., the high prevalence of *TERT* promoter mutations in both oligodendroglioma and primary glioblastoma, despite a lower prevalence in lower-grade astrocytomas).[45] However, it provides a framework to better understand some of these crucial genetic alterations along with their associated prognostic and predictive implications.

ISOCITRATE DEHYDROGENASE (*IDH*) MUTATION

Mutations in the *IDH* gene are probably early genetic abnormalities in glioma development. Although first described in tumor samples of glioblastoma,[46] they have since been found to be prevalent in most diffuse gliomas other than primary glioblastoma.

IDH mutation is a clear indicator of favorable prognosis in high-grade gliomas[17] (Fig. 14-4) and has recently been demonstrated to independently predict improved efficacy of combination chemotherapy (PCV) in patients with anaplastic

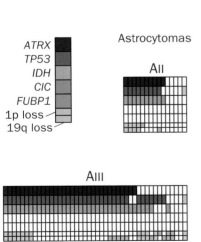

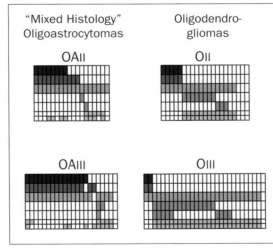

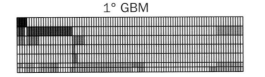

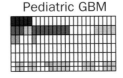

Fig. 14-3 Distribution of *ATRX, TP53, IDH, CIC*, and *FUBP1* mutations and chromosomes 1p and 19q loss in grade II to IV gliomas.

Gray cells denote analyses which were not informative or for which additional genetic material was not available for analysis.

Abbreviations: 1°, primary; 2°, secondary; AII, grade II astrocytomas; AIII, grade III astrocytomas; GBM, glioblastoma; OII, grade II oligodendrogliomas; OIII, grade III oligodendrogliomas; OAII, grade II oligoastrocytomas; OAIII, grade III oligoastrocytomas.

Reprinted from Jiao Y, Killela PJ, Reitman ZJ, et al. Frequent ATRX, CIC, FUBP1 and IDH1 mutations refine the classification of malignant gliomas. Oncotarget. Jul 2012;3(7):709-722.

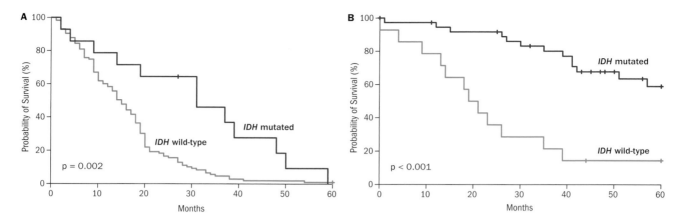

Fig. 14-4 Survival of adult patients with malignant gliomas with or without *IDH* gene mutations.

(A) For patients with glioblastomas, the median survival was 31 months for the 14 patients with mutated *IDH1* or *IDH2*, compared with 15 months for the 115 patients with wild-type *IDH1* or *IDH2*. **(B)** For patients with anaplastic astrocytomas, the median survival was 65 months for the 38 patients with mutated *IDH1* or *IDH2*, compared with 20 months for the 14 patients with wild-type *IDH1* or *IDH2*. Patients with both primary and secondary tumors were included in the analysis. For patients with secondary glioblastomas, survival was calculated from the date of the secondary diagnosis.

Reprinted with permission from Yan H, Parsons DW, Genglin J, et al. IDH1 and IDH2 Mutations in Gliomas. N Engl J Med. 2009; 360:765-773. Copyright © 2009. Massachusetts Medical Society. All rights reserved.

oligodendroglioma and anaplastic oligoastrocytoma.[18] Multivariable analysis has demonstrated that this survival advantage persists in the subset of patients who are 1p/19q non-codeleted. Of note, a germ-line single nucleotide polymorphism, the G allele of rs55705857, has recently been discovered and was found to be associated with a 6-fold increase in the risk of developing *IDH*-mutated gliomas.[12]

1p/19q CODELETION

Most oligodendrogliomas (OD) and anaplastic oligodendrogliomas (AOD)—along with many oligoastrocytomas (OA) and anaplastic oligoastrocytomas (AOA)—have been observed to have a combined loss of the short arm of chromosome 1 (1p) and the long arm of chromosome 19 (19q). This codeletion of 1p/19q

was demonstrated to be secondary to an unbalanced pericentromeric translocation event[15] and seems to be instrumental in the development of oligodendrogliomas. Several candidate genes have been identified (e.g., *CIC* [capicua transcriptional repressor], *FUBP1* [far-upstream element binding protein 1]) that may represent the genetic alteration underlying the 1p/19q codeletion.[44,47]

Many studies have demonstrated that 1p/19q codeletion is associated with a good prognosis in patients with OD/OA (Fig. 14-5).[15] More recently, 1p/19q codeletion has been determined to not only indicate a better prognosis in patients with AOD and AOA, but also predicts improved survival with combination chemotherapy (PCV) compared with patients without 1p/19 codeletion.[27,48]

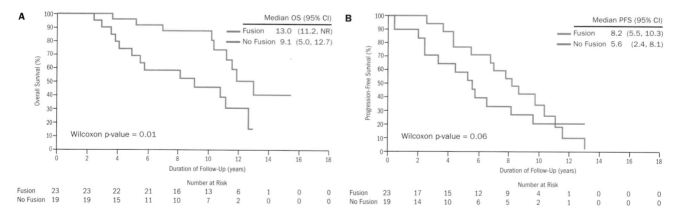

Fig. 14-5 Survival distribution in patients with low-grade oligodendroglioma/oligoastrocytoma by 1p/19q translocation (fusion) status.

Abbreviations: OS, overall survival; NR, not reported; PFS, progression-free survival.

Reprinted with permission from the American Association for Cancer Research: Jenkins RB, Blair H, Ballman KV, et al. A t(1;19)(q10;p10) mediates the combined deletions of 1p and 19q and predicts a better prognosis of patients with oligodendroglioma. Cancer Res. 2006;66(20):9852-9861.

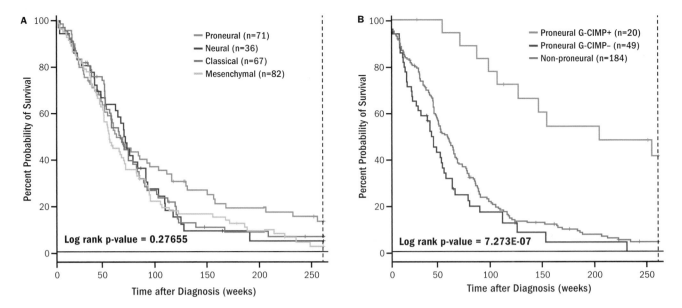

Fig. 14-6 Characterization of G-CIMP (glioma-CpG island methylator phenotype) tumors as a unique subtype of glioblastoma within the proneural gene expression subgroup.

(A) Kaplan-Meier survival curves among the four glioblastoma expression subtypes. (B) Kaplan-Meier survival curves among patients with proneural G-CIMP-positive, proneural G-CIMP-negative, and all nonproneural glioblastoma tumors.

Reprinted from Noushmehr H, Weisenberger DJ, Diefes K, et al. Identification of a CpG island methylator phenotype that defines a distinct subgroup of glioma. Cancer Cell. May 18 2010;17(5):510-522.

ATRX MUTATION

Mutations in the alpha-thalassemia/mental retardation syndrome X-linked (*ATRX*) gene are commonly seen in grade II and grade III astrocytomas and are essentially mutually exclusive with 1p/19q codeletions.[44,49] Clinical testing currently is not routinely available for *ATRX* mutations.

GENETIC ALTERATIONS IN GLIOBLASTOMA

The advent of The Cancer Genome Atlas (TCGA) has shed significant light onto the heterogeneity of the genetic landscape of glioblastoma.[50,51] Common genetic alterations include: (1) epidermal growth factor receptor (*EGFR*) mutation and amplification; (2) loss of the phosphatase and tensin homolog *(PTEN)* tumor suppressor gene; (3) retinoblastoma 1 (*RB1*) gene deletion and mutation; (4) cyclin-dependent kinase inhibitor (*CDKN2A/B*) gene deletions; and (5) neurofibromin 1 (*NF1*) gene mutations and deletions. Other abnormalities such as *TP53* mutations are also commonly observed in other diffuse gliomas.

Gene expression profiling of glioblastoma samples has identified specific subtypes of patients with differing clinical outcomes. These subtypes have been classified as proneural, classical, proliferative, and mesenchymal.[52-54] Patients with proneural subtypes have a better prognosis than those with mesenchymal or proliferative subtypes. It also appears that there is a subset of proneural glioblastoma with a distinctive pattern of DNA methylation (glioma-CpG island methylator phenotype [G-CIMP]) that has a particularly favorable prognosis (Fig. 14-6).[55] The G-CIMP pattern is strongly associated with the presence of *IDH* mutation.[51,56] Another recent report has further refined the subtypes of glioblastoma by defining six epigenetic subgroups based on methylation profiling.[57]

MGMT PROMOTER METHYLATION

MGMT is a DNA repair enzyme that plays a crucial role in DNA repair. Alkylating agents such as temozolomide lead to methylation of nucleotide bases in genomic DNA. Although some of these lesions are repaired by base excision repair, O6-methylguanine is a serious cytotoxic lesion that requires MGMT for its repair.

Hypermethylation of the *MGMT* promoter-associated CpG island has been described in approximately one-third of glioblastomas. *MGMT* promoter methylation prevents transcription of the *MGMT* gene and consequent expression of the DNA repair enzyme. Consequently, patients with *MGMT* promoter methylated tumors are expected to receive more benefit from temozolomide than patients whose tumors lack *MGMT* promoter methylation. The favorable prognosis of patients with *MGMT* promoter methylated glioblastoma is well described (Fig. 14-7), along with its association with a greater likelihood of benefit from temozolomide.[16,19,55]

KEY POINTS

■ Molecular aberrations such as *IDH* mutation, 1p/19q codeletion, and *ATRX* mutation are challenging the understanding and classification of diffuse gliomas.

■ Patients with *MGMT* promoter methylated glioblastoma have a better prognosis than patients whose tumors lack *MGMT* promoter methylation. Furthermore, *MGMT* promoter methylation predicts a greater efficacy of temozolomide in this population.

ASTROCYTOMAS

GRADE IV ASTROCYTOMA (GLIOBLASTOMA)

Grade IV astrocytomas are primarily represented by glioblastoma, the most common of the primary malignant brain tumors. Glioblastoma was classically described as glioblastoma multiforme; however, this latter term has recently fallen out of favor. Other grade IV astrocytomas include giant cell glioblastoma and gliosarcoma, however, these are much less common. Hallmark features of grade IV astrocytoma comprise not only increased cellularity, marked nuclear pleomorphism, and frequent mitoses, but also include endothelial proliferation and areas of palisading necrosis. The median age at diagnosis is approximately 65. The onset of symptoms often is abrupt and is most commonly related to mass effect and to focal neurologic symptoms. Seizures also are relatively common. Intracranial bleeding is the presenting symptom for fewer than 3% of patients.

T1-weighted MRI scans with use of gadolinium typically show a ring-enhanced mass lesion with low signal intensity in the center and surrounding the ring-enhanced component. In specimens obtained by biopsy, the central portion of the lesion often contains tumor necrosis, the ring-enhanced portion is associated with increased vascular permeability, and the surrounding low-signal component corresponds to intact brain parenchyma diffusely infiltrated by tumor cells. Studies involving the use of serial stereotactic biopsies have demonstrated isolated tumor cells well beyond any signal abnormality visible on T2-weighted scans.[13]

Molecular aberrations such as *IDH* mutations and *MGMT* promoter hypermethylation provide prognostic information for patients with glioblastoma. Patients with *IDH*-mutated glioblastoma are usually younger (median age, 32) and have a median survival of 31 months. Those with *IDH* wild-type tumors are older (median age, 59) and have a median survival of only 15 months.[17] *MGMT* promoter methylation is also associated with a prolonged survival in glioblastoma when compared to patients without methylation (18.2 vs. 12.2 months; p < 0.001).[16]

Surgery

The mainstay of treatment for glioblastoma remains surgical removal of as much tissue as possible without creating an unacceptable neurologic deficit. In general, the outcome is better for patients with a more complete surgical resection.[58] Patients with glioblastoma who do not have residual contrast-enhancing tumor after surgery have prolonged survival compared to those with incomplete resections (17.9 vs. 12.9 months; p < 0.0001).[59] Unfortunately, even in the absence of residual contrast enhancement, the extremely infiltrative nature of this tumor makes true complete surgical resection impossible. Recent analyses have indicated that a survival benefit in patients with glioblastoma is associated with a residual tumor volume of less than 5 cm^3 and at least a 70% extent of resection.[60]

Radiation

Radiation therapy has been the standard treatment for glioblastoma since the early phase III clinical trials conducted by the Brain Tumor Study Group in which postoperative radiation therapy improved survival over supportive care alone (median survival, 35 vs. 14.5 weeks).[61] Currently, radiation consisting of 60 Gy delivered in 30 fractions is considered standard. Overall survival is worse with radiation doses of less than 50 Gy[62] and no better with doses higher than 60 Gy.[63] However, a shorter course of radiation (40 Gy in 15 fractions) has been evaluated in a phase III clinical trial of elderly patients with glioblastoma because of their poorer prognosis.[64] The trial did demonstrate that a shorter course of radiation produced similar outcomes to standard radiation (60 Gy in 30 fractions) in elderly patients. Another phase III trial compared a hypofractionated course of radiation (34 Gy in 10 fractions) to standard radiation (60 Gy in 30 fractions) in elderly patients and also noted similar outcomes. However, neither of these trials utilized a noninferiority design, which would be required to definitively prove equivalence of the treatments.

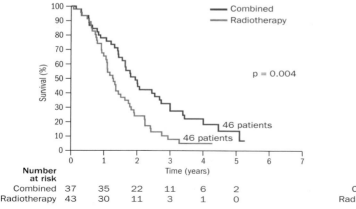 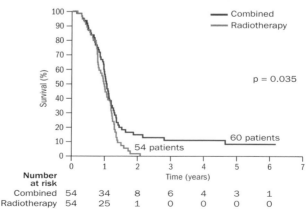

Fig. 14-7 Kaplan-Meier estimates of overall survival by methylguanine methyltransferase (*MGMT*) promoter status.

(**A**) Patients with methylated *MGMT* promoter. (**B**) Patients with unmethylated *MGMT* promoter.

Reprinted from Stupp R, Hegi ME, Mason WP, et al. Effects of radiotherapy with concomitant and adjuvant temozolomide versus radiotherapy alone on survival in glioblastoma in a randomised phase III study: 5-year analysis of the EORTC-NCIC trial. Lancet Oncol 2009; 10:459-66 with permission from Elsevier.

Multiple attempts to improve the therapeutic efficacy of radiation by using alternative fractionation schemes and radiation sensitizers have failed to produce substantially better results. Phase III randomized trials in patients with glioblastoma showed no benefit to adding either stereotactic radiosurgery or brachytherapy to radiation plus carmustine.[21,22]

Chemotherapy

Temozolomide. The benefit of adding temozolomide for patients with glioblastoma has been demonstrated convincingly. In a phase III clinical trial, patients with newly diagnosed glioblastoma were randomly assigned after surgery to receive radiotherapy alone (daily fractions of 2 Gy given 5 days per week for 6 weeks, for a total of 60 Gy) or radiotherapy plus concurrent daily temozolomide (75 mg/m² of body surface area per day, 7 days per week from the first to the last day of radiotherapy) followed by six cycles of adjuvant temozolomide (150 to 200 mg/m² of body surface area for 5 days during each 28-day cycle). Median and 2-year survival rates for patients receiving temozolomide were increased by 2.5 months (12.1 to 14.6 months) and 16.1% (10.4% to 26.5%), respectively (Fig. 14-8).[25] These results have established the current standard of care for these patients.

Moreover, a companion correlative laboratory study demonstrated that methylation of the promoter region of the *MGMT* gene in the tumor specimen is not only associated with superior survival, regardless of treatment received, but it also predicts greater efficacy of temozolomide (Fig. 14-9).[16,19] In

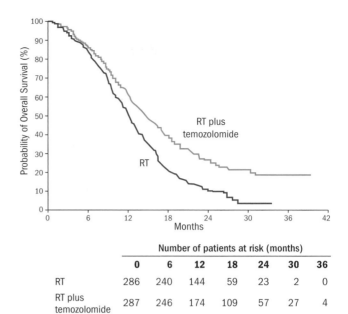

	Number of patients at risk (months)						
	0	6	12	18	24	30	36
RT	286	240	144	59	23	2	0
RT plus temozolomide	287	246	174	109	57	27	4

Fig. 14-8 Overall survival in patients with glioblastoma treated with radiation therapy (RT) alone compared with RT plus temozolomide.

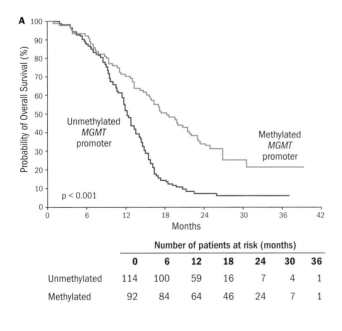

	Number of patients at risk (months)						
	0	6	12	18	24	30	36
Unmethylated	114	100	59	16	7	4	1
Methylated	92	84	64	46	24	7	1

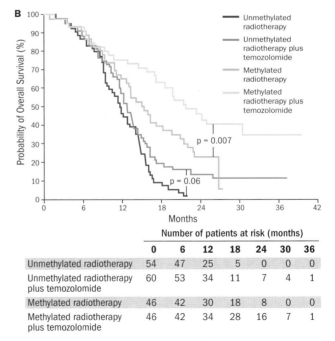

	Number of patients at risk (months)						
	0	6	12	18	24	30	36
Unmethylated radiotherapy	54	47	25	5	0	0	0
Unmethylated radiotherapy plus temozolomide	60	53	34	11	7	4	1
Methylated radiotherapy	46	42	30	18	8	0	0
Methylated radiotherapy plus temozolomide	46	42	34	28	16	7	1

Fig. 14-9 Survival in patients with glioblastoma.

(A) With and without methylation of the *MGMT* promoter as determined by methylation-specific polymerase chain reaction. (B) By *MGMT* promoter methylation status and treatment (radiation alone or radiation plus temozolomide).

Abbreviation: MGMT, methylguanine methyltransferase.

both the initial and 5-year analyses of this trial, survival differences between patients receiving radiation plus temozolomide compared to radiation alone were greatest in patients with *MGMT* promoter methylated glioblastoma (median survival, 23.4 vs. 15.3 months; p = 0.004). However, there was also a statistically significant improvement in survival in those patients without *MGMT* promoter methylation in the tumor (median survival, 12.6 vs. 11.8 months; p = 0.035).[19]

Alternative adjuvant temozolomide regimens have also been assessed but have not demonstrated superiority to the standard combined regimen. For example, a phase III randomized clinical trial compared standard adjuvant temozolomide to a dose-dense regimen of temozolomide (75 to 100 mg/m^2 on days 1 to 21 every 4 weeks).[65,66] No differences in median survival were observed, regardless of *MGMT* promoter methylation status; however, the dose-dense regimen was associated with more toxicity.

Temozolomide in elderly patients. It remains controversial as to whether elderly patients with glioblastoma experience similar benefits from the standard regimen of radiation and temozolomide. The original clinical trial excluded patients older than age 70,[25] however, patients between ages 60 and 70 did experience a significant improvement in 2-year survival with combined therapy when compared with radiation alone (21.8% vs. 5.7%).[19] Other clinical trials have demonstrated the feasibility of combined therapy in elderly patients, however, concerns have been raised regarding increased neurotoxicity in up to 40% of patients.[67,68] A phase II clinical trial has demonstrated the feasibility of a shorter course of radiation concurrent with temozolomide in elderly patients.[69] Neurotoxicity was described in only 10% of patients. An international phase III trial is currently underway to assess this regimen in elderly patients with glioblastoma.[70]

Elderly patients with poor performance status and multiple comorbidities may not be candidates for concurrent radiation and chemotherapy. Two recent phase III clinical trials have explored single-modality therapy (radiation alone compared with temozolomide alone) for patients with newly diagnosed glioblastoma.[71,72] One trial demonstrated that temozolomide alone as initial therapy is at least noninferior to standard doses of radiation alone in elderly patients (8.6 vs. 9.6 months, p [noninferiority] = 0.033). Furthermore, patients with *MGMT* promoter methylated tumors had prolonged event-free survival with temozolomide compared to radiation (8.4 vs. 4.6 months; p < 0.05), whereas the opposite was true for those with *MGMT* promoter unmethylated tumors (3.3 vs. 4.6 months; p < 0.05).[72] The second trial also noted similar overall survival between elderly patients who received temozolomide and those who received hypofractionated radiation. The second trial demonstrated an improvement in survival with temozolomide compared to standard doses of radiation (60 Gy; median survival, 8.3 vs. 6.0 months; p = 0.01), but no difference in survival when compared to a hypofractionated course of radiation (34 Gy; median survival, 8.3 vs. 7.4 months; p = 0.12).[71]

Bevacizumab. Bevacizumab is a monoclonal antibody that sequesters VEGF and is thought to reduce abnormal angiogenesis in tumors such as glioblastoma. VEGF pathway inhibitors can rapidly reduce vascular permeability, leading to a dramatic reduction in contrast enhancement around the malignant glioma that may be accompanied by reductions in T2 signal on MRI, mass effect, and clinical symptoms. A reduction in contrast enhancement with a corresponding increase in T2 signal abnormality may represent progressively infiltrating nonenhancing tumor. Hence, the use of bevacizumab can confound the interpretation of tumor progression with contrast-enhanced MRI.

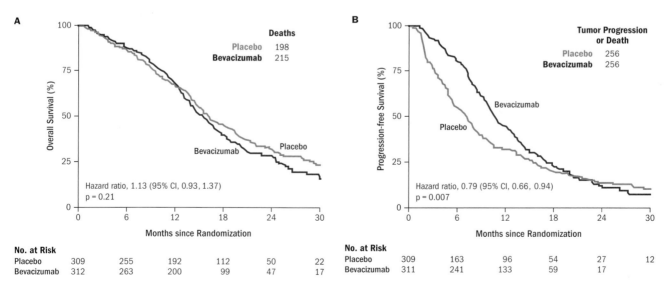

Fig. 14-10 Survival in patients with newly diagnosed glioblastoma treated with standard radiation (RT) and temozolomide (TMZ), along with either bevacizumab or placebo.

Kaplan-Meier estimates of (**A**) median overall survival and (**B**) progression-free survival.

The addition of bevacizumab to standard chemoradiation with temozolomide has recently been assessed in two large phase III clinical trials. Neither of these trials demonstrated an improvement in overall survival with bevacizumab compared with placebo (median survival, 15.7 vs. 16.1 months; p = 0.21; and 16.8 vs. 16.7 months; p = 0.10; Figs. 14-10 and 14-11).[31,32] As expected, progression-free survival was prolonged (median progression-free survival, 10.7 vs. 7.3 months; p = 0.007; and 10.6 vs. 6.2 months; p < 0.001), however, this outcome is difficult to interpret because of the impact of bevacizumab on vascular permeability. Beyond survival analyses, the studies differed on the effect of bevacizumab on quality of life. One of the studies showed improvements in several measures of quality of life,[31] while the other revealed impaired neurocognitive function and quality of life after the use of this drug.[32]

Recurrence

Treatment options for glioblastoma recurrent after radiation and temozolomide must be tailored to the individual. The value of additional radiation therapy or chemotherapy at the time of tumor progression remains under investigation. Participation in a well-designed clinical trial should be considered. Unfortunately, all standard therapies have limited benefits; symptom control with end-of-life care may be appropriate.

For patients with resectable disease along with good neurologic and performance status, a second resection can be done (with or without placement of carmustine-impregnated wafers[33]). In 2009, the FDA approved bevacizumab as treatment for recurrent glioblastoma following failure of radiation therapy and temozolomide. Phase II clinical trials of VEGF pathway inhibitors have demonstrated encouraging response rates and have shown some evidence of both increased progression-free survival at 6 months and median survival compared with historical experience (Table 15-2).[30,73-75] Nitrosoureas may also

be used to treatment recurrent glioblastoma.[76] Recent phase II data suggest that adding lomustine to bevacizumab may also be promising in recurrent glioblastoma.[77] Patients were randomly assigned to receive either bevacizumab, lomustine, or a combination of the two drugs. The 9-month survival rates were 38%, 43%, and 59%, respectively. This combination of bevacizumab and lomustine for the treatment of recurrent glioblastoma is currently being investigated in a phase III clinical trial.[78] The role of bevacizumab in combination with re-irradiation in recurrent glioblastoma is also being evaluated.[79]

NovoTTF-100A, a device that delivers alternating electromagnetic fields to electrodes placed on the shaved scalp, has been approved by the FDA. Results from a phase III randomized trial of NovoTTF-100A compared with physician's choice of chemotherapy for patients with glioblastoma recurrent following radiation therapy and temozolomide demonstrated no difference in overall survival.[80] However, the benefit of Novo-TTF-100A is debated since there is no evidence from phase III clinical trials that chemotherapy itself extends survival in this patient population.

Pseudoprogression. When the concern for tumor progression arises after first-line therapy, it is essential to consider pseudoprogression prior to initiating alternative therapy. It is now well established that pseudoprogression can mimic true tumor growth, especially in patients whose tumors exhibit *MGMT* promoter methylation.[81] On MRI, both progression and pseudoprogression are characterized by increased contrast enhancement, T2 signal abnormality, and mass effect, with or without clinical deterioration (Fig. 14-12).[82] No imaging methods can reliably distinguish the difference. For patients whose MRI scans appear worse within 1 to 3 months after completion of radiation, it is reasonable to continue adjuvant temozolomide with or without increasing corticosteroid dose, and to perform a repeat

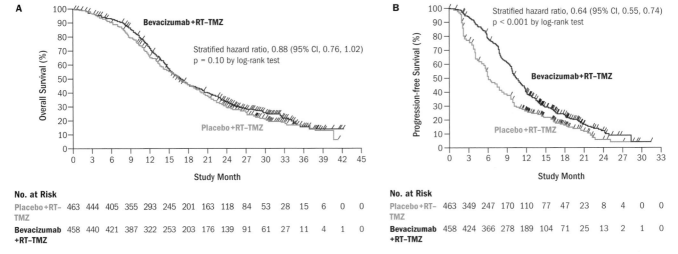

Fig. 14-11 Survival in patients with newly diagnosed glioblastoma treated with standard radiation (RT) and temozolomide (TMZ), along with either bevacizumab or placebo.

Kaplan-Meier estimates of **(A)** median overall survival and **(B)** progression-free survival.

Reprinted with permission from Chinot OL, Wick W, Mason W, et al. Bevacizumab plus radiotherapy-temozolomide for newly diagnosed glioblastoma. N Engl J Med. 2014 Feb 20;370(8):709-722. Copyright © 2014. Massachusetts Medical Society. All rights reserved.

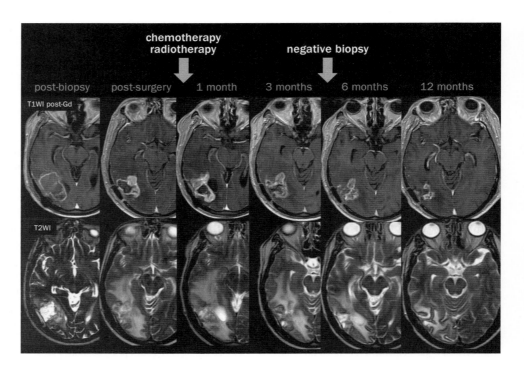

Fig. 14-12 Pseudo-progression in a 59-year-old man with glioblastoma.

MRI imaging obtained 1 month after concurrent radiation and temozolomide demonstrates an expansion of the right temporal lesion. Reductions in both the enhancing portion and the surrounding abnormal hyperintense area in the T2-weighted imaging were seen in the follow-up MRI examination.

Reprinted from Hygino da Cruz LC, Jr., Rodriguez I, Domingues RC, Gasparetto EL, Sorensen AG. Pseudoprogression and pseudoresponse: imaging challenges in the assessment of posttreatment glioma. AJNR Am J Neuroradiol. Dec 2011;32(11):1978-1985.

MRI scan in 1 to 2 months. In addition, both pseudoprogression and radiation necrosis may be ameliorated by treatment with bevacizumab (7.5 mg/kg intravenously every 3 weeks).[35] Only patients with continued deterioration in imaging should proceed to different therapy.[20]

GRADE III ASTROCYTOMA (ANAPLASTIC ASTROCYTOMA)

Anaplastic astrocytomas represent the category of grade III astrocytomas. These are differentiated from lower-grade astrocytomas by the presence of increased mitotic activity and a high propensity to transform into glioblastoma. The median age at diagnosis is approximately 55. Patients with anaplastic astrocytomas may present with seizures, focal neurologic deficit, headaches, or changes in mental status. MRI usually indicates a contrast-enhanced mass lesion, although some lesions may not be contrast-enhanced. The prognosis of patients with anaplastic astrocytoma varies significantly with *IDH* status. Patients with *IDH*-mutated tumors have a median survival of 65 to 112 months, whereas those with *IDH* wild-type tumors have a median survival of only 20 months.[17,83]

Surgery

The standard initial treatment remains maximum surgical debulking without compromising neurologic function. Removal of sufficient tissue for thorough pathologic evaluation is necessary to distinguish anaplastic astrocytoma from glioblastoma. In particular, a histologic diagnosis of anaplastic astrocytoma in a patient with a ring-enhancing mass lesion on MRI suggests that tissue representative of the true diagnosis (likely glioblastoma) has not been obtained.

Radiation

Similar to patients with glioblastoma, radiation therapy has been demonstrated to prolong survival in patients with anaplastic astrocytoma and is a standard component of treatment.[61,84] Most practitioners currently treat with 55.8 to 60 Gy in 1.8- to 2.0-Gy fractions.

Chemotherapy

The role of adjuvant chemotherapy remains controversial as outcomes from phase III trials have been mixed. A meta-analysis by the Glioma Meta-analysis Trialists' Group assessing the effect of chemotherapy in high-grade glioma[85] demonstrated a 6% absolute increase in 2-year survival for patients with anaplastic astrocytoma who received radiation plus chemotherapy compared with those who received radiation alone (37% vs. 31%). All clinical trials in this meta-analysis involved nitrosourea-based regimens. Survival outcomes from single-agent carmustine (BCNU) and PCV seem to be similar.[86] However, a large randomized trial by the Medical Research Council found no benefit of adjuvant PCV compared with radiation therapy alone (median survival, 15 vs. 13 months; 2-year survival, 42% vs. 37%; Fig. 14-13).[87] Lack of statistical significance has been attributed to insufficient power.

The role of temozolomide as an adjuvant to radiation therapy has not yet been assessed prospectively in anaplastic astrocytoma. Some retrospective analyses indicate that temozolomide may improve overall survival when administered concurrently with adjuvant radiation.[83] A phase III international trial (EORTC 26053 or CATNON) is ongoing, in which patients with anaplastic glioma without 1p/19q codeletion are randomly assigned to either radiation alone or radiation with temozolomide during radiation and/or after radiation.[88]

A phase III clinical trial has also assessed the role of chemotherapy up front in anaplastic gliomas with radiation therapy only at progression.[89] Patients were randomly assigned to three arms: radiation therapy, PCV, or temozolomide. At progression, chemotherapy arms were retreated with additional chemotherapy cycles in patients who had achieved initial disease response or stable disease. In the event of further progression (or failure of initial chemotherapy), patients were transitioned to radiation therapy. Patients on the radiation therapy arm were switched to either PCV or temozolomide at progression. In patients with anaplastic astrocytoma, up-front chemotherapy prolonged progression-free survival compared to up-front radiation therapy (18.2 vs. 10.8 months), however, there was no difference in time to treatment failure (29.4 vs. 32.0 months).

Recurrence

Chemotherapy for anaplastic astrocytoma that recurs following radiation is of benefit. Nitrosourea-based regimens have demonstrated response rates of approximately 30% in anaplastic astrocytoma.[90] Similarly, temozolomide was granted accelerated FDA approval on the basis of its activity in recurrent anaplastic astrocytoma (complete response, 6%; partial response, 28%; stable disease, 32%).[91] A randomized clinical trial compared the efficacy of PCV with temozolomide in chemotherapy-naive patients with high-grade glioma and determined that there was no difference in outcome in patients with anaplastic astrocytoma (hazard ratio [HR] 0.79; p = 0.48).[92] Bevacizumab has also demonstrated objective response in recurrent anaplastic astrocytoma (partial response, 64%; stable disease, 8%).[93]

KEY POINTS

- Anaplastic astrocytomas have a high propensity to transform into glioblastoma.
- Standard initial therapy is maximum surgical debulking followed by adjuvant radiation.
- Temozolomide is FDA-approved for the treatment of recurrent anaplastic astrocytoma.

GRADE II ASTROCYTOMAS (DIFFUSE ASTROCYTOMA)

Grade II astrocytomas mainly comprise diffuse astrocytomas, however, the group also includes other rare tumors (pilomyxoid astrocytoma and pleomorphic xanthoastrocytoma). These tumors are diffusely infiltrative and cellular. Despite a relatively indolent course, late recurrences with anaplastic transformation are relatively common.

The median age at diagnosis is approximately 45. Patients with diffuse astrocytoma typically present with seizures. Diffuse astrocytomas usually appear as lesions with low attenuation or isodensity on CT scans. These tumors may not contrast-enhance on MRI, or the contrast enhancement may be wispy and faint. Focal intense enhancement may indicate areas of anaplastic transformation. When feasible, biopsy, or preferably resection, should be performed to obtain a sample of the contrast-enhanced portion, because the prognosis is typically related to the most anaplastic part of the tumor.

Poor prognostic factors in diffuse astrocytoma include an older age (40 or older), tumor diameter of 6 cm or larger, Karnofsky performance status (KPS) less than 70, tumors that cross the midline, presence of enhancement on imaging, and neurologic deficits prior to surgery.[94,95]

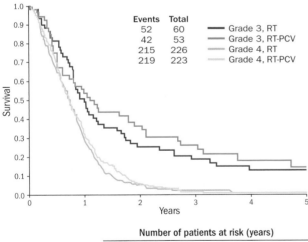

	Events	Total	
Grade 3, RT	52	60	
Grade 3, RT-PCV	42	53	
Grade 4, RT	215	226	
Grade 4, RT-PCV	219	223	

Number of patients at risk (years)						
	0	1	2	3	4	5
Grade 3, RT	60	29	15	11	6	5
Grade 3, RT-PCV	53	28	19	12	5	3
Grade 4, RT	226	64	11	5	1	1
Grade 4, RT-PCV	223	72	12	3	2	2

Fig. 14-13 Survival in patients with anaplastic astrocytoma or glioblastoma treated with radiation alone (RT) or radiation plus procarbazine, CCNU (lomustine), and vincristine (RT-PCV).

Reprinted with permission from Medical Research Council Brain Tumor Working Party. Randomized trial of procarbazine, lomustine, and vincristine in the adjuvant treatment of high-grade astrocytoma: a Medical Research Council trial. J Clin Oncol. 2001;19(2):509-18.

The treatment of diffuse astrocytoma remains controversial. Due to the relative rarity of low-grade gliomas, clinical trials have historically combined diffuse astrocytomas with other low-grade tumors such as oligodendrogliomas, oligoastrocytomas, and pilocytic astrocytomas. Consequently, the results of many current studies are difficult to interpret conclusively.

Surgery

Patients with symptomatic diffuse astrocytoma should undergo resection to debulk the tumor. Complete resection of all the tumor area with abnormal T2 signal results in superior outcomes when the risk of neurologic injury from resection is low. Retrospective single-institution data demonstrated that smaller pre- and postoperative tumor volume as measured by FLAIR sequences on MRI, as well as greater extent of resection, are associated with superior survival after adjustment for other known clinical variables.[96] Similar findings were observed in a prospective multicenter clinical trial.[97] Unfortunately, complete resection is not feasible for many patients due to tumor location. Complete resection is generally limited to a select group of patients with small unilateral tumors or tumors that do not involve critical brain structures. A practical approach is to resect as much of the abnormal tissue as possible without causing substantial neurologic deficit.

The surgical management of small asymptomatic diffuse astrocytomas is more controversial. No randomized controlled clinical trials have explored this question.[98] Either up-front surgical resection or a wait-and-watch approach may be considered.[99,100] If conservative management is planned, a biopsy is recommended in order to obtain a pathologic diagnosis.

Radiation

A phase III clinical trial has evaluated the role of immediate radiation versus delayed radiation therapy in patients with low-grade gliomas.[101] Patients were randomly assigned to receive either 54 Gy of radiation immediately after surgery or no immediate radiation. In the latter arm, radiation was administered at the time of progression. This study demonstrated that radiation therapy beginning immediately after diagnosis extends the time to recurrence compared with radiation that is delayed until the time of tumor progression (median progression-free survival, 5.3 vs. 3.4 years; p < 0.0001). However, there was no change in median overall survival (7.4 vs. 7.2 years; p = 0.87; Fig. 14-14). In the absence of an overall survival benefit, rationale exists for delaying radiation in an attempt to prevent radiation-induced neurologic damage. Prospective data had initially demonstrated that tumor growth, the use of antiepileptics, and radiation fraction sizes greater than 2 Gy are associated with neurocognitive decline.[102] However, longer periods of observation have demonstrated significant neurocognitive dysfunction in survivors of low-grade gliomas who received radiation as compared with those who had not, even if radiation fraction sizes smaller than 2 Gy were used.[103] For patients with minimal or no symptoms or for patients with seizures that are controlled with antiepileptic drugs, deferring radiation until there is evidence of symptomatic tumor growth is acceptable.

Two randomized clinical trials have explored the dose-response relationship of radiation in low-grade gliomas. The first trial compared postoperative or post-biopsy radiation doses of 45 Gy and 59.4 Gy. No differences in 5-year progression-free survival (47% vs. 50%; p = 0.94) or 5-year overall survival (58% vs. 59%; p = 0.73) were observed.[104] The second trial explored higher doses of radiation therapy (50.4 vs. 64.8 Gy). Survival was similar with higher doses of radiation (5-year overall survival, 72% vs. 64%; p = 0.48), but a higher 2-year incidence of grade 3 to 5 radiation necrosis was noted (2.5% vs. 5%).[105] In the light of the above evidence, doses of 45 Gy to 54 Gy, delivered in 1.8- to 2.0-Gy fractions, are considered acceptable.

Chemotherapy

The role of adjuvant chemotherapy for patients with low-grade astrocytomas remains under investigation. Current results from a phase III trial in which radiation alone was compared with radiation followed by chemotherapy with PCV suggest that chemotherapy is associated with superior median overall survival (13.3 vs. 7.8 years; p = 0.002; Fig. 14-15).[26,106] However, the clinical trial included patients with newly diagnosed diffuse astrocytoma, oligodendroglioma, and oligoastrocytoma. Analysis of outcomes based on genetic and molecular characterization is ongoing.

The toxicity associated with PCV has limited its general acceptability and many practitioners recommend the use of temozolomide either as initial therapy or at time of recurrence of diffuse astrocytomas. However, data supporting initial therapy with temozolomide in these tumors are limited. The European Organisation for Research and Treatment of Cancer (EORTC) recently reported early results from a phase III clinical trial in which radiation was compared to adjuvant temozolomide as initial therapy for high-risk, progressive, or symptomatic low-grade gliomas of any histologic type.[107] Patients were stratified by 1p deletion status prior to random assignment. In this study, progression-free survival did not differ between the two regimens. Post-hoc analyses suggest trends toward inferior progression-free survival in patients with 1p-intact tumors treated with temozolomide as opposed to radiation, while overall survival seems to be improved among those patients with 1p-deleted tumors assigned to treatment with temozolomide. Longer follow-up will be required to determine the reliability of these preliminary observations.

KEY POINTS

- Diffuse astrocytomas are relatively indolent tumors; however, eventual anaplastic transformation is relatively common.
- Delaying treatment modalities such as surgical resection and radiation therapy may be considered since the optimal timing for treatment remains to be determined.
- Chemotherapy with procarbazine/lomustine/vincristine (PCV) after radiation improves overall survival in high-risk, progressive, or symptomatic low-grade gliomas compared to radiation alone.

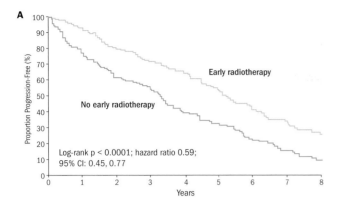
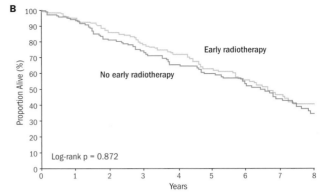

Fig. 14-14 Early compared with delayed radiotherapy for patients with low-grade astrocytoma and oligodendroglioma: intention-to-treat analyses.

(**A**) Progression-free survival by intention-to-treat analysis. Number of events: 80 for control group, 76 for early radiotherapy group. (**B**) Overall survival by intention-to-treat analysis. Number of events: 121 for control group, 96 for early radiotherapy group.

Reprinted from The Lancet, *Volume 366(9490). van den Bent MJ, Afra D, de Witte O, et al. Long-term efficacy of early versus delayed radiotherapy for low-grade astrocytoma and oligodendroglioma in adults: the EORTC 22845 randomised trial. Pages 985-990, copyright 2005. With permission from Elsevier.*

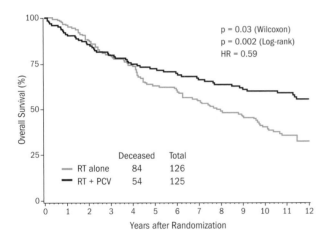

Fig. 14-15 Overall survival of patients with low-grade glioma treated with radiation alone compared with radiation followed by chemotherapy with PCV (procarbazine, lomustine, and vincristine).

Reprinted from Buckner JC, Pugh SL, Shaw EG, et al. Phase III study of radiation therapy (RT) with or without procarbazine, CCNU, and vincristine (PCV) in low-grade glioma: RTOG 9802 with Alliance, ECOG, and SWOG. J Clin Oncol. 32:5s, 2014 (suppl; abstr 2000).

GRADE I ASTROCYTOMAS

Grade I astrocytomas are relatively uncommon and include pilocytic astrocytoma and subependymal giant cell astrocytoma. These well-circumscribed tumors are typically seen in children and young adults and are associated with excellent outcomes.[108]

Pilocytic astrocytomas most frequently present in the cerebellum (40%) followed by supratentorial regions (35%). Tandem duplication at chromosome 7q34 occurs in 66% of pilocytic astrocytomas resulting in a *BRAF-KIAA1549* gene that is unique to these tumors.[109] Radiographically, pilocytic astrocytomas are frequently cystic with an associated contrast-enhancing mural nodule.[110] Contrast enhancement in these low-grade tumors is secondary to capillary proliferation with glomeruloid and hyalinized vessels. Pilocytic astrocytomas are potentially curable with complete surgical resection.

Subependymal giant cell astrocytomas (SEGA) are periventricular tumors that occur in about 1 in 10 patients with tuberous sclerosis and are the most frequent cause of decreased life expectancy in this disease.[111] Patients with tuberous sclerosis are hence recommended to undergo a brain MRI every 1 to 3 years until age 25 to screen for new occurrences.[112] Acutely symptomatic SEGA (e.g., associated with increasing ventricular enlargement) should be surgically resected. However, asymptomatic SEGA may either be surgically resected or treated with mammalian target of rapamycin complex (mTOR) inhibitors.[113]

Even if surgical resection is incomplete, grade I astrocytomas typically remain indolent. Radiation may be considered in such circumstances but is typically deferred until significant tumor progression. Chemotherapy is of uncertain value.

> **KEY POINT**
>
> - Grade I astrocytomas are more common in children and young adults. Surgical resection is usually curative.

OLIGODENDROGLIAL AND OLIGOASTROCYTIC TUMORS

Tumors containing oligodendroglial elements are relatively uncommon, accounting for only 9.5% of gliomas (Fig. 14-2). Nevertheless, they are important to note because of their unique natural history and sensitivity to chemotherapy. Characteristic molecular features of oligodendroglial tumors include 1p/19q codeletion and *IDH* mutation. Oligoastrocytic tumors seem to represent a hybrid entity as they contain both oligodendroglial and astrocytic components. At a molecular level, oligoastrocytic tumors may either have *ATRX* mutations or 1p/19q codeletion; however, 1p/19q codeletion is generally associated with superior survival outcomes compared with patients with 1p/19q non-codeleted tumors.[15]

ANAPLASTIC OLIGODENDROGLIOMAS AND ANAPLASTIC OLIGOASTROCYTOMAS

Anaplastic oligodendroglioma (AOD) and anaplastic oligoastrocytoma (AOA) are grade III gliomas and are discussed together due to the similarity in management strategy. These tumors typically demonstrate high cellularity, nuclear pleomorphism, and frequent mitoses. However, abundant endothelial proliferation and tumor necrosis may also be observed and do not automatically raise the grade of the tumor to grade IV. The median age at diagnosis is approximately 50. Mass effect or seizures are typically seen at presentation with AOD/AOA. MRI reveals a variably contrast-enhancing mass lesion in most patients.

Treatment of AOD/AOA includes optimal surgical debulking followed by radiation or by chemotherapy and radiation. Support for the use of chemotherapy and radiation after resection of AOD/AOA comes from two phase III trials, one conducted in North America and the other in Europe. In the North American trial, patients with AOD/AOA were randomly assigned to receive PCV for four cycles prior to radiation or to radiation alone. Median survival did not differ between the treatments (4.6 vs. 4.7 years; p = 0.1).

However, in the subgroup of patients with 1p and 19q deletions, median survival was 14.7 years for the PCV/radiation arm compared with 7.3 years for radiation alone.[48] In a more recent update of trial results, patients whose tumors demonstrated *IDH* mutations were found to benefit from additional PCV compared to radiation alone (median survival, 9.4 vs. 5.7 years). This relationship was independent of 1p/19q codeletion and persisted in patients with non-codeleted *IDH*-mutated tumors (5.5 vs. 3.3 years; p < 0.05). Patients with neither 1p/19q deletions nor *IDH* mutations had identical outcomes regardless of treatment received (median survival, 1.0 vs. 1.3 years; p = 0.97; Fig. 14-16).[18]

In the European trial, patients received PCV after radiation. Results were very similar to the North American results. Recently published long-term results demonstrate longer median survival in patients with 1p/19q codeleted tumors who received both radiation and PCV compared to those who received radiation alone. In contrast, patients with non-codeleted tumors did not have statistically significant improvement in overall survival with the addition of PCV.[27]

Taken together, these two randomized trials support the standard use of radiation and chemotherapy with PCV for patients with AOD/AOA with either 1p/19q codeletion or *IDH* mutation. Ongoing international trials segregate patients into 1p/19q codeleted (CODEL) and non-codeleted (CATNON) tumors.[88,114]

Prospective trials have demonstrated that temozolomide is effective in patients with recurrent AOD/AOA after radiation therapy and prior chemotherapy with PCV. One study demonstrated

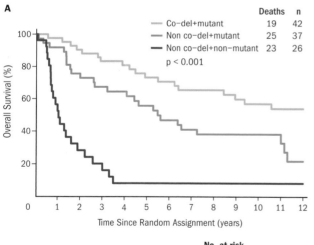
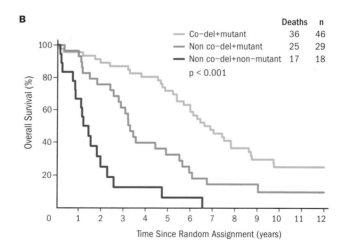

Fig. 14-16 Kaplan-Meier estimates of overall survival for patients with anaplastic oligodendroglioma or anaplastic astrocytoma whose tumors were *IDH* mutated and 1p/19q codeleted, mutated and noncodeleted, and nonmutated and noncodeleted after procarbazine/lomustine/vincristine (PCV) plus radiotherapy (RT) and RT alone.

(**A**) Median survivals after PCV plus RT were 14.7 years (95% CI 6.4, not reached), 5.5 years (95% CI 2.6, 11.0), and 1.0 years (95% CI 0.6, 1.9; p < 0.001), respectively. (**B**) Median survivals after RT alone were 6.8 years (95% CI 5.4, 8.6), 3.3 years (95% CI 2.5, 4.9), and 1.3 years (95% CI 0.8, 1.9; p < 0.001), respectively.

Reprinted from Cairncross JG, Wang M, Jenkins RB, et al. Benefit From Procarbazine, Lomustine, and Vincristine in Oligodendroglial Tumors Is Associated With Mutation of IDH. J Clin Oncol. Mar 10 2014;32(8):783-790.

an objective response rate of 44%.[115] The relatively low frequency of cumulative myelosuppression with temozolomide makes it a sound treatment option in the setting of recurrent disease.

OLIGODENDROGLIOMAS AND OLIGOASTROCYTOMAS

Oligodendrogliomas (OD) and oligoastrocytomas (OA) are both grade II gliomas with oligodendroglial elements. The median age at the time of diagnosis of oligodendroglioma is approximately 40. Patients typically present with seizures, although focal neurologic deficits, changes in mental status or personality, or symptoms of increased intracranial pressure can occur. MRI is the preferred imaging modality because these tumors may not be visible on CT scans. The tumor is most visible as increased signal intensity on T2-weighted scans. There may be a decreased signal on T1-weighted scans and occasional scant contrast enhancement. The disease course of OD and OA is even more indolent than that of grade II astrocytomas.

As earlier described (see Grade II Astrocytomas section), controversy exists regarding the optimal management of OD and OA, as these tumors have classically been studied together with other low-grade gliomas. Similar principles in surgical management, radiation therapy, and chemotherapy currently apply, however, a conservative approach is even more reasonable given the better prognosis overall (for full details, refer to the Grade II Astrocytomas section).

In summary, symptom control with antiepileptic drugs without additional antitumor therapy has been a common management strategy for small, minimally symptomatic tumors with a characteristic appearance on imaging.[98-100] However, this precludes a pathologic diagnosis. Significantly symptomatic tumors should be surgically resected as completely as possible.[96,97] Deferring radiation until disease progression or worsening symptoms is reasonable as the optimal timing remains unclear.[101] If radiation is administered, current results from a phase III clinical trial suggest that chemotherapy with PCV after radiation leads to an improvement in overall survival (13.3 vs. 7.8 years; p = 0.002).[26,106] Preliminary results from another phase III clinical trial indicate that 1p deletion in low-grade gliomas may predict a survival benefit with adjuvant temozolomide compared to adjuvant radiation.[107]

KEY POINTS

- Oligodendroglial tumors are characterized by *IDH* mutation and 1p/19q codeletion and have a more indolent course than astrocytomas.
- In patients with anaplastic oligodendroglioma or oligoastrocytoma with either 1p/19q codeletion or *IDH* mutation, chemotherapy with PCV after radiation improves overall survival.
- Patients with neither 1p/19q codeletion nor *IDH* mutations do not benefit from adjuvant PCV chemotherapy.

EPENDYMAL TUMORS

Ependymal tumors are CNS tumors that usually arise from the ependymal lining of the ventricular system of the brain or the central canal in the spinal cord. In children, this tumor is more commonly found in the posterior fossa; in adults, the tumor is somewhat more common in the spinal cord. Supratentorial lesions outside the ventricular system are infrequent.[116] Although research is ongoing into the molecular classification of ependymal tumors,[117,118] they are currently separated into four categories by the WHO classification. Subependymomas and myxopapillary ependymomas are rare grade I tumors that are usually curable with complete resection alone. Ependymomas (grade II) and anaplastic ependymomas (grade III) should be completely resected if possible.[119] Both the lower-grade and anaplastic lesions may disseminate along the leptomeningeal surfaces. Incompletely resected, anaplastic, or disseminated disease is usually treated with radiation therapy. Studies have shown that ependymomas may respond to platinum-based chemotherapy regimens, but the clinical benefit of chemotherapy remains speculative and response rates are low overall.[120,121] Many clinical trials are underway to further define the role of chemotherapy in this disease.[122,123]

MEDULLOBLASTOMA

Medulloblastoma is the most common malignant brain tumor in children, but young adults are also at risk. Medulloblastoma was previously considered to be a subset of primitive neuroectodermal tumors, however, these two entities are now known to be genetically distinct.[124] This tumor occurs in the posterior fossa. It may be located in either the cerebellar hemispheres or the vermis and may involve the fourth ventricle. Obstructive hydrocephalus is relatively common because of the proximity of the tumor to the fourth ventricle. Symptoms at presentation may include loss of balance, incoordination, diplopia, dysarthria, and signs of hydrocephalus, including headache, nausea, vomiting, and gait instability.

Molecular pathology studies have demonstrated that there are discrete subtypes of medulloblastoma with varying prognoses. The classification recommended by a recent consensus panel consists of four principal types: *WNT*, Sonic Hedgehog (*SHH*), Group 3, and Group 4 (Fig. 14-17).[125] The *WNT* group has the best prognosis, with long-term survival in more than 90% of patients. The *SHH* and Group 4 patients have an intermediate prognosis, and Group 3 patients, with overexpression of *MYC*, have the worst prognosis. Although the molecular characterization has not yet resulted in identifying specific therapies, the aberrant pathways identified may lead to targeted therapies specific for each molecularly defined entity.

MRI usually shows a contrast-enhancing mass lesion involving the cerebellum, although some medulloblastomas do not enhance. These tumors have a high propensity to seed the leptomeninges focally, as well as to spread through the subarachnoid space to involve the ventricles, cerebral convexity, and spinal leptomeningeal surfaces. MRI of the entire craniospinal axis is necessary for staging.

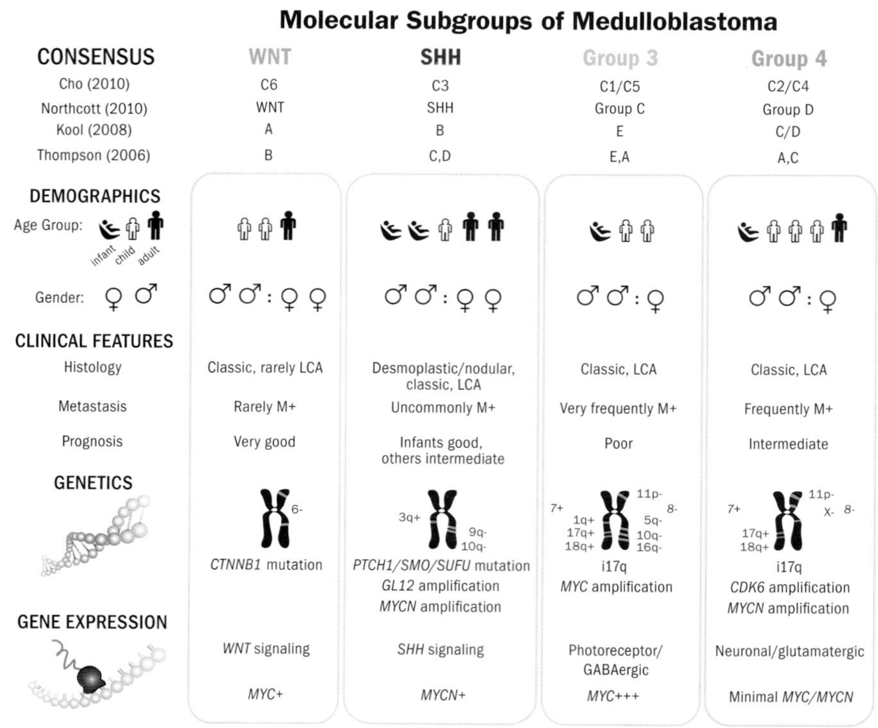

Molecular Subgroups of Medulloblastoma

	WNT	SHH	Group 3	Group 4
CONSENSUS				
Cho (2010)	C6	C3	C1/C5	C2/C4
Northcott (2010)	WNT	SHH	Group C	Group D
Kool (2008)	A	B	E	C/D
Thompson (2006)	B	C,D	E,A	A,C
DEMOGRAPHICS				
Age Group				
Gender				
CLINICAL FEATURES				
Histology	Classic, rarely LCA	Desmoplastic/nodular, classic, LCA	Classic, LCA	Classic, LCA
Metastasis	Rarely M+	Uncommonly M+	Very frequently M+	Frequently M+
Prognosis	Very good	Infants good, others intermediate	Poor	Intermediate
GENETICS	6-	3q+, 9q-, 10q-	7+, 1q+, 17q+, 18q+, 11p-, 8-, 5q-, 10q-, 16q-, i17q	7+, 17q+, 18q+, 11p-, X-, 8-, i17q
	CTNNB1 mutation	PTCH1/SMO/SUFU mutation, GL12 amplification, MYCN amplification	MYC amplification	CDK6 amplification, MYCN amplification
GENE EXPRESSION	WNT signaling	SHH signaling	Photoreceptor/GABAergic	Neuronal/glutamatergic
	MYC+	MYCN+	MYC+++	Minimal MYC/MYCN

Fig. 14-17 Comparison of the various subgroups of medulloblastoma, including their affiliations with previously published papers on medulloblastoma molecular subgrouping.

Abbreviations: SHH, Sonic Hedgehog; LCA, large cell/anaplastic; M+, metastatic.

Taylor MD, Northcott PA, Korshunov A, et al. Molecular subgroups of medulloblastoma: the current consensus. Acta Neuropathol. 2012 April;123(4):465–472.

Surgical removal of as much of the mass lesion as possible is important, because residual tumor after surgery confers a worse prognosis.[126] A worse prognosis is also associated with positive findings on cytologic analysis of the cerebrospinal fluid or the presence of leptomeningeal metastases on an MRI scan.[127] Surgery alone is not curative; surgical resection followed by radiation to the craniospinal axis with a boost to the site of the primary tumor can be curative. In addition, adjuvant chemotherapy (following radiation therapy) with a platinum drug (cisplatin or carboplatin), etoposide, and an alkylating agent (either cyclophosphamide or lomustine) plus vincristine has increased the cure rate compared with the use of radiation therapy alone. With appropriate initial therapy, 5-year event-free survival is achieved in more than 80% of patients with average-risk medulloblastoma. However, patients with disseminated disease at diagnosis fare much worse, with a 5-year event-free survival of 36%.[28] There are no robust data on the optimal treatment of patients with recurrent medulloblastoma. However, vismodegib, a small molecule inhibitor of the SHH pathway, has recently demonstrated activity in patients with recurrent SHH-type medulloblastoma,[128] and high-dose chemotherapy with autologous stem cell transplant may produce longer survival in some patients.[129,130]

VESTIBULAR SCHWANNOMA (ACOUSTIC NEUROMA)

Vestibular schwannomas, also known as acoustic neuromas, are usually benign, indolent tumors that arise from the vestibular branch of the eighth cranial nerve. Vestibular schwannomas account for approximately 6% of intracranial tumors and 85% of tumors in the cerebellopontine angle tumors.[131] The median age of diagnosis is 55.[132] Tumors are typically unilateral; bilateral vestibular schwannomas may occur in type 2 neurofibromatosis. Unilateral sensorineural hearing loss and tinnitus are the most common symptoms at presentation and are suggestive of a diagnosis of vestibular schwannoma. Patients may also have other cranial nerve deficits such as facial weakness or numbness, trigeminal neuralgia, and unsteadiness with ambulation. MRI is the imaging modality of choice and will typically reveal an enhancing mass in the vicinity of the internal auditory canal. Complete tumor resection is usually curative, however, this may not be feasible due to the proximity of several cranial nerves. Stereotactic radiosurgery is a viable option for smaller tumors. Observation may also be considered for small asymptomatic tumors. Close follow-up is needed due to the risk of progressive hearing loss.

MENINGIOMA

Meningiomas are usually benign and originate in the dura covering the brain and spinal cord. The incidence of the tumor is approximately two per 100,000 individuals. They have a female preponderance and the median age at diagnosis is approximately 65. The frequency of meningioma is increased for patients with type 2 neurofibromatosis. An association between meningioma and breast cancer has also been observed.[133] Although meningiomas can express receptors for androgen, estrogen, progesterone, and somatostatin, hormone therapies directed at these receptors have not demonstrated consistent therapeutic efficacy.[134,135]

KEY POINTS

- Medulloblastoma typically occurs in the cerebellum of children.
- Treatment for medulloblastoma includes complete surgical debulking when feasible, followed by radiation of the craniospinal axis and platinum-containing chemotherapy.

Genomic analyses have recently revealed that meningiomas fall into two broad categories (Fig. 14-18).[136] Meningiomas with NF2 mutations and/or chromosome 22 losses were more likely to be atypical, genomically unstable, and localized in the cerebral and cerebellar hemispheres. Meningiomas without NF2 mutations had an increased mutation burden in TRAF7, KLF4, AKT1, and SMO. These non–NF2-mutant tumors were more likely to have a benign clinical course and were typically situated at the medial skull base.

Patients with meningiomas may present with typical features of mass lesions in the brain, including seizures or focal neurologic deficits. Asymptomatic meningiomas may also be incidentally detected on CT or MRI scans that are obtained for other reasons. The tumors have a characteristic MRI appearance, usually consisting of uniform contrast enhancement along the dura, with distinct separation from brain parenchyma. Contrast enhancement extending from the mass lesion, known as the dural tail, is characteristic but not present in all cases. Marked parenchymal edema is seen frequently.

Many incidentally discovered meningiomas do not require treatment. For patients with an asymptomatic benign meningioma, observation may be appropriate. Epidemiologic evidence suggests that as many as two-thirds of these patients will not have symptoms over time.[137] When there is substantial mass effect with or without symptoms, the treatment of choice is usually complete resection. Surgery is often feasible if the meningioma is located over the cortical convexity, olfactory groove, anterior sagittal sinus, or posterior fossa. However, resection may be more difficult for tumors in other sites, such as sphenoid, parasagittal, orbital, tentorial, or clivus locations. Under those circumstances, external beam radiation therapy or focal stereotactic radiotherapy may be extremely useful for tumor control. No pharmaceutical interventions have reproducibly demonstrated antitumor efficacy for meningiomas, however, the abovementioned novel genetic insights[136] in benign meningiomas have opened new avenues for exploring targeted therapeutics.

Occasionally, meningiomas may have atypical histologic features or may be frankly malignant. Patients with atypical or malignant meningiomas are commonly treated with surgical resection followed by radiation therapy, either external beam or stereotactic radiosurgery. Patients who have disease relapse despite optimal surgery and radiation therapy often experience progressive debilitation and death. Although several pharmaceutical approaches have been assessed, they have minimal, if any, efficacy.[138]

PRIMARY CNS LYMPHOMA

Primary CNS lymphoma is a variant of non-Hodgkin lymphoma which involves the CNS without evidence of systemic disease. More than 95% of primary CNS lymphomas are diffuse large B-cell lymphomas. Primary CNS lymphomas constitute approximately 2% to 3% of all brain tumors in patients. The tumor is more common in men and the median age of diagnosis is approximately 55.[139] The majority of patients diagnosed with primary CNS lymphoma are immunocompetent; however, patients with a compromised immune system (e.g., solid organ transplant, congenital immunodeficiency, and HIV infection) are at increased risk for this disease. Epstein-Barr virus (EBV) is frequently associated with primary CNS lymphoma in immunocompromised individuals and EBV DNA may be found within the tumor (see Chapter 16: Lymphomas).

Patients present with a variety of symptoms characteristic of either focal or multifocal mass lesions. The MRI scan usually shows homogeneous contrast-enhanced tumors within the

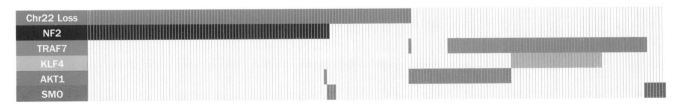

Fig. 14-18 Genomic architecture of meningiomas.

NF2, TRAF7, and SMO coding mutations along with recurrent AKT1E17K and KLF4K409Q variants reveal meningioma subtypes with mutually exclusive profiles. Analysis for chromosome 22 copy number is also shown. Each bar represents a grade I meningioma sample; 191 samples are depicted.

Reprinted from Clark VE, Erson-Omay EZ, Serin A, et al. Genomic analysis of non-NF2 meningiomas reveals mutations in TRAF7, KLF4, AKT1, and SMO. Science. Mar 1 2013;339(6123):1077-1080.

periventricular deep white matter. Multifocality is common. Heterogeneous contrast enhancement is common, especially in patients with a compromised immune system. It is extremely important to consider CNS lymphoma in the differential diagnosis of brain tumors. Administration of corticosteroids may result in complete disappearance of the contrast-enhanced lesion, making the diagnosis difficult. Consequently, when CNS lymphoma is considered in the differential diagnosis, corticosteroids should be avoided, unless mass effect is causing serious and immediate injury to the patient. Obtaining specimens of suspected lesions by biopsy is critically important because many malignant and nonmalignant CNS conditions can mimic a CNS lymphoma. Unlike systemic large cell B-cell lymphomas, for which both chemotherapy and radiation therapy are effective and treatment for localized disease is curative, CNS lymphoma usually will respond to initial therapy but then typically relapses. As with systemic lymphoma, the role of surgery is restricted primarily to obtaining appropriate tissue for diagnosis. Appropriate staging evaluation includes slit lamp examination of the eyes, MRI of the spine, lumbar puncture if there are no contraindications (such as increased intracranial pressure or coagulation concerns), and CT scan of the chest, abdomen and pelvis. Some experts recommend PET scan as well. HIV testing is also appropriate.

Standard treatment regimens for diffuse large B-cell lymphoma (e.g., rituximab/cyclophosphamide/doxorubicin/vincristine/prednisone [R-CHOP]) are not active in primary CNS lymphomas, likely due to poor blood-brain barrier penetrance.

High-dose methotrexate-based regimens have become the initial treatment of choice; however, the optimal regimen is yet to be defined. High-dose methotrexate with whole-brain radiation is associated with better outcomes than whole-brain radiation therapy alone.[140] For example, the combination of high-dose methotrexate (3.5 g/m^2, day 1) plus cytarabine has demonstrated high rates of complete remission compared to high-dose methotrexate alone in a randomized phase II trial (complete response rate, 46% vs. 18%; p = 0.009).[141] High-dose methotrexate with procarbazine, vincristine, and intraventricular methotrexate followed by whole-brain radiation demonstrated a 58% complete response rate and a median overall survival of 36.9 months.[142]

Although whole-brain radiation therapy was previously considered to play a central role in the initial treatment for this disease, this is now more controversial because of the risk of later neurotoxicity with dementia secondary to leukoencephalopathy.[143] A clinical trial is currently assessing the impact of low-dose whole-brain radiation therapy over a high-dose methotrexate-based chemotherapy regimen.[144] To avoid neurotoxicity, clinicians frequently defer whole-brain radiation therapy until recurrence if complete remission has been achieved with chemotherapy. Many studies have demonstrated that radiation may be eliminated from first-line therapy.[29,145] Chemotherapy-only regimens such as high-dose methotrexate (8 g/m^2) with temozolomide and rituximab have shown long-term survival (complete response rate, 66%; 4-year survival, 65%).[146] Intra-arterial chemotherapy following blood-brain barrier modification with mannitol has shown feasibility.[147] Clinical trials are also currently ongoing to evaluate the role of high-dose chemotherapy consolidation with stem cell transplantation.[148,149]

The doses of methotrexate described above (3.5 to 8.0 g/m^2) are potentially lethal doses if not followed by active measures to reduce associated toxicity. Multiple doses of leucovorin need to be administered starting approximately 24 hours after treatment to minimize toxicity to normal cells (leucovorin rescue) and urinary alkalinization with intravenous sodium bicarbonate is utilized to enhance methotrexate excretion. Methotrexate levels need to be monitored to confirm effective elimination. Prolonged exposure may be secondary to accumulation of methotrexate in third-space fluid collections (e.g., pleural effusions). Such fluid collections should be drained prior to treatment with methotrexate.

Strategies for treatment of recurrent disease include reinduction with high-dose methotrexate, as well as consideration of high-dose chemotherapy with stem cell transplantation, use of rituximab, combination chemotherapy, and high-dose cytarabine.

Initial therapy for patients with compromised immune systems is reduction of the cause of immunosuppression. The prognosis for such patients is usually worse than for patients who have an adequate immune system. Despite a compromised immune system, chemotherapy may still be an option for some patients; others may be able to receive only palliative radiation.

KEY POINTS

- Primary CNS lymphomas are usually diffuse large B-cell lymphomas.
- Epstein-Barr virus is frequently associated with primary CNS lymphoma in immunocompromised individuals
- High-dose methotrexate-based chemotherapy regimens are effective in primary CNS lymphoma.

METASTATIC DISEASE TO THE NERVOUS SYSTEM

BRAIN METASTASES

Metastases to the brain are the most common intracranial tumors in adults and are 10 times more common than primary brain tumors. Brain metastases are diagnosed in 8% to 10% of patients with cancer during their lifetime[150,151]; however, autopsy series suggest that the true incidence of brain metastases in adults with cancer is approximately 20%.[152] Brain metastases are most commonly associated with lung and breast cancers, melanoma, and cancer of unknown primary site. These lesions result from hematogenous spread and are most common at the junction of the gray and white matter where the caliber of blood vessels changes, thereby trapping tumor emboli. Eighty percent of the brain lesions occur in the cerebral hemispheres, 15% in the cerebellum, and 5% in the brainstem.[153] Approximately 80% of patients have a history of a systemic cancer, and 70% have multiple brain metastases that are evident on MRI scans.

The presenting signs and symptoms of these lesions are similar to those of other mass lesions in the brain. The best diagnostic test is MRI with use of a contrast medium; however, not all brain lesions in patients with cancer are metastases. In one prospective study of patients with systemic cancer who were thought to have a single brain metastasis, 11% of biopsy specimens of brain tissue showed primary brain tumors or infections.[154]

The management of brain metastases requires an individualized approach as these patients have highly heterogenous underlying disease processes. Considerations for therapy depend on multiple variables such as the number and location of the brain metastases, histology of the primary cancer, tumor molecular characteristics, degree of extracranial disease and performance status.

Two randomized prospective studies have shown that surgery plus whole-brain radiation is superior to whole-brain radiation alone in patients with one surgically accessible brain metastasis. In one trial, patients receiving surgery plus radiation survived 6 months longer than patients who received radiation alone (median survival, 40 vs. 15 weeks; p < 0.01; Fig. 14-19).[154] The second trial demonstrated similar results (median survival, 10 vs. 6 months; p = 0.04).[155,156] Multivariable analyses indicated that patients who were younger and those with inactive extracranial disease primarily benefited from surgery while those with active systemic disease did not live longer after surgical resection. Many patients with one or two brain metastases are not surgical candidates due to complicating factors such as an inaccessible tumor location.

Stereotactic radiation therapy is increasingly being used in addition to or in place of surgery for patients with one to three metastases. Local control rates with stereotactic

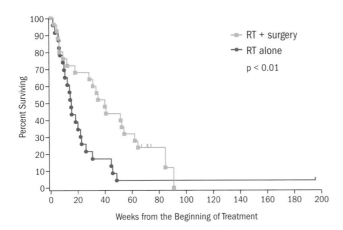

Fig. 14-19 Actuarial survival in patients with a single brain metastasis with or without surgical resection, prior to whole-brain radiation therapy.

Patients treated with surgery plus radiation (green squares) lived significantly longer after the beginning of treatment for the original brain metastasis than those treated with radiation alone (purple circles; median survival, 40 vs. 15 weeks, p < 0.01).

radiation therapy are high, ranging from 80% to 90%.[157] In a phase III clinical trial, patients with one to three brain metastases were treated with whole-brain radiation with or without a stereotactic radiosurgery boost. Patients who received stereotactic radiosurgery beyond whole-brain radiation alone were more likely to maintain a stable or higher performance score at 6 months (43% vs. 27%; p = 0.03) and those patients with a single brain metastasis also appeared to have a survival advantage (6.5 vs. 4.9 months; p = 0.04).[158] Potential advantages include the ability to treat without the risks of craniotomy, the ability to treat medically or surgically inoperable patients, and the ability to treat more than one lesion in different parts of the brain. Limitations include the inability to obtain tissue to confirm the diagnosis, limitations on the size of the tumor that can be treated safely, and the inability to lessen mass effect. In fact, stereotactic radiation may increase cerebral edema, resulting in mass effect that requires either corticosteroids or resection of radionecrotic brain tumor tissue.

In patients who have undergone a surgical resection or stereotactic radiation therapy, the role of whole-brain radiation is controversial. In a phase III clinical trial, patients with one to three brain metastases were treated with either surgery or stereotactic radiation and then randomly assigned to either whole-brain radiation (30 Gy in 10 fractions) or observation. Whole-brain radiation reduced the incidence of both intracranial progression (48% vs. 78%; p < 0.001) and neurologic death (28% vs. 44%; p < 0.002), however, overall survival was similar in the two groups (10.9 vs. 10.7 months; p = 0.89).[159] Similar results have been found in multiple other studies.[160-163] Evidence suggests that whole-brain radiation therapy added to stereotactic radiosurgery increases the time to neurocognitive decline as measured by the Mini-Mental State Examination. However, more sensitive and global measures of cognitive function and overall quality of life have not been assessed in this clinical setting.[164] Alternative studies have raised concerns regarding cognitive impairment with the addition of whole-brain radiation.[165] Recent data from a phase III clinical trial suggests that memantine concurrent with whole-brain radiation may delay cognitive decline.[166] A phase III clinical trial is currently underway to evaluate neurocognitive progression and overall survival in patients with one to four resected brain metastases who are undergoing either whole-brain radiation or stereotactic radiation.[167] Another clinical trial is evaluating hippocampal sparing during whole-brain radiation as a strategy to reduce neurocognitive decline.[168]

Definitive therapy with either surgical resection or stereotactic radiation therapy may not be an option in several situations. Patients with tumors that disseminate widely in almost all cases, such as small cell lung cancer and lymphoma, are not candidates for either surgical resection or stereotactic radiation therapy. These patients and others with multiple brain metastases should receive whole-brain radiation as standard therapy. In other situations such as brain metastases secondary to gestational trophoblastic neoplasia, surgical resection is avoided due to the high risk of intracranial hemorrhage.

Chemotherapy rarely is used as primary therapy for brain metastases. For patients with chemosensitive tumors in which chemotherapy can be curative, such as lymphoma, germ cell tumors, and gestational trophoblastic neoplasia, chemotherapy may be incorporated into the treatment plan for both brain and systemic metastatic disease, often in combination with radiation therapy. However, most tumors that metastasize to the brain (e.g., non-small cell lung cancer, carcinoma of unknown primary site, breast cancer, renal cell carcinoma, and melanoma) are not sensitive to chemotherapy or occur following failure of multiple prior therapies. Furthermore, many chemotherapy drugs have poor blood-brain barrier penetration. Nevertheless, there are reports of tumor regression in response to systemically administered chemotherapy or targeted agents in some patients. For example, the combination of lapatinib and capecitabine has demonstrated efficacy in patients with brain metastases secondary to HER2-positive breast cancer.[169] Dabrafenib is effective in *BRAF*-mutated melanoma that has metastasized to the brain.[170]

KEY POINTS

- Brain metastases are 10 times more common than primary brain tumors. The most common primary tumors are lung and breast cancers, melanoma, and cancer of unknown primary site.
- Surgical resection or stereotactic radiosurgery are of benefit to patients with a single brain metastasis who have a good Karnofsky performance score and controlled or absent primary tumor.
- The addition of whole-brain radiation to surgical resection (or stereotactic radiation) reduces intracranial progression and neurologic death compared to surgical resection (or stereotactic radiation) alone for patients with limited brain metastases, however, there is no difference in overall survival.
- Patients with *BRAF*-mutated melanoma metastatic to the brain benefit from treatment with dabrafenib.

LEPTOMENINGEAL METASTASES

Involvement of the leptomeninges occurs in approximately 5% of patients with cancer and is being recognized more commonly as patients with cancer live longer and as diagnostic studies improve.[171] The leptomeninges are most commonly involved with breast and lung cancers and melanoma. The tumor reaches the leptomeninges by hematogenous spread or by direct extension from pre-existing tumor deposits from the dura or brain parenchyma. Tumor cells are disseminated throughout the neuraxis by the flow of the cerebrospinal fluid (CSF). Patients present with signs and symptoms referable to one or more of the following:

- Local injury to nerves traveling through the spinal fluid (cranial nerve palsies, weakness, paresthesias, or pain)
- Direct invasion into the brain or spinal tissues or interruption of blood supply to those tissues (focal findings or seizures)
- Obstruction of normal cerebrospinal fluid flow pathways, increased intracranial pressure, and hydrocephalus (headache, nausea, vomiting, and dizziness)
- Interference with cognitive function (encephalopathy)

The diagnosis is made by examination of the CSF or MRI of the brain and spinal cord. Initial analysis of CSF demonstrates malignant cells in 50% of affected patients; however, in nearly 10% of patients with leptomeningeal involvement, the cytologic examination remains persistently negative.[172] Increasing the number of lumbar punctures (up to six) and the volume of CSF removed (10 cc per lumbar puncture) increases the yield of positive diagnosis. The protein concentration in the CSF usually is elevated, there is a pleocytosis, and the glucose concentration may be low. Radiographic studies may demonstrate diffuse and/or nodular contrast enhancement of the leptomeninges or hydrocephalus without a mass lesion.

Without therapy, median survival is 4 to 6 weeks, with death the result of progressive neurologic dysfunction. Often, leptomeningeal metastases are a manifestation of end-stage disease. For patients with poor performance status, significant neurologic dysfunction, and uncontrolled systemic disease, symptom management may be the most appropriate care. Corticosteroids and analgesics may offer limited temporary palliation. Radiation therapy may be considered to treat symptomatic sites. Ventriculoperitoneal shunting can be considered for palliative relief of refractory symptomatic hydrocephalus.

For patients who have minimal systemic disease, no significant neurologic deficits, and an acceptable performance status, a more aggressive approach may be considered; however, no specific treatment has definitively demonstrated an improvement in overall survival. Imaging to assess for normal CSF flow should be considered. Blockage of CSF flow by tumor deposits in the subarachnoid space reduces drug delivery and increases the risk of toxicity of intrathecal therapy. In the presence of CSF flow abnormalities, radiation therapy may be attempted to return normal CSF flow. Radiation therapy may also be used to treat areas of bulky disease and other symptomatic sites. Additionally, high-dose systemic methotrexate[173] or cytarabine[174] may be considered.

If CSF flow is normal, intrathecal therapy with methotrexate, cytarabine, or thiotepa increases the median survival to 3 to 6 months. Drugs can be administered intrathecally through an Ommaya reservoir or by repeated lumbar punctures. The major complication of intrathecal methotrexate is a necrotizing leukoencephalopathy that may develop after months of therapy for the small number of patients who do have prolonged survival. This devastating toxic effect is most common for patients who receive cranial radiation therapy prior to or concurrently with intrathecal methotrexate.

References

1. Louis DN, Ohgaki H, Wiestler OD, et al (eds). *WHO Classification of Tumours of the Central Nervous System, 4th ed.* Lyon, France: IARC Press; 2007.

2. Hartmann C, Hentschel B, Wick W, et al. Patients with IDH1 wild type anaplastic astrocytomas exhibit worse prognosis than IDH1-mutated glioblastomas, and IDH1 mutation status accounts for the unfavorable prognostic effect of higher age: implications for classification of gliomas. *Acta Neuropathol.* 2010;120(6):707-718. PMID: 21088844.

3. Ostrom QT, Gittleman H, Farah P, et al. CBTRUS statistical report: Primary brain and central nervous system tumors diagnosed in the United States in 2006-2010. *Neuro Oncol.* 2013;15 Suppl 2:ii1-56. PMID: 24137015.

4. Schwartzbaum JA, Fisher JL, Aldape KD, et al. Epidemiology and molecular pathology of glioma. *Nat Clin Pract Neurol.* 2006;2(9):494-503. PMID: 16932614.

5. Frei P, Poulsen AH, Johansen C, et al. Use of mobile phones and risk of brain tumours: update of Danish cohort study. *BMJ.* 2011;343:d6387. PMID: 22016439.

6. Wrensch M, Minn Y, Chew T, et al. Epidemiology of primary brain tumors: current concepts and review of the literature. *Neuro Oncol.* 2002;4:278-299. PMID: 12356358.

7. Melean G, Sestini R, Ammannati F, et al. Genetic insights into familial tumors of the nervous system. *Am J Med Genet C Semin Med Genet.* 2004;129C:74-84. PMID: 15264275.

8. Farrell CJ, Plotkin SR. Genetic causes of brain tumors: neurofibromatosis, tuberous sclerosis, von Hippel-Lindau, and other syndromes. *Neurol Clin.* 2007;25:925-946, viii. PMID: 17964021.

9. Wrensch M, Jenkins RB, Chang JS, et al. Variants in the CDKN2B and RTEL1 regions are associated with high-grade glioma susceptibility. *Nat Genet.* 2009;41:905-908. PMID: 19578366.

10. Shete S, Hosking FJ, Robertson LB, et al. Genome-wide association study identifies five susceptibility loci for glioma. *Nat Genet.* 2009;41:899-904. PMID: 19578367.

11. Jenkins RB, Wrensch MR, Johnson D, et al. Distinct germ line polymorphisms underlie glioma morphologic heterogeneity. *Cancer Genet.* 2011;204:13-18. PMID: 21356187.

12. Jenkins RB, Xiao Y, Sicotte H, et al. A low-frequency variant at 8q24.21 is strongly associated with risk of oligodendroglial tumors and astrocytomas with IDH1 or IDH2 mutation. *Nat Genet.* 2012;44:1122-1125. PMID: 22922872.

13. Earnest F 4th, Kelly PJ, Scheithauer BW, et al. Cerebral astrocytomas: histopathologic correlation of MR and CT contrast enhancement with stereotactic biopsy. *Radiology.* 1988;166(3):823-827. PMID: 2829270.

14. Agarwal S, Manchanda P, Vogelbaum MA, et al. Function of the blood-brain barrier and restriction of drug delivery to invasive glioma cells: findings in an orthotopic rat xenograft model of glioma. *Drug Metab Dispos.* 2013;41:33-39. PMID: 23014761.

15. Jenkins RB, Blair H, Ballman KV, et al. A t(1;19)(q10;p10) mediates the combined deletions of 1p and 19q and predicts a better prognosis of patients with oligodendroglioma. *Cancer Res.* 2006;66:9852-9861. PMID: 17047046.

16. Hegi ME, Diserens AC, Gorlia T, et al. MGMT gene silencing and benefit from temozolomide in glioblastoma. *N Engl J Med.* 2005;352:997-1003. PMID: 15758010.

17. Yan H, Parsons DW, Jin G, et al. IDH1 and IDH2 mutations in gliomas. *N Engl J Med.* 2009;360:765-773. PMID: 19228619.

18. Cairncross JG, Wang M, Jenkins RB, et al. Benefit From procarbazine, lomustine, and vincristine in oligodendroglial tumors is associated with mutation of IDH. *J Clin Oncol.* 2014;32:783-790. PMID: 24516018.

19. Stupp R, Hegi ME, Mason WP, et al. Effects of radiotherapy with concomitant and adjuvant temozolomide versus radiotherapy alone on survival in glioblastoma in a randomised phase III study: 5-year analysis of the EORTC-NCIC trial. *Lancet Oncol.* 2009;10:459-466. PMID: 19269895.

20. Brandsma D, Stalpers L, Taal W, et al. Clinical features, mechanisms, and management of pseudoprogression in malignant gliomas. *Lancet Oncol.* 2008;9:453-461. PMID: 18452856.

21. Souhami L, Seiferheld W, Brachman D, et al. Randomized comparison of stereotactic radiosurgery followed by conventional radiotherapy with carmustine to conventional radiotherapy with carmustine for patients with glioblastoma multiforme: report of Radiation Therapy Oncology Group 93-05 protocol. *Int J Radiat Oncol Biol Phys.* 2004;60:853-860. PMID: 15465203.

22. Selker RG, Shapiro WR, Burger P, et al. The Brain Tumor Cooperative Group NIH Trial 87-01: a randomized comparison of surgery, external radiotherapy, and carmustine versus surgery, interstitial radiotherapy boost, external radiation therapy, and carmustine. *Neurosurgery.* 2002;51:343-355; discussion 355-357. PMID: 12182772.

23. Fogh SE, Andrews DW, Glass J, et al. Hypofractionated stereotactic radiation therapy: an effective therapy for recurrent high-grade gliomas. *J Clin Oncol.* 2010;28:3048-3053. PMID: 20479391.

24. Pollack IF. Neuro-oncology: Therapeutic benefits of reirradiation for recurrent brain tumors. *Nat Rev Neurol.* 2010;6:533-535. PMID: 20927054.

25. Stupp R, Mason WP, van den Bent MJ, et al. Radiotherapy plus concomitant and adjuvant temozolomide for glioblastoma. *N Engl J Med.* 2005;352:987-996. PMID: 15758009.

26. National Institutes of Health. Adding chemotherapy following radiation treatment improves survival for adults with low-grade gliomas, a slow-growing type of brain tumor. 2014. http://www.nih.gov/news/health/feb2014/nci-03.htm. Accessed June 13, 2014.

27. van den Bent MJ, Brandes AA, Taphoorn MJ, et al. Adjuvant procarbazine, lomustine, and vincristine chemotherapy in newly diagnosed anaplastic oligodendroglioma: long-term follow-up of EORTC brain tumor group study 26951. *J Clin Oncol.* 2013;31:344-350. PMID: 23071237.

28. Packer RJ, Gajjar A, Vezina G, et al. Phase III study of craniospinal radiation therapy followed by adjuvant chemotherapy for newly diagnosed average-risk medulloblastoma. *J Clin Oncol.* 2006;24:4202-4208. PMID: 16943538.

29. Batchelor T, Carson K, O'Neill A, et al. Treatment of primary CNS lymphoma with methotrexate and deferred radiotherapy: a report of NABTT 96-07. *J Clin Oncol.* 2003;21:1044-1049. PMID: 12637469.

30. Friedman HS, Prados MD, Wen PY, et al. Bevacizumab alone and in combination with irinotecan in recurrent glioblastoma. *J Clin Oncol.* 2009;27:4733-4740. PMID: 19720927.

31. Chinot OL, Wick W, Mason W, et al. Bevacizumab plus radiotherapy-temozolomide for newly diagnosed glioblastoma. *N Engl J Med.* 2014;370:709-722. PMID: 24552318.

32. Gilbert MR, Dignam JJ, Armstrong TS, et al. A randomized trial of bevacizumab for newly diagnosed glioblastoma. *N Engl J Med.* 2014;370:699-708. PMID: 24552317.

33. Brem H, Piantadosi S, Burger PC, et al. Placebo-controlled trial of safety and efficacy of intraoperative controlled delivery by biodegradable polymers of chemotherapy for recurrent gliomas. The Polymer-brain Tumor Treatment Group. *Lancet.* 1995;345:1008-1012. PMID: 7723496.

34. Westphal M, Hilt DC, Bortey E, et al. A phase 3 trial of local chemotherapy with biodegradable carmustine (BCNU) wafers (Gliadel wafers) in patients with primary malignant glioma. *Neuro Oncol.* 2003;5:79-88. PMID: 12672279.

35. Levin VA, Bidaut L, Hou P, et al. Randomized double-blind placebo-controlled trial of bevacizumab therapy for radiation necrosis of the central nervous system. *Int J Radiat Oncol Biol Phys.* 2011;79:1487-1495. PMID: 20399573.

36. Tremont-Lukats IW, Ratilal BO, Armstrong T, et al. Antiepileptic drugs for preventing seizures in people with brain tumors. *Cochrane Database Syst Rev.* 2008(2):CD004424. PMID: 18425902.

37. MD Anderson Cancer Center. Lacosamide for Seizure Prophylaxis in High-Grade Gliomas. http://clinicaltrials.gov/ct2/show/NCT01432171. Accessed March 31, 2014.

38. Pulman J, Greenhalgh J, Marson AG. Antiepileptic drugs as prophylaxis for post-craniotomy seizures. *Cochrane Database Syst Rev.* 2013;2:CD007286. PMID: 23450575.

39. Wu AS, Trinh VT, Suki D, et al. A prospective randomized trial of perioperative seizure prophylaxis in patients with intraparenchymal brain tumors. *J Neurosurg.* 2013;118:873-883. PMID: 23394340.

40. Glantz MJ, Cole BF, Forsyth PA, et al. Practice parameter: anticonvulsant prophylaxis in patients with newly diagnosed brain tumors. Report of the Quality Standards Subcommittee of the American Academy of Neurology. *Neurology.* 2000;54:1886-1893. PMID: 10822423.

41. Ruff RL, Posner JB. Incidence and treatment of peripheral venous thrombosis in patients with glioma. *Ann Neurol.* 1983;13:334-336. PMID: 6303201.

42. Wen PY, Schiff D, Kesari S, et al. Medical management of patients with brain tumors. *J Neurooncol.* 2006;80:313-332. PMID: 16807780.

43. Lee AY, Levine MN, Baker RI, et al. Low-molecular-weight heparin versus a coumarin for the prevention of recurrent venous thromboembolism in patients with cancer. *N Engl J Med.* 2003;349:146-153. PMID: 12853587.

44. Jiao Y, Killela PJ, Reitman ZJ, et al. Frequent ATRX, CIC, FUBP1 and IDH1 mutations refine the classification of malignant gliomas. *Oncotarget.* 2012;3:709-722. PMID: 22869205.

45. Killela PJ, Reitman ZJ, Jiao Y, et al. TERT promoter mutations occur frequently in gliomas and a subset of tumors derived from cells with low rates of self-renewal. *Proc Natl Acad Sci U S A.* 2013;110:6021-6026. PMID: 23530248.

46. Parsons DW, Jones S, Zhang X, et al. An integrated genomic analysis of human glioblastoma multiforme. *Science.* 2008;321:1807-1812. PMID: 18772396.

47. Bettegowda C, Agrawal N, Jiao Y, et al. Mutations in CIC and FUBP1 contribute to human oligodendroglioma. *Science.* 2011;333:1453-1455. PMID: 21817013.

48. Cairncross G, Wang M, Shaw E, et al. Phase III trial of chemoradiotherapy for anaplastic oligodendroglioma: long-term results of RTOG 9402. *J Clin Oncol.* 2013;31:337-343. PMID: 23071247.

49. Kannan K, Inagaki A, Silber J, et al. Whole-exome sequencing identifies ATRX mutation as a key molecular determinant in lower-grade glioma. *Oncotarget.* 2012;3:1194-1203. PMID: 23104868.

50. Comprehensive genomic characterization defines human glioblastoma genes and core pathways. *Nature.* 2008;455:1061-1068. PMID: 18772890.

51. Brennan CW, Verhaak RG, McKenna A, et al. The somatic genomic landscape of glioblastoma. *Cell.* 2013;155:462-477. PMID: 24120142.

52. Phillips HS, Kharbanda S, Chen R, et al. Molecular subclasses of high-grade glioma predict prognosis, delineate a pattern of disease progression, and resemble stages in neurogenesis. *Cancer Cell.* 2006;9:157-173. PMID: 16530701.

53. Verhaak RG, Hoadley KA, Purdom E, et al. Integrated genomic analysis identifies clinically relevant subtypes of glioblastoma characterized by abnormalities in PDGFRA, IDH1, EGFR, and NF1. *Cancer Cell.* 2010;17:98-110. PMID: 20129251.

54. Masui K, Cloughesy TF, Mischel PS. Review: molecular pathology in adult high-grade gliomas: from molecular diagnostics to target therapies. *Neuropathol Appl Neurobiol.* 2012;38:271-291. PMID: 22098029.

55. Noushmehr H, Weisenberger DJ, Diefes K, et al. Identification of a CpG island methylator phenotype that defines a distinct subgroup of glioma. *Cancer Cell.* 2010;17:510-522. PMID: 20399149.

56. Turcan S, Rohle D, Goenka A, et al. IDH1 mutation is sufficient to establish the glioma hypermethylator phenotype. *Nature.* 2012;483:479-483. PMID: 22343889.

57. Sturm D, Witt H, Hovestadt V, et al. Hotspot mutations in H3F3A and IDH1 define distinct epigenetic and biological subgroups of glioblastoma. *Cancer Cell.* 2012;22:425-437. PMID: 23079654.

58. Laws ER, Parney IF, Huang W, et al. Survival following surgery and prognostic factors for recently diagnosed malignant glioma: data from the Glioma Outcomes Project. *J Neurosurg.* 2003;99:467-473. PMID: 12959431.

59. Stummer W, Pichlmeier U, Meinel T, et al. Fluorescence-guided surgery with 5-aminolevulinic acid for resection of malignant glioma: a randomised controlled multicentre phase III trial. *Lancet Oncol.* 2006;7:392-401. PMID: 16648043.

60. Chaichana KL, Jusue-Torres I, Navarro-Ramirez R, et al. Establishing percent resection and residual volume thresholds affecting survival and recurrence for patients with newly diagnosed intracranial glioblastoma. *Neuro Oncol.* 2014;16:113-122. PMID: 24285550.

61. Walker MD, Alexander E, Jr., Hunt WE, et al. Evaluation of BCNU and/or radiotherapy in the treatment of anaplastic gliomas. A cooperative clinical trial. *J Neurosurg.* 1978;49:333-343. PMID: 355604.

62. Coffey RJ, Lunsford LD, Taylor FH. Survival after stereotactic biopsy of malignant gliomas. *Neurosurgery.* 1988;22:465-473. PMID: 2452376.

63. Chang CH, Horton J, Schoenfeld D, et al. Comparison of postoperative radiotherapy and combined postoperative radiotherapy and chemotherapy in the multidisciplinary management of malignant gliomas. A joint Radiation Therapy Oncology Group and Eastern Cooperative Oncology Group study. *Cancer.* 1983;52:997-1007. PMID: 6349785.

64. Roa W, Brasher PM, Bauman G, et al. Abbreviated course of radiation therapy in older patients with glioblastoma multiforme: a prospective randomized clinical trial. *J Clin Oncol.* 2004;22:1583-1588. PMID: 15051755.

65. Gilbert MR, Wang M, Aldape KD, et al. Dose-dense temozolomide for newly diagnosed glioblastoma: a randomized phase III clinical trial. *J Clin Oncol.* 2013;31:4085-4091. PMID: 24101040.

66. Armstrong TS, Wefel JS, Wang M, et al. Net clinical benefit analysis of radiation therapy oncology group 0525: a phase III trial comparing conventional adjuvant temozolomide with dose-intensive temozolomide in patients with newly diagnosed glioblastoma. *J Clin Oncol.* 2013;31:4076-4084. PMID: 24101048.

67. Minniti G, De Sanctis V, Muni R, et al. Radiotherapy plus concomitant and adjuvant temozolomide for glioblastoma in elderly patients. *J Neurooncol.* 2008;88:97-103. PMID: 18250965.

68. Brandes AA, Franceschi E, Tosoni A, et al. Temozolomide concomitant and adjuvant to radiotherapy in elderly patients with glioblastoma: correlation with MGMT promoter methylation status. *Cancer.* 2009;115:3512-3518. PMID: 19514084.

69. Minniti G, Lanzetta G, Scaringi C, et al. Phase II study of short-course radiotherapy plus concomitant and adjuvant temozolomide in elderly patients with glioblastoma. *Int J Radiat Oncol Biol Phys.* 2012;83:93-99. PMID: 22079725.

70. NCIC Clinical Trials Group. NCT00482677. Radiation therapy with or without temozolomide in treating older patients with newly diagnosed glioblastoma multiforme. http://clinicaltrials.gov/ct2/show/NCT00482677. Accessed September 29, 2013.

71. Malmström A, Grønberg BH, Marosi C, et al. Temozolomide versus standard 6-week radiotherapy versus hypofractionated radiotherapy in patients older than 60 years with glioblastoma: the Nordic randomised, phase 3 trial. *Lancet Oncol.* 2012;13:916-926. PMID: 22877848.

72. Wick W, Platten M, Meisner C, et al. Temozolomide chemotherapy alone versus radiotherapy alone for malignant astrocytoma in the elderly: the NOA-08 randomised, phase 3 trial. *Lancet Oncol.* 2012;13:707-715. PMID: 22578793.

73. Batchelor TT, Sorensen AG, di Tomaso E, et al. AZD2171, a pan-VEGF receptor tyrosine kinase inhibitor, normalizes tumor vasculature and alleviates edema in glioblastoma patients. *Cancer Cell.* 2007;11:83-95. PMID: 17222792.

74. Vredenburgh JJ, Desjardins A, Herndon JE 2nd, et al. Bevacizumab plus irinotecan in recurrent glioblastoma multiforme. *J Clin Oncol.* 2007;25:4722-4729. PMID: 17947719.

75. Kreisl TN, Kim L, Moore K, et al. Phase II trial of single-agent bevacizumab followed by bevacizumab plus irinotecan at tumor progression in recurrent glioblastoma. *J Clin Oncol.* 2009;27:740-745. PMID: 19114704.

76. Brandes AA, Tosoni A, Amistà P, et al. How effective is BCNU in recurrent glioblastoma in the modern era? A phase II trial. *Neurology.* 2004;63:1281-1284. PMID: 15477552.

77. Taal W, Oosterkamp HM, Walenkamp AME, et al. A randomized phase II study of bevacizumab versus bevacizumab plus lomustine versus lomustine single agent in recurrent glioblastoma: The Dutch BELOB study. *J Clin Oncol.* 2013;31 (suppl; abstr 2001).

78. European Organisation for Research and Treatment of Cancer. NCT01290939. Bevacizumab and Lomustine for Recurrent GBM. http://clinicaltrials.gov/ct2/show/NCT01290939. Accessed April 4, 2014.

79. Radiation Therapy Oncology Group. NCT01730950. Bevacizumab With or Without Radiation Therapy in Treating Patients With Recurrent Glioblastoma. http://clinicaltrials.gov/ct2/show/NCT01730950. Accessed April 4, 2014.

80. Stupp R, Wong ET, Kanner AA, et al. NovoTTF-100A versus physician's choice chemotherapy in recurrent glioblastoma: a randomised phase III trial of a novel treatment modality. *Eur J Cancer.* 2012;48:2192-2202. PMID: 22608262.

81. Brandes AA, Franceschi E, Tosoni A, et al. MGMT promoter methylation status can predict the incidence and outcome of pseudoprogression after concomitant radiochemotherapy in newly diagnosed glioblastoma patients. *J Clin Oncol.* 2008;26:2192-2197. PMID: 18445844.

82. Hygino da Cruz LC Jr, Rodriguez I, Domingues RC, Gasparetto EL, Sorensen AG. Pseudoprogression and pseudoresponse: imaging challenges in the assessment of posttreatment glioma. *AJNR Am J Neuroradiol.* 2011;32:1978-1985. PMID: 21393407.

83. Kizilbash SH, Giannini C, Voss JS, et al. Impact of adjuvant temozolomide and IDH mutation status among patients with anaplastic astrocytoma. *J Clin Oncol.* 2013;31 (suppl; abstr 2025).

84. Kristiansen K, Hagen S, Kollevold T, et al. Combined modality therapy of operated astrocytomas grade III and IV. Confirmation of the value of postoperative irradiation and lack of potentiation of bleomycin on survival time: a prospective multicenter trial of the Scandinavian Glioblastoma Study Group. *Cancer.* 1981;47:649-652. PMID: 6164465.

85. Stewart LA. Chemotherapy in adult high-grade glioma: a systematic review and meta-analysis of individual patient data from 12 randomised trials. *Lancet.* 2002;359:1011-1018. PMID: 11937180.

86. Prados MD, Scott C, Curran WJ, Jr., et al. Procarbazine, lomustine, and vincristine (PCV) chemotherapy for anaplastic astrocytoma: A retrospective review of radiation therapy oncology group protocols comparing survival with carmustine or PCV adjuvant chemotherapy. *J Clin Oncol.* 1999;17:3389-3395. PMID: 10550132.

87. Medical Research Council Brain Tumor Working Party. Randomized trial of procarbazine, lomustine, and vincristine in the adjuvant treatment of high-grade astrocytoma: a Medical Research Council trial. *J Clin Oncol.* 2001;19:509-518. PMID: 11208845.

88. European Organisation for Research and Treatment of Cancer. NCT00626990. Radiation therapy with or without temozolomide in treating patients with anaplastic glioma. http://clinicaltrials.gov/ct2/show/NCT00626990. Accessed September 29, 2013.

89. Wick W, Hartmann C, Engel C, et al. NOA-04 randomized phase III trial of sequential radiochemotherapy of anaplastic glioma with procarbazine, lomustine, and vincristine or temozolomide. *J Clin Oncol.* 2009;27:5874-5880. PMID: 19901110.

90. Buckner JC, Brown LD, Kugler JW, et al. Phase II evaluation of recombinant interferon alpha and BCNU in recurrent glioma. *J Neurosurg.* 1995;82:430-435. PMID: 7861221.

91. Yung WK, Prados MD, Yaya-Tur R, et al. Multicenter phase II trial of temozolomide in patients with anaplastic astrocytoma or anaplastic oligoastrocytoma at first relapse. Temodal Brain Tumor Group. *J Clin Oncol.* 1999;17:2762-2771. PMID: 10561351.

92. Brada M, Stenning S, Gabe R, et al. Temozolomide versus procarbazine, lomustine, and vincristine in recurrent high-grade glioma. *J Clin Oncol.* 2010;28:4601-4608. PMID: 20855843.

93. Chamberlain MC, Johnston S. Salvage chemotherapy with bevacizumab for recurrent alkylator-refractory anaplastic astrocytoma. *J Neurooncol.* 2009;91:359-367. PMID: 18953491.

94. Pignatti F, van den Bent M, Curran D, et al. Prognostic factors for survival in adult patients with cerebral low-grade glioma. *J Clin Oncol.* 2002;20:2076-2084. PMID: 11956268.

95. Bauman G, Lote K, Larson D, et al. Pretreatment factors predict overall survival for patients with low-grade glioma: a recursive partitioning analysis. *Int J Radiat Oncol Biol Phys.* 1999;45:923-929. PMID: 10571199.

96. Smith JS, Chang EF, Lamborn KR, et al. Role of extent of resection in the long-term outcome of low-grade hemispheric gliomas. *J Clin Oncol.* 2008;26:1338-1345. PMID: 18323558.

97. Shaw EG, Berkey B, Coons SW, et al. Recurrence following neurosurgeon-determined gross-total resection of adult supratentorial low-grade glioma: results of a prospective clinical trial. *J Neurosurg.* 2008;109:835-841. PMID: 18976072.

98. Veeravagu A, Jiang B, Ludwig C, et al. Biopsy versus resection for the management of low-grade gliomas. *Cochrane Database Syst Rev.* 2013;4:CD009319. PMID: 23633369.

99. Pouratian N, Schiff D. Management of low-grade glioma. *Curr Neurol Neurosci Rep.* 2010;10:224-231. PMID: 20425038.

100. Whittle IR. What is the place of conservative management for adult supratentorial low-grade glioma? *Adv Tech Stand Neurosurg.* 2010;35:65-79. PMID: 20102111.

101. van den Bent MJ, Afra D, de Witte O, et al. Long-term efficacy of early versus delayed radiotherapy for low-grade astrocytoma and oligodendroglioma in adults: the EORTC 22845 randomised trial. *Lancet.* 2005;366:985-990. PMID: 16168780.

102. Klein M, Heimans JJ, Aaronson NK, et al. Effect of radiotherapy and other treatment-related factors on mid-term to long-term cognitive sequelae in low-grade gliomas: a comparative study. *Lancet.* 2002;360:1361-1368. PMID: 12423981.

103. Douw L, Klein M, Fagel SS, et al. Cognitive and radiological effects of radiotherapy in patients with low-grade glioma: long-term follow-up. *Lancet Neurol.* 2009;8:810-818. PMID: 19665931.

104. Karim AB, Maat B, Hatlevoll R, et al. A randomized trial on dose-response in radiation therapy of low-grade cerebral glioma: European Organization for Research and Treatment of Cancer (EORTC) Study 22844. *Int J Radiat Oncol Biol Phys.* 1996;36:549-556. PMID: 8948338.

105. Shaw E, Arusell R, Scheithauer B, et al. Prospective randomized trial of low-versus high-dose radiation therapy in adults with supratentorial low-grade glioma: initial report of a North Central Cancer Treatment Group/Radiation Therapy Oncology Group/Eastern Cooperative Oncology Group study. *J Clin Oncol.* 2002;20:2267-2276. PMID: 11980997.

106. Shaw EG, Wang M, Coons SW, et al. Randomized trial of radiation therapy plus procarbazine, lomustine, and vincristine chemotherapy for supratentorial adult low-grade glioma: initial results of RTOG 9802. *J Clin Oncol.* 2012;30:3065-3070. PMID: 22851558.

107. Baumert BG, Mason WP, Ryan G, et al. Temozolomide chemotherapy versus radiotherapy in molecularly characterized (1p loss) low-grade glioma: A randomized phase III intergroup study by the EORTC/NCIC-CTG/TROG/MRC-CTU (EORTC 22033-26033). *J Clin Oncol.* 2013; 31 (suppl; abstr 2007).

108. Burkhard C, Di Patre PL, Schüler D, et al. A population-based study of the incidence and survival rates in patients with pilocytic astrocytoma. *J Neurosurg.* 2003;98:1170-1174. PMID: 12816259.

109. Jones DT, Kocialkowski S, Liu L, et al. Tandem duplication producing a novel oncogenic BRAF fusion gene defines the majority of pilocytic astrocytomas. *Cancer Res.* 2008;68:8673-8677. PMID: 18974108.

110. Coakley KJ, Huston J, 3rd, Scheithauer BW, et al. Pilocytic astrocytomas: well-demarcated magnetic resonance appearance despite frequent infiltration histologically. *Mayo Clin Proc.* 1995;70:747-751. PMID: 7630212.

111. Goh S, Butler W, Thiele EA. Subependymal giant cell tumors in tuberous sclerosis complex. *Neurology.* 2004;63:1457-1461. PMID: 15505165.

112. Krueger DA, Northrup H, International Tuberous Sclerosis Complex Consensus Group. Tuberous sclerosis complex surveillance and management: recommendations of the 2012 International Tuberous Sclerosis Complex Consensus Conference. *Pediatr Neurol.* 2013;49:255-265. PMID: 24053983.

113. Krueger DA, Care MM, Holland K, et al. Everolimus for subependymal giant-cell astrocytomas in tuberous sclerosis. *N Engl J Med.* 2010;363:1801-1811. PMID: 21047224.

114. Alliance for Clinical Trials in Oncology. NCT00887146. Radiation Therapy With Concomitant and Adjuvant Temozolomide or Radiation Therapy With Adjuvant PCV or Temozolomide Alone in Treating Patients With Anaplastic Glioma. http://clinicaltrials.gov/ct2/show/NCT00887146. Accessed September 29, 2013.

115. Chinot OL, Honore S, Dufour H, et al. Safety and efficacy of temozolomide in patients with recurrent anaplastic oligodendrogliomas after standard radiotherapy and chemotherapy. *J Clin Oncol.* 2001;19:2449-2455. PMID: 11331324.

116. Shuangshoti S, Rushing EJ, Mena H, et al. Supratentorial extraventricular ependymal neoplasms: a clinicopathologic study of 32 patients. *Cancer.* 2005;103:2598-2605. PMID: 15861411.

117. Johnson RA, Wright KD, Poppleton H, et al. Cross-species genomics matches driver mutations and cell compartments to model ependymoma. *Nature.* 2010;466:632-636. PMID: 20639864.

118. Witt H, Mack SC, Ryzhova M, et al. Delineation of two clinically and molecularly distinct subgroups of posterior fossa ependymoma. *Cancer Cell.* 2011;20:143-157. PMID: 21840481.

119. Amirian ES, Armstrong TS, Aldape KD, et al. Predictors of survival among pediatric and adult ependymoma cases: a study using Surveillance, Epidemiology, and End Results data from 1973 to 2007. *Neuroepidemiology.* 2012;39:116-124. PMID: 22846789.

120. Gornet MK, Buckner JC, Marks RS, et al. Chemotherapy for advanced CNS ependymoma. *J Neurooncol.* 1999;45:61-67. PMID: PMID: 10728911.

121. Brandes AA, Cavallo G, Reni M, et al. A multicenter retrospective study of chemotherapy for recurrent intracranial ependymal tumors in adults by the Gruppo Italiano Cooperativo di Neuro-Oncologia. *Cancer.* 2005;104:143-148. PMID: 15912507.

122. M.D. Anderson Cancer Center. NCT01295944. Carboplatin and Bevacizumab for Recurrent Ependymoma. http://clinicaltrials.gov/ct2/show/NCT01295944. Accessed April 9, 2014.

123. Children's Oncology Group. NCT01096368. Maintenance Chemotherapy or Observation Following Induction Chemotherapy and Radiation Therapy in Treating Younger Patients With Newly Diagnosed Ependymoma. http://clinicaltrials.gov/ct2/show/NCT01096368. Accessed April 9, 2014.

124. Russo C, Pellarin M, Tingby O, et al. Comparative genomic hybridization in patients with supratentorial and infratentorial primitive neuroectodermal tumors. *Cancer.* 1999;86:331-339. PMID: 10421270.

125. Taylor MD, Northcott PA, Korshunov A, et al. Molecular subgroups of medulloblastoma: the current consensus. *Acta Neuropathol.* 2012;123(4):465-472. PMID: 22134537.

126. Zeltzer PM, Boyett JM, Finlay JL, et al. Metastasis stage, adjuvant treatment, and residual tumor are prognostic factors for medulloblastoma in children: conclusions from the Children's Cancer Group 921 randomized phase III study. *J Clin Oncol.* 1999;17:832-845. PMID: 10071274.

127. Chang CH, Housepian EM, Herbert C Jr. An operative staging system and a megavoltage radiotherapeutic technic for cerebellar medulloblastomas. *Radiology.* 1969;93:1351-1359. PMID: 4983156.

128. Gajjar AJ, Gururangan S, Qaddoumi IA, et al. A prospective phase II study to determine the efficacy of GDC 0449 (vismodegib) in adults with recurrent medulloblastoma (MB): A Pediatric Brain Tumor Consortium study (PBTC 25B). *J Clin Oncol.* 2013; 31 (suppl; abstr 2035).

129. Gill P, Litzow M, Buckner J, et al. High-dose chemotherapy with autologous stem cell transplantation in adults with recurrent embryonal tumors of the central nervous system. *Cancer.* 2008;112:1805-1811. PMID: 18300237.

130. Dunkel IJ, Gardner SL, Garvin JH, Jr., et al. High-dose carboplatin, thiotepa, and etoposide with autologous stem cell rescue for patients with previously irradiated recurrent medulloblastoma. *Neuro Oncol.* 2010;12:297-303. PMID: 20167818.

131. Nikolopoulos TP, Fortnum H, O'Donoghue G, et al. Acoustic neuroma growth: a systematic review of the evidence. *Otol Neurotol.* 2010;31:478-485. PMID: 20147867.

132. Propp JM, McCarthy BJ, Davis FG, et al. Descriptive epidemiology of vestibular schwannomas. *Neuro Oncol.* 2006;8:1-11. PMID: 16443943.

133. Wiemels J, Wrensch M, Claus EB. Epidemiology and etiology of meningioma. *J Neurooncol.* 2010;99:307-314. PMID: 20821343.

134. Chamberlain MC, Glantz MJ, Fadul CE. Recurrent meningioma: salvage therapy with long-acting somatostatin analogue. *Neurology.* 2007;69:969-973. PMID: 17785665.

135. Johnson DR, Kimmel DW, Burch PA, et al. Phase II study of subcutaneous octreotide in adults with recurrent or progressive meningioma and meningeal hemangiopericytoma. *Neuro Oncol.* 2011;13:530-535. PMID: 21558077.

136. Clark VE, Erson-Omay EZ, Serin A, et al. Genomic analysis of non-NF2 meningiomas reveals mutations in TRAF7, KLF4, AKT1, and SMO. *Science.* 2013;339:1077-1080. PMID: 23348505.

137. Go RS, Taylor BV, Kimmel DW. The natural history of asymptomatic meningiomas in Olmsted County, Minnesota. *Neurology.* 1998;51:1718-1720. PMID: 9855530.

138. Norden AD, Drappatz J, Wen PY. Advances in meningioma therapy. *Curr Neurol Neurosci Rep.* 2009;9:231-240. PMID: 19348712.

139. Miller DC, Hochberg FH, Harris NL, et al. Pathology with clinical correlations of primary central nervous system non-Hodgkin's lymphoma. The Massachusetts General Hospital experience 1958-1989. *Cancer.* 1994;74:1383-1397. PMID: 8055462.

140. Ferreri AJ, Reni M, Pasini F, et al. A multicenter study of treatment of primary CNS lymphoma. *Neurology.* 2002;58:1513-1520. PMID: 12034789.

141. Ferreri AJ, Reni M, Foppoli M, et al. High-dose cytarabine plus high-dose methotrexate versus high-dose methotrexate alone in patients with primary CNS lymphoma: a randomised phase 2 trial. *Lancet.* 2009;374:1512-1520. PMID: 19767089.

142. DeAngelis LM, Seiferheld W, Schold SC, et al. Combination chemotherapy and radiotherapy for primary central nervous system lymphoma: Radiation Therapy Oncology Group Study 93-10. *J Clin Oncol.* 2002;20:4643-4648. PMID: 12488408.

143. Abrey LE, DeAngelis LM, Yahalom J. Long-term survival in primary CNS lymphoma. *J Clin Oncol.* 1998;16:859-863. PMID: 9508166.

144. Radiation Therapy Oncology Group. NCT01399372. Rituximab, Methotrexate, Vincristine Sulfate, Procarbazine Hydrochloride, and Cytarabine With or Without Radiation Therapy in Treating Patients With Primary Central Nervous System Lymphoma. http://clinicaltrials.gov/ct2/show/NCT01399372. Accessed April 14, 2014.

145. Chamberlain MC, Johnston SK. High-dose methotrexate and rituximab with deferred radiotherapy for newly diagnosed primary B-cell CNS lymphoma. *Neuro Oncol.* 2010;12:736-744. PMID: 20511181.

146. Rubenstein JL, Hsi ED, Johnson JL, et al. Intensive chemotherapy and immunotherapy in patients with newly diagnosed primary CNS lymphoma: CALGB 50202 (Alliance 50202). *J Clin Oncol.* 2013;31:3061-3068. PMID: 23569323.

147. Doolittle ND, Miner ME, Hall WA, et al. Safety and efficacy of a multicenter study using intraarterial chemotherapy in conjunction with osmotic opening of the blood-brain barrier for the treatment of patients with malignant brain tumors. *Cancer.* 2000;88:637-647. PMID: 10649259.

148. International Extranodal Lymphoma Study Group. NCT01011920. Trial for Patients With Newly Diagnosed Primary Central Nervous System (CNS) Lymphoma. http://clinicaltrials.gov/ct2/show/study/NCT01011920. Accessed October 3, 2013.

149. Cancer and Leukemia Group B. NCT01511562. Combination Chemotherapy With or Without Autologous Stem Cell Transplant in Treating Patients With Central Nervous System B-Cell Lymphoma. http://clinicaltrials.gov/ct2/show/study/NCT01511562. Accessed October 3, 2013.

150. Schouten LJ, Rutten J, Huveneers HA, et al. Incidence of brain metastases in a cohort of patients with carcinoma of the breast, colon, kidney, and lung and melanoma. *Cancer.* 2002;94:2698-2705. PMID: 12173339.

151. Barnholtz-Sloan JS, Sloan AE, Davis FG, et al. Incidence proportions of brain metastases in patients diagnosed (1973 to 2001) in the Metropolitan Detroit Cancer Surveillance System. *J Clin Oncol.* 2004;22:2865-2872. PMID: 15254054.

152. Posner JB, Chernik NL. Intracranial metastases from systemic cancer. *Adv Neurol.* 1978;19:579-592. PMID: 570349.

153. Delattre JY, Krol G, Thaler HT, et al. Distribution of brain metastases. *Arch Neurol.* 1988;45:741-744. PMID: 3390029.

154. Patchell RA, Tibbs PA, Walsh JW, et al. A randomized trial of surgery in the treatment of single metastases to the brain. *N Engl J Med.* 1990;322:494-500. PMID: 2405271.

155. Vecht CJ, Haaxma-Reiche H, Noordijk EM, et al. Treatment of single brain metastasis: radiotherapy alone or combined with neurosurgery? *Ann Neurol.* 1993;33:583-590. PMID: 8498838.

156. Noordijk EM, Vecht CJ, Haaxma-Reiche H, et al. The choice of treatment of single brain metastasis should be based on extracranial tumor activity and age. *Int J Radiat Oncol Biol Phys.* 1994;29:711-717. PMID: 8040016.

157. Tsao MN, Lloyd NS, Wong RK, et al. Radiotherapeutic management of brain metastases: a systematic review and meta-analysis. *Cancer Treat Rev.* 2005;31:256-273. PMID: 15951117.

158. Andrews DW, Scott CB, Sperduto PW, et al. Whole brain radiation therapy with or without stereotactic radiosurgery boost for patients with one to three brain metastases: phase III results of the RTOG 9508 randomised trial. *Lancet.* 2004;363:1665-1672. PMID: 15158627.

159. Kocher M, Soffietti R, Abacioglu U, et al. Adjuvant whole-brain radiotherapy versus observation after radiosurgery or surgical resection of one to three cerebral metastases: results of the EORTC 22952-26001 study. *J Clin Oncol.* 2011;29:134-141. PMID: 21041710.

160. Patchell RA, Tibbs PA, Regine WF, et al. Postoperative radiotherapy in the treatment of single metastases to the brain: a randomized trial. *JAMA.* 1998;280:1485-1489. PMID: 9809728.

161. Aoyama H, Shirato H, Tago M, et al. Stereotactic radiosurgery plus whole-brain radiation therapy vs stereotactic radiosurgery alone for treatment of brain metastases: a randomized controlled trial. *Jama.* 2006;295:2483-2491. PMID: 16757720.

162. Tsao MN, Lloyd N, Wong R, et al. Whole brain radiotherapy for the treatment of multiple brain metastases. *Cochrane Database Syst Rev.* 2006(3):CD003869. PMID: 16856022.

163. Mehta MP, Tsao MN, Whelan TJ, et al. The American Society for Therapeutic Radiology and Oncology (ASTRO) evidence-based review of the role of radiosurgery for brain metastases. *Int J Radiat Oncol Biol Phys.* 2005;63:37-46. PMID: 16111570.

164. Aoyama H, Tago M, Kato N, et al. Neurocognitive function of patients with brain metastasis who received either whole brain radiotherapy plus stereotactic radiosurgery or radiosurgery alone. *Int J Radiat Oncol Biol Phys.* 2007;68:1388-1395. PMID: 17674975.

165. Chang EL, Wefel JS, Hess KR, et al. Neurocognition in patients with brain metastases treated with radiosurgery or radiosurgery plus whole-brain irradiation: a randomised controlled trial. *Lancet Oncol.* 2009;10:1037-1044. PMID: 19801201.

166. Brown PD, Pugh S, Laack NN, et al. Memantine for the prevention of cognitive dysfunction in patients receiving whole-brain radiotherapy: a randomized, double-blind, placebo-controlled trial. *Neuro Oncol.* 2013;15:1429-1437. PMID: 23956241.

167. North Central Cancer Treatment Group. NCT01372774. Stereotactic Radiosurgery or Whole-Brain Radiation Therapy in Treating Patients With Brain Metastases That Have Been Removed By Surgery. http://clinicaltrials.gov/show/NCT01372774. Accessed September 29, 2013.

168. Radiation Therapy Oncology Group. NCT01227954. Avoiding the Hippocampus During Whole-Brain Radiation Therapy in Treating Patients With Brain Metastases. http://clinicaltrials.gov/show/NCT01227954. Accessed April 15, 2014.

169. Lin NU, Diéras V, Paul D, et al. Multicenter phase II study of lapatinib in patients with brain metastases from HER2-positive breast cancer. *Clin Cancer Res.* 2009;15:1452-1459. PMID: 19228746.

170. Long GV, Trefzer U, Davies MA, et al. Dabrafenib in patients with Val600Glu or Val600Lys BRAF-mutant melanoma metastatic to the brain (BREAK-MB): a multicentre, open-label, phase 2 trial. *Lancet Oncol.* 2012;13:1087-1095. PMID: 23051966.

171. Pavlidis N. The diagnostic and therapeutic management of leptomeningeal carcinomatosis. *Ann Oncol.* 2004;15 Suppl 4:iv285-291.

172. Wasserstrom WR, Glass JP, Posner JB. Diagnosis and treatment of lepto-meningeal metastases from solid tumors: experience with 90 patients. *Cancer.* 1982;49(4):759-772. PMID: 6895713.

173. Glantz MJ, Cole BF, Recht L, et al. High-dose intravenous methotrexate for patients with nonleukemic leptomeningeal cancer: is intrathecal chemo-therapy necessary? *J Clin Oncol.* 1998;16:1561-1567. PMID: 9552066.

174. Frick J, Ritch PS, Hansen RM, et al. Successful treatment of meningeal leukemia using systemic high-dose cytosine arabinoside. *J Clin Oncol.* 1984;2:365-368. PMID: 6726293.

15

LEUKEMIAS

Frederick R. Appelbaum, MD

Acute myeloid leukemia

▶ The genetic landscape of acute myeloid leukemia has been more clearly defined with each case having an average of 13 mutations, eight of which are random "passenger" mutations and five of which are recurrent "driver" mutations (Ley TJ, *N Engl J Med* 2013).

▶ The evaluation of younger patients with acute myeloid leukemia should always include cytogenetics and mutational analysis of *FLT3*, *NPM1*, and *CEBPA* (Döhner H, *Blood* 2010).

▶ Progress in cord blood transplantation for adults, particularly the use of double cord grafts, has resulted in survival outcomes similar to those seen with matched, unrelated donors (Scaradavou A, *Blood* 2013).

▶ Patients with intermediate-/good-risk acute promyelocytic leukemia can be treated with all-trans retinoic acid and arsenic trioxide alone with results similar to those seen with the addition of chemotherapy (Lo-Coco F, *N Engl J Med* 2013).

Acute lymphocytic leukemia

▶ Therapy with dasatinib and prednisone alone results in complete remission in a high percentage of older patients with Philadelphia-positive acute lymphocytic leukemia without the need for concomitant chemotherapy (Foa R, *Blood* 2011).

▶ Novel therapies under investigation for adult acute lymphocytic leukemia include blinatumomab, a bispecific T-cell engager, inotuzumab ozogamicin, an immunoconjugate, and chimeric antigen receptor T cells (Hoelzer D, *Hematology Am Soc Hematol Educ Program* 2011; Grupp SA, *N Engl J Med* 2013).

Myelodysplastic syndrome

▶ *TET2*, *ASXL1*, *RUNX1*, and *TP53* are among the most commonly mutated genes in myelodysplastic syndrome (Bejar R, *N Engl J Med* 2011).

▶ Based on the available data, allogeneic hematopoietic cell transplantation prolongs survival for patients age 50 to 70 with intermediate or more advanced myelodysplastic syndrome (Koreth J, *J Clin Oncol* 2013).

Chronic myeloid leukemia

▶ Bosutinib is a third-generation tyrosine kinase inhibitor recently approved for the treatment of patients with chronic myeloid leukemia resistant or intolerant to previous therapies (Khoury HJ, *Blood* 2012).

The term leukemia is used to describe a number of related cancers of the blood-forming organ characterized by increased growth and impaired maturation. Leukemias are classically defined by their rapidity of growth (acute vs. chronic), and by the healthy cell the leukemia most resembles (myeloid vs. lymphocytic). Thus, the four major forms of leukemia are acute myeloid leukemia (AML), acute lymphocytic leukemia (ALL), chronic myeloid leukemia (CML), and chronic lymphocytic leukemia (CLL). According to the American Cancer Society (www.cancer.org), approximately 48,610 new cases of leukemia were expected to be diagnosed in the United States in 2013, with 23,720 leukemia-related deaths (Table 15-1).

ETIOLOGY
GENETIC PREDISPOSITION

The cause of leukemia is usually unknown, but some individuals have a genetic predisposition for its development. If the disease develops before age 10 in a patient with an identical twin, there is a one in five chance that the disease will develop in the unaffected twin.[1] Single germ-line mutations in *RUNX1*, *CEBPA*, and *GATA2* result in familial syndromes of acute leukemia without other manifestations.[2] Syndromes characterized by defective DNA repair, such as Fanconi anemia, ataxia telangiectasia, and Bloom syndrome, have an increased incidence of acute leukemia.[3] Bone marrow failure syndromes associated with ribosomal abnormalities, including Diamond-Blackfan, Shwachman-Diamond, and dyskeratosis congenital, also are associated with an increased incidence of acute leukemia. Germ-line mutations in *p53* and abnormalities in chromosome number, as in Klinefelter and Down syndromes, also have been associated with an increased incidence of acute leukemia.

Table 15-1 **2013 U.S. Leukemia Estimates**

	Cases	Deaths
Acute lymphocytic leukemia	6,070	1,430
Chronic lymphocytic leukemia	15,680	4,580
Acute myeloid leukemia	14,590	10,370
Chronic myeloid leukemia	5,920	610
Other	6,350	6,730

ONCOGENIC VIRUSES

Human T-cell lymphotropic virus type I is a causative agent of adult T-cell leukemia. This enveloped, single-strand RNA virus is associated with a distinct form of leukemia found in geographic clusters in southwestern Japan, the Caribbean basin, and Africa. The virus can be spread horizontally by sexual contact or through blood products; it also can be spread vertically from mother to fetus. Although the virus is endemic in the geographic clusters mentioned, adult T-cell leukemia will develop in only 2% to 4% of patients infected with the virus. The latency period is very long, estimated at 30 years or more.[4] Epstein-Barr virus is associated with the endemic African form of Burkitt lymphoma/leukemia.

KEY POINT

■ Although the cause of leukemia is unknown in most cases, the incidence of myelodysplasia and acute myeloid leukemia secondary to prior therapy is increasing as chemotherapy is used more widely to manage other diseases.

RADIATION

Ionizing radiation is leukemogenic.[5] The incidences of AML, CML, and ALL were increased in individuals who received radiation therapy for ankylosing spondylitis and in survivors of the atomic bomb blasts of Hiroshima and Nagasaki. The highest rates of leukemia were associated with higher doses of radiation, particularly if the radiation was absorbed over a shorter period of time. Younger individuals seem more susceptible to the leukemogenic effects of radiation. After radiation exposure, the incidence of leukemia seems to peak between 5 and 10 years after exposure, regardless of patient age. The incidence of chromosome aberrations has been reported to be higher than expected for individuals living in areas of high natural background radiation (often because of radon), but a higher incidence of acute leukemia has not been consistently observed.

Concern has been raised about the possible leukemogenic effects of extremely low-frequency, nonionizing electromagnetic fields emitted by high-energy wires and step-down transformers. Several studies have been conducted, and if there is any leukemogenic effect of such radiation, the magnitude of the effect seems to be small.

CHEMICALS

Extensive occupational exposure to benzene and benzene-containing compounds may lead to marrow damage that eventually can manifest as aplastic anemia, myelodysplasia, or AML. Benzene is widely used in industry—particularly for organic synthesis and as a solvent—and constitutes about 1% of unleaded gasoline. Other associations between occupational exposure to chemicals and subsequent leukemia are not as persuasive. Most studies have found a small but consistent increase in AML among cigarette smokers.

DRUG- AND THERAPY-RELATED LEUKEMIAS

Therapy with antineoplastic agents is a major identifiable cause of acute leukemia. In general, alkylating agents are the class of drugs most commonly associated with secondary leukemia.[6] Among the various alkylating agents, melphalan and the nitrosoureas seem to be particularly associated with increased risk; however, all alkylating agents are likely leukemogenic, with an increased incidence of leukemia observed after prolonged exposure and after the use of dose-intense regimens. The secondary leukemias associated with alkylating agents often present initially as a myelodysplastic syndrome (MDS) before progressing to AML; they have no other distinct morphologic features, and on cytogenetic examination, frequently exhibit whole or partial loss of chromosomes 5 or 7 and, less often, trisomy 8. These leukemias typically develop 4 to 6 years after chemotherapy and tend to have lower therapeutic response rates than does de novo disease.[7]

Patients treated with topoisomerase II inhibitors also are at risk of therapy-related leukemia. In contrast to leukemias associated with alkylating agents, disease caused by topoisomerase II inhibitors tends to have a shorter latency period (1 to 2 years), lacks a myelodysplastic phase, carries a monocytic morphology, and frequently involves abnormalities of the long arm of chromosome 11 (band q23); less commonly, translocations of 21q22 are involved.[8] Patients with lymphoma who undergo autologous hematopoietic cell transplantation (HCT) are at increased risk of leukemia, with a cumulative incidence as high as 10%.

ACUTE MYELOID LEUKEMIA
BIOLOGY, CYTOGENETICS, AND MOLECULAR GENETICS

AML, like all leukemias, is a clonal disorder with all leukemic cells arising from a common progenitor. Attempts at identifying the cell of origin, or the leukemic stem cell, generally have involved identification of the cell capable of transferring leukemia to an immunodeficient mouse. In these studies, only CD34+, CD38- blasts are capable of doing so. Such cells are relatively rare among the leukemic mass, with a frequency of 0.2 to 100/10[6] cells. In patients, the leukemia stem cell gives rise to progeny that fail to differentiate and continue to proliferate in an uncontrolled fashion, resulting in replacement of normal bone marrow by a clonal population of immature myeloid cells. The subsequent loss of normal marrow function results in the common clinical signs of AML: anemia, infection, and bleeding. If untreated, AML results in death within

several months; however, with appropriate therapy, a significant number of patients can achieve cure.

AML can be categorized according to morphology, histochemistry, cell surface markers, cytogenetics, and oncogene expression.

Morphology

AML cells are typically 12 μm to 20 μm in diameter with discrete nuclear chromatin, multiple nucleoli, and azurophilic granules in the cytoplasm. The French-American-British (FAB) group recognizes eight morphologic subtypes of AML (Fig. 15-1).[9] In an effort to incorporate etiologic, immunophenotypic, and cytogenetic characteristics, as well as the more traditional morphologic features, into the categorization of AML, the World Health Organization (WHO) has adopted the classification schema shown in Table 15-2.[10]

KEY POINTS

- In most cases of acute leukemia, a clonal abnormality in chromosome number or structure can be found. These cytogenetic abnormalities have emerged as the single most important prognostic factor in acute leukemia and are indispensable in making therapeutic decisions.
- Genome-wide sequencing has identified over 20 mutations recurrently seen in acute myeloid leukemia. Of these, testing for mutations in *FLT-3*, *NPM-1*, and *CEBPA* is important in determining how patients who enter first remission should be treated.

Histochemistry

Specific patterns of reactivity with histochemical stains are noted for the acute leukemias. Stains for myeloperoxidase react specifically with FAB types M1, M2, M3, and M4 and fail to react with lymphoid leukemias. Nonspecific esterase predominantly stains cells of monocytic lineage, specifically FAB subtypes M4 and M5.

Cell Surface Markers

Acute leukemias can be further categorized using monoclonal antibodies that are reactive with cell surface antigens. In general, these antigens are identical to antigens found on healthy immature hematopoietic cells and reflect the level of differentiation of the leukemic cells. Most cases of AML express antigens found on healthy immature myeloid cells, including CD13, CD33, and CD34.[11] AML with monocytic characteristics expresses CD14. Erythroid leukemias frequently express CD36, CD71, and the blood group H antigen, whereas megakaryocytic leukemias express CD41a and CD61. Although the antigens detected on leukemic blasts generally represent antigens found on healthy immature hematopoietic cells, they usually are present in abnormal combinations and concentrations, allowing multidimensional flow cytometry to identify abnormal leukemia

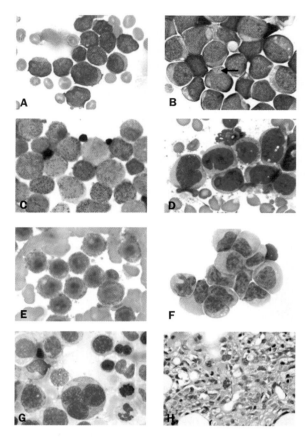

Fig. 15-1 The morphologic spectrum of the acute myeloid leukemias (AML) in bone marrow aspirates and a marrow biopsy.

(A) Acute myeloblastic leukemia with minimal (French-American-British [FAB] AML-MI) or no (FAB AML-MO) maturation. The cells are myeloblasts with dispersed chromatin and variable amounts of agranular cytoplasm. Some display medium-size, poorly defined nucleoli. (B) Acute myeloblastic leukemia with maturation (FAB AML-M2). Some of the blasts contain azurophilic granules, and there are promyelocytes. More mature neutrophils were present in other fields. Note the Auer rod (arrow). (C) Acute promyelocytic leukemia (FAB AML-M3). All of these cells are promyelocytes containing coarse cytoplasmic granules that sometimes obscure the nuclei. (D) Acute myelomonocytic leukemia (FAB AML-M4). Promonocytes with indented nuclei are present with myeloblasts. The dense nuclear staining is unusual. (E) Acute monoblastic leukemia (FAB AML-M5a). These characteristic monoblasts have round nuclei with delicate chromatin and prominent nucleoli. Cytoplasm is abundant. Nonspecific esterase staining was intense (not shown). (F) Acute monocytic leukemia (FAB AML-M5b). Most of the cells in this field are promonocytes. Monoblasts and an abnormal monocyte also are present. (G) Acute erythroid leukemia (FAB AML-M6). Dysplastic multinucleated erythroid precursors with megaloblastoid nuclei are present. (H) Acute megakaryoblastic leukemia (FAB AML-M7). In this marrow biopsy, there are large and small blasts as well as atypical megakaryocytes.

blasts in peripheral blood or marrow samples. In 10% to 20% of AML cases, the blasts also express antigens usually restricted to B- or T-cell lineages, especially CD4, CD7, and CD19. Expression of single lymphoid antigens by AML cells does not seem to influence either the natural history or therapeutic response of these leukemias.

Table 15-2 World Health Organization Classification of Acute Leukemia with Corresponding FAB Classification Subtypes (2008)[10]

Acute Myeloid Leukemia and Related Neoplasms
AML with recurrent genetic abnormalities
AML with t(8;21)(q22;q22); *RUNX1-RUNX1T1*
AML with inv(16)(p13.1;q22) or t(16;16)(p13.1;q22); *CBFB-MYH11*
APL with t(15;17)(q22;q12); *PML-RARA*
AML with t(9;11)(p22;q23); *MLLT3-MLL*
AML with t(6;9)(p23;q34); *DEK-NUP214*
AML with inv(3)(q21;q26.2) or t(3;3)(q21;q26.2); *RPN1-EVI1*
AML (megakaryoblastic) with t(1;22)(p13;q13); *RBM15-MKL1*
Provisional entity: AML with mutated NPM1
Provisional entity: AML with mutated CEBPA
AML with myelodysplasia-related changes
Therapy-related myeloid neoplasms
AML, not otherwise specified
AML with minimal differentiation
AML without maturation
AML with maturation
Acute myelomonocytic leukemia
Acute monoblastic/monocytic leukemia
Acute erythroid leukemia
Pure erythroid leukemia
Erythroleukemia, erythroid/myeloid
Acute megakaryoblastic leukemia
Acute basophilic leukemia
Acute panmyelosis with myelofibrosis
Myeloid sarcoma
Myeloid proliferations related to Down syndrome
Transient abnormal myelopoiesis
Myeloid leukemia associated with Down syndrome
Blastic plasmacytoid dendritic cell neoplasm
B Lymphoblastic Leukemia/Lymphoma
B lymphoblastic leukemia/lymphoma, not otherwise specified
B lymphoblastic leukemia/lymphoma with recurrent genetic abnormalities
B lymphoblastic leukemia/lymphoma with t(9;22)(q34;q11.2); *BCR-ABL 1*
B lymphoblastic leukemia/lymphoma with t(v;11q23); *MLL* rearranged
B lymphoblastic leukemia/lymphoma with t(12;21)(p13;q22) *TEL-AML1 (ETV6-RUNX1)*
B lymphoblastic leukemia/lymphoma with hyperdiploidy
B lymphoblastic leukemia/lymphoma with hypodiploidy
B lymphoblastic leukemia/lymphoma with t(5;14)(q31;q32) *IL3-IGH*
B lymphoblastic leukemia/lymphoma with t(1;19)(q23;p13.3); *TCF3-PBX1*
T Lymphoblastic Leukemia/Lymphoma

Abbreviations: AML, acute myeloid leukemia; APL, acute promyelocytic leukemia; FAB, French-American-British classification.

Vardiman JW, Thiele J, Arber DA, et al. The 2008 revision of the World Health Organization (WHO) classification of myeloid neoplasms and acute leukemia: rationale and important changes. Blood. 2009;114(5):937-951.

Cytogenetics and Molecular Biology

In most cases of AML, an acquired abnormality in chromosome number or structure is found. These abnormalities are clonal, involving essentially all of the malignant cells, and are not found in healthy cells. Certain abnormalities are seen repeatedly and are associated with distinct morphologic or clinical subtypes of leukemia. They may be the result of the gain or loss of a whole chromosome, but more often include translocations, deletions, or inversions (see Chapter 2: Molecular Biology).

Certain chromosome abnormalities are associated with specific syndromes in AML. Acute promyelocytic leukemia (APL; FAB subtype M3) accounts for approximately 8% of AML cases and virtually always has a translocation involving the promyelocytic leukemia *(PML)* gene on chromosome 15 and the retinoic acid receptor alpha gene *(RAR-alpha)* on chromosome 17, t(15;17)(q22;q11-12). The resultant abnormal fusion protein acts as a dominant-negative inhibitor of healthy *PML* and *RAR-alpha* function.[12] The fusion protein of *PML* and *RAR-alpha* seems to recruit nuclear corepressors and histone deacetylase, inhibiting the transcription of genes required for myeloid differentiation. Acute myelomonocytic leukemia with abnormal eosinophilia is associated with an inversion in chromosome 16 (inv[16][q13q22]), and some patients with M2 AML have a translocation between chromosomes 8 and 21, t(8;21)(q22;q22). These two translocations result in abnormalities in a transcription factor made up of core-binding factors (CBF) alpha and beta. t(8;21) results in fusion of the CBF-alpha subunit on chromosome 21 *(RUNX1T1)* with the *RUNX1* (formerly *ETO)* gene on chromosome 8, whereas inv(16) results in fusion of CBF-beta on the q arm of chromosome 16 with *MYH11* on the p arm. t(8;21) and inv(16) each account for 5% to 8% of AML cases, are more prominent among younger patients, and have a relatively favorable prognosis.[13] Some cases of t(8;21) or inv(16) AML also have mutations in the receptor tyrosine kinase gene *KIT;* such cases are associated with a less favorable outcome.[14] Translocations between the *MLL* gene located at 11q23 and any one of several partners constitute approximately 7% of adult AML cases.[15] Trisomy 8 is seen in approximately 9% of AML cases and carries an intermediate prognosis. Partial or full deletions of chromosomes 5 and 7 each account for 6% to 8% of AML cases. These abnormalities are more common in older patients with AML and in cases associated with prior exposure to alkylating agents, and they typically indicate poor prognosis. For many years, cytogenetics has formed the basis for risk categorization with t(8;21), inv(16), and t(15;17) forming the favorable group; del(5q), -5, del(7q), -7 and complex karyotypes forming the unfavorable-risk group; and all others forming the intermediate-risk group. The effect of cytogenetics on complete response rates and survival using this categorization is shown in Table 15-3 and Fig. 15-2.[16,17] More recently, it has been appreciated that any monosomy (not just -5 and -7) is associated with a poor prognosis, and having a monosomal karyotype (defined as having two or more distinct monosomies or one monosomy and another structural abnormality) is associated with a very poor prognosis (less than 4% survival at 4 years).[18]

Table 15-3 **Cytogenetics and Treatment Outcomes in Acute Myeloid Leukemia**

Risk Group	Incidence (%)	Complete Response Rate (%)	5-Year Survival (%)
Favorable	20	85	60
inv(16)			
t(8;21), t(15;17)			
Intermediate	45	76	38
Normal, +8			
Adverse	30	55	12
del(5q), -5			
del(7q), -7			
Complex, 11q23			

Modified from Cheson BD, ed. Oncology MKSAP, *2nd ed.* Philadelphia, PA: American College of Physicians, 1999.

The recurrent chromosomal abnormalities found in AML led to the initial identification and cloning of the involved genes. More recently, directed and genome-wide assays have provided a broader description of the genetic abnormalities seen in AML.[19] AML cells have an average of about 13 mutations per cell, far less than seen in epithelial cancers. In each case of AML, approximately five of the 13 mutations are in genes recurrently affected in AML, so-called driver mutations, whereas the other eight are random, so-called passenger mutations. Among the driver mutations, three, *FLT3, NPM1,* and *CEBPA,* have entered clinical practice because they affect risk assessment and may

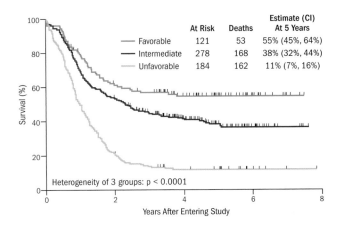

Fig. 15-2 Survival in adult acute myeloid leukemia according to cytogenetic risk group.[17]

Republished with permission of the American Society of Hematology, from Blood. *Slovak ML, Kopecky KJ, Cassileth PA, et al. Karyotypic analysis predicts outcome of preremission and postremission therapy in adult acute myeloid leukemia: a Southwest Oncology Group/Eastern Cooperative Oncology Group study.* Blood. *2000;96(13):4075-83. Permission conveyed through Copyright Clearance Center, Inc.*

guide therapy. *FLT3* is a receptor tyrosine kinase, and activating mutations in *FLT3* have been found in 20% to 40% of cases. These mutations may be internal tandem repeats (ITDs; 15% to 30%) or point mutations (5% to 10%), are somewhat more common in older patients, and are associated with a higher blast count at diagnosis, as well as a less favorable response to treatment.[20] The *FLT* ITD averages approximately 40 base pairs in length, and studies suggest that larger ITDs are associated with a less favorable prognosis. In addition, the *FLT* ITD may be biallelic, affecting both chromosomes. Having a higher ratio of abnormal to healthy alleles also seems to confer a worse prognosis. Mutations in the nucleophosmin gene *(NPM1)* have been identified in 20% to 30% of AML cases (usually those with a normal karyotype) and appear to be associated with a favorable clinical outcome.[21] Likewise, biallelic mutations in *CEBPA,* a gene encoding a leucine zipper transcription factor, exist in 4% to 15% of AML cases and are also associated with a favorable prognosis.[22] Other driver mutations include *IDH1, IDH2, DNMT3A, WT1, RUNX1, NRAS, KRAS, TP53, TET2,* and *ASXL1.* Although assays of the mutational status of these genes have not yet become standard, increasing numbers of studies suggest that such assays may provide useful prognostic, and possibly therapeutic, information.[23]

CLINICAL FEATURES

The signs and symptoms of AML are a result of decreased healthy hematopoiesis and infiltration of healthy organs by leukemic blasts. Thus, most patients present with anemia and thrombocytopenia. The white blood cell count may be elevated, normal, or low, but most patients will have granulocytopenia, and one-third will present with signs of substantial or life-threatening infection. In addition to suppressing healthy marrow function, AML cells may infiltrate healthy organs, particularly in patients with myelomonocytic or monocytic leukemias. AML cells sometimes infiltrate the skin, causing a nonpruritic raised rash (leukemia cutis), or may collect in extramedullary masses (sometimes termed myeloid sarcomas or chloromas). In 2% to 3% of cases, AML will involve the central nervous system (CNS) at the time of diagnosis.

Prognostic Factors for Untreated AML

On the basis of cytogenetic and molecular data, AML can be divided into four risk groups: favorable, intermediate-1, intermediate-2, and adverse (Table 15-4).[24] The favorable group includes the CBF AMLs, cytogenetically normal AML (CN-AML) with mutated *CEBPA,* and CN-AML with mutated *NPM1* without *FLT3* mutations. Intermediate-1 includes all patients with a normal karyotype who are not in the favorable group. Intermediate-2 includes cases with t(9;11) and those with a cytogenetic abnormality not classified as favorable or adverse, and the adverse group includes inv(3), t(6;9), *MLL* rearrangements other than t(9;11), -5, -7, del(5q), del(7q), abnl(17p), and complex cytogenetics. Other factors in addition to these cytogenetic and genetic findings influence prognosis, with a lower response rate and shorter response duration expected in older patients, those with a high white blood cell count at diagnosis, and those

Table 15-4 **Prognosis According to Cytogenetic and Molecular Genetic Data**[31]	
Genetic Group	**Subsets**
Favorable	t(8;21) inv(16) Mutated *NPM1* without *FLT3-ITD* Mutated *CEBPA*
Intermediate-1	Mutated *NPM1* with *FLT3-ITD* Wild-type *NPM1* with *FLT3-ITD* Wild-type *NPM1* without *FLT3-ITD*
Intermediate-2	t(9;11) Cytogenetic abnormality neither favorable nor adverse
Adverse	inv(3) t(6;9) t(v;11) -5 or del(5q), -7, abnl (17p), complex

Adapted from Döhner H, Estey EH, Amadori S, et al. Diagnosis and management of acute myeloid leukemia in adults: recommendations from an international expert panel, on behalf of the European LeukemiaNet. Blood. 2010;115(3):453-47.

whose disease is secondary to prior therapy or to an antecedent hematologic disorder.

TREATMENT FOR AML

The median age at diagnosis of AML is approximately 65. Because of differences in both the biology of the disease and ability to tolerate intensive therapies, most studies of AML therapy have been directed either to patients younger than age 65 or to patients older than age 65.

Initial Chemotherapeutic Approaches for Younger Patients

Induction. Standard remission induction therapy is with a combination of an anthracycline and cytarabine. With this combination, complete remission (CR) can be expected in 60% to 80% of patients up to age 65. Prospective, randomized trials have demonstrated that outcomes are better with idarubicin (10 to 12 mg/m²/day for 3 days) or a higher dose of daunorubicin (60 to 90 mg/m²/day for 3 days) than with the previous conventional daunorubicin dose of 45 mg/m²/day for 3 days.[25,26] There does not appear to be an advantage to using doses of cytarabine higher than 200 mg/m²/day for 7 days.[27] Several recent studies suggest that the addition of gemtuzumab ozogamicin may improve outcome, particularly in patients with intermediate- and good-risk disease.[28] There is no consistent evidence that adding any other drug, such as etoposide or thioguanine, improves outcomes. Use of growth factor support can diminish the period of pancytopenia after induction chemotherapy, but there is little evidence that growth factor support alters the remission rate or overall survival (OS).[29,24]

If treated with a standard induction regimen, approximately 50% of patients will still have more than 5% blasts in their marrow 1 week after the last dose of chemotherapy. Most experts would recommend beginning a second cycle of induction in such circumstances. The presence of more than 5% blasts 1 week after chemotherapy completion is associated with reduced CR rates and poorer OS.[30]

Chemotherapy after Remission. The findings of large randomized studies have demonstrated that chemotherapy administered after remission improves both disease-free survival (DFS) and OS.[31] If no therapy is administered after induction, the median duration of remission is only approximately 4 months.[32] Thus, some form of therapy is clearly indicated after remission. Based on the results of randomized trials, standard consolidation chemotherapy in fit patients younger than age 65 who are not candidates for allogeneic transplantation usually involves three to four cycles of a regimen that includes high-dose cytarabine (1 to 3 g/m^2/day for 3 to 6 days)[33-36] Low-dose maintenance therapy appears to be of no benefit in the treatment of AML.

Leukemic recurrence occurs in the CNS in less than 10% of adults with AML. The results of randomized trials have not found evidence that CNS prophylaxis improves either DFS or OS for adults with AML.[37] Whether a subgroup of patients at higher risk for CNS involvement (i.e., those with high blast counts at diagnosis and CD56+ disease) might benefit from CNS prophylaxis is unknown.

Initial Chemotherapy Approaches for Older Patients

The nature of AML changes as the age at diagnosis increases. AML in older patients is more likely to arise from a prior myelodysplastic syndrome, to have unfavorable cytogenetics, and to express multidrug resistance, all of which are associated with

a poor prognosis.[38] Older patients also are more likely to have comorbidities, possibly limiting their tolerance to aggressive chemotherapy. A trial comparing conventional-dose daunorubicin (45 mg/m^2/day for 3 days) with high-dose daunorubicin (90 mg/m^2/day for 3 days), both combined with conventional-dose cytarabine as induction therapy for AML in older adults, found that the high-dose regimen resulted in a higher CR rate and improved survival in patients up to age 65, but not patients older than 65.[39] Patients in both arms received one cycle of consolidation therapy using cytarabine at a dose of 1,000 mg/m^2 every 12 hours for 6 days. The higher doses of cytarabine that are used in younger patients frequently lead to neurotoxicity in older individuals and probably should be avoided. With high-dose induction and cytarabine consolidation, event-free survival for patients with AML older than age 65 is slightly less than 20% at 3 years from diagnosis.

Patients older than age 74 and those with a poor performance status have an increased likelihood of dying directly as a result of the toxicities of initial induction chemotherapy. Thus, consideration should be given to providing such patients with a less-intensive therapy. A randomized trial demonstrated that low-dose cytarabine (20 mg by subcutaneous injection, twice daily for 10 consecutive days) was superior to hydroxyurea both in terms of CR rates and OS.[40] Studies are evaluating the role of demethylating agent therapy (azacitidine or decitabine) either alone or combined with other agents in this difficult situation;[41] however, no randomized trials have been reported comparing these drugs with either conventional induction therapy in fit patients or low-dose cytarabine in older or infirm patients.

Chemotherapy for Recurrent Disease

The majority of patients with AML who receive conventional chemotherapy will either not go into CR (primary induction failure) or will experience disease recurrence. Patients who do not experience CR with initial induction chemotherapy have almost no chance for cure if treated with alternative chemotherapy. Consequently, allogeneic HCT is generally recommended for such patients. Although the post-transplantation relapse rate is high, the 20% to 30% OS rate with allogeneic HCT for patients with primary induction failure is better than what would be expected with further chemotherapy.[42]

For patients who experience disease relapse after achieving CR, the likelihood of achieving a second CR is higher in patients with a long first remission, in those who are younger, and in those with favorable-risk cytogenetics.[43]

Standard chemotherapy for recurrent disease has been retreatment with daunorubicin and cytarabine. Overall, this general approach yields a second CR for approximately 30% to 50% of patients, with an average remission duration of 6 months. If the initial remission was longer (more than 18 months), the rate of CR with retreatment is much higher—64% in one study—and the average duration of second remission tends to be longer (approximately 8 months).[44] Occasionally, patients retreated with daunorubicin and cytarabine may experience CR for periods beyond 3 years; rarely, a patient may experience cure. Such long second remissions usually are restricted to patients with favorable-risk cytogenetics (t[8;21] or inv[16]). If the first CR is shorter than 18 months, the chance of successful repeat induction is lower (averaging 25%), and the average duration of the second remission is only 3 months. Clofarabine, decitabine, azacitidine, and several other agents are active for recurrent disease.

The best overall approach to serving patients with recurrent AML depends on the patient's clinical characteristics and previous therapy. Patients with a long initial remission should be retreated with intensive induction with either an anthracycline and cytarabine or cytarabine in high doses. Patients with a short first remission are candidates for alternative regimens, such as clofarabine. Clofarabine is a purine nucleoside analog approved for the treatment of patients with recurrent ALL, which also has activity in recurrent AML.[45] Therapy is accompanied by pancytopenia and (not infrequently) transient elevations in liver function tests. Allogeneic HCT should be strongly considered for patients in whom a second CR is achieved by whatever means because it provides the best likelihood for long-term remission.[43] Patients with slowly evolving disease, particularly if they are older or infirm, can sometimes have a reasonable quality of life with supportive care alone; rapid and intensive induction is not always warranted for this population.

Hematopoietic Cell Transplantation

High-dose chemotherapy with or without radiation followed by HCT has become increasingly important as a therapy for AML. (Broad issues regarding transplantation are discussed in Chapter 18: Hematopoietic Cell Transplantation.) Specific issues concerning transplantation for AML are discussed here, and focus on the timing of transplantation, the source of stem cells, the choice of preparative regimen, and the form of prophylaxis used for graft-versus-host disease (GVHD).

Timing. Unless otherwise noted, the following discussion of timing concerns HCT for patients younger than age 60 who have a human leukocyte antigen (HLA)-identical sibling. If CR is not achieved with initial induction chemotherapy and the patient has an HLA-identical sibling, marrow transplantation should be strongly considered; approximately 20% of such patients can become long-term survivors, whereas second-line chemotherapy offers almost no chance of cure. For those patients in whom a first remission is achieved, the choice of continuing with chemotherapy or having allogeneic transplantation is based on the risk categorization of the AML. Several prospective comparisons have been published in which allogeneic transplantation for patients with HLA-matched siblings was compared with chemotherapy or autologous transplantation for patients without such a sibling. Meta-analyses show that OS is improved with allogeneic HCT in first remission compared with chemotherapy or autologous transplantation, with a hazard ratio of 1.15. This benefit was particularly noted for patients with poor-risk cytogenetics and was not seen for those with favorable-risk cytogenetics.[46,47] Patients with a normal leukemia karyotype can be divided into those with a more favorable risk (*CEPBA* mutated,

or *NPM1* mutated but *FLT3* wild-type) and those with less favorable risk (all others). Prospective studies demonstrated equivalent survival with chemotherapy or transplantation for the subset of patients with favorable-risk disease, but a survival advantage with transplantation for the remainder of patients.[48] Overall, allogeneic HCT from a matched sibling can be expected to result in a cure in 50% to 60% of patients undergoing transplantation in first CR.[49]

Marrow transplantation for patients in untreated first relapse and second remission results in cure in approximately 35% to 40% of cases, results that are better than those seen with conventional chemotherapy.[43] A second remission is achieved in approximately 50% of patients with AML who receive chemotherapy, and complications precluding subsequent transplantation occur in some of those patients; therefore, there seems to be little advantage to administering additional chemotherapy or attempting to achieve a second remission before marrow transplantation, if relapse is detected early and a transplant can be performed promptly.

Source of Stem Cells. The source of hematopoietic stem cells for transplantation can be defined in two ways: by their anatomic source and by the relationship of the donor and recipient. As noted in Chapter 18, the use of mobilized stem cells from the peripheral blood has largely replaced marrow as the source of stem cells for autologous transplantation because of the ease of collection and quicker engraftment. The use of peripheral blood stem cells for allogeneic transplantation from a matched sibling, when compared with the use of marrow, is associated with more rapid engraftment and an increase in chronic GVHD, but also a trend toward improved OS.[50-52] Studies comparing peripheral blood with bone marrow for unrelated donor transplantation suggest equivalent survival but more chronic GVHD with peripheral blood stem cells.[53]

The preferred source of stem cells for transplantation in AML is from an HLA-identical sibling, which can be found in approximately 30% of cases. Similar results are seen using family member donors who are single-antigen mismatches. Use of a family member donor mismatched for two or three loci has previously been associated with a poorer outcome. Recent studies using high-dose CD34+ selected stem cells or GVHD prevention with administration of high-dose cyclophosphamide (CY) post-transplant report much better outcomes than previously seen with two or three loci mismatched donors.[54]

The use of unrelated HLA-matched donors has rapidly increased, particularly since the formation of the National Marrow Donor Program. With improvements in donor selection and transplant techniques, the outcomes for transplantation using a fully matched (eight of eight antigens) unrelated donor and a matched sibling are similar, and thus the indications for transplantation should likewise be the same.[55] As noted in Chapter 18, results using a one-antigen–mismatched unrelated donor are somewhat worse than with an eight-of-eight match. Progress in the use of umbilical cord blood as a source of stem cells for unrelated donors, and particularly the use of double cord grafts, has resulted in survival outcomes similar to those seen with matched unrelated donors.[56]

The clearest indication for autologous transplantation for AML is disease in second remission. In this setting, the results of several studies have demonstrated that 30% to 35% of patients will become long-term disease-free survivors. These studies involved considerable patient selection, and no prospective study has definitively shown an advantage of autologous transplantation in second remission compared with continued chemotherapy; however, most investigators accept the premise that autologous transplantation is more likely to lead to a cure.[57] No prospective trials comparing autologous transplantation in second remission with allogeneic transplantation have been reported. A meta-analysis of contemporary randomized trials of autologous transplantation in first remission shows improved DFS, but no OS advantage, compared with chemotherapy.[58,59]

Preparative Regimen. The preparative regimen administered before transplantation for AML ideally should eradicate all disease, suppress the immune system adequately to permit sustained engraftment (in the allogeneic setting), and accomplish these goals with minimal toxicity. Commonly used regimens include CY administered at 60 mg/kg for 2 days, followed by total-body irradiation (TBI) at a dose of 10 Gy to 14 Gy administered over 3 to 6 days, or CY (120 mg/kg) with oral busulfan (16 mg/kg; CY/Bu). Although the results of a prospective, randomized study of CY plus 12 Gy TBI compared with Bu plus 120 mg/kg CY showed an advantage to the regimen that included radiotherapy, subsequent registry data evaluating large numbers of patients are not consistent with this finding.[60] In some regimens, intravenous Bu is now often substituted for the oral drug, and in other studies fludarabine is often used instead of CY, but large randomized trials supporting the advantages of these changes either are lacking or are inconsistent in their conclusions.

Graft-versus-Host Disease. GVHD considerably affects the outcome of allogeneic HCT for AML, resulting in both fewer relapses and increased nonleukemic deaths caused by GVHD and its complications. Therefore, the overall effect depends on the particular clinical situation; if the risk of recurrent leukemia is low, GVHD is likely to have a deleterious effect, but if the risk is high, mild disease may even be of some benefit. The overwhelming predictive factor for the development of this complication is the degree of patient and donor matching, with a higher incidence of GVHD found for increased degrees of mismatching. The most widely used regimens for prevention of GVHD combine methotrexate with either cyclosporine or tacrolimus.[61] The depletion of T cells in allogeneic bone marrow also is successful for decreasing the incidence of acute GVHD. In some settings, this approach has been associated with an increased incidence of both graft failure and leukemic recurrence; there is no proof that depletion of T cells can improve OS.

Allogeneic Transplantation Using Reduced-Intensity Conditioning for Older Patients. Previously, patients older than age 60 were not considered candidates for allogeneic HCT after high-dose preparative regimens because of the perception that they would be unable to tolerate the considerable toxicities associated with such therapy. On the basis of the hypothesis that much of the antileukemic effect of allogeneic transplantation derives from an allogeneic graft-versus-leukemia effect and not just the high-dose therapy, studies of reduced-intensity transplantation have been conducted. These trials demonstrate that with preparative regimens such as fludarabine plus low-dose TBI, or fludarabine plus reduced-dose Bu (with or without additional antithymocyte globulin), allogeneic engraftment can be consistently obtained.[62,63] The incidence of early toxicities associated with pancytopenia and tissue damage, such as bacterial infections, sinusoidal obstruction syndrome, and idiopathic interstitial pneumonia, are reduced compared with historical experience. However, the incidences of fungal and viral infections, as well as GVHD, are not significantly altered compared with results using high-dose preparative regimens. Preliminary results with reduced-intensity transplantation from matched siblings or from matched unrelated donors for patients age 55 to 75 with AML whose disease is in first or second remission seem quite encouraging, with DFS rates of 45% to 50% at 2 years and beyond.[64] If patients have active relapsed leukemia at the time of transplant, the results using reduced-intensity conditioning are much less encouraging, with high post-transplant relapse rates.

SPECIAL TYPES OF AML
ACUTE PROMYELOCYTIC LEUKEMIA
APL is a distinct subtype of AML, accounting for 5% to 15% of cases (average, approximately 10%), with unique clinical, morphologic, and cytogenetic features. Compared with most patients with AML, patients with APL tend to be somewhat younger (median age, 30 to 40), rarely have a myelodysplastic prodrome, and usually have a lower white blood cell count at the time of diagnosis. Among the different subtypes of AML, APL seems to be overrepresented among Hispanic patients. Whereas many of the other clinical and laboratory features are similar to other forms of AML, APL almost always presents with some of the following elements of a hemorrhagic syndrome, including hypofibrinogenemia, decreased normal coagulation factors, elevated fibrin degradation products, and increased platelet consumption. These findings are the result of both disseminated intravascular coagulation, as well as primary fibrinolysis.

As noted earlier, leukemic blasts virtually always have the characteristic translocation t(15;17)(q22;q11.12). A unique feature of APL is its sensitivity to treatment with all-trans retinoic acid (ATRA) and arsenic trioxide. As a single agent, ATRA results in complete response rates of 80% or more for patients with recurrent disease.[65] Similarly, arsenic trioxide, when used as a single agent, results in a CR for 85% of patients with recurrent disease.[66] The robust activity of these agents led to studies combining them with conventional chemotherapy as initial therapy for APL. Randomized trials have demonstrated that the addition of ATRA to conventional chemotherapy improves CR rates to approximately 90% and decreases the incidence of substantial bleeding complications. Clinical trials conducted before the availability of ATRA demonstrated that APL is particularly sensitive to anthracycline therapy.[67] Thus, substantial doses of anthracyclines were included during the consolidation treatment phase for APL. These trials also demonstrated a clear role for ATRA as maintenance therapy.[68] A large randomized trial demonstrated that the use of arsenic trioxide during consolidation therapy further improves DFS and OS in both the intermediate-/good-risk group (defined as those presenting with a white blood cell count of less than 10,000/mm³) and in poor-risk APL (defined as presenting with a white count of more than 10,000/mm³).[69] With current therapies, survival at 3 years from diagnosis can be expected for more than 85% of patients presenting with a white count of less than 10,000/mm³ and for 75% of those presenting with a white count of more than 10,000/mm³. A recent study has shown that patients with intermediate-/good-risk APL can be treated with ATRA and arsenic trioxide alone, with results similar to those seen with the addition of chemotherapy.[70] A small fraction of patients with APL morphology will have a different translocation, such as t(11;17), and will experience a poor response to ATRA and arsenic.

During induction therapy with either ATRA or arsenic trioxide, some patients will experience fever, weight gain, respiratory distress, pulmonary infiltrates, episodic hypotension, and renal failure.[71] This condition is thought to be related to the sudden maturation of promyeloblasts and usually responds to dexamethasone. Treatment with arsenic trioxide has been complicated by a prolongation of the QT interval and, rarely, by sudden death. Thus, before initiating treatment with arsenic trioxide, any electrolyte imbalances should be corrected, especially hypomagnesemia and hypocalcemia; other drugs that can prolong the QT interval should be discontinued.[72]

KEY POINTS

- The suspicion of acute promyelocytic leukemia in a newly diagnosed patient with acute myeloid leukemia should trigger the immediate administration of all-trans retinoic acid to prevent early death.
- Patients with diagnosed acute promyelocytic leukemia should receive all-trans retinoic acid and arsenic trioxide as part of induction and/or consolidation therapy.

THERAPY-RELATED MYELOID NEOPLASMS

The 2008 revision of the WHO classification of myeloid neoplasms now recommends the use of the term "therapy-related myeloid neoplasms" to describe AML, myelodysplasia, or myeloproliferative disorders that arise after treatment with alkylating agents, radiation, or topoisomerase II inhibitors. Although as noted earlier, the pattern of disease after alkylating agent exposure compared with topoisomerase II inhibitors is somewhat different (Table 15-5); in fact, most patients are exposed to both, so such a division is often not practical.

In general, the overall CR rate for treatment-related AML is lower than that seen in de novo leukemia, independent of cytogenetic risk group, averaging 35% to 40% in several large series.

Furthermore, median DFS and OS with therapy-related AML is considerably shorter than with de novo AML, and less than 10% of patients can expect to survive disease-free for more than 3 years after initiation of chemotherapy. Although the number of published studies is limited, allogeneic transplantation leads to long-term DFS for some patients with therapy-related AML.[73] Therefore, allogeneic transplantation from either a matched sibling or a matched unrelated donor should be considered for this category of AML.

ACUTE LYMPHOBLASTIC LEUKEMIA

BIOLOGY, CYTOGENETICS, AND MOLECULAR GENETICS

Like AML, ALL is a clonal disorder with all leukemic cells arising from a common progenitor. ALL can be categorized according to morphology, histochemistry, cell surface markers, cytogenetics, and molecular biology.

Morphology and Histochemistry

The leukemia cells in ALL are typically smaller than AML blasts and are devoid of granules. Three forms of ALL are recognized by the FAB (Fig. 15-3).[9] ALL blasts are typically negative for myeloperoxidase and nonspecific esterase. Periodic acid–Schiff staining is more variable, with the greatest reactivity seen in FAB subtype L1 disease.

Cell Surface Markers

Approximately 5% to 10% of all cases of adult ALL express the early B-cell antigens CD19 or CD22 and no other B-cell antigens.[74] Such cases are termed pro-B-cell ALL. In approximately 40% to 50% of adults, the leukemia expresses CD10 (the common ALL antigen [CALLA]). In approximately 10% of cases, the B-cell ALL expresses cytoplasmic immunoglobulin (Ig) but not surface Ig (pre-B-cell ALL), whereas in 5% of cases surface Ig is present (mature B-cell or Burkitt leukemia). Approximately 25% of ALL cases have a T-cell phenotype. Three subgroups of T-cell ALL are recognized: early T-precursor ALL expressing CD7 but not CD1a or CD3, thymic T-ALL expressing CD1a but not surface CD3, and mature T-ALL expressing surface CD3. The prognosis for thymic T-cell ALL is superior to the other

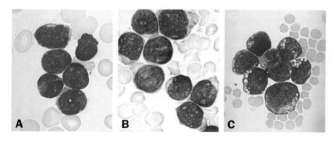

Fig. 15-3 Morphology of acute lymphoblastic leukemia (ALL) in adults.

(A) ALL childhood variant. The cells are small, homogeneous, with inconspicuous nucleoli (FAB-L1). (B) ALL adult variant. The cells are pleomorphic with some cytoplasm and prominent nucleoli (FAB-L2). (C) Burkitt-like leukemia. The cells are homogeneous with multiple nucleoli, deep blue cytoplasm, and sharply defined vacuoles (FAB-L3).

Table 15-5 Features of Therapy-Related Leukemias

	Causative Agents		
	Alkylating Agents	**Topoisomerase II Inhibitors**	**Anthracyclines, Mitoxantrone**
Chromosome abnormality	del(5q), -5	11q23	t(15;17)
	del(7q), -7	21q22	
Preleukemia phase	Myelodysplastic syndromes	None	None
FAB morphology	Not classifiable	Usually M4, M5	M3
Latency	5 to 7 years	6 months to 3 years	2 to 3 years
Response to induction therapy	Poor	Good	Good
Long-term survival	Poor	Poor	Good

Abbreviation: FAB, French-American-British.

Modified from Cheson BD, ed. Oncology MKSAP, *2nd ed.* Philadelphia, PA: American College of Physicians, 1999.

forms of T-ALL. In 25% of ALL cases, a nondefinitive (i.e., not myeloperoxidase) myeloid antigen can be detected. Although some studies suggest that such myeloid antigens are a negative prognostic factor, the bulk of evidence suggests no independent significance for their presence. As in AML, discordant combinations of antigens on leukemic blasts allow detection of small numbers of blasts in a morphologically normal marrow using multidimensional flow cytometry. Studies suggest that presence of residual disease detected by flow cytometry after induction chemotherapy can predict shorter remission durations for both AML and ALL.

In perhaps 2% to 5% of acute leukemias, definition of the disease as either myeloid or lymphoid is problematic, either because two or more distinct populations of cells exist in the same person (bilineage leukemias) or a single population co-expresses definitive myeloid and lymphoid markers (biphenotypic leukemias). In 2008, the WHO defined these diseases as mixed-phenotype acute leukemia (MPAL). Several studies suggest that patients with MPAL have a worse clinical outcome than do patients with either AML or ALL.[75]

Cytogenetics and Molecular Biology

In approximately 25% of cases of ALL, no cytogenetic abnormalities are found.[76] In approximately 10%, an alteration in chromosome number (usually hyperdiploidy) is found without any alteration in chromosome structure.[77] The most common translocation is the Philadelphia (Ph) chromosome, seen in 20% to 30% of adult ALL. The Ph chromosome results from a specific translocation, t(9;22)(q34;q11), which involves the movement of most of the *ABL* proto-oncogene from chromosome 9 adjacent to the 5′ portion of the *BCR* gene on chromosome 22. The breakpoint on chromosome 9 is highly variable and occurs anywhere over a region of 200 kilobases or more, usually within the intron 5′ of exon 2. In contrast, the breakpoints in the *BCR* gene on chromosome 22 occur within two regions: the major breakpoint cluster region (M-bcr), and the

minor breakpoint cluster region (m-bcr). Rearrangements within the M-bcr are transcribed into a chimeric messenger RNA, which produces a hybrid 210-kilodalton protein (p210[Bcr-Abl]), whereas breaks within the m-bcr express a chimeric messenger RNA that gives rise to a smaller 190-kilodalton protein (p190[Bcr-Abl]). In CML, virtually all breakpoints are mapped to the M-bcr, which has been termed the CML-type Ph chromosome. Conversely, in ALL, breakpoints are found within both the M-bcr and m-bcr, and those within the m-bcr are termed the ALL-type Ph chromosome.[78] The relative frequency of the two breakpoints in adult ALL has varied among studies, but overall, the two seem to be represented with equal frequency.[79] Ph-positive ALL with the CML-type *BCR-ABL* translocation is not simply the lymphoid blast crisis phase of CML. Patients with this disease rarely have a long prediagnostic prodrome and do not routinely have marked splenomegaly.

The other most common translocations seen in adult B-cell ALL are t(4;11)(q21;q23), which is seen in 7% of B-cell ALL, involves the *MLL* and *AF4* genes, and is associated with a poor prognosis; and t(8;14)(q24.1;q32), which is seen in 2% to 4% of adult B-cell ALL, involves *c-MYC* and the Ig heavy chain, and is the translocation associated with Burkitt leukemia. T-cell ALLs often have translocations involving chromosomes 7 or 14 at T-cell receptor enhancer gene sites. The other most common cytogenetic changes seen in adult ALL involve del(9p), seen in 5% to 9% of cases, del(6q) seen in 5% to 7%, and del(13q) seen in 3% to 5%. Cytogenetic abnormalities in ALL have important prognostic significance.

CLINICAL FEATURES

In ALL, approximately 50% of patients may have enlarged lymph nodes, hepatomegaly, or splenomegaly. Bone pain is commonly reported by patients who have acute disease, particularly by younger patients with ALL. Leukemic cells may infiltrate the skin, resulting in a raised, nonpruritic rash (leukemia cutis). Approximately 5% of patients with ALL will have involvement of the CNS at the time of diagnosis; this confers a worse prognosis. T-cell ALL is commonly associated with male sex, a mediastinal mass, and disseminated lymph node involvement.

TREATMENT FOR ALL
Induction
Standard induction therapy for adult ALL most commonly involves combination chemotherapy including vincristine, prednisone, an anthracycline, and asparaginase. Such regimens achieve a first CR in 80% to 90% of patients. Although a number of variations exist, no prospective randomized trial has identified a clearly superior regimen.[80] A number of investigators have explored the use of hematopoietic growth factors immediately after induction chemotherapy. Similar to the findings for AML, the results of such studies demonstrate accelerated myeloid recovery and a decrease in the incidence of febrile neutropenia. In some trials, the CR rate was improved, but no findings have indicated an improvement in DFS or OS.[81]

KEY POINTS

- Induction therapy in adult acute lymphoblastic leukemia (ALL) should generally include vincristine, prednisone, an anthracycline, and asparaginase. Such regimens can achieve complete remission in 80% to 90% of patients.
- Patients with Philadelphia-positive ALL should receive a tyrosine kinase inhibitor in combination with chemotherapy. Patients with mature B-cell ALL should receive rituximab in addition to chemotherapy.
- Adults with high-risk ALL, including those with Philadelphia-positive ALL or t(4;11), should receive allogeneic transplantation during first remission, if possible.

Therapy after Remission
If no further therapy is administered after achievement of CR, the duration of remission is invariably short. Therapy after achievement of remission should include CNS prophylaxis, since without prophylaxis CNS disease will develop in at least 35% of adults. Patients with a high tumor burden at diagnosis as evidenced by a high white count and elevated lactate dehydrogenase (LDH) are at highest risk. With prophylaxis, the incidence of CNS leukemia as an isolated event is less than 10%. Most clinical trials have included several cycles of intensive consolidation therapy administered over several months after CR is achieved, as well as less intensive maintenance therapy administered over a period of several years. Consolidation frequently includes combinations of high-dose methotrexate, cytarabine, CY, and an anthracycline, whereas maintenance usually comprises low-dose methotrexate, 6-mercaptopurine, vincristine, and prednisone. No single optimal regimen for CNS prophylaxis, consolidation therapy, and maintenance has been identified.

Table 15-6 **Broadly Used Prognostic Factors in Acute Lymphocytic Leukemia**[82]

	Unfavorable	Favorable
Age	> 35	≤ 35
White blood cell	> 30,000/mm³	≤ 30,000/mm³
Immunophenotype	BCP1	Other
Cytogenetics	t(9;22) t(4;11) t(1;19)	Other
Time to Complete Response	> 4 weeks	< 4 weeks

Abbreviations: BCP1, B-cell precursor.

Current trials are testing whether more intensive regimens, such as those used in pediatric ALL, are tolerable and improve outcome in adult ALL. Preliminary results suggest that such regimens are tolerated in patients younger than age 40 and may improve outcome. With current regimens, approximately 35% to 40% of adult patients with ALL will remain alive in remission at 5 years from diagnosis.[82,80]

Prognostic Factors Associated with Initial Chemotherapy
Various risk factors have been shown to affect the probability of achieving and maintaining a CR (Table 15-6). Older age and an elevated white count at diagnosis have been associated with lower CR rates and a shorter duration of remission.[81] The immunophenotype of leukemic blasts may have some prognostic value with pro-B-cell ALL, generally thought to have a somewhat worse outcome with conventional therapy. Although expression of T-cell or myeloid antigens by ALL blasts was previously associated with a worse prognosis, with modern therapy these factors have no independent prognostic importance. Failure to receive a CR within 4 weeks of the start of induction is an additional risk factor.

Cytogenetic characteristics have important prognostic and therapeutic significance (Fig. 15-4);[72] 10% to 20% of all ALL cases are Ph-positive (5% of childhood cases; 20% to 30% of adult cases), and the incidence of Ph positivity increases with age, which may explain the importance of age as a prognostic variable. In studies conducted before the availability of imatinib, the likelihood of CR was somewhat lower for patients with Ph-positive ALL, and the probability of remaining in CR was much lower. Studies designed to find molecular evidence of the *BCR-ABL* rearrangement have shown that at least 25% to 30% of adults with ALL will be *BCR-ABL*–positive. Therefore, up to 10% of cases that are Ph-negative or inadequate by cytogenetic analysis will, nonetheless, have the *BCR-ABL* rearrangement. The prognosis seems to be the same for patients who are Ph-negative by conventional cytogenetics and *BCR-ABL*–positive according to molecular studies as it is for patients who are Ph-positive. Although Ph-positive

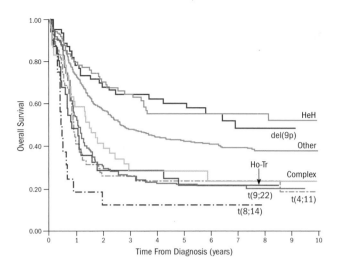

Fig. 15-4 Survival in adult acute lymphoblastic leukemia (ALL) according to cytogenetic abnormality.[77]

Abbreviations: HeH, high hyperdiploidy; Ho-Tr, hypodiploidy/near triploidy.

Republished with permission of the American Society of Hematology, from Blood. Moorman AV, Harrison CJ, Buck GAN, et al. Karyotype is an independent prognostic factor in adult acute lymphoblastic leukemia (ALL): analysis of cytogenetic data from patients treated on the Medical Research Council (MRC) UKALLXII/Eastern Cooperative Oncology Group (ECOG) 2993 trial. Blood. 2007;109(8):3189-97. Permission conveyed through Copyright Clearance Center, Inc.

ALL has a very poor prognosis when treated with conventional ALL therapy, results of trials that combined imatinib with standard induction are sufficiently encouraging to warrant inclusion of imatinib or other tyrosine kinase inhibitors (TKIs) in the initial treatment of Ph-positive ALL.[83] Other cytogenetic abnormalities of adult ALL that carry a poor prognosis (both in terms of achieving a CR and remaining in CR) include t(4;11), t(8;14), and having complex cytogenetics with five or more abnormalities. In contrast, adults with high hyperdiploidy or del(9p) seem to have a more favorable prognosis.[76,77,84]

Based on the factors listed in Table 15-6, investigators generally segregate ALL cases into standard- and high-risk. Although there are inconsistencies in the exact schemas, 5-year DFS averages about 55% for standard-risk versus 25% for high- risk patients.[80] Measurements of minimal residual disease, while informative, have not yet been broadly applied.

Hematopoietic Cell Transplantation

As with AML, the results of HCT for ALL depend largely on the remission status of the patient, the source of stem cells, and, perhaps, the choice of preparative regimen.[85] The most experience has been with the use of HLA-identical sibling donors. If such transplants are carried out for patients with disease that is resistant to conventional chemotherapy, long-term DFS can be obtained in only 10% to 20% of patients. These results are clearly superior to the results obtained with chemotherapy, but only a small fraction of patients ultimately benefit. The major cause of treatment failure is recurrent leukemia, with an actuarial relapse rate in excess of 60%. If patients undergo

transplantation during a second remission, the 5-year DFS is approximately 35%, an outcome significantly better than that seen with chemotherapy.

The best results with allogeneic transplantation have been obtained for patients in first remission, with reports ranging from 35% to 65% for long-term DFS. The largest collection of cases has been reported by the Center for International Blood and Marrow Transplant Research (CIBMTR), in which approximately 50% of patients who received a transplant remain in CR 4 years later, with an actuarial relapse rate of 25%.[86] However, considerable patient selection, both positive and negative, probably influenced the results of the registry data.

The first prospective trial to address the role of transplantation during first remission was the French LALA87 trial. In that trial, patients between age 15 and 40 were assigned to undergo allogeneic transplantation if they had a matched sibling, and were randomly assigned to undergo further chemotherapy or autologous transplantation if they did not. When patients were analyzed according to protocol intent, allogeneic transplantation was superior to chemotherapy or autologous transplantation (10-year survival, 46% vs. 31%). High-risk patients particularly benefited from allogeneic transplantation (10-year survival, 44% vs. 11%), whereas no form of therapy was particularly advantageous for patients with standard-risk disease.[87] More recently, an Eastern Cooperative Oncology Group/Medical Research Council ALL trial that included both standard- and high-risk disease demonstrated improved survival among patients with matched siblings who underwent transplantation in first remission compared with those receiving chemotherapy.[88] This large prospective study suggests that all adults younger than age 50 with ALL in first remission should be considered for an allogeneic transplant if they have a matched sibling. Transplantation has not been compared directly with pediatric-like intensive chemotherapy regimens in younger adult patients with ALL.

The best preparative regimen for transplantation for patients with ALL is uncertain. Most experience has been gained with use of the standard regimen of CY and TBI. There are suggestions that substituting etoposide for CY may offer some advantage; however, no controlled trials have been conducted to provide evidence supporting this theory.

The role of autologous transplantation in ALL is difficult to evaluate. The results for patients with multiple relapses are poor, largely owing to a high incidence of leukemic relapse. In second remission, long-term DFS has been reported for 20% to 30% of patients, and probably represents an advantage compared with conventional chemotherapy. Although no sufficiently sized randomized trials have been reported, the DFS rate for patients in first remission treated with autologous transplantation in the only prospective studies published to date has averaged approximately 30% and shows no obvious advantage compared with conventional chemotherapy.[88]

Emerging Therapies in ALL

A number of new, active therapies are being evaluated for the treatment of ALL.[89] Epratuzumab is a humanized anti-CD22 antibody, which, when combined with standard chemotherapy, appears to enhance response rates. Blinatumomab belongs to a new class of antibody-based drugs, so-called bispecific T-cell engagers, and simultaneously binds CD19 and CD3. Inotuzumab ozogamicin is an immunoconjugate composed of a humanized anti-CD22 antibody and calicheamicin. Substantial response rates in recurrent ALL have been reported with the use of both blinatumomab and inotuzumab ozogamicin as single agents. Although the number of patients reported are limited, remarkable responses have also been seen with the use of chimeric antigen receptor T-cells (CARTS) targeting CD19.[90]

SPECIAL TYPES OF ADULT ALL

As noted above, ALL associated with t(9;22) translocations has a very poor prognosis when treated with conventional chemotherapy. However, the disease is sensitive to treatment using imatinib, dasatinib, or nilotinib. Although use of these drugs as single agents can induce remissions in many patients, such remissions tend to be short-lived. Current regimens combining TKIs with conventional chemotherapy are showing more promise. Whether such combinations will substantially improve long-term cure rates and thus alleviate the need for HCT is unknown. Transplantation remains the treatment of choice, particularly for younger adults. Therapy with dasatinib and prednisone alone results in CR in a high percentage of older patients with Ph-positive ALL without the need for concomitant chemotherapy.[91]

Mature B-cell ALL (Burkitt leukemia), like Ph-positive ALL, used to be associated with a poor prognosis. However, the use of regimens containing high-dose methotrexate, high-dose cytarabine, and rituximab, along with more conventional agents, has led to dramatic improvements in prognosis for this rare subtype of ALL.[92] Nelarabine is active in the treatment of patients with recurrent T-cell ALL, achieving CR rates of 30% or higher in such patients.[93]

MYELODYSPLASTIC SYNDROMES
BIOLOGY, CYTOGENETICS, AND MOLECULAR BIOLOGY

The MDS are a group of clonal, acquired hematopoietic disorders. Clonality was originally demonstrated by studies of G6PD heterozygosity in black women and other X-linked polymorphisms, and has since been confirmed by the presence of clonal mutational and cytogenetic abnormalities. There are likely multiple steps in the development of clinically evident MDS, with an early step in its development leading to the expansion of a genetically unstable clone beginning close to, if not at, the level of the stem cell, followed by acquisition of additional mutations that may confer selective growth advantages to these clones.

G6PD studies of MDS have shown clonality not only of the myeloid lineage, but also, in some cases, of B cells and even T cells. Clonal chromosome abnormalities are detected in 40% to 70% of patients with MDS at the time of diagnosis. The frequency of clonal chromosome abnormalities varies among the subtypes of MDS and is lowest (approximately 10%) for patients with refractory anemia with ringed sideroblasts and highest (approximately 60%) for patients with refractory anemia with excess blasts. Copy number alterations in chromosome 5 (36% of patients), 7 (21%), 8 (16%), and 20 (7%) are the most frequent.

Although many of these abnormalities also are seen among patients with AML, other specific structural rearrangements that are closely associated with distinct morphologic subtypes of AML, such as inv(16), are almost never seen in MDS. Chromosome abnormalities in MDS are of prognostic importance. Abnormalities of chromosomes 5 or 7 are associated with the shortest survival; the outcome is intermediate for patients with other abnormalities, and the longest survival is associated with patients with a normal karyotype, -Y, del(5q), or del(20q) as a sole abnormality. Chromosome abnormalities also are associated with an increased risk of progression to acute leukemia.

Links between cytogenetic abnormalities and the MDS phenotype are beginning to emerge. Many cases of MDS are associated with partial deletions in 5q. One area commonly deleted is 5q31; this deletion is frequently seen in patients with therapy-related MDS and AML, and generally is associated with a poor prognosis.[94] Patients with deletions in 5q33 (the 5q- syndrome) generally have severe macrocytic anemia, a normal or elevated platelet count, and a relatively low rate of progression to AML. These patients frequently experience response with lenalidomide. Recently, RPS14 has been identified as a likely candidate gene involved in the 5q- syndrome.

Focused and genome-wide sequencing studies have revealed a number of recurrent point mutations beyond those involving cytogenetic abnormalities.[95] Among the most commonly mutated genes are TET2 (20%), ASXL1 (14%), RUNX1 (8.7%), TP53 (7.5%), EZH2 (6.4%), and NRAS (3.6%). Several of these (ASXL1, RUNX1, TP53, and EZH2) are associated with shortened survival compared with other cases of MDS. TET2, ASXL1, and EZH2 are involved with regulation of DNA methylation. SF3B1 encodes a core component of RNA splicing machinery and is frequently mutated in MDS cases with ringed sideroblasts.[95]

KEY POINT

- The three most important factors that predict outcome for patients with myelodysplasia are percentage of marrow blasts, karyotype, and number of peripheral cytopenias.

CLASSIFICATION AND PROGNOSIS

The WHO classification schema recognizes seven categories of MDS: refractory cytopenias with unilineage dysplasia, refractory anemia with ring sideroblasts, refractory anemia with multilineage dysplasia, refractory anemia with excess blasts-1, refractory anemia with excess blasts-2, MDS-unclassified, and MDS associated with del(5q) (Table 15-7).[9] In an effort to provide greater prognostic accuracy, an International Prognostic Scoring System (IPSS) was developed on the basis of outcomes for 816 patients with primary MDS.[96] In this analysis, the three major factors affecting outcome were percentage of bone marrow blasts, karyotype, and number of cytopenias (Table 15-8).

Table 15-7 World Health Organization 2008 Myelodysplastic Syndromes (MDS) Classification: Peripheral Blood and Bone Marrow Findings in MDS

Disease	Blood Findings	Bone Marrow Findings
Refractory cytopenia with unilineage dysplasia (RCUD)	Unicytopenia or bicytopenia* No or rare blasts (< 1%)†	Unilineage dysplasia: > 10% of the cells < 5% blasts
Refractory anemia with ring sideroblasts (RARS)	Anemia No blasts	≥ 15% of erythroid precursors are ring sideroblasts < 5% blasts
Refractory cytopenia with multilineage dysplasia (RCMD)	Cytopenia(s) No or rare blasts (< 1%)†	Dysplasia in ≥ 10% of the cells in ≥ 2 myeloid lineages < 5% blasts in marrow
Refractory anemia with excess blasts-1 (RAEB-1)	Cytopenia(s) < 5% blasts†	Unilineage or multilineage dysplasia 5% to 9% blasts†
Refractory anemia with excess blasts-2 (RAEB-2)	Cytopenia(s) 5% to 19% blasts§	Unilineage or multilineage dysplasia 10% to 19% blasts§
MDS—unclassified (MDS-U)	Cytopenias < 1% blasts†	Unequivocal dysplasia in < 10% of cells accompanied by a cytogenetic abnormality < 5% blasts
MDS associated with isolated del(5q)	Anemia Usually normal or increased platelet count No or rare blasts (< 1%)	Normal to increased megakaryocytes with hypolobated nuclei < 5% blasts

* Bicytopenia may occasionally be observed. Cases with pancytopenia should be classified as MDS-U.

† If the marrow myeloblast percentage is < 5% but there are 2% to 4% myeloblasts in the blood, the diagnostic classification is RAEB-1. Cases of RCUD and RCMD with 1% myeloblasts in the blood should be classified as MDS-U.

§ Cases with Auer rods and < 5% myeloblasts in the blood and < 10% in the marrow should be classified as RAEB-2. Although the finding of 5% to 19% blasts in the blood is, in itself, diagnostic of RAEB-2, cases of RAEB-2 may have < 5% blasts in the blood if they have Auer rods or 10% to 19% blasts in the marrow or both. Similarly, cases of RAEB-2 may have < 10% blasts in the marrow but may be diagnosed by the other two findings, Auer rod+ and/or 5% to 19% blasts in the blood.

Modified from Cheson BD, ed. Oncology MKSAP, 2nd ed. *Philadelphia, PA: American College of Physicians, 1999.*

On the basis of these features, patients can be categorized into four risk groups with different median survivals:[96]

- Low-risk, 5.7 years
- Intermediate-risk 1, 3.5 years
- Intermediate-risk 2, 1.2 years
- High-risk, 0.4 years

This system has since been revised to provide higher predictive power. The new revised system takes into account additional clinical and laboratory features, and results in five rather than four risk groups.[97] However, few outcomes have been published from prospective clinical studies using this new system. Findings from additional studies suggest that, stage for stage, the prognosis is somewhat worse for patients with therapy-related MDS than for patients with primary MDS.

TREATMENT

Numerous therapies have been tested for the treatment of MDS. For patients with early-stage disease (low-risk or intermediate-risk 1) or patients who are frail or elderly, supportive care with red blood cell and platelet transfusions as necessary is recommended. Lenalidomide, a 4-amino-glutarimide analog of thalidomide, has been approved for treatment of transfusion-dependent low-risk or intermediate-risk 1 MDS that is associated with chromosome 5q31-33 deletion. In a pivotal study of 148 such patients treated with lenalidomide, 64% became transfusion-independent and 75% experienced a cytogenetic response, one-half of which were CRs.[98] The mechanism of action is uncertain, but side effects include myelosuppression, pruritus, diarrhea, and urticaria.

Erythropoietin can improve the anemia associated with MDS in 20% to 30% of cases and seems to work best in patients with low endogenous erythropoietin levels.[99] For patients who do not experience a response to erythropoietin after 4 to 6 weeks, the addition of a myeloid growth factor may result in responses for 20% to 30% of patients. Myeloid growth factors, including granulocyte colony-stimulating factor (G-CSF) and granulocyte-macrophage colony-stimulating factor (GM-CSF), have been used in an effort to treat the neutropenia that sometimes accompanies MDS. The results of a randomized trial of the prophylactic use of G-CSF showed no advantage to its use

Table 15-8 International Prognostic Scoring System for Myelodysplastic Syndromes

Variable	Score Value				
	0	0.5	1.0	1.5	2.0
Percentage of bone marrow blasts	< 5	5 to 10	–	11 to 20	21 to 30
Karyotype*	Good	Intermediate	Poor	–	–
Cytopenia	0/1	2/3	–	–	–

*For karyotype values: good, -y, del(5q), del(20q); intermediate, neither good nor poor; poor, chromosome 7 abnormalities or complex abnormalities. Scores by group: low, 0; intermediate-1, 0.5 to 1.0; intermediate-2, 1.5 to 2.0; high, ≥ 2.5.

and a possible shortening of survival for patients with advanced disease.[100] Thus, myeloid growth factors should be restricted to patients with recurrent infections. Platelets have responded to low-dose interleukin-11 and to the thrombopoietin mimetic romiplostim.

Azacitidine and decitabine have both been approved by the U.S. Food and Drug Administration (FDA) for treatment of MDS. Both are thought to have utility in MDS through their DNA demethylating activity, which leads to re-expression of key genes otherwise inactivated in MDS through hypermethylation.[101,102] The effects of azacitidine were documented in a phase III trial that found improved partial responses and a longer time to AML progression than supportive care alone for patients with intermediate-risk 2 or high-risk disease.[101] Similar results have been presented with decitabine.[102] The median duration of response seen with azacitidine and decitabine is measured in months, not years, and none of the approved agents are curative. Other therapies that have been studied for the treatment of MDS include hematopoietic growth factors, immunosuppressive therapy, various biologic response modifiers, and chemotherapies other than those already mentioned.

Based on the hypothesis that the pancytopenia seen in MDS (in a manner analogous to aplastic anemia) may be the result of T cells inhibiting hematopoiesis, trials of immunosuppressive therapy have been conducted using antithymocyte globulin, cyclosporine, or the two agents in combination. Responses, sometimes enduring, have been documented for approximately one-third of patients, particularly those who express HLA-DR15.[103] A variety of biologic response modifiers have been studied in MDS, including agents developed to reduce levels of tumor necrosis factor, as well as antiangiogenesis agents, retinoic acid, amifostine, and interferon (IFN) Although responses have been seen with each of these, none have been shown in randomized trials to alter the course of the disease.

Low-dose cytarabine has been studied as a treatment option for MDS, with responses seen in 10% to 20% of cases. Patients with refractory anemia with excess blasts type I or II have, in some cases, been treated with AML-like induction chemotherapy. Although response rates are lower than the rates seen with de novo AML, complete responses in 40% to 50% of patients have been reported in some studies.[104] Whether this results in an overall improvement in survival has not been tested prospectively.

Hematopoietic Cell Transplantation

Allogeneic HCT was initially attempted for the treatment of MDS because the disease is incurable with conventional measures and transplantation can cure other forms of otherwise incurable hematologic cancer. A considerable number of studies have now shown the results of allogeneic transplantation for patients with MDS, and investigators report long-term DFS for 20% to 65% of patients, with many patients alive without evidence of disease for more than 5 years after transplantation, and some for as long as 25 years,[105,106] providing strong evidence that MDS is curable with HCT.

A major question in the management of MDS is the appropriate timing of transplantation. Patients with early-stage MDS may live for long periods without any intervention, but after MDS evolves to AML, survival is short and transplantation is less effective than if it were carried out earlier. Based primarily on a Markov decision-making analysis conducted in younger patients, an evidence-based review from the American Society of Blood and Marrow Transplantation concludes that transplantation "is recommended for patients with an IPSS score of [intermediate] 2...and for selected patients with an IPSS score of [intermediate] 1 who have poor prognostic features not included in the IPSS, including refractory cytopenias."[107] Similar results have been seen in patients age 50 to 70 with MDS.[108]

CHRONIC MYELOID LEUKEMIA
BIOLOGY, CYTOGENETICS, AND MOLECULAR GENETICS

CML was the first malignant disease found to be consistently associated with a specific cytogenetic abnormality, the Ph chromosome. The abnormal chromosome is the product of a translocation between chromosomes 9 and 22 (t[9;22] [q34;q11]), which places the *ABL* proto-oncogene from chromosome 9 contiguous with the 5' portion of the *BCR* gene on chromosome 22. The breakpoint on chromosome 9 is highly variable and occurs anywhere over a region of 200 kilobases or more, usually located in a large intron 5' of exon 2. In contrast, the breakpoint in the *BCR* gene occurs within one of two relatively short sequences. One is a 5.8-kilobase sequence, the M-bcr. This breakpoint is associated with Ph-positive CML, approximately one-half of the cases of Ph-positive ALL, and occasionally, cases of Ph-positive AML. The other breakpoint within the *BCR* gene, the m-bcr, is very rarely associated with CML, but is seen in approximately one-half of the cases of Ph-positive ALL.

Studies have shown that, in most cases of Ph-negative CML, a molecular rearrangement can still be found, even though the translocation is masked at the karyotypic level. If no chimeric *BCR-ABL* gene can be found, the disease should not be considered

CML; it should be considered a myeloproliferative disorder. The transcription of the chimeric *BCR-ABL* gene results in a hybrid messenger RNA that is translated into a hybrid p210 protein. Both the messenger RNA and the protein, which is an activated form of the ABL protein tyrosine kinase, are unique to cells of the leukemic clone. There is now definitive evidence that these changes are more than just a marker of the disease and are part of its pathogenesis. Transgenic expression of the 190-kD BCR-ABL protein in mice causes acute leukemia at birth. Retroviral transfer of *BCR-ABL* into hematopoietic stem cells of healthy mice leads to the development of a variety of acute and chronic leukemias. The BCR-ABL protein transforms hematopoietic cells so that their growth in vitro becomes cytokine-independent, protects cells from apoptotic responses to DNA damage, and increases adhesion of cells to the extracellular matrix. The persistent and increased activity of the ABL protein tyrosine kinase seems to result in the continuous activation of a number of cytoplasmic and nuclear signal transduction pathways involved in cell growth and survival, including STAT, RAS, JUN kinase, and MYC.

KEY POINTS

- Imatinib mesylate is a small molecule inhibitor of the ABL protein tyrosine kinase and is remarkably effective in newly diagnosed chronic myeloid leukemia, leading to complete hematologic and cytogenetic responses for most patients. However, continued therapy and careful follow-up are necessary.
- Second- and third-generation tyrosine kinase inhibitors, including dasatinib, nilotinib, and bosutinib, are now available for patients who develop resistance or intolerance to imatinib.

CLINICAL FEATURES

The natural history of untreated CML is a relatively benign chronic phase lasting approximately 3 years, followed by an accelerated phase lasting several months, and finally, a rapidly fatal blast crisis. At the time of diagnosis, more than 90% of patients are in the chronic phase, and as many as 50% are diagnosed incidentally during routine blood testing. Symptoms, when present, include fatigue, weight loss, bone aches, and abdominal discomfort from splenomegaly. Patients typically have leukocytosis, thrombocytosis, and anemia at the time of presentation. The marrow is virtually always hypercellular and the Ph chromosome is found in more than 90% of cases. In the remaining cases, cryptic or complex translocations can be detected by fluorescence in situ hybridization (FISH) or polymerase chain reaction (PCR) assays.

The accelerated phase is characterized by fever, night sweats, weight loss, bone pain, difficulty controlling blood counts, increased numbers of blasts and early myeloid cells in the marrow and peripheral blood, and evidence of karyotypic evolution. The most common cytogenetic changes associated with disease evolution are an additional Ph chromosome, trisomy 8, i(17q), and trisomy 19. Blast crisis is defined as having more than 30% blasts and promyelocytes in the bone marrow or peripheral blood, or the development of extramedullary blastic infiltrates. In most cases of blast crisis (more than 60%), the blasts are of myeloid lineage as determined by morphology and cell surface markers. In 25% to 30% of cases, the blasts are of lymphoid lineage, and in the remaining cases, blasts may be biphenotypic or undifferentiated. Determination of the blast lineage may be useful for selecting appropriate therapy.

TREATMENT

Before the development of specific TKIs, therapy for CML included hydroxyurea, IFN-alfa (IFN-α), and allogeneic HCT. In 1998, studies of imatinib mesylate, a small molecule inhibitor of several protein tyrosine kinases, including the ABL protein tyrosine kinase, were initiated.[109] These studies showed the agent to be remarkably effective.[110] A large randomized trial in which imatinib was compared with IFN plus low-dose cytarabine demonstrated disease progression at 6 months for 1% of patients who received imatinib compared with 10% of patients who received IFN; cytogenetic responses were seen in 63% of imatinib-treated patients compared with 10% of IFN-treated patients. Based primarily on the differences in disease progression, the authors concluded that imatinib at a daily dose of 400 mg was the nontransplant treatment of choice for patients with newly diagnosed CML.[111] With further follow-up of 6 years, the event-free survival, progression-free survival (PFS), and OS with imatinib were 83%, 93%, and 88%, respectively. For patients who were in the accelerated phase when first exposed to imatinib, the results were less encouraging, with a 37% complete hematologic response rate and a PFS rate of 40% at 3 years.[110] For patients in blast crisis, complete hematologic responses to imatinib are seen in 25%, but the duration of response is short, averaging only 7 to 10 months.[112]

Among patients in early chronic phase treated with imatinib, complete cytogenetic response will occur for approximately 75% of patients after 1 year of therapy, and major molecular response (defined as 3-log reduction in *BCR-ABL* transcripts in peripheral blood) in anywhere from 18% to 58% of patients. In approximately 15% of patients, a deep molecular response will occur, defined either as greater than a 4.5-log reduction or undetectable disease.[113] In those cases in which imatinib therapy is stopped while there is still detectable disease, rapid disease recurrence is the rule. However, among the minority of patients in whom a deep molecular response (MR$^{4.5}$) was achieved that has been maintained for at least 2 years, imatinib can be stopped and approximately 40% of these patients will remain in complete molecular remission without further therapy 1 year later.[114]

In an effort to achieve higher rates of complete cytogenetic and major molecular responses, higher doses of imatinib (600 mg or 800 mg) have been explored. Several randomized trials have compared imatinib at 400 mg/day with imatinib at 600 mg/day or 800 mg/day. Although there are some differences between studies, in most a higher complete cytogenetic response rate after 6 months of therapy was seen with the higher-dose regimen, but after 24 months, there was no difference in complete cytogenetic response rate, PFS, or OS.[115] Imatinib-related toxicities include nausea, diarrhea, muscle cramping, and peripheral edema and are more common at higher doses. Trials exploring the combination of imatinib plus cytarabine showed no benefit with the combination.[116] Trials combining imatinib and IFN have yielded inconsistent results with some showing higher major molecular response and MR[4.5] with the combination, but others showing no benefit.[116,117]

Imatinib resistance can be the result of *BCR-ABL* mutations in the kinase domain interfering with imatinib binding, *BCR-ABL* amplification or overexpression, decreased drug bioavailability, or drug efflux. In as many as 50% of cases, the reasons for resistance are unclear. Mutations in *BCR-ABL* seem to be the most common identifiable reason for resistance and can be detected in samples collected before treatment, suggesting that the delayed imatinib failure may reflect the considerable amount of time required for outgrowth of these selected clones.[72,118] Not all mutations in *BCR-ABL* have the same significance; mutations at *T315I* and those affecting the P-loop seem to confer the greatest degree of imatinib resistance, whereas others can be overcome by a dose increase or are functionally irrelevant.

Nilotinib and dasatinib are second-generation oral TKIs that result in complete cytogenetic responses in approximately 50% of patients in the chronic phase who develop resistance to imatinib. These agents are not, however, active against the *T315I* mutation. Because of their high degree of activity, prospective randomized trials have been conducted comparing either nilotinib or dasatinib with imatinib as initial therapy for CML. Therapy with nilotinib at a dose of 300 mg or 400 mg twice daily resulted in a higher rate of complete cytogenetic response and a higher rate of major molecular response after 12 months than seen with imatinib at 400 mg/day (80% vs. 65% complete cytogenetic response rates, respectively).[119] Similarly, treatment with dasatinib at a dose of 100 mg/day resulted in a higher rate of complete cytogenetic response and major molecular response after 12 months than seen with imatinib at 400 mg/day (77% vs. 66% complete cytogenetic responses, respectively).[120] Based on the presumption that the rate of complete cytogenetic response at 12 months will ultimately translate into an overall clinical benefit, both agents were approved by the FDA for the upfront treatment of newly diagnosed chronic-phase CML. However, it remains unknown whether the small benefit in early cytogenetic response rates will translate into a long-lasting survival benefit, and whether a similar benefit might be obtained with a strategy of first treating with imatinib and switching to a second-generation TKI in those with a suboptimal early response.

A third-generation oral TKI, bosutinib, has been approved for the treatment of CML in patients with resistance or intolerance to prior therapy.[121] Major cytogenetic responses can be expected in approximately 50% of patients in whom imatinib treatment failed but are still in chronic phase. If patients have experienced treatment failure with more than one TKI, or have disease in accelerated or blast crisis, response rates are substantially lower. Ponatinib, a pan-TKI, was approved by the FDA for the treatment of patients in whom previous TKI therapy failed, but because of vascular events, has been suspended from marketing by the FDA.[122] Unlike other TKIs, ponatinib is active in disease with the *T315I* mutation.

Some patients with otherwise typical chronic-phase CML will have additional chromosome abnormalities (ACA) in Ph-positive cells. The presence of ACA is predictive of a lower response rate to imatinib and shorter response duration.[123] Patients treated with imatinib can develop other chromosome abnormalities (OCA) in Ph-negative cells in 5% to 10% of cases. Approximately 50% of OCAs are trisomy 8 alone. About 10% will include trisomy 8 plus another abnormality, and an additional 15% will involve deletion of chromosome 7 alone or with other abnormalities. The implications of OCA are unclear. In some cases, particularly those involving chromosome 7, OCA has been predictive of MDS development, but in other cases, particularly those with no morphologic evidence of dysplasia, disease has remained stable or the OCA clone has disappeared.[124]

The National Comprehensive Cancer Network and the European LeukemiaNet have established milestones for response to imatinib.[125] An update of these milestones is provided in Table 15-9.[126] Failure of therapy at 3 months is defined as failure to achieve a complete hematologic response or failure to achieve any level of cytogenetic response. By 6 months, patients are expected to have achieved at least a 1-log reduction in BCR-ABL and have less than 35% Ph-positive metaphases in marrow. By 12 months, patients should have a complete cytogenetic response and have at least a 2-log reduction in BCR-ABL. Failure to achieve any of these goals is an indication to switch to a second-generation

Table 15-9 Definition of Response to Initial Tyrosine Kinase Inhibitor Therapy[127]

	Optimal	Warning	Failure
Baseline	NA	High risk or CCA/Ph+	NA
3 months	BCR-ABL ≤ 10% and/or Ph+ < 35%	BCR-ABL > 10% and/or Ph+ 36% to 95%	Non-CHR and/or Ph+ > 95%
6 months	BCR-ABL ≤ 1% and/or Ph+ 0%	BCR-ABL 1-10% and/or Ph+ 1% to 35%	BCR-ABL > 10% and/or Ph+ > 35%
12 months	BCR-ABL < 0.1%	BCR-ABL > 0.1% to 1%	BCR-ABL > 1% and/or Ph+ > 0%
> 12 months	BCR-ABL < 0.1%	CCA/Ph-	Loss of CHR Loss of CCyR Confirmed loss of MMR CCA/Ph+

Abbreviations: CCA, clonal chromosome abnormalities; CCyR, complete cytogenetic response; CHR, complete hematologic response; MMR, major molecular response; NA, not applicable; Ph, Philadelphia chromosome.

TKI. Likewise, loss of complete hematologic response or loss of a complete cytogenetic response at any time during treatment is considered as treatment failure, as is the development of additional cytogenetic changes in Ph-positive cells. Definitions of expected responses to second-line therapy have also been developed, and are relatively similar to those for first-line therapy. Failure to achieve an adequate response with second-line therapy or to lose response is an indication to proceed to hematopoietic cell transplantation. Patients in lymphoid blast crisis with disease resistant to all TKIs sometimes have a disease response to ALL-type chemotherapy, whereas AML-type induction results in temporary CR for 15% to 20% of patients in myeloid blast crisis. Allogeneic HCT, as noted in the following section, is the only known curative therapy for patients in advanced phase.

Hematopoietic Cell Transplantation

Allogeneic transplantation is the only known cure for CML. Most published studies have been limited to patients age 65 or younger. When patients undergo transplantation during blast crisis and the donor is a matched sibling, approximately 10% to 15% become long-term survivors. Transplantation for accelerated-phase CML yields somewhat better results, with cure rates of 30% to 45%. Transplantation performed during the chronic phase yielded considerably better results, with long-term survival rates of 75% to 80%.[127] The probability of relapse for such patients is approximately 10%, and the probability of death from transplant-related complications is approximately 15%. Because of the high response rate and favorable toxicity profile of imatinib and other TKIs, these drugs have become the initial treatments of choice for most patients with newly diagnosed CML, and transplantation is now reserved for patients who experience imatinib resistance or intolerance. Current guidelines suggest that patients should also be given a trial of a second-line TKI before proceeding to transplant. Prior exposure to imatinib as first-line therapy does not seem to negatively affect the outcome of transplantation for CML.[128] However, there is much less data about the effect of failure of two TKIs on transplant outcome.

Neither the best preparative regimen nor the best form of GVHD prophylaxis for transplantation in CML has been defined. However, in the setting of CML, the risk of tumor recurrence is markedly increased with T-cell depletion of donor marrow, suggesting a particularly important role for the graft-versus-tumor effect in transplantation for CML. With modern typing techniques, there is no appreciable difference in the outcome of matched-related and matched-unrelated transplants in CML.[129]

Various studies have demonstrated that *BCR-ABL* fusion messenger RNAs can be detected by PCR assays in some patients after allogeneic marrow transplantation. Of interest, in many cases, *BCR-ABL* could be detected only transiently and, with time, disappeared. In other cases, there was sustained evidence of *BCR-ABL* transcripts detected by PCR assays over several years without disease progressing to clinical relapse. Most of the current evidence suggests that detection of *BCR-ABL* transcripts during the first 3 months after transplant is not prognostically significant. In contrast, at 6 and 12 months after transplant, detection of *BCR-ABL* transcripts is associated with a 40% chance of subsequent relapse compared with a 5% chance for patients who are *BCR-ABL*–negative by the same assay.[130]

Reports suggest that several options are available for patients with chronic-phase CML who have disease recurrence after marrow transplantation. With the use of IFN-α, most patients experience a disease response, and 35% become Ph-negative. If IFN is used to treat cytogenetic relapse before the development of clinical relapse, complete cytogenetic responses have been documented for 70% of patients. Another approach to the treatment of relapse after transplantation in CML is the infusion of viable donor leukocytes. Such infusions lead to complete cytogenetic remission for approximately 75% of cases. These responses seem to be enduring, lasting more than 3 years for most patients. Donor leukocyte infusions can be complicated by marrow failure or severe GVHD. These risks can be reduced by limiting the number of leukocytes or administering them on a fractionated basis. TKIs also are effective post-transplant, particularly in patients without demonstrated resistance.[131]

CHRONIC LYMPHOCYTIC LEUKEMIA

CLL is the most prevalent adult leukemia in Western countries, with an estimated 14,570 new cases in the United States in 2011 and 4,380 deaths.[132] CLL is more common in men than in women (ratio, 1.7 to 1), with a steep age-specific incidence. There is a higher incidence in Jewish people of Russian or eastern European ancestry, but it is rare in Asian countries.

There are no known risk factors for CLL. Indeed, CLL is one of the few leukemias that does not seem to be associated with exposure to ionizing radiation, chemicals, or drugs, although data suggest a possible relationship with Agent Orange. Although single gene syndromes have not been reported, an increased familial incidence exists.[133]

DIAGNOSIS

The diagnosis of CLL requires a sustained increase in mature-appearing B lymphocytes in the peripheral blood to more than 5,000/mm³. It is not unusual that a small percentage of larger atypical cells, cleaved cells, or prolymphocytes also may be present. The predominant cell population expresses B-cell markers (CD19, CD20, and CD23) and the CD5 antigen, but not other pan-T-cell markers. The entity formerly described as T-cell CLL is now defined as T-cell prolymphocytic leukemia, and is not considered part of CLL. The B cells are monoclonal as evidenced by expressing either kappa or lambda light chains and characteristically express surface Ig, CD79b, CD20, and CD22 with low density (as opposed to mantle cell lymphoma, which usually has higher expression of CD20 and surface Ig). The bone marrow usually is infiltrated by at least 30% lymphocytes. Although a bone marrow aspirate and biopsy are not needed to make the diagnosis, they are strongly recommended if cytopenias in other cell lines are present before starting therapy. Neither lymph node biopsy nor computed tomography (CT) scanning is needed in the initial evaluation and should only be performed if clinically indicated.[134]

CYTOGENETIC AND MOLECULAR ABNORMALITIES IN CLL

Conventional banding techniques detect cytogenetic abnormalities in more than 50% of CLL cases. FISH allows for identification of cytogenetic abnormalities in more than 80% of cases.[135] The most common abnormality is deletion of 13q, which is present in 55% of cases, either alone or in combination with other abnormalities. The disease course is more benign for patients with 13q14 abnormalities, and such patients often have a normal life span. Next in frequency of abnormalities are deletions of 11q, which are identified in 15% to 20% of cases. Deletions of 11q23 are associated with massive lymphadenopathy, often out of proportion to the increase in the peripheral blood lymphocyte count. Trisomy 12 can be detected in 15% to 20% of cases. Structural abnormalities of chromosome 17 occur in at least 15% of patients when FISH testing is performed. Deletions in 17p13 lead to disruption of the *TP53* gene and are found more frequently in cases of atypical CLL, which is associated with a higher likelihood of Richter transformation, more prolymphocytes, advanced stage, resistance to chemotherapy, and a poor prognosis. More than one-third of patients have complex abnormalities.

Translocations associated with *BCL-2* (t[14;18][q32;q21]) and *BCL-3* (t[14;19][q32;q13.1]) have been detected in only 5% to 10% of cases. However, overexpression of the *BCL-2* gene is present in more than 70% of cases, even in the absence of the chromosome rearrangement. The ratio of the antiapoptotic gene *BCL-2* expression to the proapoptotic gene *BAX* is increased in CLL cells, which favors cell survival. These findings support the concept that CLL is more a disorder of prolonged cell survival than a hyperproliferative disease, although both factors probably contribute to the disease.

Lymphocytes from approximately one-half of patients with CLL are naive and have unmutated V_H genes; the other one-half contain V_H genes that are mutated, postgerminal-center B cells. These two populations are characterized by markedly different clinical outcomes, with the survival significantly shorter for the group with unmutated V_H genes. DNA microarray analyses have shown that ZAP-70 expression distinguishes the unmutated from the mutated populations of patients with CLL.[136] Increased ZAP-70 expression is associated with enhanced signal transduction

through the BCR complex, which may contribute to an aggressive course.[137] The overall incidence of genomic aberrations is similar in the mutated and unmutated V_H groups; however, the unfavorable cytogenetic abnormalities (e.g., 17p- and 11q-) occur in the unmutated group, whereas the more favorable mutations (e.g., 13q-) occur in the mutated group.[138] Lymphocytes with trisomy 12 tend to have unmutated V_H genes, whereas those with del(13q14) have evidence of somatic mutations. CD38 is expressed more commonly in CLL cells that are ZAP-70-positive and have unmutated V_H genes. Cytogenetic and molecular markers in CLL may change over time, requiring their reassessment if the tempo of disease seems to be changing. Next-generation sequencing technologies have identified recurrent mutations in CLL involving *NOTCH1* (10%), *SF3B1* (10%), and *BIRC3*.

STAGING AND PROGNOSIS

Several characteristics have been used to stratify patients with CLL into groups according to different clinical outcomes that may require different therapeutic approaches. The five-stage Rai classification is most commonly used in the United States (Table 15-10), and the three-stage Binet system is most often applied in Europe (Table 15-11). The major difference between the two systems is that Rai stage 0 and I are mostly combined into Binet stage A, and Rai stage III and IV are combined into Binet stage C.

CLINICAL FEATURES
Clinical Presentation

Most patients with CLL are generally asymptomatic at the time of presentation, and the diagnosis often is made incidentally when lymphocytosis is noted during a routine evaluation. The findings on physical examination are normal for 20% to 30% of patients, with lymphadenopathy and/or hepatosplenomegaly observed in an additional 40% to 50% of patients. However, as disease progresses, generalized lymphadenopathy and splenomegaly become common features. Involvement of other organs is unusual and should suggest the possibility of transformation to Richter syndrome.

Infections

Increased susceptibility to infections reflects the hypogammaglobulinemia that worsens with disease progression and abnormal activation of complement. Historically, the most common pathogens have been those that require opsonization for bacterial killing, such as *Streptococcus pneumoniae*, *Staphylococcus aureus*, and *Haemophilus influenzae*. The increased use of immunosuppressive agents such as fludarabine, cladribine, pentostatin, and alemtuzumab has markedly increased the number of infections with opportunistic organisms such as *Candida, Listeria, Pneumocystis jiroveci,* cytomegalovirus (CMV), *Aspergillus,* herpes viruses, and others. The prophylactic use of intravenous Igs or antimicrobial agents should be reserved for select patients with documented, repeated bacterial infections.

Aggressive Transformation

For 3% to 15% of patients with CLL, the disease will evolve into a more aggressive lymphoid malignant process, most often Richter

Table 15-10 Rai Classification for Staging Chronic Lymphocytic Leukemia

Stage	Clinical Features	Median Survival (years)
0	Lymphocytosis only	> 12.5
I	Lymphadenopathy	8.5
II	Splenomegaly with or without hepatomegaly	6
III*	Anemia	1.5
IV*	Thrombocytopenia	1.5

* The anemia or thrombocytopenia cannot be immune-mediated.

Table 15-11 Binet Classification for Staging Chronic Lymphocytic Leukemia

Stage	Symptoms	Median Survival (years)
A	< 3 node-bearing areas	> 10
B	≥ 3 node-bearing areas	5
C	Anemia and/or thrombocytopenia	2

syndrome, which characteristically presents with increasing lymphadenopathy, hepatosplenomegaly, fever, abdominal pain, weight loss, progressive anemia, and thrombocytopenia with a rapid rise in the peripheral blood lymphocyte count, and an increased serum LDH level. Evaluation of lymph node tissue obtained by biopsy may indicate a large cell lymphoma. This transformation is not clearly related to either the nature or extent of previous therapy. The large cell lymphoma shares immunologic, cytogenetic, and molecular features with the original CLL clone in one-half of cases. For patients with Richter syndrome, response to systemic therapy is poor, with a median survival of 4 to 5 months when treatment involves alkylating agents; survival may be longer after the use of nucleoside analog-based regimens.

CLL also may evolve into prolymphocytic leukemia (PLL), which is associated with progressive anemia and thrombocytopenia, with at least 55% prolymphocytes in the peripheral blood. Clinical features include lymphadenopathy, hepatosplenomegaly, wasting syndrome, and increasing resistance to therapy. Transformation to ALL, plasma cell leukemia, multiple myeloma, or Hodgkin lymphoma have been noted in anecdotal reports.

Autoimmunity

A positive Coombs antiglobulin test is present in 20% to 30% of CLL cases, with clinical hemolysis in 10% to 25% of patients. The frequency of immune thrombocytopenia seems to be approximately 2%. In most cases, these antibodies are polyclonal; therefore, they are not produced by the malignant B cells.

Autoimmune anemia or thrombocytopenia generally responds to corticosteroids such as prednisone at a dose of 60 mg/day to 100 mg/day, which may be tapered 1 or 2 weeks after evidence of response. Patients who do not experience a disease response to corticosteroids may experience a response to high-dose intravenous Igs. Rituximab and alternative immunosuppressants such as cyclosporine may also sometimes be useful. Splenectomy may be considered when systemic approaches fail. Radiation therapy to the spleen induces only transient responses.

Pure Red Cell Aplasia

Pure red cell aplasia is an uncommon occurrence in CLL. It is characterized by severe anemia without a reticulocyte response or bone marrow normoblasts and without neutropenia or thrombocytopenia. Corticosteroids, as well as cyclosporine and rituximab, may be effective.

Secondary Malignant Diseases

Secondary malignant diseases occur with increased frequency in patients with CLL, related both to the immune defects of the disease and to the consequences of therapy. The most frequent tumors are skin cancer (including melanomas), colon cancers, lung cancers, and myeloid neoplasms.

TREATMENT

CLL is not curable with currently available therapies, with the exception of allogeneic HCT, nor is there evidence that treatment of patients with early-stage disease (Rai 0 to 2 or Binet A) extends life expectancy.[139,140] Therefore, asymptomatic patients with early-stage disease should be monitored but not receive treatment unless enrolled in a clinical trial. Early-stage patients with disease-related symptoms including "B" symptoms: weight loss, pronounced fatigue, and symptoms or complications from hepatomegaly, splenomegaly or lymphadenopathy, as well as autoimmune anemia/thrombocytopenia or recurrent infections, may be candidates for treatment.[141] A rapid lymphocyte doubling time (less than 6 months) may also support the decision to treat.

Initial Therapy

The choice of initial therapy in CLL is generally based on the clinical status of the patient (fit and age younger than 70 vs. unfit and/or age older than 70) and the presence or absence of del(11q) or del(17p). For younger, fit patients without del(11q) or del(17p), there are a large number of acceptable alternatives. The most commonly used regimen is fludarabine combined with CY and rituximab (FCR).[142] However, other equally acceptable regimens include fludarabine and rituximab (without CY), pentostatin plus CY and rituximab, bendamustine plus rituximab, fludarabine plus alemtuzumab, and rituximab, CY, doxorubicin, vincristine, and prednisone (RCHOP), as well as many others.[143,144] For patients with a poorer performance status or older than age 70, similar regimens are recommended, but at reduced dosing. Other acceptable alternatives for older or infirm patients include high-dose methylprednisone with rituximab, single-agent ofatumumab (a novel anti-CD20 antibody), the combination of chlorambucil and rituximab, or the combination of obinutuzumab plus chlorambucil.[145,146] Patients with CLL with del(17p) or del(11q) have more aggressive disease and appear to benefit from the addition of CY to their regimen, and so FCR is generally recommended, although bendamustine with rituximab is an acceptable alternative.

Patients with CLL treated with either purine-analog or alemtuzumab-containing regimens become significantly immunosuppressed.[147] Thus, anti-infective prophylaxis for herpes virus (acyclovir or equivalent) and *Pneumocystis jirovecii* pneumonia (sulfamethoxazole/trimethoprim or equivalent) is recommended. For patients on alemtuzumab who are CMV seropositive, monitoring for CMV viremia and treatment for rising viral titers is generally recommended. Other expected toxicities of most regimens include moderate myelosuppression. Tumor lysis syndrome occurs in occasional patients treated for CLL, especially those with high white counts or bulky lymphadenopathy. This syndrome may be fatal and is not consistently preventable with the use of prophylactic allopurinol and/or hydration. Fludarabine may be associated with autoimmune hemolytic anemia and thrombocytopenia. Most experts recommend stopping the drug and switching to alternatives if such complications occur. Despite the profound immunosuppression associated with single-agent fludarabine, the risk of secondary malignant disease does not seem to be increased with the use of fludarabine alone. However, there may be an increased incidence of myelodysplasia when fludarabine is combined with alkylating-agent therapy.[148]

Treatment for Relapsed or Refractory Disease

Treatment is not necessarily needed for relapsed or refractory disease after initial therapy; treatment in this setting is based on the same indications as for initial treatment. The most appropriate treatment for such patients is a clinical research study. For patients who are not eligible for a trial or who are unwilling to participate in clinical research, salvage therapy is influenced by the type of primary therapy received and the duration of the initial response. In general, patients who have long first remissions can undergo retreatment with the same agents as used initially with a reasonable chance of response. Patients who experience relapse within 6 months of previous therapy should be switched to an alternative regimen. Ibrutinib, a BTK inhibitor, has recently been approved for the treatment of patients with recurrent CLL.[148a]

Hematopoietic Cell Transplantation

Initial trials of ablative allogeneic HCT for refractory CLL showed substantial nonrelapse mortality but prolonged DFS for a significant proportion of patients. For example, a study from Seattle demonstrated a 5-year DFS rate of 32% for patients with refractory CLL.[149] Studies from The University of Texas MD Anderson Cancer Center, Dana-Farber Cancer Institute, and the CIBMTR provide further evidence that prolonged DFS can be achieved in CLL with allogeneic transplantation.[150,151]

Given that the median age at diagnosis of CLL is older than 60, transplantation using high-dose preparative regimens for this disease has been limited to a minority of patients. The more

recent advent of reduced-intensity transplantation has widened the possible application of transplantation. In a study from Seattle, 64 patients with advanced CLL received a reduced-intensity regimen, with a 52% DFS rate at 2 years post-transplant.[152] Thus, reduced-intensity allogeneic transplantation seems to be a reasonable option for patients with fludarabine-refractory disease who are otherwise in reasonably good health. Patients with del(17p) have such a poor prognosis with conventional therapy that they can reasonably be considered for allogeneic transplantation, even in first remission.

Supportive Measures

Splenectomy. Splenectomy may provide important palliation for patients with CLL for whom systemic treatment has failed and who have persistent splenomegaly or cytopenia that precludes chemotherapy. The procedure also should be considered for patients with autoimmune thrombocytopenia or hemolytic anemia who do not experience a response to more conservative measures, such as corticosteroids, intravenous Ig, or rituximab.

Leukapheresis. Leukapheresis results in only transient reductions in circulating lymphocytes and is not recommended for general practice. As patients with CLL rarely experience tumor cell aggregates, regardless of the number of circulating cells, systemic treatment is usually adequate to reduce the number of circulating lymphocytes, when indicated.

Erythropoietin. Epoetin may reduce transfusion requirements for approximately two-thirds of patients with CLL, and a trial involving this agent can be considered for patients who have CLL with anemia and no other obvious correctable cause.[153] Responses are rarely seen in patients with high endogenous erythropoietin levels (more than 500 U/L).

Novel Agents in CLL

Although not yet commercially available, several novel agents show high levels of activity in phase I and II clinical trials.[154] Among the most active is idelalisib, a phosphoinositide 3-kinase (PI3K) inhibitor. In addition, not just clinical but molecular complete responses have been documented in otherwise refractory patients treated with CARTs targeted against CD19.[90]

B-PROLYMPHOCYTIC LEUKEMIA

Patients with PLL tend to be older than patients with CLL (median age, 70). At the time of presentation, the primary symptoms include abdominal discomfort, fever, and weight loss. Disease presents at an advanced stage for virtually all patients. PLL is associated with a larger spleen and a higher white blood cell count than CLL; however, there is less lymphadenopathy. PLL cells are large, with a round nucleus and a prominent nucleolus. In de novo PLL, most of the peripheral blood mononuclear cells tend to be prolymphocytes; in the setting of an aggressive transformation from CLL, there is a dimorphic population in the peripheral blood. The immunophenotype is different from CLL; the cells are positive for CD19, CD20, and

CD24, and they strongly express CD22, surface Igs, and FMC7. CD5 or CD23 is expressed in less than one-third of cases.

Patients with PLL generally receive the same regimens used to treat CLL, but response rates tend to be lower and response durations usually are shorter. Therapeutic activity with alemtuzumab and purine analogs has been noted, but tends to be transient.

HAIRY CELL LEUKEMIA

Hairy cell leukemia occurs in about 600 new patients each year in the United States, generally in older persons, with a strong predominance in men. Patients generally present with symptoms referable to cytopenias, including infections (29%) and weakness or fatigue (27%); less common presentations include pain in the left upper quadrant related to splenomegaly (5%) or bleeding related to thrombocytopenia (4%). The incidence of secondary malignant disease is increased. The most common signs include palpable splenomegaly (72% to 86%), hepatomegaly (13% to 20%), hairy cells in the peripheral blood (85% to 89%), thrombocytopenia defined as less than 100,000/mm³ (53%), anemia defined as hemoglobin of less than 12 g/dL (71% to 77%), and neutropenia defined as an absolute neutrophil count of less than 500/mm³ (32% to 39%).

> ### KEY POINTS
>
> - Hairy cell leukemia is highly responsive to cladribine or pentostatin.
> - Patients with refractory disease who require treatment may have a response to rituximab or to an anti-CD22 immunotoxin.

The cells in the peripheral blood generally have an eccentric, spongiform, kidney-shaped nucleus, with characteristic filamentous cytoplasmic projections. A bone marrow biopsy usually is needed to make the diagnosis, because an aspirate often cannot be obtained. The malignant cells are of B-cell origin, expressing CD19 and CD20, as well as the monocyte antigens CD11c and CD25. The most specific marker is CD103. The cells stain positively with tartrate-resistant acid phosphatase. It is most difficult to distinguish hairy cell leukemia from hairy cell variant; the latter is often associated with a high circulating white blood cell count, cells containing bilobed nuclei with prominent nucleoli, bone marrow with interstitial infiltration of clumped cells, and resistance to treatment with IFN-α, cladribine, and pentostatin. Mutations in *BRAF* have been found in virtually all cases of hairy cell leukemia studied so far.[155]

Treatment is indicated in the setting of massive or progressive splenomegaly, worsening blood counts, recurrent infection, more than 20,000 hairy cells/mm³ of peripheral blood, or bulky lymphadenopathy. Until the early 1980s, splenectomy was the standard treatment for hairy cell leukemia. This procedure improves symptoms related to splenomegaly and peripheral blood counts—often for prolonged periods of time—but it does not affect the disease itself. Splenectomy is now reserved for the rare occasion when a patient has disease that is refractory to treatment and has splenomegaly that is either symptomatic or is resulting in cytopenias.

IFN was the first systemic therapy to demonstrate activity in hairy cell leukemia. At doses of 2×10^6 U/m²/day or 3×10^6 U three times per week, IFN induces response in 80% of patients; however, only 10% are CRs. Although response generally occurs within 3 to 4 months, therapy may be needed for more than 1 year before a maximal effect is achieved. Hairy cell leukemia invariably recurs after IFN therapy has been discontinued, and maintenance therapy is associated with excessive toxicity and expense without any apparent survival benefit.

Purine analogs revolutionized the treatment of patients with hairy cell leukemia. Pentostatin at doses of 4 mg/m² intravenously every other week for 4 to 6 months achieves CR in 60% to 89% of previously treated or untreated disease, including in those patients for whom IFN has failed, with an overall response rate of 80% to 90%. Approximately 25% of patients experience relapse during more than 5 years of follow-up. In an intergroup trial, 350 previously untreated patients with hairy cell leukemia were randomly assigned to receive treatment with IFN or pentostatin. The CR rate was approximately 11% for IFN compared with 76% for pentostatin, with a significant advantage to the latter therapy in terms of the durability of response.[156] The lack of a survival advantage reflects the high number of patients receiving IFN who also received salvage therapy with pentostatin.

Cladribine also is highly effective for hairy cell leukemia. A 7-day infusion or a 2-hour infusion for 5 to 7 days achieves response for approximately 80% to 90% of patients, with a CR rate of 65% to 80%. The responses tend to be durable, with relapse occurring in 20% to 30% of patients during prolonged follow-up. In many cases, relapse is characterized only by an increase in hairy cells in the bone marrow, with no indication for treatment. A second durable response is achieved for most patients who need repeat treatment. The results with pentostatin are equivalent to those with cladribine. The shorter duration of treatment makes the latter drug somewhat more attractive, although it may be associated with greater toxicity.

An anti-CD22 *Pseudomonas* exotoxin immunoconjugate induces response for most patients for whom purine analog therapy has failed.[157] Rituximab also has shown promise for such patients or for patients with hairy cell variant.

CHRONIC T-CELL LEUKEMIAS

Despite considerable effort, the classification of indolent T-cell leukemias remains ambiguous with many uncommon and imperfectly defined categories.[158] Among the more common forms of chronic T-cell leukemia are T-PLL, adult T-cell leukemia/lymphoma, various subtypes of large granular lymphocytosis, and natural killer (NK)–cell leukemia. T-PLL tends to occur in older individuals (median age, 63). The presenting features include skin involvement, widespread lymphadenopathy, splenomegaly, and malignant effusions. The lymphocyte count is often more than 100,000/mm³. Anemia and thrombocytopenia are also common. T-PLL is associated with recurrent chromosome abnormalities, notably inversion of chromosome 14 with breakpoints at the long arm at q11 and q32, in 80% of patients. In more than one-half of cases, abnormalities of chromosome 8 can be identified including i(8q), trisomy 8, t(8;8)(p11;q32), or add(8)(p11). Treatment is, in general, unsatisfactory. Alemtuzumab has demonstrated impressive activity in T-PLL, with response rates of 50% to 70%.[159]

Large granular lymphocytosis can be divided into two major subsets: those that are CD3+ representing in vivo activated cytotoxic T cells (T-large granular lymphocytosis) and NK-large granular lymphocytosis that is CD3-. T-large granular lymphocytosis tends to occur in older persons, and most patients (60%) are symptomatic at diagnosis. Anemia and recurrent infections associated with neutropenia are common. The phenotype includes CD3+, CD8+, CD57+, with clonal rearrangement of T-cell receptor genes. NK-large granular lymphocytosis accounts for approximately 15% of the disease and includes aggressive NK-cell leukemia and a more indolent NK lymphocytosis. The cells are CD3-, CD8+, CD16+, CD56+, and CD57±. Rearrangements of *TCR* genes are absent. In the aggressive form of the disease, patients tend to be younger and do not have rheumatoid arthritis. Infiltration of the gastrointestinal tract and bone marrow are common. Neutropenia is modest compared with the severity of anemia and thrombocytopenia. Patients often die as a result of multiorgan failure with a coagulopathy, generally within a few months of diagnosis, despite aggressive chemotherapy. Approximately 5% of large granular lymphocytosis is a nonclonal expansion of CD3+ large granular lymphocytosis that is generally unaccompanied by lymphadenopathy or hepatosplenomegaly. The features of the cells are CD3+, CD4-, CD8-, CD16+, and CD56+. The disease is indolent, rarely requiring intervention unless accompanied by neutropenia. Prednisone and immunosuppressive agents have been used. It is not clear whether this disorder is actually neoplastic.

Adult T-cell leukemia/lymphoma is endemic in Japan, the Caribbean, parts of central Africa, and the southeastern United States. It is linked to the prevalence of human T-cell lymphotropic virus type I. There are a number of clinical variants that range from a chronic smoldering disorder to an aggressive leukemic disease. The levels of serum calcium and LDH are prognostic for outcome. The major causes of death are related to infection. Combination chemotherapy and pentostatin have had limited success.

KEY POINT

- Chronic T-cell leukemias consist of mycosis fungoides, T-cell prolymphocytic leukemia, adult T-cell leukemia/ lymphoma, various subtypes of large granular lymphocytosis, and natural killer–cell leukemia.

References

1. Buckley JD, Buckley CM, Breslow NE, et al. Concordance for childhood cancer in twins. *Med Pediatr Oncol.* 1996;26:223-229. PMID: 8600332.

2. Hahn CN, Chong CE, Carmichael CL, et al. Heritable GATA2 mutations associated with familial myelodysplastic syndrome and acute myeloid leukemia. *Nat Genet.* 2011;43:1012-1017. PMID: 21892162.

3. Owen C, Barnett M, Fitzgibbon J. Familial myelodysplasia and acute myeloid leukaemia–a review. *Br J Haematol.* 2008;140:123-132. PMID: 18173751.

4. Mortreux F, Gabet AS, Wattel E. Molecular and cellular aspects of HTLV-1 associated leukemogenesis in vivo. *Leukemia.* 2003;17:26-38. PMID: 12529656.

5. Cronkite EP, Moloney W, Bond VP. Radiation leukemogenesis: an analysis of the problem. *Am J Med.* 1960;28:673-682. PMID: 13812972.

6. Godley LA, Larson RA. Therapy-related myeloid leukemia. *Semin Oncol.* 2008;35:418-429. PMID: 18692692.

7. Kayser S, Döhner K, Krauter J, et al. The impact of therapy-related acute myeloid leukemia (AML) on outcome in 2853 adult patients with newly diagnosed AML. *Blood.* 2011;117:2137-2145. PMID: 21127174.

8. Larson RA, Le Beau MM, Ratain MJ, et al. Balanced translocations involving chromosome bands 11q23 and 21q22 in therapy-related leukemia. *Blood.* 1992;79:1892-1893. PMID: 1558980.

9. Bennett JM, Catovsky D, Daniel MT, et al. Proposals for the classification of the acute leukaemias. French-American-British (FAB) co-operative group. *Br J Haematol.* 1976;33:451-458. PMID: 188440.

10. Vardiman JW, Thiele J, Arber DA, et al. The 2008 revision of the World Health Organization (WHO) classification of myeloid neoplasms and acute leukemia: rationale and important changes. *Blood.* 2009;114:937-951. PMID: 19357394.

11. Campos L, Guyotat D, Archimbaud E, et al. Surface marker expression in adult acute myeloid leukaemia: correlations with initial characteristics, morphology and response to therapy. *Br J Haematol.* 1989;72:161-166. PMID: 2757962.

12. de Thé H, Lavau C, Marchio A, et al. The PML-RAR alpha fusion mRNA generated by the t(15;17) translocation in acute promyelocytic leukemia encodes a functionally altered RAR. *Cell.* 1991;66:675-684. PMID: 1652369.

13. Appelbaum FR, Kopecky KJ, Tallman MS, et al. The clinical spectrum of adult acute myeloid leukaemia associated with core binding factor translocations. *Br J Haematol.* 2006;135:165-173. PMID: 16939487.

14. Paschka P, Marcucci G, Ruppert AS, et al. Adverse prognostic significance of KIT mutations in adult acute myeloid leukemia with inv(16) and t(8;21): a Cancer and Leukemia Group B Study. *J Clin Oncol.* 2006;24:3904-3911. PMID: 16921041.

15. Ernst P, Wang J, Korsmeyer SJ. The role of MLL in hematopoiesis and leukemia. *Curr Opin Hematol.* 2002;9:282-287. PMID: 12042701.

16. Grimwade D, Walker H, Oliver F, et al. The importance of diagnostic cytogenetics on outcome in AML: analysis of 1,612 patients entered into the MRC AML 10 trial. The Medical Research Council Adult and Children's Leukaemia Working Parties. *Blood.* 1998;92:2322-2333. PMID: 9746770.

17. Slovak ML, Kopecky KJ, Cassileth PA, et al. Karyotypic analysis predicts outcome of preremission and postremission therapy in adult acute myeloid leukemia: a Southwest Oncology Group/Eastern Cooperative Oncology Group Study. *Blood.* 2000;96:4075-4083. PMID: 11110676.

18. Medeiros BC, Othus M, Fang M, et al. Prognostic impact of monosomal karyotype in young adult and elderly acute myeloid leukemia: the Southwest Oncology Group (SWOG) experience. *Blood.* 2010;116:2224-2228. PMID: 20562328.

19. Cancer Genome Atlas Research Network. Genomic and epigenomic landscapes of adult de novo acute myeloid leukemia. *N Engl J Med.* 2013;368:2059-2074. PMID: 23634996.

20. Fröhling S, Scholl C, Gilliland DG, et al. Genetics of myeloid malignancies: pathogenetic and clinical implications (Review). *J Clin Oncol.* 2005;23:6285-6295. PMID: 16155011.

21. Thiede C, Koch S, Creutzig E, et al. Prevalence and prognostic impact of NPM1 mutations in 1485 adult patients with acute myeloid leukemia (AML). *Blood.* 2006;107:4011-4020. PMID: 16455956.

22. Wouters BJ, Löwenberg B, Erpelinck-Verschueren CA, et al. Double CEBPA mutations, but not single CEBPA mutations, define a subgroup of acute myeloid leukemia with a distinctive gene expression profile that is uniquely associated with a favorable outcome. *Blood.* 2009;113:3088-3091. PMID: 19171880.

23. Marcucci G, Haferlach T, Döhner H. Molecular genetics of adult acute myeloid leukemia: prognostic and therapeutic implications. *J Clin Oncol.* 2011;29:475-486. PMID: 21220609.

24. Heil G, Hoelzer D, Sanz MA, et al. A randomized, double-blind, placebo-controlled, phase III study of filgrastim in remission induction and consolidation therapy for adults with de novo acute myeloid leukemia. The International Acute Myeloid Leukemia Study Group. *Blood.* 1997;90:4710-4718. PMID: 9389686.

25. Fernandez HF, Sun Z, Yao X, et al. Anthracycline dose intensification in acute myeloid leukemia. *N Engl J Med.* 2009;361:1249-1259. PMID: 19776406.

26. Ohtake S, Miyawaki S, Fujita H, et al. Randomized study of induction therapy comparing standard-dose idarubicin with high-dose daunorubicin in adult patients with previously untreated acute myeloid leukemia: the JALSG AML201 Study. *Blood.* 2011;117:2358-2365. PMID: 20693429.

27. Löwenberg B, Pabst T, Vellenga E, et al. Cytarabine dose for acute myeloid leukemia. *N Engl J Med.* 2011;364:1027-1036. PMID: 21410371.

28. Burnett AK, Hills RK, Milligan D, et al. Identification of patients with acute myeloblastic leukemia who benefit from the addition of gemtuzumab ozogamicin: results of the MRC AML15 trial. *J Clin Oncol.* 2011;29:369-377. PMID: 21172891.

29. Godwin JE, Kopecky KJ, Head DR, et al. A double-blind placebo-controlled trial of granulocyte colony-stimulating factor in elderly patients with previously untreated acute myeloid leukemia: a Southwest oncology group study (9031). *Blood.* 1998;91:3607-3615. PMID: 9572995.

30. Kern W, Haferlach T, Schoch C, et al. Early blast clearance by remission induction therapy is a major independent prognostic factor for both achievement of complete remission and long-term outcome in acute myeloid leukemia: data from the German AML Cooperative Group (AMLCG) 1992 Trial. *Blood.* 2003;101:64-70. PMID: 12393605.

31. Döhner H, Estey EH, Amadori S, et al. Diagnosis and management of acute myeloid leukemia in adults: recommendations from an international expert panel, on behalf of the European LeukemiaNet. *Blood.* 2010;115:453-474. PMID: 19880497.

32. Cassileth PA, Harrington DP, Hines JD, et al. Maintenance chemotherapy prolongs remission duration in adult acute nonlymphocytic leukemia. *J Clin Oncol.* 1988;6:583-587. PMID: 3282032.

33. Appelbaum FR. Acute myeloid leukemia in adults. In Abeloff MD, Armitage JO, Niederhuber JE, Kastan MB, McKenna WG (eds). *Clinical Oncology.* Philadelphia, PA: Elsevier Churchill Livingstone, 2004;2825-2848.

34. Mayer RJ, Davis RB, Schiffer, CA et al. Intensive postremission chemotherapy in adults with acute myeloid leukemia. Cancer and Leukemia Group B. *N Engl J Med.* 1994;331:896-903. PMID: 8078551.

35. Schaich M, Röllig C, Soucek S, et al. Cytarabine dose of 36 g/m^2 compared with 12 g/m^2 within first consolidation in acute myeloid leukemia: results of patients enrolled onto the prospective randomized AML96 study. *J Clin Oncol.* 2011;29:2696-2702. PMID: 21606413.

36. O'Donnell MR, Appelbaum FR, Baer MR, et al. Acute myeloid leukemia clinical practice guidelines in oncology. *J Natl Compr Canc Netw.* 2006;4:16-36. PMID: 16403402.

37. Morrison FS, Kopecky KJ, Head DR, et al. Late intensification with POMP chemotherapy prolongs survival in acute myelogenous leukemia—Results of a Southwest Oncology Group study of rubidazone versus adriamycin for remission induction, prophylactic intrathecal therapy, late intensification, and levamisole maintenance. *Leukemia.* 1992;6:708-714. PMID: 1625490.

38. Appelbaum FR, Gundacker H, Head DR, et al. Age and acute myeloid leukemia. *Blood.* 2006;107:3481-3485. PMID: 16455952.

39. Löwenberg B, Ossenkoppele GJ, van Putten W, et al. High-dose daunorubicin in older patients with acute myeloid leukemia. *N Engl J Med.* 2009;361:1235-1248. PMID: 19776405.

40. Burnett AK, Milligan D, Prentice AG, et al. A comparison of low-dose cytarabine and hydroxyurea with or without all-trans retinoic acid for acute myeloid leukemia and high-risk myelodysplastic syndrome in patients not considered fit for intensive treatment. *Cancer.* 2007;109:1114-1124. PMID: 17315155.

41. Cashen AF, Schiller GJ, O'Donnell MR, et al. Multicenter, phase II study of decitabine for the first-line treatment of older patients with acute myeloid leukemia. *J Clin Oncol.* 2010;28:556-561. PMID: 20026803.

42. Fung HC, Stein A, Slovak ML, et al. A long-term follow-up report on allogeneic stem cell transplantation for patients with primary refractory acute myelogenous leukemia: impact of cytogenetic characteristics on transplantation outcome. *Biol Blood Marrow Transplant.* 2003;9:766-771. PMID: 14677116.

43. Breems DA, Van Putten WL, Huijgens PC, et al. Prognostic index for adult patients with acute myeloid leukemia in first relapse. *J Clin Oncol.* 2005;23:1969-1978. PMID: 15632409.

44. Estey EH. Treatment of relapsed and refractory acute myelogenous leukemia. *Leukemia.* 2000;14:476-479. PMID: 10720145.

45. Kantarjian H, Gandhi V, Cortes J, et al. Phase 2 clinical and pharmacologic study of clofarabine in patients with refractory or relapsed acute leukemia. *Blood.* 2003;102:2379-2386. PMID: 12791647.

46. Yanada M, Matsuo K, Emi N, et al. Efficacy of allogeneic hematopoietic stem cell transplantation depends on cytogenetic risk for acute myeloid leukemia in first disease remission: a metaanalysis. *Cancer.* 2005;103:1652-1658. PMID: 15742336.

47. Koreth J, Schlenk R, Kopecky KJ, et al. Allogeneic stem cell transplantation for acute myeloid leukemia in first complete remission: systematic review and meta-analysis of prospective clinical trials. *JAMA.* 2009;301:2349-2361. PMID: 19509382.

48. Schlenk RF, Döhner K, Krauter J, et al. Mutations and treatment outcome in cytogenetically normal acute myeloid leukemia. *N Engl J Med.* 2008;358:1909-1918. PMID: 18450602.

49. Appelbaum FR. The current status of hematopoietic cell transplantation. *Annu Rev Med.* 2003;54:491-512. PMID: 12414918.

50. Bensinger WI, Martin PJ, Storer B, et al. Transplantation of bone marrow as compared with peripheral-blood cells from HLA-identical relatives in patients with hematologic cancers. *N Engl J Med.* 2001;344:175-181. PMID: 11172139.

51. Couban S, Simpson DR, Barnett MJ, et al. A randomized multicenter comparison of bone marrow and peripheral blood in recipients of matched sibling allogeneic transplants for myeloid malignancies. *Blood.* 2002;100:1525-1531. PMID: 12176866.

52. Stem Cell Trialists' Collaborative Group. Allogeneic peripheral blood stem-cell compared with bone marrow transplantation in the management of hematologic malignancies: an individual patient data meta-analysis of nine randomized trials. *J Clin Oncol.* 2005;23:5074-5087. PMID: 16051954.

53. Anasetti C, Logan BR, Lee SJ, et al. Peripheral-blood stem cells versus bone marrow from unrelated donors. *N Engl J Med.* 2012;367:1487-1496. PMID: 23075175.

54. Reisner Y, Hagin D, Martelli MF. Haploidentical hematopoietic transplantation: current status and future perspectives. *Blood.* 2011;118:6006-6017. PMID: 21921045.

55. Walter RB, Pagel JM, Gooley TA, et al. Comparison of matched unrelated and matched related donor myeloablative hematopoietic cell transplantation for adults with acute myeloid leukemia in first remission. *Leukemia.* 2010;24:1276-1282. PMID: 20485378.

56. Scaradavou A, Brunstein CG, Eapen M, et al. Double unit grafts successfully extend the application of umbilical cord blood transplantation in adults with acute leukemia. *Blood.* 2013;121:752-758. PMID: 23223509.

57. Gorin NC. Autologous stem cell transplantation in acute myelocytic leukemia. *Blood.* 1998;92:1073-1090. PMID: 9694694.

58. Levi I, Grotto I, Yerushalmi R, et al. Meta-analysis of autologous bone marrow transplantation versus chemotherapy in adult patients with acute myeloid leukemia in first remission. *Leuk Res.* 2004;28:605-612. PMID: 15120937.

59. Oliansky DM, Appelbaum F, Cassileth PA, et al. The role of cytotoxic therapy with hematopoietic stem cell transplantation in the therapy of acute myelogenous leukemia in adults: an evidence-based review. *Biol Blood Marrow Transplant.* 2008;14:137-180. PMID: 18215777.

60. Ringdén O, Labopin M, Tura S, et al. A comparison of busulphan versus total body irradiation combined with cyclophosphamide as conditioning for autograft or allograft bone marrow transplantation in patients with acute leukaemia. Acute Leukaemia Working Party of the European Group for Blood and Marrow Transplantation (EBMT). *Br J Haematol.* 1996;93:637-645. PMID: 8652385.

61. Storb R, Deeg HJ, Whitehead J, et al. Methotrexate and cyclosporine compared with cyclosporine alone for prophylaxis of acute graft versus host disease after marrow transplantation for leukemia. *N Engl J Med.* 1986;314:729-735. PMID: 3513012.

62. McSweeney PA, Niederwieser D, Shizuru JA, et al. Hematopoietic cell transplantation in older patients with hematologic malignancies: replacing high-dose cytotoxic therapy with graft-versus-tumor effects. *Blood.* 2001;97:3390-3400. PMID: 11369628.

63. Giralt S, Thall PF, Khouri I, et al. Melphalan and purine analog-containing preparative regimens: reduced-intensity conditioning for patients with hematologic malignancies undergoing allogeneic progenitor cell transplantation. *Blood.* 2001;97:631-637. PMID: 11157478.

64. Gyurkocza B, Storb R, Storer BE, et al. Nonmyeloablative allogeneic hematopoietic cell transplantation in patients with acute myeloid leukemia. *J Clin Oncol.* 2010;28:2859-2867. PMID: 20439626.

65. Warrell RP Jr, Frankel SR, Miller WH Jr, et al. Differentiation therapy of acute promyelocytic leukemia with tretinoin (all-trans-retinoic acid). *N Engl J Med.* 1991;324:1385-1393. PMID: 1850498.

66. Soignet SL, Frankel SR, Douer D, et al. United States multicenter study of arsenic trioxide in relapsed acute promyelocytic leukemia. *J Clin Oncol.* 2001;19:3852-3860. PMID: 11559723.

67. Head D, Kopecky KJ, Weick J, et al. Effect of aggressive daunomycin therapy on survival in acute promyelocytic leukemia. *Blood.* 1995;86:1717-1728. PMID: 7655004.

68. Tallman MS, Nabhan C, Feusner JH, et al. Acute promyelocytic leukemia: evolving therapeutic strategies. *Blood.* 2002;99:759-767. PMID: 11806975.

69. Powell BL, Moser B, Stock W, et al. Arsenic trioxide improves event-free and overall survival for adults with acute promyelocytic leukemia: North American Leukemia Intergroup Study C9710. *Blood.* 2010;116:3751-3757. PMID: 20705755.

70. Lo-Coco F, Avvisati G, Vignetti M, et al. Retinoic acid and arsenic trioxide for acute promyelocytic leukemia. *N Engl J Med.* 2013;369:111-121. PMID: 23841729.

71. Tallman MS, Andersen JW, Schiffer CA, et al. Clinical description of 44 patients with acute promyelocytic leukemia who developed the retinoic acid syndrome. *Blood.* 2000;95:90-95. PMID: 10607690.

72. Sanz MA, Grimwade D, Tallman MS, et al. Management of acute promyelocytic leukemia: recommendations from an expert panel on behalf of the European LeukemiaNet. *Blood.* 2009;113:1875-1891. PMID: 18812465.

73. Witherspoon RP, Deeg HJ, Storer B, et al. Hematopoietic stem-cell transplantation for treatment-related leukemia or myelodysplasia. *J Clin Oncol.* 2001;19:2134-2141. PMID: 11304765.

74. Boucheix C, David B, Sebban C, et al. Immunophenotype of adult acute lymphoblastic leukemia, clinical parameters, and outcome: an analysis of a prospective trial including 562 tested patients (LALA87). French Group on Therapy for Adult Acute Lymphoblastic Leukemia. *Blood.* 1994;84:1603-1612. PMID: 8068949.

75. Weinberg OK, Arber DA. Mixed-phenotype acute leukemia: historical overview and a new definition. *Leukemia.* 2010;24:1844-1851. PMID: 20844566.

76. Pullarkat V, Slovak ML, Kopecky KJ, et al. Impact of cytogenetics on the outcome of adult acute lymphoblastic leukemia: results of Southwest Oncology Group 9400 study. *Blood.* 2008;111:2563-2572. PMID: 18156492.

77. Moorman AV, Harrison CJ, Buck GA, et al. Karyotype is an independent prognostic factor in adult acute lymphoblastic leukemia (ALL): analysis of cytogenetic data from patients treated on the Medical Research Council (MRC) UKALLXII/Eastern Cooperative Oncology Group (ECOG) 2993 trial. *Blood.* 2007;109:3189-3197. PMID: 17170120.

78. Chan LC, Karhi KK, Rayter SI, et al. A novel abl protein expressed in Philadelphia chromosome positive acute lymphoblastic leukaemia. *Nature.* 1987;325:635-637. PMID: 3027581.

79. Radich JP, Kopecky KJ, Boldt DH, et al. Detection of BCR-ABL fusion genes in adult acute lymphoblastic leukemia by the polymerase chain reaction. *Leukemia.* 1994;8:1688-1695. PMID: 7934164.

80. Bassan R, Hoelzer D. Modern therapy of acute lymphoblastic leukemia. *J Clin Oncol.* 2011;29:532-543. PMID: 21220592.

81. Larson RA, Dodge RK, Linker CA, et al. A randomized controlled trial of filgrastim during remission induction and consolidation chemotherapy for adults with acute lymphoblastic leukemia: CALGB study 9111. *Blood.* 1998;92:1556-1564. PMID: 9716583.

82. Marks DI. Treating the "older" adult with acute lymphoblastic leukemia. *Hematology Am Soc Hematol Educ Program.* 2010;2010:13-20. PMID: 21239765.

83. Yanada M, Takeuchi J, Sugiura I, et al. High complete remission rate and promising outcome by combination of imatinib and chemotherapy for newly diagnosed BCR-ABL-positive acute lymphoblastic leukemia: a phase II study by the Japan Adult Leukemia Study Group. *J Clin Oncol.* 2006;24:460-466. PMID: 16344315.

84. Mancini M, Scappaticci D, Cimino G, et al. A comprehensive genetic classification of adult acute lymphoblastic leukemia (ALL): analysis of the GIMEMA 0496 protocol. *Blood.* 2005;105:3434-3441. PMID: 15650057.

85. Oliansky DM, Larson RA, Weisdorf D, et al. The role of cytotoxic therapy with hematopoietic stem cell transplantation in the treatment of adult acute lymphoblastic leukemia: update of the 2006 evidence-based review. *Biol Blood Marrow Transplant.* 2012;18:18-36. PMID: 21803017.

86. International Bone Marrow Transplant Registry. http://www.cibmtr.org 2013. Accessed 8 July 2014.

87. Thiebaut A, Vernant JP, Degos L, et al. Adult acute lymphocytic leukemia study testing chemotherapy and autologous and allogeneic transplantation. A follow-up report of the French protocol LALA. *Hematol Oncol Clin North Am.* 2000;14:1353-1366.

88. Goldstone AH, Richards SM, Lazarus HM, et al. In adults with standard-risk acute lymphoblastic leukemia, the greatest benefit is achieved from a matched sibling allogeneic transplantation in first complete remission, and an autologous transplantation is less effective than conventional consolidation/maintenance chemotherapy in all patients: final results of the International ALL Trial (MRC UKALL XII/ECOG E2993). *Blood.* 2008;111:1827-1833. PMID: 18048644.

89. Hoelzer, D. Novel antibody-based therapies for acute lymphoblastic leukemia. *Hematology Am Soc Hematol Educ Program.* 2011;2011;243-249. PMID: 22160041.

90. Grupp SA, Kalos M, Barrett D, et al. Chimeric antigen receptor-modified T cells for acute lymphoid leukemia. *N Engl J Med.* 2013;368:1509-1518. PMID: 23527958.

91. Foà R, Vitale A, Vignetti M, et al. Dasatinib as first-line treatment for adult patients with Philadelphia chromosome-positive acute lymphoblastic leukemia. *Blood.* 2011;118:6521-6528. PMID: 21931113.

92. Thomas DA, O'Brien S, Kantarjian HM. Monoclonal antibody therapy with rituximab for acute lymphoblastic leukemia. *Hematol Oncol Clin North Am.* 2009;23:949-971.

93. DeAngelo DJ, Yu D, Johnson JL, et al. Nelarabine induces complete remissions in adults with relapsed or refractory T-lineage acute lymphoblastic leukemia or lymphoblastic lymphoma: Cancer and Leukemia Group B study 19801. *Blood.* 2007;109:5136-5142. PMID: 17344466.

94. Ebert BL. Deletion 5q in myelodysplastic syndrome: a paradigm for the study of hemizygous deletions in cancer. *Leukemia.* 2009;23:1252-1256. PMID: 19322210.

95. Bejar R, Stevenson K, Abdel-Wahab O, et al. Clinical effect of point mutations in myelodysplastic syndromes. *N Engl J Med.* 2011;364:2496-2506. PMID: 21714648.

96. Greenberg P, Cox C, LeBeau MM, et al. International scoring system for evaluating prognosis in myelodysplastic syndromes. *Blood.* 1997;89:2079-2088. PMID: 9058730.

97. Greenberg PL, Tuechler H, Schanz J, et al. Revised international prognostic scoring system for myelodysplastic syndromes. *Blood.* 2012;120:2454-2465. PMID: 22740453.

98. List A, Kurtin S, Roe DJ, et al. Efficacy of lenalidomide in myelodysplastic syndromes. *N Engl J Med.* 2005;352:549-557. PMID: 15703420.

99. Hellström-Lindberg E, Gulbrandsen N, Lindberg G, et al. A validated decision model for treating the anaemia of myelodysplastic syndromes with erythropoietin + granulocyte colony-stimulating factor: significant effects on quality of life. *Br J Haematol.* 2003;120:1037-1046. PMID: 12648074.

100. Greenberg P, Taylor K, Larson R, et al. Phase III randomized multicenter trial of G-CSF vs. observation for MDS. *Blood.* 1993;82:196a (suppl 1; abstr).

101. Silverman LR, Demakos EP, Peterson BL, et al. Randomized controlled trial of azacitidine in patients with the myelodysplastic syndrome: a study of the cancer and leukemia group B. *J Clin Oncol.* 2002;20:2429-2440. PMID: 12011120.

102. Lübbert M, Suciu S, Baila L, et al. Low-dose decitabine versus best supportive care in elderly patients with intermediate- or high-risk myelodysplastic syndrome (MDS) ineligible for intensive chemotherapy: final results of the randomized phase III study of the European Organisation for Research and Treatment of Cancer Leukemia Group and the German MDS Study Group. *J Clin Oncol.* 2011;29:1987-1996. PMID: 21483003.

103. Molldrem JJ, Leifer E, Bahceci E, et al. Antithymocyte globulin for treatment of the bone marrow failure associated with myelodysplastic syndromes. *Ann Intern Med.* 2002;137:156-163. PMID: 12160363.

104. Estey EH, Thall PF, Cortes JE, et al. Comparison of idarubicin + ara-C-, fludarabine + ara-C-, and topotecan + ara-C-based regimens in treatment of newly diagnosed acute myeloid leukemia, refractory anemia with excess blasts in transformation, or refractory anemia with excess blasts. *Blood.* 2001;98:3575-3583. PMID: 11739159.

105. Appelbaum FR, Anderson J. Allogeneic bone marrow transplantation for myelodysplastic syndrome: outcomes analysis according to IPSS score. *Leukemia.* 1998;12 (suppl 1):S25-S29. PMID: 9777891.

106. Deeg HJ, Storer B, Slattery JT, et al. Conditioning with targeted busulfan and cyclophosphamide for hemopoietic stem cell transplantation from related and unrelated donors in patients with myelodysplastic syndrome. *Blood.* 2002;100:1201-1207. PMID: 12149198.

107. Oliansky DM, Antin JH, Bennett JM, et al. The role of cytotoxic therapy with hematopoietic stem cell transplantation in the therapy of myelodysplastic syndromes: an evidence-based review. *Biol Blood Marrow Transplant.* 2009;15:137-172. PMID: 19167676.

108. Koreth J, Pidala J, Perez WS, et al. Role of reduced-intensity conditioning allogeneic hematopoietic stem-cell transplantation in older patients with de novo myelodysplastic syndromes: an international collaborative decision analysis. *J Clin Oncol.* 2013;31:2662-2670. PMID: 23797000.

109. Savage DG, Antman KH. Imatinib mesylate–a new oral targeted therapy. *N Engl J Med.* 2002;346:683-693. PMID: 11870247.

110. Druker BJ, Talpaz M, Resta DJ, et al. Efficacy and safety of a specific inhibitor of the BCR-ABL tyrosine kinase in chronic myeloid leukemia. *N Engl J Med.* 2001;344:1031-1037. PMID: 11287972.

111. O'Brien SG, Guilhot F, Larson RA, et al. Imatinib compared with interferon and low-dose cytarabine for newly diagnosed chronic-phase chronic myeloid leukemia. *N Engl J Med.* 2003;348:994-1004. PMID: 12637609.

112. Druker BJ, Sawyers CL, Kantarjian H, et al. Activity of a specific inhibitor of the BCR-ABL tyrosine kinase in the blast crisis of chronic myeloid leukemia and acute lymphoblastic leukemia with the Philadelphia chromosome. *N Engl J Med.* 2001;344:1038-1042. PMID: 11287973.

113. Hughes TP, Kaeda J, Branford S, et al. Frequency of major molecular responses to imatinib or interferon alfa plus cytarabine in newly diagnosed chronic myeloid leukemia. *N Engl J Med.* 2003;349:1423-1432. PMID: 14534335.

114. Mahon FX, Réa D, Guilhot J, et al. Discontinuation of imatinib in patients with chronic myeloid leukaemia who have maintained complete molecular remission for at least 2 years: the prospective, multicentre Stop Imatinib (STIM) trial. *Lancet Oncol.* 2010;11:1029-1035. PMID: 20965785.

115. Cortes JE, Baccarani M, Guilhot F, et al. Phase III, randomized, open-label study of daily imatinib mesylate 400 mg versus 800 mg in patients with newly diagnosed, previously untreated chronic myeloid leukemia in chronic phase using molecular end points: tyrosine kinase inhibitor optimization and selectivity study. *J Clin Oncol.* 2010;28:424-430. PMID: 20008622.

116. Simonsson B, Gedde-Dahl T, Markevärn B, et al. Combination of pegylated IFN-2b with imatinib increases molecular response rates in patients with low- or intermediate-risk chronic myeloid leukemia. *Blood.* 2011;118:3228-3235. PMID: 21685374.

117. Cortes J, Quintás-Cardama A, Jones D, et al. Immune modulation of minimal residual disease in early chronic phase chronic myelogenous leukemia: a randomized trial of frontline high-dose imatinib mesylate with or without pegylated interferon alpha-2b and granulocyte-macrophage colony-stimulating factor. *Cancer.* 2011;117:572-580. PMID: 20886606.

118. Gorre ME, Mohammed M, Ellwood K, et al. Clinical resistance to STI-571 cancer therapy caused by BCR-ABL gene mutation or amplification. *Science.* 2001;293:876-880. PMID: 11423618.

119. Saglio G, Kim DW, Issaragrisil S, et al. Nilotinib versus imatinib for newly diagnosed chronic myeloid leukemia. *N Engl J Med.* 2010;362:2251-2259. PMID: 20525993.

120. Kantarjian H, Shah NP, Hochhaus A, et al. Dasatinib versus imatinib in newly diagnosed chronic-phase chronic myeloid leukemia. *N Engl J Med.* 2010;362:2260-2270. PMID: 20525995.

121. Khoury HJ, Cortes JE, Kantarjian HM, et al. Bosutinib is active in chronic phase chronic myeloid leukemia after imatinib and dasatinib and/or nilotinib therapy failure. *Blood.* 2012;119:3403-3412. PMID: 22371878.

122. Cortes JE, Kantarjian H, Shah NP, et al. Ponatinib in refractory Philadelphia chromosome-positive leukemias. *N Engl J Med.* 2012;367:2075-2088. PMID: 23190221.

123. O'Dwyer ME, Mauro MJ, Blasdel C, et al. Clonal evolution and lack of cytogenetic response are adverse prognostic factors for hematologic relapse of chronic phase CML patients treated with imatinib mesylate. *Blood.* 2004;103:451-455. PMID: 14512312.

124. Bacher U, Hochhaus A, Berger U, et al. Clonal aberrations in Philadelphia chromosome negative hematopoiesis in patients with chronic myeloid leukemia treated with imatinib or interferon alpha. *Leukemia.* 2005;19:460-463. PMID: 15625554.

125. Baccarani M, Cortes J, Pane F, et al. Chronic myeloid leukemia: an update of concepts and management recommendations of European LeukemiaNet. *J Clin Oncol.* 2009;27:6041-6051. PMID: 19884523.

126. Baccarani M, Deininger MW, Rosti G, et al. European LeukemiaNet recommendations for the management of chronic myeloid leukemia: 2013. *Blood.* 2013;122:872-884. PMID: 23803709.

127. Radich JP, Gooley T, Bensinger W, et al. HLA-matched related hematopoietic cell transplantation for chronic-phase CML using a targeted busulfan and cyclophosphamide preparative regimen. *Blood.* 2003;102:31-35. PMID: 12595317.

128. Oehler VG, Gooley T, Snyder DS, et al. The effects of imatinib mesylate treatment before allogeneic transplantation for chronic myeloid leukemia. *Blood.* 2007;109:1782-1789. PMID: 17062727.

129. Hansen JA, Gooley TA, Martin PJ, et al. Bone marrow transplants from unrelated donors for patients with chronic myeloid leukemia. *N Engl J Med.* 1998;338:962-968. PMID: 9521984.

130. Radich JP, Gehly G, Gooley T, et al. Polymerase chain reaction detection of the BCR-ABL fusion transcript after allogeneic marrow transplantation for chronic myeloid leukemia: results and implications in 346 patients. *Blood.* 1995;85:2632-2638. PMID: 7727789.

131. Carpenter PA, Snyder DS, Flowers ME, et al. Prophylactic administration of imatinib after hematopoietic cell transplantation for high-risk Philadelphia chromosome-positive leukemia. *Blood.* 2007;109:2791-2793. PMID: 17119111.

132. Amercian Cancer Society. *Cancer Facts and Figures 2006.* Atlanta, GA: American Cancer Society; 2006.

133. Yuille MR, Matutes E, Marossy A, et al. Familial chronic lymphocytic leukaemia: a survey and review of published studies. *Br J Haematol.* 2000;109:794-799. PMID: 10929032.

134. Hallek M, Cheson BD, Catovsky D, et al. Guidelines for the diagnosis and treatment of chronic lymphocytic leukemia: a report from the International Workshop on Chronic Lymphocytic Leukemia updating the National Cancer Institute-Working Group 1996 guidelines. *Blood.* 2008;111:5446-5456. PMID: 18216293.

135. Döhner H, Stilgenbauer S, Benner A, et al. Genomic aberrations and survival in chronic lymphocytic leukemia. *N Engl J Med.* 2000;343:1910-1916. PMID: 11136261.

136. Rosenwald A, Alizadeh AA, Widhopf G, et al. Relation of gene expression phenotype to immunoglobulin mutation genotype in B cell chronic lymphocytic leukemia. *J Exp Med.* 2001;194:1639-1647. PMID: 11733578.

137. Chen L, Widhopf G, Huynh L, et al. Expression of ZAP-70 is associated with increased B-cell receptor signaling in chronic lymphocytic leukemia. *Blood.* 2002;100:4609-4614. PMID: 12393534.

138. Kröber A, Seiler T, Benner A, et al. V(H) mutation status, CD38 expression level, genomic aberrations, and survival in chronic lymphocytic leukemia. *Blood.* 2002;100:1410-1416. PMID: 12149225.

139. CLL Trialists' Collaborative Group. Chemotherapeutic options in chronic lymphocytic leukemia: a meta-analysis of the randomized trials. CLL Trialists' Collaborative Group. *J Natl Cancer Inst.* 1999;91:861-868. PMID: 10340906.

140. Gribben JG, O'Brien S. Update on therapy of chronic lymphocytic leukemia. *J Clin Oncol.* 2011;29:544-550. PMID: 21220603.

141. Dighiero G, Hamblin TJ. Chronic lymphocytic leukaemia. *Lancet.* 2008;371:1017-1029. PMID: 18358929.

142. Robak T, Dmoszynska A, Solal-Céligny P, et al. Rituximab plus fludarabine and cyclophosphamide prolongs progression-free survival compared with fludarabine and cyclophosphamide alone in previously treated chronic lymphocytic leukemia. *J Clin Oncol.* 2010;28:1756-1765. PMID: 20194844.

143. Kay NE, Geyer SM, Call TG, et al. Combination chemoimmunotherapy with pentostatin, cyclophosphamide, and rituximab shows significant clinical activity with low accompanying toxicity in previously untreated B chronic lymphocytic leukemia. *Blood.* 2007;109:405-411. PMID: 17008537.

144. Fischer K, Cramer P, Busch R, et al. Bendamustine in combination with rituximab for previously untreated patients with chronic lymphocytic leukemia: a multicenter phase II trial of the German Chronic Lymphocytic Leukemia Study Group. *J Clin Oncol.* 2012;30:3209-3216. PMID: 22869884.

145. Bowen DA, Call TG, Jenkins GD, et al. Methylprednisolone-rituximab is an effective salvage therapy for patients with relapsed chronic lymphocytic leukemia including those with unfavorable cytogenetic features. *Leuk Lymphoma.* 2007;48:2412-2417. PMID: 18067017.

146. Wierda WG, Kipps TJ, Mayer J, et al. Ofatumumab as single-agent CD20 immunotherapy in fludarabine-refractory chronic lymphocytic leukemia. *J Clin Oncol.* 2010;28:1749-1755. PMID: 20194866.

147. Morrison VA, Rai KR, Peterson BL, et al. Impact of therapy with chlorambucil, fludarabine, or fludarabine plus chlorambucil on infections in patients with chronic lymphocytic leukemia: Intergroup Study Cancer and Leukemia Group B 9011. *J Clin Oncol.* 2001;19:3611-3621. PMID: 11504743.

148. Morrison VA, Rai KR, Peterson BL, et al. Therapy-related myeloid leukemias are observed in patients with chronic lymphocytic leukemia after treatment with fludarabine and chlorambucil: results of an intergroup study, cancer and leukemia group B 9011. *J Clin Oncol.* 2002;20:3878-3884. PMID: 12228208.

148a. Byrd JC, Brown JR, O'Brien S, et al. Ibruntinib versus ofatumumab in previously treated chronic lymphoid leukemia. *N Engl J Med.* Epub 2014 May 31. PMID: 24881631.

149. Doney KC, Chauncey T, Appelbaum FR. Allogeneic related donor hematopoietic stem cell transplantation for treatment of chronic lymphocytic leukemia. *Bone Marrow Transplant.* 2002;29:817-823. PMID: 12058231.

150. Michallet M, Archimbaud E, Bandini G, et al. HLA-identical sibling bone marrow transplantation in younger patients with chronic lymphocytic leukemia. European Group for Blood and Marrow Transplantation and the International Bone Marrow Transplant Registry. *Ann Intern Med.* 1996;124:311-315. PMID: 8554226.

151. Khouri IF, Przepiorka D, van Besien K, et al. Allogeneic blood or marrow transplantation for chronic lymphocytic leukaemia: timing of transplantation and potential effect of fludarabine on acute graft-versus-host disease. *Br J Haematol.* 1997;97:466-473. PMID: 9163617.

152. Sorror ML, Maris MB, Sandmaier BM, et al. Hematopoietic cell transplantation after nonmyeloablative conditioning for advanced chronic lymphocytic leukemia. *J Clin Oncol.* 2005;23:3819-3829. PMID: 15809448.

153. Osterborg A, Brandberg Y, Molostova V, et al. Randomized, double-blind, placebo-controlled trial of recombinant human erythropoietin, epoetin Beta, in hematologic malignancies. *J Clin Oncol.* 2002;20:2486-2494. PMID: 12011126.

154. Hillmen P. Using the biology of chronic lymphocytic leukemia to choose treatment. *Hematology Am Soc Hematol Educ Program.* 2011;2011:104-109. PMID: 22160020.

155. Tiacci E, Trifonov V, Schiavoni G, et al. BRAF mutations in hairy-cell leukemia. *N Engl J Med.* 2011;364:2305-2315. PMID: 21663470.

156. Flinn IW, Kopecky KJ, Foucar MK, et al. Long-term follow-up of remission, duration, mortality, and second malignancies in hairy cell leukemia patients treated with pentostatin. *Blood.* 2000;96:2981-2986. PMID: 11049974.

157. Kreitman RJ, Wilson WH, Bergeron K, et al. Efficacy of the anti-CD22 recombinant immunotoxin BL22 in chemotherapy-resistant hairy-cell leukemia. *N Engl J Med.* 2001;345:241-247. PMID: 11474661.

158. Jaffe ES, Harris NL, Stein H, et al. Classification of lymphoid neoplasms: the microscope as a tool for disease discovery. *Blood.* 2008;112:4384-4399. PMID: 19029456.

159. Keating MJ, Cazin B, Coutré S, et al. Campath-1H treatment of T-cell prolymphocytic leukemia in patients for whom at least one prior chemotherapy regimen has failed. *J Clin Oncol.* 2002;20:205-213. PMID: 11773171.

16

LYMPHOMAS

Oliver W. Press, MD, PhD

Updates from 2012

▶ Over 90% of patients with lymphoplasmacytic lymphomas possess a somatic mutation leading to an amino acid change (L265P) in the MYD88 protein (Treon SP, *N Engl J Med* 2012).

▶ New targeted therapies including ibrutinib (a Bruton's tyrosine kinase inhibitor) and idelalisib (a PI3 kinase delta inhibitor) have shown outstanding activity in treating patients with relapsed mantle cell lymphoma, chronic lymphocytic leukemia/small lymphocytic leukemia, lymphoplasmacytic lymphomas, and other histologies (Wang ML, *N Engl J Med* 2013; Byrd JC, *N Engl J Med* 2013).

▶ Dose-adjusted EPOCH plus rituximab has demonstrated outstanding activity in treating primary mediastinal B-cell lymphoma and Burkitt lymphoma (Dunleavy K, *N Engl J Med* 2013).

Lymphomas are among the most diverse and most curable of all human malignancies. The study of lymphomas has facilitated the identification of many basic principles of oncogenesis (acquired somatic mutations because of translocation of oncogenes) and the discovery of cell cycle regulators and effectors of apoptosis, and it has led to major breakthroughs in the management of cancer (e.g., establishment of monoclonal antibodies as effective anticancer therapies). Lymphomas are collectively responsible for an estimated 79,000 new cases of cancer and 20,000 deaths annually.[1] There are two major groups of lymphomas, Hodgkin lymphomas (HLs) and non-Hodgkin lymphomas (NHLs), as outlined below.

HODGKIN LYMPHOMA
EPIDEMIOLOGY AND ETIOLOGY

HL is a lymphoid neoplasm that is diagnosed in approximately 9,060 U.S. patients annually and causes approximately 1,090 deaths each year in the United States.[1] HL has a bimodal incidence distribution with respect to age at diagnosis with an incidence peak in young adults and a second peak in elderly individuals. The etiology of HL is not known. There is an association with the Epstein-Barr virus (EBV), and the likelihood of developing HL is increased 3-fold for people with a history of infectious mononucleosis. HL nodes show evidence of EBV DNA in the genome of the Reed-Sternberg cell in 30% to 80% of cases. However, because many cases of HL are EBV-negative, controversy remains as to whether there is a causal relationship. There is an increased frequency of the disease in patients with AIDS[2] and patients who have had bone marrow transplantation. In patients infected with HIV or AIDS, HL tends to involve extranodal sites and to exhibit an aggressive clinical course with a poor outcome. There are no clear relationships with environmental exposures, although an increase in the incidence of HL has been reported in wood workers/carpenters, farmers, and meat processors.

CLINICAL PRESENTATION AND CLASSIFICATION OF HL

HL typically presents with painless lymphadenopathy with or without splenomegaly, fevers, drenching night sweats, weight loss and pruritus, or pain in a lymph node–bearing area that is associated with alcohol consumption. The diagnosis is best established by an excisional lymph node biopsy demonstrating large, atypical lymphoblasts surrounded by a heterogeneous infiltrate of non-neoplastic inflammatory and accessory cells. The World Health Organization (WHO) classification of lymphomas distinguishes two major subtypes of HL, namely, classical HL and nodular lymphocyte predominant HL (NLPHL).

CLASSICAL HL

Classical HL currently represents 95% of all cases of HL and is characterized pathologically by the presence of bizarre monoclonal lymphoid cells that may be either mononuclear (Hodgkin cells) or multinucleate (Reed-Sternberg cells). The malignant Hodgkin and Reed-Sternberg (HRS) cells of classical HL express CD15 and CD30 surface antigens but usually not typical B-cell markers such as surface immunoglobulin, CD20, CD79a, or the common leukocyte antigen CD45.[3] The B-cell origin of HRS cells is nevertheless demonstrable by the expression of the B-cell–specific activator protein derived from the *PAX-5* gene in 90% of cases.[3] Immunoglobulin genes are rearranged in 98% of HRS cells but are not transcribed as a result of the absence of the transcription factor Oct-2 and its co-activator BOB-1. The malignant (HRS) cells are typically surrounded by a heterogeneous infiltrate of reactive T and B lymphocytes, eosinophils, macrophages, fibroblasts, and variable amounts of collagen deposition (sclerosis).[3]

Four discrete histologic subtypes of classical HL are recognized by the WHO classification based on the relative proportions of infiltrating small lymphocytes and of HRS cells and the amount of collagen (sclerosis) in the biopsy. All four subtypes of classical HL are evaluated and managed similarly, lessening the importance of subclassification of classical HL.

Nodular-Sclerosis Subtype

More than 60% of patients with classical HL present with the nodular-sclerosis subtype, which is most common in women, adolescents, and young adults. At the time of presentation, patients characteristically have an anterior mediastinal mass that may produce chest discomfort, dyspnea, or cough. The histologic pattern of nodular-sclerosis HL is at least partially nodular with fibrous bands. Diffuse areas and necrosis also may be present. HRS cells in nodular-sclerosis HL are typically giant cells with multilobulated nuclei surrounded by a clear area that is an artifact of formalin fixation, leading to their designation as lacunar variants. Nucleoli are typically less prominent than in the classical HRS cell. The tumor cells are CD30+, CD15+ or CD15- and CD45-. Epithelial membrane antigen expression is rare.

Mixed-Cellularity HL

Mixed-cellularity HL represents approximately 20% of cases and is more common in men. The histologic appearance is of a diffuse or vaguely nodular infiltrate. HRS cells are primarily of the classic variety. The cells are CD30+, CD15+ or CD15-, and CD45-. In contrast to the other histologic subtypes, EBV genomic DNA is detectable in 60% to 70% of mixed-cellularity HL. Patients tend to present with disseminated disease, and the clinical course may be aggressive; however, this subtype is still curable.

Lymphocyte-Rich Classic HL

The growth pattern in lymphocyte-rich classic HL usually is nodular but may be diffuse, with a phenotype of CD30+, CD15+ or CD15-, and CD20+ or CD20-. This subtype is more common in older males and presents at an early disease stage. Other findings are similar to NLPHL, except that patients are slightly older (age 40) at the time of diagnosis, and the presenting mass is more frequently located in the mediastinum. Late relapses are less common but more often fatal.

Lymphocyte-Depleted HL

Lymphocyte-depleted HL accounts for less than 5% of cases. It occurs more often in older men and in people who are infected with HIV. It also is more common in nonindustrialized countries. At the time of presentation, patients have a higher incidence of abdominal adenopathy and less peripheral adenopathy than is found with other types of HL. Hepatosplenomegaly may be prominent, and the bone marrow often is infiltrated with lymphoma. The histologic appearance of the lymph nodes is characterized by a diffuse infiltrate, which may appear hypocellular. HRS cells (CD30+, CD15+ or CD15-, and CD45-) are plentiful and often have a malignant appearance.

NODULAR LYMPHOCYTE PREDOMINANT HL

NLPHL is a distinctly different indolent B-cell neoplasm that is distinguished from classical HL by histologic and immunophenotypic features, including the presence of large neoplastic cells known as "popcorn" or "lymphocytic and histiocytic" cells (L and H cells) residing in large nodular meshworks of follicular dendritic cell processes filled with non-neoplastic lymphocytes. In marked contrast to the HRS cells of classical HL, the malignant L and H cells of NLPHL express typical B-cell surface antigens, including CD20 and CD79a and the common leukocyte antigen CD45, but do not express CD15 or CD30. NLPHL is responsible for approximately 5% of all cases of HL, typically affects men between age 30 and 50, usually presents with localized lymphadenopathy (stage I to II), progresses slowly, and is associated with prolonged survival despite frequent relapses.[4] Although some investigators have suggested that NLPHL should be considered a type of NHL rather than HL, genome-wide expression studies of microdissected L and H cells do not support this contention. Indeed, the gene expression signature of the L and H cells of NLPHL shows a surprising similarity to the gene expression signature of the HRS cell of classical HL and much less similarity to indolent B-cell lymphoma cells.[5]

WORKUP AND STAGING OF HL

The National Comprehensive Cancer Network has established standards for the evaluation and therapy of patients with HL.[6] Recommended diagnostic tests include a history; physical examination; excisional lymph node biopsy with evaluation for histology and immunophenotype; complete blood cell count with differential; and chemistry panel including liver function tests, albumin, lactate dehydrogenase (LDH), erythrocyte sedimentation rate, chest radiograph, computed tomography (CT) of the chest abdomen and pelvis, fluorodeoxyglucose positron emission tomography (FDG-PET), and fertility counseling. Other tests useful in selected cases include pulmonary function tests, determination of the cardiac ejection fraction, HIV testing, neck CT scans, and vaccination for encapsulated bacteria (if splenectomy or splenic irradiation is contemplated). Bone marrow biopsies are no longer considered essential for staging of HL, provided FDG-PET imaging is performed. After completion of the diagnostic workup, the extent of involvement with HL is designated using the Ann Arbor staging criteria (Table 16-1).

PROGNOSTIC FACTORS IN HL

A variety of prognostic factors have been described for patients with HL. Proven prognostic factors for patients with early-stage HL include bulky disease (greater than 10 cm in diameter or greater than one-third the mediastinal diameter), elevated erythrocyte sedimentation rate, more than two to three sites of nodal disease, presence of any extranodal sites, and elevated erythrocyte sedimentation rate.[6] For advanced HL, an international effort was organized to characterize prognostic factors in a large number of patients.[7] Data from 23 cooperative groups and treatment centers were collected for 5,141 patients with advanced disease, and patients were treated with modern therapy according to a defined protocol. Seven factors were identified, each of which reduced tumor control by 7% to 8% at 5 years (Table 16-2).

Table 16-1 Ann Arbor Staging System*§

Stage	Extent of Disease
I	Involvement of a single lymph node region or lymphoid structure
II	Involvement of two or more lymph node regions confined to one side of the diagram
III	Involvement of two or more lymph node regions on both sides of the diagram
IV	Disseminated involvement of a deep, visceral organ (bone marrow, liver, etc.)

*Each stage is subdivided into A and B substages depending on whether B symptoms (fever higher than 38° C on two or more occasions unrelated to infection, unintended loss of 10% or more of the body weight within 6 months, and/or drenching sweats) are absent (A) or present (B).

§Localized involvement of an extranodal site by direct extension from an involved lymph node is designated by the subscript "E" and does not qualify for designation as stage IV.

Table 16-2 Independent Prognostic Factors for Advanced HL[7]

- Age older than 45
- Male sex
- Stage IV disease
- Serum albumin levels less than 4.0 mg/dL
- Hemoglobin levels less than 10.5 mg/dL
- White blood count higher than 15,000/μL
- Lymphocytes less than 600/μL and/or a lymphocyte count less than 8% of the white cell count

Table 16-3 International Prognostic Factor Study Results[7]

Number of Factors	Proportion of Population	5-Year FFP
0	7%	84%
1	22%	77%
2	29%	67%
3	23%	60%
4	12%	51%
5+	7%	42%

Abbreviation: FFP, freedom from progression.

Freedom from progression (FFP) at 5 years was related to the number of factors present (Table 16-3). The 5-year FFP for patients with three or more factors (42% of the population) was 55%, compared with 74% for patients with up to two factors (58% of the population). However, the effect of the HL International Prognostic Score (IPS) developed by this working group has been less than anticipated, and its predictive value has been challenged.[8] Only 19% of patients with HL have four or more risk factors as defined by this index; the other 81% of patients have a progression-free survival (PFS) rate at least 60% with standard doxorubicin/bleomycin/vinblastine/dacarbazine (ABVD) chemotherapy. Attempts to pursue risk-adapted therapy based on the IPS have been plagued by concerns that a substantial fraction of patients will be overtreated using algorithms based on the IPS score. Recent studies have demonstrated that interim FDG-PET after two cycles of ABVD chemotherapy is superior to the IPS in predicting patient outcome (PFS, overall survival [OS]).[9]

More recently, studies have shown that heavy infiltration of HL biopsies with macrophages (detected by immunohistocytochemical staining for CD68), is associated with poor outcome, presumably because of secretion of immunosuppressive cytokines.[10] Furthermore, a 23-gene expression signature has recently been shown to have major prognostic power in patients with classical HL.[11]

FDG-PET IN EVALUATION OF HL

FDG-PET has been used in HL at diagnosis for staging, during treatment to assess response and to evaluate residual masses, and after completion of treatment for prediction of relapse.[12,13] FDG-PET is a functional imaging technique that relies on the detection of a higher rate of glucose metabolism in malignant cells compared with normal cells. Conventional radiologic methods (e.g., CT) have significant limitations in assessing response to therapy. A reduction in tumor size is used as the most important determinant; however, this is not an accurate predictor of outcome as the malignant cells in HL often comprise only a small proportion of the tumor volume, and it takes time for a reduction in tumor size to occur. Thus, size reduction cannot be used accurately for response assessment or therapy adjustment until later in the treatment course. FDG-PET evaluates metabolic changes—instead of morphologic or volume changes—providing an earlier assessment of tumor response during therapy.

Several studies have assessed the role of interim FDG-PET in HL response assessment.[12-14] One of the most influential of these studies reported the results of PET after two cycles of ABVD.[15] The scan was positive in 20 of 108 patients, of whom 17 experienced disease progression during therapy, one experienced disease relapse, and two remained in complete remission. By contrast, 85 of 88 patients (97%) with a negative scan remained in complete remission. These studies suggest that early PET is predictive of complete response and that interim assessment of response by PET is superior to assessment after completion of treatment for prediction of disease progression. Thus, FDG-PET is a strong and independent predictor of PFS and allows early identification of those patients with a suboptimal disease

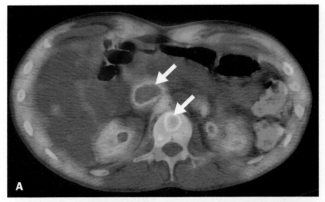

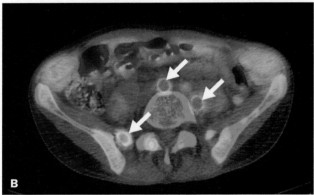

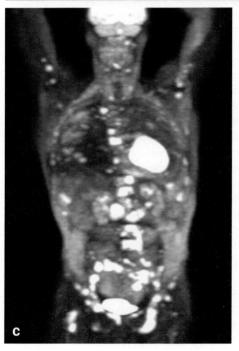

Fig. 16-1 PET/CT scans of a patient with advanced Hodgkin lymphoma showing multiple areas of hypermetabolic uptake in lymph nodes and spine.

FDG-PET fusion image of thorax and pelvis are shown in transverse sections in **A** and **B**, respectively. White arrows show several of the most conspicuous pathologic lesions. **C** shows a longitudinal view of the FDG-PET image alone, without CT scan superimposition.

Images courtesy of Gregory Wiseman, MD; Mayo Clinic.

response to initial therapy (Figs. 16-1 and 16-2). Several ongoing clinical trials are currently being conducted to determine the proper utilization of interim FDG-PET and whether early adjustment of treatment regimen intensity based on the findings of interim FDG-PET will improve patient outcomes.[16,17] In contrast to the clear utility of FDG-PET/CT in initial staging and post-treatment response assessment, and its emerging role in interim response assessment, PET has little utility in routine surveillance or monitoring of patients documented to be in complete remission at the end of therapy.

THERAPY FOR CLASSICAL HL

Stage IA and IIA

Patients with nonbulky stage IA and IIA HL are considered to have early-stage disease and typically are treated with short courses (two to four cycles) of ABVD followed by involved field radiotherapy, with a cure rate of 90% to 95%.[18] Recent randomized controlled trials suggest that as few as two cycles of ABVD followed by 20 Gy of involved field radiotherapy is sufficient for patients with two or fewer sites of disease, no masses larger than 10 cm, a normal erythrocyte sedimentation rate, and no extranodal sites of disease.[19] An alternative approach is to eliminate radiotherapy altogether and treat with three to six cycles of ABVD to avert the increased risk of secondary malignancies associated with chest radiotherapy, especially breast cancer in young women. Canellos et al treated 71 patients with early-stage, favorable HL with six cycles of ABVD without radiotherapy and achieved a 5-year failure-free survival (FFS) rate of 92%.[20]

Unfavorable prognostic factors for patients with locally advanced stage I/II HL include large tumor bulk (defined as a mass 10 cm or larger in diameter or more than one-third of the transthoracic diameter measured at the diaphragms), an erythrocyte sedimentation rate of at least 50, three or more sites of tumor involvement, the presence of B symptoms, and the presence of extranodal sites.[6] Such patients require more intensive therapy than patients with low-risk stage IA/IIA HL. A recent randomized clinical trial compared four cycles of either ABVD or bleomycin/etoposide/doxorubicin/cyclophosphamide/vincristine/procarbazine/prednisone (BEACOPP)$_{baseline}$ followed by either 20 Gy or 30 Gy of involved field radiotherapy for early-stage "unfavorable" HL. In this study, four cycles of ABVD followed by 30 Gy of radiotherapy was the best approach, affording an 85% rate of "freedom from treatment failure" and an OS rate of approximately 95% after 5 years, while maintaining a favorable toxicity profile.[21]

Stage III/IV

Patients with stage III/IV disease are considered to have advanced HL and require treatment with six to eight cycles of combination chemotherapy. The development of the mechlorethamine/vincristine/procarbazine/prednisone (MOPP) regimen in the 1960s permitted physicians to cure 50% to 60% of patients with advanced-stage HL for the first time and represented a major milestone in medical oncology.[22] However, secondary malignancies including acute myeloid leukemia (AML)

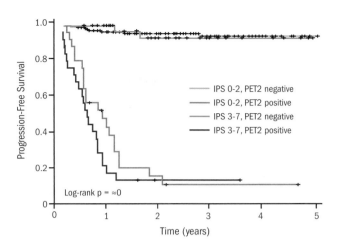

Fig. 16-2 Kaplan-Meier plot showing the progression-free survival according to IPS group and PET results after two cycles of ABVD.

Abbreviations: IPS, International Prognostic Score; PET, positron emission tomography; ABVD, doxorubicin/bleomycin/vinblastine/dacarbazine.

Reproduced with permission from Gallamini A, Hutchings M, Rigacci L, et al. Early interim 2-[18F]fluoro-2-deoxy-D-glucose positron emission tomography is prognostically superior to international prognostic score in advanced-stage Hodgkin's lymphoma: a report from a joint Italian-Danish study. J Clin Oncol. 2007;25(24):3746-3752.

and infertility were common complications of MOPP and its variants.[23] The ABVD regimen was developed by Bonadonna and colleagues in Milan in the 1970s, containing drugs considered to be non–cross-resistant with those in MOPP.[24] Randomized trials proved that ABVD was more effective and less toxic than MOPP,[25,26] with 5-year PFS rates of 60% to 70% in most studies of advanced HL. Alternating (MOPP-ABVD) and hybrid (MOPP-ABV) regimens were developed but proved to be no more effective than ABVD alone and were more toxic.[25,27-29] Based on these studies, ABVD became the standard of care in the United States and most other countries. Administration of full doses of ABVD without treatment delays, dose reductions, or growth factors appears to optimize cure rates with this regimen.[30,31]

Several groups have subsequently developed novel, augmented regimens for the treatment of advanced HL to increase the dose intensity of chemotherapy and hopefully to improve the cure rate. Stanford V is an abbreviated 12-week course of treatment in which myelosuppressive and nonmyelosuppressive treatments are alternated weekly.[32] The dose intensity of individual drugs is maintained or increased, but the cumulative doses of bleomycin (30 U/m²) and doxorubicin (150 mg/m²) are reduced in Stanford V compared with ABVD, procarbazine is omitted, and the cumulative dose of mustard is reduced to 18 mg/m² to reduce pulmonary and cardiac dysfunction, sterility, and leukemogenesis. Consolidative irradiation (36 Gy) is given to sites of bulky disease (larger than 5 cm) or macroscopic splenic disease. In a study involving 142 patients with stage III or IV disease or bulky stage I/II disease treated with Stanford V, the 5-year FFP rate was 89%, and OS was 96% after a median follow-up of 5.4 years.[32] However, three prospective, randomized multicenter clinical trials have failed to demonstrate an improvement in PFS or OS for patients treated with Stanford V compared with those treated with ABVD.[33-35] Since Stanford V is more myelotoxic than ABVD and not more effective, ABVD is preferable in the opinion of most authorities.

The BEACOPP regimen devised by the German Hodgkin Lymphoma Study Group is another augmented regimen for HL. It substitutes etoposide for dacarbazine and vinblastine and encompasses two main intensification principles: dose escalation of the putative most important drugs (cyclophosphamide, etoposide, and doxorubicin) and time intensification accomplished by shortening the respective chemotherapy cycles from 4 to 3 weeks.[36] Two different variants of BEACOPP were initially designed: BEACOPP in baseline dosage (BEACOPP-21, BEACOPP$_{baseline}$, or BEACOPP$_{standard}$) and BEACOPP in escalated dosage with granulocyte colony-stimulating factor support (escalated BEACOPP-21 or BEACOPP$_{escalated}$). A large randomized clinical trial randomly assigned 1,201 patients between ages 15 and 65 with stage IIB, III, or IV HL to either cyclophosphamide/vincristine/procarbazine/prednisone (COPP)-ABVD (considered the standard of care), BEACOPP$_{standard}$, or BEACOPP$_{escalated}$.[36,37] The majority of patients also received consolidative radiotherapy. Accrual was terminated early in the COPP-ABVD arm by the data and safety monitoring board because of inferior survival and PFS compared with the two BEACOPP arms (Table 16-4). Hematologic toxicity was similar between BEACOPP$_{standard}$ and COPP-ABVD but greatly increased with BEACOPP$_{escalated}$, with grade 4 leukopenia seen in 90% of patients assigned to receive BEACOPP$_{escalated}$, compared with 19% for COPP-ABVD. Grade 4 thrombocytopenia was seen in 47% of patients with BEACOPP$_{escalated}$ compared with 2% of patients receiving COPP-ABVD.[36] Myelodysplasia or secondary AML was seen in one of 260 evaluable patients treated with COPP-ABVD compared with seven of 469 treated with BEACOPP$_{standard}$ and 14 of 466 with BEACOPP$_{escalated}$.[37] Most patients receiving BEACOPP regimens will become infertile, compared with less than 5% of patients who receive ABVD.[23,25,38]

A subsequent randomized study in Germany (HD9) compared COPP-ABVD with BEACOPP$_{standard}$ in 75 elderly patients between ages 66 and 75.[39] There were no differences in complete remission rates (76%), OS (50% at 5 years), or freedom from treatment failure (46% at 5 years) between the two arms on this study, but 21% of elderly patients treated with BEACOPP$_{standard}$ died of acute toxicity compared with 6% treated with COPP-ABVD. The BEACOPP regimens are therefore not recommended for patients older than age 65.

Although the BEACOPP$_{escalated}$ regimen has become the standard of care for advanced HL in Germany, the regimen has been infrequently employed in the United States or other countries because of concerns about its acute and late toxicities. Although BEACOPP$_{escalated}$ may result in improved survival, it is unknown whether the increased toxicity of this regimen (3% treatment-induced mortality, 80% to 100% infertility, risk of myelodysplasia) can be justified for patients with low-risk disease. Two recent randomized controlled trials compared the efficacy of ABVD to BEACOPP$_{escalated}$ in patients with advanced-stage classical HL.[40,41] Although the findings of these studies are controversial, both studies suggest that PFS and remission duration are prolonged with BEACOPP compared to ABVD. However, toxicities were greater with BEACOPP in both studies, and OS

	COPP-ABVD	BEACOPP$_{standard}$	BEACOPP$_{escalated}$
Table 16-4 Results of a Randomized Controlled Trial of COPP-ABVD versus BEACOPP$_{standard}$ versus BEACOPP$_{escalated}$ for Advanced HL[36]			
5-year freedom from treatment failure (%)	68	76	88
5-year overall survival (%)	83	87	92
10-year freedom from treatment failure* (%)	64	70	82
10-year overall survival§ (%)	75	80	86

*$p < 0.0001$ for BEACOPP$_{escalated}$ vs. COPP-ABVD or BEACOPP$_{standard}$.

§$p = 0.19$ for COPP-ABVD vs. BEACOPP$_{standard}$; $p < 0.0001$ for BEACOPP$_{standard}$ vs. BEACOPP$_{escalated}$; $p < 0.0001$ for COPP-ABVD vs. BEACOPP$_{escalated}$.

Abbreviations: COPP-ABVD, cyclophosphamide/vincristine/procarbazine/prednisone plus doxorubicin/bleomycin/vinblastine/dacarbazine; BEACOPP, bleomycin/etoposide/doxorubicin/cyclophosphamide/vincristine/procarbazine/prednisone.

was not statistically significantly improved with the BEACOPP regimens compared to ABVD.

The Role of Radiotherapy in Advanced HL. The rationale for the use of radiation therapy to consolidate stage III and IV disease treated with induction chemotherapy has been based on observations that relapse frequently occurs in previously involved sites, even for patients with stage IV disease. In view of the reliability of radiation therapy to provide local control, many studies have utilized combined-modality therapy for stage III to IV HL. Despite this sound rationale, randomized cooperative group trials have failed to show a convincing benefit for consolidative radiation for patients in this setting, particularly if FDG-PET is negative at the conclusion of therapy. For example, in the German HD15 trial, 2,182 patients with advanced stage HL were randomly selected to receive one of three BEACOPP regimens. Patients with a persistent mass larger than 2.5 cm after chemotherapy that was positive on PET received 30 Gy of consolidative radiotherapy, whereas patients with either no residual masses (complete remission) or with persistent masses larger than 2.5 cm that were PET-negative did not receive any radiotherapy. The 5-year PFS was approximately 94% for patients in complete remission (no radiotherapy), approximately 94% for patients with "PET-negative partial remission" (no radiotherapy), and 85% for patients with "PET-positive partial remission" (30 Gy of radiotherapy).[42]

RESIDUAL MASSES IN HL

Approximately 80% of patients with bulky mediastinal or retroperitoneal disease who have an initial response to therapy will have a persistent radiographic abnormality at the conclusion of therapy. In most of these cases, the residual mass represents fibrosis rather than active tumor, and such patients do as well as patients who have a clinical complete response. FDG-PET can be useful to discriminate between fibrosis and active disease in patients with a tumor that had been positive on PET prior to therapy.[12,43] In such cases, additional therapy should not be given unless there are positive findings on biopsy or until there is clear evidence of active disease. For some patients, notably those younger than 25, the mediastinal radiographic density may actually increase within 6 months following therapy. This finding may represent regenerating thymus and can be confused with disease progression, creating a diagnostic dilemma as the thymus may be positive on PET. Careful follow-up with repeat PET or CT is necessary to confirm this possibility and to avoid unnecessary treatment. Therapy may be indicated if the mass continues to enlarge or if disease becomes apparent outside of the irradiated field. Biopsies should be performed in such circumstances to confirm persistent HL.

RELAPSED OR REFRACTORY DISEASE

Although HL is a relatively curable disease, a complete or partial response is never achieved in 10% to 20% of patients, and another 15% to 30% experience disease relapse following an initial complete response. The type of initial therapy given and the duration of the initial response play major roles in determining the appropriate second-line program. The likelihood of long-term disease-free survival (DFS) after treatment with ABVD is 50% to 80% for patients who experience relapse after radiation therapy alone. Late relapses (more than 12 months) after complete response or a durable partial response following initial chemotherapy may occasionally be treated successfully with a different combination chemotherapy. Common second-line chemotherapy regimens for relapsed HL include ifosfamide/carboplatin/etoposide[44]; gemcitabine-based combinations[45]; or chlorambucil/vinblastine/procarbazine/prednisone.[46] Disease will remain in remission after 5 years for approximately 15% of patients whose disease responds to treatment for late relapse.

High-dose therapy with autologous stem cell transplantation (ASCT) is the standard of care for patients with HL who have a disease relapse, particularly those whose disease remains sensitive to chemotherapy. This approach has been associated with a 5-year relapse-free survival rate of 20% to 50%, depending on prognostic factors such as performance status, tumor bulk, and number and type of prior chemotherapy regimens.[47-49] The likelihood of successful transplantation is higher for patients who first received ABVD than for those who received escalated BEACOPP; however, two randomized clinical trials have failed to demonstrate a benefit to up-front high-dose chemotherapy in first remission with autologous stem cell support for the initial treatment of patients with high-risk HL. A recent trial suggests that pretransplant FDG-PET is highly predictive of outcome following ASCT. In this trial, patients with a negative pretransplant PET had an event-free survival (EFS) of over 80%, compared to only 29% for patients with a positive scan (p < 0.001).[50] Non-myeloablative allogeneic stem cell transplantation (alloSCT)

has recently been shown to improve survival for patients who have a disease relapse following ASCT.[51,52]

Brentuximab vedotin is an anti-CD30 monoclonal antibody conjugated to a mitotic spindle inhibitor (auristatin E) that has shown impressive results in patients with HL whose disease recurred after ASCT or who are not candidates for ASCT.[53] In a phase II clinical trial, 96 of 102 patients with relapsed or refractory HL treated with brentuximab vedotin experienced tumor shrinkage, including 75% with objective remissions and 34% with complete remissions.[54] The major toxicity when used as a single agent was peripheral neuropathy. Caution must be used when combining this drug with regimens containing bleomycin because of an increased risk of pulmonary toxicity in this setting.

LATE COMPLICATIONS OF HL THERAPY

As cure rates for HL have steadily improved, more attention has been focused on limiting late toxicities associated with chemotherapy and radiotherapy. The types of adverse events that arise depend on the selection of HL therapy. Radiation therapy alone and ABVD alone are typically associated with a low risk of treatment-related myelodysplasia and secondary leukemia. However, secondary diffuse aggressive NHLs occur with a cumulative risk rate of 4% to 5% at 10 years. The frequency of solid tumors following first-line treatment increases from 2% at 10 years to 13% at 19 years. Radiation therapy, with or without chemotherapy, is the major contributor to the development of solid tumors (e.g., lung and breast cancers, soft tissue sarcomas, melanomas) that typically develop in the irradiated field. Breast cancers that arise following radiotherapy for HL are more often bilateral compared with breast cancers arising in women without a history of HL. Regular breast examination and magnetic resonance imaging or mammography at an early age are recommended as part of routine follow-up care for patients with HL. More than two-thirds of patients who receive mantle radiation will be diagnosed with thyroid disease, including hypothyroidism, Graves disease, silent thyrotoxicosis, and thyroid nodules, with a 2% risk rate of secondary cancer. Myelosuppression caused by radiation therapy correlates with the amount of radiated bone marrow.

Premature coronary artery disease and congestive cardiomyopathy may develop because of exposure to doxorubicin and mediastinal radiotherapy. Pulmonary fibrosis may develop as a result of bleomycin exposure and mantle radiotherapy. Long-term toxicities associated with radiation are likely to be reduced with current treatment approaches that use modern equipment, lower doses, and smaller treatment fields, such as involved site radiotherapy. Similarly, a reduction in the number of chemotherapy cycles for early-stage HL[19] and the limitation of alkylating agents in current chemotherapy regimens are anticipated to diminish the risks of late cardiopulmonary toxicities and secondary malignancies.

THERAPY FOR NLPHL

Many patients with NLPHL present with early-stage disease and can be effectively treated with local involved site radiotherapy. Alternatively, some authorities advocate two cycles of ABVD followed by local involved site radiotherapy. Late relapses are relatively common in this disease and can be treated either with additional radiotherapy (if outside the original radiotherapy field), single-agent rituximab (response rate, 70% to 100%),[55,56] or combination chemotherapy (e.g., ABVD). Disseminated NLPHL is usually treated like classical HL with ABVD chemotherapy, though rituximab has also been used effectively. In a recent study of 394 patients with NLPHL treated with these approaches, complete remission was achieved in 92% of patients with early favorable-stage NLPHL and in 77% of patients with advanced stages of NLPHL. Tumor control (freedom from treatment failure) was 88% and OS was 96% for NLPHL after a median observation period of 50 months.[4]

NON-HODGKIN LYMPHOMA
EPIDEMIOLOGY AND ETIOLOGY

NHL is the seventh most common type of cancer diagnosed annually in men in the United States and the sixth most common type in women. Approximately 70,000 new cases are diagnosed in the United States each year, with approximately 19,000 deaths annually.[1] The incidence of NHL has increased markedly in the past 50 years, presumably related to the increasing exposure to carcinogens (e.g., pesticides, herbicides) and the increasing prevalence of immunosuppressed individuals in the United States (including people with AIDS and those receiving immunosuppressive drug therapy). The greatest increases in incidence are in older individuals and in the number of cases of diffuse large B-cell lymphoma (DLBCL). The median age of patients who are diagnosed with NHL varies according to the histologic subtype, although most subtypes increase exponentially with increasing age.

The etiology of NHL is unknown for most patients. Pesticides and agricultural chemicals, smoking, hair dyes, and other toxins have been suspected but not conclusively shown to be associated with the disease. However, there is a definite

KEY POINTS

- Non-Hodgkin lymphomas (NHLs) comprise a group of heterogeneous diseases that vary widely with respect to clinical presentation, therapy, and prognosis.
- Advances in the diagnosis and classification of these diseases are facilitated by immunophenotyping and by newer molecular and genetic approaches.
- Establishing a correct diagnosis at the time of initial presentation is critical to optimal management of NHL. Therefore, an adequately sized biopsy is mandatory to permit rigorous classification. A fine-needle aspirate is virtually never adequate for establishing the initial subtype of NHL.
- Marked advances have been made in the treatment of these diseases in the past decade, largely because of the availability of monoclonal antibodies used either alone or in conjunction with chemotherapy.

Table 16-5 Infectious Agents Associated with Specific Types of Non-Hodgkin Lymphoma

Infectious Agent	Type of Non-Hodgkin Lymphoma
Epstein-Barr virus	Hodgkin lymphoma, Burkitt lymphoma, and post-transplant lymphoproliferative disorders
Human herpesvirus-8	Body cavity lymphoma, Castleman disease
Hepatitis C	Immunocytoma, splenic marginal zone lymphoma
Human T-lymphotrophic virus-1	Adult T-cell leukemia/lymphoma
Helicobacter pylori	Gastric mucosa-associated lymphoid tissue (MALT) lymphoma
Chlamydia psitacci	Orbital adnexal lymphoma
Campylobacter jejuni	Immunoproliferative small bowel disease
Borrelia burgdorferi	Cutaneous MALT lymphoma

increase in the frequency of aggressive NHL diagnosed in patients who are immunosuppressed because of drug treatments (e.g., cyclosporine, anti-CD3 antibody therapy), infections (e.g., HIV), inherited immune defects, collagen vascular diseases (e.g., rheumatoid arthritis), ASCT, or solid organ transplantation. There is also an association between a variety of infectious agents and the occurrence of lymphomas, although regional variations occur (Table 16-5).

DIAGNOSIS AND CLASSIFICATION

Most patients diagnosed with NHL initially are seen because of signs or symptoms associated with lymphadenopathy, although the enlarged nodes are usually painless. Because numerous infections, benign inflammatory conditions, and nonlymphomatous tumors also can cause enlarged nodes, precise diagnosis and classification of NHL requires evaluation of lymph node tissue obtained at biopsy. An excisional biopsy is preferred because fine-needle aspirations have a high false-negative rate.[57] Fine-needle aspirations also fail to distinguish between nodular and diffuse histologic subtypes in lesions with substantial fibrosis or sclerosis, in cases of T-cell NHL, or T-cell–rich B-cell NHL, as well as in cases in which the lymph nodes are only partially involved with disease. Although an excisional biopsy is optimal, evaluation of tissue obtained by a core-needle biopsy may be sufficient to confirm a suspected recurrence for patients with previously diagnosed lymphoma. The increased use of flow cytometry and molecular genetic studies has made it possible to diagnose a lymphoma in the mediastinal, retroperitoneal, or other deep locations through analysis of tissue obtained by core-needle biopsy.

Categorization of lymphoid neoplasms has been confounded by a long succession of different classification schemes. In 1982, the National Cancer Institute (NCI) Working Formulation

Table 16-6 Relative Frequencies of the Most Common Lymphoma Subtypes According to the World Health Organization (WHO) Classification[3]

Subtype	Aggressiveness	Frequency* (%)
B-cell malignancies		
Follicular lymphoma	Indolent	26
Mucosa-associated lymphoid tissue (MALT) lymphoma	Indolent	8
Nodal marginal zone lymphoma	Indolent	2
Splenic marginal zone lymphoma	Indolent	0.8
Chronic lymphocytic leukemia/small lymphocytic lymphoma	Indolent	11
Lymphoplasmacytic lymphoma	Indolent	1
Mantle cell lymphoma	Aggressive (variable)	6
Diffuse large B-cell lymphoma	Aggressive	33
Primary mediastinal large B-cell lymphoma	Aggessive	3
High-grade B non-Hodgkin lymphoma, not otherwise specified	Highly aggressive	2
Burkitt lymphoma	Highly aggressive	0.7
T/natural killer (NK)-cell malignancies		
Peripheral T-cell lymphoma, not otherwise specified	Aggressive	3
Angioimmunoblastic T-cell lymphoma	Aggressive	2
Extranodal NK/T-cell lymphoma	Aggressive	1
Anaplastic large cell lymphoma, anaplastic lymphoma kinase (ALK)-positive	Aggressive	0.7
Anaplastic large cell lymphoma, ALK-negative	Aggressive	0.5
Enteropathy-type T-cell lymphoma	Aggressive	0.5
Mycosis fungoides	Indolent	~1
Primary cutaneous anaplastic large cell lymphoma	Indolent	0.2
Hepatosplenic T-cell lymphoma	Highly aggressive	0.1
Adult T-cell leukemia/lymphoma	Highly aggressive	< 1
Subcutaneous panniculitis-like T-cell lymphoma	Aggressive	0.1
Unclassifiable peripheral T-cell lymphoma	Aggressive	0.2
Lymphoblastic lymphoma	Highly aggressive	< 1
Other T/NK lymphoma	Variable	1.2

*The frequency of lymphomas is based on data summarized by the WHO, and assumes 90% of lymphoid neoplasms are B-cell malignancies and 10% are T-cell malignancies. The relative frequency of lymphoma subtypes varies greatly in different geographic regions.

was adopted to facilitate communication among U.S. investigators; however, the Kiel classification remained dominant in Europe. The Revised European-American Lymphoma (REAL) Classification (1994) was used to distinguish NHLs using morphology, immunophenotype, genetic characteristics, and clinical features. The REAL Classification was modified by the WHO Classification (1999, 2008), and the latter is now universally accepted (Table 16-6).[3]

STAGING AND PROGNOSIS

The Ann Arbor staging system is used for NHL, but it is less relevant for NHL than it is for HL because NHL more often presents at an advanced stage. Staging for NHL requires PET/CT or contrast-enhanced CT of the chest, abdomen, and pelvis and an adequate bone marrow biopsy (2 cm of core tissue). Flow cytometric analysis of a biopsy specimen often is useful when immunohistochemistry studies are equivocal. FDG-PET has replaced gallium scanning for metabolic imaging because it is more sensitive and practical.[12,43] The usefulness of PET/CT imaging varies with the histologic subtype of NHL.[12,58] FDG-PET consistently identifies more sites of disease than CT in FDG-avid lymphomas when used for staging. However, stage is altered in less than one-fourth of patients, and treatment is changed on the basis of this information in only a small fraction of cases. FDG-PET is valuable in confirming stage I disease in patients being considered for radiation therapy alone. PET/CT is most useful in assessing responses in DLBCL and in HL where a complete remission may translate into cure. PET scans are less sensitive for marginal zone lymphomas and small lymphocytic lymphoma. Although interim PET scan results following one or more cycles of multi-agent chemotherapy may be predictive of outcome, there are no available data yet to suggest that altering therapy on the basis of this information has a salutary effect on patient survival.

Clinicians often group NHL subtypes into indolent (slow-growing or low-grade), aggressive (fast-growing or intermediate-grade), and highly aggressive (very rapidly growing or high-grade) categories as indicated in Table 16-6, to facilitate clinical decision-making regarding therapy and to estimate prognosis.

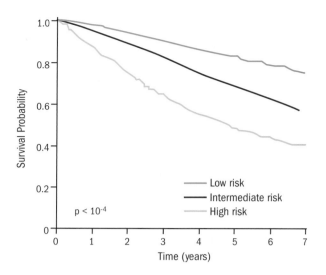

Risk Group	Number of Factors	Patients (%)	5-Year Overall Survival (%)	10-Year Overall Survival (%)
Low	0 to 1	36	90.6	70.7
Intermediate	2	37	77.8	50.9
High	3 to 5	27	52.5	35.5

Fig. 16-3 Overall survival of patients with follicular lymphoma according to the Follicular Lymphoma International Prognostic Index (FLIPI).

This research was originally published in Blood. Solal-Celigny P, Roy P, Colombat P, et al. Follicular lymphoma international prognostic index. Blood. 2004;104(5):1258-1265. © American Society of Hematology.

Index (FLIPI).[59] This index is based on age (60 or older), stage (III and IV), serum LDH level, hemoglobin, and the number of extranodal sites (Fig. 16-3). However, it is not yet clear if different therapeutic strategies should be applied to the various risk groups defined by the FLIPI index. An updated version of the FLIPI index has been introduced, known as the FLIPI2,[60] though it is little utilized. More recently, a simple prognostic index based on the baseline beta 2 microglobulin and LDH levels has been shown to be at least as prognostic as the FLIPI index and much simpler to apply.[61,62]

FOLLICULAR NHL

FL is the second most common type of lymphoma and represents the paradigm for indolent NHL. This disease is characterized by a follicular growth pattern on lymph node biopsy, although diffuse areas also may be present and should be reported by the pathologist. The characteristic immunophenotype is CD20+, CD5-, CD23-, CD10+, and usually BCL6-positive. BCL2 is overexpressed in more than 85% of patients, usually as a result of a t(14;18)(q32;q21) chromosome translocation, which can be detected by fluorescent in situ hybridization or polymerase chain reaction technology.

Approximately 10% to 15% of patients with FL have stage I or nonbulky stage II disease at the time of initial presentation. Involved field or extended field radiation therapy produces a 10-year FFS rate of 50% to 60% and an OS rate of 60% to 80%. Alternatively, such patients can be observed without treatment until disease progression, since their long-term outlook

INDOLENT NHL

The indolent histologic subtypes of NHL include follicular grades 1 (formerly follicular small cleaved cell), 2 (formerly follicular mixed), and 3A (formerly follicular large-cell lymphoma), as well as marginal zone lymphoma, lymphoplasmacytic lymphomas (LPLs; including immunocytoma and Waldenström macroglobulinemia), and small lymphocytic lymphoma. On the other hand, patients with follicular grade 3B disease have a clinical course that is more reminiscent of DLBCL and are typically treated more aggressively than the indolent histologies listed above. Prognostic groups for follicular lymphoma (FL) are best defined with the Follicular Lymphoma International Prognostic is favorable even without immediate therapy.[63] The remaining 85% to 90% of patients with follicular grade 1 or 2 NHL have advanced-stage disease (bulky stage II, or stage III or IV) at the time of presentation. The OS reported for such patients was approximately 10 years from the time of diagnosis prior to the availability of antibody-containing regimens but is now estimated to be more than 15 years by most investigators. Despite this relatively long natural history, indolent lymphomas (including FL) are typically chronic diseases characterized by multiple recurrences in most patients.

Early therapeutic interventions with alkylating agent–based therapies do not appear to prolong survival for patients with asymptomatic FL. Therefore, the conventional approach has been to "watch and wait" until therapy is indicated by the presence of increasing adenopathy, disease-related symptoms, organ compromise, or bone marrow failure. Criteria established by the Groupe d'Etude des Lymphomes Folliculaires (GELF criteria) are useful to identify patients who may benefit from earlier intervention. These criteria suggest that treatment is likely to be required for patients with a maximum lymph node diameter greater than 7 cm, more than three nodal sites greater than 3 cm in diameter, systemic symptoms, a spleen size greater than 16 cm, pleural effusions or ascites, local compressive symptoms, or cytopenias as a result of the lymphoma.[64]

The availability of an increasing number of active biologic agents, particularly monoclonal antibodies, has markedly altered the therapeutic approach for patients with NHL (Table 16-7).[65] Although some antibodies in clinical use are derived from mice (murine), newer antibody products usually are either chimeric mouse-human proteins, humanized, or fully human antibodies, which are less likely to induce the production of neutralizing human anti-mouse antibodies. CD20 is the most commonly targeted lymphoma-associated antigen.[66] This lineage-specific B-cell antigen is first expressed during the pre–B-cell stage of development and persists on B cells until terminal plasma cell differentiation. Rituximab is the chimeric anti-CD20 monoclonal antibody that has been used most extensively in the treatment of B-cell malignant diseases. When used as monotherapy for the initial treatment of patients with FL and low-grade NHL, the response rate ranges from 60% to 70%, with a median duration of response of 1.0 to 2.5 years (depending on patient selection criteria and on whether additional cycles of antibody are delivered as maintenance following the initial four-infusion induction course). The use of "extended" rituximab as maintenance treatment (as a single infusion every 2 months for 8 months, as four weekly infusions every 6 months for 2 years, or as a single infusion every 2 to 3 months for 2 years) prolongs the time to PFS and EFS following chemotherapy or rituximab plus chemotherapy induction regimens.[67-70]

Rituximab is generally well tolerated, with the major side effects being fevers and chills during infusion, although occasional patients may experience a cytokine-release syndrome that can be life-threatening. Fortunately, this side effect is rare and does not generally recur with subsequent doses of the drug. Patients with a high number of circulating malignant cells have been reported to have a rapid tumor clearance syndrome,

Table 16-7 Monoclonal Antibodies and Conjugates for the Treatment of Non-Hodgkin Lymphoma

Monoclonal Antibodies	Antigen
Rituximab	CD20
Ofatumomab	CD20
Obinutuzumab (GA101)	CD20
Veltuzumab (hA20)	CD20
Epratuzumab	CD22
Lumiliximab	CD23
Apolizumab (Hu1D10)	HLA-DR
Dacetuzumab	CD40
Alemtuzumab	CD52
Galiximab	CD80
Radioimmunoconjugates	
Iodine-131-tositumomab	CD20
Yttrium-90-ibritumomab tiuxetan	CD20
Antibody-Drug Conjugates	
Inotuzumab ozogamicin	CD22
Brentuximab vedotin	CD30
Bispecific Antibodies	
Blinatumomab (BITE)	CD19 × CD3 Bispecific antibody

with abnormal renal function, electrolyte abnormalities, and coagulopathy. Rarely, delayed neutropenia may occur following rituximab administration. The mechanism responsible for this complication remains obscure.

Several randomized studies have clearly demonstrated an advantage in PFS, EFS, and even OS from combinations of rituximab and chemotherapy regimens (e.g., cyclophosphamide/vincristine/prednisone [CVP] and cyclophosphamide/doxorubicin/vincristine/prednisone [CHOP]) compared with induction with chemotherapy alone.[71-74] The optimal regimen for the initial treatment of patients with FL is controversial and there is no consensus among experts in the field.[75] Two recent large phase III clinical trials have compared rituximab (R)-CVP, R-CHOP, and rituximab plus fludarabine-containing regimens for the treatment of grade 1 to 2 follicular lymphoma.[76,77] Both studies demonstrated superior PFS for patients treated with R-CHOP or R-fludarabine-based therapy compared with R-CVP, but OS did not differ between the three arms. Both studies also showed that regimens with fludarabine and rituximab had significantly more hematologic toxicity and a higher risk of secondary malignancies than R-CVP or R-CHOP, making fludarabine-based regimens less desirable than alkylator-based regimens. Some authorities believe these trials established R-CHOP as the preferred regimen for FL, but other lymphoma specialists are reluctant to use doxorubicin-containing regimens such as R-CHOP in patients with indolent lymphomas because of the 1% to 2% risk of cardiomyopathy. In recent years, bendamustine plus rituximab[78-80] has emerged as the preferred regimen for many oncologists treating FL, based on two randomized studies comparing R-CHOP and R-bendamustine.[81,82] Both studies concluded that R-bendamustine is at least as effective as R-CHOP and appears less toxic, although both studies have been criticized for methodologic imperfections.

Histologic Transformation of FL to Aggressive Lymphoma

Approximately 30% to 40% of patients with FL undergoes documented transformation to a more aggressive histology, typically DLBCL. The annual rate of transformation is approximately 3%, and, clinically, transformation is usually associated with the rapid growth of a single lymph node region. R-CHOP is the most appropriate therapy for patients experiencing transformation; however, the prognosis is poor despite aggressive management. Although 50% to 65% of patients presenting with de novo DLBCL are cured with R-CHOP chemotherapy, most studies suggest that less than 10% of patients with DLBCL arising by transformation from FL are cured by this intervention, with median survivals of 6 to 20 months for patients undergoing transformation.[83,84] Because of the poor outcome of treatment with R-CHOP chemotherapy alone in patients with transformed FL who have been heavily pretreated, many authorities advise high-dose therapy with ASCT or alloSCT following induction of remission with R-CHOP. Selected series suggest that long-term DFS is achieved in approximately 20% to 30% of patients undergoing transplantation for transformed FL.[85,86] Patients who present with de novo transformation of FL and have not received prior chemotherapy may be treated with R-CHOP alone, with transplantation deferred to the time of relapse. Furthermore, one recent publication suggests that survival of transformed FL may be improving, in the modern era with a reported 50-month median survival following R-CHOP, with particularly good survival in patients experiencing transformation more than 18 months after initial diagnosis of FL.[87]

RELAPSED AND REFRACTORY FOLLICULAR AND LOW-GRADE LYMPHOMA

Patients with advanced-stage indolent NHL typically experience relapse following conventional therapies, despite remissions that may last many years. The choice of salvage therapy depends on a number of factors, including the initial treatment regimen and the quality of response to that regimen, as well as patient factors such as performance status, organ function, and extent of bone marrow involvement. Rituximab (when added to induction and maintenance chemotherapy) has been demonstrated in several randomized clinical trials to prolong PFS. Although most patients have recurrence with the same histologic subtype as they do at the time of initial diagnosis, there is a constant risk of transformation to an aggressive NHL subtype. A variety of immunochemotherapy regimens have been used to treat relapsed or refractory disease (e.g., rituximab plus bendamustine, R-CVP, R-CHOP), but there is no evidence indicating a major advantage for any specific approach. New agents with promising activity include lenalidomide,[88,89] ibrutinib, idelalisib, and ABT-199. Other approaches to relapsed or refractory disease include monoclonal antibodies, radioimmunotherapy (RIT), biologic therapies, and stem cell transplantation.

Monoclonal Antibodies

The U.S. Food and Drug Administration (FDA) initially approved rituximab for the treatment of relapsed and refractory FL and low-grade NHL based on the results of a pivotal trial that evaluated 166 patients for whom previous treatment had failed. Four weekly infusions of rituximab were administered at a dose of 375 mg/m^2. The response rate was 46%, including an 8% rate of complete response and a median time to progression of approximately 1 year. The best responses to rituximab occurred in patients with FL. Only 12% of patients with small lymphocytic lymphoma had a response to a 4-week induction course in the initial pivotal trial. There is no clear advantage to eight weekly infusions compared with the standard four infusions. A second response to rituximab may be achieved in 40% of patients who have a relapse after an initial response to the antibody lasting at least 6 months. Rituximab maintenance also prolongs remission durations in patients treated with a variety of chemotherapy regimens.[69] Several humanized or fully human anti-CD20 monoclonal antibodies are being evaluated for indolent NHL, including obinutuzumab and ofatumomab, which have recently been approved for treatment of chronic lymphocytic leukemia (CLL)/small lymphocytic lymphoma (SLL).

Radioimmunotherapy

Treatment with monoclonal antibodies labeled with isotopes, such as iodine-131 (^{131}I) and yttrium-90 (^{90}Y), has provided promising results. The FDA has approved ^{90}Y-ibritumomab tiuxetan (anti-CD20) for the treatment of relapsed and refractory FL and low-grade NHL, transformed NHL, disease that has not responded to rituximab, and as consolidation for patients following initial chemotherapy. Response rates of more than 80%, with a 26% rate of complete response, were achieved for patients with relapsed and refractory indolent NHL.[90] In a randomized study, the rates of complete and overall response were higher with ^{90}Y-ibritumomab than with rituximab, but there was no difference in time to progression. In addition, a recent randomized trial showed markedly longer PFS in patients with indolent NHL who received consolidation therapy with ^{90}Y-ibritumomab tiuxetan following front-line chemotherapy.[91]

The FDA also approved ^{131}I-tositumomab (anti-CD20), with response rates for patients with relapsed or refractory FL or low-grade NHL of 50% to 80%, with an approximate 30% rate of complete response, lasting a median of 9 months.[92] In a series of 76 patients who received ^{131}I-tositumomab as initial therapy, 95% had a disease response, with a complete remission rate of 75%, and almost 60% of patients were free from disease progression at 5 years.[93] A recent study comparing six cycles of CHOP chemotherapy plus six doses of rituximab (CHOP-R) with six cycles of CHOP followed by a single dose of ^{131}I-tositumomab[94] (CHOP-RIT) has shown similar outcomes in both treatment arms. After a median follow-up of 4.9 years, the estimated 2- and 5-year PFS were 80% and 66%, respectively, with CHOP-RIT, and 76% and 60%, respectively, with CHOP-R (two-sided p = 0.11). The 2- and 5-year OS were 93% and 86%, respectively, with CHOP-RIT, and 97% and 92%, respectively, with CHOP-R (p = 0.08).[95] When administered at doses appropriate for myeloablation with stem cell support, ^{131}I-tositumomab antibody also has yielded promising results.[96]

Because these agents are myelosuppressive, patients who may be considered for treatment with them must have less than 25% lymphoma involvement in the bone marrow, cellularity of more than 15%, more than 100,000 platelets/mm^3 (more than 1,500 neutrophils/mm^3), and no history of stem cell transplantation or a failed stem cell harvest. Toxicities associated with ^{90}Y-ibritumomab tiuxetan are primarily of a myelosuppressive nature, with nadirs occurring 6 to 8 weeks after therapy. Secondary AML and myelodysplastic syndrome are partially related to previous therapy. These agents rarely cause severe nausea, vomiting, or mucositis, and the latter fact likely contributes to the low incidence of severe infections. Despite the favorable efficacy and toxicity profiles, these agents are underutilized, and the manufacturer of ^{131}I-tositumomab discontinued manufacturing of this agent in February 2014.

Other Biologic Therapies

New promising biologic approaches in development include anti-idiotype vaccines, agents targeting apoptotic pathways (e.g., BH3-only peptides), adoptive immunotherapy with chimeric-antigen receptor–modified T cells,[97] antibody-drug conjugates,[98] and inhibitors of spleen tyrosine kinase (fostamatinib disodium),[99] PI3 kinase delta,[100] and Bruton tyrosine kinase.[101,102]

Stem Cell Transplantation

The use of ASCT for treatment of relapsed or refractory indolent NHL is supported primarily by nonrandomized studies with long-term follow-up. In a collaborative study of 126 adult patients conducted by St. Bartholomew's Hospital and the Dana-Farber Cancer Institute, there was an apparent plateau in the remission duration curve of 48% at a median follow-up of 13.5 years.[103] Survival appeared to be longer among patients who received the transplant in second remission compared with patients who underwent transplantation later in their disease course. This approach also has been tested in a randomized trial involving 89 patients. Investigators observed a marked advantage in PFS and a marginal OS advantage for ASCT compared with conventional salvage chemotherapy.[104] When used as part of initial therapy for patients with high-risk disease, randomized studies demonstrate a prolongation of PFS but no increased survival.[105,106] Short- and long-term complications of ASCT include treatment-related mortality, prolonged anemia or thrombocytopenia, and a substantial increase in the incidence of secondary myelodysplasia and AML, which ranges from 7% to 19%.

The application of myeloablative allogeneic bone marrow or stem cell transplantation for the treatment of indolent NHL has been limited by high rates of morbidity and mortality and the advanced age of many patients with indolent NHL. Although myeloablative alloSCT may afford long-term DFS for approximately 40% to 50% of patients whose disease fails to respond to previous chemotherapy, transplant-related mortality rates range from 20% to 40% in most studies.[107] When alloSCT and ASCT are compared, the long-term survival rates are comparable.[107] ASCT is associated with a greater likelihood of dying from recurrent disease, whereas alloSCT results in a higher frequency of death from graft-versus-host disease (GVHD) and infection. In the past decade, nonmyeloablative and reduced-intensity alloSCT conditioning regimens have been developed to exploit the benefit of a graft-versus-lymphoma effect while minimizing transplant-related morbidity and mortality. Preliminary results of this approach are very promising.[85,108] In one study, 62 patients with indolent or transformed NHL were treated with alloSCT from related (34 patients) or unrelated (28 patients) donors after conditioning with 2 Gy of total-body irradiation with or without fludarabine.[109] Twenty patients (32%) had progressive disease after previous ASCT. The estimated OS and PFS rates at 3 years were 52% and 43%, respectively, for patients with indolent disease, and 18% and 21%, respectively, for patients with transformed disease. Patients with indolent disease and related donors (26 patients) had 3-year estimated OS and PFS rates of 67% and 54%, respectively. The incidences of grade 2 to 4 acute GVHD, grade 3 and 4 acute GVHD, and extensive chronic GVHD were 63%, 18%, and 47%, respectively. This study and others like it demonstrate that nonmyeloablative alloSCT can produce durable DFS in patients with relapsed or refractory indolent NHL and that outcomes are particularly good in patients with untransformed disease and related donors.

MARGINAL ZONE LYMPHOMAS

Marginal zone lymphomas are derived from malignant transformation of lymphocytes from the marginal zone of the spleen or lymph nodes. Several subtypes of marginal zone lymphomas have been defined, including mucosa-associated lymphoid tissue (MALT) lymphoma, nodal marginal zone lymphoma, and primary splenic marginal zone lymphoma. The immunophenotype of the malignant lymphocytes is typically CD20+, CD5-, CD10-, and CD23-. Trisomy 3 and t(11;18) have been reported in 60% of extranodal cases. Other cytogenetic abnormalities include translocations and abnormalities of 1p or 7. The t(11;18)(q21;q21) translocation is the most common of the structural abnormalities and produces a fusion between API2 on 11q21 and MLT (MALT lymphoma–associated translocation) on chromosome 18q21, also known as MALT1. IAPI2 belongs to the family of inhibitors of apoptosis, and MALT1 is a pro-caspase–like protease. BCL10 also can bind to MALT1, resulting in an increase in translocation of nuclear factor-kappa-B to the nucleus, impairing apoptosis and leading to the elaboration of a number of cytokines that favor the proliferation and longevity of the malignant cells.

Extranodal marginal zone (MALT) lymphomas affect the gastrointestinal and respiratory tracts, ocular adnexa,[110] salivary glands, kidney, prostate, and other organs. Many patients have an associated autoimmune disease, such as Sjögren syndrome or Hashimoto thyroiditis. Unlike most other indolent NHL, most patients with MALT lymphoma present with stage I or II disease, although dissemination—often to other extranodal sites—occurs in more than one-third of patients at some point in the disease course. MALT lymphomas account for approximately 80% of cases of indolent NHL of the stomach, most of which occur in association with *Helicobacter pylori* infection. MALT lymphomas of the stomach are highly responsive to double or triple antibiotic therapy (e.g., omeprazole/amoxicillin or omeprazole/metronidazole/clarithromycin), and the response is durable in more than 60% of patients.[111] Cases associated with the t(11;18)(q21;q21) translocation appear to be resistant to antibiotic therapy. For patients in whom antibiotic therapy is not successful, alternative treatment approaches include local radiation therapy,[110] single-agent rituximab, and combination chemotherapy plus rituximab. Histologic followup of gastric MALT lymphomas appears to be superior to using the polymerase chain reaction analysis in terms of identifying patients requiring additional therapy.

Nodal marginal zone NHLs represent the lymph node–based counterpart of MALT lymphomas. Patients with this disease are typically treated with the same regimens used for FL. However, the outcome following therapy is inferior to that of extranodal marginal zone lymphoma.

Patients with splenic marginal zone lymphoma typically have peripheral blood and bone marrow involvement, as well as a massively enlarged spleen, but lymph nodes are usually normal or only slightly enlarged. In some cases, circulating malignant lymphocytes may possess a distinct histologic appearance with villous cytoplasmic projections, which may be confused with hairy cell leukemia cells. Splenic marginal zone lymphomas are often associated with hepatitis C infection, and when this is the case, effective antiviral therapy (e.g., peginterferon alpha and ribavirin) may be associated with sustained clinical remission of the lymphoma in 75% of cases.[99] In other cases, splenectomy usually results in a prolonged clinical remission with correction of the cytopenias and splenic pain that frequently prompt treatment.[112,113] Single-agent rituximab and combination chemotherapy regimens are also effective temporizing measures.

LYMPHOPLASMACYTIC LYMPHOMAS

LPLs include immunocytomas and Waldenström macroglobulinemia. These lymphomas tend to occur in older people (median age, 63) and account for 1.5% of NHL. Most patients present with a monoclonal immunoglobulin M (IgM) spike, with hyperviscosity syndrome occurring in approximately 30% of patients. The disease also may be complicated by neuropathy, amyloidosis, cryoglobulinemia, and cold agglutinin disease.[114] Whole-genome sequencing has revealed that 91% of LPLs possess a point mutation leading to an amino acid change (L265P) in the MYD88 protein.[115] This mutation triggers IRAK-mediated nuclear factor-kappa-B signaling leading to a survival advantage for the transformed cells. In addition, 50% of LPLs are associated with a t(9;14)(p13;q32) translocation and rearrangement of the *PAX-5* gene encoding the B-cell–specific activator protein. An association of LPL with hepatitis C has been documented, especially for patients with mixed cryoglobulinemia. Treatment of LPL is indicated for symptomatic hyperviscosity as a result of high serum IgM levels, enlarging organomegaly, or other disease-related symptoms. Plasmapheresis may provide acute, symptomatic relief for hyperviscosity symptoms. More durable systemic therapeutic options include rituximab either alone or combined with cyclophosphamide, bortezomib, thalidomide, lenalidomide, or dexamethasone.[114-117] In addition, the Bruton tyrosine kinase inhibitor ibrutinib is highly active in relapsed and refractory LPL. Fludarabine-based regimens are effective but have fallen out of favor because of prolonged cytopenias, hematopoietic stem cell damage, and an increased risk of acute leukemia. The median survival in many LPL series is 5 to 10 years from diagnosis. Although the disease is initially responsive to therapy, relapse is inevitable, and most patients die from the disease. In selected patients, nonmyeloablative alloSCT can yield durable complete remissions and possibly cures.[114] The prognosis is worse for patients whose disease transforms to large-cell NHL (approximately 24% of cases).

KEY POINTS

- Aggressive non-Hodgkin lymphomas (NHLs) typically grow rapidly and nearly always require prompt initiation of therapy soon after the diagnosis is established to ameliorate symptoms, avert rapid progression of the disease, and optimize survival.
- Calculation of the International Prognostic Index for a patient at the time of diagnosis with aggressive NHL permits estimation of projected survival based on individual clinical characteristics.
- Multi-agent chemotherapy regimens are nearly always employed in the treatment of aggressive lymphomas. Doxorubicin appears to be the critical drug in curative regimens.
- Stage I to II aggressive lymphomas are often treated with short courses of chemotherapy (three to four cycles) followed by consolidative radiotherapy, whereas patients with more advanced disease (stages III to IV) usually receive six to eight cycles of chemotherapy without radiotherapy.
- Diffuse large B-cell lymphoma (DLBCL) is the most common aggressive NHL and is usually treated with R-CHOP with a cure rate of approximately 60%.
- Central nervous system prophylaxis is necessary for patients with DLBCL presenting with high-risk features and for all patients with Burkitt lymphoma, lymphoblastic lymphoma, or HIV-associated aggressive lymphomas.

Risk Group	Risk Factors	Distribution of Patients (%)	Complete Response Rate (%)	Relapse-Free Survival 2-Year Rate (%)	Relapse-Free Survival 5-Year Rate (%)	Survival 2-Year Rate (%)	Survival 5-Year Rate (%)
Low	0 or 1	35	87	79	70	84	73
Low-intermediate	2	27	67	66	50	66	51
High-intermediate	3	22	55	59	49	54	43
High	4 or 5	16	44	58	40	34	26

*The total number of patients includes 1,385 in a training sample and 646 in a validation sample.

SMALL LYMPHOCYTIC LYMPHOMA

SLL, the tissue counterpart of CLL, is characterized by an accumulation of small, mature-appearing lymphocytes in the blood, bone marrow, and lymph nodes. The classic immunophenotypic profile of CLL/SLL is expression of CD5, CD19, and CD23, with low-level expression of surface immunoglobulin and CD20. CLL and SLL are usually distinguished arbitrarily by whether the number of circulating clonal B cells is more than 5,000/mm^3 (CLL) or less (SLL). Thus, the diagnosis of SLL can be made in the absence of blood or bone marrow involvement. Although SLL often is included in clinical trials with FL and other low-grade NHLs, its biology and response to various therapies differ enough from those of the other indolent NHLs that it is better treated as CLL (see Chapter 15: Leukemias).[118]

DIFFUSE LARGE B-CELL LYMPHOMA

DLBCL is the most common form of NHL in the United States, accounting for 30% to 35% of all cases, and represents the prototype for aggressive NHL. In up to 40% of patients with DLBCL, the disease initially presents in an extranodal site—most commonly in the gastrointestinal tract but also in the central nervous system (CNS), genitourinary or reproductive tracts, lung, and other sites. Morphologically, DLBCL typically effaces the normal architecture of the lymph node. The characteristic immunophenotype of this lymphoma consists of expression of CD19 and CD20 without expression of CD5 or CD23. *BCL2* and *BCL6* are variably expressed in many, but not all, cases. Disease that expresses CD10 appears to be of germinal center origin. Multiple recurrent somatic mutations have been identified in the germinal center B-cell (e.g., in the *EZH2*, *TNFRSF14*, *MEF2B*, *GNA13*, and *SGK1* genes) and activated B-cell (CD79b, MYD88) subtypes of DLBCL, offering hope that specifically targeted therapies can be applied addressing the specific molecular derangements in the future.

The International Prognostic Index (IPI) is widely used to classify patients with aggressive B-cell NHL into four groups according to risk: low, low-intermediate, high-intermediate, and high (Table 16-8).[119] The identified parameters include:

- Age (younger or older than 60)
- Serum LDH level (normal or increased)
- Performance status (0 to 1 or 2 to 4)
- Number of extranodal sites (none or one compared with more than one)
- Tumor stage (I or II compared with III or IV)

The IPI was derived from a database containing only patients treated in the pre-rituximab era. A revised schema for patients treated with rituximab has been proposed.[120] Although the IPI separates DLBCL into clinically meaningful risk groups, there is considerable heterogeneity within those groups. Studies using DNA microarray analyses suggest that there are at least three distinct subgroups within DLBCL—namely a germinal center–like B cell, an activated B-cell type, and a primary mediastinal B-cell NHL. The activated B-cell type is associated with a worse prognosis even within subgroups of the IPI.[121] Gene expression profiling studies have also shown that survival after treatment of DLBCL is influenced by differences in immune cells, fibrosis, and angiogenesis in the tumor microenvironment. A prognostically favorable stromal-1 signature reflects extracellular-matrix deposition and histiocytic infiltration, whereas a prognostically unfavorable stromal-2 signature reflects tumor blood-vessel density.

Limited Disease

Approximately 20% of patients with DLBCL have limited disease (stage I or nonbulky stage II) at the time of presentation. The likelihood of cure is more than 80% for patients with clinical stage I disease when treated with either involved field or extended field radiation therapy. However, one-third to one-half of patients with stage II disease treated with radiation therapy alone subsequently experience relapse. A study conducted by the Southwest Oncology Group (SWOG) suggested a survival advantage for three cycles of CHOP followed by involved field radiation compared with eight cycles of CHOP alone; however, the curves merge at year 10.[122] More recent studies from this group suggest that the addition of rituximab to this regimen further improves the outcome of patients with limited DLBCL, with a 4-year PFS of 88%.[123] However, a Groupe d'Etude des

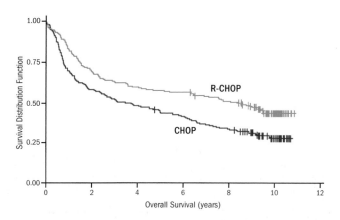

Fig. 16-4 Overall survival of 399 patients, age 60 to 80, with stage II to IV diffuse large B-cell lymphoma (DLBCL), treated with either R-CHOP or CHOP, with a median follow-up time of 10 years (p < 0.0001).

Abbreviations: CHOP, cyclophosphamide/doxorubicin/vincristine/prednisone; R, rituximab.

This research was originally published in Blood. Coiffier B, Thieblemont C, Van Den Neste E, et al. Long-term outcome of patients in the LNH-98.5 trial, the first randomized study comparing rituximab-CHOP to standard CHOP chemotherapy in DLBCL patients: a study by the Groupe d'Etudes des Lymphomes de l'Adulte. Blood. 2010;116(12):2040-2045. © American Society of Hematology.

Lymphomes de l'Adulte (GELA) study has challenged the importance of radiotherapy in the management of early-stage aggressive lymphoma. Their study compared four cycles of CHOP with or without involved field radiation for older patients with stage I to II aggressive NHL. The study failed to demonstrate a benefit from the addition of radiation, even in patients with bulky tumors[124]; however, the outcomes in both arms of this study were poor compared to other clinical trials investigating early-stage DLBCL, with only an approximate 60% to 65% 5-year EFS rate. This raises questions regarding the validity of basing treatment recommendations on this study.

Advanced Disease

The first major progress in the treatment of advanced, aggressive B-cell NHL resulted from the addition of doxorubicin to CVP to form the regimen now known as CHOP. Complete response was achieved in 50% to 70% of patients, with a plateau on the DFS curve at approximately 30%. Other combination regimens—including various doses and schedules of other standard agents—failed to demonstrate benefit compared with CHOP and were more toxic and expensive.[125] Thus, CHOP remained the standard treatment for more than a decade. Single-agent activity with rituximab, as well as promising phase II data for R-CHOP, led to randomized studies in which this combination was compared with CHOP alone. GELA randomly assigned 399 patients (ages 60 to 80) to receive either CHOP alone or R-CHOP.[124] The rates of complete response, time to progression, and OS were markedly better for patients treated with R-CHOP (Fig. 16-4), although this effect was most pronounced for patients in the low-risk category. Several trials have now confirmed the benefit of rituximab in the treatment of DLBCL.[126,127] A dose-intensified 14-day R-CHOP

schedule was not superior to the conventional, less-toxic 21-day schedule in three randomized clinical trials.[128,129]

Wilson at the NCI has developed a novel, infusional regimen (EPOCH) that involves administration of etoposide, vincristine, and doxorubicin by continuous infusion for 96 hours with bolus doses of cyclophosphamide and oral prednisone.[130] The doses of etoposide, doxorubicin, and cyclophosphamide are adjusted by 20% each cycle to achieve a nadir absolute neutrophil count below 0.5×10^9/L. Phase II trials of dose-adjusted EPOCH with rituximab (DA-EPOCH-R) have achieved impressive results both in single-institution[130] and cooperative group settings,[131] and a phase III trial is currently being conducted to determine if DA-EPOCH-R is superior to standard R-CHOP-21. The role of ASCT in front-line therapy of DLBCL remains controversial,[132,133] although a recent SWOG trial suggests that patients with high-risk DLBCL (IPI of 4 to 5) have improved survival if consolidated with ASCT in first complete remission.[134]

CNS Prophylaxis

DLBCL disseminates to the leptomeninges and/or brain in 2% to 10% of cases, usually with devastating consequences. Several risk factors have been identified that predict for CNS dissemination, including initial presentation of DLBCL in the paranasal sinuses, testicles, or epidural space; bone marrow involvement with large-cell lymphoma, HIV positivity, or the presence of two extranodal sites and an elevated LDH. Management of such cases is very controversial,[135] although national guidelines recommend CNS prophylaxis with four to eight doses of intrathecal methotrexate or cytosine arabinoside or administration of high-dose methotrexate (3 to 8 g/m²).[136]

Relapsed or Refractory Disease

R-CHOP cures approximately 60% to 65% of patients with advanced DLBCL. Because 10% to 25% of patients who have late recurrence have an indolent histologic subtype (e.g., FL), a repeat biopsy is necessary to plan appropriate treatment. Therapy for patients with relapsed or refractory DLBCL remains unsatisfactory. Several combination salvage regimens have been studied (e.g., rituximab/ifosfamide/carboplatin/etoposide, and dexamethasone/high-dose cytarabine/cisplatin). These second-line regimens typically produce objective remissions in 50% to 70% of patients with DLBCL, including 20% to 50% complete remissions, but remissions are usually of short duration and few patients are cured.[137] High-dose chemotherapy with autologous stem cell support results in long-term DFS of 20% to 50% of patients with chemosensitive, relapsed DLBCL,[138] but this treatment is much less effective for patients with primary refractory disease or for patients whose disease relapsed following induction regimens containing rituximab.[137] The outlook is unfavorable for patients who experience a relapse after ASCT. Single-agent rituximab induces response in 30% of patients, but the response duration is brief. Approximately 20% to 40% of patients with DLBCL relapsing after ASCT can achieve long-term DFS with nonmyeloablative alloSCT, particularly if the procedure is conducted in a setting of minimal residual disease.[85,139]

MANTLE CELL LYMPHOMA

Mantle cell lymphoma comprises approximately 6% of NHL. The malignant cells characteristically express CD20 and CD5—features shared with CLL. However, mantle cell lymphoma does not express CD23 (a feature of CLL) or CD10 (found on most cases of FL). Mantle cell lymphoma is usually associated with the t(11;14)(q13;q32) translocation resulting in overexpression of cyclin D1.[140] Patients with mantle cell lymphoma may present with diffuse bowel involvement (lymphomatous polyposis). CNS involvement has been noted in almost 20% of cases at some stage in the disease course, but this is usually a late feature. Mantle cell lymphoma is an incurable lymphoma with a variable clinical course.[141] A small subset of patients with mantle cell lymphoma have an indolent clinical course, and their disease can be managed initially with observation alone.[142] Short-course chemotherapy followed by involved field radiotherapy, or radiotherapy alone, is effective for the 10% to 15% of patients who present with localized stage I to II disease.[141,143] Combination chemotherapy regimens induce disease responses in as many as 80% to 90% of patients, with complete response occurring in more than one-half of patients; however, responses are not durable, with a median survival in most series of 3.5 to 4 years. The addition of rituximab to CHOP for initial therapy improves complete remission rates but does not clearly prolong survival.[144] Studies in Europe suggest that regimens alternating R-CHOP with a regimen containing high-dose cytarabine (e.g. R-DHAP) improves the durability of remissions, especially if consolidated with ASCT. Bendamustine plus rituximab has also emerged as a popular and effective induction regimen for mantle cell lymphoma, particularly in elderly patients, based on a randomized phase III study demonstrating at least equal efficacy and less toxicity than R-CHOP in this setting.[81] An aggressive acute leukemia-like regimen, cyclophosphamide/vincristine/doxorubicin/dexamethasone alternating with high-dose methotrexate and high-dose cytarabine (hyperCVAD), given with rituximab, appears to improve complete response rates, remission durations, and survival but does not appear to be curative.[145] Several recent trials suggest that ASCT in first remission following induction therapy with hyperCVAD or other regimens containing high-dose cytarabine can produce long-term DFS in many patients.[146,147] For elderly patients who are not candidates for ASCT, maintenance rituximab may reduce the risk of disease progression or death.[148]

For patients who experience relapse, a regimen of rituximab plus fludarabine/cyclophosphamide/mitoxantrone with rituximab maintenance improves response rates and produces an apparent prolongation of survival.[149] Bortezomib has been approved for relapsed and refractory mantle cell lymphoma, with several published studies showing response rates of 30% to 50%.[150] More recently, the oral Bruton tyrosine kinase inhibitor ibrutinib has demonstrated outstanding single-agent activity in patients with relapsed or refractory mantle cell lymphoma, with an overall response rate of 68%, a complete response rate of 21%, and a median response duration of more than 17 months.[102] Lenalidomide is another option for relapsed mantle cell lymphoma, inducing remissions in approximately 28% of such patients.[151]

Other promising therapies include temsirolimus and idelalisib. Provocative results have also been reported for reduced intensity alloSCT for patients with relapsed mantle cell lymphoma, with 60% to 80% of patients reported to be alive and disease free 2 years after transplant in selected series of patients.[152,153]

LYMPHOBLASTIC LYMPHOMA

Lymphoblastic lymphoma is a very aggressive neoplasm that typically presents in young men (median age, 16) with mediastinal masses. The tumor exhibits an immature T-cell immunophenotype, with expression of CD7, cytoplasmic CD3, and Tdt. Rearrangements of the T-cell receptor genes are virtually always present, and activating *Notch* mutations are present in the majority of cases. The clinical distinction between lymphoblastic lymphoma and T-cell acute lymphoblastic leukemia (T-ALL) is based on an arbitrary definition assigning diagnosis as T-ALL if the bone marrow contains more than 25% lymphoblasts, and lymphoblastic lymphoma if it contains less than 25%. The presence of an elevated serum LDH level and bone marrow or CNS involvement confers an unfavorable prognosis. Complete remission can be achieved in more than 90% of patients treated with intensive, multi-agent chemotherapy regimens, such as hyperCVAD.[154,155] Involvement of sanctuary sites such as the testes and CNS is common, mandating incorporation of intrathecal chemotherapy and testicular irradiation into treatment regimens. The role of mediastinal radiotherapy is controversial. Recent series suggest that such intensive "leukemia-type" chemotherapy regimens produce long-term DFS rates of 73% to 90% in children and 45% to 72% in adults.[155] A role for high-dose therapy during first complete remission is under investigation for patients with high-risk disease.[156] Long-term survival rates are 63% for patients who undergo ASCT during first complete remission, 31% for patients undergoing transplantation during second complete remission, and only 15% for patients undergoing transplantation with resistant disease. Nelarabine has recently demonstrated impressive single-agent activity in patients with relapsed lymphoblastic lymphoma.[157]

BURKITT LYMPHOMA

Classical Burkitt lymphoma is a highly aggressive tumor characterized by an exceptionally high proliferation rate (Ki67 score of approximately 100%), a mature B-cell immunophenotype (monoclonal surface IgM, CD10, CD19, CD20, CD22, BCL6, CD38, and CD43 expression), and a histologic appearance demonstrating diffuse infiltration with a "starry-sky" pattern of macrophages phagocytosing apoptotic tumor cells. All cases of classical Burkitt lymphoma possess a translocation of the *c-Myc* oncogene at band 8q24, most commonly associated with a t(8;14) translocation, although t(2;8) and t(8;22) translocations also occur. The disease occurs endemically in Africa, where it typically presents with jaw tumors in children and is almost invariably associated with EBV. Sporadic cases occur elsewhere in the world, often presenting with ileocecal masses and associated with EBV in less than 30% of cases. Burkitt lymphoma is one of the most common types of lymphoma occurring in patients with AIDS. High-risk features of Burkitt

Table 16-9 Features Associated with AIDS-Related Lymphoma (ARL)

Lymphoma Type	Frequency of ARL	Virus (%)	Comment
Classic Burkitt lymphoma	30%	EBV (30%)	Neoplastic cells may be found circulating in peripheral blood. Frequently associated with leptomeningeal and bone marrow involvement. Seen most frequently in earlier stages of HIV infection.
Burkitt with plasmacytoid differentiation	20%	EBV (50%-70%)	
Burkitt-like (atypical)	< 10%	EBV (30%-50%)	
Diffuse large B-cell lymphoma			
Centroblastic	25%	EBV (30%)	Most often associated with primary central nervous system lymphoma.
Immunoblastic	10%	EBV (> 90%)	
CD30+ anaplastic large cell	< 5%	EBV (30%)	
Primary effusion lymphoma/ body cavity lymphoma	< 5%	HHV-8 (90%)	May be associated with Castleman disease and KS. Malignant effusions contain large pleomorphic cells which stain for CD45 and plasma cell markers, but usually negative for B-cell markers. Occurs in late stages of HIV infection.
Plasmablastic lymphoma	< 5%	HHV-8 (10%)	Rare tumor with aggressive phenotype and plasmacytoid features.

Abbreviations: EBV, Epstein-Barr virus; HHV-8, human herpesvirus-8; KS, Kaposi sarcoma.

lymphoma include involvement of the CNS and/or bone marrow and a markedly elevated LDH.

Burkitt lymphomas are characterized by a rapid growth rate, and treatment may be associated with a potentially fatal tumor lysis syndrome, renal failure, hyperuricemia, and hyperkalemia. Biochemical abnormalities should be corrected rapidly before treatment, and patients should receive prophylactic rasburicase or xanthine oxidase inhibitors and hydration. Chemotherapy for Burkitt lymphoma has traditionally involved intensive therapy with regimens such as R-hyperCVAD or cyclophosphamide/vincristine/doxorubicin/methotrexate alternating with ifosfamide/etoposide/high-dose cytarabine (CODOX-M/IVAC), using treatment principles reminiscent of those employed for ALL, including routine CNS prophylaxis.[158-160] The rate of complete response with R-hyperCVAD or R-CODOX-M/IVAC is 85% to 95%, with 47% to 80% FFS at 5 years in various series, depending on patient selection factors. The OS rate is 74% for adults treated with aggressive chemotherapy and CNS prophylaxis. Addition of rituximab to aggressive chemotherapy regimens appears to increase the response rate and duration, although randomized clinical trials in this disease are lacking.

Recently, investigators at the NCI have suggested that less intense regimens may also achieve excellent outcomes in Burkitt lymphoma.[161] Dunleavy et al treated 30 consecutive patients with infusional EPOCH-R regimens, including 19 patients with HIV-negative disease treated with DA-EPOCH-R and 11 patients with HIV-positive disease treated with a short-course (SC) regimen incorporating a double dose of rituximab (SC-EPOCH-RR). The rates of freedom from progression of disease and OS were, respectively, 95% and 100% with DA-EPOCH-R and 100% and 90% with SC-EPOCH-RR.

Patients with Burkitt lymphoma that relapses after initial therapy are typically treated with aggressive salvage chemotherapy regimens followed by attempts at stem cell transplantation, but outcomes are poor in this setting.

B-CELL LYMPHOMA UNCLASSIFIABLE, WITH FEATURES INTERMEDIATE BETWEEN DLBCL AND BURKITT LYMPHOMA

It has long been recognized that some patients present with morphologic, clinical, and molecular features intermediate between DLBCL and Burkitt lymphoma. In the past, these cases have been called atypical Burkitt lymphoma, Burkitt-like lymphomas, or gray zone lymphomas.[3,162] Microscopically, such cases usually contain a mixture of medium-sized cells (resembling those of Burkitt lymphoma) and larger cells (resembling DLBCL). The Ki67 proliferation index in such cases is typically 80% to 100%, and c-Myc rearrangements are often present. Establishing a diagnosis is difficult and not highly reproducible, although DNA microarray analysis may facilitate categorizing these tumors.[163] Recently it has been appreciated that many lymphomas previously considered Burkitt-like are "double-hit" lymphomas containing two separate translocations, one of which affects the MYC/8q24 locus and the second breakpoint rearranging either BCL2 or BCL6.[164-166] Such double-hit lymphomas are highly aggressive, and the most appropriate treatment regimen has not yet been established, although regimens such as R-hyperCVAD, CODOX-M/IVAC and front-line stem cell transplantation are usually advised. These patients usually present with poor prognostic features, including an elevated LDH, bone marrow and CNS involvement, and a high IPI score. Virtually all series of patients with double-hit lymphomas report poor outcomes with a median survival of 0.2 to 1.5 years, even if treated with aggressive chemotherapy regimens and stem cell transplantation in first remission.[164-166]

PRIMARY CNS LYMPHOMA

Primary CNS lymphoma (PCNSL) may occur de novo or in the setting of immunodeficiency (as in patients who are HIV-positive receiving immunosuppressive drugs following solid organ transplantation) or with immunologic or rheumatologic disorders. The disease presents at a median age of 60 with focal neurologic deficits, personality change, seizures, and headache.[167] Intraocular involvement is seen in 10% to 20% of cases. The factors most consistently predictive of improved outcome include age younger than 50 and good performance status at presentation.[168] Historically, the standard approach has been radiation therapy, with no additional benefit from regimens such as CHOP. However, more recent studies have convincingly demonstrated that high-dose methotrexate with or without high-dose cytarabine[167] produces superior results (median survival, 51 months) compared with radiotherapy.[167,169,170] The current role of whole-brain radiotherapy is controversial and many authorities suggest it should be deferred in patients who are in remission until recurrence, because of an unacceptable incidence of devastating leukoencephalopathy, particularly in patients older than 60. The roles of rituximab, temozolomide, and ASCT for consolidation of first remission are currently under investigation. Further details of the management of CNS lymphomas are provided in Chapter 14: Central Nervous System Tumors.

HIV-ASSOCIATED LYMPHOMAS

The profound immunosuppression associated with HIV infection predisposes patients to both opportunistic infections and the development of malignancies, including a 60- to 200-fold increase in incidence of NHLs. The evolution of HIV-associated lymphomas is believed to involve chronic antigen stimulation due to opportunistic infections resulting in B-cell stimulation and expansion, the presence of co-infecting oncogenic viruses (e.g., EBV, human herpesvirus-8), the acquisition of somatic mutations, cytokine dysregulation, and the abrogation of immune surveillance due to T-cell depletion.[171] The most common lymphoma subtypes observed in patients with HIV include DLBCL, Burkitt lymphoma, PCNSL, primary effusion lymphoma (PEL), plasmablastic lymphoma (PBL), and HL (Table 16-9). Since the widespread introduction of highly active antiretroviral therapy (HAART), the risk of developing HIV-associated lymphomas has decreased, and there has been a shift in the relative frequency of the various histologic subtypes observed. Patients treated with HAART are less likely to develop PCNSL and PEL, which typically occur in patients with the profound immunosuppression associated with extremely low CD4 counts (< 50 per μL), whereas the relative frequency of Burkitt lymphoma and HL, which often occur in patients with higher CD4 counts and better immune function, have increased.

Management of HIV-associated lymphomas has changed dramatically in the past 15 years. In the pre-HAART era, patients with AIDS-related lymphomas were commonly treated with either palliative care alone or attenuated doses of chemotherapy because of their poor performance status, cytopenias, and the frequent occurrence of life-threatening infections. Since the introduction of HAART, patients generally have a better performance status, have higher CD4 counts, and are better able to withstand full-dose therapies. The current standard of care for DLBCL—the most common subtype of HIV-associated lymphoma—is to administer full-dose EPOCH-R or R-CHOP. Most HIV experts currently favor the infusional EPOCH-R regimen based on very promising single-institution results published by investigators at the NCI[172,173] and multicenter studies conducted through the AIDS Malignancy Consortium.[174] A pooled analysis of two consecutive trials compared the outcomes of 99 patients with HIV-associated lymphomas who received R-CHOP with 51 patients treated with EPOCH-R. Patients treated with EPOCH-R had higher complete remission rates, better EFS after 2 years (~75% vs. 45%), and better OS after 2 years (~75% vs. ~50%) than the historical group treated with R-CHOP.[175] Treatment-associated death occurred in 6% of patients with CD4 counts greater than 50 per μL when treated with R-CHOP or EPOCH-R, compared to a 37% rate of treatment related mortality for patients with CD4 less than 50 per μL (p < 0.01). Recently, a SC EPOCH-R regimen has been described in which patients were treated for just one cycle of chemotherapy beyond achievement of stable radiographic and FDG-PET scans but received two doses of rituximab per treatment cycle. With this approach, 79% of patients received only three cycles of EPOCH-R with a PFS at 5 years of 84%.[171] CNS prophylaxis (e.g., intrathecal methotrexate) should be administered to patients with HIV who have aggressive B-cell lymphomas because of a high risk of CNS disease in the absence of such therapy. Most authorities advise concomitant administration of HAART while patients are receiving chemotherapy; the NCI group prefers to withhold HAART during chemotherapy and then promptly administer it at the completion of treatment. Caution should be exercised in administering rituximab to patients who have HIV and lymphoma with CD4 counts less than 50 per μL due to an apparent increase in infection-related deaths attributable to rituximab in this setting.[176]

PEL and PBL are unusual, aggressive variants of DLBCL, and their management remains poorly defined. PEL is invariably associated with both EBV and human herpesvirus-8 and typically presents with pleural effusions and ascites without demonstrable mass legions. PEL cells typically lack expression of CD20, CD79a, PAX5, or other B lymphocyte surface markers, although CD30, CD38, CD45, and CD138 are often expressed. Patients with PEL are usually treated with anthracycline-based combination chemotherapy, but outcomes are poor, with a median survival of only 6 months. PBL is also associated with both HIV and EBV infections and has a marked tropism for the oral cavity where it may be confused with periodontal disease, cellulitis, Kaposi sarcoma, or melanoma.[177] PBL is characterized by weak or absent expression of CD20 and other B-cell markers, although it typically expresses plasma cell antigens such as CD38, CD138, MUM-1, and VS38c. Rearrangements of the *MYC* oncogene are seen in about half of the cases. Most patients have been treated with CHOP, although recent guidelines advocate

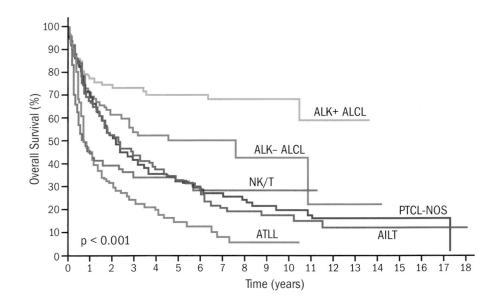

Fig. 16-5 Survival of patients with the common subtypes of peripheral T-cell lymphoma.

Abbreviations: ALK+ ALCL, anaplastic lymphoma kinase expressing anaplastic large cell lymphoma; ALK- ALCL, anaplastic large cell lymphoma that does not express ALK; NK/T, natural killer/T-cell lymphomas; PCTL-NOS, peripheral T-cell lymphoma, not otherwise specified; AILT, angioimmunoblastic T-cell lymphoma; ATLL, adult T-cell leukemia lymphoma.

This research was originally published in Blood. Foss FM, Zinzani PL, Vose JM, et al. Peripheral T-cell lymphoma. Blood. 2011;117(25):6756-6767. © American Society of Hematology.

more intensive regimens such as DA-EPOCH-R, hyperCVAD, or CODOX-M/IVAC. Unfortunately, the prognosis is poor with any of these approaches, with a median OS of 14 months in a recent systematic analysis.[177] Novel approaches are needed and investigations have begun incorporating treatment of the underlying viral infections with cidofovir and administration of agents targeting plasma cells (e.g., bortezomib).

AIDS-associated Burkitt lymphoma has been imperfectly studied. In many series, patients with DLBCL and Burkitt lymphoma have been combined in small series and treated identically, confounding analysis of outcomes. The NCI group recently reported excellent outcomes for HIV-associated Burkitt lymphoma with SC, low-dose EPOCH-R[161] as described above in the section on Burkitt lymphoma. More traditional Burkitt lymphoma regimens such as R-CODOX-M/IVAC or R-hyperCVAD have also been used successfully with HIV-associated Burkitt lymphoma.

PERIPHERAL T-CELL LYMPHOMAS

The term peripheral T-cell lymphoma (PTCL) refers to a diverse group of post-thymic T-cell tumors that have a mature T-cell phenotype. Patients tend to have higher scores on the IPI, more B symptoms, advanced-stage disease, and higher serum beta 2-microglobulin than comparable patients with DLBCL. Patients with PTCL usually have inferior treatment responses, a high rate of relapse, and few sustained remissions when treated with multi-agent chemotherapy regimens such as CHOP. The Prognostic Index for PTCL (PIT) includes patient age, LDH level, performance status, and presence of bone marrow involvement.[178] Poor prognosis is also associated with p53 expression, a high Ki67 proliferation index (> 25%), adverse chemokine expression patterns (CXCR3-positive/CCR4-negative), and expression of CD30 and CD56, BCL2, or BCL$_{XL}$. A full exposition of the details of this diverse group of disorders is beyond the scope of this chapter, but excellent recent reviews are available.[179,180] Brief descriptions of the most common entities follow.

PTCL Not Otherwise Specified

PTCL not otherwise specified (PTCL-NOS) is the most common of the nodal T-cell lymphomas, representing 25% to 30% of all T-cell lymphomas worldwide.[179,180] PTCL usually presents with paracortical or diffuse nodal infiltration of malignant lymphoid cells expressing T-cell markers including CD2, CD3, TCR, and usually CD4, often with down-regulation of CD5 and CD7.[181] The median age of patients with PTCL is 60, with a male to female ratio of 1.9:1. The majority of patients present with advanced-stage disease (69%), and two-thirds of the patients have extranodal disease in addition to adenopathy. Historically, patients have usually been treated with doxorubicin-based chemotherapy regimens such as CHOP, but outcomes have been poor, with only 56% achieving complete remission, 36% surviving 5 years, and 22% remaining failure-free after 5 years with this management strategy (Fig. 16-5).[180] Retrospective subset analyses suggest that the addition of etoposide to the CHOP regimen (CHOEP) may improve outcomes for patients younger than 60 with PTCL. Pralatrexate and romidepsin are recent additions to the therapeutic armamentarium that have considerable activity in patients with relapsed PTCL.[182,183] If the tumors express CD30, brentuximab vedotin may be of value. The role of ASCT or alloSCT in first remission appears promising but is controversial.[178,182]

Angioimmunoblastic T-Cell Lymphoma

Angioimmunoblastic T-cell lymphoma (AITL) accounts for 18.5% of T-cell NHL worldwide[179] and typically presents with generalized lymphadenopathy, fevers, weight loss, and rash, with autoimmune features including hypergammaglobulinemia and a positive Coombs test. The disease is derived from follicular helper T-cells (T$_{FH}$), with malignant cells typically expressing CD10, BCL6, PD1, and CXCL13, in addition to typical T-cell markers (CD2, CD3, CD5, and CD4). The disease course is typically complicated by serious and often fatal infections. EBV-associated B-cell lymphoma often develops during the course of treatment for AITL, apparently derived from EBV-infected B-cell blasts present in the tumor. Recent retrospective studies suggest that patients with AITL may have improved outcomes if they undergo ASCT in first remission.[184,185]

Anaplastic Large-Cell Lymphoma

Anaplastic large-cell lymphoma (ALCL) is a malignancy of large pleomorphic mature T lymphocytes that express the CD30 antigen (Ki-1) as well as T-cell surface markers such as CD2, CD4, and CD5. Curiously, the pan-T-cell antigen CD3 is negative in more than 75% of cases. Nodal ALCL typically is associated with a cytogenetic abnormality, t(2;5)(p23;q35), leading to expression of a nucleophosmin-anaplastic lymphoma kinase (NPM-ALK) fusion protein, which is associated with a favorable outcome. ALK-positive ALCL usually presents in the first 3 decades of life, with advanced stage III/IV disease and B symptoms. ALK-positive ALCL is one of the more favorable histologic subtypes of aggressive NHL. Chemotherapy regimens such as CHOP induce complete responses in more than 70% of patients, with 50% to 80% remaining alive and disease free after 5 years. Patients with ALK-negative nodal ALCL have a prognosis intermediate between ALK-positive ALCL and PTCL-NOS.[180] ALK-negative ALCL confined to the skin appears to be a different disease than systemic ALCL; it usually presents in elderly individuals and typically has a favorable prognosis even with conservative therapy (excision, local radiation). Patients with ALCL who experience relapse following front-line therapy can be effectively salvaged with brentuximab vedotin, with 86% of patients achieving objective remissions, many of which are durable.[186]

Enteropathy-Associated T-Cell Lymphoma

Enteropathy-associated T-cell lymphoma (EATL) accounts for approximately 5% of T-cell lymphomas and is more common in geographic areas with a higher incidence of celiac disease, including North America and Europe. Patients typically present with pain, weight loss, and bowel perforation.[187] Cases associated with celiac disease typically exhibit a pleomorphic histology and express CD3 and CD7 but not CD56, whereas patients without celiac disease often display a monomorphic histology and express CD56. Up to 70% of cases of EATL contain gains at chromosome 9q33-q34. Conventional therapy consists of CHOP, with a median OS of only 10 months in a recent international series of 62 patients, with a median FFS of only 6 months.[188] The presence of clinical sprue and an adverse PIT score both predicted independently for poor survival. One recent study suggests outcomes with EATL may be improved by inducing remission with a novel regimen of ifosfamide/etoposide/epirubicin alternating with intermediate-dose methotrexate followed by consolidation with ASCT.[189] This approach yielded a 5-year PFS of 52% and OS of 60% among 26 patients who underwent transplant.

Extranodal Nasal Natural Killer/T-Cell Lymphoma

Extranodal nasal natural killer (NK)/T-cell lymphoma is an angioinvasive, necrotizing lymphoma derived from cytotoxic NK or T cells that is almost invariably associated with EBV infection and typically presents in the nasal cavity, nasopharynx, or paranasal sinuses of Asian men. In occasional cases, NK/T-cell lymphoma can also affect skin, the gastrointestinal tract, or testes. Nasal obstruction, bleeding, and ulceration are typical; hence the previous designation of this disease as lethal midline granuloma. The malignant lymphoid cells of nasal NK/T-cell lymphoma typically express CD2, CD56, and cytoplasmic CD3-epsilon (but not surface CD3), as well as cytotoxic molecules such as TIA1, granzyme B, and perforin. The disease often presents at an early stage; nevertheless, outcome has been variable, with best results reported when radiotherapy is given up front to patients with early-stage disease, either preceding or concurrent with chemotherapy.[190] The disease is relatively resistant to CHOP-type chemotherapy but appears more sensitive to intense regimens such as dexamethasone (steroid)/methotrexate/ifosfamide/L-asparaginase/etoposide (SMILE).[191]

Hepatosplenic Gamma-Delta T-Cell Lymphoma

Hepatosplenic gamma-delta T-cell lymphoma is a rare disease of young males derived from immature or nonactivated gamma-delta T-cells possessing an isochromosome 7q abnormality. This lymphoma typically infiltrates the liver, spleen, and marrow sinusoids, with minimal adenopathy. Patients often present with fever, chills, and other systemic symptoms. Cytopenias, especially thrombocytopenia, are typical and often accompanied by a fatal hemophagocytic syndrome. Outcome is poor regardless of management, although many authorities recommend aggressive chemotherapy followed by stem cell transplantation in first remission.

Panniculitis-Like T-Cell Lymphomas

Panniculitis-like T-cell lymphomas typically present in men with subcutaneous nodules that may become necrotic. Up to 20% of patients have associated autoimmune diseases, such as systemic lupus erythematosus. Biopsies of lesions reveal rim-like infiltrates of neoplastic T cells expressing CD3 and CD8 (but not CD4) that surround fat cells in the subcutaneous tissues. The more common T-cell receptor alpha-beta panniculitis-like lymphomas have a favorable prognosis, whereas cases with a gamma-delta immunophenotype have a worse outcome. Both single-agent and combination chemotherapy (CHOP) have been employed successfully,[180] although more conservative immunosuppressive regimens (cyclosporine, prednisone) also have been reported to be effective for the alpha-beta lymphomas.[192]

Overall, outcomes for T-cell lymphomas remain suboptimal, perhaps because they traditionally have been treated using paradigms developed for B-cell lymphomas. Improved outcomes will likely only be attained with regimens designed specifically for T-NHL, which may incorporate novel new drugs such as pralatrexate, romidepsin, nelarabine, denileukin diftitox, gemcitabine, and antibodies targeting T-cell–associated antigens including siplizumab (CD2), zanolimumab (CD4), LMB-2 (CD25), brentuximab vedotin (CD30), alemtuzumab (CD52), KW-0761 (CCR4), and bevacizumab (VEGF).

Cutaneous T-Cell Lymphomas

Cutaneous T-cell lymphomas (CTCL) are a heterogeneous group of lymphomas characterized by infiltration of the skin and other organs by mature T cells.[193] In the WHO classification, these disorders are considered indolent T-cell malignancies and include mycosis fungoides and Sézary syndrome. In most cases of mycosis fungoides, the diagnosis is made after a prolonged period of ill-defined skin disease or parapsoriasis. Subsequently, patches or plaques characteristic of mycosis fungoides develop. At the time of diagnosis, less than one-half of patients have limited plaques, one-third have extensive plaques, and 10% to 15% have generalized erythroderma. The spleen, liver, and lymph nodes also may be involved, especially in patients with advanced skin disease and circulating malignant cells. When the peripheral blood becomes extensively involved with the malignant T cells and erythroderma develops, the condition is called Sézary syndrome.

Most patients with CTCL initially are treated with topical measures, including corticosteroids, photochemotherapy with oral methoxypsoralen therapy followed by ultraviolet light, mechlorethamine, bexarotene, or electron beam radiation (either localized or total skin).[193] Systemic therapy is needed when these approaches fail or when patients develop major organ involvement, diffuse lymphadenopathy, or transformation to large-cell NHL. Treatment options for advanced CTCL include extracorporeal photopheresis, interferon-alpha, bexarotene, denileukin diftitox, liposomal doxorubicin, nucleoside analogs (e.g., gemcitabine), alemtuzumab, or combination chemotherapy. Histone deacetylate inhibitors such as vorinostat and romidepsin have shown major activity in this condition,[194] as has pralatrexate, and these drugs are being increasingly employed earlier in the disease course. Patients with CTCL often die from infections, and as such, good skin care and oral antibiotics are important adjuncts to therapy. The only known curative therapy for mycosis fungoides is alloSCT, although this approach is only appropriate for a minority of patients.[195]

References

1. Siegel R, Naishadham D, Jemal A. Cancer statistics, 2013. *CA Cancer J Clin*. 2013;63:11-30. PMID: 23335087.

2. Bohlius J, Schmidlin K, Boué F, et al. HIV-1-related Hodgkin lymphoma in the era of combination antiretroviral therapy: incidence and evolution of CD4+ T-cell lymphocytes. *Blood*. 2011;117:6100-6108. PMID: 21368291.

3. Swerdlow SH, Campo E, Harris NL, et al. *WHO Classification of Tumours of Haematopoietic and Lymphoid Tissues*. Lyon: International Agency for Research on Cancer; 2008.

4. Nogová L, Reineke T, Brillant C, et al. Lymphocyte-predominant and classical Hodgkin's lymphoma: a comprehensive analysis from the German Hodgkin Study Group. *J Clin Oncol*. 2008;26:434-439. PMID: 18086799.

5. Brune V, Tiacci E, Pfeil I, et al. Origin and pathogenesis of nodular lymphocyte-predominant Hodgkin lymphoma as revealed by global gene expression analysis. *J Exp Med*. 2008;205:2251-2268. PMID: 18794340.

6. Hoppe RT, Advani RH, Ambinder RF, et al. Hodgkin disease/lymphoma. *J Natl Compr Canc Netw*. 2008;6:594-622. PMID: 18597713.

7. Hasenclever D, Diehl V. A prognostic score for advanced Hodgkin's disease. International Prognostic Factors Project on Advanced Hodgkin's Disease. *N Engl J Med*. 1998;339:1506-1514. PMID: 9819449.

8. Hasenclever D. The disappearance of prognostic factors in Hodgkin's disease. *Ann Oncol*. 2002;13 Suppl 1:75-78. PMID: 12078907.

9. Gallamini A, Hutchings M, Rigacci L, et al. Early interim 2-[18F]fluoro-2-deoxy-D-glucose positron emission tomography is prognostically superior to international prognostic score in advanced-stage Hodgkin's lymphoma: a report from a joint Italian-Danish study. *J Clin Oncol*. 2007;25:3746-3752. PMID: 17646666.

10. Steidl C, Lee T, Shah SP, et al. Tumor-associated macrophages and survival in classic Hodgkin's lymphoma. *N Engl J Med*. 2010;362:875-885. PMID: 20220182.

11. Scott DW, Chan FC, Hong F, et al. Gene expression-based model using formalin-fixed paraffin-embedded biopsies predicts overall survival in advanced-stage classical Hodgkin lymphoma. *J Clin Oncol*. 2013;31:692-700. PMID: 23182984.

12. Cheson BD. Role of functional imaging in the management of lymphoma. *J Clin Oncol*. 2011;29:1844-1854. PMID: 21482982.

13. Seam P, Juweid ME, Cheson BD. The role of FDG-PET scans in patients with lymphoma. *Blood*. 2007;110:3507-3516. PMID: 17709603.

14. Terasawa T, Nagai H. Current clinical evidence on interim fluorine-18 fluorodeoxy glucose positron emission tomography for advanced-stage Hodgkin lymphoma and diffuse large B-cell lymphoma to predict treatment outcomes. *Leuk Lymphoma*. 2009;50:1750-1752. PMID: 19863179.

15. Gallamini A, Rigacci L, Merli F, et al. The predictive value of positron emission tomography scanning performed after two courses of standard therapy on treatment outcome in advanced stage Hodgkin's disease. *Haematologica*. 2006;91:475-481. PMID: 16585014.

16. Gallamini A, Patti C, Viviani S, et al. Early chemotherapy intensification with BEACOPP in advanced-stage Hodgkin lymphoma patients with a interim-PET positive after two ABVD courses. *Br J Haematol*. 2011;152:551-560. PMID: 21166786.

17. Armitage JO. PET scans: when and how? *Blood*. 2011;118:2-3. PMID: 21737605.

18. Fermé C, Eghbali H, Meerwaldt JH, et al. Chemotherapy plus involved-field radiation in early-stage Hodgkin's disease. *N Engl J Med*. 2007;357:1916-1927. PMID: 17989384.

19. Engert A, Plütschow A, Eich HT, et al. Reduced treatment intensity in patients with early-stage Hodgkin's lymphoma. *N Engl J Med*. 2010;363:640-652. PMID: 20818855.

20. Canellos GP, Abramson JS, Fisher DC, et al. Treatment of favorable, limited-stage Hodgkin's lymphoma with chemotherapy without consolidation by radiation therapy. *J Clin Oncol*. 2010;28:1611-1615. PMID: 20159818.

21. Eich HT, Diehl V, Görgen H, et al. Intensified chemotherapy and dose-reduced involved-field radiotherapy in patients with early unfavorable Hodgkin's lymphoma: final analysis of the German Hodgkin Study Group HD11 trial. *J Clin Oncol*. 2010;28:4199-4206. PMID: 20713848.

22. DeVita VT Jr, Simon RM, Hubbard SM, et al. Curability of advanced Hodgkin's disease with chemotherapy. Long-term follow-up of MOPP-treated patients at the National Cancer Institute. *Ann Intern Med*. 1980;92:587-595. PMID: 6892984.

23. van der Kaaij MA, Heutte N, Le Stang N, et al. Gonadal function in males after chemotherapy for early-stage Hodgkin's lymphoma treated in four subsequent trials by the European Organisation for Research and Treatment of Cancer: EORTC Lymphoma Group and the Groupe d'Etude des Lymphomes de l'Adulte. *J Clin Oncol*. 2007;25:2825-2832. PMID: 17515571.

24. Santoro A, Bonfante V, Bonadonna G. Salvage chemotherapy with ABVD in MOPP-resistant Hodgkin's disease. *Ann Intern Med*. 1982;96:139-143. PMID: 6174060.

25. Canellos GP, Anderson JR, Propert KJ, et al. Chemotherapy of advanced Hodgkin's disease with MOPP, ABVD, or MOPP alternating with ABVD. *N Engl J Med*. 1992;327:1478-1484. PMID: 1383821.

26. Canellos GP, Niedzwiecki D, Johnson JL. Long-term follow-up of survival in Hodgkin's lymphoma. *N Engl J Med*. 2009;361:2390-2391. PMID: 20007568.

27. Connors JM, Klimo P, Adams G, et al. Treatment of advanced Hodgkin's disease with chemotherapy–comparison of MOPP/ABV hybrid regimen with alternating courses of MOPP and ABVD: a report from the National Cancer Institute of Canada clinical trials group. *J Clin Oncol*. 1997;15:1638-1645. PMID: 9193364.

28. Johnson PW, Radford JA, Cullen MH, et al. Comparison of ABVD and alternating or hybrid multidrug regimens for the treatment of advanced Hodgkin's lymphoma: results of the United Kingdom Lymphoma Group LY09 Trial (ISRCTN97144519). *J Clin Oncol*. 2005;23:9208-9218. PMID: 16314615.

29. Duggan DB, Petroni GR, Johnson JL, et al. Randomized comparison of ABVD and MOPP/ABV hybrid for the treatment of advanced Hodgkin's

disease: report of an intergroup trial. *J Clin Oncol*. 2003;21:607-614. PMID: 12586796.

30. Boleti E, Mead GM. ABVD for Hodgkin's lymphoma: full-dose chemotherapy without dose reductions or growth factors. *Ann Oncol*. 2007;18:376-380. PMID: 17071938.

31. Evens AM, Cilley J, Ortiz T, et al. G-CSF is not necessary to maintain over 99% dose-intensity with ABVD in the treatment of Hodgkin lymphoma: low toxicity and excellent outcomes in a 10-year analysis. *Br J Haematol*. 2007;137:545-552. PMID: 17459049.

32. Horning SJ, Hoppe RT, Breslin S, et al. Stanford V and radiotherapy for locally extensive and advanced Hodgkin's disease: mature results of a prospective clinical trial. *J Clin Oncol*. 2002;20:630-637. PMID: 11821442.

33. Gobbi PG, Levis A, Chisesi T, et al. ABVD versus modified stanford V versus MOPPEBVCAD with optional and limited radiotherapy in intermediate- and advanced-stage Hodgkin's lymphoma: final results of a multicenter randomized trial by the Intergruppo Italiano Linfomi. *J Clin Oncol*. 2005;23:9198-9207. PMID: 16172458.

34. Hoskin PJ, Lowry L, Horwich A, et al. Randomized comparison of the stanford V regimen and ABVD in the treatment of advanced Hodgkin's Lymphoma: United Kingdom National Cancer Research Institute Lymphoma Group trial ISRCTN 64141244. *J Clin Oncol*. 2009;27:5390-5396. PMID: 19738111.

35. Gordon LI, Hong F, Fisher RI, et al. A randomized phase III trial of ABVD vs. stanford V ± radiation therapy in locally extensive and advanced stage Hodgkin's lymphoma: an intergroup study coordinated by the Eastern Cooperative Oncology Group (E2496). *Blood*. 2010;116 (abstr 415).

36. Diehl V, Franklin J, Pfreundschuh M, et al. Standard and increased-dose BEACOPP chemotherapy compared with COPP-ABVD for advanced Hodgkin's disease. *N Engl J Med*. 2003;348:2386-2395. PMID: 12802024.

37. Engert A, Diehl V, Franklin J, et al. Escalated-dose BEACOPP in the treatment of patients with advanced-stage Hodgkin's lymphoma: 10 years of follow-up of the GHSG HD9 study. *J Clin Oncol*. 2009;27:4548-4554. PMID: 19704068.

38. Sieniawski M, Reineke T, Nogova L, et al. Fertility in male patients with advanced Hodgkin lymphoma treated with BEACOPP: a report of the German Hodgkin Study Group (GHSG). *Blood*. 2008;111:71-76. PMID: 17890456.

39. Ballova V, Rüffer JU, Haverkamp H, et al. A prospectively randomized trial carried out by the German Hodgkin Study Group (GHSG) for elderly patients with advanced Hodgkin's disease comparing BEACOPP baseline and COPP-ABVD (study HD9elderly). *Ann Oncol*. 2005;16:124-131. PMID: 15598949.

40. Viviani S, Zinzani PL, Rambaldi A, et al. ABVD versus BEACOPP for Hodgkin's lymphoma when high-dose salvage is planned. *N Engl J Med*. 2011;365:203-212. PMID: 21774708.

41. Carde PP, Karrasch M, Fortpied C, et al. ABVD (8 cycles) versus BEACOPP (4 escalated cycles ≥ 4 baseline) in stage III-IV high-risk Hodgkin lymphoma (HL): First results of EORTC 20012 Intergroup randomized phase III clinical trial. *J Clin Oncol*. 2012;30:(suppl; abstr 8002).

42. Engert A, Haverkamp H, Kobe C, et al. Reduced-intensity chemotherapy and PET-guided radiotherapy in patients with advanced stage Hodgkin's lymphoma (HD15 trial): a randomised, open-label, phase 3 non-inferiority trial. *Lancet*. 2012;379:1791-1799. PMID: 22480758.

43. Juweid ME, Stroobants S, Hoekstra OS, et al. Use of positron emission tomography for response assessment of lymphoma: consensus of the Imaging Subcommittee of International Harmonization Project in Lymphoma. *J Clin Oncol*. 2007;25:571-578. PMID: 17242397.

44. Moskowitz CH, Bertino JR, Glassman JR, et al. Ifosfamide, carboplatin, and etoposide: a highly effective cytoreduction and peripheral-blood progenitor-cell mobilization regimen for transplant-eligible patients with non-Hodgkin's lymphoma. *J Clin Oncol*. 1999;17:3776-3785. PMID: 10577849.

45. Bartlett NL, Niedzwiecki D, Johnson JL, et al. Gemcitabine, vinorelbine, and pegylated liposomal doxorubicin (GVD), a salvage regimen in relapsed Hodgkin's lymphoma: CALGB 59804. *Ann Oncol*. 2007;18:1071-1079. PMID: 17426059.

46. Vose JM, Bierman PJ, Anderson JR, et al. CHLVPP chemotherapy with involved-field irradiation for Hodgkin's disease: favorable results with acceptable toxicity. *J Clin Oncol*. 1991;9:1421-1425. PMID: 2072145.

47. Moskowitz CH, Kewalramani T, Nimer SD, et al. Effectiveness of high dose chemoradiotherapy and autologous stem cell transplantation for patients with biopsy-proven primary refractory Hodgkin's disease. *Br J Haematol*. 2004;124:645-652. PMID: 14871252.

48. Gutierrez-Delgado F, Holmberg L, Hooper H, et al. Autologous stem cell transplantation for Hodgkin's disease: busulfan, melphalan and thiotepa compared to a radiation-based regimen. *Bone Marrow Transplant*. 2003;32:279-285. PMID: 12858199.

49. Schmitz N, Pfistner B, Sextro M, et al. Aggressive conventional chemotherapy compared with high-dose chemotherapy with autologous haemopoietic stem-cell transplantation for relapsed chemosensitive Hodgkin's disease: a randomised trial. *Lancet*. 2002;359:2065-2071. PMID: 12086759.

50. Moskowitz CH, Matasar MJ, Zelenetz AD, et al. Normalization of pre-ASCT, FDG-PET imaging with second-line, non-cross-resistant, chemotherapy programs improves event-free survival in patients with Hodgkin lymphoma. *Blood*. 2012;119:1665-1670. PMID: 22184409.

51. Sarina B, Castagna L, Farina L, et al. Allogeneic transplantation improves the overall and progression-free survival of Hodgkin lymphoma patients relapsing after autologous transplantation: a retrospective study based on the time of HLA typing and donor availability. *Blood*. 2010;115:3671-3677. PMID: 20220116.

52. Corradini P, Sarina B, Farina L. Allogeneic transplantation for Hodgkin's lymphoma. *Br J Haematol*. 2011;152:261-272. PMID: 21155760.

53. Younes A, Bartlett NL, Leonard JP, et al. Brentuximab vedotin (SGN-35) for relapsed CD30-positive lymphomas. *N Engl J Med*. 2010;363:1812-1821. PMID: 21047225.

54. Younes A, Gopal AK, Smith SE, et al. Results of a pivotal phase II study of brentuximab vedotin for patients with relapsed or refractory Hodgkin's lymphoma. *J Clin Oncol*. 2012;30:2183-2189. PMID: 22454421.

55. Schulz H, Rehwald U, Morschhauser F, et al. Rituximab in relapsed lymphocyte-predominant Hodgkin lymphoma: long-term results of a phase 2 trial by the German Hodgkin Lymphoma Study Group (GHSG). *Blood*. 2008;111:109-111. PMID: 17938252.

56. Ekstrand BC, Lucas JB, Horwitz SM, et al. Rituximab in lymphocyte-predominant Hodgkin disease: results of a phase 2 trial. *Blood*. 2003;101:4285-4289. PMID: 12586628.

57. Hehn ST, Grogan TM, Miller TP. Utility of fine-needle aspiration as a diagnostic technique in lymphoma. *J Clin Oncol*. 2004;22:3046-3052. PMID: 15284254.

58. Elstrom R, Guan L, Baker G, et al. Utility of FDG-PET scanning in lymphoma by WHO classification. *Blood*. 2003;101:3875-3876. PMID: 12531812.

59. Solal-Céligny P, Roy P, Colombat P, et al. Follicular lymphoma international prognostic index. *Blood*. 2004;104:1258-1265. PMID: 15126323.

60. Federico M, Bellei M, Marcheselli L, et al. Follicular lymphoma international prognostic index 2: a new prognostic index for follicular lymphoma developed by the international follicular lymphoma prognostic factor project. *J Clin Oncol*. 2009;27:4555-4562. PMID: 19652063.

61. Press OW, Unger JM, Rimsza LM, et al. Phase III randomized intergroup trial of CHOP plus rituximab compared with CHOP chemotherapy plus (131)iodine-tositumomab for previously untreated follicular non-Hodgkin lymphoma: SWOG S0016. *J Clin Oncol*. 2013;31:314-320. PMID: 23233710.

62. Press OW, Unger JM, Rimsza LM, et al. A comparative analysis of prognostic factor models for follicular lymphoma based on a phase III trial of CHOP-rituximab versus CHOP + 131iodine–tositumomab. *Clin Cancer Res*. 2013;19:6624-6632. PMID: 24130072.

63. Advani R, Rosenberg SA, Horning SJ. Stage I and II follicular non-Hodgkin's lymphoma: long-term follow-up of no initial therapy. *J Clin Oncol*. 2004;22:1454-1459. PMID: 15024027.

64. Brice P, Bastion Y, Lepage E, et al. Comparison in low-tumor-burden follicular lymphomas between an initial no-treatment policy, prednimustine, or interferon alfa: a randomized study from the Groupe d'Etude des Lymphomes Folliculaires. Groupe d'Etude des Lymphomes de l'Adulte. *J Clin Oncol*. 1997;15:1110-1117. PMID: 9060552.

65. Cheson BD, Leonard JP. Monoclonal antibody therapy for B-cell non-Hodgkin's lymphoma. *N Engl J Med*. 2008;359:613-626. PMID: 18687642.

66. Alduaij W, Illidge TM. The future of anti-CD20 monoclonal antibodies: are we making progress? *Blood*. 2011;117:2993-3001. PMID: 21209380.

67. Ghielmini M, Schmitz SF, Cogliatti SB, et al. Prolonged treatment with rituximab in patients with follicular lymphoma significantly increases event-free survival and response duration compared with the standard weekly x 4 schedule. *Blood*. 2004;103:4416-4423. PMID: 14976046.

68. Hochster HS, Weller E, Gascoyne RD, et al. Maintenance rituximab after CVP results in superior clinical outcome in advanced follicular lymphoma (FL): results of the E1496 phase III trial from the Eastern Cooperative Oncology Group and the Cancer and Leukemia Group B. *Blood*. 2005;106:106a (abstr 349).

69. Hainsworth JD. First-line and maintenance treatment with rituximab for patients with indolent non-Hodgkin's lymphoma. *Semin Oncol*. 2003;30:9-15. PMID: 12652459.

70. Salles G, Seymour JF, Offner F, et al. Rituximab maintenance for 2 years in patients with high tumour burden follicular lymphoma responding to rituximab plus chemotherapy (PRIMA): a phase 3, randomised controlled trial. *Lancet.* 2011;377:42-51. PMID: 21176949.

71. Hiddemann W, Kneba M, Dreyling M, et al. Frontline therapy with rituximab added to the combination of cyclophosphamide, doxorubicin, vincristine, and prednisone (CHOP) significantly improves the outcome for patients with advanced-stage follicular lymphoma compared with therapy with CHOP alone: results of a prospective randomized study of the German Low-Grade Lymphoma Study Group. *Blood.* 2005;106:3725-3732. PMID: 16123223.

72. Herold M, Haas A, Srock S, et al. Rituximab added to first-line mitoxantrone, chlorambucil, and prednisolone chemotherapy followed by interferon maintenance prolongs survival in patients with advanced follicular lymphoma: an East German Study Group Hematology and Oncology Study. *J Clin Oncol.* 2007;25:1986-1992. PMID: 17420513.

73. van Oers MH, Van Glabbeke M, Giurgea L, et al. Rituximab maintenance treatment of relapsed/resistant follicular non-Hodgkin's lymphoma: long-term outcome of the EORTC 20981 phase III randomized intergroup study. *J Clin Oncol.* 2010;28:2853-2858. PMID: 20439641.

74. Marcus R, Imrie K, Solal-Celigny P, et al. Phase III study of R-CVP compared with cyclophosphamide, vincristine, and prednisone alone in patients with previously untreated advanced follicular lymphoma. *J Clin Oncol.* 2008;26:4579-4586. PMID: 18662969.

75. Press OW, Palanca-Wessels MC. Selection of first-line therapy for advanced follicular lymphoma. *J Clin Oncol.* 2013;31:1496-1498. PMID: 23530108.

76. Salles G, Seymour JF, Offner F, et al. Rituximab maintenance for 2 years in patients with high tumour burden follicular lymphoma responding to rituximab plus chemotherapy (PRIMA): a phase 3, randomised controlled trial. *Lancet.* 2011;377:42-51. PMID: 21176949.

77. Federico M, Luminari S, Dondi A, et al. R-CVP versus R-CHOP versus R-FM for the initial treatment of patients with advanced-stage follicular lymphoma: results of the FOLL05 trial conducted by the Fondazione Italiana Linfomi. *J Clin Oncol.* 2013;31:1506-1513. PMID: 23530110.

78. Friedberg JW, Cohen P, Chen L, et al. Bendamustine in patients with rituximab-refractory indolent and transformed non-Hodgkin's lymphoma: results from a phase II multicenter, single-agent study. *J Clin Oncol.* 2008;26:204-210. PMID: 18182663.

79. Friedberg JW. The emerging role of bendamustine in follicular lymphoma. *Leuk Lymphoma.* 2009;50:317-318. PMID: 19347722.

80. Cheson BD, Rummel MJ. Bendamustine: rebirth of an old drug. *J Clin Oncol.* 2009;27:1492-1501. PMID: 19224851.

81. Rummel MJ, Niederle N, Maschmeyer G, et al. Bendamustine plus rituximab versus CHOP plus rituximab as first-line treatment for patients with indolent and mantle-cell lymphomas: an open-label, multicentre, randomised, phase 3 non-inferiority trial. *Lancet.* 2013;381:1203-1210. PMID: 23433739.

82. Flinn IW, Van der Jagt RH, Kahl BS, et al. An open-label, randomized study of bendamustine and rituximab (BR) compared with rituximab, cyclophosphamide, vincristine, and prednisone (R-CVP) or rituximab, cyclophosphamide, doxorubicin, vincristine, and prednisone (R-CHOP) in first-line treatment of patients with advanced indolent non-Hodgkin's lymphoma (NHL) or mantle cell lymphoma (MCL): the Bright Study. *American Society of Hematology Annual Meeting.* 2013 (abstr 902).

83. Montoto S, Davies AJ, Matthews J, et al. Risk and clinical implications of transformation of follicular lymphoma to diffuse large B-cell lymphoma. *J Clin Oncol.* 2007;25:2426-2433. PMID: 17485708.

84. Al-Tourah AJ, Gill KK, Chhanabhai M, et al. Population-based analysis of incidence and outcome of transformed non-Hodgkin's lymphoma. *J Clin Oncol.* 2008;26:5165-5169. PMID: 18838711.

85. Rezvani AR, Norasetthada L, Gooley T, et al. Non-myeloablative allogeneic haematopoietic cell transplantation for relapsed diffuse large B-cell lymphoma: a multicentre experience. *Br J Haematol.* 2008;143:395-403. PMID: 18759762.

86. Williams CD, Harrison CN, Lister TA, et al. High-dose therapy and autologous stem-cell support for chemosensitive transformed low-grade follicular non-Hodgkin's lymphoma: a case-matched study from the European Bone Marrow Transplant Registry. *J Clin Oncol.* 2001;19:727-735. PMID: 11157024.

87. Link BK, Maurer MJ, Nowakowski GS, et al. Rates and outcomes of follicular lymphoma transformation in the immunochemotherapy era: a report from the University of Iowa/MayoClinic Specialized Program of Research Excellence Molecular Epidemiology Resource. *J Clin Oncol.* 2013;31:3272-3278. PMID: 23897955.

88. Friedberg JW, Vose JM, Kelly JL, et al. The combination of bendamustine, bortezomib, and rituximab for patients with relapsed/refractory indolent and mantle cell non-Hodgkin lymphoma. *Blood.* 2011;117:2807-2812. PMID: 21239695.

89. Fowler N, Kahl BS, Lee P, et al. Bortezomib, bendamustine, and rituximab in patients with relapsed or refractory follicular lymphoma: the phase II VERTICAL study. *J Clin Oncol.* 2011;29:3389-3395. PMID: 21810687.

90. Cheson BD. Radioimmunotherapy of non-Hodgkin's lymphomas. *Curr Drug Targets.* 2006;7:1293-1300. PMID: 17073591.

91. Morschhauser F, Radford J, Van Hoof A, et al. Phase III trial of consolidation therapy with yttrium-90-ibritumomab tiuxetan compared with no additional therapy after first remission in advanced follicular lymphoma. *J Clin Oncol.* 2008;26:5156-5164. PMID: 18854568.

92. Fisher RI, LeBlanc M, Press OW, et al. New treatment options have changed the survival of patients with follicular lymphoma. *J Clin Oncol.* 2005;23:8447-8452. PMID: 16230674.

93. Kaminski MS, Tuck M, Estes J, et al. 131I-tositumomab therapy as initial treatment for follicular lymphoma. *N Engl J Med.* 2005;352:441-449. PMID: 15689582.

94. Press OW, Unger JM, Braziel RM, et al. Phase II trial of CHOP chemotherapy followed by tositumomab/iodine I-131 tositumomab for previously untreated follicular non-Hodgkin's lymphoma: five-year follow-up of Southwest Oncology Group Protocol S9911. *J Clin Oncol.* 2006;24:4143-4149. PMID: 16896003.

95. Press OW, Unger JM, Rimsza L, et al. A phase III randomized intergroup trial of CHOP chemotherapy plus rituximab compared with CHOP chemotherapy plus (131)iodine-tositumomab for previously untreated follicular non-Hodgkin lymphoma: SWOG S0016. *J Clin Oncol.* 2013;31:314-320.

96. Press OW, Eary JF, Gooley T, et al. A phase I/II trial of iodine-131-tositumomab (anti-CD20), etoposide, cyclophosphamide, and autologous stem cell transplantation for relapsed B-cell lymphomas. *Blood.* 2000;96:2934-2942. PMID: 11049969.

97. Kochenderfer JN, Rosenberg SA. Treating B-cell cancer with T cells expressing anti-CD19 chimeric antigen receptors. *Nat Rev Clin Oncol.* 2013;10:2267-276. PMID: 23546520.

98. Palanca-Wessels MC, Press OW. Advances in the treatment of hematologic malignancies using immunoconjugates. *Blood.* 2014;123:2293-2301.

99. Friedberg JW, Sharman J, Sweetenham J, et al. Inhibition of Syk with fostamatinib disodium has significant clinical activity in non-Hodgkin lymphoma and chronic lymphocytic leukemia. *Blood.* 2010;115:2578-2585. PMID: 19965662.

100. Lannutti BJ, Meadows SA, Herman SE, et al. CAL-101, a p110delta selective phosphatidylinositol-3-kinase inhibitor for the treatment of B-cell malignancies, inhibits PI3K signaling and cellular viability. *Blood.* 2011;117:591-594. PMID: 20959606.

101. Byrd JC, Furman RR, Coutre SE, et al. Targeting BTK with ibrutinib in relapsed chronic lymphocytic leukemia. *N Engl J Med.* 2013;369:32-42. PMID: 23782158.

102. Wang ML, Rule S, Martin P, et al. Targeting BTK with ibrutinib in relapsed or refractory mantle-cell lymphoma. *N Engl J Med.* 2013;369:507-516. PMID: 23782157.

103. Rohatiner AZ, Nadler L, Davies AJ, et al. Myeloablative therapy with autologous bone marrow transplantation for follicular lymphoma at the time of second or subsequent remission: long-term follow-up. *J Clin Oncol.* 2007;25:2554-2559. PMID: 17515573.

104. Schouten HC, Qian W, Kvaloy S, et al. High-dose therapy improves progression-free survival and survival in relapsed follicular non-Hodgkin's lymphoma: results from the randomized European CUP trial. *J Clin Oncol.* 2003;21:3918-3927. PMID: 14517188.

105. Lenz G, Dreyling M, Schiegnitz E, et al. Myeloablative radiochemotherapy followed by autologous stem cell transplantation in first remission prolongs progression-free survival in follicular lymphoma: results of a prospective, randomized trial of the German Low-Grade Lymphoma Study Group. *Blood.* 2004;104:2667-2674. PMID: 15238420.

106. Deconinck E, Foussard C, Milpied N, et al. High-dose therapy followed by autologous purged stem-cell transplantation and doxorubicin-based chemotherapy in patients with advanced follicular lymphoma: a randomized multicenter study by GOELAMS. *Blood.* 2005;105:3817-3823. PMID: 15687232.

107. van Besien K, Loberiza FR Jr., Bajorunaite R, et al. Comparison of autologous and allogeneic hematopoietic stem cell transplantation for follicular lymphoma. *Blood.* 2003;102:3521-3529. PMID: 12893748.

108. Khouri IF, McLaughlin P, Saliba RM, et al. Eight-year experience with allogeneic stem cell transplantation for relapsed follicular lymphoma after nonmyeloablative conditioning with fludarabine, cyclophosphamide, and rituximab. *Blood.* 2008;111:5530-5536. PMID: 18411419.

109. Rezvani AR, Storer B, Maris M, et al. Nonmyeloablative allogeneic hematopoietic cell transplantation in relapsed, refractory, and transformed indolent non-Hodgkin's lymphoma. *J Clin Oncol.* 2008;26:211-217. PMID: 18056679.

110. Stefanovic A, Lossos IS. Extranodal marginal zone lymphoma of the ocular adnexa. *Blood.* 2009;114:501-510. PMID: 19372259.

111. Stathis A, Chini C, Bertoni F, et al. Long-term outcome following Helicobacter pylori eradication in a retrospective study of 105 patients with localized gastric marginal zone B-cell lymphoma of MALT type. *Ann Oncol.* 2009;20:1086-1093. PMID: 19193705.

112. Iannitto E, Tripodo C. How I diagnose and treat splenic lymphomas. *Blood.* 2011;117:2585-2595. PMID: 21119113.

113. Thieblemont C, Felman P, Berger F, et al. Treatment of splenic marginal zone B-cell lymphoma: an analysis of 81 patients. *Clin Lymphoma.* 2002;3:41-47. PMID: 12141954.

114. Treon SP. How I treat Waldenström macroglobulinemia. *Blood.* 2009;114:2375-2385. PMID: 19617573.

115. Treon SP, Xu L, Yang G, et al. MYD88 L265P somatic mutation in Waldenström's macroglobulinemia. *N Engl J Med.* 2012;367:826-833. PMID: 22931316.

116. Treon SP, Ioakimidis L, Soumerai JD, et al. Primary therapy of Waldenström macroglobulinemia with bortezomib, dexamethasone, and rituximab: WMCTG clinical trial 05-180. *J Clin Oncol.* 2009;27:3830-3835. PMID: 19506160.

117. Dimopoulos MA, Anagnostopoulos A, Kyrtsonis MC, et al. Primary treatment of Waldenström macroglobulinemia with dexamethasone, rituximab, and cyclophosphamide. *J Clin Oncol.* 2007;25:3344-3349. PMID: 17577016.

118. Gribben JG. How I treat CLL up front. *Blood.* 2010;115:187-197. PMID: 19850738.

119. A predictive model for aggressive non-Hodgkin's lymphoma. The International Non-Hodgkin's Lymphoma Prognostic Factors Project. *N Engl J Med.* 1993;329:987-994. PMID: 8141877.

120. Sehn LH, Berry B, Chhanabhai M, et al. The revised International Prognostic Index (R-IPI) is a better predictor of outcome than the standard IPI for patients with diffuse large B-cell lymphoma treated with R-CHOP. *Blood.* 2007;109:1857-1861. PMID: 17105812.

121. Lenz G, Staudt LM. Aggressive lymphomas. *N Engl J Med.* 2010;362:1417-1429. PMID: 20393178.

122. Miller TP, Dahlberg S, Cassady JR, et al. Chemotherapy alone compared with chemotherapy plus radiotherapy for localized intermediate- and high-grade non-Hodgkin's lymphoma. *N Engl J Med.* 1998;339:21-26. PMID: 9647875.

123. Persky DO, Unger JM, Spier CM, et al. Phase II study of rituximab plus three cycles of CHOP and involved-field radiotherapy for patients with limited-stage aggressive B-cell lymphoma: Southwest Oncology Group study 0014. *J Clin Oncol.* 2008;26:2258-2263. PMID: 18413640.

124. Bonnet C, Fillet G, Mounier N, et al. CHOP alone compared with CHOP plus radiotherapy for localized aggressive lymphoma in elderly patients: a study by the Groupe d'Etude des Lymphomes de l'Adulte. *J Clin Oncol.* 2007;25:787-792. PMID: 17228021.

125. Fisher RI, Gaynor ER, Dahlberg S, et al. Comparison of a standard regimen (CHOP) with three intensive chemotherapy regimens for advanced non-Hodgkin's lymphoma. *N Engl J Med.* 1993;328:1002-1006. PMID: 7680764.

126. Coiffier B, Thieblemont C, Van Den Neste E, et al. Long-term outcome of patients in the LNH-98.5 trial, the first randomized study comparing rituximab-CHOP to standard CHOP chemotherapy in DLBCL patients: a study by the Groupe d'Etudes des Lymphomes de l'Adulte. *Blood.* 2010;116:2040-2045. PMID: 20548096.

127. Pfreundschuh M. How I treat elderly patients with diffuse large B-cell lymphoma. *Blood.* 2010;116:5103-5110. PMID: 20805363.

128. Delarue R, Tilly H, Mounier N, et al. Dose-dense rituximab-CHOP compared with standard rituximab-CHOP in elderly patients with diffuse large B-cell lymphoma (the LNH03-6B study): a randomised phase 3 trial. *Lancet Oncol.* 2013;14:525-533. PMID: 23578722.

129. Cunningham D, Hawkes EA, Jack A, et al. Rituximab plus cyclophosphamide, doxorubicin, vincristine, and prednisolone in patients with newly diagnosed diffuse large B-cell non-Hodgkin lymphoma: a phase 3 comparison of dose intensification with 14-day versus 21-day cycles. *Lancet.* 2013;381:1817-1826. PMID: 23615461.

130. Wilson WH, Grossbard ML, Pittaluga S, et al. Dose-adjusted EPOCH chemotherapy for untreated large B-cell lymphomas: a pharmacodynamic approach with high efficacy. *Blood.* 2002;99:2685-2693. PMID: 11929754.

131. Wilson WH, Jung SH, Porcu P, et al. A Cancer and Leukemia Group B multicenter study of DA-EPOCH-rituximab in untreated diffuse large B-cell lymphoma with analysis of outcome by molecular subtype. *Haematologica.* 2012;97:758-765. PMID: 22133772.

132. Strehl J, Mey U, Glasmacher A, et al. High-dose chemotherapy followed by autologous stem cell transplantation as first-line therapy in aggressive non-Hodgkin's lymphoma: a meta-analysis. *Haematologica.* 2003;88:1304-1315. PMID: 14607760.

133. Stiff PJ, Micallef I, Nademanee AP, et al. Transplanted CD34(+) cell dose is associated with long-term platelet count recovery following autologous peripheral blood stem cell transplant in patients with non-Hodgkin lymphoma or multiple myeloma. *Biol Blood Marrow Transplant.* 2011;17:1146-1153. PMID: 21126595.

134. Stiff PJ, Unger JM, Cook JR, et al. Autologous transplantation as consolidation for aggressive non-Hodgkin's lymphoma. *N Engl J Med.* 2013;369:1681-1690. PMID: 24171516.

135. Bernstein SH, Unger JM, Leblanc M, et al. Natural history of CNS relapse in patients with aggressive non-Hodgkin's lymphoma: a 20-year follow-up analysis of SWOG 8516 -- the Southwest Oncology Group. *J Clin Oncol.* 2009;27:114-119. PMID: 19047289.

136. Zelenetz AD, Abramson JS, Advani RH, et al. Non-Hodgkin's lymphomas. *J Natl Compr Canc Netw.* 2011;9:484-560. PMID: 21550968.

137. Gisselbrecht C, Glass B, Mounier N, et al. Salvage regimens with autologous transplantation for relapsed large B-cell lymphoma in the rituximab era. *J Clin Oncol.* 2010;28:4184-4190. PMID: 20660832.

138. Philip T, Armitage JO, Spitzer G, et al. High-dose therapy and autologous bone marrow transplantation after failure of conventional chemotherapy in adults with intermediate-grade or high-grade non-Hodgkin's lymphoma. *N Engl J Med.* 1987;316:1493-1498. PMID: 3295541.

139. van Kampen RJ, Canals C, Schouten HC, et al. Allogeneic stem-cell transplantation as salvage therapy for patients with diffuse large B-cell non-Hodgkin's lymphoma relapsing after an autologous stem-cell transplantation: an analysis of the European Group for Blood and Marrow Transplantation Registry. *J Clin Oncol.* 2011;29:1342-1348. PMID: 21321299.

140. Pérez-Galán P, Dreyling M, Wiestner A. Mantle cell lymphoma: biology, pathogenesis, and the molecular basis of treatment in the genomic era. *Blood.* 2011;117:26-38. PMID: 20940415.

141. Ghielmini M, Zucca E. How I treat mantle cell lymphoma. *Blood.* 2009;114:1469-1476. PMID: 19556426.

142. Martin P, Chadburn A, Christos P, et al. Outcome of deferred initial therapy in mantle-cell lymphoma. *J Clin Oncol.* 2009;27:1209-1213. PMID: 19188674.

143. Leitch HA, Gascoyne RD, Chhanabhai M, et al. Limited-stage mantle-cell lymphoma. *Ann Oncol.* 2003;14:1555-1561. PMID: 14504058.

144. Lenz G, Dreyling M, Hoster E, et al. Immunochemotherapy with rituximab and cyclophosphamide, doxorubicin, vincristine, and prednisone significantly improves response and time to treatment failure, but not long-term outcome in patients with previously untreated mantle cell lymphoma: results of a prospective randomized trial of the German Low Grade Lymphoma Study Group (GLSG). *J Clin Oncol.* 2005;23:1984-1992. PMID: 15668467.

145. Romaguera JE, Fayad L, Rodriguez MA, et al. High rate of durable remissions after treatment of newly diagnosed aggressive mantle-cell lymphoma with rituximab plus hyper-CVAD alternating with rituximab plus high-dose methotrexate and cytarabine. *J Clin Oncol.* 2005;23:7013-7023. PMID: 16145068.

146. Till BG, Gooley TA, Crawford N, et al. Effect of remission status and induction chemotherapy regimen on outcome of autologous stem cell transplantation for mantle cell lymphoma. *Leuk Lymphoma.* 2008;49:1062-1073. PMID: 18452065.

147. Geisler CH, Kolstad A, Laurell A, et al. Long-term progression-free survival of mantle cell lymphoma after intensive front-line immunochemotherapy with in vivo-purged stem cell rescue: a nonrandomized phase 2 multicenter study by the Nordic Lymphoma Group. *Blood.* 2008;112:2687-2693. PMID: 18625886.

148. Kluin-Nelemans HC, Hoster E, Hermine O, et al. Treatment of older patients with mantle-cell lymphoma. *N Engl J Med.* 2012;367:520-531. PMID: 22873532.

149. Forstpointner R, Unterhalt M, Dreyling M, et al. Maintenance therapy with rituximab leads to a significant prolongation of response duration after salvage therapy with a combination of rituximab, fludarabine, cyclophosphamide, and mitoxantrone (R-FCM) in patients with recurring and refractory follicular and mantle cell lymphomas: Results of a prospective randomized study of the German Low Grade Lymphoma Study Group (GLSG). *Blood.* 2006;108:4003-4008. PMID: 16946304.

150. Fisher RI, Bernstein SH, Kahl BS, et al. Multicenter phase II study of bortezomib in patients with relapsed or refractory mantle cell lymphoma. *J Clin Oncol.* 2006;24:4867-4874. PMID: 17001068.

151. Goy A, Sinha R, Williams ME, et al. Single-agent lenalidomide in patients with mantle-cell lymphoma who relapsed or progressed after or were refractory to bortezomib: phase II MCL-001 (EMERGE) study. *J Clin Oncol.* 2013;31:3688-3695. PMID: 24002500.

152. Maris MB, Sandmaier BM, Storer BE, et al. Allogeneic hematopoietic cell transplantation after fludarabine and 2 Gy total body irradiation for relapsed and refractory mantle cell lymphoma. *Blood.* 2004;104:3535-3542. PMID: 15304387.

153. Khouri IF, Lee MS, Saliba RM, et al. Nonablative allogeneic stem-cell transplantation for advanced/recurrent mantle-cell lymphoma. *J Clin Oncol.* 2003;21:4407-4412. PMID: 14645431.

154. Thomas DA, O'Brien S, Cortes J, et al. Outcome with the hyper-CVAD regimens in lymphoblastic lymphoma. *Blood.* 2004;104:1624-1630. PMID: 15178574.

155. Cortelazzo S, Intermesoli T, Oldani E, et al. Results of a lymphoblastic leukemia-like chemotherapy program with risk-adapted mediastinal irradiation and stem cell transplantation for adult patients with lymphoblastic lymphoma. *Ann Hematol.* 2012;91:73-82. PMID: 21559811.

156. Song KW, Barnett MJ, Gascoyne RD, et al. Primary therapy for adults with T-cell lymphoblastic lymphoma with hematopoietic stem-cell transplantation results in favorable outcomes. *Ann Oncol.* 2007;18:535-540. PMID: 17158775.

157. Gökbuget N, Basara N, Baurmann H, et al. High single-drug activity of nelarabine in relapsed T-lymphoblastic leukemia/lymphoma offers curative option with subsequent stem cell transplantation. *Blood.* 2011;118:3504-3511. PMID: 21715318.

158. Thomas DA, Faderl S, O'Brien S, et al. Chemoimmunotherapy with hyper-CVAD plus rituximab for the treatment of adult Burkitt and Burkitt-type lymphoma or acute lymphoblastic leukemia. *Cancer.* 2006;106:1569-1580. PMID: 16502413.

159. Magrath I, Adde M, Shad A, et al. Adults and children with small non-cleaved-cell lymphoma have a similar excellent outcome when treated with the same chemotherapy regimen. *J Clin Oncol.* 1996;14:925-934. PMID: 8622041.

160. Mead GM, Barrans SL, Qian W, et al. A prospective clinicopathologic study of dose-modified CODOX-M/IVAC in patients with sporadic Burkitt lymphoma defined using cytogenetic and immunophenotypic criteria (MRC/NCRI LY10 trial). *Blood.* 2008;112:2248-2260. PMID: 18612102.

161. Dunleavy K, Pittaluga S, Shovlin M, et al. Low-intensity therapy in adults with Burkitt's lymphoma. *N Engl J Med.* 2013;369:1915-1925. PMID: 24224624.

162. Salaverria I, Siebert R. The gray zone between Burkitt's lymphoma and diffuse large B-cell lymphoma from a genetics perspective. *J Clin Oncol.* 2011;29:1835-1843. PMID: 21482997.

163. Dave SS, Fu K, Wright GW, et al. Molecular diagnosis of Burkitt's lymphoma. *N Engl J Med.* 2006;354:2431-2442. PMID: 16760443.

164. Johnson NA, Savage KJ, Ludkovski O, et al. Lymphomas with concurrent BCL2 and MYC translocations: the critical factors associated with survival. *Blood.* 2009;114:2273-2279. PMID: 19597184.

165. Aukema SM, Siebert R, Schuuring E, et al. Double-hit B-cell lymphomas. *Blood.* 2011;117:2319-2331. PMID: 21119107.

166. Snuderl M, Kolman OK, Chen YB, et al. B-cell lymphomas with concurrent IGH-BCL2 and MYC rearrangements are aggressive neoplasms with clinical and pathologic features distinct from Burkitt lymphoma and diffuse large B-cell lymphoma. *Am J Surg Pathol.* 2010;34:327-340. PMID: 20118770.

167. Ferreri AJ. How I treat primary CNS lymphoma. *Blood.* 2011;118:510-522. PMID: 21613254.

168. Abrey LE, Ben-Porat L, Panageas KS, et al. Primary central nervous system lymphoma: the Memorial Sloan-Kettering Cancer Center prognostic model. *J Clin Oncol.* 2006;24:5711-5715. PMID: 17116938.

169. Gavrilovic IT, Hormigo A, Yahalom J, et al. Long-term follow-up of high-dose methotrexate-based therapy with and without whole brain irradiation for newly diagnosed primary CNS lymphoma. *J Clin Oncol.* 2006;24:4570-4574. PMID: 17008697.

170. Ferreri AJ, Reni M, Pasini F, et al. A multicenter study of treatment of primary CNS lymphoma. *Neurology.* 2002;58:1513-1520. PMID: 12034789.

171. Dunleavy K, Little RF, Pittaluga S, et al. The role of tumor histogenesis, FDG-PET, and short-course EPOCH with dose-dense rituximab (SC-EPOCH-RR) in HIV-associated diffuse large B-cell lymphoma. *Blood.* 2010;115:3017-3024. PMID: 20130244.

172. Dunleavy K, Wilson WH. How I treat HIV-associated lymphoma. *Blood.* 2012;119:3245-3255. PMID: 22337719.

173. Little RF, Pittaluga S, Grant N, et al. Highly effective treatment of acquired immunodeficiency syndrome-related lymphoma with dose-adjusted EPOCH: impact of antiretroviral therapy suspension and tumor biology. *Blood.* 2003;101:4653-4659. PMID: 12609827.

174. Sparano JA, Lee JY, Kaplan LD, et al. Rituximab plus concurrent infusional EPOCH chemotherapy is highly effective in HIV-associated B-cell non-Hodgkin lymphoma. *Blood.* 2010;115:3008-3016. PMID: 20023215.

175. Barta SK, Lee JY, Kaplan LD, et al. Pooled analysis of AIDS malignancy consortium trials evaluating rituximab plus CHOP or infusional EPOCH chemotherapy in HIV-associated non-Hodgkin lymphoma. *Cancer.* 2012;118:3977-3983. PMID: 22180164.

176. Kaplan LD, Lee JY, Ambinder RF, et al. Rituximab does not improve clinical outcome in a randomized phase 3 trial of CHOP with or without rituximab in patients with HIV-associated non-Hodgkin lymphoma: AIDS-Malignancies Consortium Trial 010. *Blood.* 2005;106:1538-1543. PMID: 15914552.

177. Castillo JJ, Reagan JL. Plasmablastic lymphoma: a systematic review. *ScientificWorldJournal.* 2011;11:687-696. PMID: 21442146.

178. Gallamini A, Stelitano C, Calvi R, et al. Peripheral T-cell lymphoma unspecified (PTCL-U): a new prognostic model from a retrospective multicentric clinical study. *Blood.* 2004;103:2474-2479. PMID: 14645001.

179. Vose J, Armitage J, Weisenburger D. International peripheral T-cell and natural killer/T-cell lymphoma study: pathology findings and clinical outcomes. *J Clin Oncol.* 2008;26:4124-4130. PMID: 18626005.

180. Foss FM, Zinzani PL, Vose JM, et al. Peripheral T-cell lymphoma. *Blood.* 2011;117:6756-6767. PMID: 21493798.

181. Weisenburger DD, Savage KJ, Harris NL, et al. Peripheral T-cell lymphoma, not otherwise specified: a report of 340 cases from the International Peripheral T-cell Lymphoma Project. *Blood.* 2011;117:3402-3408. PMID: 21270441.

182. Piekarz RL, Frye R, Prince HM, et al. Phase 2 trial of romidepsin in patients with peripheral T-cell lymphoma. *Blood.* 2011;117:5827-5834. PMID: 21355097.

183. O'Connor OA, Pro B, Pinter-Brown L, et al. Pralatrexate in patients with relapsed or refractory peripheral T-cell lymphoma: results from the pivotal PROPEL study. *J Clin Oncol.* 2011;29:1182-1189. PMID: 21245435.

184. Reimer P, Rüdiger T, Geissinger E, et al. Autologous stem-cell transplantation as first-line therapy in peripheral T-cell lymphomas: results of a prospective multicenter study. *J Clin Oncol.* 2009;27:106-113. PMID: 19029417.

185. Kyriakou C, Canals C, Goldstone A, et al. High-dose therapy and autologous stem-cell transplantation in angioimmunoblastic lymphoma: complete remission at transplantation is the major determinant of Outcome-Lymphoma Working Party of the European Group for Blood and Marrow Transplantation. *J Clin Oncol.* 2008;26:218-224. PMID: 18182664.

186. Pro B, Advani R, Brice P, et al. Brentuximab vedotin (SGN-35) in patients with relapsed or refractory systemic anaplastic large-cell lymphoma: results of a phase II study. *J Clin Oncol.* 2012;30:2190-2196. PMID: 22614995.

187. Sieniawski MK, Lennard AL. Enteropathy-associated T-cell lymphoma: epidemiology, clinical features, and current treatment strategies. *Curr Hematol Malig Rep.* 2011;6:231-240. PMID: 21912848.

188. Delabie J, Holte H, Vose JM, et al. Enteropathy-associated T-cell lymphoma: clinical and histological findings from the international peripheral T-cell lymphoma project. *Blood.* 2011;118:148-155. PMID: 21566094.

189. Sieniawski M, Angamuthu N, Boyd K, et al. Evaluation of enteropathy-associated T-cell lymphoma comparing standard therapies with a novel regimen including autologous stem cell transplantation. *Blood.* 2010;115:3664-3670. PMID: 20197151.

190. Yamaguchi M, Tobinai K, Oguchi M, et al. Phase I/II study of concurrent chemoradiotherapy for localized nasal natural killer/T-cell lymphoma: Japan Clinical Oncology Group Study JCOG0211. *J Clin Oncol.* 2009;27:5594-5600. PMID: 19805668.

191. Yamaguchi M, Suzuki R, Kwong YL, et al. Phase I study of dexamethasone, methotrexate, ifosfamide, L-asparaginase, and etoposide (SMILE) chemotherapy for advanced-stage, relapsed or refractory extranodal natural killer (NK)/T-cell lymphoma and leukemia. *Cancer Sci.* 2008;99:1016-1020. PMID: 18294294.

192. Willemze R, Jansen PM, Cerroni L, et al. Subcutaneous panniculitis-like T-cell lymphoma: definition, classification, and prognostic factors: an EORTC Cutaneous Lymphoma Group Study of 83 cases. *Blood.* 2008;111:838-845. PMID: 17934071.

193. Prince HM, Whittaker S, Hoppe RT. How I treat mycosis fungoides and Sézary syndrome. *Blood.* 2009;114:4337-4353. PMID: 19696197.

194. Duvic M, Talpur R, Ni X, et al. Phase 2 trial of oral vorinostat (suberoylanilide hydroxamic acid, SAHA) for refractory cutaneous T-cell lymphoma (CTCL). *Blood.* 2007;109:31-39. PMID: 16960145.

195. Duvic M, Donato M, Dabaja B, et al. Total skin electron beam and non-myeloablative allogeneic hematopoietic stem-cell transplantation in advanced mycosis fungoides and Sezary syndrome. *J Clin Oncol.* 2010;28:2365-2372. PMID: 20351328.

17

MULTIPLE MYELOMA

S. Vincent Rajkumar, MD

Updates from 2012

▶ From the outset, there is significant clonal heterogeneity in myeloma and there are varying dominant clones that emerge during the course of the disease (Keats JJ, *Blood* 2012).

▶ Clonal plasma cell involvement of 60% or more of the marrow is considered multiple myeloma even in the absence of end-organ damage (Rajkumar SV, *N Engl J Med* 2011).

▶ The presence of trisomies ameliorates the adverse prognosis associated with high-risk cytogenetic abnormalities (Kumar S, *Blood* 2012).

▶ A randomized controlled trial demonstrated an overall survival benefit in patients with high-risk smoldering multiple myeloma with lenalidomide and low-dose dexamethasone compared with observation alone (Mateos MV, *N Engl J Med* 2013).

▶ Preliminary results of a randomized controlled trial from Italy demonstrated a survival benefit with lenalidomide maintenance therapy (Boccardoro M, *J Clin Oncol* 2013).

▶ Pomalidomide and carfilzomib are approved by the U.S. Food and Drug Administration for the treatment of relapsed and refractory myeloma (Siegel DS, *Blood* 2012; Lacy MQ, *J Clin Oncol* 2009).

▶ Pomalidomide is a new oral immunomodulatory agent that is active in patients with disease that is refractory to bortezomib and lenalidomide (Lacy MQ, *J Clin Oncol* 2009; Lacy MQ, *Blood* 2011).

▶ Carfilzomib is a new proteasome inhibitor that is active in patients with disease that is refractory to bortezomib and lenalidomide (Siegel DS, *Blood* 2012).

▶ New investigational agents with single-agent activity in myeloma include ARRY-520 (a kinesin spindle protein inhibitor), monoclonal antibodies to CD38, and cyclin dependent kinase inhibitors (Rajkumar SV, *Am J Hematol* 2013).

Multiple myeloma is a plasma cell malignancy characterized by osteolytic bone lesions, anemia, hypercalcemia, and renal failure.[1,2] Over 20,000 new cases and 10,000 myeloma deaths are estimated to occur in the United States each year.[3] The disease is generally considered incurable, and the clinical course is typically characterized by remissions and relapses, with a decrease in the remission duration with each successive therapy.[4] However, the survival of patients with multiple myeloma has improved dramatically in recent years, with an increase in the 3-year survival rate from 42% with melphalan/prednisone to over 80% today. This improvement can be attributed to incorporation of drugs such as thalidomide,[5] bortezomib,[6] lenalidomide,[7,8] carfilzomib,[9] and pomalidomide[10,11] into the overall treatment strategy,

Table 17-1 Diagnostic Criteria for Plasma Cell Disorders

Disorder	Disease Definition
Monoclonal gammopathy of undetermined significance (MGUS)[15]	All three criteria must be met: ■ Serum monoclonal (M) protein < 3 g/dL ■ Clonal bone marrow plasma cells < 10% ■ Absence of end-organ damage such as hypercalcemia, renal insufficiency, anemia, and bone lesions (CRAB) that can be attributed to the plasma cell proliferative disorder; or in the case of immunoglobulin (Ig) M MGUS, no evidence of anemia, constitutional symptoms, hyperviscosity, lymphadenopathy, or hepatosplenomegaly that can be attributed to the underlying lymphoproliferative disorder
Smoldering multiple myeloma (SMM; also referred to as asymptomatic multiple myeloma)[15]	Both criteria must be met: ■ Serum M protein (IgG or IgA) ≥ 3 g/dL and/or clonal bone marrow plasma cells ≥ 10% ■ Absence of end-organ damage such as lytic bone lesions, anemia, hypercalcemia, or renal failure that can be attributed to a plasma cell proliferative disorder

Multiple myeloma[15,16]	All three criteria must be met except as noted:
	
	■ Clonal bone marrow plasma cells ≥ 10% and/or biopsy proven plasmacytoma
	■ Presence of serum and/or urinary M protein (except in patients with true nonsecretory multiple myeloma)
	■ Presence of ≥ 60% clonal bone marrow plasma cells or presence of end-organ damage that can be attributed to the underlying plasma cell proliferative disorder, specifically
	  □ Hypercalcemia: Serum calcium ≥ 11.5 mg/dL or
	  □ Renal insufficiency: Serum creatinine > 173 micromoles/L (or > 2 mg/dL) or estimated creatinine clearance less than 40 mL/minute
	  □ Anemia: Normochromic, normocytic with a hemoglobin value of > 2 g/dL below the lower limit of normal or a hemoglobin value < 10 g/dL
	  □ Bone lesions: Lytic lesions, severe osteopenia or pathologic fractures

IgM monoclonal gammopathy of undetermined significance (IgM MGUS)[17-21]	All three criteria must be met: ■ Serum IgM M protein < 3 g/dL ■ Bone marrow lymphoplasmacytic infiltration < 10% ■ No evidence of anemia, constitutional symptoms, hyperviscosity, lymphadenopathy, or hepatosplenomegaly that can be attributed to the underlying lymphoproliferative disorder
Smoldering Waldenström macroglobulinemia (also referred to as indolent or asymptomatic Waldenström macroglobulinemia)[17-21]	Both criteria must be met: ■ Serum IgM M protein ≥ 3 g/dL and/or bone marrow lymphoplasmacytic infiltration ≥ 10% ■ No evidence of anemia, constitutional symptoms, hyperviscosity, lymphadenopathy, or hepatosplenomegaly that can be attributed to the underlying lymphoproliferative disorder
Waldenström macroglobulinemia[17-21]	All three criteria must be met: ■ IgM monoclonal gammopathy (regardless of the size of the M protein) ■ ≥ 10% bone marrow lymphoplasmacytic infiltration (usually intertrabecular) by small lymphocytes that exhibit plasmacytoid or plasma cell differentiation and a typical immunophenotype (eg., surface IgM+, CD5+/-, CD10-, CD19+, CD20+, CD23-) that satisfactorily excludes other lymphoproliferative disorders including chronic lymphocytic leukemia and mantle cell lymphoma ■ Evidence of anemia, constitutional symptoms, hyperviscosity, lymphadenopathy, or hepatosplenomegaly that can be attributed to the underlying lymphoproliferative disorder
Light chain MGUS[22]	All four criteria must be met: ■ Abnormal free light chain (FLC) ratio (< 0.26 or > 1.65) ■ Increased level of the appropriate involved light chain (increased kappa FLC in patients with ratio > 1.65 and increased lambda FLC in patients with ratio < 0.26) ■ No immunoglobulin heavy chain expression on immunofixation ■ Absence of end-organ damage such as lytic bone lesions, anemia, hypercalcemia, or renal failure that can be attributed to a plasma cell proliferative disorder

Table 17-1 continued

	All four criteria must be met:
Solitary plasmacytoma[23,24]	▪ Biopsy-proven solitary lesion of bone or soft tissue with evidence of clonal plasma cells ▪ Normal bone marrow with no evidence of clonal plasma cells ▪ Normal skeletal survey and magnetic resonance imaging (MRI) of spine and pelvis (except for the primary solitary lesion) ▪ Absence of end-organ damage such as hypercalcemia, renal insufficiency, anemia, or bone lesions (CRAB) that can be attributed to a lymphoplasma cell proliferative disorder
Systemic light chain (AL) amyloidosis[25]	All four criteria must be met: ▪ Presence of an amyloid-related systemic syndrome (such as renal, liver, heart, gastrointestinal tract, or peripheral nerve involvement) ▪ Positive amyloid staining by Congo red in any tissue (e.g., fat aspirate, bone marrow, or organ biopsy) ▪ Evidence that amyloid is light chain–related established by direct examination of the amyloid (possibly using mass spectrometry [MS]-based proteomic analysis, or immuno-electronmicroscopy; note that immunohistochemistry results to type amyloid may be unreliable) ▪ Evidence of a monoclonal plasma cell proliferative disorder (serum or urine M protein, abnormal FLC ratio, or clonal plasma cells in the bone marrow)
	Note: Approximately 2% to 3% of patients with AL amyloidosis will not meet the requirement for evidence of a monoclonal plasma cell disorder listed above; the diagnosis of AL amyloidosis must be made with caution in these patients.

POEMS syndrome[26,27]	All four criteria must be met:
	
	▪ Polyneuropathy
	▪ Monoclonal plasma cell proliferative disorder (almost always lambda)
	▪ Any one of the following three other <u>major</u> criteria:
	  1. Sclerotic bone lesions
	  2. Castleman disease
	  3. Elevated levels of vascular endothelial growth factor (VEGF)*
	▪ Any one of the following six <u>minor</u> criteria
	  1. Organomegaly (splenomegaly, hepatomegaly, or lymphadenopathy)
	  2. Extravascular volume overload (edema, pleural effusion, or ascites)
	  3. Endocrinopathy (adrenal, thyroid, pituitary, gonadal, parathyroid, pancreatic)**
	  4. Skin changes (hyperpigmentation, hypertrichosis, glomeruloid hemangiomata, plethora, acrocyanosis, flushing, white nails)
	  5. Papilledema
	  6. Thrombocytosis/polycythemia

	Note: Not every patient meeting the above criteria will have POEMS syndrome; the features should have a temporal relationship to each other and no other attributable cause. Anemia and/or thrombocytopenia are distinctively unusual in this syndrome unless Castleman disease is present.

*The source data do not define an optimal cut-off value for considering elevated VEGF level as a major criterion. One recommendation is that VEGF measured in the serum or plasma should be at least 3- to 4-fold higher than the normal reference range for the laboratory that is doing the testing to be considered a major criteria.
** In order to consider endocrinopathy as a minor criterion, an endocrine disorder other than diabetes or hypothyroidism is required, since these two disorders are common in the general population.
Modified from Kyle RA, Rajkumar SV. Criteria for diagnosis, staging, risk stratification and response assessment of multiple myeloma. Leukemia. 2009;23:3-9. PMID: 18971951.

as well as the use of autologous stem cell transplantation (ASCT) in selected patients and improvements in supportive care, particularly bisphosphonates.

DISEASE DEFINITION

Multiple myeloma is defined by the presence of 10% or more clonal plasma cells on bone marrow examination or biopsy-proven plasmacytoma, monoclonal (M) protein in serum and/or urine (except in the case of nonsecretory myeloma), and evidence of hypercalcemia, renal insufficiency, anemia, or bone lesions that can be attributed to the plasma cell

proliferative disorder.[12] In addition, patients with 60% or greater involvement of the bone marrow with clonal plasma cells are considered to have multiple myeloma regardless of the presence or absence of end-organ damage.[13,14] There is ongoing research to identify highly specific biomarkers that can be used to identify myeloma prior to the onset of end-organ damage. Patients with multiple myeloma must be differentiated from those with monoclonal gammopathy of undetermined significance (MGUS), smoldering multiple myeloma (SMM), and other related plasma cell disorders (Table 17-1).[15-27] MGUS is an asymptomatic premalignant phase of multiple myeloma.[28,29] The risk of progression of MGUS to myeloma or a related disorder is fixed at approximately 1% per year.[29] SMM is a more advanced intermediate stage, defined by the presence of a serum M protein greater than 3 g/dL or greater than 10% clonal plasma cells in the marrow, but without end-organ damage. SMM is not a unique biologic stage of disease evolution, but is an intermediate *clinical* entity that must be differentiated from MGUS and multiple myeloma (Table 17-1), primarily for prognostic and management reasons.[30] In a study of 276 patients with SMM, the risk of progression to multiple myeloma in the first 5 years following diagnosis was 10% per year, 3% per year over the next 5 years, and 1% per year thereafter.[31]

EPIDEMIOLOGY AND RISK FACTORS

Multiple myeloma accounts for 1% of all malignant disease and slightly more than 10% of hematologic malignancies. The annual incidence, age-adjusted to the 2000 U.S. population, is 4.3 per 100,000.[3] In 2013, approximately 22,350 new cases were expected to occur in the United States, and 10,710 deaths will be attributable to myeloma.[3] Myeloma is twice as common in the black population compared with the white population.[32] The median age of patients at diagnosis is about 65. There is no known etiology. Exposure to radiation, benzene, and other organic solvents, herbicides, and insecticides may play a role. There is a slight increase in the incidence of multiple myeloma in first-degree relatives of patients with the disease.

KEY POINTS

- The diagnosis of myeloma requires evidence of hypercalcemia, renal insufficiency, anemia, or bone lesions that can be attributed to the plasma cell proliferative disorder. An exception to this is the presence of 60% or more involvement of the bone marrow with clonal plasma cells; such patients are considered to have myeloma regardless of the presence or absence of end-organ damage.
- Monoclonal gammopathy of undetermined significance and smoldering multiple myeloma are asymptomatic plasma cell proliferative disorders that should be distinguished from myeloma.
- Multiple myeloma accounts for 1% of all cancers and approximately 10% of hematologic cancers.
- Myeloma is twice as common in the black population compared with the white population.

PATHOGENESIS

Multiple myeloma is preceded by a premalignant phase referred to as MGUS.[33] However, because MGUS is asymptomatic and can be detected only through specific laboratory testing, most patients with multiple myeloma do not have a history of MGUS. The pathogenesis of multiple myeloma involves two initial steps: 1) development of the premalignant MGUS stage, and 2) progression of MGUS to multiple myeloma. The evolution of a normal plasma cell to a MGUS clone is likely triggered by an abnormal response to antigenic stimulation. This results in the development of primary cytogenetic abnormalities in the affected plasma cells. In approximately 40% to 50% of MGUS cases, the primary cytogenetic abnormality is a reciprocal translocation involving the immunoglobulin (Ig) heavy chain (IgH) locus on chromosome 14q32 (IgH-translocated MGUS) and one of five recurrent partner chromosome loci: 11q13 (cyclin D1 gene [*CCND1*]), 4p16.3 (*FGFR-3* and *MMSET*), 6p21 (cyclin D3 gene [*CCND3*]), 16q23 (*c-maf*), and 20q11 (*mafB*; Table 17-2).[34] In most of the remaining patients with MGUS, the primary abnormality is the development of trisomies of one or more of the odd-numbered chromosomes, often resulting in hyperdiploidy (referred to as hyperdiploid MGUS or IgH-nontranslocated MGUS).[35] In a small proportion of cases, neither trisomies nor IgH translocations are found, and in some patients both types of abnormalities are found in the same clone.

Once an MGUS clone is established, the second step of progression to multiple myeloma follows a simple, random, two-hit genetic model of malignancy. Although several alterations, such as abnormalities involving the *myc* family of oncogenes, *Ras* mutations, *p16* methylation, and *p53* mutations, have been associated with malignant transformation of MGUS to multiple myeloma, the specific pathogenetic steps are unknown. Recent studies indicate that there is significant clonal heterogeneity in myeloma, with a different dominant clone emerging through the course of various treatments.[36]

KEY POINTS

- Myeloma is preceded by a premalignant phase, clinically referred to as monoclonal gammopathy of undetermined significance (MGUS).
- The two principal pathogenetic steps in the development of multiple myeloma are: 1) transition from a normal plasma cell to a MGUS, and 2) transition from MGUS to myeloma.
- The onset of MGUS is associated with hyperdiploidy in about 50% of the cases and immunoglobulin heavy chain translocations in the remaining 50% of cases.
- Progression of MGUS to multiple myeloma is associated with overexpression of receptor activator of nuclear factor kappa-B ligand (RANKL), reduction in the level of its decoy receptor, osteoprotegerin (OPG), and osteoblast inhibition that together lead to bone destruction.

Table 17-2 Cytogenetic Categories of Monoclonal Gammopathy of Undetermined Significance (MGUS) and Multiple Myeloma (MM)

Cytogenetic Type	Gene(s) Involved	Comment
I. Hyperdiploid (trisomic) MGUS or MM	Unknown; Likely many	Characterized by trisomies of one or more odd-numbered chromosomes; in patients with myeloma, hyperdiploidy is considered standard risk
II. *IgH*-translocated (nonhyperdiploid) MGUS or MM		Reciprocal translocation involving the immunoglobulin heavy chain (*IgH*) gene on chromosome 14q32 and a variety of partner chromosomes
t(11;14)	*CCND1* (cyclin D1)	
t(4;14) MM	*FGFR-3* and *MMSET*	
t(14;16) MM	*C-MAF*	Considered to indicate high-risk disease in setting of MM
t(6;14) MM	*CCND3* (cyclin D3)	
t(14;20) MM	*MAFB*	Considered to indicate high-risk disease in setting of MM
III. Unclassified MGUS or MM		

Progression of MGUS to myeloma is typically accompanied by an increase in receptor activator of nuclear factor kappa-B ligand (RANKL) expression by osteoblasts and a reduction in the level of its decoy receptor, osteoprotegerin (OPG).[37] This leads to an increased RANKL/OPG ratio, a key factor for osteoclast activation and subsequent bone resorption. Increased levels of macrophage inflammatory protein–1-alpha (MIP-1-alpha), stromal derived factor alpha (SDF-alpha), interleukin (IL)-3, IL-1 beta, and IL-6 may also play a role in osteoclast activation. At the same time, increased levels of IL-3, IL-7, and dickkopf1 (DKK1) contribute to inhibition of osteoblast differentiation. This combination of osteoclast activation and osteoblast suppression leads to the pure osteolytic bone disease that is the hallmark of multiple myeloma.

PREVENTION

Prevention of myeloma is hampered by the low likelihood of progression in patients with the premalignant MGUS stage. If deaths due to unrelated competing causes are taken into account, only 10% of patients with MGUS will ever develop myeloma. In SMM, the risk of progression in the first 5 years is considerably higher at approximately 50%. Thus, preventive strategies for multiple myeloma are currently focused on preventing progression of high-risk patients with newly diagnosed SMM. A randomized trial conducted by the Spanish Myeloma Group in patients with high-risk SMM found improved progression-free and overall survival with early use of lenalidomide plus dexamethasone versus observation.[38] However, the multiparametric flow cytometric methods used to identify high-risk SMM in this trial is not standardized, and more data are needed. Therefore, for most patients with SMM, observation remains the standard of care.[39]

KEY POINT

■ Early intervention with lenalidomide has shown promise in the treatment of smoldering multiple myeloma (SMM). Additional clinical trials are ongoing to determine the role of preventive therapy in SMM.

CLINICAL PRESENTATION AND DIAGNOSIS

The most common presenting symptoms of multiple myeloma are fatigue and bone pain.[40] Osteolytic bone lesions and/or compression fractures are hallmarks of the disease and can be detected on routine radiographs, magnetic resonance imaging (MRI), or computed tomography (CT) scans in approximately 70% of patients.[37] Anemia occurs in 70% of patients at diagnosis and is the primary cause of weakness and fatigue. Hypercalcemia is found in 15% of patients. Other symptoms may result from acute renal failure, radiculopathy, or infection.

When multiple myeloma is suspected, patients should be tested for the presence of M proteins by serum protein electrophoresis (SPEP), serum immunofixation (SIFE), urine protein electrophoresis (UPEP), and urine immunofixation (UIFE). The serum free light chain (FLC) assay can be used for screening in place of the urine studies mentioned above.[41] The serum FLC assay and urine studies help identify the subset of patients with multiple myeloma who lack M protein heavy chain expression (light chain multiple myeloma). Only 82% of patients with multiple myeloma have an M protein that is detectable on SPEP, whereas SIFE will identify an M protein in 93% of

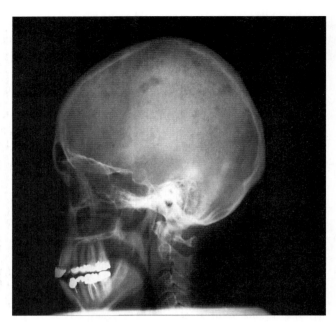

Fig. 17-1 Skull x-ray showing multiple osteolytic lesions.

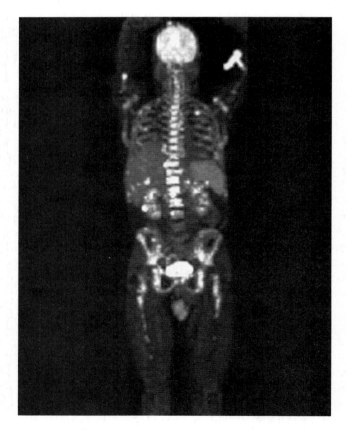

Fig. 17-2 Positron emission tomography (PET) scan showing multiple bone lesions with increased uptake of fluorodeoxyglucose (FDG) consistent with active myeloma.

There is also extramedullary involvement within the liver, gallbladder, kidney, and pancreas.

patients.[40] Combining serum studies with either urine studies or the serum FLC assay will reveal an M protein in 97% to 98% of patients with multiple myeloma.[40,41] Patients with serum M protein less than 1 g/dL and urine M protein less than 200 mg per day are considered to have oligosecretory myeloma. In addition, approximately 2% to 3% of patients with multiple myeloma have true nonsecretory disease with no evidence of an M protein on serum or urine immunofixation and have a normal serum FLC ratio.[40]

Other essential tests required are complete blood count (CBC), serum creatinine, calcium, beta-2 microglobulin, albumin, and lactate dehydrogenase. A unilateral bone marrow aspiration and biopsy is needed for the diagnosis. The monotypic nature of marrow plasma cells must be established by an abnormal kappa:lambda ratio by immunohistochemistry or flow cytometry. Myeloma cells typically stain positive for CD38, CD56, and CD138. Bone marrow plasma cells should also be studied with fluorescent in situ hybridization (FISH) and/or karyotyping to enable risk stratification (see Staging and Risk Stratification section below).[42] FISH studies do not require dividing cells and hence are considerably more informative in myeloma than conventional karyotyping, which requires the presence of metaphases.

Plain radiographic examination of all bones (skeletal survey) is required for detecting lytic bone lesions (Fig. 17-1). MRI and/or fluorodeoxyglucose positron emission tomography (FDG-PET) combined with CT (PET-CT) may be performed if symptomatic areas show no abnormality on routine radiographs (Fig. 17-2). MRI and PET-CT are also useful in assessing extramedullary disease, and whenever there is a concern that the adequacy of disease assessment may be inadequate with plain radiographs and M protein assessments alone.

DIFFERENTIAL DIAGNOSIS

Myeloma should be differentiated from MGUS, SMM, solitary plasmacytoma, Waldenström macroglobulinemia, and light chain (AL) amyloidosis using the criteria listed on Table 17-1.[12] Note that patients with MGUS may have symptoms from unrelated conditions, and that to make the diagnosis of multiple myeloma, the observed end-organ damage (anemia, hypercalcemia, renal failure, or bone lesions) must be felt to be attributable to the underlying plasma cell disorder.

MONITORING

Once multiple myeloma is diagnosed, patients require periodic measurements of CBC, serum creatinine, serum calcium, and M protein by SPEP and UPEP to assess treatment response, and monitor for relapse. In patients with oligosecretory myeloma (serum M protein less than 1 g/dL and urine M protein less than 200 mg/24 hours), the serum FLC assay can be used to monitor response to therapy, provided the FLC ratio is abnormal and the level of the involved FLC is 10 mg/dL or higher.[43] In patients with oligosecretory myeloma who have lower levels of FLC and in patients with true nonsecretory myeloma, monitoring is more difficult and requires periodic radiographic studies and bone marrow examinations. Serum and urine tests for

Table 17-3 **International Myeloma Working Group (IMWG) Uniform Response Criteria for Multiple Myeloma**[44]

Response Subcategory	Response Criteria
Complete response* (CR)	■ Negative immunofixation of serum and urine, and ■ Disappearance of any soft tissue plasmacytomas, and ■ < 5% plasma cells in bone marrow
Stringent complete response (sCR)**	CR as defined above plus ■ Normal free light chain (FLC) ratio, and ■ Absence of clonal plasma cells by immunohistochemistry or 2-4 color flow cytometry
Very good partial response (VGPR)*	■ Serum and urine monoclonal (M)-component detectable by immunofixation but not on electrophoresis, or ■ ≥ 90% or greater reduction in serum M-component plus urine M-component < 100 mg per 24 hours
Partial response (PR)	■ ≥ 50% reduction of serum M-protein and reduction in 24-hour urinary M-protein by ≥ 90% or to < 200 mg per 24 hours ■ If the serum and urine M-protein are unmeasurable a ≥ 50% decrease in the difference between involved and uninvolved FLC levels is required in place of the M-protein criteria ■ If serum and urine M-protein are unmeasurable, and serum free light assay is also unmeasurable, ≥ 50% reduction in bone marrow plasma cells is required in place of M-protein, provided baseline percentage was ≥ 30% ■ In addition to the above criteria, if present at baseline, ≥ 50% reduction in the size of soft tissue plasmacytomas is also required
Stable disease (SD)	■ Not meeting criteria for CR, VGPR, PR, or PD

Progressive disease (PD)**	■ Increase of 25% from lowest response value in any one or more of the following:
	  □ Serum M-component (absolute increase must be ≥ 0.5 g/dL) and/or
	  □ Urine M-component (absolute increase must be ≥ 200 mg/24 hours) and/or
	  □ Only in patients without measurable serum and urine M-protein levels: the difference between involved and uninvolved FLC levels (absolute increase must be > 10 mg/L)
	  □ Only in patients without measurable serum and urine M-protein levels and without measurable disease by FLC levels, bone marrow plasma cell percentage (absolute percentage must be ≥ 10%)
	■ Definite development of new bone lesions or soft tissue plasmacytomas or definite increase in the size of existing bone lesions or soft tissue plasmacytomas
	■ Development of hypercalcemia (corrected serum calcium > 11.5 mg/dL) that can be attributed solely to the plasma cell proliferative disorder

All response categories (CR, sCR, VGPR, PR, and PD) require two consecutive assessments made any time before the institution of any new therapy; CR, PR, and SD categories also require no known evidence of progressive or new bone lesions if radiographic studies were performed. VGPR and CR categories require serum and urine studies regardless of whether disease at baseline was measurable on serum, urine, both, or neither. Radiographic studies are not required to satisfy these response requirements. Bone marrow assessments need not be confirmed.

*Note clarifications to IMWG criteria for coding CR and VGPR in patients in whom the only measurable disease is by serum FLC levels: CR in such patients requires a normal FLC ratio of 0.26 to 1.65 in addition to CR criteria listed above. VGPR in such patients requires a > 90% decrease in the difference between involved and uninvolved FLC levels.

** Note clarifications to IMWG criteria for coding PD: Bone marrow criteria for PD are to be used only in patients without measurable disease by M protein and by FLC levels. Clarified that "25% increase" refers to M protein, FLC, and bone marrow results, and does not refer to bone lesions, soft tissue plasmacytomas, or hypercalcemia. Note that the "lowest response value" does not need to be a confirmed value.

Reproduced from Kyle RA, Rajkumar SV. Criteria for diagnosis, staging, risk stratification and response assessment of multiple myeloma. Leukemia. 2009;23:3-9. PMID: 18971951.

monitoring are done monthly during active therapy and once every 3 to 4 months thereafter. Radiographic tests are done every 6 to 12 months depending on response to treatment, as well as when symptoms indicate their need. Bone marrow studies are repeated if needed to confirm complete response or when clinically indicated to assess relapse. Response to therapy is assessed using the International Myeloma Working Group uniform response criteria (Table 17-3).[44]

STAGING AND RISK STRATIFICATION

There are two methods of staging multiple myeloma: the Durie–Salmon Staging system (DSS),[45] and the International Staging

Table 17-4 Staging Systems for Myeloma

Stage	Durie-Salmon Staging System*	International Staging System
Stage I	All of the following: ▪ 0-1 bone lesion, ▪ Hemoglobin > 10 g/dL, ▪ Normal calcium, and ▪ Low monoclonal protein production	Serum β-2 microglobulin < 3.5 mg/L and albumin ≥ 3.5 g/dL
Stage II	Not fitting stage I or III	Not fitting stage I or III
Stage III	One or more of the following: ▪ Advanced bone lesions, ▪ Hemoglobin < 8.5 g/dL, ▪ Increased calcium, or ▪ High monoclonal protein production	Serum β-2 microglobulin ≥ 5.5 mg/L

*Each stage in the Durie-Salmon Staging system is additionally coded with "A" if the serum creatinine < 2.0 mg/dL and with "B" if the serum creatinine is ≥ 2.0 mg/dL

Table 17-5 Risk Stratification of Myeloma Based on Baseline Cytogenetics

Standard risk	1. Trisomies 2. Translocation t(11;14) 3. Translocation t(6;14)
Intermediate risk	1. Translocation t(4;14)
High risk	1. 17p deletion 2. Translocation t(14;16) 3. Translocation t(14;20)

System (ISS; Table 17-4).[46] Both staging systems are useful for estimating prognosis but not for choosing therapy, and both have limitations. The DSS is complex and relies on the assessment of extent of bone disease, which is subjective. The ISS does not correlate with disease burden and is nonspecific for multiple myeloma. Besides stage, age, and performance status, prognosis in multiple myeloma is dictated by the underlying disease biology. The baseline disease biology and aggressiveness is best assessed by the underlying cytogenetics of the disease (Table 17-5).[42,47] For example, median survival is greater than 7 years in standard-risk multiple myeloma compared with 2 to 3 years in high-risk disease. The t(4;14) translocation has been associated with adverse prognosis, but outcomes are improving with bortezomib-based therapy, and such patients are considered as intermediate-risk. In addition to providing additional information on prognosis, cytogenetic risk stratification can also aid in choosing therapy. For example, patients with intermediate risk have better outcomes when treated early in the disease course with bortezomib in combination with ASCT.[42]

THERAPEUTIC MANAGEMENT

INITIAL THERAPY

The overall approach to therapy in patients with newly diagnosed multiple myeloma is shown in Fig. 17-3. The most commonly used regimens for the treatment of newly diagnosed multiple myeloma are lenalidomide plus low-dose dexamethasone (Rd), bortezomib plus dexamethasone (VD), bortezomib plus thalidomide and dexamethasone (VTD), lenalidomide plus bortezomib and dexamethasone (RVD), cyclophosphamide plus bortezomib and dexamethasone (VCd), bortezomib plus melphalan and prednisone (VMP), and melphalan plus prednisone with thalidomide (MPT).[1] Table 17-6 provides a list of the most commonly used treatment regimens in multiple myeloma.[48-59] Table 17-7 provides the results of recent randomized trials with these regimens in multiple myeloma.[49,50,52-56,60-66] Although these regimens are considered superior to older regimens such as vincristine plus doxorubicin and dexamethasone (VAD) or thalidomide plus dexamethasone (TD), with few exceptions, these modern regimens have not been compared against each other in randomized trials, and most recommendations are based on nonrandomized data and expert opinion.[4]

Initial therapy for myeloma is determined by eligibility for stem cell transplantation. In general, eligibility for stem cell transplantation is determined by age, performance status, and coexisting comorbidities. In the United States, the upper age limit for ASCT may be as high as 75, as long as patients are in good functional status without significant comorbidities. In most European countries, patients age 65 and older are not considered candidates for ASCT. Patients who are not

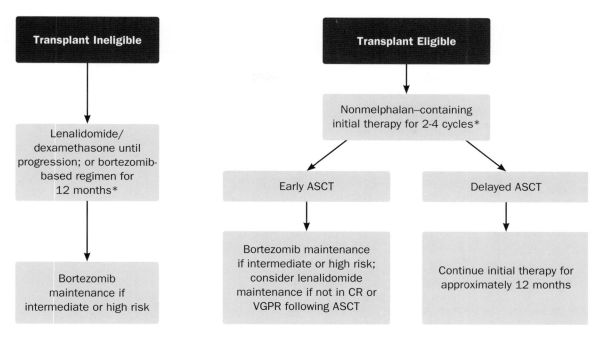

Fig. 17-3 Treatment approach for newly diagnosed patients with myeloma.

*Bortezomib-containing regimens preferred for patients with intermediate- or high-risk myeloma.

Abbreviations: ASCT, autologous stem cell transplantation; CR, complete response; VGPR, very good partial response.

candidates for ASCT are treated for approximately 12 to 18 months with one of many possible treatment regimens (Table 17-6). Patients who are considered potential candidates for ASCT are first treated with two to four cycles of nonmelphalan-containing treatment regimens followed by a stem cell harvest (Fig. 17-3).[42] After stem cell harvest, most patients proceed to ASCT (early ASCT approach), while some may choose to continue the initial treatment regimen and delay ASCT for relapse (delayed ASCT approach).

TREATMENT FOR PATIENTS WHO ARE NOT CANDIDATES FOR ASCT

For patients who are not candidates for ASCT, the standard treatment for decades was melphalan plus prednisone (MP). However, randomized trials have shown that the addition of thalidomide to MP (MPT) is superior compared with MP alone.[52,53,62-64] In four of these trials, there was a significant prolongation of progression-free survival with MPT and in three trials, an overall survival advantage was also seen. Similarly, VMP also improves overall survival compared with MP.[65,66] Neuropathy is a substantial risk of MPT or VMP therapy. The risk of bortezomib-induced neuropathy can be greatly decreased by using a once-weekly schedule of bortezomib,[54,67] as well as a subcutaneous route of administration.[68] In contrast to MPT and VMP, TD has inferior overall survival compared with MP in elderly patients and is not recommended as initial therapy in these patients.[69] Similarly, the addition of lenalidomide to MP (MPR) has shown no survival benefit over MP alone and is not recommended.[55] Preliminary results from an Italian randomized trial suggest that overall survival may be improved further

by using a four-drug combination of VMP plus thalidomide; however, it is impossible to interpret the value of the additional drug to induction since the trial also had differences in maintenance between the two treatment arms.[70]

Regimens such as Rd, RVD, and VCd that were initially developed for patients who were candidates for ASCT appear equally effective and less toxic than MPT and VMP, and are increasingly used in elderly patients as well.[1,42] VCd is similar to VMP, but uses cyclophosphamide instead of melphalan and is probably less marrow-toxic and more predictable to manage than VMP. Similarly, in elderly patients, Rd is better tolerated than many of the melphalan-containing regimens. In two recent studies, the 3-year overall survival rate with Rd was 70% in patients age 70 or older, comparable with those seen with MPT and VMP.[71,72] Preliminary results also suggest superiority of Rd over MPT in a large, randomized, controlled trial.

The specific regimen used for initial therapy varies widely, and there is no clear standard. The author prefers Rd for low-risk, VCd for intermediate-risk, and a modified version of RVD for high-risk patients based on efficacy, toxicity, convenience, and cost considerations.

TREATMENT FOR CANDIDATES FOR ASCT

The overall approach to initial therapy of patients who are candidates for ASCT is shown in Fig. 17-3. Two randomized trials found TD to be superior to dexamethasone alone, leading to the approval of thalidomide for newly diagnosed multiple myeloma in the United States, but TD has fallen out of favor because the toxicity and early mortality rates are unacceptably high compared with other regimens such as Rd, VCd, and RVD.[48,49] TD

Table 17-6 **Common Treatment Regimens in Multiple Myeloma**

Regimen	Suggested Starting Doses*	Overall Response Rate (%)	Estimated CR plus VGPR Rate (%)
Thalidomide/dexamethasone (TD)**[48,49]	■ Thalidomide 200 mg oral days 1–28 ■ Dexamethasone 40 mg oral days 1, 8, 15, 22 ■ Repeated every 4 weeks	65	30
Lenalidomide/ dexamethasone (Rd)[50]	■ Lenalidomide 25 mg oral days 1–21 every 28 days ■ Dexamethasone 40 mg oral days 1, 8, 15, 22 every 28 days ■ Repeated every 4 weeks	70	40
Bortezomib/dexamethasone (VD)**[51]	■ Bortezomib 1.3 mg/m^2 intravenous days 1, 8, 15, 22 ■ Dexamethasone 20 mg on day of and day after bortezomib (or 40 mg days 1, 8, 15, 22) ■ Repeated every 4 weeks	80	40
Melphalan/prednisone/ thalidomide (MPT)[52,53]	■ Melphalan 0.25 mg/kg oral days 1–4 (use 0.20 mg/kg/day oral on days 1–4 in patients older than age 75) ■ Prednisone 2 mg/kg oral days 1–4 ■ Thalidomide 100-200 mg oral days 1–28 (use 100-mg dose in patients older than age 75) ■ Repeated every 6 weeks	70	30
Bortezomib/melphalan/ prednisone (VMP)**[54]	■ Bortezomib 1.3 mg/m^2 intravenous days 1, 8, 15, 22 ■ Melphalan 9 mg/m^2 oral days 1–4 ■ Prednisone 60 mg/m^2 oral days 1–4 ■ Repeated every 35 days	70	40
Melphalan/prednisone/ lenalidomide (MPR)[55]	■ Melphalan 0.18 mg/kg oral days 1–4 ■ Prednisone 2 mg/kg oral days 1–4 ■ Lenalidomide 10 mg oral days 1–21 ■ Repeated every 4 weeks	67	33
Bortezomib/thalidomide/ dexamethasone (VTD)**[56]	■ Bortezomib 1.3 mg/m^2 intravenous days 1, 8, 15, 22 ■ Thalidomide 100-200 mg oral days 1–21 ■ Dexamethasone 20 mg on day of/after bortezomib (or 40 mg days 1, 8, 15, 22) ■ Repeated every 4 weeks x four cycles as pretransplant induction therapy	95	60
Bortezomib/ cyclophosphamide/ dexamethasone (VCd)**[57]	■ Cyclophosphamide 300 mg/m^2 orally on days 1, 8, 15 and 22 ■ Bortezomib 1.3 mg/m^2 intravenously on days 1, 8, 15, 22 ■ Dexamethasone 40 mg orally on days on days 1, 8, 15, 22 ■ Repeated every 4 weeks	90	70
Bortezomib/lenalidomide/ dexamethasone (VRD)**[58,59]	■ Bortezomib 1.3 mg/m^2 intravenous days 1, 8, 15 ■ Lenalidomide 25 mg oral days 1–14 ■ Dexamethasone 20 mg on day of and day after bortezomib (or 40 mg days 1, 8, 15, 22) ■ Repeated every 3 weeks	100	70

*Doses of dexamethasone and bortezomib reduced from initial trial reports to once-weekly schedules.

** All of these regimens used high-dose pulsed dexamethasone, which is no longer recommended. The dosing of dexamethasone recommended in this table is the low-dose schedule.

Abbreviations: CR, complete response; VGPR, very good partial response.

Reproduced from Rajkumar SV. Treatment of Multiple Myeloma. Nature Rev Clin Oncol. 2011;8:479-91. PMID: 21522124.

remains an option when lenalidomide or bortezomib are not available for initial therapy, and in these circumstances it is usually combined with cyclophosphamide.[73]

Lenalidomide is a safer and more effective analog of thalidomide; it also has the added convenience of being an oral agent. Thus, Rd has become one of the commonly used regimens for initial therapy in multiple myeloma.[7,74] A randomized trial by the Eastern Cooperative Oncology Group (ECOG) found that lenalidomide plus low-dose dexamethasone (40 mg of dexamethasone once a week) was superior to lenalidomide plus high-dose dexamethasone (40 mg of dexamethasone on days 1 to 4, 9 to 12, and 17 to 20) in terms of overall survival.[50] Based on this

Trial	Regimen	Number of Patients	Overall Response Rate (%)	CR plus VGPR (%)	Median PFS (months)	p-value for PFS	3-Year OS Rate (%)*	p-value for OS
Rajkumar et al. (2008)[49]	D	235	46	16	7	< 0.001	40	NS
	TD	235	23	44	15		60	NS
Rajkumar et al. (2010)[50]	RD	223	81	50	19	0.026	75	NS
	Rd	222	70	40	25		74	NS
Harousseau et al. (2010)[60]	VAD	242	63	15	30	0.06	77	NS
	VD	240	79	38	36		81	NS
Cavo et al. (2010)[56]	TD	238	79	28	40	0.006	84	NS
	VTD	236	93	62	NR		85	NS
Moreau et al. (2010)[61]	VD	99	81	35	NA	NA	NA	NS
	VTD	100	90	51	NA		NA	NS
Facon et al. (2007)[52]	MP	196	35	7	17.8	< 0.001	48	< 0.001
	Mel 100	126	65	43	19.4		52	
	MPT	125	76	47	27.5		66	
Hulin et al. (2009)[53]	MP + placebo	116	31	7	18.5	0.001	40	0.028
	MPT	113	62	21	24.1		55	
Wijermans et al. (2010)[62]	MP	168	45	10	9	< 0.001	43	0.05
	MPT	165	66	27	13		55	
Palumbo et al. (2006)[63]	MP	164	48	11	14.5	0.004	65	0.79
	MPT	167	69	29	21.8		65	
Waage et al. (2010)[64]	MP + placebo	175	33	7	14	NS	43	0.16
	MPT	182	34	23	15		43	
San Miguel et al. (2008)[65]; Mateos et al. (2010)[66]**	MP	331	35	8	16.6	< 0.001	54	< 0.001
	VMP	337	71	41	24		69	
Mateos et al. (2010)[54]	VMP	130	80	32	34	0.10	74	0.3
	VTP	130	81	36	25		65	
Palumbo et al. (2012)[55]	MP	154	50	12	13	< 0.001	66	NS
	MPR	153	68	33	14		62	
	MPR-R	152	77	33	31		70	
Moreau et al. (2010)[61]	VD	99	81	35	NA	NA	NA	NS
	VTD	100	90	51	NA		NA	NS

*Estimated from survival curves when not reported.

**Progression-free survival not reported, numbers indicate time to progression.

Abbreviations: CR, complete response; D, dexamethasone; Mel 100, reduced-intensity stem cell transplantation using melphalan 100 mg/m^2; MP, melphalan/prednisone; MPR, melphalan/prednisone/lenalidomide; MPR-R, melphalan/prednisone/lenalidomide followed by maintenance lenalidomide; MPT, melphalan/prednisone/thalidomide; NA, not available; NR, not reached; NS, not significant; OS, overall survival; PFS, progression-free survival; Rd, lenalidomide/low-dose dexamethasone; RD, lenalidomide/high-dose dexamethasone; TD, thalidomide/dexamethasone; VAD, vincristine/doxorubicin/dexamethasone; VD, bortezomib/dexamethasone; VGPR, very good partial response; VMP, bortezomib/melphalan/prednisone; VTD, bortezomib/thalidomide/dexamethasone; VTP, bortezomib/thalidomide/prednisone.

Modified from Rajkumar SV. Treatment of multiple myeloma. Nature Rev Clin Oncol. 2011;8:479-91. PMID: 21522124 trial, the use of high-dose dexamethasone is no longer recommended in newly diagnosed multiple myeloma. Rd can impair collection of peripheral blood stem cells in some patients when granulocyte colony-stimulating factor (G-CSF) alone is used for stem cell mobilization.[75] Stem cell mobilization in these patients is usually successful with a chemotherapy-containing mobilization regimen such as cyclophosphamide and G-CSF, or with the use of plerixafor, a CXCR4 inhibitor.

Another option for initial therapy is VD, which results in better response rates compared with the old VAD regimen.[60] The major advantage of VD over Rd is absence of deep vein thrombosis (DVT) risk, and the lack of any adverse effect on stem cell mobilization. The major disadvantage, however, is the risk of neurotoxicity. VD and similar bortezomib-based regimens are of particular value in patients presenting with acute renal failure[76] and in patients with high-risk multiple myeloma. Rd and VD have not been compared directly in a randomized trial.

Three-drug combinations such as VTD, VCd, and RVD produce better overall response rates, deeper and higher complete response rates, and longer progression-free survival compared with VD and Rd, but no overall survival benefit has been demonstrated so far.[57-59,61] VCd may be less toxic than VD because it allows the administration of bortezomib and dexamethasone at lower doses. Recent studies show that the combination of carfilzomib, lenalidomide, and dexamethasone (CRd) is highly active in newly diagnosed myeloma.[77] However, carfilzomib is significantly more expensive and cumbersome compared with bortezomib; therefore, CRd is not recommended as initial therapy outside the context of clinical trials. An ongoing randomized trial coordinated by ECOG is evaluating RVD versus CRd in patients newly diagnosed with myeloma.

In patients with very aggressive disease (plasma-cell leukemia or extramedullary disease), combination chemotherapy such as bortezomib with dexamethasone, thalidomide, cisplatin, doxorubicin, cyclophosphamide, and etoposide (VDT-PACE) is usually used as initial therapy to achieve rapid disease control.[78] Numerous other combinations have been developed, but randomized controlled trials have not shown a clear effect on long-term endpoints compared with the regimens discussed above.

As for patients who are not candidates for ASCT, the regimen of choice for initial therapy in candidates for transplant varies widely, and the author prefers Rd for low-risk, VCd for intermediate-risk, and VRd for high-risk patients based on efficacy, toxicity, convenience, and cost considerations.

AUTOLOGOUS STEM CELL TRANSPLANTATION

ASCT is not curative for multiple myeloma, but prolongs median overall survival by approximately 12 months.[79,80] The treatment-related mortality rate is very low (1% to 2%), and 40% to 50% of ASCT can be done entirely on an outpatient basis.[81] Melphalan (at a dose of 200 mg/m^2) is used as the standard conditioning regimen, and trials are underway trying to improve the efficacy of the conditioning regimen. ASCT can be done immediately following initial therapy or can be delayed until first relapse. In either case, stem cells must be collected early in the disease course. Three randomized trials show that overall survival is similar whether ASCT is performed early (after induction therapy) or late (at first relapse).[82-84] Therefore, patient and physician preference plays an important role in deciding the timing of ASCT. Although some randomized trials show benefit with two ASCTs done back to back ("tandem ASCT"),[85-87] the benefit of a second ASCT is primarily seen in patients whose disease fails to achieve a complete response or very good partial response with the first transplant.

ALLOGENEIC STEM CELL TRANSPLANTATION

Conventional myeloablative allogeneic transplantation has a limited role in multiple myeloma because of high treatment-related mortality. One study found a significant overall survival advantage with ASCT followed by nonmyeloablative allogeneic transplantation compared with ASCT alone.[88,89] However, other trials have not shown such a benefit.[90-92] At present, allogeneic transplantation is generally not recommended for the treatment of multiple myeloma outside of clinical trials, except in selected high-risk patients.

MAINTENANCE THERAPY

Maintenance therapy with interferon-alfa, corticosteroids, and thalidomide results in relatively modest benefit compared with cost and toxicity.[93] Bortezomib (administered twice per month) following ASCT has shown benefit and may be considered for patients with high- or intermediate-risk cytogenetics.[94] Two randomized studies have shown superior progression-free survival with lenalidomide maintenance post-ASCT, but there was a significant increased risk of second cancers (approximately 7% in the lenalidomide group compared with 3% in the placebo group; p < 0.01; Table 17-8).[95,96] Both hematologic cancers (acute myeloid leukemia, Hodgkin lymphoma) and nonhematologic cancers (gastrointestinal, breast, etc.) were increased. In one of the two studies, an overall survival benefit was seen.[95] Preliminary results of a more recent randomized trial also suggested a survival benefit with lenalidomide maintenance.[97] However, there are several limitations to these trials including study design issues, follow-up, and access to lenalidomide in the control arms at the time of initial relapse.[98] More data are needed to make definitive conclusions, and until a clear overall survival benefit is seen, routine therapy with lenalidomide post-ASCT remains controversial.

TREATMENT OF RELAPSED DISEASE

Almost all patients with multiple myeloma eventually experience relapse, and with each relapse, the remission duration decreases progressively.[99,100] In general, patients can be retreated with regimens that have been effective in the past, if the initial remission duration was longer than 6 months. Alternatively, regimens that contain active drugs that the patient has not received before can also be tried (Table 17-6). As in newly diagnosed disease, the presence of extramedullary plasmacytomas or plasma cell leukemia may require therapy with a multidrug regimen such as VDT-PACE for 1 to 2 months to obtain maximum disease control. Patients who experience remission duration of longer than 18 months with initial ASCT can also be considered for a second ASCT as salvage therapy.

Table 17-8 Results of Randomized Phase III Trials of Lenalidomide Maintenance in Myeloma following Autologous Stem Cell Transplantation

Trial	Regimen	Number of Patients	Median PFS (months)	p-value for PFS	3-Year OS Rate (%)*	Median OS	p-value for OS	Second Cancers (%)‡	Reported p-value for Second Cancer Incidence
McCarthy et al. (2012)[95]	Placebo	229	27	< 0.001	80	NR	0.03§	2.6	0.008
	Lenalidomide maintenance	231	46		88	NR		7.7	
Attal et al. (2012)[96]	Placebo	307	23	< 0.001	84	NR	0.70	3.0	0.002
	Lenalidomide maintenance	307	41		80	NR		7.5	

*Estimated from survival curves when not reported.
‡Excludes nonmelanoma skin cancers.
§Derived from Cox proportional hazard model; not clear if two-tailed or if adjustment for covariates were done or not.
Abbreviations: OS, overall survival; PFS, progression-free survival; NR, not reported.
Modified from Rajkumar SV. Lenalidomide maintenance- perils of a premature denouement. Nat Rev Clin Oncol. 2012; 9:372-374. PMID: 22665364

Newer options for patients with relapsed refractory myeloma include pomalidomide (an analogue of lenalidomide)[10,11] and carfilzomib (a new proteasome inhibitor).[9] Both drugs have a response rate of approximately 20% when used as single agents in patients whose disease is refractory to both lenalidomide and bortezomib (dual-refractory). The combination of pomalidomide plus low-dose dexamethasone results in response rates of approximately 35% in the same patient population.

Patients with relapsed refractory myeloma should also be considered for clinical trials. The advances in myeloma in the last decade have been made possible by participation of patients in clinical trials. Many ongoing clinical trials include drugs that have already shown clinical activity. Promising investigational agents with documented single-agent activity in myeloma include ixazomib (also referred to as MLN 9708; oral proteasome inhibitor), marizomib (proteasome inhibitor), ARRY-520 (kinesin spindle protein inhibitor), daratumumab and SAR650984 (monoclonal antibodies to CD38), and dinaciclib (cyclin dependent kinase inhibitor). Several clinical trials are ongoing with these agents. Additional agents with potential activity when combined with standard anti-myeloma agents include panobinostat (histone deacetylase inhibitor) and elotuzumab (anti–CS-1 antibody). Panobinostat has shown promise in combination with bortezomib in a phase III trial. Elotuzumab has shown promising activity when used in combination with lenalidomide and low-dose dexamethasone, and is in phase III clinical trials in both newly diagnosed and relapsed refractory disease.

TREATMENT OF COMPLICATIONS AND PALLIATIVE CARE
TREATMENT OF DISEASE COMPLICATIONS
Patients with multiple myeloma should receive bisphosphonates (pamidronate or zoledronic acid) once per month for 1 to 2 years to prevent bone disease.[101-103] A recent trial showed improved overall survival in multiple myeloma with the use of zoledronic acid as prophylactic therapy.[73] Calcium supplementation and daily vitamin D supplementation is needed for patients receiving bisphosphonates. Surgical fixation of fractures or impending fractures of long bones can be done as needed; however, local radiation should be limited to patients with disabling pain that has not responded to analgesics and systemic therapy. Vertebroplasty and kyphoplasty may be useful to decrease pain.[104] Some patients with multiple myeloma can develop severe hypercalcemia. This is a medical emergency and requires treatment with hydration, corticosteroids, and either pamidronate (60 mg to 90 mg intravenously over 2 to 4 hours) or zoledronic acid (4 mg intravenously over 15 minutes).

Renal failure is common in multiple myeloma and can be multifactorial. Volume depletion, nonsteroidal anti-inflammatory agents, infection, and radiographic contrast media may also contribute to renal failure. The most common cause of acute renal failure is light chain cast nephropathy, which requires prompt therapy to lower serum light chain levels. The role of plasmapheresis is controversial.[105,106]

Other disease-related complications include anemia, infections, and hyperviscosity syndrome. Anemia usually improves with treatment of the underlying multiple myeloma, but some patients may require transfusions or erythropoietin. Patients who are being treated with bortezomib are at high risk for reactivation of herpes zoster, and routine prophylaxis with acyclovir is recommended. Intravenous gammaglobulin is indicated only if patients have recurrent serious infections associated with severe hypogammaglobulinemia. Hyperviscosity syndrome manifests with symptoms such as epistaxis, mucosal bleeding, headache, and blurred vision. Hyperviscosity syndrome requires emergent plasmapheresis.

MANAGEMENT OF DRUG TOXICITY

The major side effects with thalidomide are sedation, constipation, and peripheral neuropathy. In contrast, the major side effects of lenalidomide are anemia, neutropenia, and thrombocytopenia. Both drugs cause fatigue. Due to the risk of teratogenicity, the use of any of the immunomodulatory agents (thalidomide, lenalidomide, and pomalidomide) in pregnant patients is absolutely contraindicated. Further, to prevent teratogenicity, there are strict requirements that must be met before these drugs can be prescribed. Patients receiving thalidomide, lenalidomide, and pomalidomide are also at significant risk of venous and arterial thrombotic events and require thromboprophylaxis with aspirin, low molecular-weight heparin, or warfarin.[107,108] Thalidomide and lenalidomide can cause a skin rash that can be serious in a small proportion of patients. Medications such as sulfonamides and allopurinol may increase the risk and severity of skin toxicity and should be avoided. Treatment with thalidomide, lenalidomide, and pomalidomide can lead to thyroiditis and subsequent hypothyroidism. Thyroid function tests should be performed at baseline and every 3 to 4 months thereafter while on therapy. Approximately 10% to 15% of patients taking prolonged lenalidomide can develop severe diarrhea. The treatment is cessation of therapy and standard antimotility agents. Lenalidomide requires dose reduction in patients with renal failure; the starting dose should be reduced to 10 mg per day in patients with creatinine clearance of 30 mL/min to 60 mL/min, 15 mg every other day with creatinine clearance less than 30 mL/min, and 5 mg per day for patients on dialysis.

The major side effects of bortezomib are gastrointestinal toxicity, thrombocytopenia, and neuropathy. The best way to reduce the risk of neuropathy is to use bortezomib in the once-weekly schedule instead of the twice-weekly schedule, and subcutaneous instead of intravenous administration. Major side effects of carfilzomib include fatigue, nausea, cytopenias, and shortness of breath.[109]

Because steroids play a major role in the treatment of multiple myeloma, patients often develop major steroid-related side effects. These are best prevented by using the lowest possible dose of steroids. During the first few months of therapy, dexamethasone at 40 mg once per week is sufficient.[50] Some patients require a lower dose even from the outset. After the first few months, an attempt should be made to rapidly reduce the dose of steroids.

Bisphosphonate therapy is associated with a risk of osteonecrosis of the jaw, and dental hygiene should be assessed prior to initiation of bisphosphonate therapy. Other drug-induced complications are a result of the myelosuppressive effects of the various chemotherapy agents used and long-term risk of second cancers.

RELATED DISORDERS
MONOCLONAL GAMMOPATHY OF UNDETERMINED SIGNIFICANCE

MGUS is a premalignant precursor of multiple myeloma.[28,29] It is defined by a serum M protein concentration lower than 3 g/dL, less than 10% clonal plasma cells in the bone marrow,

KEY POINTS

- Patients who are not candidates for autologous stem cell transplantation (ASCT) are treated with Rd until progression or with a bortezomib-based regimen such as VCd or VRd for approximately 12 months.
- Patients who are considered potential candidates for an ASCT are first treated with two to four cycles of nonmelphalan-containing treatment regimens such as Rd, VCd, or VRd, followed by a stem cell harvest. After stem cell harvest, patients can either proceed to early ASCT or continue initial treatment regimen and delay ASCT for relapse.
- Patients with myeloma should receive prophylactic bisphosphonates to prevent bone disease.
- Severe hypercalcemia is a medical emergency and requires treatment with hydration, corticosteroids, and intravenous bisphosphonates.
- The most common cause of acute renal failure is light chain cast nephropathy, which requires prompt therapy to lower serum light chain levels.
- Patients receiving thalidomide, lenalidomide, and pomalidomide have an increased risk of venous and arterial thrombotic events and require routine thromboprophylaxis.
- The best way to reduce the risk of neuropathy is to use bortezomib in the once-weekly schedule instead of the twice-weekly schedule, and subcutaneous instead of intravenous administration.
- The standard dose of steroids to be used in myeloma therapy should not usually exceed dexamethasone at 40 mg once per week (or equivalent) unless there is a need for emergent response.

and absence of lytic bone lesions, anemia, hypercalcemia, and renal insufficiency that can be attributed to a plasma cell disorder.[12] MGUS is present in over 3% of the population older than age 50.[28] MGUS risk is significantly higher in the black population compared with the white population.[110] The risk of MGUS is also higher in first-degree relatives of patients with MGUS or multiple myeloma,[111] and in those exposed to certain pesticides.[112]

MGUS is asymptomatic, but in a small subset of patients may be associated with sensorimotor peripheral neuropathy (MGUS neuropathy), membranoproliferative glomerulonephritis (MPGN), lichen myxedematosus (papular mucinosis, scleromyxedema), pyoderma gangrenosum, or necrobiotic xanthogranuloma. The main clinical significance of MGUS is its lifelong risk of transformation to multiple myeloma or related malignancy at a rate of 1% per year.[29] The size and type of the M protein at diagnosis of MGUS and an abnormal serum FLC ratio are prognostic factors for progression.[113] There is no treatment needed for MGUS. Patients should be followed at 6 months and if stable, yearly thereafter.

LIGHT CHAIN MGUS

Light chain MGUS is a premalignant clonal plasma cell disorder characterized by the presence of monoclonal immunoglobulin light chains without expression of heavy chains.[22] It is defined by an abnormal serum FLC ratio, elevated level of the respective FLC, absence of heavy chain expression on serum immunofixation, less than 10% clonal plasma cells in the bone marrow, and absence of lytic bone lesions, anemia, hypercalcemia, and renal insufficiency that can be attributed to a plasma cell disorder. It is prevalent in approximately 1% of the general population over age 50, and carries a risk of progression to light chain multiple myeloma. No therapy is indicated unless progression to malignancy occurs.

SMOLDERING MULTIPLE MYELOMA

SMM is defined by the presence of an M protein level greater than 3 g/dL in serum or 10% or more plasma cells in bone marrow in the absence of anemia, renal insufficiency, hypercalcemia, or skeletal lesions.[12,31] It is differentiated from MGUS and light chain MGUS based on the size of the M protein and the level of marrow involvement. The risk of progression to multiple myeloma or a related plasma cell disorder is 10-fold higher than with MGUS. The current standard of care for most patients with SMM is observation every 3 to 4 months. A recent randomized trial found improved progression-free and overall survival with early use of lenalidomide plus dexamethasone versus observation in patients with high-risk SMM.[38] This trial incorporated a definition for high-risk SMM that included a multiparametric flow cytometry method that is not yet standardized, and more data are required before the results of this trial can be generalized for clinical practice. At present, certain ultra-high-risk patients should be considered for early intervention, including those with markedly elevated FLC ratio (≥ 100) or more than one focal lesion identified by MRI scanning.[39]

SOLITARY PLASMACYTOMA

Solitary plasmacytoma is an early-stage plasma cell malignancy that is in between MGUS/SMM and multiple myeloma along the spectrum of plasma cell disorders. It is defined by the presence of a single biopsy-proven plasmacytoma (bony or extramedullary) and a normal bone marrow examination.[12] An M protein may be present in serum or urine at diagnosis but is usually resolved with therapy. Treatment consists of radiation therapy at 40 Gy to 50 Gy to the involved site. Unlike multiple myeloma, approximately 50% of patients with solitary plasmocytoma can be cured.

PLASMA CELL LEUKEMIA

Plasma cell leukemia is an aggressive form of multiple myeloma characterized by circulating clonal plasma cells in the peripheral blood and extramedullary disease. Treatment of plasma cell leukemia is unsatisfactory and requires the use of a combination of treatment approaches including multidrug chemotherapy, stem cell transplantation, and maintenance. An aggressive initial treatment with a regimen such as VDT-PACE for two to three cycles followed by ASCT and subsequent maintenance therapy is a reasonable strategy.

IMMUNOGLOBULIN LIGHT CHAIN AMYLOIDOSIS

Amyloid is a proteinaceous substance that consists of rigid, linear, nonbranching fibrils, that are 7.5 nm to 10 nm in width and aggregated in a beta-pleated sheet conformation.[114] It is detected on Congo Red staining based on the classic apple-green birefringence. There are several types of amyloidosis, classified based on the major protein component of the amyloid. In AL amyloidosis, the fibrils consist of the variable portion of a monoclonal light chain. AL amyloidosis is an infrequent consequence of clonal plasma cell disorders and may be seen with MGUS, SMM, or multiple myeloma. It is a systemic disease that can affect numerous organs such as the tongue (macroglossia), heart, liver, kidney, peripheral nerves, and lungs. The standard treatment is melphalan plus dexamethasone or a bortezomib-based regimen (e.g., VCd) for approximately 1 year. Eligible patients can also be considered for ASCT.[115]

WALDENSTRÖM MACROGLOBULINEMIA

Waldenström macroglobulinemia is a malignancy of plasma cells that have not yet undergone switch recombination. It might better be considered a lymphoproliferative disorder, pathologically and clinically similar to low-grade lymphomas, in which an immunoglobulin (Ig) M paraprotein is present. The neoplastic cells in Waldenström macroglobulinemia secrete IgM M protein, and have a morphologic appearance that is in between

---

KEY POINTS

- Monoclonal gammopathy of undetermined significance can progress to myeloma or related malignancy at a rate of 1% per year.
- The risk of progression to myeloma or related plasma cell disorder in smoldering multiple myeloma is 10-fold higher than with monoclonal gammopathy of undetermined significance.
- Solitary plasmacytoma is defined by the presence of a single biopsy-proven plasmacytoma (bony or extramedullary) and a normal bone marrow examination. Treatment consists of radiation therapy (40 Gy to 50 Gy) to the involved site.
- Plasma cell leukemia is an aggressive form of myeloma characterized by circulating clonal plasma cells in the peripheral blood and extramedullary disease.
- Immunoglobulin AL amyloidosis is a systemic plasma cell proliferative disorder that can affect numerous organs such as the tongue (macroglossia), heart, liver, kidney, peripheral nerves, and lungs.
- Waldenström macroglobulinemia is a malignancy of plasma cells that secrete IgM M protein.
- POEMS syndrome is a rare plasma cell disorder characterized by **p**olyneuropathy, **o**rganomegaly, **e**ndocrinopathy, **M** protein, and **s**kin changes.

lymphocytes and true plasma cells commonly referred to as "lymphoplasmacytic." The disease definition requires presence of an IgM M protein, 10% or greater bone marrow involvement, and a typical immunophenotype (e.g., surface IgM+, CD10−, CD19+, CD20+, CD23−) that would exclude other lymphoproliferative disorders.[12] The main symptoms are weakness, fatigue, and hyperviscosity. In contrast to multiple myeloma, lytic bone lesions are not seen. Treatment should consist of single-agent rituximab, or rituximab in combination with any one of the following agents: cyclophosphamide, fludarabine, cladribine, or bortezomib.[116] There is a risk of a "tumor flare" if single-agent rituximab is used, resulting in a rapid rise in IgM levels. Therefore, combination therapy is preferred for patients with high IgM M protein levels. A common regimen used in initial therapy is rituximab plus cyclophosphamide and dexamethasone.

POEMS SYNDROME

This syndrome is characterized by **p**olyneuropathy, **o**rganomegaly, **e**ndocrinopathy, **M** protein, and **s**kin changes (POEMS).[27] Patients with POEMS syndrome usually have osteosclerotic bone lesions or Castleman disease (a rare polyclonal lymphoproliferative disorder). The major clinical problem in POEMS is a severe chronic inflammatory-demyelinating polyneuropathy with predominantly motor features. If the osteosclerotic lesions are in a limited area, radiation therapy is the treatment of choice. If there are widespread osteosclerotic lesions, treatment is similar to that of multiple myeloma.

References

1. Rajkumar SV. Multiple myeloma: 2013 update on diagnosis, risk-stratification, and management. *Am J Hematol.* 2013;88:226-235. PMID: 23440663.

2. Kyle RA, Rajkumar SV. Multiple myeloma. *N Engl J Med.* 2004;351:1860-1873. PMID: 15509819.

3. Siegel R, Naishadham D, Jemal A. Cancer statistics, 2013. *CA Cancer J Clin.* 2013;63:11-30. PMID: 23335087.

4. Rajkumar SV, Gahrton G, Bergsagel PL. Approach to the treatment of multiple myeloma: a clash of philosophies. *Blood.* 2011;118:3205-3211. PMID: 21791430.

5. Singhal S, Mehta J, Desikan R, et al. Antitumor activity of thalidomide in refractory multiple myeloma. *N Engl J Med.* 1999;341:1565-1571. PMID: 10564685.

6. Richardson PG, Sonneveld P, Schuster MW, et al. Bortezomib or high-dose dexamethasone for relapsed multiple myeloma. *N Engl J Med.* 2005;352:2487-2498. PMID: 15958804.

7. Rajkumar SV, Hayman SR, Lacy MQ, et al. Combination therapy with lenalidomide plus dexamethasone (Rev/Dex) for newly diagnosed myeloma. *Blood.* 2005;106:4050-4053. PMID: 16118317.

8. Richardson PG, Blood E, Mitsiades CS, et al. A randomized phase 2 study of lenalidomide therapy for patients with relapsed or relapsed and refractory multiple myeloma. *Blood.* 2006;108:3458-3464. PMID: 16840727.

9. Siegel DS, Martin T, Wang M, et al. A phase 2 study of single-agent carfilzomib (PX-171-003-A1) in patients with relapsed and refractory multiple myeloma. *Blood.* 2012;120:2817-2825. PMID: 22833546.

10. Lacy MQ, Hayman SR, Gertz MA, et al. Pomalidomide (CC4047) plus low-dose dexamethasone as therapy for relapsed multiple myeloma. *J Clin Oncol.* 2009;27:5008-5014. PMID: 19720894.

11. Lacy MQ, Allred JB, Gertz MA, et al. Pomalidomide plus low-dose dexamethasone in myeloma refractory to both bortezomib and lenalidomide: comparison of 2 dosing strategies in dual-refractory disease. *Blood.* 2011;118:2970-2975. PMID: 21690557.

12. Kyle RA, Rajkumar SV. Criteria for diagnosis, staging, risk stratification and response assessment of multiple myeloma. *Leukemia.* 2009;23:3-9. PMID: 18971951.

13. Rajkumar SV, Merlini G, San Miguel JF. Haematological cancer: Redefining myeloma. *Nat Rev Clin Oncol.* 2012;9:494-496. PMID: 22850755.

14. Rajkumar SV, Larson D, Kyle RA. Diagnosis of smoldering multiple myeloma. *N Engl J Med.* 2011;365:474-475. PMID: 21812699.

15. International Myeloma Working Group. Criteria for the classification of monoclonal gammopathies, multiple myeloma and related disorders: a report of the International Myeloma Working Group. *Br J Haematol.* 2003;121:749-757. PMID: 12780789.

16. Rajkumar SV, Kyle RA. Multiple myeloma: diagnosis and treatment. *Mayo Clinic Proceedings.* 2005;80:1371-1382. PMID: 16212152.

17. Kyle RA, Therneau TM, Rajkumar SV, et al. Long-term follow-up of IgM monoclonal gammopathy of undetermined significance. *Blood.* 2003;102:3759-3764. PMID: 12881316.

18. Gobbi PG, Baldini L, Broglia C, et al. Prognostic validation of the international classification of immunoglobulin M gammopathies: a survival advantage for patients with immunoglobulin M monoclonal gammopathy of undetermined significance? *Clin Cancer Res.* 2005;11:1786-1790. PMID: 15756000.

19. Kyle RA, Therneau TM, Rajkumar SV, et al. Long-term follow-up of IgM monoclonal gammopathy of undetermined significance. *Semin Oncol.* 2003;30:169-171. PMID: 12720130.

20. Baldini L, Goldaniga M, Guffanti A, et al. Immunoglobulin M monoclonal gammopathies of undetermined significance and indolent Waldenstrom's macroglobulinemia recognize the same determinants of evolution into symptomatic lymphoid disorders: proposal for a common prognostic scoring system. *J Clin Oncol.* 2005;23:4662-4668. PMID: 16034042.

21. Owen RG, Treon SP, Al-Katib A, et al. Clinicopathological definition of Waldenstrom's macroglobulinemia: consensus panel recommendations from the Second International Workshop on Waldenstrom's Macroglobulinemia. *Semin Oncol.* 2003;30:110-115. PMID: 12720118.

22. Dispenzieri A, Katzmann JA, Kyle RA, et al. Prevalence and risk of progression of light-chain monoclonal gammopathy of undetermined significance: a retrospective population-based cohort study. *Lancet.* 2010;375:1721-1728. PMID: 20472173.

23. Dimopoulos MA, Moulopoulos LA, Maniatis A, et al. Solitary plasmacytoma of bone and asymptomatic multiple myeloma. *Blood.* 2000;96:2037-2044. PMID: 10979944.

24. Dimopoulos MA, Kiamouris C, Moulopoulos LA. Solitary plasmacytoma of bone and extramedullary plasmacytoma. *Hematol Oncol Clin North Am.* 1999;13:1249-1257. PMID: 10626148.

25. Rajkumar SV, Dispenzieri A, Kyle RA. Monoclonal gammopathy of undetermined significance, Waldenström macroglobulinemia, AL amyloidosis, and related plasma cell disorders: diagnosis and treatment. *Mayo Clinic Proceedings.* 2006;81:693-703. PMID: 16706268.

26. Dispenzieri A, Kyle RA, Lacy MQ, et al. POEMS syndrome: definitions and long-term outcome. *Blood.* 2003;101:2496-2506. PMID: 12456500.

27. Dispenzieri A. POEMS syndrome. *Blood Rev.* 2007;21:285-299. PMID: 17850941.

28. Kyle RA, Therneau TM, Rajkumar SV, et al. Prevalence of monoclonal gammopathy of undetermined significance. *N Engl J Med.* 2006;354:1362-1369. PMID: 16571879.

29. Kyle RA, Therneau TM, Rajkumar SV, et al. A long-term study of prognosis in monoclonal gammopathy of undetermined significance. *N Engl J Med.* 2002;346:564-569. PMID: 11856795.

30. Rajkumar SV. Prevention of progression in monoclonal gammopathy of undetermined significance. *Clin Cancer Res.* 2009;15:5606-5608. PMID: 19737944.

31. Kyle RA, Remstein ED, Therneau TM, et al. Clinical course and prognosis of smoldering (asymptomatic) multiple myeloma. *N Engl J Med.* 2007;356:2582-2590. PMID: 17582068.

32. Landgren O, Weiss BM. Patterns of monoclonal gammopathy of undetermined significance and multiple myeloma in various ethnic/racial groups: support for genetic factors in pathogenesis. *Leukemia.* 2009;23:1691-1697. PMID: 19587704.

33. Landgren O, Kyle RA, Pfeiffer RM, et al. Monoclonal gammopathy of undetermined significance (MGUS) consistently precedes multiple myeloma: a prospective study. *Blood.* 2009;113:5412-5417. PMID: 19179464.

34. Bergsagel PL, Kuehl WM. Chromosome translocations in multiple myeloma. *Oncogene.* 2001;20:5611-5622. PMID: 11607813.

35. Fonseca R, Barlogie B, Bataille R, et al. Genetics and cytogenetics of multiple myeloma: a workshop report. *Cancer Res.* 2004;64:1546-1558. PMID: 14989251.

36. Keats JJ, Chesi M, Egan JB, et al. Clonal competition with alternating dominance in multiple myeloma. *Blood.* 2012;120:1067-1076. PMID: 22498740.

37. Roodman GD. Pathogenesis of myeloma bone disease. *Leukemia.* 2009;23:435-441. PMID: 19039321.

38. Mateos MV, Hernández MT, Giraldo P, et al. Lenalidomide plus dexamethasone for high-risk smoldering multiple myeloma. *N Engl J Med.* 2013;369:438-447. PMID: 23902483.

39. Rajkumar SV, Kyle RA. Haematological cancer: Treatment of smoldering multiple myeloma. *Nat Rev Clin Oncol.* 2013;10:554-555. PMID: 23999214.

40. Kyle RA, Gertz MA, Witzig TE, et al. Review of 1027 patients with newly diagnosed multiple myeloma. *Mayo Clin Proc.* 2003;78:21-33. PMID: 12528874.

41. Katzmann JA, Dispenzieri A, Kyle RA, et al. Elimination of the need for urine studies in the screening algorithm for monoclonal gammopathies by using serum immunofixation and free light chain assays. *Mayo Clin Proc.* 2006;81:1575-1578. PMID: 17165636.

42. Mikhael JR, Dingli D, Roy V, et al. Management of newly diagnosed symptomatic multiple myeloma: updated Mayo Stratification of Myeloma and Risk-Adapted Therapy (mSMART) consensus guidelines 2013. *Mayo Clin Proc.* 2013;88:360-376. PMID: 23541011.

43. Dispenzieri A, Kyle R, Merlini G, et al. International Myeloma Working Group guidelines for serum-free light chain analysis in multiple myeloma and related disorders. *Leukemia.* 2009;23:215-224. PMID: 19020545.

44. Durie BG, Harousseau JL, Miguel JS, et al. International uniform response criteria for multiple myeloma. *Leukemia.* 2006;20:1467-1473. PMID: 16855634.

45. Durie BG, Salmon SE. A clinical staging system for multiple myeloma. Correlation of measured myeloma cell mass with presenting clinical features, response to treatment, and survival. *Cancer.* 1975;36:842-854. PMID: 1182674.

46. Greipp PR, San Miguel J, Durie BG, et al. International staging system for multiple myeloma. *J Clin Oncol.* 2005;23:3412-3420. PMID: 15809451.

47. Kumar S, Fonseca R, Ketterling RP, et al. Trisomies in multiple myeloma: impact on survival in patients with high-risk cytogenetics. *Blood.* 2012;119:2100-2105. PMID: 22234687.

48. Rajkumar SV, Blood E, Vesole D, et al. Phase III clinical trial of thalidomide plus dexamethasone compared with dexamethasone alone in newly diagnosed multiple myeloma: a clinical trial coordinated by the Eastern Cooperative Oncology Group. *J Clin Oncol.* 2006;24:431-436. PMID: 16365178.

49. Rajkumar SV, Rosiñol L, Hussein M, et al. Multicenter, randomized, double-blind, placebo-controlled study of thalidomide plus dexamethasone versus dexamethasone as initial therapy for newly diagnosed multiple myeloma. *J Clin Oncol.* 2008;26:2171-2177. PMID: 18362366.

50. Rajkumar SV, Jacobus S, Callander NS, et al. Lenalidomide plus high-dose dexamethasone versus lenalidomide plus low-dose dexamethasone as initial therapy for newly diagnosed multiple myeloma: an open-label randomised controlled trial. *Lancet Oncol.* 2010;11:29-37. PMID: 19853510.

51. Harousseau JL, Attal M, Leleu X, et al. Bortezomib plus dexamethasone as induction treatment prior to autologous stem cell transplantation in patients with newly diagnosed multiple myeloma: results of an IFM phase II study. *Haematologica.* 2006;91:1498-1505. PMID: 17043025.

52. Facon T, Mary JY, Hulin C, et al. Melphalan and prednisone plus thalidomide versus melphalan and prednisone alone or reduced-intensity autologous stem cell transplantation in elderly patients with multiple myeloma (IFM 99-06): a randomised trial. *Lancet.* 2007;370:1209-1218. PMID: 17920916.

53. Hulin C, Facon T, Rodon P, et al. Efficacy of melphalan and prednisone plus thalidomide in patients older than 75 years with newly diagnosed multiple myeloma: IFM 01/01 trial. *J Clin Oncol.* 2009;27:3664-3670. PMID: 19451428.

54. Mateos MV, Oriol A, Martínez-López J, et al. Bortezomib, melphalan, and prednisone versus bortezomib, thalidomide, and prednisone as induction therapy followed by maintenance treatment with bortezomib and thalidomide versus bortezomib and prednisone in elderly patients with untreated multiple myeloma: a randomised trial. *Lancet Oncol.* 2010;11:934-941. PMID: 20739218.

55. Palumbo A, Hajek R, Delforge M, et al. Continuous lenalidomide treatment for newly diagnosed multiple myeloma. *N Engl J Med.* 2012;366:1759-1769. PMID: 22571200.

56. Cavo M, Tacchetti P, Patriarca F, et al. Bortezomib with thalidomide plus dexamethasone compared with thalidomide plus dexamethasone as induction therapy before, and consolidation therapy after, double autologous stem-cell transplantation in newly diagnosed multiple myeloma: a randomised phase 3 study. *Lancet.* 2010;376:2075-2085. PMID: 21146205.

57. Reeder CB, Reece DE, Kukreti V, et al. Cyclophosphamide, bortezomib and dexamethasone induction for newly diagnosed multiple myeloma: high response rates in a phase II clinical trial. *Leukemia.* 2009;23:1337-1341. PMID: 19225538.

58. Richardson PG, Weller E, Lonial S, et al. Lenalidomide, bortezomib, and dexamethasone combination therapy in patients with newly diagnosed multiple myeloma. *Blood.* 2010;116:679-686. PMID: 20385792.

59. Kumar SK, Flinn I, Noga SJ, et al. Bortezomib, dexamethasone, cyclophosphamide and lenalidomide combination for newly diagnosed multiple myeloma: phase 1 results from the multicenter EVOLUTION study. *Leukemia.* 2010;24:1350-1356. PMID: 20508619.

60. Harousseau JL, Attal M, Avet-Loiseau H, et al. Bortezomib plus dexamethasone is superior to vincristine plus doxorubicin plus dexamethasone as induction treatment prior to autologous stem-cell transplantation in newly diagnosed multiple myeloma: results of the IFM 2005-01 phase III trial. *J Clin Oncol.* 2010;28:4621-4629. PMID: 20823406.

61. Moreau P, Facon T, Attal M, et al. Comparison of reduced-dose bortezomib plus thalidomide plus dexamethasone (vTD) to bortezomib plus dexamethasone (VD) as induction treatment prior to ASCT in de novo multiple myeloma (MM): Results of IFM2007-02 study. *J Clin Oncol.* 2010;28:15s (suppl; abstr 8014).

62. Wijermans P, Schaafsma M, Termorshuizen F, et al. Phase III study of the value of thalidomide added to melphalan plus prednisone in elderly patients with newly diagnosed multiple myeloma: the HOVON 49 Study. *J Clin Oncol.* 2010;28:3160-3166. PMID: 20516439.

63. Palumbo A, Bringhen S, Caravita T, et al. Oral melphalan and prednisone chemotherapy plus thalidomide compared with melphalan and prednisone alone in elderly patients with multiple myeloma: randomised controlled trial. *Lancet.* 2006;367:825-831. PMID: 16530576.

64. Waage A, Gimsing P, Fayers P, et al. Melphalan and prednisone plus thalidomide or placebo in elderly patients with multiple myeloma. *Blood.* 2010;116:1405-1412. PMID: 20448107.

65. San Miguel JF, Schlag R, Khuageva NK, et al. Bortezomib plus melphalan and prednisone for initial treatment of multiple myeloma. *N Engl J Med.* 2008;359:906-917. PMID: 18753647.

66. Mateos MV, Richardson PG, Schlag R, et al. Bortezomib plus melphalan and prednisone compared with melphalan and prednisone in previously untreated multiple myeloma: updated follow-up and impact of subsequent therapy in the phase III VISTA trial. *J Clin Oncol.* 2010;28:2259-2266. PMID: 20368561.

67. Palumbo A, Bringhen S, Rossi D, et al. Bortezomib-melphalan-prednisone-thalidomide followed by maintenance with bortezomib-thalidomide compared with bortezomib-melphalan-prednisone for initial treatment of multiple myeloma: a randomized controlled trial. *J Clin Oncol.* 2010;28:5101-5109. PMID: 20940200.

68. Moreau P, Pylypenko H, Grosicki S, et al. Subcutaneous versus intravenous administration of bortezomib in patients with relapsed multiple myeloma: a randomised, phase 3, non-inferiority study. *Lancet Oncol.* 2011;12:431-440. PMID: 21507715.

69. Ludwig H, Hajek R, Tóthová E, et al. Thalidomide-dexamethasone compared with melphalan-prednisolone in elderly patients with multiple myeloma. *Blood.* 2009;113:3435-3442. PMID: 18955563.

70. Palumbo A, Bringhen S, Rossi D, et al. Overall survival benefit for bortezomib-melphalan-prednisone-thalidomide followed by maintenance with bortezomib-thalidomide (VMPT-VT) versus bortezomib-melphalan-prednisone (VMP) in newly diagnosed multiple myeloma patients. *ASH Annual Meeting Abstracts.* 2012;120 (abstr 200).

71. Jacobus S, Callander N, Siegel D, et al. Outcome of elderly patients 70 years and older with newly diagnosed myeloma in the ECOG randomized trial of lenalidomide/high-dose dexamethasone (RD) versus lenalidomide/low-dose dexamethasone (Rd). *Haematologica.* 2010;95:149 (suppl 2; abstr 0370).

72. Gay F, Hayman S, Buadi F, et al. Safety and efficacy of lenalidomide plus dexamethasone in elderly newly diagnosed multiple myeloma patients 70 years of age and older. *Haematologica.* 2010;95:153 (suppl; abstr 0379).

73. Morgan GJ, Davies FE, Gregory WM, et al. First-line treatment with zoledronic acid as compared with clodronic acid in multiple myeloma (MRC Myeloma IX): a randomised controlled trial. *Lancet.* 2010;376:1989-1999. PMID: 21131037.

74. Zonder JA, Crowley J, Hussein MA, et al. Lenalidomide and high-dose dexamethasone compared with dexamethasone as initial therapy for multiple myeloma: a randomized Southwest Oncology Group trial (S0232). *Blood.* 2010;116:5838-5841. PMID: 20876454.

75. Kumar S, Dispenzieri A, Lacy MQ, et al. Impact of lenalidomide therapy on stem cell mobilization and engraftment post-peripheral blood stem cell transplantation in patients with newly diagnosed myeloma. *Leukemia.* 2007;21:2035-2042. PMID: 17581613.

76. San-Miguel J, Harousseau JL, Joshua D, et al. Individualizing treatment of patients with myeloma in the era of novel agents. *J Clin Oncol.* 2008;26:2761-2766. PMID: 18427148.

77. Jakubowiak AJ, Dytfeld D, Griffith KA, et al. A phase 1/2 study of carfilzomib in combination with lenalidomide and low-dose dexamethasone as a front-line treatment for multiple myeloma. *Blood*. 2012;120:1801-1809. PMID: 22665938.

78. Barlogie B, Anaissie E, van Rhee F, et al. Incorporating bortezomib into upfront treatment for multiple myeloma: early results of total therapy 3. *British Journal of Haematology*. 2007;138:176-185. PMID: 17593024.

79. Attal M, Harousseau JL, Stoppa AM, et al. A prospective, randomized trial of autologous bone marrow transplantation and chemotherapy in multiple myeloma. Intergroupe Français du Myélome. *N Engl J Med*. 1996;335:91-97. PMID: 8649495.

80. Child JA, Morgan GJ, Davies FE, et al. High-dose chemotherapy with hematopoietic stem-cell rescue for multiple myeloma. *N Engl J Med*. 2003;348:1875-1883. PMID: 12736280.

81. Gertz MA, Ansell SM, Dingli D, et al. Autologous stem cell transplant in 716 patients with multiple myeloma: low treatment-related mortality, feasibility of outpatient transplantation, and impact of a multidisciplinary quality initiative. *Mayo Clin Proc*. 2008;83:1131-1138. PMID: 18828972.

82. Barlogie B, Kyle RA, Anderson KC, et al. Standard chemotherapy compared with high-dose chemoradiotherapy for multiple myeloma: final results of phase III US Intergroup Trial S9321. *J Clin Oncol*. 2006;24:929-936. PMID: 16432076.

83. Facon T, Mary JY, Harousseau JL, et al. Front-line or rescue autologous bone marrow transplantation (ABMT) following a first course of high dose melphalan (HDM) in multiple myeloma (MM). Preliminary results of a prospective randomized trial (CIAM) protocol. *Blood*. 1996;88:685a (suppl 1).

84. Fermand JP, Ravaud P, Chevret S, et al. High-dose therapy and autologous peripheral blood stem cell transplantation in multiple myeloma: up-front or rescue treatment? Results of a multicenter sequential randomized clinical trial. *Blood*. 1998;92:3131-3136. PMID: 9787148.

85. Attal M, Harousseau JL, Facon T, et al. Double Autologous Transplantation Improves Survival of Multiple Myeloma Patients: Final Analysis of a Prospective Randomized Study of the Intergroupe Francophone du Myelome (IFM 94). *Blood*. 2002;100:5a.

86. Cavo M, Cellini C, Zamagni E, et al. Superiority of double over single autologous stem cell transplantation as first-line therapy for multiple myeloma. *Blood*. 2004;104:155a (abstr 536).

87. Regelink JC, van Roessel CH, van Galen KP, et al. Long-term follow-up of tandem autologous stem-cell transplantation in multiple myeloma. *J Clin Oncol*. 2010;28:e741-e743. PMID: 20160027.

88. Bruno B, Rotta M, Patriarca F, et al. A comparison of allografting with autografting for newly diagnosed myeloma 10.1056/NEJMoa065464. *N Engl J Med*. 2007;356:1110-1120. PMID: 17360989.

89. Björkstrand B, Iacobelli S, Hegenbart U, et al. Tandem autologous/reduced-intensity conditioning allogeneic stem-cell transplantation versus autologous transplantation in myeloma: long-term follow-up. *J Clin Oncol*. 2011;29:3016-3022. PMID: 21730266.

90. Garban F, Attal M, Michallet M, et al. Prospective comparison of autologous stem cell transplantation followed by dose-reduced allograft (IFM99-03 trial) with tandem autologous stem cell transplantation (IFM99-04 trial) in high-risk de novo multiple myeloma. *Blood*. 2006;107:3474-3480. PMID: 16397129.

91. Rosiñol L, Pérez-Simón JA, Sureda A, et al. A prospective PETHEMA study of tandem autologous transplantation versus autograft followed by reduced-intensity conditioning allogeneic transplantation in newly diagnosed multiple myeloma. *Blood*. 2008;112:3591-3593. PMID: 18612103.

92. Krishnan A, Pasquini MC, Logan B, et al. Autologous haemopoietic stem-cell transplantation followed by allogeneic or autologous haemopoietic stem-cell transplantation in patients with multiple myeloma (BMT CTN 0102): a phase 3 biological assignment trial. *Lancet Oncol*. 2011;12:1195-1203. PMID: 21962393.

93. Attal M, Harousseau JL, Leyvraz S, et al. Maintenance therapy with thalidomide improves survival in patients with multiple myeloma. *Blood*. 2006;108:3289-3294. PMID: 16873668.

94. Sonneveld P, Schmidt-Wolf IG, van der Holt B, et al. Bortezomib induction and maintenance treatment in patients with newly diagnosed multiple myeloma: results of the randomized phase III HOVON-65/GMMG-HD4 trial. *J Clin Oncol*. 2012;30:2946-2955. PMID: 22802322.

95. McCarthy PL, Owzar K, Hofmeister CC, et al. Lenalidomide after stem-cell transplantation for multiple myeloma. *N Engl J Med*. 2012;366:1770-1781. PMID: 22571201.

96. Attal M, Lauwers-Cances V, Marit G, et al. Lenalidomide maintenance after stem-cell transplantation for multiple myeloma. *N Engl J Med*. 2012;366:1782-1791. PMID: 22571202.

97. Boccadoro M, Cavallo F, Gay FM, et al. Melphalan/prednisone/lenalidomide (MPR) versus high-dose melphalan and autologous transplantation (MEL200) plus lenalidomide maintenance or no maintenance in newly diagnosed multiple myeloma (MM) patients. *J Clin Oncol*. 2013;31 (suppl; abstr 8509).

98. Rajkumar SV. Haematological cancer: Lenalidomide maintenance—perils of a premature denouement. *Nat Rev Clin Oncol*. 2012;9:372-374. PMID: 22665364.

99. Kumar SK, Therneau TM, Gertz MA, et al. Clinical course of patients with relapsed multiple myeloma. *Mayo Clinic Proceedings*. 2004;79:867-874. PMID: 15244382.

100. Kumar S, Blade J, Crowley J, et al. Outcome of patients with myeloma relapsing after IMiD and bortezomib therapy: a multicenter study from the International Myeloma Foundation Working Group. *Haematologica*. 2010;95:151 (suppl 2; abstr 0376).

101. Berenson JR, Lichtenstein A, Porter L, et al. Efficacy of pamidronate in reducing skeletal events in patients with advanced multiple myeloma. Myeloma Aredia Study Group. *N Engl J Med*. 1996;334:488-493. PMID: 8559201.

102. Berenson JR, Rosen LS, Howell A, et al. Zoledronic acid reduces skeletal-related events in patients with osteolytic metastases. *Cancer*. 2001;91:1191-1200. PMID: 11283917.

103. Rosen LS, Gordon D, Kaminski M, et al. Zoledronic acid versus pamidronate in the treatment of skeletal metastases in patients with breast cancer or osteolytic lesions of multiple myeloma: a phase III, double blind, comparative trial. *Cancer J*. 2001;7:377-387. PMID: 11693896.

104. Fourney DR, Schomer DF, Nader R, et al. Percutaneous vertebroplasty and kyphoplasty for painful vertebral body fractures in cancer patients. *J Neurosurg*. 2003;98:21-30. PMID: 12546384.

105. Johnson WJ, Kyle RA, Pineda AA, et al. Treatment of renal failure associated with multiple myeloma. Plasmapheresis, hemodialysis, and chemotherapy. *Arch Intern Med*. 1990;150:863-869. PMID: 2183734.

106. Burnette BL, Leung N, Rajkumar SV. Renal improvement in myeloma with bortezomib plus plasma exchange. *New Engl J Med*. 2011;364:2365-2366. PMID: 21675906.

107. Palumbo A, Cavo M, Bringhen S, et al. Aspirin, warfarin, or enoxaparin thromboprophylaxis in patients with multiple myeloma treated with thalidomide: a phase III, open-label, randomized trial. *J Clin Oncol*. 2011;29:986-993. PMID: 21282540.

108. Palumbo A, Rajkumar SV, Dimopoulos MA, et al. Prevention of thalidomide- and lenalidomide-associated thrombosis in myeloma. *Leukemia*. 2008;22:414-423. PMID: 18094721.

109. Kortuem KM, Stewart AK. Carfilzomib. *Blood*. 2013;121:893-897. PMID: 23393020.

110. Landgren O, Katzmann JA, Hsing AW, et al. Prevalence of monoclonal gammopathy of undetermined significance among men in Ghana. *Mayo Clin Proc*. 2007;82:1468-1473. PMID: 18053453.

111. Vachon CM, Kyle RA, Therneau TM, et al. Increased risk of monoclonal gammopathy in first-degree relatives of patients with multiple myeloma or monoclonal gammopathy of undetermined significance. *Blood*. 2009;114:785-790. PMID: 19179466.

112. Landgren O, Kyle RA, Hoppin JA, et al. Pesticide exposure and risk of monoclonal gammopathy of undetermined significance in the Agricultural Health Study. *Blood*. 2009;25:6386-6391. PMID: 19387005.

113. Rajkumar SV, Kyle RA, Therneau TM, et al. Serum free light chain ratio is an independent risk factor for progression in monoclonal gammopathy of undetermined significance. *Blood*. 2005;106:812-817. PMID: 15855274.

114. Rajkumar SV, Gertz MA. Advances in the treatment of amyloidosis. *N Engl J Med*. 2007;356:2413-2415. PMID: 17554124.

115. Gertz MA. Immunoglobulin light chain amyloidosis: 2013 update on diagnosis, prognosis, and treatment. *Am J Hematol*. 2013;88:416-425. PMID: 23605846.

116. Ansell SM, Kyle RA, Reeder CB, et al. Diagnosis and management of Waldenström macroglobulinemia: Mayo stratification of macroglobulinemia and risk-adapted therapy (mSMART) guidelines. *Mayo Clin Proc*. 2010;85:824-833. PMID: 20702770.

18

HEMATOPOIETIC CELL TRANSPLANTATION

Frederick R. Appelbaum, MD

Updates from 2012

▶ Compared with transplants from matched related donors, transplantation using matched unrelated donors is associated with higher rates of acute and chronic graft-versus-host disease (GVHD), but similar overall survival (Horowitz MM, *Best Pract Res Clin Haematol* 2012).

▶ Compared to bone marrow, use of peripheral blood as the stem cell source for matched unrelated transplantation following standard high-dose conditioning is associated with higher rates of chronic GVHD with no survival benefit (Anasetti C, *N Engl J Med* 2012).

▶ When a single umbilical cord unit of adequate cell dose is not available, double unit grafts are an acceptable substitute, thereby extending access to nearly all patients (Scaradavou A, *Blood* 2013).

▶ Reduced-intensity conditioning is associated with increased relapse rates but reduced toxicity, making transplantation an option for patients into their 70s and for those with significant comorbidities (Storb R, *J Clin Oncol* 2013; Ringdén O, *J Clin Oncol* 2009).

B one marrow transplantation was the term originally used to describe the process of transferring the lymphohematopoietic system from one individual to another. With the demonstration that peripheral blood and umbilical cord blood also can serve as sources of hematopoietic stem cells, the term hematopoietic cell transplantation (HCT) may be more appropriate. HCT can be used to replace an abnormal but nonmalignant hematopoietic system with one from a normal donor. HCT is also used to treat a variety of malignancies because it allows administration of higher doses of chemotherapy and radiotherapy than would otherwise be possible, and, in the setting of allogeneic transplantation, it confers an immunologic graft-versus-tumor effect. Worldwide, more than 65,000 patients received HCTs in 2012.[1] This chapter focuses on general principles of HCT, including stem cell source, preparative regimens, and complications. The role of transplantation in the treatment of specific diseases is discussed in greater detail in the chapters focused on those illnesses.

INDICATIONS
IMMUNODEFICIENCY STATES
Allogeneic transplantation can successfully establish a normal immune system for patients with severe combined immunodeficiency disorders; it also can correct the abnormalities associated with Wiskott-Aldrich syndrome and other immunodeficiency states.[2,3]

NONMALIGNANT DISORDERS OF HEMATOPOIESIS

The most data and best outcomes of transplantation for nonmalignant disorders of hematopoiesis are reported for severe aplastic anemia and thalassemia, with a growing experience for sickle cell anemia. Ninety percent of patients with severe aplastic anemia can be cured with allogeneic HCT from a matched sibling[4]; results are slightly less favorable if a matched unrelated donor is used.[5] Allogeneic HCT cures 70% to 90% of patients with thalassemia major, with the best results seen in patients who received the transplant before the development of hepatomegaly or portal fibrosis.[6] Although data for sickle cell disease are more limited, current reports document 5-year survival and disease-free survival of 93% and 84%, respectively.[7,8] Cures also have been obtained for other nonmalignant disorders of hematopoiesis, including Fanconi anemia,[9] Blackfan-Diamond syndrome,[10] chronic granulomatous disease,[11] Kostmann syndrome, and leukocyte adhesion deficiency.[12] However, as allogeneic transplantation still has significant and unpredictable complications, treatment recommendations should be based on identifying patients at high risk from their underlying diseases for whom the risk of HCT is justified.

ENZYMATIC DISORDERS

Allogeneic HCT can replace the abnormal enzyme systems and result in cure for patients with mucopolysaccharidosis and Gaucher disease. Prior damage caused by the enzyme abnormality may not be reversible, arguing for early transplantation for the more severe syndromes.

MALIGNANT DISEASES

The most frequent use of HCT has been for the treatment of malignant diseases. In the United States, the leading indications for allogeneic transplantation are acute myeloid leukemia (AML; approximately 50%), followed by acute lymphoblastic leukemia (ALL) and myelodysplasia (MDS). Transplantation consistently achieves 5-year disease-free survival rates of 50% to 70% when performed for AML and ALL in first remission.[13] Meta-analyses of studies comparing the outcome of matched sibling allogeneic HCT compared with conventional chemotherapy for adult patients with these disorders show improved survival with HCT.[14-16] The advantages of transplantation are most apparent in patients with higher-risk leukemia and less apparent in those with lower-risk disease. If transplantation is withheld until second remission, results are less favorable, with cure rates of 25% to 40%. Cure rates of 30% to 60% have been reported for patients with MDS who are treated with allogeneic HCT.[17] Because patients with early-stage MDS often live for long periods without treatment, HCT is generally reserved for patients with advanced-stage disease.[18,19] Although more than 70% of patients with chronic myeloid leukemia (CML) in chronic phase can be cured with allogeneic HCT, transplantation is usually restricted to patients whose disease has progressed following initial therapy with a tyrosine kinase inhibitor.[20] Allogeneic transplantation is also used in the treatment of patients with recurrent chronic lymphocytic leukemia and non-Hodgkin lymphoma with marrow involvement.[21]

The leading indication for autologous transplantation in the United States is multiple myeloma, followed by non-Hodgkin lymphoma and Hodgkin lymphoma. Prospective randomized trials have shown that autologous transplantation used as part of initial therapy prolongs life for patients with multiple myeloma.[22,23] Autologous HCT is curative for 40% to 50% of patients with non-Hodgkin lymphoma or Hodgkin lymphoma that recurred following first-line therapy; these results are superior to what would be expected with additional chemotherapy.[24] Randomized trials suggest that autologous HCT may improve survival of patients with high-risk non-Hodgkin lymphoma if used in first remission. Autologous HCT also is used to treat chemosensitive solid tumors, with the largest experience with testicular cancer and neuroblastoma.[25]

SOURCE OF STEM CELLS

Hematopoietic stem cells used for transplantation can be categorized according to the relationship between the donor and the recipient or according to anatomic source. In those rare cases where the patient has an identical (syngeneic) twin, HCT can be conducted without the risks of graft rejection or graft-versus-host disease (GVHD), because the individuals are genetically identical throughout the genome.

When the marrow of a patient is clearly abnormal (as in aplastic anemia and for most leukemia cases), allogeneic transplantation from a human leukocyte antigen (HLA)-identical sibling usually is preferred. HLA molecules display both exogenous peptides (e.g., from an infecting organism) and endogenous peptides, presenting them to T cells to initiate an immune response. If two persons are HLA non-identical, T cells from one person will react vigorously to the mismatched HLA molecules on the surface of cells from the second individual. The HLA molecules themselves are termed major HLA determinants. Even though non-twin siblings may be HLA-matched, the endogenous peptides presented by the HLA antigens will differ, resulting in T-cell responses against minor HLA determinants. The genes encoding HLA class I *(HLA-A, HLA-B,* and *HLA-C)* and class II *(HLA-DP, HLA-DQ,* and *HLA-DR)* are located on chromosome 6, are tightly linked, are codominantly expressed, and tend to be inherited as haplotypes with low recombination frequency (Fig. 18-1). Thus, for any given patient, the likelihood that a full sibling will be HLA-matched with the patient is 25%. The likelihood of finding a matched sibling for a patient can be calculated by the formula $x = 1 - 0.75^n$, where "x" equals the probability of finding a matched sibling, and "n" equals the number of siblings. Given the size of families in the United States, the chance that a matched sibling can be identified for any patient is approximately 30%. Since hematopoietic stem cells do not express ABO, HCT can be carried out across ABO

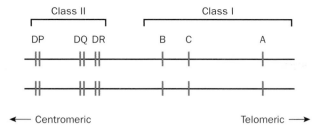

Class II | Class I

DP   DQ DR   B   C   A

← Centromeric   Telomeric →

Fig. 18-1 Genes associated with human leukocyte antigen (HLA) typing.

The genes encoding HLA class I (*HLA-A, HLA-B, and HLA-C*) and class II (*HLA-DP, HLA-DQ,* and *HLA-DR*) are located on chromosome 6, are tightly linked, are codominantly expressed, and tend to be inherited as haplotypes with low recombination frequency. Thus, for any given patient, the likelihood that a full sibling will be HLA-matched with the patient is 25%.

blood group barriers by removing incompatible red blood cells and/or isoagglutinins from the donor graft.

Family members who are genotypically identical to the patient for one HLA haplotype and are either phenotypically identical or partially matched on the other HLA haplotype have been used as donors. Use of one-antigen mismatched related donors results in a marginal increase in graft rejection, GVHD, and transplant-related mortality.[26] If patients are undergoing transplantation for leukemia in remission, this degree of mismatching appears to result in a slightly worse outcome. However, if patients are undergoing transplantation for higher-risk leukemia, the increased graft-versus-tumor effect associated with a single mismatch appears to balance the negative effect.[25] If donors are mismatched for two or three antigens, the incidences of GVHD and graft rejection are higher, and the results are considerably worse (Table 18-1).[26-28] Novel techniques specifically designed to allow transplantation from haplotype-mismatched donors are under study and include the use of T-replete bone marrow with post-transplant high-dose cyclophosphamide to eradicate reactive T cells, and the use of T-depleted bone marrow and peripheral blood containing high CD34+ cell doses.[29,30]

KEY POINTS

- Both graft rejection and graft-versus-host disease (GVHD) are more common with the use of cells from unrelated donors than with the use of cells from matched siblings, even when individuals are HLA-identical, because of increased disparities in minor histocompatibility antigens. However, survival rates appear similar.
- When compared to bone marrow, use of granulocyte colony-stimulating factor (G-CSF)–mobilized peripheral blood for allogeneic transplantation is associated with faster engraftment and less infection. However, such transplantation is associated with a higher risk of chronic GVHD.

Table 18-1 Effect of Human Leukocyte Antigen (HLA) Matching on Graft Rejection and Graft-versus-Host Disease (GVHD) following Transplantation for Leukemia[26-28]

HLA Match	Graft Failure (%)	Acute GVHD (Grade III or more)*(%)
Genotypic match	2	7
Phenotypic match	7	7
Mismatch of 1 locus	9	32
Mismatch of 2 or 3 loci	21	62
Matched, unrelated	3	36
Mismatch of 1 locus, unrelated	5	51

*See Table 18-4 for definition of grades.
Modified with permission from Cheson BD, ed. Oncology MKSAP, 2nd ed. Philadelphia, PA: American College of Physicians; 1999.

Donors who are completely unrelated to the patient but are matched for *HLA-A, HLA-B, HLA-C,* and *HLA-DR* have been used in an increasing number of cases with promising results. Since the formation of the National Marrow Donor Program and other international registries, more than 20 million healthy individuals have volunteered to serve as stem cell donors. When compared with the outcome of matched sibling transplantation, transplants from unrelated donors matched with the patient at *HLA-A, -B, -C,* and *-DRB1* are associated with greater morbidity, mostly from GVHD, but survival at 3 to 5 years post-transplant is very similar.[31] A single antigen mismatch is associated with more GVHD, higher treatment-related mortality, and lower survival.[32] In a study of 3,857 unrelated transplants, which largely involved bone marrow as the source of stem cells, mismatches at *HLA-A* or *-DRB1* were less well tolerated than mismatches at *HLA-B* or *HLA-C.* Mismatching at two loci was associated with even greater risk.[33] Once HLA is taken into account, other donor factors, including age, sex, parity, and cytomegalovirus (CMV) serology have no apparent effect on outcome.[34] If peripheral blood rather than marrow is the source of unrelated stem cells, mismatching for *HLA-C* appears to be less well tolerated.[35] With modern typing methods, the difference in outcome between matched sibling and fully matched unrelated donor transplants has greatly diminished, and in most settings, the indications for transplantation are the same using a matched related or matched unrelated donor. It is estimated that a matched unrelated donor can be found for more than 60% of individuals, with higher rates for white individuals and decreased rates for both Hispanic and black individuals, in part because of under-representation of these groups in the registries, but also because of greater HLA diversity in these populations.[36] On average, the period of time between initiating the search for an unrelated matched donor and performing the transplant is 3 to 4 months; however, in urgent circumstances donors can sometimes be identified and grafts procured within 6 weeks.

The use of a patient's own (autologous) stem cells for transplantation also is possible. Autologous transplantation was initially used for the treatment of lymphoma and other tumors in which marrow was not overtly involved in the disease. The technique also has been explored as a treatment option for patients with AML and ALL, using stem cells collected during remission. In the cases of AML and ALL, enough patients have received transplants with either allogeneic or autologous marrow to allow for comparisons of the two therapies. In general, autologous transplantation is associated with fewer complications; GVHD does not occur, and the incidence of infectious complications, idiopathic pneumonia syndrome, and sinusoidal obstruction syndrome (formerly termed veno-occlusive hepatic disease) are lower. However, the risk of tumor recurrence is higher with autologous transplantation, likely because of a lack of a graft-versus-tumor effect and tumor contamination of the re-infused stem cell product. Gene marking studies have demonstrated that tumor cells within the transplanted marrow can contribute to relapse.[37] Ex vivo treatment of autologous stem cell collections to remove contaminating cells—although based on sound preclinical models—has never been adequately tested in prospective randomized clinical studies.

BONE MARROW

Because bone marrow is rich in hematopoietic stem cells, it was used first as the source of stem cells for transplantation. Marrow for transplantation usually is obtained through multiple aspirations from the posterior and sometimes from the anterior iliac crests. To obtain as many marrow cells with as little peripheral blood contamination as possible, the collection from each aspiration site is normally limited to 5 mL to 10 mL, and a total collection usually comprises approximately 1 L to 1.5 L of marrow from a healthy adult donor.[38] The marrow is heparinized and filtered through screens to remove osseous spicules and fat globules before either being infused to the patient or cryopreserved for later transplantation. In some studies, the marrow has been treated before infusion or cryopreservation to test whether removal of T cells, or T-cell subsets, from allogeneic marrow can improve outcome by reducing GVHD or whether tumor cells can be removed prior to autologous transplantation.[39] The risks associated with marrow donation are minimal. Of the first 1,220 marrow donations in Seattle, Washington, no donor died and there were only six complications, mostly local hematomas or infection that required hospitalization.[40] More recent reviews confirm the relative, although not absolute, safety of the procedure.[41]

PERIPHERAL BLOOD

Hematopoietic stem cells circulate in the peripheral blood, albeit in small numbers. During recovery from drug-induced cytopenias or after exposure to hematopoietic growth factors, such as granulocyte macrophage-colony stimulating factor (GM-CSF) or granulocyte-colony stimulating factor (G-CSF), the number of hematopoietic progenitor cells in the peripheral blood increases considerably. With the use of these mobilizing techniques, followed by leukapheresis, it is possible to collect sufficient stem cells from the peripheral blood to permit successful transplantation. Because peripheral blood has a higher proportion of T cells than marrow, the first trials of peripheral blood stem cell transplantation were performed in the autologous setting, in which GVHD was not a concern. These studies demonstrated that such transplantation is not only possible but also results in faster engraftment than is seen with marrow.[42] When more than 5.0×10^6 CD34+ cells/kg are infused, recovery to 0.5×10^3 granulocytes/µL and 20×10^3 platelets/µL is generally seen less than 2 weeks after transplantation. Because of the increased safety and decreased costs associated with peripheral blood stem cell transplantation, it has largely replaced marrow as the source of stem cells for autologous transplantation.

Given the rapid recovery associated with the use of autologous peripheral blood stem cells, pilot studies of allogeneic peripheral blood stem cell transplantation using HLA-identical sibling donors were performed.[43] The results of these studies demonstrated rapid engraftment without an increase in the incidence of acute GVHD; randomized trials have confirmed these findings.[44] In most studies, the incidence of chronic GVHD associated with allogeneic peripheral blood stem cell transplantation is higher, but both disease-free and overall survival rates appear to be improved, particularly for patients who received transplants for more advanced-stage diseases.[45] In the unrelated donor setting, a large randomized study comparing marrow with peripheral blood after myeloablative conditioning showed faster engraftment but more chronic GVHD with peripheral blood and equivalent survival, thus favoring the use of marrow in this setting.[46]

Stromal cell–derived factor 1, also termed CXCL12, produced by marrow stromal cells is a key regulator of hematopoietic stem cell homing and retention in the marrow by interacting with the alpha-chemokine receptor CXCR4 found on stem cells. Plerixafor, an antagonist of CXCR4, results in mobilization of CD34+ cells and may be useful when added to G-CSF in the 10% to 20% of patients who experience failure in the mobilization of adequate numbers of cells when treated with G-CSF alone.[47]

UMBILICAL CORD BLOOD

Umbilical cord blood also is rich in hematopoietic stem cells, and studies have shown that cord blood can serve as a source of stem cells for transplantation. Cord blood has relatively few mature T cells; as a result, the risk of GVHD with cord blood appears to be somewhat less than the risk associated with similarly matched marrow, although the risk of graft rejection or failure may be greater. Cord blood is sometimes used as a source of stem cells to treat family members suffering from hematologic disorders, with survival essentially equivalent to that seen following matched sibling bone marrow transplantation.[48] By far the most common use of cord blood has been in the treatment of unrelated recipients who lack matched related or unrelated donors. Because of the paucity of mature T cells in cord blood, matching criteria can be less stringent, allowing treatment of one- or two-antigen mismatched patients. In an analysis of 1,061 recipients of transplants from unrelated cord blood, the number of cells per kilogram infused was found to have a considerable influence on the outcome, as did patient age and degree of match with donors, with improved survival associated with higher cell dose, younger patient age, and greater degree of matching.[49] A low dose of cord-blood cells increases the risk of graft failure, delayed hematopoietic engraftment, and delayed immune recovery, which previously limited cord-blood transplantation to children and smaller adults.[50] Trials exploring the use of double-cord transplants demonstrate that even though only one cord ultimately engrafts, the use of two cords reduces the risk of graft failure and is associated with an enhanced graft-versus-tumor effect.[51,52]

PREPARATIVE REGIMEN

The form of treatment administered to patients directly before transplantation depends on the disease being treated and on the source of stem cells. Patients with severe combined immunodeficiency diseases often require no therapy before transplantation because there is no abnormal cell population that must be eradicated and because their immune system is so severely compromised that the infused marrow rarely is rejected if the donor is an HLA-matched sibling. In contrast, patients with aplastic anemia are sufficiently immunocompetent to reject allogeneic marrow if no pretransplant immunosuppression is given. Thus, high-dose cyclophosphamide alone or combined with antithymocyte globulin (ATG) often is used as the preparative regimen for allogeneic transplantation. When transplantation is applied to the treatment of leukemia or other malignant diseases, the regimen must be both immunosuppressive (in the setting of allogeneic transplantation) and capable of eradicating the malignant disease. Commonly used regimens involve high doses of cyclophosphamide, etoposide, busulfan, melphalan, and total-body radiation therapy, in various combinations. The choice of specific regimens is discussed more completely in chapters focused on the particular diseases for which transplantation is used.

Although high-dose myeloablative preparative regimens have traditionally been used in transplantation for malignant diseases, the observation that some of the antitumor effects following allogeneic transplantation are the result of a graft-versus-tumor response has led to investigations of whether reduced-intensity regimens might be as effective and less toxic. Evidence for the existence of a graft-versus-tumor effect includes the finding that relapse rates following allogeneic marrow transplantation are the lowest when acute and chronic

> ## KEY POINT
>
> - The purpose of the preparative regimen used prior to hematopoietic cell transplantation is to help eliminate the underlying disease and, in the case of allogeneic transplantation, to provide sufficient immunosuppression to allow the donor cells to engraft.

GVHD develops, greater if no GVHD develops, and greater still if syngeneic or T-cell–depleted allogeneic marrow is used.[53,54] Additional evidence of a potent graft-versus-tumor effect comes from the use of viable donor lymphocyte infusions. The simple transfusion of as few as 1×10^7 viable donor lymphocytes/kg as treatment for patients whose disease relapsed after allogeneic transplantation can result in complete remission for as many as 70% of patients with CML and for a smaller but still substantial portion of patients with AML, MDS, or multiple myeloma.[55]

Currently used preparative regimens for allogeneic transplantation can be placed in three general categories: myeloablative, which cause irreversible marrow aplasia and require replacement of the hematopoietic system; nonmyeloablative, which cause minimal marrow suppression; and reduced-intensity conditioning, which cause cytopenias of intermediate duration.[56] Compared with high-dose preparative regimens, nonmyeloablative and reduced-intensity regimens result in shorter duration of pancytopenias with reduced transfusion needs, fewer bacterial infections, and a lower incidence of direct toxicities to the lung and liver.[57] Relapse rates are generally higher with reduced-dose regimens.[58] Although definitive studies are yet to be reported, reduced-intensity conditioning is generally selected for older patients and those with significant comorbidities, while high-dose regimens are preferred for younger, fit patients.

ENGRAFTMENT

Following administration of a myeloablative preparative regimen and the infusion of stem cells, a period of profound myelosuppression ensues. Within 1 to 2 weeks after transplantation, the peripheral leukocyte count begins to increase, signifying engraftment. When stem cells are procured from marrow and no hematopoietic growth factors are used after transplantation, the granulocyte count reaches $0.1 \times 10^3/\mu L$ by approximately day 16 and $1.0 \times 10^3/\mu L$ by day 26. Administration of G-CSF or GM-CSF to the recipient can accelerate the recovery of peripheral granulocyte counts by as much as 1 week. The platelet count recovers simultaneously with or shortly after recovery of granulocytes.

When peripheral blood is the source of stem cells, engraftment is more rapid, with a granulocyte count of $0.5 \times 10^3/\mu L$ and a platelet count of $20 \times 10^3/\mu L$ achieved by day 12, on average. Engraftment following cord blood transplantation is typically delayed by approximately 1 week compared with marrow. Engraftment of allogeneic stem cells can be documented using fluorescence in situ hybridization of sex chromosomes if donor and recipient are of opposite sex, or DNA-based assays of short tandem repeat loci; with these techniques the donor-versus-recipient origin of populations of cells can now be determined in virtually all cases.

COMPLICATIONS OF MARROW TRANSPLANTATION

Both the nature and the degree of complications associated with HCT depend on the age and health of the patient, the specific preparative regimen used, and the source of stem cells. The frequency of complications is higher and the rate of survival is lower for patients with a Karnofsky performance score of less than 80% and for patients with significant comorbidities.[59] GVHD is normally seen only after allogeneic transplantation and is associated with an increased incidence of infection. The extent of other specific organ toxicities is largely dependent on the specific preparative regimen used. Figure 18-2 illustrates the approximate timing of possible toxicities after allogeneic transplantation using a typical intensive preparative regimen. Scoring systems have been developed that can predict the overall likelihood of mortality following HCT.[60] The following sections discuss the major complications of HCT.

GRAFT FAILURE

In some instances, the transplanted graft functions briefly, but, after a period of days or weeks, marrow function is lost and myeloid elements are absent on evaluation of marrow obtained by biopsy. In the setting of allogeneic transplantation, failure of the graft usually is the result of residual host immune elements rejecting the donor marrow, a phenomenon termed graft rejection. Following transplantation involving an HLA-identical donor, graft rejection occurs most commonly when the patient has received multiple transfusions prior to transplantation, little prior chemotherapy, and when the preparative regimen is less immunosuppressive, such as with the use of cyclophosphamide monotherapy before transplantation for aplastic anemia. In general, the greater the disparity in HLA antigens between donor and recipient, the higher the chance of rejection. Also, because donor T cells react with and help eliminate host immune-competent cells not eradicated by the preparative regimen, T-cell depletion of donor marrow prior to transplantation can lead to persistence of host immunity, resulting in an increased chance of graft rejection.

Graft failure occurs rarely in recipients of autologous transplants. A single cause often is difficult to identify, but several have been implicated, including prior exposure to stem cell poisons, marrow damage during in vitro processing and cryopreservation, drug toxicity after transplantation, and viral infections.

Patients with graft failure (but not immunologically mediated graft rejection) sometimes have a response to treatment with a hematopoietic growth factor, such as GM-CSF, with an increase in the granulocyte count that may be sustained even after discontinuation of the growth factor. If persistent host lymphocytes are detected, which documents graft rejection, a second marrow transplant following an immunosuppressive preparative regimen may be successful.[61]

GRAFT-VERSUS-HOST DISEASE

GVHD is a complication usually restricted to allogeneic transplants and is the result of allogeneic T cells that were transfused with the graft reacting against targets on the genetically different host. A National Institutes of Health Consensus Report recognized two categories of GVHD, each with two subcategories (Table 18-2).[62] Acute GVHD classically develops within the first 3 months after allogeneic HCT and typically presents with an erythematous or maculopapular rash (Fig. 18-3), nausea, vomiting, anorexia, diarrhea (sometimes profuse), ileus, or cholestatic jaundice. Symptoms of acute GVHD sometimes may occur beyond 3 months from transplant (late-onset GVHD) or only when immunosuppression is withdrawn.

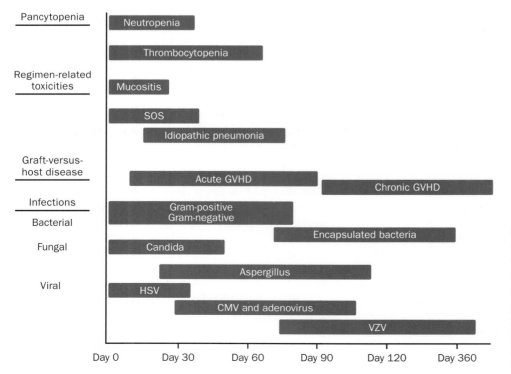

Fig. 18-2 The approximate timing of possible toxicities after allogeneic transplantation using a typical intensive preparative regimen.

Abbreviations: CMV, cytomegalovirus; HSV, herpes simplex virus; GVHD, graft-versus-host disease; SOS, sinusoidal obstruction syndrome; VZV, Varicella-Zoster virus.

rejection and tumor recurrence following transplantation, especially in the setting of CML. Factors associated with an increased risk of moderate or severe acute GVHD include HLA-mismatching, older age of patient and donor, a multiparous woman as the donor, and exposure to more intensive conditioning regimens.

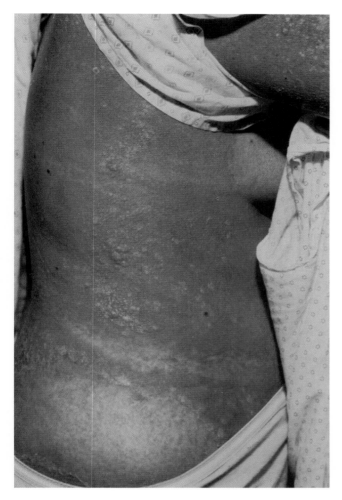

Fig. 18-3 Acute graft-versus-host disease.

Acute graft-versus-host disease classically develops within the first 3 months after allogeneic HCT and typically presents with an erythematous or maculopapular rash.

Reproduced from John Wiley & Sons, Inc., copyright 2009: Appelbaum FR, Forman SJ, Negrin R, Blume KG. (eds). Thomas' Hematopoietic Cell Transplantation, 4th Edition. Oxford, UK: Wiley Blackwell Publishing Ltd., 2009.

Acute GVHD usually is staged and graded using a modification of the original Seattle system (Tables 18-3 and 18-4). The most commonly used regimens to prevent GVHD include a combination of an antimetabolite (methotrexate or mycophenolate mofetil) and a calcineurin inhibitor (cyclosporine or tacrolimus).

If no evidence of acute GVHD develops, these drugs usually are continued for approximately 3 months and then tapered until discontinuation at 6 months. With these regimens, moderate GVHD requiring therapy occurs in approximately 30% of patients who have undergone transplants from a matched sibling donor. Lethal acute GVHD is uncommon for patients who have had transplants from an HLA-identical donor, occurring in less than 5% of patients.

Another approach to preventing acute GVHD is the removal of T cells from the donor marrow. Although effective, this approach has been associated with an increased risk of graft

Table 18-2 Categories of Acute and Chronic GVHD[62]

Category	Time of Symptoms after HCT	Presence of Acute GVHD Features	Presence of Chronic GVHD Features
Acute GVHD			
Classic acute	≤ 100 days	Yes	No
Late-onset	> 100 days	Yes	No
Chronic GVHD			
Classic chronic	No time limit	No	Yes
Overlap	No time limit	Yes	Yes

Abbreviations: GVHD, graft-versus-host disease; HCT, hematopoietic cell transplantation.

Reprinted from the Biol Blood Marrow Transplant, Volume 11(12). Filipovich AH, Weisdorf D, Pavletic S. National Institutes of Health Consensus Development Project on Criteria for Clinical Trials in Chronic Graft-versus-Host Disease: I. Diagnosis and Staging Working Group Report. Pages 945-955, copyright 2005. With permission from Elsevier.

Table 18-3 Clinical Staging of Acute Graft-versus-Host Disease[26]

Clinical Stage	Skin (Erythematous Rash)	Liver (Serum Bilirubin)	Gut (Diarrhea)
1	25% of body surface	2-3 mg/dL	500–1,000 mL per day
2	25% to 50% of body surface	3-6 mg/dL	1,000–1,500 mL per day
3	Generalized	6-15 mg/dL	> 1,500 mL per day
4	Desquamation and bullae	> 15 mg/dL	(Pain or ileus)

Modified with permission from Cheson BD, ed. Oncology MKSAP, 2nd ed. Philadelphia, PA: American College of Physicians; 1999.

Table 18-4 Clinical Grading of Acute Graft-versus-Host Disease[26]

Clinical Grade	Skin	Liver	Gut
I (Mild)	1 or 2	0	0
II (Moderate)	3	1	1
III (Severe)	1, 2, or 3	2 or 3	2, 3, or 4
IV (Life-threatening)	4	4	

Modified with permission from Cheson BD, ed. Oncology MKSAP, 2nd ed. Philadelphia, PA: American College of Physicians; 1999.

Responses have been reported after many different therapies for established acute GVHD, and none have proven superior (Table 18-5).

Chronic GVHD affects 20% to 40% of matched sibling transplant recipients and resembles a collagen vascular disease involving skin, liver, eyes, mouth, upper respiratory track, esophagus, and, less frequently, serosal surfaces, female genitalia, and fascia.[62,63] Chronic GVHD also may appear as an overlap syndrome in which features of chronic and acute GVHD appear together.

Chronic GVHD is seen more frequently with HLA mismatching, with the use of peripheral blood stem cells instead of marrow, in older patients, and in patients who have had prior episodes of acute GVHD. If chronic GVHD develops while the calcineurin inhibitor is being tapered, increasing the inhibitor to therapeutic levels may be effective. Mild chronic GVHD can sometimes be managed using local therapies alone (e.g., topical steroids to the skin and cyclosporine eye drops). More severe disease is usually treated with prednisone alone or in combination with a calcineurin inhibitor, which can control chronic GVHD in 50% to 70% of cases. Randomized trials exploring alternative approaches to primary therapy have so far failed to identify a better approach.[63] Patients for whom primary treatment of chronic GVHD fails are sometimes treated with mycophenolate mofetil, sirolimus, or extracorporeal photopheresis. Eventually, immunosuppression can be tapered and discontinued in 80% to 90% of patients, but many months to several years of immunosuppression may be required before tolerance develops. The median duration of treatment is 2 to 3 years. Bacterial infection frequently occurs in patients with chronic GVHD, and prophylactic treatment with antibiotics should be administered while patients are receiving immunosuppressive therapy. A commonly used regimen includes trimethoprim/sulfamethoxazole plus penicillin, which provides protection against both *Pneumocystis jirovecii* and encapsulated organisms.

As noted earlier, the incidence of both acute and chronic GVHD is increased in recipients of transplants from mismatched or unrelated donors (Table 18-1). A mild syndrome, similar to

GVHD, that involves the skin and gastrointestinal system develops in some patients after autologous transplantation. The syndrome nearly always resolves with a short course of prednisone, does not appear to have an antitumor effect, and does not affect overall transplant outcome. Following allogeneic transplantation, in 3% to 5% of cases, an autoimmune disorder will develop, most commonly autoimmune hemolytic anemia or idiopathic thrombocytopenia purpura. Unrelated donor source and chronic GVHD are risk factors. Treatment is with cyclosporine, prednisone, or rituximab.[64]

INFECTIOUS COMPLICATIONS

Infection is a major risk for nearly all transplant recipients. Recipients of autologous transplants are at risk for the early bacterial and fungal infections common to all patients with granulocytopenia. Recipients of allogeneic hematopoietic grafts, particularly patients in whom GVHD develops, also are at risk for late-onset bacterial, fungal, and viral diseases.

During the early neutropenic period following transplantation, patients are likely to become febrile, and in approximately 50% of febrile neutropenic patients, a bacterial source can be identified. Therefore, at most transplant centers, antibiotic treatment is initiated once patients become granulocytopenic, even if they are afebrile. Prophylaxis with fluconazole or voriconazole reduces the incidence of both superficial and invasive fungal infections and improves overall survival. Patients who become or remain febrile despite treatment with broad-spectrum antibiotics and who have no obvious source of infection usually are treated with additional antifungal agents (voriconazole, micafungin, or amphotericin, depending on the clinical situation).[65]

Although laminar airflow isolation and prophylactic granulocyte transfusions can prevent early infection, neither action influences overall survival, and thus, neither approach is recommended. With current methods of supportive care, the risk of death as a result of infection during the early granulocytopenic period after transplantation is less than 3% for recipients of either allogeneic or autologous transplants.

Herpes simplex infection, which can contribute to the severity of oral mucositis, can be prevented with the use of systemic acyclovir (250 mg/m^2 every 8 hours intravenously), beginning 1 week before transplant and continuing for 1 month after transplantation.[66]

In the past, symptomatic CMV infection, which typically involves either the gastrointestinal tract or the lungs, occurred in approximately 25% of patients who received allogeneic transplant and led to death (typically from CMV pneumonia) in 10% to 15% of patients. Primary CMV infection in the setting in which both donor and recipient are without latent CMV infection (as evidenced by having no detectable antibodies to CMV before transplantation) can be prevented by using only blood products that come from donors without latent CMV, or by using blood products that have been filtered to remove all leukocytes. For patients with evidence of latent CMV before transplantation, the use of prophylactic ganciclovir, starting either at the time of initial engraftment or at the time of CMV reactivation, can substantially reduce the risk of CMV disease.

Table 18-5 **Treatment Options for Graft-versus-Host Disease**	
Acute Graft-versus-Host Disease	▪ Prednisone ▪ Antithymocyte globulin (ATG) ▪ Calcineurin inhibitor ▪ Mycophenolate mofetil ▪ Rapamycin ▪ Monoclonal antibodies against T cells
Chronic Graft-versus-Host Disease	▪ Calcineurin inhibitor ▪ Prednisone ▪ Extracorporeal phototherapy ▪ Mycophenolate mofetil ▪ Sirolimus

KEY POINTS

- In patients beginning transplantation without latent cytomegalovirus (CMV) infection (as evidenced by lack of antibodies to CMV), death from CMV infection can be prevented by using only blood products from donors similarly without latent CMV or blood products depleted of white blood cells. In patients beginning transplantation with latent CMV infection, death also can be substantially reduced by administering ganciclovir at the time of CMV reactivation.
- GVHD results from T cells in the donor graft reacting against allogeneic targets on the genetically different host. It can be prevented in many cases by removing T cells from the donor graft or by administering various combinations of immunosuppressants for several months after transplantation.

Prophylactic ganciclovir is not without toxicities, however, and granulocytopenia is more common for patients receiving prophylactic ganciclovir than for patients in control groups.[67] The granulocytopenia seen with ganciclovir usually responds to G-CSF treatment. Prophylactic ganciclovir generally is not recommended for patients who have an autologous transplant, except for cases in which T cells are removed from the stem cell inoculum. Foscarnet is effective for some patients in whom CMV infection develops despite the use of ganciclovir, as well as for patients who cannot tolerate ganciclovir. Foscarnet can, however, be associated with severe electrolyte wasting.

Pneumonia as a result of *Pneumocystis jirovecii,* previously seen in 5% to 10% of transplant recipients, can be prevented by treatment with oral trimethoprim/sulfamethoxazole for 1 week before transplantation and resuming prophylaxis once the granulocyte count exceeds $0.5 \times 10^3/\mu L$. Treatment 2 days per week while patients are receiving immunosuppressive drugs after transplantation usually is sufficient to prevent pneumocystis disease. Allergic reactions to trimethoprim/sulfamethoxazole are common but usually can be managed with desensitization. Additionally, dapsone or atovaquone can serve as a substitute for trimethoprim/sulfamethoxazole.

Community-acquired viral infections, including respiratory syncytial virus (RSV), influenza virus, and parainfluenza virus, can cause lethal pneumonias in the transplant patient. Pre-transplant patients with upper respiratory symptoms should be screened by nasopharyngeal lavage for viral infections before proceeding to HCT. If RSV, influenza virus, or parainfluenza virus is found, the transplant should be delayed. Ribavirin and anti-RSV antibody may be effective in treating established RSV infection in the transplant patient.

Late infections, occurring more than 3 months post-transplant, usually are restricted to Varicella-Zoster virus (VZV) or, for patients with chronic GVHD, to recurrent bacterial or fungal infections. The use of prophylactic trimethoprim/sulfamethoxazole, penicillin, or other agents can reduce the incidence of late-onset bacterial infections for patients with chronic GVHD. Reactivation of VZV can be prevented by the use of prophylactic acyclovir.

Antibody titers to vaccine-preventable diseases decline after allogeneic or autologous HCT if the recipient is not revaccinated. The U.S. Centers for Disease Control and Prevention have developed recommendations for revaccination of patients who have undergone HCT. These include vaccination against tetanus, diphtheria, Haemophilus influenza, and polio (using inactivated polio virus vaccine) starting at 12 months post-transplant, vaccination against pneumococcal pneumonia using PPV23 at 12 and 24 months, and vaccination against measles, mumps, and rubella (MMR) and VZV (and possibly pertussis) at 24 months.[68]

CHEMORADIOTHERAPY TOXICITIES

Following most standard preparative regimens, immediate toxicities, such as nausea, vomiting, fever, and mild skin erythema, are common. Unusual toxicities associated with high-dose cyclophosphamide include hemorrhagic cystitis and, rarely, acute hemorrhagic carditis. Parotiditis commonly is seen in patients undergoing total-body radiation therapy.

Oral mucositis requiring narcotic analgesia typically develops 5 to 7 days following transplantation using high-dose preparative regimens. Patient-controlled analgesia provides the greatest patient satisfaction and results in lower cumulative doses of narcotics. Keratinocyte growth factor (palifermin) significantly shortens the duration of severe mucositis following high-dose autologous transplant regimens.[69]

Sinusoidal obstruction syndrome (SOS; previously termed veno-occlusive hepatic disease) can develop within 1 to 4 weeks of treatment with many high-dose preparative regimens, and its symptoms include weight gain, ascites, tender hepatomegaly, and jaundice. The overall incidence of SOS is approximately 5%, but this rate varies according to the preparative regimen. In general, the incidence is higher for patients with abnormal results of liver function tests before transplant and for patients with an active infection at the time of transplant.[70] No therapy for SOS has proven effective, although the results of studies with defibrotide may hold promise.[71] Prophylaxis with ursodeoxycholic acid may decrease the incidence of SOS, and randomized studies have shown decreased rates of acute GVHD and better survival.

Idiopathic pneumonia syndrome (IPS), which is thought to be a toxicity directly related to chemoradiotherapy, occurs 30 to 90 days after transplant in up to 5% of patients. As with other toxicities, the incidence of IPS is dependent, in part, on the preparative regimen, occurring more frequently following administration of regimens that include high doses of total-body radiation therapy. Pre-existing lung disease, prior radiation therapy to the thorax, and increased age also seem to be associated with an increased risk of IPS, whereas fractionated radiation instead of single-dose radiation appears to decrease this risk. The mortality rate associated with IPS is approximately 50%, and no available treatments are clearly effective, although early results with tumor necrosis factor blockade may be favorable.[72]

Late complications attributable to the preparative regimen include decreased growth velocity in children and delayed development of secondary sexual characteristics. Most postpubescent women will experience ovarian failure, and few men regain spermatogenesis following HCT using high-dose preparative regimens. However, occasional patients will regain fertility following even myeloablative conditioning regimens, and patients should be counseled about this possibility.[73] Cataracts occur in as many as one-third of patients, with an increased risk in patients receiving high doses of total-body irradiation and patients requiring steroids for treatment of GVHD. Thyroid dysfunction, usually well-compensated, also may occur. Patients treated with high-dose chemoradiotherapy and HCT are at an increased risk for the development of second cancers and posttransplant lymphoproliferative disorders (PTLD). The risk for Epstein-Barr virus–associated PTLD is highest for patients receiving T-cell–depleted allogeneic transplants and for patients who receive multiple cycles of highly immunosuppressive drugs to treat GVHD.[74] An increase in solid tumors has been reported after transplantation, with a 3% 10-year cumulative rate which is 2 to 3 times the age-adjusted general population rate. A high incidence of MDS (nearly 10%) has been reported following autologous transplantation for lymphoma, but whether MDS is a complication of transplantation or is the long-term effect of chemotherapy used before transplantation is unknown.[75]

LONG-TERM SURVIVORSHIP

Case-control studies of patients who survive more than 5 years after undergoing transplant show that survivors are symptomatically similar to control patients, reporting approximately equal rates of osteoporosis, hypothyroidism, employment, marital satisfaction, divorce, and psychologic conditions. Transplant survivors do report an increased incidence of musculoskeletal problems and sexual dysfunction.[76] However, among those surviving more than 5 years after transplant, mortality rates remain higher than expected, yielding an estimated 30% lower life expectancy compared with that of the general population.[77] The leading causes of excess deaths in 5-year survivors are, in order, recurrent disease, second malignancy, chronic GVHD, respiratory ailments, and cardiovascular events.

RELAPSE AFTER TRANSPLANTATION

There is a substantial risk of recurrent malignant disease after transplantation, particularly when transplantation is performed after failure of conventional therapy rather than earlier in the course of the disease. The appropriate management of relapse after transplantation depends on the disease and type of transplant. Patients in whom disease recurs after autologous transplantation may have a response to subsequent chemotherapy, and occasionally such responses are surprisingly complete and prolonged, particularly if the duration of remission after transplantation was long. Reduced-intensity allogeneic HCT has been found to be tolerable (and sometimes effective) for patients whose disease relapsed following an autologous transplant.[78]

Patients taking immunosuppressive drugs who have recurrent disease after allogeneic transplantation will, on occasion, have a second complete remission after discontinuation of immunosuppressive therapy. Infusions of viable lymphocytes from the original stem cell donors can result in complete remission for many patients. In a European study involving 135 patients, the rate of complete response was 70% for patients with chronic-phase CML, 12% for patients with advanced-phase CML, 29% for patients with AML or MDS, and 0% for patients with ALL.[55] Occasionally, patients with myeloma and non-Hodgkin lymphoma also have a disease response. Most experts recommend that patients with recurrent acute leukemia undergo reinduction chemotherapy prior to donor lymphocyte infusions to decrease the leukemia cell burden and provide sufficient time for a graft-versus-tumor effect to develop. Some form of GVHD develops in approximately 60% of patients after infusion of donor lymphocytes; of those patients, 50% require therapy for GVHD, and 15% experience life-threatening GVHD. In addition, marrow aplasia occurs in 35% of patients, and the overall mortality associated with infusion of donor lymphocytes is 20%. Limiting the dose of CD3+ lymphocytes to less than 10×10^7 can decrease the risk of GVHD and life-threatening complications without impairing the graft-versus-leukemia effect.[79] For patients with CML who experience disease relapse after transplant, the disease appears to be sensitive to interferon therapy, with complete cytogenetic responses reported for 35% of patients treated for hematologic relapse and 70% for patients treated for cytogenetic relapse. Tyrosine kinase inhibitors are also highly effective for patients who have not previously had disease resistance to them before transplantation.[80]

A number of patients have had a second allogeneic transplant as treatment for relapse after the first transplant. Such transplants, if performed within 1 year of the original transplant, have been associated with a high risk of severe or fatal transplant-related toxicities, including SOS and idiopathic interstitial pneumonia. However, the results are better when the second transplant is performed more than 1 year after the original transplant, with prolonged subsequent remissions reported for as many as 25% of patients.[78]

References

1. Center for International Blood and Marrow Transplant Research. www.cibmtr.org. Accessed September 8, 2013.
2. Buckley RH, Schiff SE, Schiff RI, et al. Hematopoietic stem-cell transplantation for the treatment of severe combined immunodeficiency. N Engl J Med. 1999;340:508-516. PMID: 10021471.
3. Grunebaum E, Mazzolari E, Porta F, et al. Bone marrow transplantation for severe combined immune deficiency. JAMA. 2006;295:508-518. PMID: 16449616.
4. Storb R, Blume KG, O'Donnell MR, et al. Cyclophosphamide and antithymocyte globulin to condition patients with aplastic anemia for allogeneic marrow transplantations: the experience in four centers. Biol Blood Marrow Transplant. 2001;7:39-44. PMID: 11215697.
5. Deeg HJ, O'Donnell M, Tolar J, et al. Optimization of conditioning for marrow transplantation from unrelated donors for patients with aplastic anemia after failure of immunosuppressive therapy. Blood. 2006;108:1485-1491. PMID: 16684959.
6. Lucarelli G, Galimberti M, Polchi P, et al. Marrow transplantation in patients with thalassemia responsive to iron chelation therapy. N Engl J Med. 1993;329:840-844. PMID: 8355742.

7. Panepinto JA, Walters MC, Carreras J, et al. Matched-related donor transplantation for sickle cell disease: report from the Center for International Blood and Transplant Research. *Br J Haematol.* 2007;137:479-485. PMID: 17459050.

8. Hsieh MM, Kang EM, Fitzhugh CD, et al. Allogeneic hematopoietic stem-cell transplantation for sickle cell disease. *N Engl J Med.* 2009;361:2309-2317. PMID: 20007560.

9. Ayas M, Saber W, Davies SM, et al. Allogeneic hematopoietic cell transplantation for Fanconi anemia in patients with pretransplantation cytogenetic abnormalities, myelodysplastic syndrome, or acute leukemia. *J Clin Oncol.* 2013;31:1669-1676. PMID: 23547077.

10. MacMillan ML, Hughes MR, Agarwal S, et al. Cellular therapy for Fanconi anemia: the past, present, and future. *Biol Blood Marrow Transplant.* 2011;17:S109-S114. PMID: 21195298.

11. Segal BH, Veys P, Malech H, et al. Chronic granulomatous disease: lessons from a rare disorder. *Biol Blood Marrow Transplant.* 2011;17:S123-S131. PMID: 21195301.

12. Ozsahin H, Cavazzana-Calvo M, Notarangelo LD, et al. Long-term outcome following hematopoietic stem-cell transplantation in Wiskott-Aldrich syndrome: collaborative study of the European Society for Immunodeficiencies and European Group for Blood and Marrow Transplantation. *Blood.* 2008;111:439-445. PMID: 17901250.

13. Armand P, Gibson CJ, Cutler C, et al. A disease risk index for patients undergoing allogeneic stem cell transplantation. *Blood.* 2012;120:905-913. PMID: 22709687.

14. Yanada M, Matsuo K, Suzuki T, et al. Allogeneic hematopoietic stem cell transplantation as part of postremission therapy improves survival for adult patients with high-risk acute lymphoblastic leukemia: a metaanalysis. *Cancer.* 2006;106:2657-2663. PMID: 16703597.

15. Yanada M, Matsuo K, Emi N, et al. Efficacy of allogeneic hematopoietic stem cell transplantation depends on cytogenetic risk for acute myeloid leukemia in first disease remission: a metaanalysis. *Cancer.* 2005;103:1652-1658. PMID: 15742336.

16. Koreth J, Schlenk R, Kopecky KJ, et al. Allogeneic stem cell transplantation for acute myeloid leukemia in first complete remission: systematic review and meta-analysis of prospective clinical trials. *JAMA.* 2009;301:2349-2361. PMID: 19509382.

17. Deeg HJ, Storer B, Slattery JT, et al. Conditioning with targeted busulfan and cyclophosphamide for hemopoietic stem cell transplantation from related and unrelated donors in patients with myelodysplastic syndrome. *Blood.* 2002;100:1201-1207. PMID: 12149198.

18. Cutler CS, Lee SJ, Greenberg P, et al. A decision analysis of allogeneic bone marrow transplantation for the myelodysplastic syndromes: delayed transplantation for low-risk myelodysplasia is associated with improved outcome. *Blood.* 2004;104:579-585. PMID: 15039286.

19. Koreth J, Pidala J, Perez WS, et al. Role of reduced-intensity conditioning allogeneic hematopoietic stem-cell transplantation in older patients with de novo myelodysplastic syndromes: an international collaborative decision analysis. *J Clin Oncol.* 2013;31:2662-2670. PMID: 23797000.

20. Baccarani M, Deininger MW, Rosti G, et al. European LeukemiaNet recommendations for the management of chronic myeloid leukemia: 2013. *Blood.* 2013;122:872-884. PMID: 23803709.

21. Dreger P, Döhner H, Ritgen M, et al. Allogeneic stem cell transplantation provides durable disease control in poor-risk chronic lymphocytic leukemia: long-term clinical and MRD results of the German CLL Study Group CLL3X trial. *Blood.* 2010;116:2438-2447. PMID: 20595516.

22. Attal M, Harousseau JL, Stoppa AM, et al. A prospective, randomized trial of autologous bone marrow transplantation and chemotherapy in multiple myeloma. Intergroupe Français du Myélome. *N Engl J Med.* 1996;335:91-97. PMID: 8649495.

23. Child JA, Morgan GJ, Davies FE, et al. High-dose chemotherapy with hematopoietic stem-cell rescue for multiple myeloma. *N Engl J Med.* 2003;348:1875-1883. PMID: 12736280.

24. Philip T, Guglielmi C, Chauvin F, et al. Autologous bone marrow transplantation (ABMT) versus (vs) conventional chemotherapy (DHAP) in relapsed non-Hodgkin lymphoma (NHL): Final analysis of the PARMA randomized study (216 patients). *Proc Am Soc Clin Oncol.* 1995;14:390 (suppl; abstr 1220).

25. Einhorn LH, Williams SD, Chamness A, et al. High-dose chemotherapy and stem-cell rescue for metastatic germ-cell tumors. *N Engl J Med.* 2007;357:340-348. PMID: 17652649.

26. Anasetti C, Amos D, Beatty PG, et al. Effect of HLA compatibility on engraftment of bone marrow transplants in patients with leukemia or lymphoma. *N Engl J Med.* 1989;320:197-204. PMID: 2643045.

27. Kanda Y, Chiba S, Hirai H, et al. Allogeneic hematopoietic stem cell transplantation from family members other than HLA-identical siblings over the last decade (1991-2000). *Blood.* 2003;102:1541-1547. PMID: 12714500.

28. Szydlo R, Goldman JM, Klein JP, et al. Results of allogeneic bone marrow transplants for leukemia using donors other than HLA-identical siblings. *J Clin Oncol.* 1997;15:1767-1777. PMID: 9164184.

29. Reisner Y, Hagin D, Martelli MF. Haploidentical hematopoietic transplantation: current status and future perspectives. *Blood.* 2011;118:6006-6017. PMID: 21921045.

30. Brunstein CG, Fuchs EJ, Carter SL, et al. Alternative donor transplantation after reduced intensity conditioning: results of parallel phase 2 trials using partially HLA-mismatched related bone marrow or unrelated double umbilical cord blood grafts. *Blood.* 2011;118:282-288. PMID: 21527516.

31. Horowitz MM. Does matched unrelated donor transplantation have the same outcome as matched sibling transplantation in unselected patients? *Best Pract Res Clin Haematol.* 2012;25:483-486. PMID: 23200546.

32. Spellman SR, Eapen M, Logan BR, et al. A perspective on the selection of unrelated donors and cord blood units for transplantation. *Blood.* 2012;120:259-265. PMID: 22596257.

33. Lee SJ, Klein J, Haagenson M, et al. High-resolution donor-recipient HLA matching contributes to the success of unrelated donor marrow transplantation. *Blood.* 2007;110:4576-4583. PMID: 17785583.

34. Confer DL, Abress LK, Navarro W, et al. Selection of adult unrelated hematopoietic stem cell donors: beyond HLA. *Biol Blood Marrow Transplant.* 2010;16:S8-S11. PMID: 19892026.

35. Woolfrey A, Klein JP, Haagenson M, et al. HLA-C antigen mismatch is associated with worse outcome in unrelated donor peripheral blood stem cell transplantation. *Biol Blood Marrow Transplant.* 2011;17:885-892. PMID: 20870028.

36. Chell JW. Hematopoietic cell donor registries. In Blume KG, Forman SJ, Appelbaum FR (eds). *Thomas' Hematopoietic Cell Transplantation, 3rd ed.* Oxford, United Kingdom: Blackwell Publishing Ltd., 2004;624-631.

37. Brenner MK, Rill DR, Moen RC, et al. Gene-marking to trace origin of relapse after autologous bone-marrow transplantation. *Lancet.* 1993;341:85-86. PMID: 8093407.

38. Goldman JM. A special report: bone marrow transplants using volunteer donors–recommendations and requirements for a standardized practice throughout the world–1994 update. The WMDA Executive Committee. *Blood.* 1994;84:2833-2839. PMID: 7949160.

39. Gribben JG, Freedman AS, Neuberg D, et al. Immunologic purging of marrow assessed by PCR before autologous bone marrow transplantation for B-cell lymphoma. *N Engl J Med.* 1991;325:1525-1533. PMID: 1944436.

40. Martin PJ, Rowley SD, Anasetti C, et al. A phase I-II clinical trial to evaluate removal of CD4 cells and partial depletion of CD8 cells from donor marrow for HLA-mismatched unrelated recipients. *Blood.* 1999;94:2192-2199. PMID: 10498588.

41. Pulsipher MA, Chitphakdithai P, Logan BR, et al. Acute toxicities of unrelated bone marrow versus peripheral blood stem cell donation: results of a prospective trial from the National Marrow Donor Program. *Blood.* 2013;121:197-206. PMID: 23109243.

42. Bensinger WI, Longin K, Appelbaum F, et al. Peripheral blood stem cells (PBSCs) collected after recombinant granulocyte colony stimulating factor (rhG-CSF): an analysis of factors correlating with the tempo of engraftment after transplantation. *Br J Haematol.* 1994;87:825-831. PMID: 7527244.

43. Bensinger WI, Weaver CH, Appelbaum FR, et al. Transplantation of allogeneic peripheral blood stem cells mobilized by recombinant human granulocyte colony-stimulating factor. *Blood.* 1995;85:1655-1658. PMID: 7534140.

44. Bensinger WI, Martin PJ, Storer B, et al. Transplantation of bone marrow as compared with peripheral-blood cells from HLA-identical relatives in patients with hematologic cancers. *N Engl J Med.* 2001;344:175-181. PMID: 11172139.

45. Stem Cell Trialists' Collaborative Group. Allogeneic peripheral blood stem-cell compared with bone marrow transplantation in the management of hematologic malignancies: an individual patient data meta-analysis of nine randomized trials. *J Clin Oncol.* 2005;23:5074-5087. PMID: 16051954.

46. Anasetti C, Logan BR, Lee SJ, et al. Peripheral-blood stem cells versus bone marrow from unrelated donors. *N Engl J Med.* 2012;367:1487-1496. PMID: 23075175.

47. Calandra G, McCarty J, McGuirk J, et al. AMD3100 plus G-CSF can successfully mobilize CD34+ cells from non-Hodgkin's lymphoma, Hodgkin's disease and multiple myeloma patients previously failing mobilization with chemotherapy and/or cytokine treatment: compassionate use data. *Bone Marrow Transplant.* 2008;41:331-338. PMID: 17994119.

48. Locatelli F, Kabbara N, Ruggeri A, et al. Outcome of patients with hemoglobinopathies given either cord blood or bone marrow transplantation from an HLA-identical sibling. *Blood.* 2013;122:1072-1078. PMID: 23692854.

49. Barker JN, Scaradavou A, Stevens CE. Combined effect of total nucleated cell dose and HLA match on transplantation outcome in 1061 cord blood recipients with hematologic malignancies. *Blood.* 2010;115:1843-1849. PMID: 20029048.

50. Rocha V, Labopin M, Sanz G, et al. Transplants of umbilical-cord blood or bone marrow from unrelated donors in adults with acute leukemia. *N Engl J Med.* 2004;351:2276-2285. PMID: 15564544.

51. Scaradavou A, Brunstein CG, Eapen M, et al. Double unit grafts successfully extend the application of umbilical cord blood transplantation in adults with acute leukemia. *Blood.* 2013;121:752-758. PMID: 23223509.

52. Delaney C, Gutman JA, Appelbaum FR. Cord blood transplantation for haematological malignancies: conditioning regimens, double cord transplant and infectious complications. *Br J Haematol.* 2009;147:207-216. PMID: 19796270.

53. Appelbaum FR. Haematopoietic cell transplantation as immunotherapy. *Nature.* 2001;411:385-389. PMID: 11357147.

54. Horowitz MM, Gale RP, Sondel PM, et al. Graft-versus-leukemia reactions after bone marrow transplantation. *Blood.* 1990;75:555-562. PMID: 2297567.

55. Kolb HJ, Schattenberg A, Goldman JM, et al. Graft-versus-leukemia effect of donor lymphocyte transfusions in marrow grafted patients. *Blood.* 1995;86:2041-2050. PMID: 7655033.

56. Bacigalupo A, Ballen K, Rizzo D, et al. Defining the intensity of conditioning regimens: working definitions. *Biol Blood Marrow Transplant.* 2009;15:1628-1633. PMID: 19896087.

57. Storb R, Gyurkocza B, Storer BE, et al. Graft-versus-host disease and graft-versus-tumor effects after allogeneic hematopoietic cell transplantation. *J Clin Oncol.* 2013;31:1530-1538. PMID: 23478054.

58. Ringdén O, Labopin M, Ehninger G, et al. Reduced intensity conditioning compared with myeloablative conditioning using unrelated donor transplants in patients with acute myeloid leukemia. *J Clin Oncol.* 2009;27:4570-4577. PMID: 19652066.

59. Sorror ML, Sandmaier BM, Storer BE, et al. Comorbidity and disease status based risk stratification of outcomes among patients with acute myeloid leukemia or myelodysplasia receiving allogeneic hematopoietic cell transplantation. *J Clin Oncol.* 2007;25:4246-4254. PMID: 17724349.

60. Parimon T, Au DH, Martin PJ, et al. A risk score for mortality after allogeneic hematopoietic cell transplantation. *Ann Intern Med.* 2006;144:407-414. PMID: 16549853.

61. Gyurkocza B, Cao TM, Storb RF, et al. Salvage allogeneic hematopoietic cell transplantation with fludarabine and low-dose total body irradiation after rejection of first allografts. *Biol Blood Marrow Transplant.* 2009;15:1314-1322. PMID: 19747640.

62. Filipovich AH, Weisdorf D, Pavletic S, et al. National Institutes of Health consensus development project on criteria for clinical trials in chronic graft-versus-host disease: I. Diagnosis and staging working group report. *Biol Blood Marrow Transplant.* 2005;11:945-956. PMID: 16338616.

63. Socie G, Ritz J, Martin PJ. Current challenges in chronic graft-versus-host disease. *Biol Blood Marrow Transplant.* 2010;16:S146-S151. PMID: 19836455.

64. Daikeler T, Labopin M, Ruggeri A, et al. New autoimmune diseases after cord blood transplantation: a retrospective study of EUROCORD and the Autoimmune Disease Working Party of the European Group for Blood and Marrow Transplantation. *Blood.* 2013;121:1059-1064. PMID: 23247725.

65. Marr KA, Seidel K, Slavin MA, et al. Prolonged fluconazole prophylaxis is associated with persistent protection against candidiasis-related death in allogeneic marrow transplant recipients: long-term follow-up of a randomized, placebo-controlled trial. *Blood.* 2000;96:2055-2061. PMID: 10979947.

66. Wade JC, Newton B, Flournoy N, et al. Oral acyclovir for prevention of herpes simplex virus reactivation after marrow transplantation. *Ann Intern Med.* 1984;100:823-828. PMID: 6326632.

67. Zaia JA. Prevention and management of CMV-related problems after hematopoietic stem cell transplantation. *Bone Marrow Transplant.* 2002;29:633-638. PMID: 12180106.

68. Centers for Disease Control and Prevention, Infectious Disease Society of America, American Society of Blood and Marrow Transplantation. Guidelines for preventing opportunistic infections among hematopoietic stem cell transplant recipients. *MMWR Recomm Rep.* 2000;49:1-125. PMID: 11718124.

69. Spielberger R, Stiff P, Bensinger W, et al. Palifermin for oral mucositis after intensive therapy for hematologic cancers. *N Engl J Med.* 2004;351:2590-2598. PMID: 15602019.

70. DeLeve LD, Shulman HM, McDonald GB. Toxic injury to hepatic sinusoids: sinusoidal obstruction syndrome (veno-occlusive disease). *Semin Liver Dis.* 2002;22:27-42. PMID: 11928077.

71. Richardson PG, Murakami C, Jin Z, et al. Multi-institutional use of defibrotide in 88 patients after stem cell transplantation with severe veno-occlusive disease and multisystem organ failure: response without significant toxicity in a high-risk population and factors predictive of outcome. *Blood.* 2002;100:4337-4343. PMID: 12393437.

72. Crawford SW, Hackman RC. Clinical course of idiopathic pneumonia after bone marrow transplantation. *Am Rev Respir Dis.* 1993;147:1393-1400. PMID: 8503550.

73. Loren AW, Chow E, Jacobsohn DA, et al. Pregnancy after hematopoietic cell transplantation: a report from the late effects working committee of the Center for International Blood and Marrow Transplant Research (CIBMTR). *Biol Blood Marrow Transplant.* 2011;17:157-156. PMID: 20659574.

74. Witherspoon RP, Fisher LD, Schoch G, et al. Secondary cancers after bone marrow transplantation for leukemia or aplastic anemia. *N Engl J Med.* 1989;321:784-789. PMID: 2671734.

75. Metayer C, Curtis RE, Vose J, et al. Myelodysplastic syndrome and acute myeloid leukemia after autotransplantation for lymphoma: a multicenter case-control study. *Blood.* 2003;101:2015-2023. PMID: 12393427.

76. Syrjala KL, Langer SL, Abrams JR, et al. Late effects of hematopoietic cell transplantation among 10-year adult survivors compared with case-matched controls. *J Clin Oncol.* 2005;23:6596-6606. PMID: 16170167.

77. Martin PJ, Counts GW Jr, Appelbaum FR, et al. Life expectancy in patients surviving more than 5 years after hematopoietic cell transplantation. *J Clin Oncol.* 2010;28:1011-1016. PMID: 20065176.

78. Baron F, Storb R, Storer BE, et al. Factors associated with outcomes in allogeneic hematopoietic cell transplantation with nonmyeloablative conditioning after failed myeloablative hematopoietic cell transplantation. *J Clin Oncol.* 2006;24:4150-4157. PMID: 16896000.

79. Bar M, Sandmaier BM, Inamoto Y, et al. Donor lymphocyte infusion for relapsed hematological malignancies after allogeneic hematopoietic cell transplantation: prognostic relevance of the initial CD3+ T cell dose. *Biol Blood Marrow Transplant.* 2013;19:949-957. PMID: 23523892.

80. Carpenter PA, Snyder DS, Flowers ME, et al. Prophylactic administration of imatinib after hematopoietic cell transplantation for high-risk Philadelphia chromosome-positive leukemia. *Blood.* 2007;109:2791-2793. PMID: 17119111.

19

CANCER IN ELDERLY PATIENTS

Arati V. Rao, MD, and Harvey Jay Cohen, MD

Updates from 2012

▶ Comprehensive geriatric assessment (CGA) provides valuable information essential to the care of elderly patients with cancer (Hurria A, *J Clin Oncol* 2011).

▶ Chemotherapy toxicity risk can be predicted by parameters that are typically included in a CGA (Hurria A, *J Clin Oncol* 2012).

▶ Geriatric assessment predicts survival in older adults with acute myeloid leukemia receiving induction chemotherapy (Klepin HD, *Blood* 2013).

▶ Multiple oral and targeted agents, including ibrutinib, ofatumumab, and obinutuzumab, have recently been approved for use in chronic lymphocytic leukemia and are attractive options as an alternative to chemotherapy in elderly patients (Byrd JC, *N Engl J Med* 2013; Shanafelt T, *Cancer* 2013; Goede V, *N Engl J Med* 2014).

▶ Elderly patients with multiple myeloma have more therapeutic options with newer agents such as pomalidomide and carfilzomib (Dimopoulous MA, *Leukemia* 2014; Jakubowiak AJ, *Leukemia* 2013).

▶ Personalized cancer therapy using afatinib and crizotinib in elderly patients with non-small cell lung cancer may improve efficacy and decrease toxicity (Katakami M, *J Clin Oncol* 2013; Shaw AT, *N Engl J Med* 2013).

Geriatric medicine is a subspecialty that deals with care of elderly individuals. Although there is no consensus on the chronologic age that defines the geriatric patient population, age 65 and older is generally accepted. Cancer, a major problem for elderly individuals, is the second leading cause of death after heart disease in the United States. Age is the single most important risk factor for developing cancer, with approximately 60% of all newly diagnosed malignant tumors and 70% of all cancer deaths occurring in persons age 65 or older.[1] It has been estimated that by the year 2030, 20% of the U.S. population (70 million people) will be older than age 65. The median age range for diagnosis for most major tumors, common to both men and women, is 68 to 74, and the median age range at death is 70 to 79.[2,3] For most malignancies, the death rate is disproportionately higher for the elderly population. Possible explanations include an altered natural history of some cancers, competing comorbid medical conditions, decreased physiologic reserve compromising the ability to tolerate therapy, physicians' reluctance to provide aggressive therapy, and barriers in the elderly person's access to care. Communication between health care providers and elderly patients may be hampered by deficits in hearing, vision, and cognition. The elderly patient with cancer often has an elderly caregiver, and the diagnosis of cancer often affects the health-related quality of life of both individuals. All of these challenges contribute to defining geriatric oncology as a true subspecialty and has led to the development of guidelines by the National Comprehensive Cancer Network (NCCN) that address special considerations in older patients with cancer.[4]

The costs of cancer care to Medicare are substantial and vary by tumor site, phase of care, stage at diagnosis, and survival. In a 2008 Surveillance, Epidemiology, and End Results (SEER) database review, the mean net costs of care were highest in the initial and last-year-of-life phases of care and lowest in the continuing phase. Mean 5-year net costs varied widely, from less than $20,000 for patients with breast cancer or melanoma of the skin to more than $40,000 for patients with brain or other nervous system, esophageal, gastric, or ovarian cancers or lymphoma. In patients with acute myeloid leukemia (AML), 80% of the costs are related to inpatient hospitalization. In 2004, the 5-year net costs of elderly cancer care to Medicare were approximately $21.1 billion.[5] However, with the advent of several new targeted agents, the cost of anticancer agents has more than doubled compared with a decade ago, from $4,500 to more than $10,000 per month.[6] Of the 12 anticancer drugs approved by the U.S. Food and Drug Administration (FDA) in 2012, only three prolonged survival (two of them by less than 2 months), and nine of were priced at more than $10,000 per month. Many targeted agents have been priced between $6,000 and $12,000 per month, or approximately $70,000 to $115,000 per patient annually. The high cost may prevent all elderly patients from being able to procure the medication and can lead to noncompliance.[7] This is turn results in costs in excess of $100 billion annually, due to increased health services utilization, hospital admission, and adverse drug events associated with nonadherence.[8] The economic impact of cancer survivorship is considerable; the cost can remain high years after a cancer diagnosis, and affects both young and elderly cancer survivors similarly.[9]

An understanding of the biology of aging, an appreciation of the effect of comorbidities, use of comprehensive geriatric assessment (CGA), and a willingness to spend time with the patient and his or her family are essential to providing care for older patients. This chapter discusses many of the general relationships of oncology and aging. It focuses on the epidemiologic, basic etiologic, and biologic relationships between the processes of aging and neoplasia. It also establishes the importance of CGA in treatment decision-making and prediction of chemotherapy toxicity in the elderly patient with cancer. The clinical management of individual malignancies is discussed only as an example of general principles and the approach to specific malignancies is covered in chapters related to the appropriate organ system.

Ultimately, the goal of intervention is to add "life to years," rather than just "years to life."

RELATIONSHIP OF AGING AND NEOPLASIA

The molecular, cellular, and physiologic changes that contribute to the aging process also predispose patients to the development of cancer. Carcinogenesis is a multistep process that includes initiation, followed by promotion and progression to disease. Various theories link aging and cancer[10-14]:

1. Longer duration of carcinogenic exposure: It is possible that aging simply allows the time necessary for the accumulation of cellular events to develop into a clinical neoplasm. Somatic mutations are believed to occur at the rate of approximately one in 10 cell divisions, with approximately 10 cell divisions occurring in a lifetime of a human being.
2. Altered susceptibility of aging cells to carcinogens.
3. Decreased ability to repair DNA: It is possible that damage, once initiated, is more difficult to repair in older cells.
4. Oncogene activation or amplification or decrease in tumor suppressor gene activity: These processes might be increased in the older host, resulting either in increased action or promotion or in differential clonal evolution.
5. Telomere shortening and genetic instability: The function of telomeres and the enzyme telomerase appears to be intimately involved in both the senescence and neoplasia processes. Telomeres, the terminal end of all chromosomes, shorten progressively as cells age. This functional decline begins at age 30 and continues at a loss of approximately 1% per year. This shortening appears to be causally related to controlled cell proliferation and limitation of population doubling. It is thought that each time a cell divides, 30 to 200 base pairs are lost from the end of that cell's telomeres. Because the major function of telomeres is to protect the stability of the more internal coding sequences (i.e., allow cells to divide without losing genes), the loss of this function may lead to genetic instability, which may promote mutations in oncogenic or tumor-suppressor gene sequences. Without telomeres, chromosome ends could fuse together and degrade the cell's genetic blueprint, making the cell malfunction, become cancerous, or even die. Telomere length is a predictor of mortality in people age 60 or older. The enzyme telomerase is responsible for adding back telomeric repeats to the ends of chromosomes (i.e., regenerate the telomeres). This enzyme is generally not expressed in normal cells, but it is activated in malignant cells. While telomerase can reverse replicative cell senescence, the indiscriminate expression of this enzyme might increase the likelihood of tumor formation.
6. Microenvironment alterations: Older people accumulate senescent cells and have higher levels of interleukin (IL)-6, the "geriatric cytokine" which is one of the causes of frailty.

Senescent cells can compromise tissue renewal capacity, and secrete multiple factors (e.g., IL-1, matrix metalloproteinase [MMP]-3) that alter tissue homeostasis and create a tissue environment that synergizes with mutation accumulation to facilitate the progression of malignancies.

7. Decreased immune surveillance: There is a considerable amount of evidence in animal models for a loss of tumor-specific immunity with progressive age.

Overall, there are several interactions of these factors, resulting in initiation, then cumulative promoting events, including mutations and other alterations in critical genes, which alternately exceed a threshold of host resistance factors, which have been progressively reduced during the aging process. Cellular senescence suppresses cancer by arresting cells at risk of malignant transformation.[15] However, senescence is a double-edged sword, since these senescent cells also secrete molecules that can stimulate premalignant cells to proliferate and form tumors, suggesting that the senescence response is antagonistically pleiotropic. Thus, cellular senescence-induced suppression of malignant transformation, a function important for the organism in early life (through the reproductive period), may be selected for, despite the fact that cellular senescence may be quite injurious in later life. In this case, senescence could be viewed as the price we pay in later life for the rigorous attempt to control proliferation to avoid neoplasia early on.

AGE-RELATED PHYSIOLOGIC CHANGES

A decline in physiologic functioning begins at age 30 and continues at a rate of approximately 1% per year. The aging process occurs at a different rate in each person, and the loss of individual organ reserve occurs at different rates within the same person.[16,17] In most cases, these physiologic changes are clinically imperceptible. However, the delicate balance of functioning can be disrupted by an illness and the consequent medical intervention. Once this balance is upset, the patient's physiology may not return to its baseline.

The physiologic changes of aging that lead to decreased functional reserve affect every organ system. The percentage of body fat increases and the total body water and muscle mass decrease. Hormone dysfunction can be measured as decreases in renin, aldosterone, dehydroepiandrosterone (DHEA), sex hormones, and triiodothyronine; however, insulin, norepinephrine, parathyroid hormone (PTH), vasopressin, and atrial natriuretic peptide levels increase. Senescence of hormone production results in a decrease in protein synthesis and contributes to age-related loss of strength and muscle mass, known as sarcopenia.[18] The integument of the skin changes, becoming increasingly dry as sweat glands are lost. The thinning of skin and loss of subcutaneous connective tissue and fat expose blood vessels and contribute to tears and bruising.

Functional decline in the gastrointestinal tract manifests as a decrease in motility and absorption. As blood flow and liver mass decrease, hepatic function declines. Metabolism through the cytochrome P450 microsomal enzyme system also decreases, impairing the body's ability to convert some drugs to their active metabolite and compromising the elimination of other drugs.[19] In the kidney, renal blood flow decreases, and both kidney mass and glomeruli are lost and replaced by fat and fibrotic tissue. These changes cause a decrease in the kidney's ability to concentrate urine, excrete water, and eliminate toxins.

The senescent brain undergoes a number of changes. The weight of the brain, blood flow, and the amount of produced neurotransmitters all decline with age. This decrease in neurotransmitters may explain the high incidence of Parkinson disease in the older population; it has been estimated that clinical evidence of this disease is present in 30% of individuals older than age 70. Both speed of walking and truncal stability correlate with longevity and the development of geriatric problems, including depression and dementia.[20,21] With increasing age, gait speed slows as the stride length shortens and individuals increasingly lean forward. It is speculated that these changes reflect a decline in the number of Purkinje cells within the cerebellum. Gait is a complex motor process that is an indicator of the integrity of other physiologic processes.

Neuronal loss may also lead to decreased levels of neuroreceptors, such as mu and delta. The loss of these receptors provides one potential mechanism for enhanced sensitivity to opioid analgesics in older individuals. The loss of sensory neurons contributes to a decreased ability to perceive pain and also may contribute to compromised wound healing.

The changes in the immune system are more complicated than a mere decline in lymphocyte functioning and are most consistent with an immunologic dysregulation. Declines in both thymic mass and thymic hormones lead to a decrease in the number of naive lymphocytes and an increase in memory cells. The total lymphocyte count remains normal, but the response to mitogens decreases.[12] The levels of inflammatory cytokines IL-6 and IL-1-beta, C-reactive protein (CRP), and transforming growth factor (TGF)-beta all increase with age. Elevations of IL-6 and D-dimer have been associated with both shorter survival and increased functional dependency.[22] The level of IL-2 decreases with age, contributing to a loss of lymphocyte proliferation. Although the etiology for the increased levels of cytokines is uncertain, it has been proposed that incompletely healed inflammatory reactions throughout a lifetime result in an accumulation of certain cytokines. These cytokines contribute to an overall catabolic state and to sarcopenia. The levels of immunoglobulins increase, but antibody response decreases. This immunologic dysregulation leads to increasing susceptibility to infection and may be responsible for the altered natural history of certain malignant diseases in the older population.

In general, breast and prostate cancers have a more indolent course for older patients. However, hematologic malignancies tend to be more aggressive and less responsive to therapy, possibly because of the increases in the level of IL-6. In the older population, the levels of hemoglobin, the number of white blood cells, and platelet counts are usually within the normal range, despite the fact that marrow mass is lost over time and is then replaced by fat. The marrow reserve is compromised, and with the stress of illness or treatment, blood counts can decline disproportionately compared with counts in younger patients.

Anemia is more common with age; it occurs in 10% of patients over age 65 and 20% of patients over age 85, according to the National Health and Nutrition Examination Survey (NHANES).[23]

COMPREHENSIVE GERIATRIC ASSESSMENT

Aging is a heterogeneous process that is not captured by chronologic age. Thus, a CGA has been demonstrated to be very useful, since it is designed to capture the functional age of an older adult. This identifies those older adults who have a diminished life expectancy and/or are at risk for hospitalization and functional decline. Traditionally in oncology, performance status (PS) is used as an attempt to quantify a patient's general well-being and is also used to determine whether a patient can receive chemotherapy. The most commonly used measure, the Eastern Cooperative Oncology Group (ECOG) PS, runs from 0 to 5, with 0 denoting perfect health and 5, death. However, in the geriatric oncology population, it has been demonstrated that ECOG PS alone is not sufficient, and CGA adds substantial information to the functional assessment of elderly patients with cancer, including patients with a good ECOG PS. CGA includes assessment tools to predict the functional age of patients with cancer based on functional status, comorbidities that may interfere with cancer therapy, nutritional status, polypharmacy, psychological and cognitive status, socioeconomic issues, and geriatric syndromes. There are a series of abbreviated screening instruments available as described in Table 19-1.[24] The assessment that is increasingly being used in North America was designed by Hurria et al as described in Table 19-2.[25] The measures included in this brief geriatric assessment were chosen for their reliability, validity, brevity, and prognostic ability to determine risk for morbidity or mortality in an older patient. The geriatric assessment tool primarily consists of self-reported measures, which are completed by the patient; three items are completed by the health care professional. The median time to complete the CGA tool is 22 minutes, and 87% of patients complete their portion without assistance.

CGA has proved useful in studies in elderly patients with cancer to predict for chemotherapy toxicity. In one study conducted by by the Cancer and Aging Research Group (CARG), geriatric assessment variables along with sociodemographic information, tumor/treatment variables, and laboratory test results were incorporated into a model that would predict for chemotherapy toxicity in older adults.[26] Five hundred older patients with cancer were followed through their chemotherapy course to capture grade 3 (severe), grade 4 (life-threatening or disabling), and grade 5 (death) toxicity. A scoring system in which the median risk score was 7 (range, 0 to 19) was utilized to risk-stratify patients (risk score: percent incidence of grade 3 to 5 toxicity). This identified older adults at low (0 to 5 points; 30%), intermediate (6 to 9 points; 52%), or high risk (10 to 19 points; 83%) of chemotherapy toxicity (p < 0 .001).

Table 19-1 Comparisons of Comprehensive Geriatric Assessment (CGA) Methodologies[24]

Instrument	Method	Scoring	Interpretation	Remarks
G8	Interview	Total score: 17	■ Score 0 to 14: Presence of geriatric risk profile ■ Score > 14: Absence of geriatric risk profile	Takes 2 to 3 minutes to complete screening
Groningen Frailty Indicator (GFI)	Conducting screening tests on patient	Total score: 15	■ Score 0 to 3: Absence of geriatric risk profile ■ Score 4 to 15: Presence of geriatric risk profile	Circle answers and use specific scoring rules set by the test
Vulnerable Elders Survey-13 (VES-13)	Self-report and interview	Total score: 10	■ Score 0 to 2: Absence of vulnerability ■ Score 3 to 10: Presence of vulnerability	Takes less than 5 minutes to complete
Senior Adult Oncology Program 2 (SAOP2)	Self-report and interview	N/A	■ If one item is positive: Respective specialist consulted ■ If several items impaired: Geriatric referral for MDT	Clinic staff administers last page of interview
Abbreviated CGA (aCGA)	Interview: ■ Four questions from the GDS ■ Three questions about ADL ■ Four questions about IADL ■ Four questions from the MMSE		■ GDS score ≥ 2: Complete full 15-item GDS ■ Any impairment of ADL: Complete full ADL ■ Any impairment of IADL: Complete full IADL ■ Cognitive screening score ≤ 6: Complete full MMSE	

Abbreviations: ADL, Activities of Daily Living; GDS, Geriatric Depression Scale; IADL, Instrumental Activities of Daily Living; MDT, multidisciplinary team; MMSE, Mini Mental State Examination.

Table 19-2 Domains for Cancer-Specific Comprehensive Geriatric Assessment (CGA)[25]

Domain with Measure	Number of Items	Description
Functional Status		
MOS physical health	10	Measures limitations in a wide range of physical functions (from bathing/dressing to vigorous activities such as running)
Instrumental Activities of Daily Living (IADL, subscale of the OARS)	7	Measures ability to complete activities required to maintain independence in the community (i.e., meal preparation, shopping, making telephone calls, money management)
Karnofsky performance status*	1	Global indicator of patient function determined by the health care professional on a scale of 0 to 100
Numbers of falls in past 6 months	1	Number of times patient has fallen in the past 6 months
Timed Up and Go*	1	Performance-based measure of functional status: Amount of time it takes for seated patient to rise from a chair, walk 10 feet, walk back, and sit down
MOS social activities	4	Measures ability to participate in social activities and degree to which health status limits normal social activities
Comorbid Medical Conditions		
Physical health section (subscale of the OARS)	15	List of comorbid illnesses and the degree to which they impair daily activities; patient can add additional comorbid illnesses not listed; rating of eyesight and hearing
Psychological State		
Hospital Anxiety and Depression Scale	14	Measures of anxiety and depression
Social Support		
MOS social support survey: Emotional/informational and tangible subscales	12	Perceived availability of social support
Nutritional Status		
Body mass index	1	Weight/height
Percent unintentional weight loss in past 6 months	1	Unintentional weight loss in the past 6 months/baseline body weight x 100
Cognition		
Blessed Orientation-Memory-Concentration Test*	6	Gross measure of cognitive function
Medications		
Comprehensive list of medications	1	List of medications including prescribed, herbal, and over-the-counter medications

*Items completed by the health care professional.
Abbreviations: MOS, Medical Outcomes Study; OARS, Older American Resources and Services.

In another study of 518 elderly patients with cancer, 24 parameters including geriatric assessment were incorporated to create the CRASH (Chemotherapy Risk Assessment Scale for High-Age Patients) score to predict grade 4 hematologic or grade 3/4 nonhematologic toxicity.[27] Based on the scores, risk categories were created and those patients with low-risk scores had only a 7% chance of hematologic and 33% chance of nonhematologic toxicity compared to high-risk patients, who had a 100% risk of hematologic and 93% risk of nonhematologic toxicity from chemotherapy. One limitation of these two studies was the small numbers of patients with hematologic malignancies (these patients tend to have lower bone marrow reserve, making them especially vulnerable to hematologic toxicities) and the inability to predict for grade 2 toxicities, which can also affect an elderly patient's quality of life significantly.

CGA has also been used to aid the treating oncologist in the decision-making process. In the ELCAPA01 study, 375 elderly patients with cancer were assessed by geriatricians using the CGA to identify factors associated with changes in the cancer treatment: intensification, decrease, or delay of more than 2 weeks.[28] Multivariate assessment revealed that functional status assessed by the ADL (activity of daily living) score, and the presence of malnutrition, were independently associated with changes in cancer treatment. CGA has also been utilized in the Pre-Operative Assessment of Cancer in the Elderly (PACE) trial to determine suitability of older patients for surgery.[29] PACE incorporated a battery of validated instruments including the CGA, Brief Fatigue Inventory, ECOG PS, and American Society of Anesthesiologists (ASA) grade in a large study of 460 elderly patients with cancer prior to receiving elective surgery. Of these, 83% were observed to have at least one comorbidity, the most common being hypertension (53.5%). In a multivariate analysis, moderate to severe fatigue, a dependent instrumental activities of daily living (IADL) score, and poor PS were identified as independent predictors of postoperative complications. Finally, one recent study has demonstrated that CGA predicts survival for older adults receiving induction chemotherapy for AML.[30] In this study of 74 patients with AML (median age, 70), overall survival was significantly shorter in patients who screened positive for impairment in cognition and objectively measured physical function.

CONCEPT OF FRAILTY

A position statement from the American Medical Association defined the term frailty as characterizing "the group of patients that presents the most complex and challenging problems to the physician and all health care professionals," because these are the individuals who have a higher susceptibility to adverse outcomes, such as mortality and institutionalization. Currently, two main models of frailty exist: the phenotype model and the cumulative deficit model.[31]

PHENOTYPE MODEL

The phenotype model of frailty was based on a landmark study wherein secondary analysis by Fried et al evaluated 5,210 men and women age 65 and older within the large prospective Cardiovascular Health Study.[32] A frailty phenotype was established with five variables:

1. Unintentional weight loss
2. Self-reported exhaustion
3. Low energy expenditure
4. Slow gait speed
5. Weak grip strength

Individuals with three or more of the five factors were judged to be frail, those with one or two factors as pre-frail, and those with no factors as not frail or robust elderly people. At a 3-and 5-year follow-up, people categorized as frail were reported to have more adverse outcomes in terms of disability and mortality than the other two groups. Mortality at 7 years was 12%, 23%, and 43% for the not frail, pre-frail, and frail groups, respectively.

CUMULATIVE DEFICIT MODEL

The cumulative deficit frailty index was developed as part of the CSHA study, which was a large 5-year prospective cohort study (10,263 patients) designed to investigate the epidemiology and burdens of dementia in elderly people in Canada (mean age, 82).[33] Ninety-two baseline variables of symptoms, signs, and abnormal laboratory values, disease states, and disabilities (collectively referred to as deficits) were used to define frailty. The frailty index was a simple calculation of the presence or absence of each variable as a proportion of the total (e.g., 20 deficits present of a possible 92 gives a frailty index of $20 \div 92 = 0.22$). Frailty was defined as the cumulative effect of individual deficits or simply, "the more individuals have wrong with them, the more likely they are to be frail."

FRAILTY IN CANCER

Although frailty models provide important prognostic information for the geriatric population at large, to the best of current knowledge, data applicable to patients with cancer are lacking. Mohile et al analyzed a national sample of 12,480 community-based elderly individuals using the 2003 Medicare Current Beneficiary Survey.[34] Eighteen percent reported a history of cancer. Among those with cancer, 60.3% reported one or more geriatric syndromes compared with 53.2% of those without cancer (p < 0.001). Overall, those with cancer had a statistically significantly higher prevalence of hearing trouble, urinary incontinence, falls, depression, and osteoporosis than those without cancer. Analysis of specific cancer subtypes showed that lung cancer was associated with vision, hearing, and eating trouble; prostate cancer was associated with incontinence and falls; cervix/uterine cancer was associated with falls and osteoporosis; and colon cancer was associated with depression and osteoporosis.

BIOLOGIC MARKERS OF FRAILTY

Aging is associated with increased levels of circulating cytokines and proinflammatory markers. Aged-related changes in the immune system (i.e., immunosenescence) and increased secretion of cytokines by adipose tissue can lead to a state of

---

KEY POINTS

- The comprehensive geriatric assessment (CGA) assists in defining physiologic reserve.
- Comorbid medical conditions increase the physiologic age.
- Aging is associated with an increase in proinflammatory cytokines such as tumor necrosis factor-α and interleukin-6, which contribute to frailty.
- Frailty defines a severe loss of functional reserve and lack of tolerance to intervention.
- Eastern Cooperative Oncology Group or Karnofsky performance status alone may not provide an accurate measure of an older patient's functional status.
- CGA has been utilized in the CARG and CRASH scores to predict for chemotherapy toxicity in the older patient with cancer.

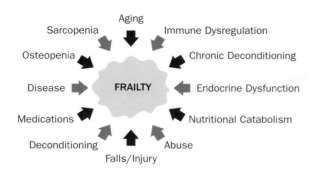

Fig. 19-1 Factors contributing to the development of frailty. Many factors contribute to the development of frailty, which is determined by clinical assessment of the elderly patient.

chronic inflammation, or "inflamm-aging." High levels of IL-6, IL-1, tumor necrosis factor (TNF)-α, and CRP in elderly people are associated with increased risk of morbidity and mortality. In particular, cohort studies in elderly participants have indicated that increased TNF-α and IL-6 levels are associated with frailty.[22] These biomarkers of frailty have now been evaluated in elderly and nonelderly patients with cancer in several studies of many tumor types (e.g., colon cancer, AML, multiple myeloma) and have all demonstrated increased levels of pro-inflammatory cytokines in these patients. These frailty cytokines have not only been thought to play a role in carcinogenesis (e.g., AML and multiple myeloma) but in fact are also responsible for several cancer-related symptom complexes including cancer cachexia, fatigue, poor performance status, and cognitive issues. Figure 19-1 describes the many factors which contribute to the development of frailty, which is determined by clinical assessment of the elderly patient.

TREATMENT APPROACHES
SURGERY
Surgery and other invasive procedures are frequently involved in initial diagnostic as well as in therapeutic approaches to the elderly patient with cancer. An increased number of comorbid medical conditions, decreased wound healing, and lack of physiologic reserve contribute to both prolonged hospital stay and rehabilitation following operative treatment. All phases of healing are compromised by the aging process. Both the inflammatory and proliferative responses are decreased, remodeling occurs to a lesser degree, and the collagen formed is qualitatively different from that in younger individuals. Normally, the repair process initiated by inflammation requires intact sensory nerves that stimulate increased blood flow and growth factor production. The loss of sensory neurons and the coexistence of other medical conditions, such as diabetes and vascular disease, contribute to delayed wound healing. Additionally, complications are more common when surgical intervention is performed on an emergency basis. Often, it is more appropriate to perform an operation as a preventive measure when dealing with older populations; for example, a hemicolectomy may

be performed—even for patients with advanced colorectal cancer—to prevent the need for an emergency operation to treat bowel perforation or obstruction. The American Geriatrics Society Task Force and the American College of Surgeons provide general guidelines for older adults undergoing surgery and these may be applied to older patients with cancer undergoing surgery.[35]

RADIATION THERAPY
Radiation therapy (RT) can be used in the older patient with cancer with both curative and palliative intent. RT is also used as an effective adjunct to surgery, chemotherapy, or both. The International Society of Geriatric Oncology (SIOG) Task Force has put forth guidelines for best practices in radiation oncology in elderly patients with cancer.[36] Per these guidelines, patient selection should include comorbidity and geriatric evaluation. In elderly patients with breast cancer, shorter courses of hypofractionated whole-breast RT are safe and effective. In patients with non-small cell lung cancer (NSCLC), conformal radiotherapy and involved field radiotherapy (IFRT) techniques without elective nodal irradiation have improved outcomes without increasing toxicity. If comorbidities preclude surgery, stereotactic body radiotherapy (SBRT) is an option for early-stage NSCLC and pancreas cancer. In patients with lymphoma, IFRT may be based on pretreatment positron emission tomography (PET) data to reduce toxicity. In patients with intermediate-risk prostate cancer, 4 to 6 months of hormone therapy combined with external beam radiotherapy (EBRT) may be an option. Short-course EBRT is an alternative to combined-modality therapy in older patients with rectal cancer without significant comorbidities. Endorectal RT may be an option for early disease. For primary brain tumors, shorter courses of postoperative RT following maximal debulking provides equivalent survival to longer schedules. Stereotactic RT provides an alternative to whole-brain RT in patients with limited brain metastases. Intensity-modulated RT provides an excellent technique to reduce doses to the carotids in head and neck cancer and improves locoregional control in esophageal cancer. It is crucial to monitor older patients receiving radiation since the effects of radiation on normal tissue may be enhanced by 10% to 15% in the elderly patient. Radiation to the oral pharynx and oral cavity can produce a loss of taste, dryness of mucous membranes, and involution of salivary glands; when combined with a precarious nutritional intake in a frail and elderly individual these toxicities might be lethal, or certainly may contribute a considerable amount of morbidity, if not recognized. Moreover, if daily treatment is tolerated poorly owing to nausea or weakness, treatment may be compromised because of the decreased daily doses, the patient's unscheduled absences, or decrease in the total planned dose. Pulmonary complications such as severe radiation pneumonitis have been noted in one study to occur more frequently in elderly patients with lung cancer than in younger patients, regardless of radiation field size and concurrent therapies. Depression and cognitive decline are side effects of whole-brain RT.

SYSTEMIC THERAPY: CHEMOTHERAPY AND TARGETED AGENTS

There continues to be a lack of data to make evidence-based decisions with regard to chemotherapy for elderly patients, due to the minimal participation of older patients in clinical trials. Prospective data for elderly patients, particularly for those patients older than 80, is almost entirely lacking. The SIOG Task Force has published guidelines for dose modification of chemotherapy in elderly patients with renal insufficiency and has reviewed the use of certain classes of drugs (alkylators, antimetabolites, anthracyclines, taxanes, camptothecins, and epipodophyllotoxins) in elderly patients with cancer.[37,38] When oral agents are used, despite delayed gastric emptying, absorption is adequate, but the physician must pay attention to concomitant medications such as H2 blockers, antacids, and proton pump inhibitors. Caution must be exercised when administering cytotoxic drugs such as methotrexate, bleomycin, cisplatin, and ifosfamide. Both a decrease in the number of nephrons and a decline in the glomerular filtration rate may contribute to excess toxicity. Also, there is a decrease in lean body mass in elderly people, thus, adjusting the dose based on a creatinine clearance and not merely the creatinine is very important. In addition, concomitant administration of drugs such as nonsteroidal anti-inflammatory drugs may compromise renal function. Although the reasons are unclear, acute toxicities such as nausea and vomiting occur less frequently in older patients; however, the lack of functional reserve can lead to catastrophic outcomes quickly (i.e., dehydration, renal insufficiency). Neurotoxicity secondary to taxanes, platinum agents, vincristine, high-dose cytarabine, and bortezomib, cardiotoxicity from doxorubicin, and mucositis from 5-fluorouracil are all more common and severe in elderly patients. Whether the risk of myelotoxicity increases with age remains a controversial issue, but studies do indicate longer duration of neutropenia in elderly patients. As described previously, CGA is helpful when incorporated with other parameters to predict for the risk of toxicity in elderly patients.

There has been an increased use of targeted therapeutic agents in the past decade, including antiangiogenic agents, tyrosine kinase inhibitors (TKIs), and monoclonal antibodies.[39,40] Bevacizumab, an antiangiogenic agent, is now routinely used. Pooled data from five randomized trials in three different tumor types found that arterial thromboembolic complications are significantly higher for patients age 65 and older.[41] Many of the TKIs are oral agents and thus an attractive option for elderly patients. However, these drugs are metabolized by the cytochrome P450 liver enzymes and thus have significant drug interactions when taken concomitantly with P450 inhibitors or inducers. One study demonstrated that comorbidities and polypharmacy impacted cytogenetic response rates in elderly patients with chronic myeloid leukemia.[42] In addition, while these drugs have a favorable safety profile compared to chemotherapy, there is still a higher risk of toxicity, leading to a higher rate of dose reduction and discontinuation when compared to younger patients.

HEMATOPOIETIC STEM CELL TRANSPLANTATION

Hematopoietic stem cell transplantation (HSCT) is applied to high-risk hematologic diseases to overcome poor outcomes from non-HSCT approaches. Historically, the associated morbidity and mortality limited the use of allogeneic SCT to individuals younger than age 50. However, autologous SCT for lymphoma and myeloma has been performed in patients age 65 to 70. There are no guidelines for HSCT in the elderly population, so patient selection, choice of conditioning regimen, immunosuppression, and stem cell source are arbitrary and may be based on cardiopulmonary and hepatorenal function. Risk-assessment tools such as CGA and comorbidity measures have recently been applied to facilitate decisions regarding HSCT eligibility and tolerance. Reduced-intensity conditioning (RIC) for allogeneic HCT has improved tolerance, decreased mortality, and removed traditional age barriers.[43] RIC regimens may vary in the degree of immunosuppression and myeloablation and transplant-related mortality is typically lower than with myeloablative approaches. Another important issue is donor selection for older recipients. Older patients tend to have older human leukocyte antigen (HLA)-matched siblings, raising issues about the upper age or health limitations for donor collection, as older donor age slightly diminishes hematopoietic stem cell yields. Numerous other geriatric domains such as nutrition, caregiver support, and cognitive assessment have not been evaluated in the setting of HSCT. For example, delirium occurs in up to 50% of allogeneic HSCT recipients and likely more often among older adults, and needs further study.[44] More specific details are covered in Chapter 18: Hematopoietic Cell Transplantation.

SUPPORTIVE CARE MEASURES

Elderly patients may require substantial supportive care since the effects of cancer and its treatment may be devastating. The goal of such therapy is to maximize the ability of patients to tolerate the treatment in order to prevent dose reductions and delays in therapy. Many of the specific aspects of supportive care are covered in Chapter 20: Symptom Management and are only mentioned here to stress their importance for the management of the elderly patient with cancer. These include the effective management of pain, anxiety, and depression, maintenance of nutritional support, and the importance of patient, physician, and family discussions concerning decisions regarding terminal care and other issues and the utility of hospice care. There are several established guidelines on the prevention and treatment of mucositis, use of antiemetics, and growth factors.

The risk of chemotherapy-induced neutropenia is reduced by 60% to 75% with hematopoietic growth factors, thus reducing the risk of febrile neutropenia and documented infections. This in turn prevents dose reductions that can compromise the effectiveness of the therapy. The ASCO guidelines for use of hematopoietic growth factors (granulocyte-colony stimulating factor, granulocyte-macrophage colony stimulating factor) recommends routine prophylactic use of these growth factors in persons age 70 or older receiving treatment with cyclophosphamide/doxorubicin/vincristine/prednisone (CHOP) or a drug combination of similar dose intensity (cyclophosphamide/doxorubicin/5-fluorouracil [CAF], 5-fluorouracil/epirubicin/cyclophosphamide [FEC100], cyclophosphamide/doxorubicin [CA]), and for patients age 60 or older receiving induction or consolidation chemotherapy for AML.[45] Antiemetic prophylaxis with a 5-HT3-receptor antagonist in combination with a steroid is recommended in patients receiving moderately to highly emetogenic chemotherapy or radiotherapy.[46] Use of stool softeners to prevent constipation from vincristine- and vinblastine-induced bowel wall neuropathy is important.

Another significant problem resulting from either the cancer itself or therapy for the cancer is the occurrence of fatigue in elderly patients.[47] This is one of the most common symptoms and significantly affects a patient's quality of life. In one systematic review, the prevalence of fatigue was 40% to 90% during treatment and 19% to 80% after completion of treatment. The etiology of fatigue is multifold, ranging from immobility and deconditioning to anemia, depression, pain, poor nutrition, drugs, and metabolic causes. Fatigue is usually managed by treating the underlying causes (e.g., treat anemia with hematinics, iron, B12, folate). Exercise programs can play a very positive role in the treatment of cancer-related fatigue. Drugs like methylphenidate and modafinil have been used to treat cancer-related fatigue, but have yet to be studied specifically in older patients with cancer.

END-OF-LIFE ISSUES

The geriatric population is unique in that people expect and have a realistic approach to the fact that they are nearing the end of life. Older patients and their families are more open to discussions about their disease and the potential consequences. In one landmark study of patients age 60 or older who were terminally ill, the authors noted that if the outcome was survival but with either severe functional impairment or cognitive impairment, 74.4% and 88.8% of participants, respectively, would not choose treatment.[48] These issues are discussed in further detail in Chapter 21: Palliative and End-of-Life Care.

KEY POINTS

- The American Geriatrics Society Task Force and the American College of Surgeons provide general guidelines for older adults undergoing surgery. These recommendations may be applied to older patients with cancer undergoing surgery.
- The delivery, duration, and dosage of radiotherapy must be carefully planned based on organ functioning, comorbidity, and geriatric evaluation, since side effects may be more pronounced in elderly patients.
- Chemotherapy should be dosed based on creatinine clearance, with use of colony stimulating growth factors when indicated.
- Oral targeted agents may have several drug interactions in the older patient with polypharmacy.

SPECIAL CONSIDERATIONS IN COMMON MALIGNANT DISEASES

The randomized controlled trial is the gold standard for investigating new therapies, yet older patients are consistently underrepresented in clinical trials, and much of the treatment data for this population are derived from subset analyses of large studies. Overall survival (OS) is a primary endpoint in many clinical trials; however, for the older population, survival may be compromised more as a result of comorbid conditions than because of the cancer itself. A recent SIOG and European Organisation for the Research and Treatment of Cancer task force has put forth suggestions for clinical trial design and clinical endpoints in geriatric oncology research.[49] They suggest that all clinical trials in oncology should be without an upper age limit to allow entry of eligible older adults, should include measures of quality of life, and should note decreases in cancer-related symptoms. Older patients may wish to receive cancer therapy when an intervention can prolong life, but not at the expense of compromising their quality of life. When possible, patients should be encouraged to participate in trials designed to answer cancer management questions. This chapter aims to cover only "elderly-specific" issues from trials in some common cancers types that are relevant to the practicing oncologist.

BREAST CANCER

Almost 50% of all breast cancers develop in women age 65 or older, and 13% develop in women older than age 80. Recognized prognostic factors, such as estrogen receptor (ER) status, histologic grade, ploidy, p53 status, epidermal growth factor receptor status, and HER2 status, suggest that tumors should become less aggressive with advancing age.[50,51] However, women older than age 75 often have higher mortality rates, even with early-stage breast cancer, than their younger counterparts. Triple-negative breast cancer may occur in 15% to 25% of older women and carries a poor prognosis, similar to what is seen in younger patients.[52] Resection of the primary tumor and administration of tamoxifen may be appropriate for select women with small, ER-positive breast cancers and for patients with a limited life expectancy.[53,54] Since aromatase inhibitors are associated with greater progression-free survival (PFS) and less thrombotic and uterine carcinogenic toxicity, they often are used in lieu of tamoxifen in the adjuvant setting. Few adjuvant chemotherapy trials have been designed to answer questions specific to the elderly population. The first U.S. adjuvant chemotherapy trial in elderly patients randomly assigned women age 65 or older with localized breast cancer to receive six cycles of single-agent capecitabine or to receive either CA or cyclophosphamide/methotrexate/5-fluorouracil (CMF). With a median follow-up of 2.4 years, both relapse-free survival and OS rates were better with combination chemotherapy. This trial confirms the importance of combination chemotherapy in improving outcomes for older women.[55,56] Thus, in the absence of severe comorbidities, the guidelines for adjuvant therapy are the same as those for younger women. An Oncotype DX Recurrence Score may be helpful in guiding the need for chemotherapy in addition to endocrine therapy in women with ER-positive, HER2-negative disease. The Adjuvant! Online program is a valuable tool for weighing the potential benefits of adjuvant therapy with the effect of comorbidities on survival.

In elderly patients with advanced breast cancer, targeted agents like the m-TOR inhibitor everolimus, in combination with exemestane, have been demonstrated to be effective.[57] For patients with HER2-positive advanced breast cancer, trastuzumab emtansine (T-DM1) has improved both PFS and OS with lower toxicity compared to lapatinib plus capecitabine.[58] Subgroup analysis from the CLEOPATRA trial suggested that older patients with HER2-positive advanced breast cancer who received pertuzumab plus trastuzumab and docetaxel had better survival than those patients who received placebo plus trastuzumab and docetaxel.[59] Diarrhea, fatigue, asthenia, decreased appetite, vomiting, and dysgeusia were reported more frequently in patients older than age 65, but neutropenia and febrile neutropenia were reported less frequently in the older age group.

Screening

Controlled trials of screening mammography have excluded older women. The efficacy of screening can be assessed only from observational trials, and these data suggest a decrease in breast cancer–related mortality for women age 70 to 79. The American Geriatrics Society recommends annual screening mammography for women up to age 85 if their life expectancy is at least 4 years.[60,61]

Chemoprevention

The Breast Cancer Prevention Trial concluded that tamoxifen use reduces the incidence of hormone receptor–positive breast cancer. However, in patients older than age 55, the potential benefit from chemoprevention is outweighed, at least in part, by an increased risk of endometrial cancer and thrombosis. Raloxifene is as effective as tamoxifen for preventing invasive breast cancers and has a lower incidence of thromboembolic events, cataracts, and endometrial cancer.[62]

LUNG CANCER
Non-Small Cell Lung Cancer

The median age of patients with newly diagnosed NSCLC is 70. The prognosis for lung cancer is related to the stage of disease, performance status, sex, and the patient's ability to tolerate adequate treatment.[63] Controlled trials involving patients age 70 or older confirm a small benefit from chemotherapy for patients with extensive-stage disease. The ELVIS trial compared single-agent vinorelbine with best supportive care for patients age 70 or older. The primary endpoint of improvement in quality of life was achieved in the vinorelbine arm. Patients in the treatment arm also experienced a significant improvement in median survival (28 vs. 21 weeks; p = 0.03), associated with a reduced relative hazard of death (hazard ratio [HR] 0.64, 95% CI 0.45, 0.93).[64,65] Similarly, compared with docetaxel plus gemcitabine, single-agent docetaxel improved the time to progression (but not OS) for older patients and for patients with a performance status higher than 2.[66] A retrospective subset analysis

of ECOG4599 found that patients age 65 or older who received bevacizumab in addition to carboplatin and paclitaxel experienced more grade 3 and 4 toxicities than younger patients. Compared with carboplatin and paclitaxel, the addition of bevacizumab produced a higher response rate but no improvement in PFS or OS.[67] The combination of carboplatin and paclitaxel was compared with single-agent vinorelbine or gemcitabine in 451 patients age 70 to 89 with locally advanced or metastatic NSCLC. After a 30-month follow up, OS was significantly longer for those receiving combination therapy (6.2 vs. 10.3 months; p < 0.0001) but at the cost of more asthenia and myelosuppression.[68] Oral erlotinib is an attractive option as first-line therapy for patients age 70 and older who have extensive-stage disease. Toxicity is mild and the 10.9-month median survival reported is comparable with other single-agent trials in this population.[69] As second- or third-line therapy, single-agent erlotinib demonstrated a similar effect on PFS and OS across all ages. However, patients age 70 or older experienced more toxicity and thus more dose interruptions.[70] More recently, afatinib, an irreversible ErbB-family blocker, has been approved for use in patients with late-stage metastatic lung cancer whose tumors express epidermal growth factor receptor (EGFR) gene mutation.[71] In addition, crizotinib, an oral tyrosine kinase inhibitor targeting the anaplastic lymphoma kinase gene (ALK), has been shown to be superior to standard chemotherapy in patients with previously treated advanced NSCLC with ALK rearrangement.[72] These oral agents have also demonstrated better control of symptoms of lung cancer and greater improvement in global quality of life, and thus may be an attractive option for older patients.

One-third of older patients present with locally advanced disease (stages IIIA and IIIB). The 5-year survival benefit of adjuvant vinorelbine and cisplatin in the National Cancer Institute of Canada BR10 trial was observed for patients both younger and older than age 65.[73] Available data for the use of concurrent chemotherapy and radiation therapy suggest that the "fit older patient" benefits from combined-modality therapy. However, the frequency of grade 4 toxicity—notably hematologic toxicity—is higher for older patients.

Small Cell Lung Cancer

Similar results of the benefit of combination chemotherapy (cisplatin and etoposide) have been demonstrated in elderly patients with small cell lung cancer (SCLC). A recent SEER database study identified 1,926 patients age 70 or older with limited-stage SCLC; 7.2% patients received prophylactic cranial irradiation (PCI).[74] The authors concluded that PCI remained an independent predictor of OS among patients age 75 to 79, but not among patients age 80 or older. Given the poor prognosis of SCLC, there are little to no data on the long-term effects of PCI on cognition and mood of elderly patients.

COLORECTAL CANCER

The median age at diagnosis of colorectal cancer is 71. For older patients, lesions are more likely to develop on the right side, and anemia is more likely to occur (compared with pain).[75] Surgical resection of the primary tumor has been the mainstay of treatment. Perforation, bleeding, and obstruction may develop if the primary tumor is not removed, and emergency surgical intervention may be needed. Because the rates of morbidity and mortality associated with emergency operations are higher than expected for patients older than age 70, surgery may be advisable for palliative purposes, even for patients with advanced disease.[76] Preoperative chemoradiation is used only in patients with rectal cancer to downstage the tumor and allow for sphincter-preserving surgery. This remains controversial in patients older than age 70 due to excessive side effects, dose reductions, and treatment interruptions. Patients with colon cancer who receive adjuvant chemotherapy are less likely to die of colorectal cancer. Unfortunately, not only is adjuvant chemotherapy offered less frequently to older patients, up to 30% will discontinue treatment prematurely, and many are treated at substantially reduced and ineffective doses.[77] Yet adjuvant therapy with a fluoropyrimidine provides the same survival benefit for patients age 70 and older as it does for younger patients.[78] Oxaliplatin-based chemotherapy is increasingly used in the adjuvant setting, but its benefit in older patients has recently been challenged, especially since older patients experience more neurotoxicity with this agent. A pooled data analysis from six adjuvant therapy trials found that oxaliplatin does not improve OS or relapse-free survival compared with 5-fluorouracil/leucovorin in patients older than age 70. Despite this, the utility of oxaliplatin in older patients continues to be a topic of debate.[79]

In the metastatic setting, one study compared the outcome of liver resection for colorectal metastases in elderly patients with that of younger patients. The 3-year OS was 57% in elderly patients and 60% in younger patients, with similar outcomes in patients age 70 to 75, 75 to 80, or at least 80. Chemotherapy offers a survival benefit to elderly patients with recurrent and/or metastatic disease. Capecitabine has been shown to be better tolerated and as effective as bolus 5-fluorouracil in elderly patients.[80] Because older patients experience more diarrhea and hand-foot syndrome, a starting dose of 1,000 mg/m² is recommended. First-line treatment in metastatic disease generally includes bevacizumab, which is as efficacious in older patients as in younger ones, with improvements in PFS and OS. However, hypertension and arterial thrombotic events are more common in older individuals. One phase II study demonstrated that cetuximab was safe and moderately active when used as a first-line single agent in fit patients with metastatic colorectal cancer. Subgroup analysis of the pivotal panitumumab trial and the CRYSTAL study suggests that the benefit in elderly individuals is comparable to what was observed in younger patients.[81]

Screening

Colonoscopy has been established as a cost-effective screening tool. In average-risk individuals, screening colonoscopy should be performed every 10 years beginning at age 50. The USPSTF recommends against routine screening for colorectal cancer in adults age 76 to 85.[82]

ACUTE MYELOID LEUKEMIA

The median age of diagnosis of AML is 68. This is a malignancy with a more aggressive biology in elderly patients. Elderly patients with AML present with higher numbers of poor-risk karyotypes, underlying myelodysplastic syndrome, and increased expression of the multidrug resistance genes.[83] One study has demonstrated an increased probability of *RAS*, *Src*, and *TNF* pathway activation in elderly patients with AML when compared to their younger counterparts.[84] Induction therapy for AML with 7+3 (cytarabine plus anthracycline) has resulted in complete response (CR) rates ranging from 39% to 63%, with poor OS and high rates of relapse. The 30-day induction mortality is approximately 10% to 14% across all elderly age groups (age 55 to 80) if patients have good ECOG PS. However, mortality can be as high as 50% in older patients with a poor PS.

Induction therapy with intensified anthracycline or cytarabine doses has not consistently been associated with improved outcomes in elderly patients with AML. In a study by Löwenberg et al, subgroup analysis showed that in patients age 60 to 65, the arm that received escalated-dose daunorubicin (90 mg/m²) had higher complete remission rates than those patients in the standard-dose (45 mg/m²) arm.[85] More recently, the ALFA-0701 study concluded that the use of fractionated lower doses of an anti-CD33 monoclonal antibody, gemtuzumab ozogamicin, in combination with chemotherapy was safe and led to better response rates and survival in elderly patients with AML.[86] Post-remission therapy continues to be controversial in elderly patients with AML. A landmark CALGB trial has shown that cytarabine at high doses of 3 g/m² as consolidation therapy improved disease-free survival when compared to low- or intermediate-dose cytarabine in patients age 60 or younger with AML. However, this benefit was not seen in patients older than 60 and large numbers of elderly patients were not able to complete therapy due to toxicity.[87] Further, at least three studies have now dismissed the benefit of consolidation chemotherapy in elderly patients with AML. However, fit elderly patients with poor-risk cytogenetics and *FLT3* AML should be offered a consultation for reduced-intensity conditioning allogeneic SCT.[87]

In patients who are unfit or have poor PS, are older than 70, or have too many comorbidities, epigenetic therapy with hypomethylating agents (decitabine or azacitidine) is an option. In fact, one study analyzed 671 patients age 65 or older with newly diagnosed AML treated with intensive chemotherapy or epigenetic (i.e., azacitidine- or decitabine-based) therapy.[88] The CR rates with chemotherapy and epigenetic therapy were 42% and 28%, respectively (p = 0.001), and the 8-week mortality was 18% and 11%, respectively (p = 0.075). The 2-year relapse-free survival (28% vs. 39%; p = 0.843) and median survival (6.7 vs. 6.5 months; p = 0.413) were similar in both groups. Decitabine was associated with improved median overall survival compared with azacitidine (5.5 vs. 8.8 months, respectively; p = 0.03). Epigenetic therapy may be an attractive option for some elderly patients since it is usually administered in the outpatient setting compared to the intense 4- to 6-week inpatient stay with traditional induction therapy. Patients typically have delayed responses, with median time to CR being 4.5 cycles of therapy. Importantly, in view of the serious complications of AML therapy and the high treatment-related mortality, older patients should be treated in centers skilled in the management and supportive care of AML.

CHRONIC LYMPHOCYTIC LEUKEMIA

Chronic lymphocytic leukemia (CLL) is the most prevalent lymphoid malignancy in the United States, with a median age at diagnosis of 70. Most patients who need treatment are 75 or older.[89] Traditional risk factors, such as chromosomal aberrations detected by interphase fluorescence in situ hybridization (FISH), analysis of somatic hypermutation (mutation status) of *IGHV*, and measurement of expression of protein markers such as zeta-associated protein (ZAP)-70 and CD38, have been shown to predict time to first treatment but not OS. CGA may assist in identifying fit elderly patients.[90] These fit patients with non-17p13 CLL should be offered chemoimmunotherapy with a purine analogue and rituximab. Bendamustine plus rituximab also is a good option for older untreated fit patients with CLL as demonstrated by the German CLL study group.[91] More recently, several targeted agents have shown benefit in CLL and received FDA approval. Obinutuzumab, a type 2 glycoengineered antibody, was administered in combination with chlorambucil in patients with CLL with multiple comorbidities. The median age in this study was 73; obinutuzumab was superior to rituximab when each was combined with chlorambucil.[92] Ofatumumab, a fully human anti-CD20 monoclonal antibody, combined with pentostatin and cyclophosphamide has been well tolerated in untreated patients with CLL. It is currently approved for patients with CLL in whom fludarabine or alemtuzumab have failed.[93] In CLL, the PI3K pathway is constitutively activated and dependent on PI3Kδ. Idelalisib, an oral PI3Kδ isoform–selective inhibitor that promotes apoptosis in primary CLL cells, has been combined with rituximab as a frontline therapy and led to high overall response rates with relatively few side effects.[94] Finally, Bruton's tyrosine kinase (BTK) plays a role in the signal transduction of the B-cell receptor. Ibrutinib, an orally active small molecule inhibiting BTK, has shown high response rates with modest toxicity in patients with relapsed CLL, including those with advanced-stage and high-risk (17p-deleted) disease.[95]

MULTIPLE MYELOMA

The median age at diagnosis for multiple myeloma (MM) is 70, with 35% of patients younger than 65, 28% age 65 to 74, and 37% older than 75.[96] For many years, melphalan and prednisone (MP) was the only option for older patients with MM. More recently, the addition of thalidomide (MPT) was associated with significantly superior response rates and PFS, but at the cost of toxicity (i.e., constipation, fatigue, neuropathy, cytopenias, infection, and deep venous thrombosis).[97] The second-generation immunomodulatory agent lenalidomide is better tolerated. In a large double-blind multicenter randomized study, induction therapy with MP/lenalidomide followed by lenalidomide maintenance (MPR-R) significantly prolonged PFS in patients

age 65 or older who were ineligible for transplantation.[98] Approximately 25% of elderly patients with MM have cytogenetic abnormalities that are associated with a high risk of disease progression and very poor prognosis. High-risk cytogenetic profiles include del(17p), t(4;14), and/or t(14;16).[99] Bortezomib (V)-based combinations have also been evaluated as initial and maintenance therapy in elderly patients. In the VISTA trial of VMP versus MP, patients with high-risk cytogenetic profiles, including the presence of a t(4;14), t(14;16), and/or del(17p), had the same CR rate and similar time to progression and OS times as patients with standard-risk cytogenetics, suggesting that the addition of bortezomib to MP was able to overcome the poor prognosis of these patients.[100] However, the small numbers and the lack of reproducibility in subsequent Italian and Spanish trials led to the conclusion that the first generation of novel agents do not overcome the negative prognosis of high-risk cytogenetic abnormalities in newly diagnosed elderly patients with MM.[101]

Recently, an expert panel provided recommendations for the appropriate use of pomalidomide, the most recently approved immunomodulatory agent in MM.[102] They recommended no dose changes for the drug in elderly patients and, based on current studies, the use of pomalidomide plus low-dose dexamethasone is appropriate in patients with high-risk cytogenetics. The second-generation proteasome inhibitor carfilzomib has been combined with lenalidomide/dexamethasone (CRd) in a pilot phase I/II trial in patients with newly diagnosed MM.[103] Subgroup analysis of 23 elderly patients with MM showed impressive efficacy (100% overall response rate, with 65% stringent CR), and an acceptable toxicity profile with 13% grade 1 to 2 peripheral neuropathy. Finally, while high-dose therapy followed by autologous SCT is the treatment approach for younger patients, this has not yet been established for elderly patients. This is partly due to the lack of consensus on what constitutes transplant eligibility in elderly patients.

LYMPHOMA

Older patients tend to present with more aggressive histologic subtypes of lymphoma. The International Prognostic Index (IPI) identifies age of 60 or older as an independent poor prognostic factor. Regardless of age, prognosis is favorable for patients with stage I and II disease who are treated with chemotherapy and radiation therapy.[104] The landmark practice-changing GELA study established rituximab (a chimeric anti-CD20 monoclonal antibody) plus CHOP (R-CHOP) as the standard of care for patients age 65 or older with diffuse large B-cell lymphoma. In this study, CHOP was compared to R-CHOP in elderly patients.[105] Elderly patients on the R-CHOP arm had a highly significant advantage in response rate, failure-free survival, and OS, and this benefit has now held up over follow-up period of more than 10 years. The StiL study demonstrated that in patients with previously untreated indolent lymphoma and mantle-cell lymphoma, bendamustine plus rituximab (BR) may be the preferred first-line treatment approach over R-CHOP because of increased PFS and fewer toxic effects.[106] Owing to its better toxicity profile, BR reduced the cost of treating adverse events by over £1,000 per patient compared with R-CHOP in one study.[107] More recently, in a phase II study of patients with relapsed mantle-cell lymphoma with a median age of 68, the oral BTK inhibitor ibrutinib has shown durable single-agent efficacy.[108]

References

1. Smith BD, Smith GL, Hurria A. Future of cancer incidence in the United States: burdens upon an aging, changing nation. *J Clin Oncol.* 2009;27:2758-2765. PMID: 19403886.

2. Warren JL, Mariotto AB, Meekins A, et al. Current and future utilization of services from medical oncologists. *J Clin Oncol.* 2008;26:3242-3247. PMID: 18591559.

3. Yancik R. Cancer burden in the aged: an epidemiologic and demographic overview. *Cancer.* 1997;80:1273-1283. PMID: 9317180.

4. National Comprehensive Cancer Network (NCCN) guidelines for Senior Adult Oncology version 2.2014. www.nccn.org/professionals/physician_gls/f_guidelines.asp#age. Accessed June 18, 2014.

5. Yabroff KR, Lamont EB, Mariotto A, et al. Cost of care for elderly patients with cancer in the United States. *J Natl Cancer Inst.* 2008;100:630-641. PMID: 18445825.

6. Kantarjian HM, Fojo T, Mathisen M et al. Cancer drugs in the United States: Justum Pretium–the just price. *J Clin Oncol.* 2013;31:3600-3604. PMID: 23650428.

7. Dusetzina SB, Winn AN, Abel GA, et al. Cost sharing and adherence to tyrosine kinase inhibitors for patients with chronic myeloid leukemia. *J Clin Oncol.* 2014;32:306-311. PMID: 24366936.

8. Aitkin M, Valkova S. Avoidable Costs in U.S. Healthcare: The $200 Billion Opportunity from Using Medicines More Responsibly. www.imshealth.com/deployedfiles/imshealth/Global/Content/Corporate/IMS%20Institute/RUOM-2013/IHII_Responsible_Use_Medicines_2013.pdf. Accessed June 18, 2014.

9. Guy GP Jr, Ekwueme DU, Yabroff KR, et al. Economic burden of cancer survivorship among adults in the United States. *J Clin Oncol.* 2013;31:3749-3757. PMID: 24043731.

10. Cohen HJ. Biology of aging as related to cancer. *Cancer.* 1994;74:2092-2100 PMID: 8087776.

11. Hanahan D, Weinberg RA. The hallmarks of cancer. *Cell.* 2000;100:57-70. PMID: 10647931.

12. Staiano-Coico L, Darzynkiewicz Z, Hefton JM, et al. Increased sensitivity of lymphocytes from people over 65 to cell cycle arrest and chromosomal damage. *Science.* 1983;219:1335-1337 PMID: 6828861.

13. Trosko JE, Chu EH. The role of DNA repair and somatic mutation in carcinogenesis. *Adv Cancer Res.* 1975;21:391-425. PMID: 174398.

14. Wright WE, Shay JW. Telomere biology in aging and cancer. *J Am Geriatr Soc.* 2005;53:S292-S294. PMID: 16131355.

15. Campisi J. Senescent cells, tumor suppression, and organismal aging: good citizens, bad neighbors. *Cell.* 2005;120:513-522. PMID: 15734683.

16. Harman D. The aging process. *Proc Natl. Acad Sci. U S A.* 1981;78:7124-7128. PMID: 6947277.

17. Gilchrest BA, Bohr VA. Aging processes, DNA damage, and repair. *FASEB J.* 1997;11:322-330. PMID: 9141498.

18. Melton LJ 3rd, Khosla S, Crowson CS, et al. Epidemiology of sarcopenia. *J Am Geriatr Soc.* 2000;48:625-630. PMID: 10855597.

19. Sotaniemi EA, Arranto AJ, Pelkonen O, et al. Age and cytochrome P450-linked drug metabolism in humans: an analysis of 226 subjects with equal histopathologic conditions. *Clin Pharmacol Ther.* 1997;61:331-339. PMID: 9091249.

20. Hajjar I, Yang F, Sorond F, et al. A novel aging phenotype of slow gait, impaired executive function, and depressive symptoms: relationship to blood pressure and other cardiovascular risks. *J Gerontol A BiolSci Med Sci.* 2009;64:994-1001. PMID: 19535785.

21. Verghese J, Holtzer R, Lipton RB, et al. Quantitative gait markers and incident fall risk in older adults. *J Gerontol A BiolSci Med Sci.* 2009;64:896-901. PMID: 19349593.

22. Harris TB, Ferrucci L, Tracy RP, et al. Associations of elevated interleukin-6 and C-reactive protein levels with mortality in the elderly. *Am J Med.* 1999;106:506-512. PMID: 10335721.

23. Guralnik JM, Eisenstaedt RS, Ferrucci L, et al. Prevalence of anemia in persons 65 years and older in the United States: evidence for a high rate of unexplained anemia. *Blood.* 2004;104:2263-2268. Epub 2004 Jul 6. PMID: 15238427.

24. Extermann M, Aapro M, Bernabei R et al. Use of comprehensive geriatric assessment in older patients with cancer: recommendations from the task force on CGA of the International Society of Geriatric Oncology (SIOG). *Crit Rev Oncol Hematol.* 2005;55:241-252. PMID: 16084735.

25. Hurria A, Cirrincione CT, Muss HB, et al. Implementing a geriatric assessment in cooperative group clinical cancer trials: CALGB 360401. *J Clin Oncol.* 2011;29:1290-1296. PMID: 21357782.

26. Hurria A, Togawa K, Mohile SG, et al. Predicting chemotherapy toxicity in older adults with cancer: a prospective multicenter study. *J Clin Oncol.* 2011;29:3457-3465. PMID: 21810685.

27. Extermann M, Boler I, Reich RR, et al. Predicting the risk of chemotherapy toxicity in older patients: the Chemotherapy Risk Assessment Scale for High-Age Patients (CRASH) score. *Cancer.* 2012;118:3377-3386. PMID: 22072065.

28. Caillet P, Canoui-Poitrine F, Vouriot J, et al. Comprehensive geriatric assessment in the decision-making process in elderly patients with cancer: ELCAPA study. *J Clin Oncol.* 2011;29:3636-3642. PMID: 21709194.

29. Pope D, Ramesh H, Gennari R, et al. Pre-operative assessment of cancer in the elderly (PACE): a comprehensive assessment of underlying characteristics of elderly patients with cancer prior to elective surgery. *Surg Oncol.* 2006;15:189-197. PMID: 17531743.

30. Klepin HD, Geiger AM, Tooze JA, et al. Geriatric assessment predicts survival for older adults receiving induction chemotherapy for acute myelogenous leukemia. *Blood.* 2013;121:4287-4294. PMID: 23550038.

31. Clegg A, Young J, Iliffe S, et al. Frailty in elderly people. *Lancet.* 2013;381:752-762. PMID: 23395245.

32. Fried LP, Tangen CM, Walston J, et al. Frailty in older adults: evidence for a phenotype. *J Gerontol A Biol Sci Med Sci.* 2001;56:M146-156. PMID: 11253156.

33. Song X, Mitnitski A, Rockwood K. Prevalence and 10-year outcomes of frailty in older adults in relation to deficit accumulation. *J Am Geriatr Soc.* 2010;58:681-687. PMID: 20345864.

34. Mohile SG, Fan L, Reeve E, et al. Association of cancer with geriatric syndromes in older Medicare beneficiaries. *J Clin Oncol.* 2011;29:1458-1464. PMID: 21402608.

35. Chow WB, Rosenthal RA, Merkow RP, et al. Optimal preoperative assessment of the geriatric surgical patient: a best practices guideline from the American College of Surgeons National Surgical Quality Improvement Program and the American Geriatrics Society. *J Am Coll Surg.* 2012;215:453-466. PMID: 22917646.

36. Kunkler IH, Audisio R, Belkacemi Y, et al. Review of current best practice and priorities for research in radiation oncology for elderly patients with cancer: the International Society of Geriatric Oncology (SIOG) task force. *Ann Oncol.* Epub 2014 Mar 13. PMID: 24625455.

37. Lichtman SM, Wildiers H, Chatelut E, et al. International Society of Geriatric Oncology Chemotherapy Taskforce: evaluation of chemotherapy in older patients–an analysis of the medical literature. *J Clin Oncol.* 2007;25:1832-1843. PMID: 17488981.

38. Lichtman SM, Wildiers H, Launay-Vacher V, et al. International Society of Geriatric Oncology (SIOG) recommendations for the adjustment of dosing in elderly patients with cancer with renal insufficiency. *Eur J Cancer.* 2007;43:14-34. PMID: 17222747.

39. Breccia M, Tiribelli M, Alimena G. Tyrosine kinase inhibitors for elderly chronic myeloid leukemia patients: a systematic review of efficacy and safety data. *Crit Rev Oncol Hematol.* 2012;84:93-100 PMID: 22280914.

40. Rao AV, Schmader K. Monoclonal antibodies as targeted therapy in hematologic malignancies in older adults. *Am J Geriatr Pharmacother.* 2007;5:247-262. PMID: 17996665.

41. Scappaticci FA, Skillings JR, Holden SN, et al. Arterial thromboembolic events in patients with metastatic carcinoma treated with chemotherapy and bevacizumab. *J Natl Cancer Inst.* 2007;99:1232-1239. PMID: 17686822.

42. Iurlo A, Ubertis A, Artuso S, et al. Comorbidities and polypharmacy impact on complete cytogenetic response in chronic myeloid leukaemia elderly patients. *Eur J Intern Med.* 2014;25:63-66. PMID: 24309387.

43. Koreth J, Pidala J, Perez WS et al. Role of reduced-intensity conditioning allogeneic hematopoietic stem-cell transplantation in older patients with de novo myelodysplastic syndromes: an international collaborative decision analysis. *J Clin Oncol.* 2013;31:2662-2670. PMID: 23797000.

44. Fann JR, Hubbard RA, Alfano CM, et al. Pre- and post-transplantation risk factors for delirium onset and severity in patients undergoing hematopoietic stem-cell transplantation. *J Clin Oncol.* 2011;29:895-901. PMID: 21263081.

45. Smith TJ, Khatcheressian J, Lyman GH, et al. 2006 update of recommendations for the use of white blood cell growth factors: an evidence-based clinical practice guideline. *J Clin Oncol.* 2006;24:3187-3205. PMID: 16682719.

46. Basch E, Prestrud AA, Hesketh PJ, et al. Antiemetics: American Society of Clinical Oncology clinical practice guideline update. *J Clin Oncol.* 2011;29:4189-4198. PMID: 21947834.

47. Rao AV, Cohen HJ. Fatigue in older patients with cancer: etiology, assessment, and treatment. *Semin Oncol.* 2008;35:633-642. PMID: 19027467.

48. Fried TR, Bradley EH, Towle VR, et al. Understanding the treatment preferences of seriously ill patients. *N Engl J Med.* 2002;346:1061-1066. PMID: 11932474.

49. Wildiers H, Mauer M, Pallis A, et al. End points and trial design in geriatric oncology research: a joint European organisation for research and treatment of cancer–Alliance for Clinical Trials in Oncology–International Society Of Geriatric Oncology position article. *J Clin Oncol.* 2013;31:3711-3718. PMID: 24019549.

50. Diab SG, Elledge RM, Clark GM. Tumor characteristics and clinical outcome of elderly women with breast cancer. *J Natl Cancer Inst.* 2000;92:550-556. PMID: 10749910.

51. Basche M, Byers T. Re: Tumor characteristics and clinical outcome of elderly women with breast cancer. *J Natl Cancer Inst.* 2001;93:64-65; author reply 65-66. PMID: 11136846.

52. Aapro M, Wildiers H. Triple-negative breast cancer in the older population. *Ann Oncol.* 2012;23 Suppl 6:vi52-vi55. PMID: 23012304.

53. Fyles AW, McCready DR, Manchul LA, et al. Tamoxifen with or without breast irradiation in women 50 years of age or older with early breast cancer. *N Engl J Med.* 2004;351:963-970. PMID: 15342804.

54. Hughes KS, Schnaper LA, Berry D, et al. Lumpectomy plus tamoxifen with or without irradiation in women 70 years of age or older with early breast cancer. *N Engl J Med.* 2004;351:971-977. PMID: 15342805.

55. Muss HB, Berry DA, Cirrincione CT, et al. Adjuvant chemotherapy in older women with early-stage breast cancer. *N Engl J Med.* 2009;360:2055-2065. PMID: 19439741.

56. Muss HB, Woolf S, Berry D, et al. Adjuvant chemotherapy in older and younger women with lymph node-positive breast cancer. *JAMA.* 2005;293:1073-1081. PMID: 15741529.

57. Pritchard KI, Burris HA 3rd, Ito Y, et al. Safety and efficacy of everolimus with exemestane vs. exemestane alone in elderly patients with HER2-negative, hormone receptor-positive breast cancer in BOLERO-2. *Clin Breast Cancer.* 2013;13:421-432. PMID: 24267730.

58. Verma S, Miles D, Gianni L, et al. Trastuzumab emtansine for HER2-positive advanced breast cancer. *N Engl J Med.* 2012;367:1783-1791. PMID: 23020162.

59. Swain SM, Kim SB, Cortés J, et al. Pertuzumab, trastuzumab, and docetaxel for HER2-positive metastatic breast cancer (CLEOPATRA study): overall survival results from a randomised, double-blind, placebo-controlled, phase 3 study. *Lancet Oncol.* 2013;14:461-471. PMID: 23602601.

60. Breast cancer screening in older women. American Geriatrics Society Clinical Practice Committee. *J Am Geriatr Soc.* 2000;48:842-844. PMID: 10894327.

61. American Geriatrics Society Ethics Committee. Health screening decisions for older adults: AGS position paper. *J Am Geriatr Soc.* 2003;51:270-271. PMID: 12558727.

62. Vogel VG, Costantino JP, Wickerham DL, et al. Effects of tamoxifen vs raloxifene on the risk of developing invasive breast cancer and other disease outcomes: the NSABP Study of Tamoxifen and Raloxifene (STAR) P-2 trial. *JAMA.* 2006;295:2727-2741. PMID: 16754727.

63. Johnson DH. Treatment of the elderly patient with small-cell lung cancer. *Chest.* 1993;103:72S-74S. PMID: 8380138.

64. Effects of vinorelbine on quality of life and survival of elderly patients with advanced non-small cell lung cancer. The Elderly Lung Cancer Vinorelbine Italian Study Group. *J Natl Cancer Inst.* 1999;91:66-72. PMID: 9890172.

65. Frasci G, Lorusso V, Panza N, et al. Gemcitabine plus vinorelbine versus vinorelbine alone in elderly patients with advanced non-small-cell lung cancer. *J Clin Oncol.* 2000;18:2529-2536. PMID: 10893283.

66. Hainsworth JD, Spigel DR, Farley C, et al. Weekly docetaxel versus docetaxel/gemcitabine in the treatment of elderly or poor performance status patients with advanced nonsmall cell lung cancer: a randomized phase 3 trial of the Minnie Pearl Cancer Research Network. *Cancer.* 2007;110:2027-2034. PMID: 17823908.

67. Ramalingam SS, Dahlberg SE, Langer CJ, et al. Outcomes for elderly, advanced-stage non small-cell lung cancer patients treated with bevacizumab in combination with carboplatin and paclitaxel: analysis of Eastern Cooperative Oncology Group Trial 4599. *J Clin Oncol.* 2008;26:60-65. PMID: 18165641.

68. Quoix E, Zalcman G, Oster JP, et al. Carboplatin and weekly paclitaxel doublet chemotherapy compared with monotherapy in elderly patients with advanced non-small-cell lung cancer: IFCT-0501 randomised, phase 3 trial. *Lancet.* 2011;378:1079-1088. PMID: 21831418.

69. Jackman DM, Yeap BY, Lindeman NI, et al. Phase II clinical trial of chemotherapy-naive patients ≥ 70 years of age treated with erlotinib for advanced non-small-cell lung cancer. *J Clin Oncol.* 2007;25:760-766. PMID: 17228019.

70. Wheatley-Price P, Ding K, Seymour L, et al. Erlotinib for advanced non-small-cell lung cancer in the elderly: an analysis of the National Cancer Institute of Canada Clinical Trials Group Study BR.21. *J Clin Oncol.* 2008;26:2350-2357. PMID: 18467727.

71. Katakami N, Atagi S, Goto K, et al. LUX-Lung 4: a phase II trial of afatinib in patients with advanced non-small-cell lung cancer who progressed during prior treatment with erlotinib, gefitinib, or both. *J Clin Oncol.* 2013;31:3335-3341. PMID: 23816963.

72. Shaw AT, Kim DW, Nakagawa K, et al. Crizotinib versus chemotherapy in advanced ALK-positive lung cancer. *N Engl J Med.* 2013;368:2385-2394. PMID: 23724913.

73. Pepe C, Hasan B, Winton TL, et al. Adjuvant vinorelbine and cisplatin in elderly patients: National Cancer Institute of Canada and Intergroup Study JBR.10. *J Clin Oncol.* 2007;25:1553-1561. PMID: 17442999.

74. Eaton BR, Kim S, Marcus DM, et al. Effect of prophylactic cranial irradiation on survival in elderly patients with limited-stage small cell lung cancer. *Cancer.* 2013;119:3753-3760. PMID: 23921891.

75. Mulcahy HE, Patchett SE, Daly L, et al. Prognosis of elderly patients with large bowel cancer. *Br J Surg.* 1994;81:736-738. PMID: 8044567.

76. Vivi AA, Lopes A, Cavalcanti Sde F, et al. Surgical treatment of colon and rectum adenocarcinoma in elderly patients. *J Surg Oncol.* 1992;51:203-206. PMID: 1434647.

77. Hubbard J, Thomas DM, Yothers G, et al. Benefits and adverse events in younger versus older patients receiving adjuvant chemotherapy for colon cancer: findings from the Adjuvant Colon Cancer Endpoints data set. *J Clin Oncol.* 2012;30:2334-2339. PMID: 22614981.

78. Neugut AI, Matasar M, Wang X, et al. Duration of adjuvant chemotherapy for colon cancer and survival among the elderly. *J Clin Oncol.* 2001;24:2368-2375. PMID: 16618946.

79. McCleary NJ, Meyerhardt JA, Green E, et al. Impact of age on the efficacy of newer adjuvant therapies in patients with stage II/III colon cancer: findings from the ACCENT database. *J Clin Oncol.* 2013;31:2600-2606. PMID: 23733765.

80. Hoff PM, Ansari R, Batist G, et al. Comparison of oral capecitabine versus intravenous fluorouracil plus leucovorin as first-line treatment in 605 patients with metastatic colorectal cancer: results of a randomized phase III study. *J Clin Oncol.* 2001;19:2282-2292. PMID: 11304782.

81. Van Cutsem E, Peeters M, Siena S, et al. Open-label phase III trial of panitumumab plus best supportive care compared with best supportive care alone in patients with chemotherapy-refractory metastatic colorectal cancer. *J Clin Oncol.* 2007;25:1658-1664. PMID: 17470858.

82. Colon cancer screening (USPSTF recommendation). U.S. Preventive Services Task Force. *J Am Geriatr Soc.* 2000;48:333-335. PMID: 10733063.

83. Appelbaum FR, Gundacker H, Head DR, et al. Age and acute myeloid leukemia. *Blood.* 2006;107:3481-3485. PMID: 16455952.

84. Rao AV, Valk PJ, Metzeler KH, et al. Age-specific differences in oncogenic pathway dysregulation and anthracycline sensitivity in patients with acute myeloid leukemia. *J Clin Oncol.* 2009;27:5580-5586. PMID: 19858393.

85. Löwenberg B, Ossenkoppele GJ, van Putten W et al. High-dose daunorubicin in older patients with acute myeloid leukemia. *N Engl J Med.* 2009;361:1235-1248. PMID: 19776405.

86. Castaigne S, Pautas C, Terré C, et al. Effect of gemtuzumab ozogamicin on survival of adult patients with de-novo acute myeloid leukaemia (ALFA-0701): a randomised, open-label, phase 3 study. *Lancet.* 2012;379:1508-1516. PMID: 22482940.

87. Rowe JM. Optimal induction and post-remission therapy for AML in first remission. *Hematology Am Soc Hematol Educ Program.* 2009;396-405. PMID: 20008225.

88. Quintás-Cardama A, Ravandi F, Liu-Dumlao T, et al. Epigenetic therapy is associated with similar survival compared with intensive chemotherapy in older patients with newly diagnosed acute myeloid leukemia. *Blood.* 2012;120:4840-4845. PMID: 23071272.

89. Shanafelt T. Treatment of older patients with chronic lymphocytic leukemia: key questions and current answers. *Hematology Am Soc Hematol Educ Program.* 2013;2013:158-167. PMID: 24319177.

90. Shanafelt TD, Rabe KG, Kay NE, et al. Age at diagnosis and the utility of prognostic testing in patients with chronic lymphocytic leukemia. *Cancer.* 2010;116:4777-4787. PMID: 20578179.

91. Fischer K, Cramer P, Busch R, et al. Bendamustine in combination with rituximab for previously untreated patients with chronic lymphocytic leukemia: a multicenter phase II trial of the German Chronic Lymphocytic Leukemia Study Group. *J Clin Oncol.* 2012;30:3209-3216. PMID: 22869884.

92. Goede V, Fischer K, Busch R et al. Obinutuzumab plus chlorambucil in patients with CLL and coexisting conditions. *N Engl J Med.* 2014;370:1101-1110. PMID: 24401022.

93. Shanafelt T, Lanasa MC, Call TG, et al. Ofatumumab-based chemoimmunotherapy is effective and well tolerated in patients with previously untreated chronic lymphocytic leukemia (CLL). *Cancer.* 2013;119:3788-3796. PMID: 23922059.

94. Furman RR, Sharman JP, Coutre SE, et al. Idelalisib and rituximab in relapsed chronic lymphocytic leukemia. *N Engl J Med.* 2014;370:997-1007. PMID: 24450857.

95. Byrd JC, Furman RR, Coutre SE, et al. Targeting BTK with ibrutinib in relapsed chronic lymphocytic leukemia. *N Engl J Med.* 2013;369:32-42. PMID: 23782158.

96. Palumbo A, Mina R. Management of older adults with multiple myeloma. *Blood Rev.* 2013;27:133-142. PMID: 23623929.

97. Fayers PM, Palumbo A, Hulin C, et al. Thalidomide for previously untreated elderly patients with multiple myeloma: meta-analysis of 1685 individual patient data from 6 randomized clinical trials. *Blood.* 2011;118:1239-1247. PMID: 21670471.

98. Mateos MV, Hernández MT, Giraldo P, et al. Lenalidomide plus dexamethasone for high-risk smoldering multiple myeloma. *N Engl J Med.* 2013;369: 438-447. PMID: 23902483.

99. Bergsagel PL, Mateos MV, Gutierrez NC, et al. Improving overall survival and overcoming adverse prognosis in the treatment of cytogenetically high-risk multiple myeloma. *Blood.* 2013;121:884-892. PMID: 23165477.

100. Mateos MV, San Miguel JF. How should we treat newly diagnosed multiple myeloma patients? *Hematology Am Soc Hematol Educ Program.* 2013;488-495. PMID: 24319223.

101. Harousseau JL, Palumbo A, Richardson PG, et al. Superior outcomes associated with complete response in newly diagnosed multiple myeloma patients treated with nonintensive therapy: analysis of the phase 3 VISTA study of bortezomib plus melphalan-prednisone versus melphalan-prednisone. *Blood.* 2010;116:3743-3750. PMID: 20628153.

102. Dimopoulos MA, Leleu X, Palumbo A, et al. Expert panel consensus statement on the optimal use of pomalidomide in relapsed and refractory multiple myeloma. *Leukemia.* Epub 2014 Feb 5. PMID: 24496300.

103. Jakubowiak AJ, Siegel DS, Martin T, et al. Treatment outcomes in patients with relapsed and refractory multiple myeloma and high-risk cytogenetics receiving single-agent carfilzomib in the PX-171-003-A1 study. *Leukemia.* 2013;27:2351-2356. PMID: 23670297.

104. Pfreundschuh M. How I treat elderly patients with diffuse large B-cell lymphoma. *Blood.* 2010;116:5103-5110. PMID: 20805363.

105. Coiffier B, Lepage E, Briere J, et al. CHOP chemotherapy plus rituximab compared with CHOP alone in elderly patients with diffuse large-B-cell lymphoma. *N Engl J Med.* 2002;346:235-242. PMID: 11807147.

106. Rummel MJ, Niederle N, Maschmeyer G, et al. Bendamustine plus rituximab versus CHOP plus rituximab as first-line treatment for patients with indolent and mantle-cell lymphomas: an open-label, multicentre, randomised, phase 3 non-inferiority trial. *Lancet.* 2013;381:1203-1210. PMID: 23433739.

107. Dewilde S, Woods B, Castaigne JG, et al. Bendamustine-rituximab: a cost-utility analysis in first-line treatment of indolent non-Hodgkin's lymphoma in England and Wales. *J Med Econ.* 2014;17:111-124. PMID: 24308372.

108. Wang ML, Rule S, Martin P, et al. Targeting BTK with ibrutinib in relapsed or refractory mantle-cell lymphoma. *N Engl J Med.* 2013;369:507-516. PMID: 23782157.

20

SYMPTOM MANAGEMENT

Charles L. Loprinzi, MD

Hot flashes

▶ Paroxetine is now approved by the U.S. Food and Drug Administration for the treatment of hot flashes.

Nausea and vomiting

▶ Intravenous fosaprepitant, for 1 day, decreases chemotherapy-induced nausea and vomiting as well as 3 days of oral aprepitant (Grunberg S, *J Clin Oncol* 2011).

▶ Fosaprepitant causes vein toxicity in an appreciable number of patients receiving doxorubicin-based chemotherapy (Fujii T, *J Clin Oncol* 2013; Leal AD, *Support Care Cancer* 2014).

▶ Antiemetic guidelines have now established that palonosetron is more effective than other 5-hydroxytryptamine-3 receptor antagonists (Basch E, *J Clin Oncol* 2012).

▶ An olanzapine-based regimen is now endorsed by the 2014 National Comprehensive Cancer Network guidelines for preventing nausea/vomiting from moderately and highly emetogenic regimens.

▶ In 2013, the European Medicines Agency's Committee for Medicinal Products for Human Use recommended that metoclopramide be curtailed due to serious neurologic side effects.

Chemotherapy-induced neuropathy

▶ It has now been shown that intravenous calcium and magnesium are not helpful for preventing oxaliplatin-associated neuropathy (Loprinzi C, *J Clin Oncol* 2013).

▶ Duloxetine moderately decreases established oxaliplatin-associated neuropathic pain (Smith E, *JAMA* 2013).

Cancer fatigue

▶ Ginseng moderately decreases cancer-associated fatigue (Barton D, *J Clin Oncol* 2012; Barton D, *J Natl Compr Canc Netw* 2013).

Mucositis

▶ A doxepin mouthwash moderately decreases oral mucosal pain associated with radiation therapy–induced mucositis (Miller RC, *J Clin Oncol* 2014).

▶ Multinational Association for Supportive Care in Cancer guidelines now recommend low-level laser therapy for oral mucositis prevention in adults receiving high-dose chemotherapy in preparation for hematopoietic stem cell transplantation with or without irradiation. The same has been recommended for the prevention of radiotherapy-induced oral mucositis (Migliorati C, *Support Care Cancer* 2013).

Efforts to alleviate common symptoms related to cancer and/or cancer therapy are important aspects of ideal oncologic patient care. The following symptoms/issues are discussed in this chapter:

- Nausea and vomiting associated with cytotoxic agents
- Management of estrogen-deprivation symptoms
- Oral mucositis and esophagitis associated with treatment
- Malignant ascites
- Anorexia and cachexia
- Diarrhea associated with cancer or cancer therapy
- Cancer fatigue
- Skin rashes from cytotoxic agents
- Chemotherapy-induced peripheral neuropathy
- Sexual health
- Bone health
- Anemia
- Prevention and treatment of thromboembolic complications
- Alopecia

Although these symptoms do not encompass all toxicities of cancer and cancer therapy, others, such as pain, dyspnea, and constipation, are discussed in Chapter 21: Palliative and End-of-Life Care.

NAUSEA AND VOMITING ASSOCIATED WITH CYTOTOXIC AGENTS

Vomiting is a natural protective mechanism to rid the body of toxic substances. However, in the setting of cancer chemotherapy and radiation therapy, nausea and vomiting become toxicities of major concern. For patients, nausea and vomiting are one of the most feared toxicities related to cancer treatment—an observation described in surveys conducted in the 1980s and confirmed in the 1990s—even after the introduction of antiemetic agents that are considered highly effective. Protracted emesis can lead to dehydration, electrolyte imbalance, and other metabolic derangements. Patient refusal to continue chemotherapy also may result. In view of the psychological and social implications, as well as the physical detriments associated with nausea and vomiting, appropriate and effective management of this problem continues to be of major importance.

The emetic response can be conceptualized as a brainstem-based reflex arc. The final common pathway begins in the emetic center, a diffuse neural complex located in the brainstem near the nucleus tractus solitarius. Efferent neuronal pathways from the emetic center activate and coordinate the many muscle groups necessary for an effective vomiting response. This reflex arc has multiple afferent pathways that lead to the vomiting center. The chemoreceptor trigger zone, located in the area postrema adjacent to the fourth ventricle, can be activated by humoral mediators that enter the cerebrospinal fluid. Activation signals are then transmitted to the emetic center. The peripheral pathways begin at nerve endings in the upper gastrointestinal tract itself. Vagal pathways, which terminate in the brainstem, allow activation of the emetic center. Other afferent pathways include cerebral cortical-signaling pathways (learned emesis) and vestibular pathways related to motion sickness.

The emetic reflex arc includes synaptic sites through which signals are relayed to receptors by various neurotransmitters. Identification and blockade of these key neurotransmitter receptors have been the major strategies for the development of effective antiemetic agents. Dopaminergic, serotonergic, and neurokinin receptors have been considered to be of major importance in acute vomiting. Other receptors, such as cannabinoid and opiate receptors, also may have a role in emetic pathways.

Emetic potential can be affected by patient characteristics. Of these features, poor control with prior chemotherapy is particularly important. Emesis tends to be more severe in younger patients than in older patients and in women. A history of motion sickness and/or a history of morning sickness during pregnancy also appear to directly correlate with chemotherapy-induced nausea and vomiting. Findings from several retrospective and prospective studies have suggested that the risk for emesis is lower for patients with a history of excessive alcohol intake than for patients with no such history. However, biochemical and genetic differences that explain these risk factors have not been firmly established.

There are three different types of nausea and vomiting related to chemotherapy: acute (within 24 hours from chemotherapy), delayed (after 24 hours from chemotherapy), and anticipatory (prior to a subsequent chemotherapy dose).

ACUTE NAUSEA AND VOMITING

Acute nausea and vomiting induced by chemotherapy has been defined as that which occurs within the first 24 hours after administration of a chemotherapy agent. This type is generally the most prominent clinical nausea and vomiting problem.

DELAYED NAUSEA AND VOMITING

Some chemotherapy drugs, such as cisplatin and cyclophosphamide, may cause delayed nausea and vomiting, which is defined as occurring 2 to 5 days after administration of chemotherapy. This delayed emesis is often less intense and occurs in fewer patients, but it can be of longer duration than acute emesis. In addition, it may appear independent of the acute emetic response. However, the lack of control of acute emesis is a risk factor for the development of delayed emesis. The relative role of central (as opposed to peripheral) sites of activation for both acute and delayed emesis is controversial. However, the fact that the antiemetic agents that are effective for managing delayed vomiting differ from the agents that are effective for managing acute emesis suggests that different neurotransmitter mechanisms—if not different physical sites—are involved in these two forms of emesis. Delayed nausea and emesis remains a challenge to manage. With the use of available agents, vomiting has been decreased, but nausea has been less influenced. The risk factors are the same as for acute nausea and vomiting and include chemotherapy-related factors and patient characteristics.

ANTICIPATORY NAUSEA AND VOMITING

Anticipatory (learned) emesis is a conditioned reflex that can be rapidly established by poor antiemetic protection during an early course of chemotherapy. It can be triggered by numerous stimuli that come to be associated with chemotherapy and can occur at any time. Anticipatory emesis is similar to conditioned taste aversions that are also sometimes seen in patients with cancer. Although there are treatment strategies for this problem, the best protection against anticipatory emesis is prevention of the conditioning event itself. Thus, appropriately aggressive antiemetic therapy initiated with the first course of chemotherapy is best for an optimal overall antiemetic response.

TREATMENT ACCORDING TO EMETOGENIC POTENTIAL OF CHEMOTHERAPY

In 1999, ASCO convened a multidisciplinary panel to classify the emetogenic potential of chemotherapy agents and to provide recommendations to manage nausea and vomiting.[1] Following an extensive review of the literature and guided by clinical experience, the panel categorized agents based on the incidence with which each chemotherapy regimen caused emesis.[2,3] Regimens causing vomiting in more than 90% of patients receiving such therapy when antiemetics were not employed were classified as high risk. For regimens causing emesis in 30% to 90% of patients, the risk is moderate. The intermediate-risk category in the present classification includes agents that produced emesis in 10% to 30% of patients; the low-risk category includes agents that produced emesis in fewer than 10% of patients.

Combination doxorubicin/cyclophosphamide chemotherapy—although initially considered to be a moderately emetogenic regimen—is now identified as a highly emetogenic regimen.

TREATMENT OF NAUSEA AND VOMITING

The best strategy for managing emesis is prevention. Ideally, other than with the low-risk category, prevention should begin with the first course of chemotherapy, because once emesis occurs, it is far more difficult to control. Effective management of emesis reduces medical complications that can result from protracted vomiting. An added benefit is that control of emesis decreases the possibility of a patient prematurely discontinuing chemotherapy.

Most of the antiemetic agents developed in the 1960s and 1970s were antidopaminergic drugs specifically targeted at the dopamine-2 receptor. These agents include the phenothiazines (e.g., prochlorperazine), the butyrophenones (e.g., haloperidol), and the substituted benzamides (e.g., metoclopramide).

A dose-response curve for efficacy for phenothiazines and butyrophenones indicates that these two classes of agents have a low therapeutic index. Antidopaminergic toxicity, including extrapyramidal reactions, agitation, and depression, is dose-dependent and can be limiting for the use of these agents. Therefore, phenothiazines and butyrophenones generally are used in relatively low doses only to control mildly emetogenic chemotherapy.

The substituted benzamide metoclopramide blocks the dopamine-2 receptor and, at high doses, the 5-hydroxytryptamine (HT)-3 receptor as well. Development of the high-dose metoclopramide regimen (2 mg/kg intravenously every 2 hours for five doses) in 1981 was a breakthrough in antiemetic therapy and provided the first effective treatment for control of emesis induced by high-dose cisplatin. However, antidopaminergic toxicity is a major limiting factor with high-dose metoclopramide. In general, metoclopramide has been replaced with 5-HT3 receptor antagonists because of their improved toxicity profiles. In 2013, the European Medicines Agency's Committee for Medicinal Products for Human Use recommended that metoclopramide be curtailed because of serious neurologic side effects.[4]

Antiemetic agents with a high therapeutic index include 5-HT3 receptor antagonists and corticosteroids (Table 20-1). 5-HT3 receptor antagonists became available in the 1990s and have become a cornerstone of modern antiemetic therapy for highly emetogenic and moderately emetogenic chemotherapy regimens.

Clinical trials have shown that the efficacy is similar for the three 5-HT3 receptor antagonists that have been available in clinical practice for some time: ondansetron, granisetron, and dolasetron. The classic dose-response curve of 5-HT3 receptor antagonists approximates a logarithmic shape; that is, a steep and linear dose response is present until a threshold (shoulder) value is reached, after which, increasing the dose does not further increase efficacy (plateau effect). Although the modest side effect profile of 5-HT3 receptor antagonists allows for dose escalation without a substantial increase in side effects, the most cost-effective dose will be one close to the threshold value; that is, the lowest dose that provides maximum antiemetic protection. However, this value is affected by the emetic potential of the chemotherapy administered; therefore, the threshold value varies for different classes of chemotherapy agents and for high-dose (compared with standard-dose) regimens. As a group, 5-HT3 receptor antagonists have a mild side effect profile, including mild headache, transient and asymptomatic elevation of transaminase levels, and constipation. Additionally, they can cause QTc prolongation, which may be important if used with other newer oral agents such as pazopanib, which may exacerbate this risk. The newest 5-HT3 receptor antagonist, palonosetron, has a longer half-life and a higher receptor-binding affinity than the other three agents. Palonosetron has been established as being more effective than other 5-HT3 receptor antagonists.[5]

Corticosteroids can be useful either as a single agent or in combination with a 5-HT3 receptor antagonist or a

Table 20-1 Antiemetic Agents	
Therapeutic Index	**Agents**
High	5-HT3 receptor antagonists (ondansetron, granisetron, dolasetron, and palonosetron); corticosteroids (dexamethasone and methylprednisolone); neurokinin-1 receptor antagonist (aprepitant)
Limited	Dopamine-2 receptor antagonist (metoclopramide); phenothiazines (chlorpromazine and prochlorperazine); butyrophenones (haloperidol)
Adjunctive	Benzodiazepines (anxiolytics); antihistamines

dopamine-receptor antagonist. Generally, a corticosteroid (e.g., dexamethasone) is recommended whenever a 5-HT3 receptor antagonist is given. A small- to moderate-sized randomized, placebo-controlled, cross-over clinical trial was performed to look at the beneficial effects (e.g., decreased nausea/vomiting) compared with known toxicities of dexamethasone, given on day 2 and 3 postchemotherapy; it showed that significant differences were not found in patient preference, quality of life, or symptoms between the study arms.[6] These results support the opportunity to stop dexamethasone in subsequent chemotherapy courses if the patient develops too many side effects from this drug (e.g., glucose intolerance or insomnia).

The neurokinin-1 receptor antagonist aprepitant was a major advance in the prevention of both acute and delayed nausea and vomiting, especially delayed.[7] In the recent past, it was most commonly prescribed as a 3-day oral treatment. It has now been demonstrated that a single day of intravenous fosaprepitant controls nausea and vomiting as well as 3 days of oral aprepitant.[8] The 2006 ASCO guidelines recommended its use for patients receiving highly emetogenic chemotherapy, including combination doxorubicin/cyclophosphamide chemotherapy.[9]

New data have supported that intravenous fosaprepitant causes substantial venous toxicity when administered through peripheral veins, especially with doxorubicin-based chemotherapy.[10]

The 2014 version of the National Comprehensive Cancer Network (NCCN) guidelines recommend that an olanzapine-containing regimen is an option for preventing nausea and vomiting in patients receiving moderately to highly emetogenic chemotherapy, based on a series of trials supporting its use.[11-14] This regimen consists of oral olanzapine 10 mg on days 1 to 4 along with palonosetron 0.25 mg and dexamethasone 20 mg, both intravenously on day 1. The guidelines also recommend olanzapine as a breakthrough medication in patients who develop nausea/vomiting after chemotherapy.

Studies show that cannabinoids have a low therapeutic index. In addition, their role is limited by side effects such as dizziness, sedation, hypotension, and dysphoria, especially in older adults. Occasionally, adjunctive agents, such as benzodiazepines and antihistamines, are a helpful addition to the antiemetic regimen. If the patient is particularly anxious, an anxiolytic agent such as a benzodiazepine may be helpful, especially 1 to 12 hours prior to therapy. Of the benzodiazepines, lorazepam is used most often; its contribution probably results from its anxiolytic properties.

Management options for anticipatory nausea and vomiting include:

- Prevention by the appropriate use of prophylactic antiemetic use
- Behavioral desensitization
- Distraction
- Focusing on enjoyable things
- Benzodiazepines
- Relaxation

GUIDELINES

Perhaps the best way to ensure the appropriate use of antiemetic agents for patients receiving chemotherapy is to apply guidelines in clinical practice. In addition to ASCO guidelines, last updated in 2012,[5] several other guidelines are available.[15-18]

RADIATION THERAPY–INDUCED NAUSEA AND VOMITING

As with chemotherapy, radiation therapy can cause nausea and vomiting, the treatment field being one of the major determinants of risk. The dose of radiation therapy administered per fraction and the pattern of fractionation are also important risk factors but are less well defined. As with chemotherapy, the risk can be classified as high, intermediate, or low.

The 2006 ASCO guidelines[9] addressed this issue by stating that 5-HT3 receptor antagonists are considered the mainstay of therapy for patients receiving radiation with more than a minimal emetogenic risk. Nonetheless, there is a dearth of data regarding this subject, and more information is desired. In practice, many radiation oncologists do not treat all patients with prophylactic therapy; rather, they treat patients if nausea and vomiting become an issue.

For patients receiving radiation with low emetogenic risk, either a 5-HT3 receptor antagonist or a dopamine-receptor antagonist (e.g., prochlorperazine) can be used as needed and continued prophylactically for each remaining day of radiation treatment. Because the difference in efficacy between dopamine receptor antagonists and 5-HT3 receptor antagonists is smaller in this setting, dopamine receptor antagonists are recommended (based on expense), with 5-HT3 receptor antagonists reserved for rescue.

KEY POINTS

- There are three types of chemotherapy-induced nausea and vomiting: acute, delayed, and anticipatory.
- Serotonin-3 (5-HT3) receptor antagonists are helpful medications for patients receiving emetogenic chemotherapy. When 5-HT3 receptor antagonists are used, corticosteroids also are recommended.
- Oral aprepitant and intravenous fosaprepitant are neurokinin-1 receptor antagonists that are particularly efficacious for preventing delayed nausea and vomiting, and are recommended for patients receiving highly emetogenic chemotherapy.
- Knowledge of the emetogenic potential of chemotherapy agents and the use of antiemetic guidelines is critical to treating patients.

MANAGEMENT OF ESTROGEN-DEPRIVATION SYMPTOMS

HOT FLASHES

Menopausal symptoms, including hot flashes, are highly prevalent among patients with breast cancer and other premenopausal women who undergo ovarian function suppression.

Approximately 75% of men undergoing androgen-deprivation therapy will have substantial discomfort because of hot flashes. Many times, these hot flashes are severe and may last for a considerable time.[19]

Treatment

Estrogens and androgens can alleviate hot flashes for women and men, respectively. Clearly, there is concern about giving estrogen to women who have had breast cancer.[20] Similarly, the administration of androgens to men with prostate cancer defeats the purpose of androgen-deprivation therapy. The consensus among experts is that estrogen-replacement therapy should not generally be recommended for women with a history of breast cancer. In contrast to this recommendation, some data suggest that estrogen therapy is not associated with adverse events for most survivors.[20,21] This means that estrogen can be used by certain women for relief of symptoms, provided they understand the potential risks associated with treatment. Nonetheless, alternative agents are available to control hot flashes for this patient population (Table 20-2).

Progesterone analogs appear to alleviate hot flashes about as effectively as estrogen, with low doses of megestrol acetate or medroxyprogesterone acetate (MPA) decreasing hot flashes by approximately 80%.[22] Despite this efficacy, there is concern regarding the use of any hormone for patients with breast or prostate cancer. Although megestrol acetate is used at times to manage metastatic prostate cancer, men who receive low doses of megestrol acetate may have a marked and prolonged decrease in prostate-specific antigen (PSA) levels when low doses of the drug are withdrawn. This effect is somewhat similar to withdrawal of flutamide, which causes a reduction of prostate cancer activity. Other side effects from megestrol acetate include increased appetite, weight gain, and venous thrombosis; however, these have been largely seen with drug doses that are

many-fold higher than the doses used for the treatment of hot flashes. It is not clear that the same side effects are seen with the low doses used for hot flash management.

An alternative way to give a progesterone analog is to use intramuscular MPA. The results of randomized studies show that intramuscular MPA injections of 400 mg to 500 mg control hot flashes for a prolonged period in breast cancer survivors.[23,24] Because this modality can control hot flashes for a prolonged period, relatively short-term progesterone analog therapy is possible, alleviating the concern about long-term, continuous hormone therapy.

Given that there has been a desire to find nonhormonal agents to treat hot flashes, a number of clinical studies have been conducted to explore this possibility. Selective serotonin receptor reuptake inhibitors and serotonin-norepinephrine receptor reuptake inhibitors, antidepressant medications, have been found to be effective for the treatment of hot flashes (Table 20-2). Pilot studies demonstrated that low doses of venlafaxine decreased hot flash intensity and frequency both in breast cancer survivors and in men receiving androgen-deprivation therapy. The results of a randomized, placebo-controlled trial confirmed these findings in women, demonstrating a dose-response effect with as much as 75 mg daily of venlafaxine (target dose, noting that patients should be started on a 37.5 mg/day dose for a week). This dose resulted in a 60% reduction in the frequency of hot flashes, compared with a 27% reduction for the placebo.[25] Paroxetine (10 mg to 20 mg daily) was associated with a similar reduction in the number of hot flashes in a randomized, placebo-controlled trial.[26] More recently, in randomized, double-blind, placebo-controlled trials, citalopram,[27] escitalopram,[28] and desvenlafaxine[29] decreased hot flashes to a similar degree. Fluoxetine (20 mg daily) and sertraline (50 mg daily) appear to reduce hot flashes slightly more than placebo, but these agents appear to be less effective than the other antidepressants noted above.[30,31] Paroxetine, fluoxetine, and sertraline decrease the metabolism of tamoxifen to its active metabolite, endoxifen, by the enzyme CYP2D6. Therefore, these agents should be avoided for patients receiving tamoxifen. Venlafaxine and citalopram do not alter tamoxifen metabolism as much as some other antidepressants.[32] A meta-analysis confirmed that multiple antidepressants moderately decrease hot flashes.[33]

Data from pilot and randomized clinical trials demonstrate that relatively low doses of gabapentin also decrease the frequency of hot flashes, to a degree similar to that of the newer antidepressant agents.[34-37] Gabapentin should be started at 100 mg to 300 mg daily. After 3 days, the dosing frequency can be titrated upward. Doses of 900 mg daily decrease hot flashes by approximately 50%. Although some data suggest that higher doses may be more efficacious, this has not been proven.

One clinical trial did look at the efficacy of gabapentin compared with venlafaxine utilizing patient preference as its primary endpoint. Patients were randomly assigned to receive venlafaxine or gabapentin in relatively standard doses recommended by previous placebo-controlled clinical hot flash trials. Patients were treated for 4 weeks followed by a 2-week

Table 20-2	**Pharmacologic Treatment of Hot Flashes (Agents Other Than Estrogen)**	
Progesterone Analogs	Megestrol acetate: 20 mg to 40 mg orally per day
	Medroxyprogesterone acetate: 400 mg to 500 mg intramuscular injection (once)
Nonhormonal Agents	Venlafaxine: 37.5 mg orally per day for 1 week, then 75 mg orally per day
	Paroxetine: 10 mg orally per day
	Citalopram: 10 mg to 20 mg orally per day
	Desvenlafaxine: 50 mg orally per day for 1 week, then 100 mg orally per day
	Escitalopram: 10 mg to 20 mg orally per day
	Gabapentin: titrate oral doses up to 900 mg per day
	Clonidine: 0.1 mg orally per day

washout period, before being crossed over to the alternate treatment. Although both agents appeared to reduce hot flashes to similar extents (approximately a 65% reduction) and had similar amounts of toxicities, 68% of patients preferred venlafaxine compared with only 32% of patients who preferred gabapentin (p = 0.01).[38] The authors concluded that venlafaxine was preferred as an initial treatment, but that some patients experienced a better outcome with gabapentin, supporting a trial of this medication if venlafaxine is not sufficiently efficacious.

The results from well-powered, randomized, placebo-controlled trials indicate that the antihypertensive medication clonidine inhibits hot flashes more than placebo (p = 0.0006).[39] However, clonidine causes substantially more toxicity (e.g., hypotension, drowsiness, dry mouth, and constipation) than placebo. Because patients were just as likely to choose placebo as they were clonidine in a randomized, double-blind, cross-over clinical trial, enthusiasm for this agent is tempered.

Although the findings from a number of pilot studies suggested that soy products could alleviate hot flashes, the majority of results from large, placebo-controlled clinical trials do not demonstrate any benefit from a phytoestrogen product for breast cancer survivors.[40,41] Likewise, well-conducted studies have not demonstrated any benefit from black cohosh. Limited data support that vitamin E can decrease hot flashes slightly more than a placebo.[42,43] Lastly, a recent placebo-controlled trial reported that flaxseed did not alter hot flashes.[44]

Several nonpharmacologic options to prevent hot flashes have been studied for otherwise healthy postmenopausal women. Although pilot information supports the use of paced respirations,[39] the more established of these nonpharmacologic approaches to date is hypnosis; randomized trials of clinical hypnosis compared with a structured attention control arm demonstrated a decrease in hot flashes by both patient diary and physiologic measurements of hot flashes[45,46] supporting the use of this approach by experienced personnel.

VAGINAL DRYNESS

Vaginal dryness from urogenital atrophy is another major symptom of estrogen depletion for some women. It can contribute to pain with intercourse, as well as itching and irritation. Non-estrogen–containing vaginal lubricants are helpful for alleviating symptoms.[47] Nonetheless, these products appear to be less efficacious than topical estrogen therapy.[48]

Given that women with estrogen receptor–positive breast cancer benefit from the use of aromatase inhibitors, which lower postmenopausal estrogen levels, and that all vaginal preparations appear to be absorbed to some degree, there is heightened concern about giving vaginal estrogen. Patients must be informed of the risks of vaginal estrogen therapy, and should be allowed to balance the desire for controlled symptoms against presumably small potential risks. However, it does not make much sense to use vaginal estrogens in women on aromatase inhibitors, given that the goal of the latter is to lower estrogen levels as much as possible. There is less theoretical concern in patients on tamoxifen, since tamoxifen works in premenopausal women.

There are intriguing data that dehydroepiandrosterone (DHEA) can decrease vaginal dryness and reduce discomfort during sexual activity without leading to increased systemic estrogen levels in women with vaginal dryness who do not have a history of breast cancer.[49,50] A randomized, double-blind, placebo-controlled clinical trial in patients with a history of breast cancer has completed accrual and results should be available soon.

ORAL MUCOSITIS AND ESOPHAGITIS ASSOCIATED WITH TREATMENT

Oral mucositis and esophagitis are common complications of chemotherapy and radiation therapy. The overall incidence of oral mucositis is approximately 40% for patients who receive standard-dose chemotherapy. The incidence varies with the chemotherapy agents used and increases substantially for patients who receive dose-intensified regimens. Mucositis and esophagitis are common in patients receiving radiation to susceptible areas, and both can be exacerbated by concomitant chemotherapy. Dental evaluation prior to therapy should be encouraged if poor oral hygiene is seen on exam. Mucositis may occur as a result of direct injury from cytotoxic chemotherapy or radiation therapy, secondary infections from treatment-induced myelosuppression, or graft-versus-host disease.

The severity of mucositis is dose- and treatment-specific. Mucositis typically starts 5 to 7 days after the initiation of chemotherapy. It often presents first as erythema on the soft palate, the buccal mucosa, the ventral surface of the tongue, and the floor of the mouth. These symptoms may progress to a generalized desquamation, commonly reaching a maximum on days 11 to 14. More than 90% of ulcerations are localized on nonkeratinized mucosa. Mucositis resulting from chemotherapy can resolve within a few days or last as long as 2 to 3 weeks; oral mucositis caused by radiation therapy typically lasts an average of 6 weeks.

Chemotherapy agents frequently associated with mucositis include the antimetabolites fluorouracil and methotrexate and high-dose or prolonged infusions of chemotherapy. Radiation therapy to the oral cavity frequently causes a host of oral complications, including mucositis, xerostomia, dental caries, tissue necrosis, and taste alterations.

PREVENTION OF CHEMOTHERAPY-ASSOCIATED MUCOSITIS

The Multinational Association of Supportive Care in Cancer (MASCC) has developed clinical practice guidelines for the prevention and treatment of cancer therapy–induced oral and gastrointestinal mucositis.[51] The prevention of oral mucositis is an important goal because, once present, it can make ingestion of fluids, nutrition, and medications difficult. Two general approaches have been taken to try to prevent this condition (Table 20-3). Numerous agents have been proposed to prevent chemotherapy-induced mucositis, but most have not been shown to be effective when compared with a placebo. Such agents include sucralfate, allopurinol, chamomile tea, glutamine, and vitamin E. One treatment that has been shown in clinical trials to effectively prevent mucositis is oral cryotherapy—sucking on ice chips during administration of chemotherapy. This treatment produces temporary vasoconstriction and appears to reduce the delivery of bolus-dose fluorouracil chemotherapy to the oral mucosa. Results from several controlled clinical trials indicated that oral cryotherapy reduces oral mucositis resulting from such treatment by approximately 50%.[52,53] Phase II evidence suggests that oral cryotherapy also decreases edatrexate-associated mucositis.[54-56]

Palifermin,[57-59] a keratinocyte growth factor, has been recommended by guidelines to decrease severe mucositis for patients undergoing autologous stem cell transplantation with total-body irradiation conditioning regimens.

Palifermin also has been studied in a placebo-controlled trial for patients receiving 5-fluorouracil; results suggest that it decreased mucositis more than placebo. The results, however, were not overly promising, and the patients enrolled in

this trial were not given oral cryotherapy to alleviate mucositis. This, and the expense of the drug, precludes its use for preventing fluorouracil-induced mucositis, pending data from subsequent trials.[60]

MASCC guidelines now recommend low-level laser therapy for oral mucositis prevention in adults receiving high-dose chemotherapy in preparation for hematopoietic stem cell transplantation with or without irradiation.[61] This is only applicable for institutions that are geared to give this therapy.

PREVENTION OF RADIATION-ASSOCIATED ORAL MUCOSITIS

A dental evaluation before the initiation of radiation therapy to the oral cavity is recommended. Fluoride carriers can provide fluoride for maintaining tooth integrity and, if worn during treatments, may help prevent radiation scatter from metal dental work, decreasing the inappropriately high radiation dose to buccal mucosa in the vicinity of metal dental work.

Effective management of established oral mucositis includes general measures, such as oral hygiene and dietary modification, topical local anesthetics, and systemic analgesics. MASCC guidelines now recommend low-level laser for the prevention of radiotherapy-induced oral mucositis.[61]

PREVENTION OF RADIATION-ASSOCIATED ESOPHAGITIS

The results of a placebo-controlled trial showed no benefit from the use of sucralfate for the prevention of radiation-associated esophagitis.[62] Some evidence suggests that amifostine can mildly decrease radiation-induced esophagitis but at the cost of moderate toxicity, inconvenience, and expense.[63,64] These data do not support the use of amifostine.

TREATMENT OF ESTABLISHED MUCOSITIS

General measures to treat oral mucositis include good oral hygiene and dietary modification. Patients should brush gently with a soft-bristled toothbrush and fluoride toothpaste two to three times daily. Gentle flossing daily is encouraged to remove food and bacteria build-up. The mouth can be rinsed every 4 hours with a diluted saline and baking soda solution (one-half teaspoon of salt plus one-half teaspoon of baking soda in a cup of warm water). This treatment has been reported to be soothing and is thought to be cleansing. Also, dentures should be removed, particularly at night. It is noteworthy that these recommendations have not been validated by controlled clinical trials but intuitively appear reasonable for recommendation.

The maintenance of adequate caloric intake in the presence of mucositis can be a challenge. The length of time food is allowed to come in contact with the oral mucosa should be limited. The diet should consist of food that requires little or no chewing. Foods that irritate the mucosa (chemically or mechanically) should be avoided, including foods that are acidic, spicy, salty, coarse, or dry.

Adequate relief of pain associated with mucositis should be sought with pharmacologic agents. Recent double-blind, placebo-controlled trial data have supported that a liquid

Table 20-3	**Steps to Prevent Oral Mucositis**	
Step	**Rationale**	**Example**
Alter the mucosal delivery and excretion of individual chemotherapy agents	Mucous membranes have less exposure to the cytotoxic agent	Oral cryotherapy
Modify the epithelial proliferative capabilities of the mucosa	Rate of basal epithelial cell proliferation correlates with the susceptibility of mucosal tissues to the toxic effects of chemotherapy	Palifermin

doxepin preparation decreased oral mucosal pain associated with radiation therapy.[65] Alternatively, local anesthetic agents, such as viscous lidocaine, provide some pain relief, but the effects last for a few hours at best. The use of hydroxypropyl cellulose films as a mechanical barrier has shown some success, but effectiveness lasts only a few hours. Most cancer centers have some type of "magic mouthwash" that typically includes a mixture of diphenhydramine, viscous lidocaine, magnesium hydroxide/aluminum hydroxide, nystatin, and corticosteroids.[66] Although not adequately studied, one randomized trial suggested no benefit of magic mouthwash compared with oral saline and soda mouth rinse.[67] In one small trial of patients receiving combined chemotherapy and radiation to the oral cavity, the use of an oral liquid morphine solution led to a 3.5-day decrease in oral pain when compared with a magic mouthwash preparation.[68] Another small randomized, double-blind, placebo-controlled, cross-over trial also supported benefit for an oral morphine mouthwash.[69] Chlorhexidine is not effective and causes some morbidity, likely associated with its alcohol base. There are a number of other mouthwash preparations that have been proposed as being helpful, but not yet proven.

KEY POINTS

- There are multiple causes of mucositis related to cytotoxic therapy.
- Oral cryotherapy is useful for patients receiving bolus-dose fluorouracil therapy. Several other drugs have been suggested as being helpful for preventing standard chemotherapy-induced mucositis, but the results of randomized trials generally have shown these agents to be ineffective and/or associated with some toxicity.
- Palifermin decreased oral mucositis in patients receiving a bone marrow–ablative chemotherapy regimen associated with a high incidence of mucositis.
- Treatment of established mucositis involves the use of analgesics, a saline and baking soda solution mouthwash, and modification of food consistency.
- A doxepin mouthwash decreases mucosal pain associated with radiation therapy–induced mucositis.

MALIGNANT ASCITES
ETIOLOGY AND DIAGNOSIS

Ascites, the accumulation of fluid in the abdominal cavity, is a common cause of distress for patients with advanced cancer. More than 80% of patients in whom malignant ascites develop have epithelial cancers, particularly of the ovaries, endometrium, breast, colon, gastrointestinal tract, and pancreas.

Under physiologic conditions, intravascular and extravascular hydrostatic and colloid osmotic pressures are in balance, preventing the accumulation of extravascular fluid. Ascites develops when the influx of abdominal fluid increases or the outflow decreases, causing an accumulation of fluid in the peritoneal space. Ascites may indicate conditions that elevate hydrostatic pressure (e.g., congestive heart failure or cirrhosis), conditions that decrease osmotic pressure (e.g., nephrotic syndrome or malnutrition), or conditions in which fluid production exceeds resorptive capacity (e.g., infections and malignant diseases).

Because of the different pathophysiologic features and treatments, physicians must first distinguish between malignant and nonmalignant ascites. It should not be assumed that cancer is the cause until other common etiologies, such as cirrhosis, heart failure, or peritonitis, have been considered.

Clinical determination of the presence or absence of ascites has the advantages of speed, convenience, and cost savings. A focused history and physical examination may identify the signs and symptoms of ascites. The clinical history can distinguish patients with high and low probabilities for ascites. For example, the development of ascites is unlikely for patients who report no increase in abdominal girth and for men who report no history of ankle swelling.

During a physical examination, signs supporting ascites include bulging flanks, dullness over the flanks on percussion, shifting dullness, and the presence of a fluid wave. Diagnostic imaging may help diagnose ascites, particularly if the physical examination is equivocal, when there is a relatively small amount of fluid, or when loculation is present. Ultrasound or computed tomography (CT) of the abdomen may identify even small amounts of free fluid.[70]

When diagnostic confirmation of ascites is needed, analysis of fluid obtained by paracentesis can help determine its cause. Ultrasound guidance is helpful if the fluid is difficult to obtain or loculation is suspected. The most specific test to determine whether the ascites is the result of a malignant process is cytologic analysis; however, the absence of malignant cells does not exclude cancer. The fluid should be evaluated for color, cell count, and total protein concentration; a serum-ascites albumin gradient also should be determined (Table 20-4).

Ascitic fluid indicates a likely malignant etiology when the following are present:

- Blood;
- Positive findings on cytologic analysis;
- Low (negligible) absolute neutrophil count; and/or
- Total protein concentration of at least 2.5 g/dL.

TREATMENT

Once a diagnosis of malignant ascites is established, treatment is largely directed at relieving symptoms such as dyspnea, abdominal pain, fatigue, anorexia or early satiety, and reduced exercise tolerance. Although treatment is not required for patients with a small amount of ascitic fluid, intervention may be needed to relieve symptoms when a larger amount is present. Because each treatment has adverse effects that must be taken into account for the individual patient, the physician should discuss the prognosis, expected response to treatment, and treatment preferences with the patient before making a treatment plan.

Table 20-4 Analysis of Fluid Obtained by Paracentesis		
Characteristics	**Interpretation**	**Comment**
White, milky color	Chylous ascites	
Reddish (bloody) color	Malignant disease	Blood also may be caused by abdominal tuberculosis
Cytologic analysis	Malignant cells indicate cancer	Absence of malignant cells does not exclude cancer
Absolute neutrophil count of greater than 250/μL	Bacterial peritonitis	
Total protein concentration of 2.5 g/dL or less	Transudative ascites (less likely to have malignant cells)	
Serum-ascites albumin gradient of 11 g/L or greater	Portal hypertension	

Table 20-5 Treatment Options for Ascites	
Therapeutic Approach	**Comment**
Sodium restriction	Potential benefits and burdens of sodium restriction, as well as other treatment options, should first be discussed with the patient
Chemotherapy	For patients with cancers that are responsive to chemotherapy, such as lymphoma, breast, or ovarian cancer
Diuretics	Well-tolerated and particularly useful for patients with cancer in whom ascites arises at least partially from nonmalignant causes; must be used carefully (see text)
Paracentesis	For ascites that is associated with respiratory distress or for symptomatic ascites that is resistant to diuretics
Intraperitoneal catheters	For patients who need recurrent paracenteses

Therapeutic interventions for malignant ascites should be carefully selected (Table 20-5), including the use of chemotherapy for patients with potentially chemotherapy-sensitive diseases. Diuretics can be used for select patients. The goal of diuretic therapy is to reduce the fluid accumulation. Diuretics should not be administered to render the patient free of edema and ascites; rather, they should remove only enough fluid to ensure the patient's comfort. Diuresis should be slow and gradual, not to exceed the patient's capacity to mobilize ascitic fluid. Overly aggressive management of ascites for a patient with liver disease may lead to the hepatorenal syndrome and death.

It is usually best to start with a diuretic that works to block the effect of increased aldosterone activity at the distal nephron. Spironolactone often is used as first-line treatment, starting with a daily dose of 25 mg to 50 mg in the morning. Spironolactone may be associated with painful gynecomastia, and as such, amiloride at 5 mg daily is an alternative. If the response is suboptimal despite maximal use of distal diuretics, a low dose of a loop diuretic may be added, such as 20 mg of furosemide daily.

The initial dose of the diuretic may be gradually increased until the desired symptomatic relief is achieved. It may take several weeks for a given dose of diuretic to achieve its ultimate effect. Sometimes, very large doses of diuretics are needed to produce an adequate diuresis.

As with any drug therapy in the supportive care setting, the patient's symptoms and lifestyle should be evaluated to consider the benefits and burdens of the treatment before deciding on medical management of ascites. Diuretic therapy is likely to be burdensome for patients who have limited mobility or urinary tract outflow symptoms, such as hesitancy or frequency, poor appetite or poor oral intake, or difficulties related to polypharmacy.

Diuretic therapy is frequently associated with more disadvantages than benefits for patients with advanced cancer and a poor performance status. In these situations, therapy can result in incontinence, can lead to sleep deprivation, and may cause problems related to self-esteem, skin care, safety, fatigue, hyponatremia, hypokalemia, or symptomatic postural hypotension.

Therapeutic paracentesis may provide symptomatic relief with minimal morbidity and mortality. It may be the only therapeutic modality that is effective for patients with malignant ascites, and it provides symptomatic relief more rapidly than diuretics. As much as 5 L of fluid may safely be removed during a single session. Paracentesis can be performed either in the outpatient clinic setting or in the individual's home. Ascitic fluid, however, may reaccumulate within 1 to 4 days. The frequency of the subsequent drainage depends on the patient's subjective reports of shortness of breath, activity intolerance, or dyspnea on exertion.

A variety of intraperitoneal catheters have been used in patients for whom repeated large-volume paracentesis is needed for comfort and for whom the prognosis warrants a surgical procedure. These include Tenckhoff, Port-a-Cath, and PleurX catheters.[71] Surgical treatment of malignant ascites is associated with risks and, therefore, is rarely recommended.

Anecdotal information suggests that octreotide may be helpful for patients with malignant ascites.[72] A small randomized, placebo-controlled clinical trial of this subject sponsored by the North Central Cancer Treatment Group (NCCTG) of the National Cancer Institute (NCI) was not able to confirm benefit but had low power.[73]

Having reviewed all of the treatment options for malignant ascites, it should be noted that ascites often can be a marker of disease progression. It may be appropriate to have a discussion with these patients that focuses on realistic goals and options, such as supportive care and hospice.

ANOREXIA AND CACHEXIA

Involuntary weight loss has long been recognized as an adverse prognostic factor for patients with cancer. It has been reported to occur in 15% to 40% of patients at the time of presentation and in as many as 80% of patients with advanced cancer. Anorexia contributes to the wasting seen in cancer-related cachexia, but it is not the complete cause. The etiology of involuntary weight loss for patients with cancer is believed to be multifactorial.

In 1980, Dewys et al reported that decreased survival was a consequence of cancer-associated cachexia. A retrospective analysis of 3,047 patients with 11 different tumor types demonstrated a relationship between tumor type and incidence, as well as between tumor type and degree of weight loss. For each tumor type, survival times were shorter for patients who lost weight compared with patients who had not.[74] In addition to survival, there are several other consequences of involuntary weight loss, including decreased response to and tolerance of radiation therapy and chemotherapy, increased frequency of surgical complications, weakness, fatigue, loss of energy, and inability to perform everyday tasks.

Cachexia is the physical wasting of lean body tissue. In 2011, a consensus opinion was reported regarding the definition of cancer cachexia.[75] It is commonly accompanied by anorexia, early satiety, chronic nausea, asthenia, changes in body image, involuntary weight loss, impaired immune function, poor performance status, and fatigue. Cancer-related cachexia differs from simple starvation because there is a disproportionate loss of lean body mass among patients with cancer-induced cachexia. Data support that lean muscle mass measurement by abdominal CT scans can be helpful for defining patients with cancer cachexia, supporting that some patients with cancer cachexia are actually obese. A host of metabolic alterations are thought to play an important role, including tumor products, such as lipolytic and proteolytic factors; humoral factors, such as serotonin and bombesin; and cytokines, such as tumor necrosis factor (TNF), interleukin (IL)-1, IL-6, and interferon-alfa.

The end result is a reduction in the synthesis of lipids and proteins and an increase in lipolysis.[76]

Anorexia is a multidimensional symptom that usually results from multiple contributing factors, some of which are directly related to the presence of the tumor and some of which are related to reversible comorbid factors. The potential causes of anorexia/cachexia include constipation, emesis, mucositis, depression, decreased gastric emptying, dysphagia, food aversions, and fat malabsorption. One of the challenges in the clinical assessment of patients with anorexia is to characterize all of the different contributors so that a targeted treatment approach can be implemented.

The intensity of symptoms varies among patients. Although anorexia may be a major problem for many patients, it is not a major concern for all of them, even if cachexia is prominent. The lack of eating is often a bigger problem for the family than for the patient, because the patient may not be bothered by a lack of appetite. When patients abstain from eating, the family loses a chance to nurture their loved one. Teaching the family to substitute other nurturing activities (e.g., help with bathing, massage) may help to relieve their concerns about the patient's lack of appetite. For some patients, it may be best not to offer medications; anorexia may be one of many symptoms that will promote discussion of the goals of care and lead to a shift to a greater focus on symptom management, supportive care, or hospice.

TREATMENT OF CANCER-RELATED ANOREXIA AND CACHEXIA

Numerous prospective randomized clinical trials have been conducted to ascertain whether nutritional support would improve outcomes for patients with cancer. In general, the results of these studies have shown that if there is such an effect, it is likely a small one or it is confined to a small subset of patients. Nutritional counseling alone is capable of improving daily caloric intake by approximately 450 calories. However, this advantage is generally short-lived and does not appear to translate into improved patient weight, quality of life, or survival.

The use of parenteral nutrition does not have a major role for most patients with advanced cancer.[77] However, it may provide some benefit for selected patients with cancer, such as patients unable to maintain adequate nutrition because of bowel obstruction but who do not have another life-threatening problem. Parenteral nutrition also may benefit cachectic patients who have a potentially curable tumor and who require short-term nutritional support. In addition, parenteral nutrition is useful preoperatively for patients who will have tumor resection. In this latter indication, parenteral nutrition has been shown—in some situations—to decrease surgical complications and to possibly increase survival.

Enteral nutrition, usually through a gastrostomy tube that has been placed endoscopically or by an interventional radiologist, may be considered when food intake is inadequate but the gastrointestinal tract is functionally intact. This technique often is used for patients with upper aerodigestive

Table 20-6 **Advantages of Enteral Nutrition Compared with Parenteral Nutrition**
▪ Fewer risks and complications
▪ Less expensive
▪ More easily carried out at home by most patients
▪ Delivers nutrients in a more physiologic manner

tract cancer who may have temporary disruption of eating and swallowing while undergoing radiation therapy. Enteral nutrition offers several advantages compared with parenteral nutrition (Table 20-6). The major serious complication associated with enteral nutrition is aspiration, with the risk of this complication increasing for patients with delayed gastric emptying. The risk can be reduced by frequent aspiration of the gastric contents during the first days of infusion, to decrease stasis. If stasis is found, metoclopramide or domperidone can be given to increase gastric emptying, understanding that, in 2013, the European Medicines Agency's Committee for Medicinal Products for Human Use recommended that metoclopramide use be curtailed because of serious neurologic side effects. Alternatively, a duodenal tube can be inserted as an alternate route of nutritional support; however, there is no good evidence that placing a tube in the duodenum or jejunum (rather than in the stomach) helps prevent aspiration. All are associated with an increased risk for aspiration pneumonia (as evidenced in dementia studies). Other side effects associated with enteral nutrition include diarrhea or constipation, nausea and vomiting, and abdominal cramping, bloating, or distension.

Fat malabsorption may occur in patients with pancreatic disease, in patients who have had gastric resection or bone marrow transplantations, or in patients who have short-bowel syndrome or chronic radiation enteritis. If there is increased stool odor, an empiric trial of exogenous pancreatic enzyme should be considered. Eight thousand units of lipase should be administered for every 5 g to 7 g of fat in a meal.

Drugs that have been demonstrated to be helpful for the treatment of cancer anorexia/cachexia are listed in Table 20-7.

Megestrol acetate is the drug most widely studied in cancer-related anorexia and cachexia, with at least 12 completed controlled clinical trials. In these studies, megestrol acetate was administered daily throughout periods ranging from 1 week to longer than 12 weeks. Increases in appetite and/or body weight were documented in the vast majority of the studies.[78] Megestrol acetate, at a dosage of 160 mg to 1,600 mg daily, provides benefits for appetite, caloric intake, and weight gain. In one clinical trial, the effect appeared to plateau at 800 mg, suggesting that this amount should be the maximum dose. The weight gained with the use of megestrol is predominantly adipose tissue, not lean body mass.[79]

Benefits of megestrol acetate should not be overestimated. Although randomized, placebo-controlled trials have shown that as many as 70% of patients assigned to the megestrol arm gained weight, so did 44% of those assigned to the placebo group. In addition, there was no effect of megestrol on either survival or quality of life in these studies. The NCCTG conducted a randomized, placebo-controlled trial of megestrol compared with placebo in 243 patients with non-small cell lung cancer and found that those receiving megestrol had a median survival of 8.2 months compared with a 10.2-month median survival in patients on placebo. Jatoi et al estimated that only about 20% of patients receiving megestrol for treatment of anorexia/cachexia will derive benefit.[80-82]

Megestrol acetate is commercially available in the United States as 20-mg and 40-mg tablets and as a 40-mg/mL oral suspension. A 160-mg tablet is available in Canada. Several factors should be considered in dose selection:

▪ Side effects may be dose related.
▪ High doses are expensive. The oral suspension is the preferred delivery mode, as it is less expensive and more bioavailable than the tablets.
▪ Lower doses are effective in stimulating appetite; therefore, it is reasonable to start with a daily dose of 400 mg, with the dose titrated to clinical response.
▪ There is a newer micronized megestrol acetate formulation that reportedly allows for better drug absorption in the fasting state, but it is more expensive than other forms of this drug.[83]

Table 20-7 **Treatment of Cancer-Related Anorexia**		
Drug	**Function**	**Dosing**
Megestrol acetate	Improves appetite, increases caloric intake, decreases nausea and vomiting	Activity seen with range of 160 mg/day to 1,600 mg/day; recommended maximum dose, 800 mg/day
Medroxyprogesterone acetate	Stimulates appetite	Activity seen with range of 300 mg to 1,000 mg/day; generally well tolerated with a side effect profile similar to that of megestrol acetate
Dexamethasone	Increases appetite and food intake and improves the sense of well-being and performance status, generally only for a short period of time	2 mg to 4 mg per day

Megestrol acetate generally is well tolerated, with side effects occurring infrequently and likely in relation to the dose administered. In clinical trials, patients receiving megestrol acetate generally are no more likely to discontinue treatment because of side effects than patients receiving placebo. The side effect of greatest concern is thromboembolic complications. Because of this possibility, megestrol acetate is relatively contraindicated for patients with a history of thromboembolic disease. Also, because the drug can cause adrenal-axis suppression, adrenal insufficiency may occur either while a patient is using the medication or shortly after discontinuing treatment. Thus, in the event of infection, surgery, or trauma, stress doses of corticosteroids should be given. Furthermore, anecdotal experience suggests that megestrol acetate may alter glucose control for patients with diabetes mellitus who require insulin. Of note, this agent has antiemetic efficacy; the findings from randomized, placebo-controlled clinical trials have demonstrated less nausea and vomiting for patients receiving the drug compared with patients receiving placebo preparations.[81,84]

MPA is another progestational agent that stimulates appetite, but it has been less widely studied than megestrol acetate. It is generally well tolerated, with a side effect profile similar to megestrol acetate.

At least five randomized clinical trials have been conducted with various corticosteroids, and the results have indicated that these drugs increase appetite and food intake and enhance the patient's sense of well-being and performance status.[78,85]

To compare the activity and tolerability of megestrol acetate and a corticosteroid, a randomized controlled study was conducted in which patients with cancer-related anorexia and cachexia were randomly assigned to receive 800 mg of megestrol acetate daily or 0.75 mg of dexamethasone four times daily. Patients were followed at monthly intervals. Both drugs produced similar appetite enhancement and changes in non-fluid weight, with a trend favoring megestrol acetate. Drug discontinuation because of toxicity or patient refusal was significantly higher with dexamethasone than with megestrol acetate (36% vs. 25%; p = 0.03). However, deep vein thrombosis was more common with megestrol acetate (5% vs. 1%; p = 0.06).[86]

Several factors should be considered when deciding whether to use megestrol acetate or corticosteroids for the treatment of cancer-related cachexia. Megestrol acetate is favored when cachexia is the main symptom, whereas corticosteroids may be useful when other symptoms, such as pain, also are present. Megestrol acetate is preferable for long-term use or when weight gain is desired. Corticosteroids are particularly useful for patients with limited survival expectancy in whom weight gain is not an anticipated outcome. Corticosteroids should not be used longer than several weeks because longer-term use is associated with unacceptable side effects, such as edema, muscle weakness, dysphoria, hypokalemia, hyperglycemia, and immune suppression. There is no known advantage to using corticosteroids and megestrol acetate concomitantly.

Cyproheptadine is a serotonin antagonist that has been available for longer than 20 years. It has been used in Latin America and Europe as an appetite stimulant for patients with cancer. In a large randomized controlled study, oral cyproheptadine, at a dose of 8 mg three times daily, produced a mild increase in appetite and food intake but had no effect on progressive weight loss.[87] As a result of its side effects (notably sedation) and lack of much efficacy, cyproheptadine is not recommended for patients with cancer-related cachexia.

Many other agents have been suggested for the treatment of cancer-related anorexia and cachexia, but none of these agents have been beneficial when tested in controlled clinical trials. These drugs include hydrazine sulfate, eicosapentaenoic acid, pentoxifylline, and dronabinol.[88-91] Reports of trials involving antibodies against TNF (otherwise known as cachectin), such as etanercept and infliximab, suggest that these drugs also are not helpful.[92] Newer drugs being tested as potential therapies for cancer cachexia include olanzapine (an antipsychotic agent that increases appetite), gherelin (a growth hormone-related analog), enobosarm (an androgenic preparation), and myostatin inhibitors.

KEY POINTS

- Anorexia is a prominent clinical problem for many patients with advanced cancer. For patients with far-advanced cancer who are not undergoing therapy, anorexia needs to be treated only if the patient considers it to be a substantially bothersome symptom.
- The two classes of medications that have been demonstrated to be helpful for cancer-related anorexia and cachexia are corticosteroids and progesterone analogs. Progesterone analogs (e.g., megestrol acetate) are generally better tolerated than corticosteroids when given for long periods of time.
- Deep vein thrombosis and adrenal suppression are two notable side effects of megestrol acetate.
- Total parenteral nutrition should be used for carefully selected patients only.
- Anorexia may cause emotional problems for family members because of a perception of a lost nurturing opportunity. Teaching the family to substitute other nurturing activities (e.g., help with bathing, massage) may be beneficial.

DIARRHEA ASSOCIATED WITH CANCER OR CANCER THERAPY

Cancer and cancer therapy can cause diarrhea from any one of a large number of mechanisms. Careful evaluation is required to determine the most effective therapy for the patient. Nonpharmacologic and pharmacologic steps often are required for the management of acute treatment-related diarrhea, and several nonpharmacologic measures can be carried out in clinical practice to manage subacute diarrhea (Table 20-8).[93] Rehydration is important for patients with diarrhea severe enough to cause dehydration. Usually, an increased intake of clear liquids

Table 20-8 Steps in the Treatment of Patients with Diarrhea

- Conduct a comprehensive evaluation of the patient at the first report of diarrhea.
- Obtain information about the onset and duration of diarrhea and the number and characteristics of the stool.
- Ask the patient about other symptoms, such as fever, abdominal pain, dizziness, and weakness, that could indicate the cause of diarrhea and the risk of dehydration and infection.
- Review the patient's diet and medication usage to identify any foods or medicines that may be causing or contributing to the diarrhea.
- Advise the patient to eat frequent small meals and to avoid foods that irritate the intestines or stimulate its motility.
- Encourage the patient to drink 8 to 10 large glasses of clear liquid per day in order to maintain adequate hydration and to prevent potential dehydration.
- Taper or eliminate medications that may cause or exacerbate diarrhea, if medically possible.

Table 20-9 Incidence of Diarrhea for Irinotecan and Topotecan

Drug	Diarrhea	
	Any Grade (%)	Grade 3 or 4 (%)
Irinotecan		
Early-onset diarrhea	50	10
Late-onset diarrhea	90	30
Topotecan	30	5

will suffice, but parenteral administration of fluids and electrolytes may be necessary for some patients.

CHEMOTHERAPY-INDUCED DIARRHEA

Etiology and Incidence

Chemotherapy can cause diarrhea by irritating or damaging the crypt and villous cells of the intestinal mucosa. The incidence and severity of chemotherapy-induced diarrhea depends on a number of factors, including the treatment regimen and drug doses. In general, diarrhea is most common with regimens that include antimetabolites. Of these agents, fluorouracil (5-FU) is the most studied agent. The risk for diarrhea from 5-FU increases when leucovorin is given as a modulating agent. Of note, capecitabine provides long-term exposure to 5-FU similar to infusional 5-FU and has similar toxicities.

Diarrhea also is common with other antimetabolites, such as irinotecan and topotecan. With irinotecan, diarrhea may occur immediately after administration through a cholinergic mechanism (early-onset diarrhea), or a more severe, potentially life-threatening form of diarrhea may develop days after administration (late-onset diarrhea). The severity of late-onset diarrhea correlates with peak plasma levels of the irinotecan metabolite, SN38. The incidence of diarrhea associated with these two drugs for patients with metastatic cancer of the colon or rectum ranges from 5% to 90% (Table 20-9).[93] It is important to note that patients who have received antibiotics or cisplatin-based therapy may have a *Clostridium difficile* infection and that patients with neutropenia might develop typhlitis.

Treatment

The choice of effective pharmacologic measures is limited despite the availability of many types of anti-diarrheal agents. Atropine can be used to treat the acute-onset diarrhea with irinotecan. Opioid-like medications often are useful for other types of therapy-related diarrhea, understanding that they are relatively contraindicated with infectious causes of diarrhea. Of these agents, loperamide and diphenoxylate are most commonly used for treating acute diarrhea caused by a variety of conditions. Octreotide also is effective and is generally well tolerated. Loperamide has been compared with octreotide for the treatment of fluorouracil-induced diarrhea. In one clinical trial, 41 patients, with grade 2 or greater diarrhea (according to the NCI Common Terminology Criteria for Adverse Events) resulting from fluorouracil-containing chemotherapy, were randomly assigned to receive 0.1 mg of subcutaneous octreotide twice daily for 3 days or 4 mg of oral loperamide initially and then 2 mg every 6 hours for 3 days. Diarrhea resolved in 19 of the 21 patients (91%) in the octreotide arm compared with three of the 20 patients (15%) in the loperamide arm (p = 0.005). No side effects were observed in either treatment arm.[94] An alternative to starting octreotide upon the failure of the doses of loperamide utilized in this randomized trial is to give higher doses of loperamide (i.e., 4 mg initially and then 2 mg every 2 hours) until the patient has been diarrhea-free for 12 hours.

A randomized, double-blind clinical trial of octreotide was conducted in patients receiving cisplatin. All of the patients enrolled in the study had experienced diarrhea as a result of a prior course of cisplatin therapy. Forty-three patients were randomly assigned to receive octreotide (0.1 mg) or placebo (1 cc of saline solution) by subcutaneous injection 15 minutes before and 6 hours after cisplatin therapy. Diarrhea, defined as more than two loose bowel movements per day, occurred in 75% of patients who received placebo and in 5% of patients who received octreotide (p = 0.01). Side effects were minimal. These findings suggest that octreotide is useful for the secondary prevention of cisplatin-induced diarrhea for patients with a history of diarrhea during prior courses of cisplatin.[95]

Treatment of chemotherapy-induced diarrhea can follow an algorithmic approach, as shown in Table 20-8 and Fig. 20-1.[93]

RADIATION-INDUCED DIARRHEA

Etiology and Incidence

Diarrhea is the most common adverse effect of pelvic radiation therapy. Such therapy damages the mucosa of the small and large intestines and thereby can produce secretory diarrhea. The incidence and severity increases with the addition of fluorouracil. For example, in one study, the combination of

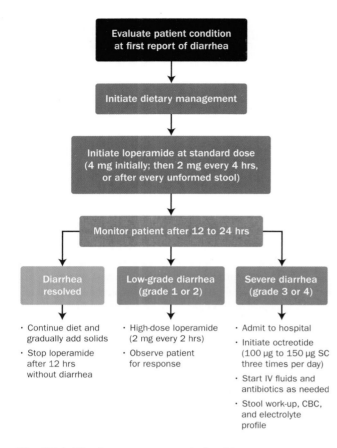

Fig. 20-1 Diarrhea management algorithm.

Abbreviations: hrs, hours; SC, subcutaneously; IV, intravenous; CBC, complete blood count.

fluorouracil and radiation therapy produced a significantly higher rate of acute diarrhea at any time during treatment than radiation therapy alone (79% vs. 41%; p = 0.001). The difference between the two groups was also observed for grade 3 and 4 diarrhea (22% vs. 4%; p = 0.001).[96]

Treatment

A number of placebo-controlled clinical trials have been unable to identify a drug that can be used to prevent diarrhea induced by pelvic radiation therapy. The findings from one trial involving olsalazine suggested that the use of this agent increased diarrhea.[97] Similar findings were seen with recently seen with sulfasalazine.[65]

Another trial demonstrated that cholestyramine decreased diarrhea but at the cost of other toxicities that negated the benefit.[98] Trials of sucralfate have provided mixed results that preclude its recommendation for clinical practice use.[99,100] Glutamine did not improve diarrhea in a double-blinded clinical trial.[101] A randomized, double-blind, placebo-controlled clinical trial was unable to demonstrate any benefit for octreotide as an agent to prevent radiation-induced diarrhea.[102]

Preliminary evidence suggests that octreotide, however, may have a role in the treatment of diarrhea induced by pelvic radiation therapy. Thirty-two patients with grade 2 or 3 diarrhea associated with pelvic radiation therapy were randomly assigned to receive 0.1 mg of subcutaneous octreotide three times daily or 10 mg of oral diphenoxylate (with atropine) daily. Diarrhea resolved within 3 days for 13 of the 16 patients in the octreotide arm and for three of the 16 patients in the diphenoxylate arm (81% vs. 19%; p = 0.005).[103]

The most important lesson to be learned from clinical trials designed to evaluate diarrhea prevention for patients receiving pelvic radiation therapy is that the use of pharmacologic agents, on an ad hoc basis outside of a clinical trial, may be inappropriate. Virtually all of the various categories of agents evaluated in clinical trials consistently failed to show a benefit with an acceptable safety profile. Thus, using seemingly benign drugs to prevent diarrhea during pelvic radiation therapy may expose patients to toxicity without any corresponding benefit.

GRAFT-VERSUS-HOST DISEASE–ASSOCIATED DIARRHEA

For patients who have received a bone marrow transplant, diarrhea may result from graft-versus-host disease (GVHD) or from infections related to the use of immunosuppressive therapy. The epithelial damage caused by high-dose chemotherapy can serve as a stimulus for activation of alloreactive cytotoxic T cells, which release a cascade of inflammatory cytokines that contribute to necrosis of epithelial crypt cells.

At the first sign of acute gastrointestinal symptoms that may signify a graft-versus-host reaction, a stool specimen should be evaluated for bacterial, fungal, and viral pathogens, and supportive management should be initiated. In addition, the general measures for managing diarrhea should be used (Table 20-8). Consultation with a gastroenterologist should be considered.

If the findings on stool evaluation are positive for pathologic bacteria, a course of appropriate antibiotics should be started. For patients with a diagnosis of GVHD (established by biopsy), corticosteroids should be used, and prophylactic immunosuppressive therapy should be continued. Octreotide should be considered at an intravenous dose of 500 mcg three times daily. If the patient has a response within 4 days, octreotide should be discontinued to avoid ileus. However, if there is no response to octreotide, second-line therapy with antithymocyte globulin or with infliximab should be considered. Alternatively, participation in a clinical trial regarding this problem is reasonable, as there is no uniform agreement on the ideal treatment for this problem.

CANCER-ASSOCIATED DIARRHEA

Cancer itself, rather than its treatment, may cause diarrhea. For example, in pancreas cancer, the presence of inadequate digestive enzymes may lead to osmotic diarrhea. For patients who have an increased stool odor, an empiric trial of exogenous pancreatic enzyme should be considered. There are various forms of pancreatic enzymes that contain various amounts of lipase, protease, and amylase. Doses need to be individualized and modified based on results.

Secretory diarrhea may occur in medullary thyroid cancer as a result of the overproduction of calcitonin and prostaglandins, in carcinoid syndrome as a result of the increased secretion of prostaglandins and serotonin, and with pancreatic islet cell cancers. In these situations, octreotide generally is the best option for controlling diarrhea. Cyproheptadine also may be helpful for carcinoid syndrome–related diarrhea.

CANCER FATIGUE

Fatigue is one of the most bothersome symptoms in patients with cancer.[104,105] It affects patients receiving adjuvant chemotherapy or radiation therapy and those with advanced disease. Fatigue has been noted to occur in anywhere from 60% to 90% of patients receiving chemotherapy and in 65% to 100% of patients receiving radiation therapy. The NCCN has defined cancer fatigue as "a persistent subjective sense of tiredness related to cancer or cancer treatment that interferes with usual functioning." This problem is often not relieved with rest.

Evaluation of this problem should consist of a history, physician examination, and screening blood work, including a complete blood count and chemistry evaluation of renal function, thyroid function, liver function, calcium, and electrolytes. Adrenal function tests also may be indicated in selected situations, and screening for depression also is appropriate. If any abnormalities are noted from the screening evaluation, reasonable attempts to correct these abnormalities are recommended.

Exercise is a commonly recommended therapy for cancer-related fatigue.[106-113] Psychostimulants such as methylphenidate and modafinil have been studied, but the bulk of evidence suggests that they are not very helpful.[114-117] Ginseng also has been studied, based on preliminary clinical information and animal data.[118-122] Two randomized, placebo-controlled trials

support that ginseng is helpful for alleviating cancer-related fatigue.[123,124] The recommended dose from these studies is 2,000 mg per day, divided into two doses of 1,000 mg each at breakfast and lunch. It is probably best to take both doses before noon just to better ensure that it does not have a negative effect on sleep. The two studies evaluated American ginseng and used a pure ground root product. It may be important to use pure ground root as opposed to extracted ginseng that could have ethanol. The use of ethanol-derived extracts has been found, in preclinical studies, to exhibit estrogenic characteristics and, therefore, would be contraindicated for most breast cancer survivors and patients with other estrogen-sensitive cancers. If American ginseng is purchased in a store or online, it is important to buy pure ground root, preferably 5% ginsenoside content, as opposed to ginseng extract, because under most circumstances, it will not be obvious what was used to make the extract. It might be best to obtain the manufactured product that was used in the actual clinical trials (which can be obtained online), given the unregulated status of herbal preparations in some countries.

SKIN RASHES FROM TARGETED AGENTS AND CAPECITABINE

RASHES ASSOCIATED WITH EPIDERMAL GROWTH FACTOR RECEPTOR INHIBITORS AND OTHER TARGETED AGENTS

Epidermal growth factor receptor (EGFR) inhibitors are approved by the U.S. Food and Drug Administration (FDA) for use in various cancers.[125-128] One of the most common toxicities of EGFR inhibitors is a prominent skin rash, affecting as many as 50% of patients treated with these drugs.[128-130] This rash has acne-like characteristics, but is not considered acne (Fig. 20-2). Other targeted drugs that are associated with a similar rash include inhibitors of the mammalian target of rapamycin (mTOR), such as everolimus and temsirolimus, and multikinase inhibitors such as sorafenib and sunitinib.

Although there are many anecdotal therapies that may be useful in this situation, there are a paucity of clinical trial data to appropriately guide therapeutic choices. Three randomized, double-blind, placebo-controlled clinical trials have looked at tetracycline or a tetracycline derivative as a potential means for preventing this rash for patients initiating EGFR inhibitor

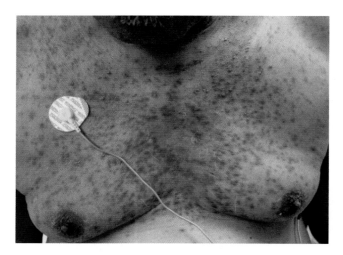

Fig. 20-2 Representative papular rash in a patient receiving an epidermal growth factor receptor (EGFR) antagonist.

therapy. Two of these trials suggested that tetracycline or minocycline use moderately decreased rash severity,[131,132] although the third trial did not support this finding.[133]

A manuscript[134] has reported that a combination therapy approach decreased EGFR inhibitor (i.e., panitumumab) skin toxicity when compared with a control group. The treatment consisted of skin moisturizers, sunscreen, a topical steroid preparation (1% hydrocortisone cream), and doxycycline (100 mg twice daily). Despite the treatment groups being randomly assigned, the control arm did not receive placebo preparations, so there was no attempt to blind the patients or their attending physicians. Although the data from this pilot randomized trial are, thus, not definitive, they nonetheless were associated with a markedly decreased incidence in reported grade 2 or worse skin toxicity (62% vs. 29%).

Given the paucity of definitive clinical trials regarding the management of this rash, the therapeutic options are based on clinical experience and expert opinions. Consultation with a dermatologist is recommended for patients with moderate to severe rashes. Agents that have been recommended for use include sunscreen (despite a placebo-controlled trial that was unable to prove benefit),[135] skin moisturizers, steroid creams, topical clindamycin, and oral doxycycline. For severe rashes, investigation of potential infections is appropriate.

In addition to the acneiform rash, these drugs can also cause a large number of other dermatologic problems including periungual disease, photosensitivity, pruritus, xerosis, Stevens-Johnson syndrome, and skin cancers. Of note, there are extensive data supporting that patients who develop a rash appear to have more antitumor activity with the EGFR inhibitor than patients who do not develop a rash.[136-139] This may be related to pharmacogenetic factors.

CAPECITABINE AND LIPOSOMAL DOXORUBICIN RASHES

One of capecitabine's dose-limiting toxicities is a prominent rash labeled palmar-plantar erythrodysesthesia, also known as hand-foot syndrome. This problem can be seen, usually to a lesser extent, from other chemotherapy agents, such as infusional 5-FU. Symptoms from this problem usually begin with erythema and proceed to pain and then to desquamation. If the drug is used for too long, this syndrome can lead to substantial morbidity to the point that patients may be incapacitated, are unable to use their hands well, and/or are unable to walk. Patients also may develop ulcers that do not heal well.

Anecdotal information had suggested that vitamin B6 was helpful for alleviating this problem, but a large placebo-controlled study was unable to show any benefit for this approach.[140] Another proposed antidote consisted of a urea-lactic acid cream, but a placebo-controlled NCCTG trial suggested that it actually caused more skin troubles than did a placebo.[141]

At this time, it is recommended that patients are carefully educated to immediately stop taking their planned multiday cycle of capecitabine if they develop tenderness of their palms or soles. Doses from the next cycle should be appropriately attenuated.

Liposomal doxorubicin also causes palmar-plantar erythrodysesthesia, affecting about 20% of patients at the FDA-approved dose of 50 mg/m². Although topical emollients have been commonly used for symptom management, there are no good studies to demonstrate benefit; dose reduction is helpful to decrease risk in subsequent cycles.

KEY POINTS

- Epidermal growth factor receptor (EGFR) inhibitors commonly cause rashes.
- Patients with rashes may be more likely to have EGFR inhibitor–induced tumor regression or stability.
- Capecitabine-induced palmar-plantar erythrodysesthesia is best managed by dose attenuation.

CHEMOTHERAPY-INDUCED PERIPHERAL NEUROPATHY

Chemotherapy-induced peripheral neuropathy (CIPN) is a common clinical problem, especially with platinum agents, taxanes, vinca alkaloids, and epothilones. These agents can cause numbness, tingling, and pain, usually in a stocking-glove distribution. Additionally, data strongly support that the acute pain syndrome caused by paclitaxel, which has classically been identified as "arthralgias and myalgias," is not from an injury to muscles or joints; rather, it appears to be a manifestation of an acute neuropathy.[142,143]

ASCO guidelines have recently interrogated the value of such agents for preventing CIPN and for treating established CIPN.[144] Table 20-10 provides the results of this work.

SEXUAL HEALTH

As highlighted in an article in the "Art of Oncology" section of the *Journal of Clinical Oncology*, "The Sounds of Silence: Sexuality

Table 20-10 **Summary Recommendations from ASCO Guideline on Prevention and Management of Chemotherapy-Induced Peripheral Neuropathy (CIPN)**[144]

Guideline Question

What are the optimum prevention and treatment approaches in the management of chemotherapy-induced neuropathies in adult cancer survivors?

Target Population
- Adult cancer survivors with chemotherapy-induced neuropathies

Target Audience
- Health care practitioners who provide care to cancer survivors

Recommendations
- The following recommendations are evidence-based, informed by small randomized controlled trials, and guided by clinical experience. The recommendations were developed by a multidisciplinary group of experts.

Prevention of CIPN
- There are no established agents recommended for the prevention of CIPN in patients with cancer undergoing treatment with neurotoxic agents. This is based on the paucity of high-quality, consistent evidence and a balance of benefits versus harms.
- Clinicians should not offer the following agents for the prevention of CIPN to patients with cancer undergoing treatment with neurotoxic agents:
  - Acetyl-L-carnitine (ALC)
  - Amifostine
  - Amitriptyline
  - Calcium/magnesium (CaMg) for patients receiving oxaliplatin-based chemotherapy
  - Diethyldithiocarbamate (DDTC)
  - Glutathione (GSH) for patients receiving paclitaxel/carboplatin chemotherapy
  - Nimodipine
  - ORG 2766
  - All-trans retinoic acid
  - RhuLIF (recombinant human leukemia inhibitory factor)
  - Vitamin E

  Venlafaxine is not recommended for routine use in clinical practice. While the venlafaxine data support its potential utility, the data were not strong enough to recommend its use in clinical practice until additional supporting data become available.

  No recommendations can be made on the use of N-acetylcysteine, carbamazepine, glutamate, or glutathione for patients receiving cisplatin or oxaliplatin-based chemotherapy, goshajinkigan (GJG), omega-3 fatty acids, or oxcarbazepine for the prevention of CIPN at this time.

Treatment of CIPN
- For patients with cancer experiencing CIPN, clinicians may offer duloxetine.

  No recommendations can be made on the use of:
  - Acetyl-L-carnitine, noting that a positive phase III abstract supported its value, but this work has not yet been published in a peer-reviewed journal and a prevention trial suggested that this agent was associated with worse outcomes.
  - Tricyclic antidepressants; however, based on the limited options that are available for this prominent clinical problem and the demonstrated efficacy of these drugs for other neuropathic pain conditions, it is reasonable to try a tricyclic antidepressant (e.g., nortriptyline or desipramine) in patients suffering from CIPN following a discussion with the patients about the limited scientific evidence for CIPN, potential harms, benefits, cost, and patient preferences.
  - Gabapentin, noting that the available data were limited regarding its efficacy for treating CIPN. However, the panel felt that this agent is reasonable to try for selected patients with CIPN pain given that only a single negative randomized trial for this agent was completed, given the established efficacy of gabapentin and pregabalin for other forms of neuropathic pain, and given the limited CIPN treatment options. Patients should be informed about the limited scientific evidence for CIPN, potential harms, benefits, and costs.
  - A topical gel treatment containing baclofen (10 mg), amitriptyline hydrochloride (40 mg), and ketamine (20 mg), noting that a single trial supported that this product did decrease CIPN symptoms. Given the available data, this agent is reasonable to try for selected patients with CIPN pain. Patients should be informed about the limited scientific evidence for the treatment of CIPN, potential harms, benefits, and costs.

Reprinted from Hershman DL, Lacchetti C, Dworkin RH, et al. Prevention and management of chemotherapy-induced peripheral neuropathy in survivors of adult cancers: American Society of Clinical Oncology Clinical Practice Guideline. J Clin Oncol. 2014;32:1941-1967. PMID: 24733808.

Information for Cancer Patients,"[145] discussion of sexual health is not something that often happens in oncologists' offices. There are at least two reasons this topic rarely is addressed. First, oncologists have limited experience and/or comfort with discussing this issue, and second, there are limited proven therapies available for patients with cancer who have sexuality concerns—at least regarding those therapies that an oncologist can administer. However, it is recommended that oncologists take a sexual history, with referral to appropriate specialists if a problem is identified.[145]

A study examining sexuality issues in patients with cancer evaluated transdermal testosterone administration in women with complaints of decreased libido. A number of prior trials in women who did not have cancer had evaluated testosterone in a similar dose and formulation. The results of these trials were positive, suggesting that testosterone improved libido, at least to some degree.[146,147] However, the results of the randomized, double-blind, placebo-controlled trial of transdermal testosterone in women with cancer were negative.[148] A potential explanation for the negative trial in patients with cancer is that the women involved in this trial were postmenopausal and did not receive supplemental estrogen. In all of the previous trials in other patient groups, women had been premenopausal and/or had also been receiving estrogen replacement therapy.

KEY POINTS

- Sexual health concerns are common in patients with cancer.
- Sexual health is not commonly discussed by oncologists.
- Testosterone, without the addition of estrogen replacement therapy, does not appear to help libido in postmenopausal women with cancer.

BONE HEALTH

Bone health issues in the general population are receiving more attention with the recognition of fracture problems associated with osteopenia/osteoporosis, the aging population, and the availability of treatment options for prevention and/or treatment of this situation. Women with breast cancer and men with prostate cancer have more bone loss issues than patient populations with most other cancers.

BREAST CANCER

Women with breast cancer are at an increased risk for osteoporotic troubles because of treatment-induced menopause. Treatment-induced menopause can occur as a result of chemotherapy or from oophorectomies performed for therapeutic or preventative reasons. In addition, aromatase inhibitors lower estrogen levels for postmenopausal women and, by this means,

this class of drugs increases the risk of osteoporosis and subsequent fractures.

Given these heightened risks, ASCO guidelines recommend interval bone mineral density screening for women with breast cancer after they have experienced menopause.[149]

Current recommendations in women with osteopenia or osteoporosis include weight-bearing physical activity, a calcium intake of 1,200 mg to 1,500 mg per day (in diet and supplements), and vitamin D intake of 1,000 IU per day. Smoking cessation and moderate or lessened alcohol intake is suggested. Bisphosphonates, available in intravenous or oral formulations, or denosumab also are recommended for woman diagnosed with osteoporosis.

A number of clinical trials have been developed to examine bone loss issues in women with breast cancer. More than 200 premenopausal women receiving adjuvant chemotherapy for breast cancer were enrolled in a clinical trial that randomly assigned the participants to receive calcium and vitamin D or the same supplements plus oral weekly risedronate. This trial demonstrated that risedronate did not substantially attenuate the bone loss for these patients.[150] Another similar trial, however, demonstrated that intravenous zoledronate decreased bone loss for these patients.[151] Nonetheless, there is no published evidence yet that these interventions decrease osteoporotic bone fractures in this setting. Thus, bisphosphonates are not routinely recommended for treatment of premenopausal women receiving adjuvant chemotherapy for breast cancer.

Many trials also have examined the prevention of bone loss associated with aromatase inhibitor therapy. Large trials of women receiving aromatase inhibitors have been conducted in which patients were randomly assigned to receive a bisphosphonate (either intravenous zoledronic acid or oral risedronate) or no treatment. These trials have demonstrated that bisphosphonate therapy attenuates the bone loss seen with use of an aromatase inhibitor.[152] Similar findings have been observed in patients randomly assigned to denosumab, an antibody targeted against RANK ligand and given by subcutaneous injections, compared with a placebo.[153]

However, a substantial reduction in bone fractures has not been reported from these trials; therefore, it is not routinely recommended that such patients receive a bisphosphonate or denosumab as part of standard therapy, unless a patient has osteoporosis or marked osteopenia.

A randomized trial compared denosumab with zoledronic acid in 1,026 patients with metastatic breast cancer.[154] This study supported that denosumab, compared with zoledronate, increased the time to skeletal-related events (p = 0.01), had better reductions in bone turnover markers, caused more hypocalcemia, had less renal toxicities and acute phase reaction troubles, and was associated with similar survival rates, times to disease progression, and incidences of osteonecrosis of the jaw. According to a 2011 updated ASCO guideline, there is not enough evidence to recommend either a bisphosphonate or denosumab compared with the other (Table 20-11).[149]

PROSTATE CANCER

It has been well understood that men with prostate cancer receiving androgen ablation therapy have an increased risk for bone loss. Studies have randomly assigned men receiving androgen ablation therapy to a bisphosphonate or to no treatment. The results from these trials demonstrate an attenuation of bone loss with the use of a bisphosphonate. Similar data were seen in a trial comparing denosumab with a placebo, involving 1,468 men.[155] No clear evidence of decreased bone fractures, however, has been reported.[156] Thus, the recommendations for patients with prostate cancer include screening for bone density and treatment with a bone antiresorptive agent if they become markedly osteopenic or osteoporotic.

Data support that bisphosphonates will decrease skeletal-related events in patients with metastatic prostate cancer. Denosumab decreases skeletal-related events slightly better and decreases markers of bone turnover more than a bisphosphonate, although it is not related to improved survival rates and it comes at an increased economic cost.[157] Thus, as with metastatic breast cancer, there is no clearly preferred agent (Table 20-11).[158]

MULTIPLE MYELOMA AND OTHER SOLID CANCERS

Similar data are available for bisphosphonates and denosumab in patients with myeloma and other solid cancers with bone metastases (Table 20-11). Notable differences are that patients with non-small cell lung cancer had a suggestion of improved survival rates with zoledronate compared with denosumab, while the opposite was seen in patients with multiple myeloma.[159]

OSTEONECROSIS OF THE JAW AND BRITTLE BONE FRACTURES

A serious side effect of intravenous bisphosphonate therapy and denosumab is osteonecrosis of the jaw.[160, 161] This condition is relatively uncommon but can be clinically devastating when it occurs. It is particularly problematic in patients with poor dentition and/or for patients requiring dental work.

Somewhat similar to the problem of osteonecrosis of the jaw are reports of brittle bone fractures in patients on long-term bisphosphonate therapy. Although this phenomenon has not yet been established with the use of bisphosphonates in patients taking this therapy for osteoporosis, there may be a higher risk for this problem in patients with cancer who are receiving higher-dose, longer-term bone antiresorptive therapy.

There has been substantial interest in the frequency and duration of antiresorptive bone therapy for patients with cancer. Oncologists question the routine use of long-term therapy for patients with cancer, based on concern about this toxicity. The safest and most effective interval for treatment with these agents is yet to be defined. The 2011 updated ASCO guidelines state that there is no proof that therapy longer than 1 year is more beneficial than 1 year of therapy.[149]

Table 20-11	Results of Phase III Randomized Trials Comparing Zoledronic Acid with Denosumab					
	Time to First SRE					
Primary Cancer Site Evaluated by Trial	**Median (months)***	**HR**	**95% CI**	**p-value**	**Overall Survival**	**Summary of AEs of Interest (trends and statistically significant; unadjusted)**
Solid tumors (not breast or prostate) and myeloma[159]	20.6 vs. 16.3	0.84	0.71, 0.98	< 0.001 (noninferiority)	No difference in overall population	Zoledronic acid: more acute phase reaction symptoms, renal AEs
				0.06 adjusted (superiority)	NSCLC: HR 0.79, 95% CI 0.66, 0.95	Denosumab: more hypocalcemia
					Myeloma: HR 2.26, 95% CI 1.13, 4.50	
Breast cancer[154]	NR vs. 26.4	0.82	0.71, 0.95	< 0.001 (noninferiority)	No difference	Zoledronic acid: more acute phase reaction symptoms, renal AEs
				0.01 (superiority)		Denosumab: more hypocalcemia, ONJ
Prostate cancer[155]	20.7 vs. 17.1	0.82	0.71, 0.95	< 0.001 (noninferiority)	No difference	Zoledronic acid: more acute phase reaction symptoms, renal AEs
				0.008 adjusted (superiority)		Denosumab: more hypocalcemia, ONJ

Abbreviations: SREs, skeletal-related events; CI, confidence interval; HR, hazard ratio; AEs, adverse effects; NSCLC, non–small cell lung cancer; NR, not reached; ONJ, osteonecrosis of the jaw.

*The first number refers to denosumab and the second to zoledronic acid.

Reproduced with permission from West H. Denosumab for prevention of skeletal-related events in patients with bone metastases from solid tumors: incremental benefit, debatable value. J Clin Oncol. 2011;29(9):1095-1098.

A recently conducted clinical trial randomly assigned patients with bone metastases to receive a 3-year course of 4 mg of intravenous zoledronate every month compared with every 3 months to evaluate the risks and benefits with each option. Accrual has been completed and data are maturing.

VITAMIN D

There has been much discussion about the use of vitamin D for patients with advanced cancer. At this time, it is clear that many patients have low vitamin D serum concentrations and that these low concentrations can be increased with oral vitamin D supplementation. What is not clear is whether vitamin D concentrations should be routinely measured in patients with advanced cancer and/or whether vitamin D supplementation increases quality or length of life. The 2011 version of the ASCO breast cancer metastatic bone disease guidelines recommends the use of calcium and vitamin D in patients receiving antiresorptive bone therapy, in doses that are common for patients who do not have cancer but are receiving antiresorptive bone therapy.[149]

KEY POINTS

- Bone loss is common in women with estrogen depletion and in men receiving androgen ablation therapy.
- Although both bisphosphonates and denosumab can decrease bone loss caused by hormone deprivation, their use should be reserved for patients with osteoporosis or with marked osteopenia with risk factors for bone fractures.
- Although both bisphosphonates and denosumab can decrease skeletal-related events in patients with bone metastases and denosumab is slightly superior to zoledronate, available guidelines at this time do not recommend one compared with the other.
- There is no proof that longer than 1 year of bone antiresorptive therapy is better than 1 year of such in patients with bone metastases.
- Oral doses of calcium and vitamin D and weight-bearing exercise are recommended for patients at risk for bone loss.
- Bisphosphonates and denosumab can cause osteonecrosis of the jaw.

ANEMIA

Anemia is a common problem for patients with cancer. Multiple causes for anemia include myelophthisis, bleeding, hemolysis, deficiency of a micronutrient (e.g., iron, folate, or vitamin B12), anemia of chronic disease, and other causes from chemotherapy and radiation therapy.

Anemia can cause many symptoms, including fatigue, shortness of breath, and angina. Appropriate evaluation of patients with anemia is important and includes evaluation for sites of blood loss, hemolysis, or deficiencies of iron, folate, and/or vitamin B12.

Erythropoietic agents, such as erythropoietin and darbepoetin, have been used to treat chemotherapy-induced anemia. Although they appear to be helpful for increasing hemoglobin concentrations for patients with cancer-associated (as opposed to chemotherapy-associated) anemia, there is evidence that these agents stimulate tumor growth and decrease survival for some patients; therefore, this indication is not approved by the FDA. For chemotherapy-associated anemia treatment, there is no convincing evidence that one agent is particularly better than the other agent—both erythropoietin and darbepoetin increase hemoglobin levels as well as decrease transfusion requirements. The compilation of available data do not suggest that they substantially improve quality of life, although there is a trend that they may do so slightly.[162]

There are data to demonstrate that erythropoietic agents increase the risk for thromboembolic complications, and there are data to suggest that this might be a problem with higher hemoglobin levels.[162] For this reason, use of erythropoietic agents should be stopped when hemoglobin levels reach 12 mg/dL or higher. Rare cases of red cell aplasia have been reported in conjunction with use of some erythropoietic agents. It is now well established that erythropoietic agents adversely affect survival, particularly in patients who are not receiving concomitant chemotherapy and have a baseline hemoglobin level greater than 12 mg/dL.[162]

There are risks and benefits for deciding to use erythropoietic agents compared with red blood cell transfusions. Erythropoietic agents can increase the incidence of blood clots and may stimulate cancer growth and/or decrease survival; the main advantage is that they decrease the need for red blood cell transfusions. On the other hand, transfusions cause transfusion reactions, viral infections, and autoantibodies and can increase the incidence of fluid and/or iron overload; the advantage is that they cause a more rapid increase in hemoglobin and may improve symptoms faster.

Given the high profile of erythropoietic products in 2008, the FDA provided additional guidance regarding the use of erythropoietic products, including the following recommendations:

- Use these agents only for patients receiving chemotherapy.
- Initiate use only when hemoglobin levels are 10.0 g/dL or lower.
- Administer the lowest possible doses that will gradually increase hemoglobin levels to a degree that will avoid transfusion requirements.
- Cease use when there is no longer a likelihood for needing transfusions.
- Avoid administering to patients for whom cure is the goal of therapy.

The Risk Evaluation and Mitigation Strategy (REMS) program, termed APPRISE (Assisting Providers and Cancer Patients with Risk Information for the Safe Use of ESAs [erythropoietic stimulating agents]) was approved by the FDA in

Table 20-12 Summary Recommendations and Evidence Regarding ASCO Guidelines for Thromboembolic Treatment[163]

Patient Group	Role of VTE Prophylaxis	Evidence
Hospitalized patients with cancer	Patients with cancer should be considered candidates for VTE prophylaxis with anticoagulants (UFH, LMWH, or fondaparinux) in the absence of bleeding or other contraindications to anticoagulation.*	Multiple RCTs of hospitalized medical patients with subgroups of patients with cancer. The 2004 ACCP guidelines strongly recommend (1A) prophylaxis with either low-dose heparin or LMWH for bedridden patients with active cancer.
Ambulatory patients with cancer without VTE receiving systemic chemotherapy	Routine prophylaxis with an antithrombotic agent is not recommended except as noted below.	Routine prophylaxis in ambulatory patients receiving chemotherapy is not recommended due to conflicting trials, potential bleeding, the need for laboratory monitoring and dose adjustment, and the relatively low incidence of VTE.
	LMWH or adjusted-dose warfarin (INR ~ 1.5) is recommended in patients with myeloma on thalidomide or lenalidomide plus chemotherapy or dexamethasone.	This recommendation is based on nonrandomized trial data and extrapolation from studies of postoperative prophylaxis in orthopedic surgery and a trial of adjusted-dose warfarin in breast cancer.
Patients with cancer undergoing surgery	All patients undergoing major surgical intervention[†] for malignant disease should be considered for thromboprophylaxis with low-dose UFH, LMWH, or fondaparinux starting as early as possible, for at least 7 to 10 days unless contraindicated.*	RCTs of UFH and those comparing the effects of LMWH and UFH on DVT rates in patients with cancer indicate broadly similar prophylactic efficacies for these two agents.[146,150,152]
	Mechanical methods may be added to anticoagulation in very high-risk patients but should not be used alone unless anticoagulation is contraindicated.*	Based on a Cochrane review of 19 studies.[153]
	LMWH for up to 4 weeks may be considered after major abdominal/pelvic surgery with residual malignant disease, obesity, and a previous history of VTE.	Recent RCTs suggest that prolonging prophylaxis up to 4 weeks is more effective than short-course prophylaxis in reducing postoperative VTE.[149,154]
Treatment of patients with established VTE to prevent recurrence	LMWH is the preferred approach for the initial 5 to 10 days in a patient with cancer with established VTE.	LMWH for 3 to 6 months is more effective than vitamin K antagonists given for a similar duration for preventing recurrent VTE.[147,155]
	LMWH for at least 6 months is preferred for long-term anticoagulant therapy. Vitamin K antagonists with a targeted INR of 2 to 3 are acceptable when LMWH is not available.	The CLOT study demonstrated a relative risk reduction of 49% with LMWH vs. a vitamin K antagonist.[75] Dalteparin sodium was approved by the FDA in 2007 for extended treatment of symptomatic VTE to reduce risk of recurrence of VTE in patients with cancer.
	Anticoagulation for an indefinite period should be considered for patients with active cancer (metastatic disease; continuing chemotherapy).	In the absence of clinical trials, benefits and risks of continuing LMWH beyond 6 months is a clinical judgment in the individual patient. Caution is urged in elderly patients and those with intracranial malignancy.
	Inferior vena cava filters are reserved for those with contraindications to anticoagulation or PE despite adequate long-term LMWH.	Consensus recommendation because of a lack of data in cancer-specific populations.
Anticoagulants in the absence of established VTE to improve survival	Anticoagulants are not currently recommended to improve survival in patients with cancer without VTE.	RCTs and meta-analyses of warfarin, UFH, and LMWH have reported encouraging but variable results, generally showing clinical benefit only in subgroup analyses.[148]

*Relative contraindications to anticoagulation include, among other conditions: active, uncontrollable bleeding; active cerebrovascular hemorrhage; dissecting or cerebral aneurysm; bacterial endocarditis; pericarditis, active peptic or other GI ulceration; severe, uncontrolled, or malignant hypertension; severe head trauma; pregnancy (warfarin); heparin-induced thrombocytopenia (heparin, LMWH); and epidural catheter placement.

[†]Laparotomy, laparoscopy, or thoracotomy lasting longer than 30 minutes.

Abbreviations: ACCP, American College of Chest Physicians; CLOT, Randomized Comparison of Low-Molecular-Weight Heparin Versus Oral Anticoagulant Therapy for the Prevention of Recurrent Venous Thromboembolism in Patients with Cancer; DVT, deep venous thrombosis; FDA, U.S. Food and Drug Administration; INR, international normalized ratio; LMWH, low molecular-weight heparin; PE, pulmonary embolism; RCT, randomized controlled trial; UFH, unfractionated heparin; VTE, venous thromboembolism.

Reproduced with permission from Lyman GH, Khorana AA, Falanga A, et al. American Society of Clinical Oncology Guideline: Recommendations for Venous Thromboembolism Prophylaxis and Treatment in Patients with Cancer. J Clin Oncol. 2007;24(34):5490-5505.

February 2010. Per this communication, hospitals and physicians prescribing erythropoietic agents need to undergo educational training, maintain registration on a REMS program, and document in writing prior to an initiation of an erythropoietic agent to an individual patient that there was a discussion regarding the risks for blood clots, stroke, heart failure, heart attack, tumor progression, and/or death.

> ## KEY POINTS
>
> - Anemia is common in patients with cancer.
> - Anemia is caused by multiple factors including anticancer therapy with chemotherapy, radiation therapy, or surgery.
> - Transfusions are recommended for patients with symptomatic anemia.
> - For less severe anemia, erythropoietic agents decrease transfusion requirements and increase hemoglobin levels.
> - Both darbepoetin and erythropoietin are relatively similar regarding efficacy and safety.
> - Current recommendations are to cease use of erythropoietin products when the hemoglobin level is greater than or equal to 12 g/dL.

THROMBOEMBOLIC THERAPY PREVENTION AND TREATMENT

ASCO guidelines regarding the use of anticoagulants for preventing and treating venous thromboembolic problems recommend that patients with cancer who are hospitalized should be considered for prophylaxis with anticoagulants if they do not have evidence of bleeding or other contraindications.[163] They also recommend that outpatients should not be routinely anticoagulated, with the exception of considering such in patients receiving thalidomide or lenalidomide. The guidelines state that patients undergoing major surgery for cancer should be considered for anticoagulation; low molecular-weight heparin is preferred compared with coumadin. These recommendations are summarized in Table 20-12.

Newer agents, such as the oral direct factor Xa inhibitors apixaban and rivaroxaban, have been demonstrated to be noninferior to standard anticoagulant therapy.[164-167] Although some clinicians are using these drugs in patients with cancer, some investigators and clinicians feel that more specific studies should be completed in patients with cancer-related blood clots prior to more widespread use in patients with cancer.

ALOPECIA

Since the 1970s, scalp hypothermia (cryotherapy) has been reported to improve alopecia, a major untoward toxicity of many chemotherapy regimens. The results from initial efforts at this therapy were less than ideal and it largely went out of favor because of limited efficacy and concerns about patients potentially facilitating scalp metastases, because cryotherapy prevented chemotherapy from getting to the scalp.

Nonetheless, cryotherapy has had a resurgence of popularity in recent years. There have been, to date, more than 50 published trials, many of them nonrandomized but a few are randomized trials.[168,169] Efficacy has improved since this treatment was first developed. Published trials, since 1995, support that about 75% of patients are satisfied with the maintenance of their hair when they use the scalp cryotherapy. Scalp cryotherapy is relatively well tolerated. However, the therapy can be time-intensive and cumbersome. In addition, some patients can develop headaches and get too cold. Thus, this therapy is not universally employed.

The incidence of scalp metastases in patients with cancer is quite low, although it may be higher in patients with hematologic malignancies.[170,171] In one retrospective trial, the incidence of scalp metastases in patients receiving scalp cryotherapy was 0.45% (2 of 442 patients).[172] In another retrospective cohort study, scalp metastases were seen in 1.1% of patients who did get scalp hypothermia compared with 1.2% of patients who did not get scalp hypothermia.[173] A Dutch registry trial, involving 1,411 patients, reported that they had not observed a scalp metastasis within this cohort.[174] Ongoing work is further evaluating cryotherapy methods, trying to increase efficacy and decrease the burdensomeness of this approach. Of note on a related topic, fingertip cryotherapy has been shown to decrease docetaxel-caused nail toxicity.[168]

References

1. Gralla RJ, Osoba D, Kris MG, et al. Recommendations for the use of antiemetics: evidence-based, clinical practice guidelines. American Society of Clinical Oncology. *J Clin Oncol.* 1999;17:2971-2994. PMID: 10561376.
2. Hesketh PJ. Comparative review of 5-HT3 receptor antagonists in the treatment of acute chemotherapy-induced nausea and vomiting. *Cancer Invest.* 2000;18:163-173. PMID: 10705879.
3. Hesketh PJ, Kris MG, Grunberg SM, et al. Proposal for classifying the acute emetogenicity of cancer chemotherapy. *J Clin Oncol.* 1997;15:103-109. PMID: 8996130.
4. European Medicines Agency. European Medicines Agency recommends changes to the use of metoclopramide. www.ema.europa.eu/ema/index.jsp?curl=pages/news_and_events/news/2013/07/news_detail_001854.jsp&mid=WC0b01ac058004d5c1. Accessed July 9, 2014.
5. Basch E, Prestrud AA, Hesketh PJ, et al. Antiemetics: American Society of Clinical Onconology clinical practice guideline update. *J Clin Oncol.* 2012;29:4189-4198. PMID: 21947834.
6. Vardy J, Chiew KS, Galica J, et al. Side effects associated with the use of dexamethasone for prophylaxis of delayed emesis after moderately emetogenic chemotherapy. *Br J Cancer.* 2006;94:1011-1015. PMID: 16552437.
7. Poli-Bigelli S, Rodrigues-Pereira J, Carides AD, et al. Addition of the neurokinin 1 receptor antagonist aprepitant to standard antiemetic therapy improves control of chemotherapy-induced nausea and vomiting. Results from a randomized, double-blind, placebo-controlled trial in Latin America. *Cancer.* 2003;97:3090-3098. PMID: 12784346.
8. Grunberg S, Chua D, Maru A, et al. Single-dose fosaprepitant for the prevention of chemotherapy-induced nausea and vomiting associated with cisplatin therapy: randomized, double-blind study protocol–EASE. *J Clin Oncol.* 2011;29:1495-1501. PMID: 21383291.
9. American Society of Clinical Oncology, Kris MG, Hesketh PJ, et al. American Society of Clinical Oncology guideline for antiemetics in oncology: update 2006. *J Clin Oncol.* 2006;24:2932-2947. PMID: 16717289.
10. Leal AD, Kadakia KC, Looker S, et al. Fosaprepitant-induced phlebitis: a focus on patients receiving doxorubicin/cyclophosphamide therapy. *Support Care Cancer.* 2014;22:1313-1317. Epub 2014 Jan 9. PMID:24402411.

11. Navari RM, Nagy CK, Gray SE. The use of olanzapine versus metoclopramide for the treatment of breakthrough chemotherapy-induced nausea and vomiting in patients receiving highly emetogenic chemotherapy. *Support Care Cancer*. 2013;21:1655-1663. PMID: 23314603.

12. Navari RM, Gray SE, Kerr AC. Olanzapine versus aprepitant for the prevention of chemotherapy-induced nausea and vomiting: a randomized phase III trial. *J Support Oncol*. 2011;9:188-195. PMID: 22024310.

13. Navari RM, Einhorn LH, Loehrer PJ Sr, et al. A phase II trial of olanzapine, dexamethasone, and palonosetron for the prevention of chemotherapy-induced nausea and vomiting: a Hoosier oncology group study. *Support Care Cancer*. 2007;15:1285-1291. PMID: 17375339.

14. Passik SD, Navari RM, Jung SH, et al. A phase I trial of olanzapine (Zyprexa) for the prevention of delayed emesis in cancer patients: a Hoosier Oncology Group study. *Cancer Invest*. 2004;22:383-388. PMID: 15493359.

15. Loprinzi CL, Alberts SR, Christensen BJ, et al. History of the development of antiemetic guidelines at Mayo Clinic Rochester. *Mayo Clin Proc*. 2000;75:303-309. PMID: 10725961.

16. Roila F, Herrstedt J, Aapro M, et al. Guideline update for MASCC and ESMO in the prevention of chemotherapy- and radiotherapy-induced nausea and vomiting: results of the Perugia consensus conference. *Ann Oncol*. 2010;21 Suppl 5:v232-v243. PMID: 20555089.

17. Gralla RJ, Roila F, Tonato M. The 2004 Perugia Antiemetic Consensus Guideline process: methods, procedures, and participants. *Support Care Cancer*. 2005;13:77-79. PMID: 15605253.

18. Kris MG, Hesketh PJ, Herrstedt J, et al. Consensus proposals for the prevention of acute and delayed vomiting and nausea following high-emetic-risk chemotherapy. *Support Care Cancer*. 2005;13:85-96. PMID: 15565277.

19. Charig CR, Rundle JS. Flushing. Long-term side effect of orchiectomy in treatment of prostatic carcinoma. *Urology*. 1989;33:175-178. PMID: 2465644.

20. Vassilopoulou-Sellin R, Zolinski C. Estrogen replacement therapy in women with breast cancer: a survey of patient attitudes. *Am J Med Sci*. 1992;304:145-149. PMID: 1476153.

21. O'Meara ES, Rossing MA, Daling JR, et al. Hormone replacement therapy after a diagnosis of breast cancer in relation to recurrence and mortality. *J Natl Cancer Inst*. 2001;93:754-762. PMID: 11353785.

22. Loprinzi CL, Michalak JC, Quella SK, et al. Megestrol acetate for the prevention of hot flashes. *N Engl J Med*. 1994;331:347-352. PMID: 8028614.

23. Barton D, Loprinzi C, Quella S, et al. Depomedroxyprogesterone acetate for hot flashes. *J Pain Symptom Manage*. 2002;24:603-607. PMID: 12551811.

24. Loprinzi CL, Levitt R, Barton D, et al. Phase III comparison of depomedroxyprogesterone acetate to venlafaxine for managing hot flashes: North Central Cancer Treatment Group Trial N99C7. *J Clin Oncol*. 2006;24:1409-1414. PMID: 16505409.

25. Loprinzi CL, Kugler JW, Sloan JA, et al. Venlafaxine in management of hot flashes in survivors of breast cancer: a randomised controlled trial. *Lancet*. 2000;356:2059-2063. PMID: 11145492.

26. Stearns V, Beebe KL, Iyengar M, et al. Paroxetine controlled release in the treatment of menopausal hot flashes: a randomized controlled trial. *JAMA*. 2003;289:2827-2834. PMID: 12783913.

27. Barton DL, LaVasseur BI, Sloan JA, et al. Phase III, placebo-controlled trial of three doses of citalopram for the treatment of hot flashes: NCCTG trial N05C9. *J Clin Oncol*. 2010;28:3278-3283. PMID: 20498389.

28. Carpenter JS, Guthrie KA, Larson JC, et al. Effect of escitalopram on hot flash interference: a randomized, controlled trial. *Fertil Steril*. 2012;97:1399-1404. PMID: 22480818.

29. Archer DF, Seidman L, Constantine GD, et al. A double-blind, randomly assigned, placebo-controlled study of desvenlafaxine efficacy and safety for the treatment of vasomotor symptoms associated with menopause. *Am J Obstet Gynecol* 2009;200:172.e1-e10. PMID: 19110224.

30. Loprinzi CL, Sloan JA, Perez EA, et al. Phase III evaluation of fluoxetine for treatment of hot flashes. *J Clin Oncol*. 2002;20:1578-1583. PMID: 11896107.

31. Kimmick GG, Lovato J, McQuellon R, et al. Randomized, double-blind, placebo-controlled, crossover study of sertraline (Zoloft) for the treatment of hot flashes in women with early stage breast cancer taking tamoxifen. *Breast J*. 2006;12:114-122. PMID: 16509835.

32. Borges S, Desta Z, Li L, et al. Quantitative effect of CYP2D6 genotype and inhibitors on tamoxifen metabolism: implication for optimization of breast cancer treatment. *Clin Pharmacol Ther*. 2006;80:61-74. PMID: 16815318.

33. Loprinzi CL, Sloan J, Stearns V, et al. Newer antidepressants and gabapentin for hot flashes: an individual patient pooled analysis. *J Clin Oncol*. 2009;27:2831-2837. PMID: 19332723.

34. Guttuso T Jr, Kurlan R, McDermott MP, et al. Gabapentin's effects of hot flashes in postmenopausal women: a randomized controlled trial. *Obstet Gynecol*. 2003;101:337-345. PMID: 12576259.

35. Pandya KJ, Morrow GR, Roscoe JA, et al. Gabapentin for hot flashes in 420 women with breast cancer: a randomised double-blind placebo-controlled trial. *Lancet*. 2005;366:818-824. PMID: 16139656.

36. Butt DA, Lock M, Lewis JE, et al. Gabapentin for the treatment of menopausal hot flashes: a randomized controlled trial. *Menopause*. 2008;15:310-318. PMID: 17917611.

37. Reddy SY, Warner H, Guttuso T Jr, et al. Gabapentin, estrogen, and placebo for treating hot flashes: a randomized controlled trial. *Obstet Gynecol*. 2006;108:41-48. PMID: 16816054.

38. Bordeleau L, Pritchard KI, Loprinzi CL, et al. Multicenter, randomized, cross-over clinical trial of venlafaxine versus gabapentin for the management of hot flashes in breast cancer survivors. *J Clin Oncol*. 2010;28:5147-5152. PMID: 21060031.

39. Goldberg RM, Loprinzi CL, O'Fallon JR, et al. Transdermal clonidine for ameliorating tamoxifen-induced hot flashes. *J Clin Oncol*. 1994;12:155-158. PMID: 8270972.

40. Quella SK, Loprinzi CL, Barton DL, et al. Evaluation of soy phytoestrogens for the treatment of hot flashes in breast cancer survivors: A North Central Cancer Treatment Group Trial. *J Clin Oncol*. 2000;18:1068-1074. PMID: 10694559.

41. Nelson HD, Vesco KK, Haney E, et al. Nonhormonal therapies for menopausal hot flashes: systematic review and meta-analysis. *JAMA*. 2006;295:2057-2071. PMID: 16670414.

42. Barton DL, Loprinzi CL, Quella SK, et al. Prospective evaluation of vitamin E for hot flashes in breast cancer survivors. *J Clin Oncol*. 1998;16:495-500. 9469333.

43. Ziaei S, Kazemnejad A, Zareai M. The effect of vitamin E on hot flashes in menopausal women. *Gynecol Onstet Invest*. 2007;64:204-207. PMID: 17664882.

44. Pruthi S, Qin R, Terstreip SA, et al. A phase III, randomized, placebo-controlled, double-blind trial of flaxseed for the treatment of hot flashes: North Central Cancer Treatment Group N08C7. *Menopause*. 2012;19:48-53. PMID: 21900849.

45. Elkins G, Marcus J, Stearns V, et al. Randomized trial of a hypnosis intervention for treatment of hot flashes among breast cancer survivors. *J Clin Oncol*. 2008;26:5022-5026. PMID: 18809612.

46. Elkins GR, Fisher WI, Johnson AK, et al. Clinical hypnosis in the treatment of postmenopausal hot flashes: a randomized controlled trial. *Menopause*. 2013;20:291-298. PMID: 23435026.

47. Loprinzi CL, Abu-Ghazaleh S, Sloan JA, et al. Phase III randomized double-blind study to evaluate the efficacy of a polycarbophil-based vaginal moisturizer in women with breast cancer. *J Clin Oncol*. 1997;15:969-973. PMID: 9060535.

48. Bygdeman M, Swahn ML. Replens versus dienoestrol cream in the symptomatic treatment of vaginal atrophy in postmenopausal women. *Maturitas*. 1996;23:259-263. PMID: 8794418.

49. Labrie F, Archer D, Bouchard C, et al. Effect of intravaginal dehydroepiandrosterone (Prasterone) on libido and sexual dysfunction in postmenopausal women. *Menopause*. 2009;16:923-931. PMID: 19424093.

50. Labrie F, Archer D, Bouchard C, et al. Serum steroid levels during 12-week intravaginal dehydroepiandrosterone administration. *Menopause*. 2009;16:897-906. PMID: 19436226.

51. Lalla RV, Ashbury FD. The MASCC/ISOO Mucositis Guidelines: dissemination and clinical impact. *Support Care Cancer*. 2013;21:3161-3163. PMID: 23942597.

52. Mahood DJ, Dose AM, Loprinzi CL, et al. Inhibition of fluorouracil-induced stomatitis by oral cryotherapy. *J Clin Oncol*. 1991;9:449-452. PMID: 1999715.

53. Cascinu S, Fedeli A, Fedeli SL, et al. Oral cooling (cryotherapy), an effective treatment for the prevention of 5-fluorouracil-induced stomatitis. *Eur J Cancer B Oral Oncol*. 1994;30B:234-236. PMID: 7950836.

54. Edelman MJ, Gandara DR, Perez EA, et al. Phase I trial of edatrexate plus carboplatin in advanced solid tumors: amelioration of dose-limiting mucositis by ice chip cryotherapy. *Invest New Drugs*. 1998;16:69-75. PMID: 9740546.

55. Gandara DR, Edelman MJ, Crowley JJ, et al. Phase II trial of edatrexate plus carboplatin in metastatic non-small-cell lung cancer: a Southwest Oncology Group study. *Cancer Chemother Pharmacol*. 1997;41:75-78. PMID: 9443617.

56. Dreicer R, Propert KJ, Kuzel T, et al. A phase II trial of edatrexate in patients with advanced renal cell carcinoma. An Eastern Cooperative Oncology Group study. *Am J Clin Oncol.* 1997;20:251-253. PMID: 9167747.

57. Spielberger R, Stiff P, Bensinger W, et al. Palifermin for oral mucositis after intensive therapy for hematologic cancers. *N Engl J Med.* 2004;351:2590-2598. PMID: 15602019.

58. Loprinzi CL, Martenson JA. Keratinocyte growth factor: not yet ready for prime time. *J Clin Oncol.* 2003;21:1429-1430. PMID: 12697863.

59. Loprinzi CL, Barton DL, Sloan JA. Whose opinion counts? *J Clin Oncol.* 2006;24:5183-5185. PMID: 17075108.

60. Rosen LS, Abdi E, Davis ID, et al. Palifermin reduces the incidence of oral mucositis in patients with metastatic colorectal cancer treated with flu-orouracil-based chemotherapy. *J Clin Oncol.* 2006;24:5194-5200. PMID: 17075109.

61. Migliorati C, Hewson I, Lalla RV, et al. Systematic review of laser and other light therapy for the management of oral mucositis in cancer patients. *Support Care Cancer.* 2013;21:333-341. PMID:23001179.

62. McGinnis WL, Loprinzi CL, Buskirk SJ, et al. Placebo-controlled trial of sucralfate for inhibiting radiation-induced esophagitis. *J Clin Oncol.* 1997;15:1239-1243. PMID: 9060568.

63. Komaki R, Lee JS, Kaplan B, et al. Randomized phase III study of chemora-diation with or without amifostine for patients with favorable performance status inoperable stage II-III non-small cell lung cancer: preliminary re-sults. *Semin Radiat Oncol.* 2002;12:46-49. PMID: 11917284.

64. Antonadou D, Coliarakis N, Synodinou M, et al. Randomized phase III trial of radiation treatment +/- amifostine in patients with advanced-stage lung cancer. *Int J Radiat Oncol Biol Phys.* 2001;51:915-922. PMID: 11704311.

65. Miller RC, Leenstra J, Qun R, et al. N09C6 (Alliance) – A phase 3, random-ized, double-blind study of doxepin rinse versus placebo in the treat-ment of acute oral mucositis pain in patients receiving head and neck radiation therapy with or without chemotherapy. *Int J Radiat Oncol Biol Phys.* 2013;85:21.

66. Chan A, Ignoffo RJ. Survey of topical oral solutions for the treatment of che-mo-induced oral mucositis. *J Oncol Pharm Pract.* 2005;11:139-143. PMID: 16595065.

67. Dodd MJ, Dibble SL, Miaskowski C, et al. Randomized clinical trial of the effectiveness of 3 commonly used mouthwashes to treat chemotherapy-induced mucositis. *Oral Surg Oral Med Oral Pathol Oral Radiol Endod.* 2000;90:39-47. PMID: 10884634.

68. Cerchietti LC, Navigante AH, Bonomi MR, et al. Effect of topical morphine for mucositis-associated pain following concomitant chemoradiother-apy for head and neck carcinoma. *Cancer.* 2002;95:2230-2236. PMID: 12412178.

69. Vayne-Bossert P, Escher M, de Vautibault CG, et al. Effect of topical mor-phine (mouthwash) on oral pain due to chemotherapy- and/or radiother-apy-induced mucositis: a randomized double-blinded study. *J Palliat Med.* 2010;13:125-128. PMID: 19827964.

70. Williams JW, Jr., Simel DL. The rational clinical examination. Does this patient have ascites? How to divine fluid in the abdomen. *JAMA.* 1992;267:2645-2648. PMID: 1573734.

71. Fleming ND, Alvarez-Secord A, Von Gruenigen V, et al. Indwelling catheters for the management of refractory malignant ascites: a systematic litera-ture overview and retrospective chart review. *J Pain Symptom Manage.* 2009;38:341-349. PMID: 19328648.

72. Cairns W, Malone R. Octreotide as an agent for the relief of malignant ascites in palliative care patients. *Palliat Med.* 1999;13:429-430. PMID: 10659116.

73. Jatoi A, Nieva JJ, Qin R, et al. A pilot study of long-acting octreotide for symp-tomatic malignant ascites. *Oncology.* 2012;82:315-320. PMID: 22572824.

74. Dewys WD, Begg C, Lavin PT, et al. Prognostic effect of weight loss prior to chemotherapy in cancer patients. Eastern Cooperative Oncology Group. *Am J Med.* 1980;69:491-497. PMID: 7424938.

75. Fearon K, Strasser F, Anker SD, et al. Definition and classification of can-cer cachexia: an international consensus. *Lancet Oncol.* 2011;12:489-495. PMID: 21296615.

76. Tisdale MJ. Biology of cachexia. *J Natl Cancer Inst.* 1997;89:1763-1773. PMID: 9392617.

77. McGeer AJ, Detsky AS, O'Rourke K. Parenteral nutrition in cancer patients undergoing chemotherapy: a meta-analysis. *Nutrition.* 1990;6:233-240. PMID: 2152097.

78. Jatoi A, Loprinzi C. Loss of appetite and weight. In: Fish MJ, Bruera E (Eds). *The Cambridge Handbook of Advanced Cancer Care.* Cambridge, UK: Cam-bridge University Press; 2003: 369-373.

79. Loprinzi CL, Schaid DJ, Dose AM, et al. Body-composition changes in pa-tients who gain weight while receiving megestrol acetate. *J Clin Oncol.* 1993;11:152-154. PMID: 8418227.

80. Jatoi A, Kumar S, Sloan JA, et al. On appetite and its loss. *J Clin Oncol.* 2003;21:79s-81s. PMID: 12743203.

81. Rowland KM Jr, Loprinzi CL, Shaw EG, et al. Randomized double-blind placebo-controlled trial of cisplatin and etoposide plus megestrol acetate/placebo in extensive-stage small-cell lung cancer: a North Central Cancer Treatment Group study. *J Clin Oncol.* 1996;14:135-141. PMID: 8558188.

82. Mateen F, Jatoi A. Megestrol acetate for the palliation of anorexia in ad-vanced, incurable cancer patients. *Clin Nutr.* 2006;25:711-715. PMID: 16867306.

83. Deschamps B, Musaji N, Gillespie JA. Food effect on the bioavailability of two distinct formulations of megestrol acetate oral suspension. *Int J Nano-medicine.* 2009;4:185-192. PMID: 19774117.

84. Loprinzi CL, Ellison NM, Schaid DJ, et al. Controlled trial of megestrol ac-etate for the treatment of cancer anorexia and cachexia. *J Natl Cancer Inst.* 1990;82:1127-1132. PMID: 2193166.

85. Moertel CG, Schutt AJ, Reitemeier RJ, et al. Corticosteroid therapy of preter-minal gastrointestinal cancer. *Cancer.* 1974;33:1607-1609. PMID: 4135151.

86. Loprinzi CL, Kugler JW, Sloan JA, et al. Randomized comparison of meges-trol acetate versus dexamethasone versus fluoxymesterone for the treat-ment of cancer anorexia/cachexia. *J Clin Oncol.* 1999;17:3299-3306. PMID: 10506633.

87. Kardinal CG, Loprinzi CL, Schaid DJ, et al. A controlled trial of cypro-heptadine in cancer patients with anorexia and/or cachexia. *Cancer.* 1990;65:2657-2662. PMID: 2187585.

88. Loprinzi CL, Kuross SA, O'Fallon JR, et al. Randomized placebo-controlled evaluation of hydrazine sulfate in patients with advanced colorectal cancer. *J Clin Oncol.* 1994;12:1121-1125. PMID: 8201373.

89. Loprinzi CL, Goldberg RM, Su JQ, et al. Placebo-controlled trial of hydrazine sulfate in patients with newly diagnosed non-small-cell lung cancer. *J Clin Oncol.* 1994;12:1126-1129. PMID: 8201374.

90. Goldberg RM, Loprinzi CL, Mailliard JA, et al. Pentoxifylline for treatment of cancer anorexia and cachexia? A randomized, double-blind, placebo-controlled trial. *J Clin Oncol.* 1995;13:2856-2859. PMID: 7595749.

91. Jatoi A, Windschitl HE, Loprinzi CL, et al. Dronabinol versus megestrol ac-etate versus combination therapy for cancer-associated anorexia: a North Central Cancer Treatment Group study. *J Clin Oncol.* 2002;20:567-573. PMID: 11786587.

92. Jatoi A, Dakhil S, Kugler JW, et al. A placebo-controlled trial of etanercept, a tumor necrosis factor (TNF) inhibitor, in patients with the cancer anorex-ia/weight loss syndrome: a North Central Cancer Treatment Group study (NCCTG) trial N00C1. *J Clin Oncol.* 2006;24:18s (suppl; abstr 8534).

93. Wadler S, Benson AB 3rd, Engelking C, et al. Recommended guide-lines for the treatment of chemotherapy-induced diarrhea. *J Clin Oncol.* 1998;16:3169-3178. PMID: 9738589.

94. Cascinu S, Fedeli A, Fedeli SL, et al. Octreotide versus loperamide in the treatment of fluorouracil-induced diarrhea: a randomized trial. *J Clin On-col.* 1993;11:148-151. PMID: 8418225.

95. Gebbia V, Carreca I, Testa A, et al. Subcutaneous octreotide versus oral lop-eramide in the treatment of diarrhea following chemotherapy. *Anticancer Drugs.* 1993;4:443-445. PMID: 8400346.

96. Miller RC, Martenson JA, Sargent DJ, et al. Acute treatment-related diarrhea during postoperative adjuvant therapy for high-risk rectal carcinoma. *Int J Radiat Oncol Biol Phys.* 1998;41:593-598. PMID: 9635707.

97. Martenson JA Jr, Hyland G, Moertel CG, et al. Olsalazine is contraindi-cated during pelvic radiation therapy: results of a double-blind, random-ized clinical trial. *Int J Radiat Oncol Biol Phys.* 1996;35:299-303. PMID: 8635937.

98. Heusinkveld RS, Manning MR, Aristizabal SA. Control of radiation-induced diarrhea with cholestyramine. *Int J Radiat Oncol Biol Phys.* 1978;4:687-690. PMID: 101491.

99. Henriksson R, Arevärn M, Franzen L, et al. Beneficial effects of sucralphate in radiation induced diarrhea. An open randomized study in gynecological cancer patients. *Eur J Gynaecol Oncol.* 1990;11:299-302. PMID: 2245814.

100. Martenson JA, Bollinger JW, Sloan JA, et al. Sucralfate in the prevention of treatment-induced diarrhea in patients receiving pelvic radiation therapy: A North Central Cancer Treatment Group phase III double-blind placebo-controlled trial. *J Clin Oncol.* 2000;18:1239-1245. PMID: 10715293.

101. Kozelsky TF, Meyers GE, Sloan JA, et al. Phase III double-blind study of glutamine versus placebo for the prevention of acute diarrhea in patients receiving pelvic radiation therapy. *J Clin Oncol.* 2003;21:1669-1674. PMID: 12721240.

102. Martenson JA, Halyard MY, Sloan JA, et al. Phase III, double-blind study of depot octreotide versus placebo in the prevention of acute diarrhea in patients receiving pelvic radiation therapy: results of North Central Cancer Treatment Group N00CA. *J Clin Oncol.* 2008;26:5248-5253. PMID: 18768432.

103. Yavuz MN, Yuvuz AA, Ilis E, et al. A randomized study of the efficacy of octreotide versus diphenoxylate on radiation-induced diarrhea. *Proc Am Soc Clin Oncol.* 2000;19:602a (suppl; abstr 2370).

104. Mock V. Fatigue management: evidence and guidelines for practice. *Cancer.* 2001;92:1699-1707. PMID: 11598890.

105. Fulton C, Knowles G. Cancer fatigue. *Eur J Cancer Care (Engl).* 2000;9:167-171. PMID: 11881726.

106. Mock V, Burke MB, Sheehan P, et al. A nursing rehabilitation program for women with breast cancer receiving adjuvant chemotherapy. *Oncol Nurs Forum.* 1994;21:899-907; discussion 908. PMID: 7937251.

107. Schwartz AL, Mori M, Gao R, et al. Exercise reduces daily fatigue in women with breast cancer receiving chemotherapy. *Med Sci Sports Exerc.* 2001;33:718-723. PMID: 11323538.

108. Mock V, Pickett M, Ropka ME, et al. Fatigue and quality of life outcomes of exercise during cancer treatment. *Cancer Pract.* 2001;9:119-127. PMID: 11879296.

109. Stevinson C, Lawlor DA, Fox KR. Exercise interventions for cancer patients: systematic review of controlled trials. *Cancer Causes Control.* 2004;15:1035-1056. PMID: 15801488.

110. Stricker CT, Drake D, Hoyer KA, et al. Evidence-based practice for fatigue management in adults with cancer: exercise as an intervention. *Oncol Nurs Forum.* 2004;31:963-976. PMID: 15378097.

111. Galvão DA, Newton RU. Review of exercise intervention studies in cancer patients. *J Clin Oncol.* 2005;23:899-909. PMID: 15681536.

112. Knols R, Aaronson NK, Uebelhart D, et al. Physical exercise in cancer patients during and after medical treatment: a systematic review of randomized and controlled clinical trials. *J Clin Oncol.* 2005;23:3830-3842. PMID: 15923576.

113. Schmitz KH, Holtzman J, Courneya KS, et al. Controlled physical activity trials in cancer survivors: a systematic review and meta-analysis. *Cancer Epidemiol Biomarkers Prev.* 2005;14:1588-1595. PMID: 16030088.

114. Stankoff B, Waubant E, Confavreux C, et al. Modafinil for fatigue in MS: a randomized placebo-controlled double-blind study. *Neurology.* 2005;64:1139-1143. PMID: 15824337.

115. Morrow G, Jean-Pierre P, Roscoe JA, et al. A phase III randomized, placebo-controlled, double-blind trial of a eugeroic agents for 642 cancer patients reporting fatigue during chemoptheray: a URCC CCOP Study. *J Clin Oncol.* 2008;15s (suppl; abstr 9512).

116. Moraska AR, Sood A, Dakhil SR, et al. Phase III, randomized, double-blind, placebo-controlled study of long-acting methylphenidate for cancer-related fatigue: North Central Cancer Treatment Group NCCTG-N05C7 trial. *J Clin Oncol.* 2010;28:3673-3679. PMID: 20625123.

117. Bruera E, Yennurajalingam S, Palmer JL, et al. Methylphenidate and/or a nursing telephone intervention for fatigue in patients with advanced cancer: a randomized, placebo-controlled, phase II trial. *J Clin Oncol.* 2013;31:2421-2427. PMID: 23690414.

118. Tadano T, Nakagawasai O, Niijima F, et al. The effects of traditional tonics on fatigue in mice differ from those of the antidepressant imipramine: a pharmacological and behavioral study. *Am J Chin Med.* 2000;28:97-104. PMID: 10794121.

119. Banerjee U, Izquierdo JA. Antistress and antifatigue properties of Panax ginseng: comparison with piracetam. *Acta Physiol Lat Am.* 1982;32:277-285. PMID: 6892267.

120. Younus J, Collins A, Wang X, et al. A double-blind, placebo-controlled pilot study to evaluate the effect of ginseng on fatigue and quality of life in adult chemo-native cancer patients. *J Clin Oncol.* 2003;22:733 (suppl; abstr 2947).

121. Engels HJ, Fahlman MM, Wirth JC. Effects of ginseng on secretory IgA, performance, and recovery from interval exercise. *Med Sci Sports Exerc.* 2003;35:690-696. PMID: 12673155.

122. Engels HJ, Kolokouri I, Cieslak TJ 2nd, et al. Effects of ginseng supplementation on supramaximal exercise performance and short-term recovery. *J Strength Cond Res.* 2001;15:290-295. PMID: 11710653.

123. Barton D, Liu H, Dakhil S, et al. Phase III evaluation of American ginseng (panax quinquefolius) to improve cancer-related fatigue: NCCTG Trial N07C2. *J Clin Oncol.* 2012;30:15s (suppl; abstr 9001).

124. Barton DL, Liu H, Dakhil SR, et al. Wisconsin Ginseng (Panax quinquefolius) to improve cancer-related fatigue: a randomized, double-blind trial, N07C2. *J Natl Cancer Inst.* 2013;105:1230-1238. PMID: 23853057.

125. Baselga J, Rischin D, Ranson M, et al. Phase I safety, pharmacokinetic, and pharmacodynamic trial of ZD1839, a selective oral epidermal growth factor receptor tyrosine kinase inhibitor, in patients with five selected solid tumor types. *J Clin Oncol.* 2002;20:4292-4302. PMID: 12409327.

126. Fukuoka M, Yano S, Giaccone G, et al. Multi-institutional randomized phase II trial of gefitinib for previously treated patients with advanced non-small-cell lung cancer (The IDEAL 1 Trial) [corrected]. *J Clin Oncol.* 2003;21:2237-2246. PMID: 12748244.

127. Cohen EE, Rosen F, Stadler WM, et al. Phase II trial of ZD1839 in recurrent or metastatic squamous cell carcinoma of the head and neck. *J Clin Oncol.* 2003;21:1980-1987. PMID: 12743152.

128. Herbst RS, Maddox AM, Rothenberg ML, et al. Selective oral epidermal growth factor receptor tyrosine kinase inhibitor ZD1839 is generally well-tolerated and has activity in non-small-cell lung cancer and other solid tumors: results of a phase I trial. *J Clin Oncol.* 2002;20:3815-3825. PMID: 12228201.

129. Kris MG, Natale RB, Herbst RS, et al. Efficacy of gefitinib, an inhibitor of the epidermal growth factor receptor tyrosine kinase, in symptomatic patients with non-small cell lung cancer: a randomized trial. *JAMA.* 2003;290:2149-2158. PMID: 14570950.

130. Saltz LB, Meropol NJ, Loehrer PJ Sr, et al. Phase II trial of cetuximab in patients with refractory colorectal cancer that expresses the epidermal growth factor receptor. *J Clin Oncol.* 2004;22:1201-1208. PMID: 14993230.

131. Jatoi A, Rowland K, Sloan JA, et al. Tetracycline to prevent epidermal growth factor receptor inhibitor-induced skin rashes: results of a placebo-controlled trial from the North Central Cancer Treatment Group (N03CB). *Cancer.* 2008;113:847-853. PMID: 18543329.

132. Scope A, Agero AL, Dusza SW, et al. Randomized double-blind trial of prophylactic oral minocycline and topical tazarotene for cetuximab-associated acne-like eruption. *J Clin Oncol.* 2007;25:5390-5396. PMID: 18048820.

133. Jatoi A, Dakhil SR, Sloan JA, et al. Prophylactic tetracycline does not diminish the severity of epidermal growth factor receptor (EGFR) inhibitor-induced rash: results from the North Central Cancer Treatment Group (Supplementary N03CB). *Support Care Cancer.* 2011;19:1601-1607. PMID: 20820817.

134. Lacouture ME, Mitchell EP, Piperdi B, et al. Skin toxicity evaluation protocol with panitumumab (STEPP), a phase II, open-label, randomized trial evaluating the impact of a pre-Emptive Skin treatment regimen on skin toxicities and quality of life in patients with metastatic colorectal cancer. *J Clin Oncol.* 2010;28:1351-1357. PMID: 20142600.

135. Jatoi A, Thrower A, Sloan JA, et al. Does sunscreen prevent epidermal growth factor receptor (EGFR) inhibitor-induced rash? Results of a placebo-controlled trial from the North Central Cancer Treatment Group (N05C4). *The Oncologist.* 2010;15:1016-1022. PMID: 20798191.

136. Peréz-Soler R, Saltz L. Cutaneous adverse effects with HER1/EGFR-targeted agents: is there a silver lining? *J Clin Oncol.* 2005;23:5235-5246. PMID:16051966.

137. Fiala O, Pesek M, Finek J, et al. Skin rash as useful marker of erlotinib efficacy in NSCLC and its impact on clinical practice. *Neoplasma.* 2013;60:26-32. PMID: 23067213.

138. Stintzing S, Kapaun C, Laubender RP, et al. Prognostic value of cetuximab-related skin toxicity in metastatic colorectal cancer patients and its correlation with parameters of the epidermal growth factor receptor signal transduction pathway: results from a randomized trial of the GERMAN AIO CRC Study Group. *Int J Cancer.* 2013;132:236-245. PMID:22644776.

139. Petrelli F, Borgonovo K, Cabiddu M, et al. Relationship between skin rash and outcome in non-small-cell lung cancer patients treated with anti-EGFR tyrosine kinase inhibitors: a literature-based meta-analysis of 24 trials. *Lung Cancer.* 2012;78:8-15. PMID: 22795701.

140. Lee S, Lee Y, Chun M, et al. Pyridoxine is not effective for the prevention of hand foot syndrome (HFS) associated with capecitabine therapy: results of a randomized double-blind placebo-controlled study. *J Clin Oncol.* 2007;25:18s (suppl; abstr 9007).

141. Wolf SL, Qin R, Menon SP, et al. Placebo-controlled trial to determine the effectiveness of a urea/lactic acid-based topical keratolytic agent for prevention of capecitabine-induced hand-foot syndrome: North Central Cancer Treatment Group Study N05C5. *J Clin Oncol.* 2010;28:5182-5187. PMID: 21060036.

142. Loprinzi CL, Maddocks-Christianson K, Wolf SL, et al. The paclitaxel acute pain syndrome: sensitization of nociceptors as the putative mechanism. *Cancer J.* 2007;13:399-403. PMID: 18032978.

143. Loprinzi CL, Reeves BN, Dakhil SR, et al. Natural history of paclitaxel-associated acute pain syndrome: prospective cohort study NCCTG N08C1. *J Clin Oncol.* 2011;29:1472-1478. PMID: 21383290.

144. Hershman DL, Lacchetti C, Dworkin RH, et al. Prevention and management of chemotherapy-induced peripheral neuropathy in survivors of adult cancers: American Society of Clinical Oncology Clinical Practice Guideline. J Clin Oncol. 2014;32:1941-1967. PMID: 24733808.

145. Katz A. The sounds of silence: sexuality information for cancer patients. J Clin Oncol. 2005;23:238-241. PMID: 15625380.

146. Shifren JL, Braunstein GD, Simon JA, et al. Transdermal testosterone treatment in women with impaired sexual function after oophorectomy. N Engl J Med. 2000;343:682-688. PMID: 10974131.

147. Nathorst-Böös J, Flöter A, Jarkander-Rolff M, et al. Treatment with percutaneous testosterone gel in postmenopausal women with decreased libido--effects on sexuality and psychological general well-being. Maturitas. 2006;53:11-18. PMID: 16183220.

148. Barton DL, Wender DB, Sloan JA, et al. Randomized controlled trial to evaluate transdermal testosterone in female cancer survivors with decreased libido; North Central Cancer Treatment Group protocol N02C3. J Natl Cancer Inst. 2007;99:672-679. PMID: 17470735.

149. Van Poznak CH, Temin S, Yee GC, et al. American Society of Clinical Oncology executive summary of the clinical practice guideline update on the role of bone-modifying agents in metastatic breast cancer. J Clin Oncol. 2011;29:1221-1227. PMID: 21343561.

150. Hines SL, Mincey BA, Sloan JA, et al. Phase III randomized, placebo-controlled, double-blind trial of risedronate for the prevention of bone loss in premenopausal women undergoing chemotherapy for primary breast cancer. J Clin Oncol. 2009;27:1047-1053. PMID: 19075260.

151. Hershman DL, McMahon DJ, Crew KD, et al. Zoledronic acid prevents bone loss in premenopausal women undergoing adjuvant chemotherapy for early-stage breast cancer. J Clin Oncol. 2008;26:4739-4745. PMID: 18711172.

152. Brufsky A. Management of cancer-treatment-induced bone loss in postmenopausal women undergoing adjuvant breast cancer therapy: a Z-FAST update. Semin Oncol. 2006;33:S13-S17. PMID: 16730272.

153. Ellis GK, Bone HG, Chlebowski R, et al. Randomized trial of denosumab in patients receiving adjuvant aromatase inhibitors for nonmetastatic breast cancer. J Clin Oncol. 2008;26:4875-4882. PMID: 18725648.

154. Stopeck AT, Lipton A, Body JJ, et al. Denosumab compared with zoledronic acid for the treatment of bone metastases in patients with advanced breast cancer: a randomized, double-blind study. J Clin Oncol. 2010;28:5132-5139. PMID: 21060033.

155. Smith MR, Saad F, Egerdie B, et al. Effects of denosumab on bone mineral density in men receiving androgen deprivation therapy for prostate cancer. J Urol. 2009;182:2670-2675. PMID: 19836774.

156. Smith MR, Eastham J, Gleason DM, et al. Randomized controlled trial of zoledronic acid to prevent bone loss in men receiving androgen deprivation therapy for nonmetastatic prostate cancer. J Urol. 2003;169:2008-2012. PMID: 12771706.

157. Fizazi K, Carducci M, Smith M, et al. Denosumab versus zoledronic acid for treatment of bone metastases in men with castration-resistant prostate cancer: a randomised, double-blind study. Lancet. 2011;377:813-822. PMID: 21353695.

158. West H. Denosumab for prevention of skeletal-related events in patients with bone metastases from solid tumors: incremental benefit, debatable value. J Clin Oncol. 2011;29:1095-1098. PMID: 21343550.

159. Henry DH, Costa L, Goldwasser F, et al. Randomized, double-blind study of denosumab versus zoledronic acid in the treatment of bone metastases in patients with advanced cancer (excluding breast and prostate cancer) or multiple myeloma. J Clin Oncol. 2011;29:1125-1132. PMID: 21343556.

160. Ruggiero SL, Mehrotra B, Rosenberg TJ, et al. Osteonecrosis of the jaws associated with the use of bisphosphonates: a review of 63 cases. J Oral Maxillofac Surg. 2004;62:527-534. PMID: 15122554.

161. Woo SB, Hellstein JW, Kalmar JR. Narrative [corrected] review: bisphosphonates and osteonecrosis of the jaws. Ann Intern Med. 2006;144:753-761. PMID: 16702591.

162. Tonia T, Mettler A, Robert N, et al. Erythropoietin or darbepoetin for patients with cancer. Cochrane Database Syst Rev. 2012;12:CD003407. PMID: 23235597.

163. Lyman GH, Khorana AA, Falanga A, et al. American Society of Clinical Oncology guideline: recommendations for venous thromboembolism prophylaxis and treatment in patients with cancer. J Clin Oncol. 2007;25:5490-5505. PMID: 17968019.

164. EINSTEIN Investigators, Bauersachs R, Berkowitz SD, et al. Oral rivaroxaban for symptomatic venous thromboembolism. N Engl J Med. 2010;363:2499-2510. PMID: 21128814.

165. EINSTEIN-PE Investigators, Buller HR, Prins MH, et al. Oral rivaroxaban for the treatment of symptomatic pulmonary embolism. N Engl J Med. 2012;366:1287-1297. PMID: 22449293.

166. Agnelli G, Buller HR, Cohen A, et al. Oral apixaban for the treatment of acute venous thromboembolism. N Engl J Med. 2013;369:799-808. PMID: 23808982.

167. Agnelli G, Buller HR, Cohen A, et al. Apixaban for extended treatment of venous thromboembolism. N Engl J Med. 2013;368:699-708. PMID: 23216615.

168. Kadakia KC, Rozell SA, Butala AA, et al. Supportive cryotherapy: a review from head to toe. J Pain Symptom Manage. 2014;47:1100-1115. Epub 2013 Nov 7. PMID: 24210702.

169. Grevelman EG, Breed WP. Prevention of chemotherapy-induced hair loss by scalp cooling. Ann Oncol. 2005;16:352-358. PMID: 15642703.

170. Witman G, Cadman E, Chen M. Misuse of scalp hypothermia. Cancer Treatment Reports 1981;65:507-508. PMID: 7237471.

171. Forsberg SA. Scalp cooling therapy and cytotoxic treatment. Lancet. 2001;357:1134. PMID: 11303618.

172. Christodoulou C, Tsakalos G, Galani E, et al. Scalp metastases and scalp cooling for chemotherapy-induced alopecia prevention. Ann Oncol. 2006;17:350. PMID: 16166175.

173. Lemieux J, Amireault C, Provencher L, et al. Incidence of scalp metastases in breast cancer: a retrospective cohort study in women who were offered scalp cooling. Breast Cancer Res Treat. 2009;118:547-552. PMID: 19241158.

174. van den Hurk CJ, Peerbooms M, van de Poll-Franse LV, et al. Scalp cooling for hair preservation and associated characteristics in 1411 chemotherapy patients - results of the Dutch Scalp Cooling Registry. Acta oncologica. 2012;51:497-504. PMID: 22304489.

21

PALLIATIVE AND END-OF-LIFE CARE

Arif H. Kamal, MD, and Amy P. Abernethy, MD, PhD

Updates from 2012

▶ Advanced care planning and end-of-life (EOL) discussions early in the course of advanced cancer reduce the aggressiveness of EOL care and increase timely utilization of hospice (Mack JW, *J Clin Oncol* 2012).

▶ Oncologists should acknowledge the efforts of informal caregivers, because the degree of support patients receive predicts some important outcomes, including hospital readmission and survival (Aizer AA, *J Clin Oncol* 2013).

▶ Regular comprehensive symptom and emotional well-being assessments are key to improving quality of life and timely symptom management (Kamal AH, *J Oncol Pract* 2013; Seow H, *J Oncol Pract* 2012).

In oncology, palliative care focuses on relief of suffering and improvement in quality of life for the patient with cancer and his or her caregivers, who may include family members and other loved ones. As currently conceptualized, the needs addressed by palliative care encompass four dimensions: physical, psychological (emotional), social (including both relational and logistical), and spiritual/existential. To address these dimensions throughout the disease trajectory, palliative care begins at the time of diagnosis and extends throughout the course of cancer care, often in conjunction with treatment for the disease, but also extending beyond the conclusion of active treatment. Most simply stated, palliative care is about living life to the fullest when faced with the reality of life-threatening illness. The palliative focus requires specific considerations that must be part of an ongoing, carefully documented conversation about the individual's preferences (and values underpinning those preferences) for care in the context of his or her life.

Although palliative care is relevant throughout the disease trajectory, and is not synonymous with end-of-life (EOL) care, to avoid overlap with other chapters, this chapter focuses on palliation after discontinuation of active anticancer therapy, when the patient may be approaching the EOL. Here the goals of care shift from cure and disease-free survival to optimization of physical comfort, psychosocial well-being, and quality of life. In this phase of care, symptom management should address the full range of the patient's experiences—including physical symptoms, cognitive effects, and psychosocial concerns—that may diminish the patient's comfort and erode quality of life.

There is increasing recognition that palliative care serves a vital role earlier in the cancer illness trajectory than originally conceived. Palliative care can—and should—be delivered simultaneously with antineoplastic treatment when the aim of that therapy is not explicitly curative; ideally, oncologists and palliative care clinicians should work together on a day-to-day basis. This approach is supported by recent evidence that palliative care improves not only traditional symptom-focused and quality-of-life outcomes, but also survival. A randomized controlled trial suggested that early application of palliative care improved life expectancy of patients with metastatic lung cancer by more than 2 months (a magnitude of benefit that has allowed many expensive targeted therapies to become licensed for use), improved quality of care, and reduced costs.[1] This high-profile study heightened awareness that the health care delivery system should make palliative care available to address the needs of patients who are suffering from serious life-limiting illness before their last few days of life to improve overall survival and quality of life, as well as health care utilization. This research is complemented by work demonstrating the health and survival benefits of palliative care to caregivers long after they have relinquished their role.[2,3] A Provisional Clinical Opinion released in March 2012 by ASCO recommends early palliative care for people with metastatic lung cancer, consideration of a similar approach in other advanced cancer scenarios, and improved access to palliative care even when people are not in the hospital or not yet ready for hospice.[4]

MANAGEMENT OF PHYSICAL SYMPTOMS

Management of the physical symptoms of cancer is of primary importance for patients during all stages of care. This management starts with standardizing approaches for routine symptom assessment, which then informs timely management. Frequent comprehensive symptom assessments coupled with assessments of emotional well-being (e.g., depression, anxiety) predict higher quality of life.[5] Further, researchers have shown that increased documentation of symptom severity using standardized approaches results in more timely clinical actions taken to alleviate moderate or severe symptoms.[6]

Typically, patients experience multiple physical symptoms in a sometimes complex and shifting pattern, rather than in a discrete or sequential way. The palliative management of physical concerns for the patient with advanced cancer begins with a comprehensive assessment of symptoms (e.g., a review of systems), attends to all existing issues within the overall context of the patient's well-being, and requires regular monitoring to ensure relief and comfort, adjusting treatment as the landscape of symptoms changes. When developing an initial care plan and throughout its iterative adjustment, the clinician should include not only the patient's perspective, but also that of the patient's family and other caregivers.

CANCER-RELATED PAIN

Pain is one of the most prevalent cancer-related symptoms. Between 50% and 90% of patients with advanced cancer experience moderate to severe pain.[7-9] In the context of palliative and EOL care, where the focus of care is on relief of suffering, adequate pain management is imperative.

Of primary importance for the patient receiving palliative or EOL care is a solid basic pharmacotherapeutic approach that achieves the best possible pain relief through a combination of nonopioid and opioid analgesics, based on individual circumstances. The World Health Organization (WHO) three-step

ladder for cancer pain relief remains the starting point for clinical management (Fig. 21-1). The WHO approach employs three categories of agents: opioid analgesics, nonopioid analgesics, and adjuvant therapies. An individualized combination of opioid and nonopioid drugs constitutes the foundation of pain management; to this foundation the clinician adds tailored care, selecting from a broad array of adjuvant interventions to achieve maximum comfort for the patient. Guidelines are available to assist the clinician in determining a foundation of treatment; for example, the National Comprehensive Cancer Network (NCCN) and American Pain Society both maintain publicly available guidelines that serve as excellent sources for cancer pain management.[10,11]

Palliative pain management begins with a comprehensive diagnostic assessment that addresses the medical, psychological, and social components of pain.[12] Location and severity of the pain should be defined; common approaches use either a numeric rating scale (e.g., 0 to 10, with 0 representing no pain and 10 representing worst possible pain) or a visual depiction such as the Wong-Baker FACES Pain Rating Scale or the Iowa Pain Thermometer scale.[13,14]

Pain should be classified as acute or chronic. Acute pain is characterized by a well-defined temporal pattern of onset, generally associated with subjective and objective physical signs and with hyperactivity of the autonomic nervous system. Usually self-limited, acute pain responds to treatment with analgesic drug therapy and to treatment of its precipitating cause. There are numerous specific acute cancer pain syndromes associated with diagnostic and therapeutic procedures or specific antitumor therapies (e.g., pain related to bone marrow biopsy). Acute pain can be further subdivided into subacute and episodic. Subacute pain occurs throughout several days, and presents a pattern of symptom progression. Episodic or intermittent pain occurs during confined periods of time, on a regular or irregular basis. Management of cancer-related acute pain

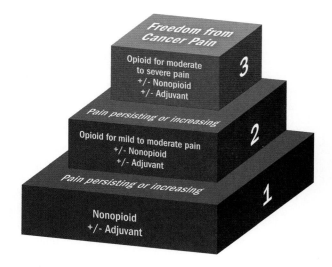

Fig. 21-1 World Health Organization Pain Relief Ladder.

Modified with permission from the World Health Organization. WHO's Pain Relief Ladder, www.who.int/cancer/palliative/painladder/en.

syndromes is similar to any other acute pain management approach, following usual standards of care.

Chronic pain persists for longer than 3 months, with a less well-defined temporal onset and without the objective signs common to acute pain; most cancer-related pain treatment in the palliative care setting is chronic. Treatment of chronic pain in the patient with cancer requires a careful assessment of not only the intensity of pain but also its broad multidimensional aspects. Baseline pain is the average pain intensity experienced for 12 or more hours during a 24-hour period. Breakthrough pain is a transient increase in pain to greater-than-moderate intensity, occurring on top of a baseline pain. Various epidemiologic studies have reported prevalence of breakthrough pain in 23% to 90% of patients with cancer.[15-18] The transitory increase in pain can mark onset or worsening of pain at the end of a dosing interval or with a regularly scheduled analgesic. When caused by an action of the patient, it is termed "incident pain."

According to the WHO ladder, pain treatment begins with nonopioid drugs alone or in combination (Table 21-1). First treatment options are acetaminophen and nonsteroidal anti-inflammatory agents. If these drugs are successful in achieving pain relief, no further therapy is necessary. However, if nonopioid drugs fail to provide adequate relief, the clinician can judiciously select from among multiple opioid options

including morphine—the WHO drug of choice—or congeners of morphine, including hydromorphone, codeine, oxycodone, methadone, and fentanyl. The choice of agent depends upon the clinician's comfort with using the drug, route of delivery, availability, cost, and patient factors such as age, renal function, comorbidities, and other drugs currently being taken. Adjuvant, or coanalgesic, drugs are nonopioid medications that enhance the analgesia provided by opioids; their addition to an opioid regimen can result in better pain control and/or fewer adverse effects (Table 21-2).[12]

Because most pain managed in the cancer-related palliative care setting is chronic, the palliative approach should include an "around-the-clock" management strategy for continuous baseline pain, supplemented with additional medications for breakthrough or incident pain. Generally, long-acting sustained-release products and routine scheduled dosing are matched with short-acting "rescue" doses for breakthrough events. When opioids are prescribed, the breakthrough dose usually should be 10% to 20% of the total daily around-the-clock sustained-release dose (except in the case of short-acting fentanyl products, for which the short-acting dose is established by independent titration until analgesic efficacy is achieved). Further, because the maximal analgesic effect is reached at 1 hour, clinicians may prescribe short-acting oral opioids to be taken as needed every

Table 21-1 Nonopioid Analgesics for Mild to Moderate Pain

Class	Generic Name	Half-Life (hours)	Dosing Schedule	Recommended Starting Dose (mg)	Maximum Daily Dose (mg)
Salicylates	Aspirin	3-12	q4-6h	2,400*	6,000
	Choline magnesium trisalicylate	9-17	q12h	200§	600
	Diflunisal	8-12	q12h	1,500 for the first dose, then 1,000 q12h	4,000
p-Aminophenol derivative	Acetaminophen (paracetamol)	2-4	q4-6h	2,600*	4,000
Propionic acids	Ibuprofen	1.8-2	q4-8h	1,200§	3,200
	Fenoprofen	2-3	q4-6h	800*	3,200
	Ketoprofen	2-3	q6-8h	150§	300
	Naproxen	13	q12h	550§	1,100
	Naproxen sodium	13	q12h	550§	1,100
Acetic acids	Etodolac	7	q6-8h	600§	1,200
	Ketorolac	4-7	q6h	15-30 q6h IV, IM	120 IV, IM
				10 q6h PO	40 PO
Fenamates	Meclofenamic acid	1.3	q6-8h	150§	400
	Mefenamic acid	2	q6h	500 for the first dose, then 250 q6h	1,000
COX2 inhibitor	Celecoxib	11	qd-q12h	100§	200

*Recommended daily starting dose.
§Recommended individual starting dose.
Abbreviations: h, hours; IM, intramuscularly; IV, intravenously; PO, orally; q, every; qd, every day.

Table 21-2 Coanalgesic Therapy for Common Cancer Pain Syndromes

Cancer Pain Syndrome	Coanalgesic Therapy
Bone metastases, soft tissue infiltration, arthritis, serositis, and other inflammatory pain	Oral NSAIDs • Choline magnesium trisalicylate 1,500 mg PO BID • Ibuprofen 800 mg PO TID • Naproxen 500 mg PO TID
Postoperative pain (plus arthritis, serositis, and other inflammatory pain syndromes in patients who cannot use oral NSAIDs)	Parenteral or enteral NSAIDs • Ketorolac 15-30 mg IV every 6 hours (< 5 days) • Indomethacin 50 mg PR every 6-8 hours
Acute nerve compression, visceral distention, increased intracranial pressure, soft tissue infiltration	Corticosteroids • Dexamethasone 4-8 mg PO BID/TID • Methylprednisolone 16-32 mg PO BID/TID
Acute spinal cord compression, severe increased intracranial pressure	Corticosteroids • Dexamethasone 10-20 mg IV every 6 hours • Methylprednisolone 40-80 mg IV every 6 hours
Neuropathic pain	Tricyclic antidepressants[a] • Nortriptyline 100-150 mg PO at bedtime • Desipramine 100-300 mg PO at bedtime Anticonvulsants[b,c] • Gabapentin 300-900 mg PO at TID/QID • Carbamazepine 200 mg PO BID/QID • Clonazepam 0.25-0.5 mg PO TID Antispasticity drug • Baclofen 5-30 mg PO BID/TID Local anesthetic • Topical lidocaine 1-3 patches daily, 12 hours on and 12 hours off
Bone pain from metastases	• Pamidronate 90 mg IV every 3-4 weeks • Zoledronic acid 4 mg IV every 4-6 weeks • Calcitonin 200 IU IV or intranasal BID
Bowel spasm from obstruction	• Scopolamine 0.4 mg IV or SC every 4 hours • Octreotide 50-100 mcg SQ BID/TID

[a] Starting dose of nortriptyline and desipramine should be 25 mg PO at bedtime (10 mg if patient is frail or older) and increased by one tablet every 3 to 7 days to target dose as tolerated. Serum drug levels should be checked at target dose or at maximum tolerated dose to assess patient adherence and prevent unexpected toxicity. Onset of pain relief should be expected at 1 to 2 weeks and mood elevation at 4 to 6 weeks of maximum tolerated or target dose.

[b] Serum drug levels should be followed with carbamazepine to assess compliance and prevent unexpected toxicity. The multiple drug–drug interactions noted require review of all medications before initiation.

[c] Possible severe bone marrow suppression requires blood counts to be followed closely.

Abbreviations: BID, twice daily; IV, intravenously; NSAID, nonsteroidal anti-inflammatory drug; PO, orally; PR, as needed; QID, four times daily; SC, subcutaneously; TID, three times daily.

1 to 2 hours. This is especially helpful in two scenarios: when actively titrating oral opioids to better understand total opioid need, or during the active dying phase when opioid requirements are often dynamic.

Morphine continues to be the mainstay of opioid treatment, although its potential adverse effects can limit utility. Because many patients can tolerate morphine without adverse effects, morphine is the most cost-efficient and practical first-line opioid choice in most situations. Oxycodone is a practical alternative that does not have the same metabolite challenges as morphine and, therefore, may be a better choice for patients with advanced age, poor hepatic or renal function, or other comorbidities. Long-acting and short-acting products are available for both morphine and oxycodone; typically, a sustained-release preparation is combined with "as needed" doses of an immediate-release preparation, dosed at 10% to 20% of the total daily opioid dose. Consideration of coadministration of nonopioid and adjuvant drugs, as suggested by the WHO ladder, may help achieve optimal pain control with the least amount of constipation, sedation, and confusion.

If short-acting alternatives to morphine or oxycodone are needed (and for patients in whom morphine provides insufficient analgesia and/or causes intolerable adverse effects) hydromorphone is a useful alternative treatment. Because it has a short half-life, hydromorphone is commonly used in elderly patients. Its high solubility and availability in high-potency parenteral form (10 mg/mL) make it a practical choice for chronic subcutaneous administration. High doses may induce myoclonus, possibly as a result of accumulation of its metabolites (3'-0 methyl glucuronide and hydromorphone-6-glucuronide).[19] A systematic review, originally published in 2002 and updated in 2009, reported little difference between morphine and hydromorphone in terms of analgesic efficacy, adverse effects, or patient preference, although evidence remains limited.[20] In prior studies, patients receiving hydromorphone exhibited less-favorable cognitive performance but reported better mood than did patients receiving morphine.[21,22]

Oxymorphone, an active metabolite of morphine, is available in oral, oral sustained-release, intravenous, and rectal preparations. Oxymorphone serves as an alternative to morphine and its other congeners. Because of its reduced histamine effect, oxymorphone may benefit patients who complain of headache or itchiness after administration of other opioids. Levorphanol has high bioavailability but a long plasma half-life (12 to 16 hours); it should be used cautiously even in the palliative care setting because accumulation can occur with repeated administration.

Previously considered a late-line option for pain management, methadone is used with increasing frequency as the second- or even first-line drug for patients with cancer. There are a few unique characteristics about methadone that require expert oversight in its prescribing and monitoring. First, pharmacokinetic properties of methadone differ from those of morphine (Table 21-3); notably, it has a higher bioavailability and longer half-life.[23] The parenteral-to-oral ratio of methadone is 1:2, compared with 1:6 for morphine. Note that although the plasma half-life of methadone is long, with reports of up to 50 hours in some patients with cancer, the duration of analgesia is 4 to 8 hours. By comparison, the half-lives of morphine, hydromorphone, and fentanyl are 2 to 4 hours, 2 to 3 hours, and 4 hours, respectively, and half-lives are more commensurate with analgesia.[24] The discrepancy between the analgesic duration and plasma half-life of methadone requires careful titration, and makes it a difficult drug to use in a treatment-naive patient. Second, methadone interacts adversely with numerous other drugs and agents (e.g., selective serotonin reuptake inhibitors [SSRIs], antifungal agents, antibiotics, calcium channel blockers, anticonvulsants, corticosteroids, grapefruit juice, and alcohol).

Conversion from other opiates to methadone is one of the most challenging aspects of methadone use. Studies of interindividual differences in response to opioid analgesics have demonstrated that significantly reduced dosages of methadone can affect analgesia for patients taking morphine or hydromorphone on a chronic basis. Conversion from morphine to methadone is most common (compared with conversion from other opioids); a 1:1 ratio is typically reported in single-dose studies, although this conversion ratio does not apply to continuous dosing. As a result of methadone's pharmacokinetic properties (i.e., extensive bioavailability, long half-life, lipophilicity, and incomplete cross-tolerance), higher dose ratios are usually necessary, and close monitoring is warranted.[25]

Consensus guidelines to assist clinicians with dose conversion from other opioids to methadone have been developed by a panel of experts in pain and palliative care, oncology, pharmacology, cardiology, and hospice (Table 21-4). These guidelines concur with specific dose ratios previously developed by Ripamonti et al in a prospective study.[26] From that study, the authors suggested that, for patients taking 30 mg to 90 mg of morphine, the dose ratio is 4:1; for patients taking 90 mg to 300 mg daily, 6:1; and for 300 mg or more, 8:1. Based on survey data, Bruera et al developed a similar ratio for hydromorphone[27] that advises a dose ratio of 1.6:1.0 for patients receiving more than 330 mg of hydromorphone and a dose ratio of 0.95:1.0 for patients receiving less than 300 mg. Current research is attempting to better elucidate the clinical pharmacology of methadone to facilitate its broader use.

Meperidine should not be used to manage chronic pain in the advanced cancer setting. It is available in oral and intramuscular preparations, with a parenteral-to-oral ratio of 1:4. Repetitive intramuscular administration is associated with local tissue fibrosis and sterile abscess. Repetitive dosing of

Table 21-3 **General Comparison of Pharmacokinetic Properties of Methadone and Morphine**		
Characteristic	**Methadone**	**Morphine**
Oral bioavailability	80%	35%
Protein binding	60%-90%	35%
Elimination half-life	30 hours	3-4 hours
Active metabolites	No	Yes
Influenced by kidney disease	Slightly	Highly
Influenced by liver disease	Highly	Slightly

Modified from Ripamonti C, Bianchi M. The use of methadone for cancer pain. Hematol Oncol Clin North Am. 2002 Jun;16:543-55.

Table 21-4 **Conversion Table from Oral Morphine to Intravenous Methadone for Chronic Administration**		
Total Daily Baseline Oral Morphine Dose (mg)	**Estimated Daily Oral Methadone Requirement as Percent of Total Daily Morphine Dose (%)**	**Estimated Daily IV Methadone as Percent of Total Daily Oral Morphine Dose* (%)**
< 100	20-30	10-15
100 to 300	10-20	5-10
300 to 600	8-12	4-6
600 to 1,000	5-10	3-5
> 1,000	< 5	< 3

*The total daily methadone dose derived from the table may then be divided to reflect the intended dosing schedule (i.e., for administration every 8 hours, divide the daily methadone dose by 3).
Abbreviation: IV, intravenous.
Reproduced with permission from Wolters-Kluwer Health. Wickersham RM, Novak KK, managing eds. Drug Facts and Comparisons. St. Louis, MO: Wolters Kluwer Health, Inc.; 2005.

meperidine (more than 250 mg/day) can lead to accumulation of normeperidine, an active metabolite that can produce central nervous system (CNS) hyperexcitability.[28] This hyperirritability is characterized by subtle mood effects followed by tremors, multifocal myoclonus, and occasional seizures. It occurs most commonly in patients with renal disease, but also can occur after repeated administration in patients with normal renal function. Naloxone does not reverse meperidine-induced seizures, and its use in meperidine toxicity is controversial. Case reports have suggested that the use of naloxone has precipitated generalized seizures for some patients. In rare instances, CNS toxicity characterized by hyperpyrexia, muscle rigidity, and seizure has been reported after the administration of a single dose of meperidine to patients receiving treatment with monoamine oxidase inhibitors.

Transdermal patches offer a good option for pain control in the palliative or EOL setting when oral administration of drugs is difficult or undesirable; by maintaining constant plasma drug levels, transdermal systems may provide better sustained pain relief and reduce the incidence of adverse effects.[29] Fentanyl, an opioid analgesic, is the drug most readily available in a transdermal patch form. Newer opioid preparations are forthcoming; notably, transdermal buprenorphine was recently registered with the U.S. Food and Drug Administration for chronic pain, and is routinely prescribed in Australia and Europe for cancer pain management, although its mixed agonist/antagonist activity, dosage ceiling, and high affinity to the opiate receptor limits its use to those patients requiring large daily doses of opioids.[30]

Fentanyl is used effectively to manage both acute and chronic cancer-related pain. A multicenter prospective randomized controlled study enrolling patients with advanced cancer who required strong opioids found transdermal fentanyl to be comparable to oral morphine and oral methadone in effectiveness and tolerability; patients randomly assigned to receive the three drugs also required similar quantities of symptomatic drugs and coanalgesics.[29,31] The half-life of fentanyl is 1 to 2 hours. Kornick et al have drafted guidelines for fentanyl use summarizing all currently available data.[32] The uniqueness of the transdermal preparation facilitates management in patients who are unable to take drugs by mouth, allowing continuous opioid analgesia with minimal associated distress. Patches—available in 12.5 μg/hour to 100 μg/hour doses—are changed every 72 hours. When a patient begins using the fentanyl patch, there is as long as a 12- to 15-hour delay in the onset of analgesia, and alternate approaches must be used to maintain the patient's pain control during this period. Specific guidelines for switching to the fentanyl patch after an intravenous infusion of fentanyl have been developed and are based on use of a 1:1 conversion ratio. Fentanyl also can be used as an anesthetic premedication, as well as intravenously and epidurally for pain control.

Oral transmucosal fentanyl formulations have demonstrated effectiveness in treating breakthrough pain in 0.2- to 1.6-mg doses, providing onset of pain relief in as few as 5 minutes. Transbuccal and effervescent fentanyl products may be superior. Transmucosal, transbuccal, and intranasal fentanyl in dose-titration trials have been shown to be safe and effective, with the effective dose being a variable requiring titration in the majority of patients (Table 21-5).

If severe pain persists or if the adverse effects of drugs are not tolerated, the physician should consider switching analgesics (e.g., from oral morphine to methadone), changing the route of administration (e.g., from oral to subcutaneous), or performing a procedural intervention (e.g., nerve block) for localized pain. A trial of an adjuvant drug together with the opioid and nonopioid drug may also be helpful. Adjuvants appropriate in this setting include anticonvulsants (gabapentin, pregabalin, carbamazepine, valproate) and antidepressants (amitriptyline, nortriptyline, imipramine, duloxetine), especially when the patient is experiencing neuropathic pain.[33] More often, adjuvant agents are being administered as the primary pain therapy, sometimes leading to complete response without requiring opioids (and thereby eliminating the problem of opioid adverse effects).

For patients in whom opioids induce excessive sedation or confusion, the use of a neurostimulant or haloperidol can adequately treat this side effect while maintaining the patient's analgesia. Alternatively, excessive adverse effects resulting from systemic opioid delivery, such as confusion or sedation, may warrant a switch to epidural or intrathecal opioids. For localized pain, neurolytic blocks are indicated. For severe pain, unilateral and below-the-waist cordotomy may be appropriate.

Table 21-5 Opioid Analgesics Commonly Used in Cancer Pain Management

Drug*	Half-Life (hours)	Duration of Action (hours)
Codeine	2-3	2-4
Dihydrocodeine	2-3	2-4
Oxycodone	2-3	2-4
Propoxyphene	2-3	2-4
Morphine	2-3	3-4
Hydromorphone	2-3	2-4
Methadone	15-190	4-8
Meperidine	2-3	2-4
Oxymorphone	2-3	3-4
Levorphanol	12-15	4-8
Fentanyl (parenteral)	1-2	1-3
Fentanyl (transdermal system)†	–	48-72
Fentanyl (transmucosal and transbuccal)	1-2	1-2

*Oxycodone, hydromorphone, and morphine available in slow-release preparations.
†Transdermal fentanyl, 100 μg/hour; morphine, 4 mg/hour.

For the patient receiving palliative or EOL care, pain must be both proactively and aggressively managed to ensure that the patient neither suffers nor dies with unrelieved pain. At this stage, it is especially important to educate family members and caregivers that addiction is not a concern, and to reiterate the shared goal of maximizing the patient's comfort. Consultation with pain specialists and/or a multidisciplinary approach is warranted to ensure best care. Behavioral approaches, such as guided imagery, may be integrated and used along with pharmacologic approaches. For example, cognitive behavioral therapy in the form of brief relaxation and distraction audiotapes have proven effective in relieving pain in the short term, although pain relief may not be sustained (e.g., for weeks post-intervention).[34]

KEY POINTS

- Best possible pain control in the patient receiving palliative and end-of-life care is of paramount importance.
- The World Health Organization three-step ladder provides the basis for good pain management.
- Morphine and oxycodone are the mainstays of opioid treatment, given the low cost and ready availability of oral long-acting preparations.
- Hydromorphone, with a short half-life but comparable analgesia to morphine, is useful in this population; fentanyl patches have the advantages of ease of application and long-acting effect.
- Methadone often may be a good choice for the home-based patient with advanced cancer.
- Transmucosal, transbuccal, and effervescent fentanyl products are useful alternatives for episodic breakthrough pain.

DYSPNEA

Dyspnea (shortness of breath) is a highly subjective symptom defined by a combination of underlying pathology, the signaling of neural pathways, and the patient's perceived sensation of breathlessness.[35] Patients' descriptions of dyspnea vary widely; the patient's disease, ethnic/racial background, previous experiences, and emotional state contribute to these variations. Patients often report dyspnea that seems out of proportion to known underlying disease or other physiologic etiologies. Dyspnea that does not improve despite maximal treatment for the underlying illness is termed "refractory dyspnea."

A host of pharmacologic and nonpharmacologic interventions have been studied for relief of breathlessness. A systematic review conducted in 2008 searched for randomized controlled trials assessing all pharmacologic and nonpharmacologic interventions for dyspnea palliation in patients with cancer, and included 18 studies: seven assessed opioids (primarily morphine), five oxygen, one helium-enriched air, and one furosemide. Four trials evaluated nonpharmacologic interventions

(e.g., nursing-led programs based on breathlessness rehabilitation techniques, acupuncture). Results clearly supported the use of opioids for dyspnea relief in patients with cancer, but not the use of furosemide. Although oxygen was no more effective than air in most studies, those that included patients with cancer who were hypoxemic and terminally ill did show a significant effect on dyspnea.[36] Helium-enriched air showed promise, but requires further study.

In the EOL setting, opioids (either oral or parenteral) and oxygen are the most frequently used interventions for dyspnea. The mechanism of action for opioids in reducing dyspnea is poorly understood; these agents may act centrally, peripherally, or by reducing anxiety.[35] Opioids reduce ventilatory response to carbon dioxide,[37] hypoxia,[38,39] inspiratory flow-resistive loading,[39,40] and exercise.[41] Additionally, morphine decreases oxygen consumption both at rest and with exercise in healthy individuals.[41]

Opioids, particularly morphine, seem well tolerated when used as interventions to alleviate dyspnea. Morphine has been found neither to depress the respiratory rate nor to result in severe sedation or obtundation.[42] As with any use of opioids, constipation should be anticipated and preventively treated. For the person who cannot take morphine, it is unclear whether the efficacy of morphine for the management of breathlessness can be generalized to other opioids (e.g., oxycodone), but, in general, most clinicians are comfortable with generalizing the morphine evidence to other opioids when needed.

As a practical starting point, the clinician can consider 2.5 mg to 10 mg of morphine orally every 4 hours as needed for the opioid-naive patient.[11] If less-frequent dosing is desirable, a 20-mg starting dose of once-daily sustained-release morphine can be used, assuming no contraindication. If the once-daily product is not available, a 15-mg twice-daily formulation can be prescribed, initially administered once per day and increasing to twice per day after 3 to 5 days if the patient tolerates the medication and has residual breathlessness. When the patient has a contraindication to morphine, long-acting oxycodone can be used, starting at 10 mg once per day and increased to twice per day; no objective data are available to support this practice, and approaches are generalized from the morphine data. If an opioid-tolerant patient is already receiving a regular dose of morphine or another opioid, consider sequentially increasing the opioid by 20% of the total daily dose every 3 to 5 days until the patient's breathlessness is relieved or adverse effects occur.[43]

Palliative oxygen often is prescribed to relieve refractory dyspnea in patients with cancer who do not meet criteria for long-term home oxygen therapy. Although palliative oxygen is indicated for severely hypoxemic patients, it does not confer greater benefit than air does for mildly hypoxemic or nonhypoxemic patients.[34] A multinational randomized controlled trial that enrolled patients with refractory dyspnea and PaO_2 greater than 55 mmHg established that palliative oxygen provides no significantly greater dyspnea relief than does air when both gases are delivered from a canister through a nasal cannula. Results also indicated that the burden of oxygen therapy, which includes cost, tubing, confinement to a concentrator, and exaggeration of the "sick role," may outweigh its benefit for certain patients.[44]

Potential nonpharmacologic interventions include a fan, lower room temperatures, stress management, relaxation therapy, and physical comfort measures to help alleviate the sensation of breathlessness. Additionally, because anxiety can exacerbate dyspnea (and may be among the causes of dyspnea, setting up a worsening spiral of cause and effect), the role of benzodiazepines for anxiety should be considered; the starting dose for a benzodiazepine-naive patient is 0.5 mg to 1.0 mg of lorazepam orally every 4 hours as needed.[11] Importantly, the role of benzodiazepines for management of dyspnea is highly debated, and should not be considered standard of care.

KEY POINTS

- Assessment of dyspnea is complicated by its highly subjective nature.
- Oral and parenteral opioids have a highly statistically significant effect on the sensation of breathlessness.
- Morphine alleviates the sensation of breathlessness without reducing respiratory rate; as with morphine use in cancer pain, constipation is a predictable side effect that should be prevented.
- Anxiety should be treated for its potential role in intensifying the experience of dyspnea.
- Palliative oxygen may alleviate dyspnea symptoms for hypoxemic patients, but is not superior to moving air for patients with dyspnea whose PaO_2 is greater than 55 mmHg.
- Nonpharmacologic interventions, such as a fan or relaxation therapy, offer useful adjuncts to opioids and oxygen.

NUTRITION AND HYDRATION

Nutrition and hydration often become important issues for families caring for a loved one with a potentially life-limiting illness. Fearing that withdrawal of nutrition or hydration will result in death by starvation, many families request that the patient—even the terminally ill patient—receive nutrition and hydration support. These are some of the last therapies to be withdrawn at the EOL.[45,46]

Although clinicians frequently provide nutritional supplementation for patients nearing the EOL, the evidence does not suggest that it benefits these patients by preventing aspiration, improving survival, increasing activity capacity, or alleviating cachexia.[47,48] As patients progress toward death, it is quite common to eat less; hunger is not an issue for the majority of patients.[49] Observational studies of dying patients who are no longer receiving hydration or nutrition have not demonstrated an increase in discomfort.[50,51] Therefore, nutritional supplementation in dying patients is not recommended,[52]

except in select scenarios such as gastrointestinal complications (especially involving bowel obstruction) when there also is limited spread of cancer to other vital organs.[53] Because of the emotional charge that frequently surrounds the issue of nutritional supplementation, the family or other informal caregivers should be educated by informing them that patients who are dying typically do not experience hunger and thirst; patients with advanced cancer may not be able to metabolize nutritional supplements; risks of artificial nutrition include fluid overload, infection, and hastened death; and withdrawal of intravenous or nasogastric tube feeding is ethically acceptable, will not exacerbate symptoms, and may improve certain symptoms.[11]

The prevalence of thirst in patients at the EOL has been estimated to be between 25% to 83%.[54,55] However, the association between thirst and dehydration at the EOL has been controversial in the recent past.[54,56] Proponents of the use of artificial hydration had argued that the use of judicious hydration may improve the excretion of drug metabolites, thereby alleviating or preventing symptoms such as delirium, agitation, nausea, and myoclonus.[57-59] A multicenter study evaluating terminally ill patients found no difference in myoclonus, confusion, or agitation for patients receiving hydration compared with patients who did not receive hydration.[60] More recently, a well-conducted, placebo-controlled, double-blind, randomized trial, by a previous strong proponent of intravenous hydration, also did not support any benefit for this approach.[61] Another recent study using a randomized, placebo-controlled trial of normal saline hydration coupled with qualitative interviews of patients and families reached the same conclusions of lack of efficacy. Importantly, the authors found that patients in both arms reported continued hope in prolonging life, enhancing life, and promoting comfort. Although the clinical trial results did not find a significant, measurable benefit with hydration, it remains important to recognize the high expectations and hope given to it by patients and caregivers.[61]

Arguments exist regarding the potential harms of hydration at the EOL.[62] These include worsening pulmonary congestion, peripheral edema, ascites, and increased need for voiding and diuretic use.[60,63] To maintain enteral, intravenous, or subcutaneous access, increased use of restraints often is required, subjecting patients to the prospect of injury or discomfort.[64] Lastly, although there is little evidence that hydration prolongs life for dying patients, terminal hydration may artificially prolong the dying process.[65,66]

For acutely dying patients, routine use of artificial hydration generally is not recommended. Instead, providers should discuss prognosis, goals of care, and possible benefits and harms of hydration and nutritional therapy with the patient, family members, and other caregivers involved. Through the use of good mouth care and small offerings of liquid or ice chips, patients who do not receive hydration are likely to experience comfort before death. Focus should remain on the patient's goals and preferences, while heeding distress and concern among family members; clinicians should discuss alternative ways in which family members can care for the patient, and make emotional support available to them. In situations where patients or families insist on therapies that are unlikely to be beneficial, the clinician can suggest a time-limited trial with explicit, objective criteria for desired outcomes. When supplemental hydration must be used, subcutaneously administered enteroclysis may be an option that allows patients to receive fluid at home without intravenous access.[67]

KEY POINTS

- Evidence does not suggest benefit of nutritional supplementation for patients with advanced cancer.
- Hydration at the end of life is generally not recommended.
- Family/caregiver distress is a common reason for continuation of nutrition and hydration support; clinicians should discuss the goals of care with these individuals, explaining the lack of evidence to suggest benefit of these treatments and reassuring them that hunger is generally not a concern of patients at this stage.
- Comfort with respect to thirst can often be achieved through alternative measures such as sips of water, ice chips, and good oral care.

DYSPHAGIA

Dysphagia affects 23% of patients with advanced cancer, and as many as 46% of patients with cancer in the last week of life.[68,69] Although most commonly associated with upper and lower gastrointestinal cancers and head and neck cancers, dysphagia is not limited to these malignancies.[70] Appearance of dysphagia threatens to compromise the patient's nutrition, hydration, and quality of life. Basic nursing care and management of dysphagia-related anxiety are paramount. For the patient who is expected to live longer than 2 months but with progressive nutrition-related problems, a percutaneous gastrostomy tube may be appropriate. Suction of oral secretions may assist with comfort, especially for the person unable to swallow them. To date, few clinical trials of the best management strategies for dysphagia have been conducted.

NAUSEA AND VOMITING

Nausea and vomiting associated with chemotherapy and/or radiation therapy are thoroughly addressed in Chapter 20: Symptom Management. Some patients continue to experience nausea for extended periods after treatment has been discontinued as a result of response failure. At this point, the primary goal of controlling nausea is to ease the patient's discomfort; efforts should be made to determine underlying causes and an appropriate course of treatment.

Among terminally ill patients, nausea may be the result of a number of contributing factors, including opioid pain medications, autonomic failure, peptic ulcer disease, constipation,

bowel obstruction, metabolic abnormalities, and increased intracranial pressure.[71] Ideally, the therapeutic agent is matched to the etiology. When bowel obstruction is not a factor, metoclopramide might be helpful for controlling chronic nausea, especially when the nausea is opioid-related; a randomized, blinded, crossover trial of a controlled-release formulation of metoclopramide (40 mg every 12 hours) compared with placebo in patients with advanced cancer found significantly reduced nausea in the metoclopramide group.[72] However, in 2013, the European Medicines Agency's Committee on Medical Products for Human Use recommended that metoclopramide be limited in response to serious neurologic side effects.[73] Dexamethasone and other corticosteroids can be administered to augment the antiemetic effects of metoclopramide, 5-HT3 antagonists, and other agents.[74,75] Data support that megestrol acetate[76] and olanzapine[77-83] have antiemetic properties in patients with nausea/vomiting associated with advanced cancer. A recommended ordering of interventions to desired effect is: (1) dopamine receptor antagonist (e.g., metoclopramide or prochlorperazine); (2) 5-HT3 antagonist (e.g., ondansetron) possibly with an antihistamine (e.g., meclizine), anticholinergic (e.g., scopolamine), or cannabinoid; (3) corticosteroid, olanzapine, or megestrol acetate; (4) continuous infusion and/or opioid rotation; (5) alternative therapies (e.g., cognitive behavioral therapy or hypnosis).[11] If bowel obstruction is present, a centrally active drug such as dimenhydrinate can be used; insufficient evidence is available to support use of haloperidol for nausea and vomiting in patients receiving palliative care, according to a 2009 Cochrane review.[84] Octreotide and other agents that minimize gut motility seem to help control nausea and vomiting when the bowel is obstructed.[85] Refractory nausea also may respond to palliative sedation with midazolam.[86-88]

NCCN guidelines recommend the following general approaches to management of nausea and vomiting (medication-induced or nonspecific) in patients with advanced cancer in the palliative and EOL care settings: discontinue unnecessary medications; check blood levels of necessary medications; initiate opioid rotation and/or reduce opioid requirement by prescribing coanalgesics; treat with medications in the order described above; add lorazepam (0.5 mg to 1.0 mg every 4 hours as needed) if anxiety is a contributing factor.[11] Oral formulations of medications are preferable, but when the oral route is not feasible, rectal, subcutaneous, or intravenous administration are options.

BOWEL ISSUES
Constipation

Constipation, which broadly refers to slowed small intestinal transit and the difficult passage of feces, is a common symptom in patients with advanced cancer[89]; rates in terminally ill patients have been reported from 50% to 87%.[90-93] A 2005 study of patients in hospice reported that 65% were constipated despite laxative treatment. Constipation can be physically, emotionally, and socially stressful for the patient and caregivers; additionally, it can lead to an array of concomitant concerns including headache, fatigue, abdominal swelling and pain, nausea and vomiting, hemorrhoids, and urinary complications.[90,94,95]

Although constipation can cause significant distress in patients with advanced disease, clinicians often approach it as a relatively minor concern for various reasons, not least of which is the lack of clear guidance for diagnosing and managing constipation in the context of critical illness.[96,97] Consensus on assessment exists in the Rome criteria, but this schema's requirement that symptoms be present for at least 3 months[98] limits its application to the palliative care setting.[99] Management of constipation for the patient with advanced cancer is further complicated by the symptom's largely subjective nature.

Communication between patients and medical staff regarding constipation can be difficult; patients often struggle to characterize symptoms that may be highly relative and complex in their presentation. Because determining what constitutes "normal" bowel habits is a complicated process for both clinician and patient, there may be a tendency to under-report constipation. Fallon and O'Neill found that although only one-half of patients receiving palliative care complain of constipation, about 80% require administration of laxatives,[100] which often takes place only after constipation has become a significant problem.[101]

Severe constipation can have serious quality-of-life repercussions, with some patients becoming excessively preoccupied with their bowels,[102] some reporting it to be more distressing than pain,[103,104] and some refusing to accept analgesic treatment.[90,93,105] The severity of constipation correlates negatively with perceived quality of life[106]; conversely, prevention and effective management of constipation leads to improved quality of life and to better adherence to medication regimens.[105]

Best supportive care for the patient with advanced cancer emphasizes prevention and treatment of constipation, guided by regular assessment of not only objective criteria but also the patient's subjective experience of the symptom and its relative significance.[99,102] The latter is important because common assessment approaches may not fully capture patients' perceptions of constipation.[107]

In the context of advanced illness, the cause of constipation is often multifactorial. Although the relative contribution of each factor is difficult to determine, the onset of constipation is frequently iatrogenic, resulting from the administration of chemotherapy, tricyclic antidepressants, and opioid analgesics. Among the approximately 500,000 patients who die as a result of cancer annually in the United States, more than half receive opioid agents in the terminal stages of disease,[90,97] with 50% to 87% of patients who receive opioids also requiring laxative medication.[90,93] Constipation may also result from the tumor itself, the secondary effects of major illness (reduced fiber and fluid intake, inactivity, lack of privacy, unfamiliar toilet arrangements), and pathologic changes associated with the disease.[90,97,99,102,108]

Constipation frequently results from the action of opioid drugs at multiple sites in the gastrointestinal tract and in the spinal cord, causing a decrease in intestinal secretions and peristalsis, which leads to dry stool. In anticipation of this possible chain of events, when initiating opioid analgesics the clinician should initiate a regular bowel regimen that includes a stimulant laxative and stool softener, such as bisacodyl and senna with or without docusate (two tablets per night).[11] Polyethylene glycol (PEG) has long been used for short-term treatment of occasional constipation, and has been found effective and safe for long-term treatment in patients with chronic constipation.[109] A Cochrane meta-analysis established the superiority of PEG compared with the common alternative osmotic laxative, lactulose.[110]

Peripheral opioid antagonists are playing a growing role in the management of opioid-induced constipation. Methylnaltrexone has been shown to be well tolerated and to relieve constipation for patients receiving chronic opioid medications (without reversing the analgesic effect of the opioids); immediate large-volume laxation may result.[111] It is available as a subcutaneous injection, but is contraindicated in bowel obstruction.[112] Another peripheral opioid antagonist, alvimopan, is indicated for postoperative ileus.[113] Alvimopan is available in a convenient oral formulation and has a similar efficacy profile to methylnaltrexone; however, it does not have an indication for opioid-induced constipation because of concerns of potential cardiac adverse effects. A recent study demonstrates that amidotrizoate is an effective, convenient, well-tolerated, and inexpensive breakthrough medication, inducing bowel movement in 45% of patients with advanced cancer whose symptoms were unresponsive to common laxatives.[114] Early evidence suggests possible efficacy of low-dose subcutaneous neostigmine for relieving severe and refractory constipation in patients with advanced cancer.[115] Oral naloxone has been shown to be effective in treating constipation, but its use is variable dependent on the degree of the patient's opioid exposure.[116]

Anecdotal surveys suggest that laxative doses far higher than those used for routine bowel management are needed for patients with opioid-induced or refractory constipation. Tolerance to effect often eventually develops, but the process is relatively slow.

Nonpharmacologic approaches to constipation management should be employed where possible. Increase in fluids,

KEY POINTS

- Although often neglected by oncologists, prevention and management of constipation leads to improved quality of life and better adherence to medication regimens, especially analgesics.
- Evidence-based bowel regimens supported by clinical experience and current guidelines include senna derivatives, polyethylene glycol, and bisacodyl.
- Evidence suggests that methylnaltrexone is safe and effective for alleviating opioid-related constipation without diminishing analgesic efficacy; other peripheral opioid antagonists may also be helpful.

fiber intake, and exercise can help alleviate constipation, although feasibility is limited in patients with advanced cancer. Pilot evidence suggests that aromatherapy massage can relieve constipation in patients with advanced cancer, while also improving physical and supportive domains of quality of life; however, further study is warranted.[117]

Gastrointestinal Tract Obstruction

Gastrointestinal tract obstruction arises commonly in patients with advanced cancers, especially those with cancers of pelvic or abdominal origin. Reported frequencies range from 5% to 42% in advanced ovarian cancer and from 4% to 24% in advanced colorectal cancer.[118-126]

Gastrointestinal tract obstruction can be caused by multiple and often coexisting etiologies, such as intraluminal masses, direct infiltration of the bowel wall (colon cancer), external compression of the lumen, carcinomatosis causing dysmotility (ovarian cancer), intra-abdominal adhesion (resulting from postoperative changes), constipation, vascular infarcts, and intussusception. Symptoms result from partial or total occlusion of the bowel lumen, alteration of normal peristaltic motion, and alterations in physiologic intestinal fluid secretion and absorption. The site of obstruction varies, and multiple areas of the tract may be involved.

Although the definitive management of gastrointestinal obstruction differs by cause of obstruction, the symptom complex is similar. Approximately 90% of patients experience continuous abdominal pain.[118,119,121,127] Pain is generally less severe, and more intermittent, when the large bowel is affected.[128] Augmenting the continuous pain, peristaltic waves against the obstruction and consequent additional distention of the intestine causes intermittent pain ("colic") in approximately 75% of patients.[118,119,121,127] The inflammatory response to obstruction in or around the bowel wall may further exacerbate fluid secretion through prostaglandin-mediated increases in membrane permeability with or without additional cellular breakdown. Local inflammation may cause edema and contribute directly to increased tumor bulk, thereby precipitating or exacerbating the obstruction. Most patients with gastrointestinal tract obstruction experience nausea and vomiting.

Control of symptoms caused by gastrointestinal tract obstruction in patients with advanced cancer presents a considerable challenge. The first step in treating patients who present with abdominal pain, distension, vomiting, or decreased bowel movement is to evaluate the patient for possible ileus caused by treatment (e.g., vinca alkaloids), antiemetics (e.g., 5-HT$_3$ antagonists), opioids, inactivity, and/or decreased oral fluid intake. If obstruction is present, the clinician should rule out rectal impaction that may respond to a suppository or enema and may render a nasogastric tube unnecessary.

Repeated episodes of emesis may warrant medical management with intravenous fluids and intermittent nasogastric tube suction. Decompression of the gas and fluid accumulation in the stomach and intestine is the primary goal of nasogastric tube placement; this treatment can be initiated while an assessment for operability is being made. A nasogastric tube can be clamped when the nasogastric volume decreases to 100 cc; the tube may be removed if there is no subsequent nausea/vomiting or at the patient's request. Use of a nasogastric tube can be intrusive and distressing to patients, and, thus, should be minimized.

Patients with gastrointestinal tract obstruction often are malnourished and debilitated; the operative mortality risk is high for such patients (12% to 33%),[129] providing further impetus for avoiding unhelpful surgery. Surgery is appropriate for select patients, although not for most who have opted for palliative care. Select patients who are not candidates for surgery may be evaluated for placement of a stent across the site of obstruction. Endoscopic stenting can relieve symptoms in patients for whom esophageal, gastric, and pancreatic cancers cause upper tract obstruction, or for patients with rectal cancers that have caused distal blockage. In general, candidates for stent placement have an isolated site of partial obstruction that is approachable by endoscopic means. Although generally safe, the treatment can result in perforation, bleeding, pain, or migration of the stent; severe complications arise in as many as 10% (mean, 1%) of patients and minor complications occur in up to 30% (mean, 26%).[130,131] Ultrasound-guided placement of vents, either percutaneously or surgically, is an option for more permanent decompression of the obstruction and prevention of emesis (if the patient is deemed not a candidate for operative management).

Often a nasogastric tube, stent, or venting gastrostomy produces insufficient relief. In many cases, emptying the gastric contents alone is not effective in alleviating the obstructive symptoms. A nasogastric tube is uncomfortable, and its ongoing presence increases the risk of iatrogenic complications. Although data supporting venting gastrostomy are more favorable, many patients with advanced disease choose not to have this (or any other) surgical procedure to control their symptoms.[132]

Pharmacologic management of gastrointestinal tract obstruction can be an effective approach to symptom relief, supported by a growing body of clinical experience. Octreotide, a synthetic analogue of somatostatin, is commonly used to treat symptoms related to gastrointestinal obstruction. Somatostatin functions as a neurotransmitter and a neurohormone, with regulatory effects in the gastrointestinal tract, including both endocrine and exocrine outcomes on the pancreas. It inhibits the glandular secretion of growth hormone, thyrotropin, corticotropin, and prolactin and slows the release of gastrin, cholecystokinin, insulin, glucagon, gastric acid, and pancreatic enzymes. It also may prevent neurotransmission in the peripheral nerves of the gastrointestinal tract, leading to diminished peristalsis and a decrease in splanchnic blood flow. There also is some indication that somatostatin inhibits the function of activated immune cells and may have a central opioid-like function. Somatostatin is the naturally occurring precursor hormone of octreotide; octreotide is marketed, available, and frequently prescribed for bowel obstruction. Its duration of action is 8 hours and it is generally well tolerated. Many palliative care specialists recommend treatment with octreotide be initiated soon after diagnosis of gastrointestinal tract obstruction, at a dose of 100 µg to 300 µg subcutaneously two to three times daily or 10- to 40-µg per hour continuous subcutaneous/intravenous infusion.

Doses may be titrated every 24 hours to control nausea and vomiting. In early-phase studies and retrospective analyses, the use of octreotide has been associated with cessation of nausea and vomiting, removal of nasogastric tubes, and, in some cases, the ability of the patient to resume modest oral intake.[133-135] That being said, an adequately powered randomized controlled trial of optimal medical management with and without octreotide was recently completed; conference proceedings suggest that octreotide did not increase the likelihood of controlling the symptoms of bowel obstruction compared with optimal management with regular ranitidine, dexamethasone, and parenteral hydration, with the results manuscript under review.[136]

Antiemetics may be used to relieve nausea associated with gastrointestinal obstruction, mostly for cases of incomplete bowel obstruction. Among these, parenteral metoclopramide has been frequently used in patients with mainly functional bowel obstruction; it is not recommended for patients with complete mechanical bowel obstruction as it may increase colic, nausea, and vomiting as well as pain resulting from increasing motility against a fixed obstruction.[118,137,138] Prochlorperazine is not very effective in this setting, controlling nausea for only a minority of patients. Corticosteroids, which can relieve nausea through both central and peripheral antiemetic effects, have been recommended to decrease the inflammatory response and resultant edema. Corticosteroid effectiveness may result from reduced volume of intestinal fluid caused by either the tumor's disruption of cellular integrity or the inflammatory response. A Cochrane review, updated through 2006, reported a statistically nonsignificant trend that intravenous corticosteroids (dose range, 6 mg to 16 mg of dexamethasone) may lead to resolution of bowel obstruction.[139] Olanzapine has also been reported to be useful for decreasing nausea in patients with partial bowel obstruction.[140]

Opioid analgesics control continuous pain for many patients with gastrointestinal obstruction, but may not be effective for intermittent colicky pain. The mechanism of such pain is thought to be spasms of smooth muscle, as well as bowel-wall distension in response to peristaltic waves converging on the site of obstruction. Thus, antimuscarinic anticholinergic agents can be used in addition to opioids to help manage this symptom complex. Atropine, a racemic mixture of dextrohyoscyamine and levohyoscyamine, is the prototypic gastrointestinal antimuscarinic agent and can be administered intravenously, subcutaneously, or orally every 4 hours. Its usefulness is limited by its adverse effects, which include xerostomia, blurred vision, cycloplegia, mydriasis, photophobia, anhidrosis, urinary retention, tachycardia, palpitations, constipation, mental confusion, and delirium. Scopolamine, another antimuscarinic anticholinergic drug, is available in both parenteral and transdermal preparations in the United States. Intravenous or subcutaneous doses in the range of 5 μg to 100 μg every hour have been reported to be effective. However, because this agent is available only as the hydrobromide salt that penetrates the CNS, it carries potential for significant side effects. Glycopyrrolate, a quaternary ammonium compound, has clinical effects similar to scopolamine but, unlike scopolamine, does not carry risk of

inducing delirium or other CNS-related side effects.[141] The recommended dose is 0.1 mg to 0.2 mg subcutaneously or intravenously three to four times daily. It is compatible with prochlorperazine, promethazine, lorazepam, midazolam, morphine, and other opioids including fentanyl, hydromorphone, and levorphanol, but should not be administered in conjunction with diazepam, methylprednisolone, dexamethasone, dimenhydrinate, and phenobarbital.[142]

KEY POINTS

- Malignant bowel obstruction can have multiple etiologies related to the tumor itself or to adhesions from prior abdominal surgery.
- Patients should be evaluated initially for possible ileus caused by treatment, antiemetics, opioids, inactivity, and/or decreased oral fluid intake.
- A nasogastric tube with suction is the usual first treatment for patients with bowel obstruction, but its duration should be minimized to respect patients' comfort.
- Endoscopic placement of a stent and venting gastrostomy are additional options for mechanical relief of the blockage and, hence, symptoms.
- Medical management with octreotide should be considered.
- Symptom control with steroids, metoclopramide, antiemetics, scopolamine, or glycopyrrolate can supplement medical management and procedural strategies.

Diarrhea

Although cancer-related diarrhea is most frequently associated with chemotherapy and radiation therapy, it can afflict patients with advanced cancer who are receiving only palliative care. In these cases, the cancer itself may cause diarrhea. In patients with pancreatic cancer, the presence of inadequate digestive enzymes may lead to osmotic diarrhea; if these patients have an increased stool odor, the clinician should consider administering exogenous pancreatic enzyme. For patients with thyroid cancer, secretory diarrhea may result from the overproduction of calcitonin and prostaglandins. Patients with carcinoid syndrome as a result of the increased secretion of prostaglandins and serotonin may benefit from octreotide; cyproheptadine also may be helpful for carcinoid syndrome-related diarrhea. (See Chapter 20: Symptom Management for a more detailed discussion of diarrhea management.)

SLEEP/WAKE DISTURBANCES

Various physical and/or psychological issues can cause sleep disorders at or near the EOL, diminishing the patient's quality of life and potentially contributing to symptoms such as pain, fatigue, and distress.[143] The clinician should inquire about the adequacy of the patient's sleep, and if the patient indicates dissatisfaction, should evaluate the type and severity of sleep disturbance. Factors such as pain, delirium, depression, anxiety, and nausea can all contribute to sleep/wake disturbances; hence, good symptom control is a first step in treating these issues. Similarly, medication adverse effects or effects of withdrawal from medications and other substances (e.g., corticosteroids, anticonvulsants, barbiturates, tricyclic antidepressants, caffeine, alcohol) can have deleterious effects on sleep and daytime wakefulness. These effects should be closely monitored when weaning the patient off of unnecessary medications.

Many sleep/wake disturbances can be managed satisfactorily with oral pharmacologic agents. For insomnia, zolpidem (5 mg to 10 mg orally at bedtime, with a second dose available if the patient wakes in the middle of the night) and lorazepam (0.5 mg to 1.0 mg at bedtime) are effective for most patients. Potentially sedating medications, such as opioids and anticholinergics, can be scheduled to promote sleep; conversely, steroids and other medications that inhibit sleep should be timed so that they do not interfere with regular sleep routines. To counteract daytime sedation, methylphenidate and modafinil have been used, but randomized trials have not clarified benefit from this approach and some suggest that they result in net harm.[11] Especially with daytime drowsiness, it is important to discuss treatment of the sleep/wake disturbance with the patient, to ascertain whether the patient wants treatment for this symptom. When psychological distress is suspected to be largely responsible for the disturbance, the clinician should consider referral to a psychologist or other mental health professional; cognitive behavioral therapy, for example, may be of help to the patient.

MANAGEMENT OF COGNITIVE AND PSYCHOSOCIAL SYMPTOMS

Increasingly, cognitive and psychosocial symptoms are recognized as important targets of care for patients with cancer. Guidelines such as the NCCN Guidelines v1.2011 Distress Management[144] offer resources for managing complex psychosocial issues in patients with cancer, providing, for example, a definition of cancer-related distress, treatment guidelines, and suggestions for screening tools and appropriate referrals. Although patients undergoing active treatment, survivors in the posttreatment phase, and patients with advanced cancer share many similar psychosocial concerns, the population of patients in the palliative and dying phases has its own constellation of concerns.

COMMUNICATION

Communicating bad news to patients and families is a critical but challenging aspect of providing supportive care for terminally ill patients. The provision of accurate information to patients and caregivers can facilitate collaborative decision-making. Not only the content of the discussion, but the manner in which the clinician delivers difficult news can have repercussions for the emotional health of both patients and their loved ones.[145]

Discussion of advanced care planning is an important starting point for conversations at or near the EOL, and truly, for any patient with advanced and potentially life-limiting disease. Components of advanced care planning, which the patient may or may not have completed in written form, include advanced care directives, health care proxies or powers of attorney, living wills, and do-not-resuscitate (DNR) orders. Where these documents exist, they can be used as the basis of discussion about the patient's values and preferences for EOL care. Where they have not been completed, the clinician can enlist the assistance of an appropriate individual (e.g., a social worker or member of the palliative care team) to help the family complete forms, after he or she has introduced the concept, explained the purpose, and discussed the benefits and process of advanced care planning with the patient and any relevant family members or caregivers. In many cases, the patient with very advanced cancer will not be capable of medical decision-making him- or herself; here, an assessment should confirm this status, and, thereafter, a surrogate should be identified. Options for palliative care, including hospice, should be described at this time. Conversations should elicit the patient's and family's values, feelings, and preferences with respect to decision-making on EOL care.

Good communication in palliative and EOL care should begin with (1) assessment of the patient's and family's understanding of the likely course of the disease, the patient's capacity for decision-making or need for a surrogate, and the patient's and family's communication style; (2) clarification of how much information the patient would like, and how much information should be given to the family; and (3) discussion of the patient's and family's preferences for care and quality of life. This approach, which emphasizes "asking permission" before embarking on a difficult discussion or addressing an important topic, is an important step to help in building rapport and keeping communication lines open.[146] It should initiate an ongoing process of clear and consistent discussion with the patient and family regarding treatment, changes of status, prognosis, EOL, and patient and family needs. Timely advanced care planning discussions and readdressing of planning needs during disease transitions remain major predictors of aggressiveness of EOL care and hospice utilization, further reinforcing the role of these conversations in optimizing appropriate, patient-centered advanced cancer care.[147] When appropriate, the palliative care team and/or hospice providers can be introduced to assist with these conversations.

Evidence demonstrates that many patients with metastatic cancer incorrectly perceive chemotherapy as being likely to cure them of disease, reflecting the gaps between clinicians' intentions and patients' perceptions. Underscoring this, a recent study from Weeks and colleagues demonstrated that more than 50% of patients with metastatic colon and lung cancer perceive their chemotherapy as being likely to cure their disease.[148] Discussing intent and potential benefits of cancer-directed therapies should be considered an integral component of the informed consent process, alongside the usual conversations of risk and potential side effects of antineoplastic therapy.

Physicians sometimes knowingly provide an overly optimistic evaluation of a patient's prognosis,[149,150] or alternatively, provide no prognostic information until the patient nears death.[151,152] Additionally, patients often interpret prognostic information in an optimistic way; many patients exhibit a tendency to believe that they will be an exception, the one to "beat the odds."[153] Patients' perceptions of prognosis and their choices regarding therapy are demonstrably influenced by the way in which they receive information from their physicians.[154,155] Information presented from a positive perspective (such as percentage of patients with a given condition who survive to 5 years) is perceived to be better than the same information delivered in negative terms (such as percent of patients with this same condition who do not survive to 5 years). Patients who harbor falsely optimistic perceptions often opt for aggressive medical therapy, despite evidence that aggressive care—compared with palliative measures only—confers no survival benefit for terminally ill patients.[156]

Many physicians express concern that an accurate prognosis may undermine a patient's hope.[157,158] The value of hope is rated very highly by both patients and caregivers who emphasize that they do not want doctors to lessen hope, even at the EOL.[159,160] In terminal illness, however, physicians can redefine hope—without implying a cure—by helping patients come to a realistic understanding of their prognosis and by setting realistic goals such as reduction of pain, alleviation of distress, and achievement of closure with family members.[145] Similarly, many people worry that an accurate prognosis will diminish the patient's "fighting spirit," especially when there is coexisting depression. Although it is essential to address any presenting psychiatric illness, little evidence exists to suggest that a fighting spirit improves morbidity or mortality.[161] In reality, many patients struggle to cope with news of a poor prognosis; this struggle is often apparent in seemingly contradictory expressions of unrealistic hope for longevity alongside awareness of prognosis (e.g., by discussing funeral plans).[162]

Although most existing guidelines for delivering bad news to patients and families do not have empirical evidence to support their use, they are based on viable communication principles and consensus expert opinion, and, therefore, have good face validity.[163,164] A formal discussion of bad news might best be preceded by thorough preparation. Clinicians should discuss how patients would like to receive prognostic information (and whether they actually desire it) before starting any conversation involving bad news. The physician should take into account that patients and families hold different views about who should participate in such discussions, what information should be included, the appropriate setting, and who should convey the information. Clinicians should ideally endeavor to be prepared with accurate, up-to-date information and to deliver the news themselves. If possible, the setting should be private and free from distractions.

To evaluate the patient's and family's levels of understanding and to anticipate their reactions, the clinician should initiate any discussion of bad news by asking them about what they already know. This enables the patient and family to determine the level of information they seek and how to best convey that information. The physician can then deliver the information, but also should pause frequently to verify understanding and to allow for questions; a reasonable approach is to provide no more than three items of information before pausing to ensure that the patient and his or her family understand and do not have questions. At the end of the discussion, the clinician should confirm that the patient and family have a sound understanding, for example, by asking them to summarize the information in their own words. Finally, a clear agenda should be established, covering what the patient and family will do, what the physician will do, and when the next contact will occur.

Recently, cross-cultural reviews have helped expand the literature related to communication in palliative and EOL care; these perspectives are particularly relevant to clinicians treating increasingly heterogeneous populations. An Indian review reported on collusion in palliative care communications resulting in, for example, nearly one-half of patients with cancer in India being unaware of their diagnosis and treatment.[165] Similar cultural norms with respect to truth-telling and withholding of information have been reported in Chinese culture.[166] In both instances, strong family values include a central role for family members in managing the patient's disease, communication, and health care at or near the EOL. Of relevance to the U.S. oncologist, these studies suggest the importance of (a) being aware that patients with a background in other cultures may have different expectations for communication, and (b) explaining and discussing the communication plan with the patient and family members to establish common expectations. Where available, an interpreter or other cultural liaison may be of help in facilitating effective communications.

PSYCHOLOGICAL DISTRESS
Patient
Death is a process fraught with emotional charge for patients as well as for family members, other informal caregivers, and health care providers, all of whom have a unique relationship to the dying patient. Although psychosocial concerns frequently arise at the EOL, they can be difficult to detect or diagnose. Certain psychological states that may resemble depression are in fact normal at the EOL; physical symptoms normally experienced by the patient at the EOL may otherwise constitute somatic diagnostic criteria for psychiatric illnesses. Nevertheless, health care providers must remain vigilant for signs and symptoms of distress, which include concerns about illness, sadness, anger, feelings of loss of control, poor sleep, poor appetite, poor concentration, and preoccupation with thoughts of illness and death. Awareness of psychological concerns takes on greater importance for clinicians treating terminally ill patients, for whom psychological distress may increase as death approaches.[167]

Estimates suggest that as many as 82% of terminally ill patients experience some form of psychiatric illness,[168,169] including adjustment disorder (10% to 16%),[170,171] depressive disorders (3% to 82%),[170,171] and anxiety disorders (7% to 79%).[168,171] Risk factors for distress in patients with cancer include cognitive impairment, communication barriers (e.g., language, literacy), history of psychiatric disorder, history of substance abuse, history of depression or suicidality, psychosocial issues (e.g., family conflict, young/dependent children, financial concerns, limited social support, living alone), and uncontrolled symptoms.

Although the EOL is frequently marked by psychiatric symptoms, physicians often struggle to address emotional concerns during the medical interview. Many physicians report feeling uncertain about their ability to effectively discuss emotional topics, especially those that accompany bad news.[163,172] Reimbursement restrictions and the typical structure of the medical interview further discourage some clinicians from freely discussing psychosocial issues.[173] Physicians often fear that discussions that address emotional content will take too much time or elicit powerful feelings on the part of the patient that they will be unable to manage. The evidence, however, should dispel this concern: Research demonstrates that medical encounters are actually shorter when the physician openly acknowledges the patient's emotional concerns.[174]

Distress in patients with advanced cancer can be identified using a simple screening tool such as the NCCN Distress Thermometer (Fig. 21-2), which asks the patient to rate his or her distress on a 0 to 10 visual scale from "no distress" (0) to "extreme distress" (10). Many other distress assessment instruments exist; a recent systematic review identified 33 instruments of varying lengths examined in 106 validation studies. In patients receiving palliative care, the Combined Depression Questions performed best of the ultra-short measures (one to four items). Among the short instruments (five to 20 items), the Hospital Anxiety and Depression Scale (HADS) and the Center for Epidemiologic Studies Depression Scale demonstrated adequate psychometric properties. Long instruments (21 to 50 items) are also available but are often less clinically feasible in the palliative care setting; ones exhibiting robust psychometrics are the Beck Depression Inventory (BDI), General Health Questionnaire—28, Psychosocial Screen for Cancer, Questionnaire on Stress in Cancer Patients—Revised, and Rotterdam Symptom Checklist.[175]

For patients who report significant distress, appropriate referral to psychiatric care, psychotherapy, counseling or social work services, or chaplaincy is warranted.

Caregiver/Family

Psychosocial problems are not limited to the patient with a terminal illness. Studies have found that 32% to 70% of caregivers (primarily family members, but also including other informal caregivers) of patients with advanced cancer experience a level of distress or depressive symptoms high enough to suggest clinical depression.[176-178] Caregivers often are unprepared for the various commitments—financial, emotional, and physical—that are involved in caring for a dying loved one.[179] Furthermore, many caregivers lack the medical knowledge and skills necessary to anticipate the needs of the patient. Because of the multiple demands of caregiving, family members often are forced to leave their jobs or to work part-time, which adds financial worries to a period that is already emotionally challenging. Moreover, by attending to the needs of their dying loved one, caregivers often neglect their own health and emotional needs.[180]

Certain characteristics of caregivers are associated with negative effect of caregiving. These include age of the caregiver, ethnicity, sex, socioeconomic status, and caregiver health and functional status. Individuals who are younger, non-white, women, and less affluent tend to experience greater negative effect such as distress or depressive symptoms. Other factors associated with negative effect include the duration and intensity of caregiving, mood and physical health of the caregiver, a recurrence of the patient's illness, and the caregiver's subjective sense of burden.[181]

Providing effective symptom relief is a primary way in which physicians can help both caregivers and terminally ill patients.[182] Just as treating depression can improve pain control, control of both pain and non-pain symptoms has been shown to help alleviate or prevent depression.[183,184] Patients who have higher levels of symptom distress or depression are more likely to have caregivers with greater depressive symptoms and negative perceptions of their own health.[185-187] When a terminally ill patient experiences a reduction in distress, it also can help decrease the caregiving burden and the psychological effects of terminal illness on caregivers.

Support of caregivers has become an important topic within oncology. The latest data report that as many as 40% of all U.S. adults are now caring for a sick or elderly family member. These caregivers are having important effects on the treatment and outcomes of the patients they care for. For example, one recent retrospective cohort study of a large cancer registry by Aizer et al found that patients with spouses were less likely to present with metastatic disease, more likely to receive curative therapy, and less likely to die from cancer after adjusting for demographics, stage, and treatment.[188] Another study

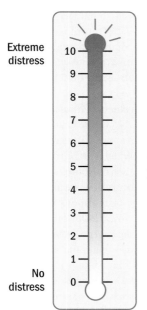

Fig. 21-2 National Comprehensive Cancer Network Distress Thermometer.

Reproduced with permission from the NCCN Clinical Practice Guidelines in Oncology (NCCN Guidelines®) for Distress Management V.1.2013. Available at www.nccn.org. Accessed August 2012. ©National Comprehensive Cancer Network, 2012. To view the most recent and complete version of the Guideline, go online to www.nccn.org.

Instructions:
First please circle the number (0 to 10) that best describes how much distress you have been experiencing in the past week, including today.

Extreme distress

No distress

demonstrated that the quality and frequency of interactions between patients and caregivers predicts hospital readmission, an important measure of care quality.[189] As many patients with advanced cancer experience an unplanned hospital admission in the last months of life, caregiver support is increasingly recognized as a way oncology teams can further patient-centered, resource-efficient care.

In offering supportive care at the EOL, the clinician exerts a powerful therapeutic effect simply by being present. By being available, by communicating openly about difficult topics, and by addressing symptoms that are causing distress, the physician can provide significant support. Caregivers particularly value the support and respect of their health care providers; those who report that physicians listen to their opinions and concerns are less likely to report depressive symptoms.[190,191] Good communication, which includes anticipatory guidance and clear explanations of what to expect, is an essential therapeutic tool. By providing appropriate referrals to assistance agencies, such as hospice, physicians can greatly support family members.[3] In all cases, effective communication, listening, and availability contribute substantially to alleviating suffering at the EOL.

KEY POINTS

- Although psychological distress is normal among terminally ill patients, clinicians should remain alert for signals of true psychiatric illness.
- A majority of dying patients experience psychological distress. Therefore, physicians must be prepared to address related issues using both medical and psychosocial means, and to make appropriate referrals.
- Family members and caregivers also frequently experience significant psychological distress.
- Physicians can provide a substantial measure of psychological relief for all concerned through effective management of the patient's symptoms.
- The presence of a sympathetic, responsive, and well-informed clinician with good communication skills has a powerful therapeutic effect for patients and caregivers alike.

SPIRITUAL/EXISTENTIAL SUFFERING

As the patient nears the EOL, the spiritual needs of the patient, family members, and other caregivers typically become heightened. Good care of the spirit is essential to high-quality EOL care. Care of the spirit involves helping the patient and loved ones address existential issues that may arise, such as questions like, "What is the meaning of life?", "Why am I here?", "What have I achieved in my life?", "How do I fit into the universe?", and "What will happen to 'me' after my death?". The clinician should recognize that the religious belief systems of all parties concerned, as well as their personal belief systems regarding our spiritual nature, will influence how they react to these broad spiritual questions.

Although physicians typically are not trained to provide spiritual care, patients and families often assume that their health care professionals will be able to adequately introduce and discuss issues surrounding care of the spirit. Many people consider an expected death to be a valuable opportunity to address any outstanding spiritual issues, and they expect that this work will take place in the context of their loved one's medical care. Yet, for many clinicians, the prospect of providing spiritual care to someone at the EOL presents a formidable challenge.

Cancer care at the EOL, perhaps more than in any other phase of illness, involves multidisciplinary efforts. Each member of the EOL care team must possess the key competency of being comfortable with exploring and discussing spiritual issues. Because spiritual concerns may be broached by patients and their families at any time, each care team member should be ready and able to discuss spiritual care, both in a manner appropriate for the specific context and professionally. Although certain issues may need to be referred to an appropriate person in the pastoral care team, many spiritual issues can be explored safely by the team member with whom they are first raised. To be able to converse meaningfully with patients about their beliefs and concerns, clinicians must have contemplated important spiritual and existential questions. However, during spiritual conversations with patients, clinicians should not attempt to share their own perspectives; rather, the clinician's attention should be on trying to understand the depths and nuances of the patient's orientation toward this potentially complex area of life. This understanding will assist clinicians in identifying needs that other professionals (e.g., chaplains, psychotherapists) should address; the oncologist's responsibility is to guide the delivery of compassionate care, and to incorporate insights about the patient's spiritual/existential status into clinical decisions to best treat the patient as a whole person.

Many people, especially in developed nations, encounter death infrequently; they may even be well into adulthood before they are first confronted by death. As a person observes the death of a loved one, especially when it is the first time they have witnessed this process, his or her reckoning with mortality can be profound. This personal experience can manifest in a variety of emotions such as anger, fear, or powerlessness. At times these feelings can be directed toward clinical staff as well as toward family members, the dying person, a deity, or some other construct. As death nears, many patients are forced to confront questions that they might otherwise prefer to ignore. Chief among these are questions concerning the nature and purpose of suffering, and the injustice of a painful or premature death.

As patients articulate their beliefs and interpretations about spiritual issues with family members, the emotional rawness of dying and death can become magnified. Long-ignored or contentious issues often emerge in a family at this time. When these situations arise, clinicians can help by refocusing family members on the real purpose of spiritual care: to support patients as they explore and express their spirituality at the EOL, to the extent that they wish and in the manner most meaningful and comfortable for them. Containing or managing family conflict is crucial to ensuring that patients can approach death with calm and in a context of full support for their medical, psychosocial, and spiritual needs.

Clinicians may tend to refer to a patient's, family's, or caregiver's belief system (e.g., religious affiliation) to evaluate their orientation toward spirituality, life, dying, and death. However, although patients may name a particular belief system, one cannot assume that particular interpretations or beliefs apply, even if they are commonly associated with the declared religion or belief system. Although a religion may provide a broad frame of reference for a person's beliefs, it cannot supply the detail required to understand the ways in which a patient may respond to arising spiritual concerns or to determine how to best support him or her with spiritual care. Belief systems may help structure broad conversations that occur around life and death; however, clinicians should remember that spirituality and religion are different. A patient need not adhere to any particular system of belief to successfully resolve existential or spiritual issues. One also must recognize that belief systems may either relieve or worsen anxiety and fear as death approaches. Both fear induced by a lack of faith and fear of losing faith in the face of the unknown can exacerbate anxiety. At times, a patient's belief system is tested at the EOL either by the disease (e.g., "Only bad people get this disease, and I have been good") or by the mode of death (e.g., "No one should suffer like this").

Many people value the opportunity to make peace with God, the universe, a deity, or a belief system as death approaches. Those who are dying, their families, and caregivers will appreciate the clinician's efforts to ensure that they have the space, quiet, encouragement, and support to explore spiritual issues that are important to them.

KEY POINTS

- Care team members must be prepared to competently address spiritual issues at any time in the dying process.
- Clinicians should be adequately conversant in spiritual matters, but should primarily adopt a stance of listening, understanding, and supporting spiritual exploration.
- Appropriate referrals (e.g., to a chaplain, pastor, or rabbi) can be made when the patient is receptive.
- The goal of spiritual discussion is to elicit the spiritual concerns of the patient, family, and caregivers in order to better orchestrate whole-person care.
- Care team members must take care to approach a patient's identified religion or belief system only as a broad index of his or her spiritual orientation; no assumptions should be made.
- The dying process can be a fulfilling experience in which spiritual resolution is achieved by and among dying patients and their loved ones.

DEPRESSION

Identifying and differentiating between preparatory grief and depression in a dying patient can be quite difficult, even for seasoned clinicians. In general, depressed patients tend to remain in a persistent state of sadness, to have a poor view of themselves, to sustain a sense of hopelessness, and to derive little pleasure from new situations or from memories of past events.[192,193] By contrast, patients with normal grief reactions typically experience a progression of feelings, are able to maintain a realistic view of themselves, and can modify their health care goals to maintain hope. Diagnosing depression at the EOL is of paramount importance; studies have demonstrated that untreated depression results in an increase in morbidity and sequelae including suicide. Depression, as well as hopelessness, loss of meaning in life, and loss of interest in activities, ranks among the risk factors for the desire to hasten death.[145,194] Patients whose psychosocial needs are acknowledged are less likely to persist in their desire for death.[50] When a patient expresses a desire to hasten death, requests should be addressed explicitly, and should prompt a reassessment of symptom control, psychosocial issues such as relationship strain or fear of caregiver burden, spiritual/existential suffering, and psychological issues such as depression. The care plan should be clarified with renewed attention to how best to relieve physical, psychological, interpersonal, and spiritual suffering.[11]

Studies in patients with cancer in palliative settings report rates of general depression and depressive mood ranging from 21% to 37%.[169,195] Median prevalence of major depressive disorder in patients with advanced cancer has been reported at 15%.[196] Several instruments have been created or adapted to help identify depression in the terminally ill. Well-recognized and validated instruments include the BDI-Short Form (BDI-SF),[197] HADS,[198] Edmonton Symptom Assessment Scale,[199] Edinburgh Depression Scale, and Brief Edinburgh Depression Scale.[200] Considerable effort has been devoted to developing simple one- and two-item verbal screens for depression, but Bayesian meta-analysis has found that, although these brief methods perform well at excluding depression in the nondepressed person, they perform poorly at identifying depression; two-item measures are superior to single-item screens, but neither is sufficient for depression assessment.[201] Clinicians may elect to use these brief assessments for convenience and as an initial screen, but should not rely exclusively on them. Assessment of terminally ill patients for symptoms of depression is a critical component of care, and warrants a more thorough assessment using a well-validated instrument.

Guidelines established for the general care of psychiatric illness may be applied to the treatment of depression for terminally ill patients, but with certain adjustments. Referral should be made to an appropriate clinician, ideally a palliative care expert, psychiatrist, or psychologist with expertise in management of psychological disorders who can tailor care to this stage of illness. Treatments, particularly pharmacologic therapies, must take into account the patient's prognosis. For example, when the patient has a limited life expectancy, SSRIs may not exert an effect quickly enough; psychostimulants may offer a more realistic treatment strategy.

DELIRIUM

Characterized by disturbance of consciousness, cognition, and perception, delirium occurs in 28% to 83% of patients as death approaches; it often provokes considerable distress among patients, families, caregivers, and providers who are witnessing the patient's transition toward death.[202,203] Delirium is generally an indirect result of various factors associated with the patient's underlying cancer, such as adverse treatment effects, metabolic disorder, nutritional deficiency, or infection; adverse effects of medications (particularly opioids) seem to be the most common cause of delirium for patients near the EOL.[204]

Two types of delirium are observed in the palliative care population: agitated/hyperactive delirium and hypoactive delirium. In either case, onset is signaled by an acute change in the patient's level of arousal, which can manifest as disorientation, visual or auditory hallucinations, a change in speech patterns, memory or language alteration, or upset of the sleep/wake cycle. Symptoms typically wax and wane over time.[205]

For clinical diagnosis, delirium is assessed at the bedside using instruments such as the Delirium Rating Scale,[206] Confusion Assessment Method,[207] Delirium Symptom Interview,[208] Memorial Delirium Assessment Scale,[209] or the more general and widely recognized Mini-Mental State Examination.[210]

To manage delirium, the first step is to screen for and treat any underlying reversible causes; these may include CNS events, bladder outlet or bowel obstruction, hypoxia, metabolic disorder, and medication/substance effects or withdrawal. If these potential causes are ruled out, the clinician typically discontinues all medications (especially psychoactive ones) that are not absolutely necessary. Reorienting the patient to time and place, ensuring that family and other familiar individuals are available, and restoring normal surroundings and routine can be very helpful. Thereafter, the goal of treating delirium is to restore patients to a condition that more closely reflects their baseline mental state, rather than to suppress agitation or to sedate them.[52] For patients receiving palliative care, intravenous or oral haloperidol is the drug of choice and is titrated upward, as necessary, from a starting dose of 0.5 mg twice daily; haloperidol's antiemetic effect can have supplemental benefit. For more severe delirium, or persistent symptoms despite haloperidol, alternative agents include olanzapine (2.5 mg to 7.5 mg/day intramuscularly every 2 to 4 hours as needed or 5 mg to 20 mg/day orally) or chlorpromazine (25 mg to 100 mg/day intramuscularly/intravenously every 4 hours as needed); for mild to moderate delirium, alternative agents include risperidone (0.5 mg to 1.0 mg orally twice daily), and quetiapine fumarate (25 mg to 200 mg orally/sublingually twice daily).[11] However, data do not suggest that these medications are more effective or safer than haloperidol, and they are generally more expensive. Although they may help calm the delirious patient, benzodiazepines (e.g., lorazepam, midazolam) are generally avoided; they can worsen delirium by further sedating and disinhibiting the patient or by causing agitation.

When terminal delirium is severe, especially in the actively dying patient, an alternative strategy is to sedate the patient through continuous infusion of a benzodiazepine or barbiturate (midazolam or pentobarbital are most commonly used).[211,212]

However, this approach should be reserved for the most extreme cases, when the patient and/or family exhibit considerable distress, and implemented in monitored surroundings. A palliative medicine specialist should be involved if terminal sedation is considered.

The effectiveness of medical approaches may be enhanced by the presence of family and friends, familiar surroundings, consistent care staff, and a tranquil setting. Satisfactory management of delirium results in adequate control of delirium symptoms, reduction in patient and family distress, regaining of a sense of control, relief of caregiver burden, and improved quality of life. Reassessment should be iteratively conducted to ensure ongoing and adequate management of this troubling symptom.

MANAGEMENT OF THE LAST DAYS OF LIFE

Clinicians should actively recognize the process of dying as a result of cancer. The diagnosis is supported by a continued deterioration of a person's overall condition with increasing lethargy, decreasing levels of consciousness, and at times, increasing confusion, increasing time asleep, less spontaneous movement, and changes in patterns of respiratory effort. For many people, systemic signs can include progressive hypotension, diminishing oxygenation, and progressive loss of peripheral perfusion.

Alternatively, the terminal phase of cancer may be signaled by a sudden change in condition: an intracerebral bleed, a pulmonary embolus, a perforated viscous, or overwhelming sepsis. When this change is superimposed on an already moribund condition, continued symptom control becomes the primary goal. Understanding patients' wishes—often through conversations they have had with their families both throughout the course of their illness and during the course of life—will help determine the best course of action. Many people, in the event of a catastrophic change in their condition, may wish to focus on comfort; others may wish to try to achieve functional improvement, however limited at this phase of life.

Whether the EOL approaches as an expected deterioration or as an unexpected catastrophic decline, the issue of comfort is paramount. Clinicians should ensure that all clinical actions contribute to the comfort of the person who is dying.

PHYSICAL CARE

Attention to the nursing care of the dying patient is crucial. Regular check of vital signs should be replaced, at this stage, with regular (e.g., every 4 hours) check of symptoms. Mouth care, to ensure that the dying person's mouth is clean and moist, will aid comfort. Proper skin care includes regular repositioning of the patient to relieve musculoskeletal pain from inertia and to avoid the excruciating (and difficult to control) pain of skin tears and pressure sores. Use of a pressure-relieving mattress is advised. An air mattress will facilitate shifting of the person's weight. The head of the bed can be elevated to help reduce noisy upper respiratory tract secretions. Urinary retention and fecal impaction should be evaluated and treated, if present.

DEATH RATTLE

Noisy ventilation ("death rattle" or "terminal secretions"), caused by oscillatory movements of accumulated bronchial mucosa and salivary secretions, is common among patients who are dying and are unable to clear secretions by coughing or swallowing.[213] The symptom usually occurs after patients are unconscious, though it may nonetheless cause considerable distress to families and caregivers. Previous observational studies have estimated that death rattle occurs in up to 92% of unconscious dying patients.[55]

Intervention to reduce secretions is often instituted to alleviate the distress of attendant family members, even when the patient seems settled. Standard non-pharmacologic practices for alleviating death rattle include suctioning, positioning, reducing parenteral and enteral fluids, and explanation to the patient's family or other caregiver(s).

The mainstay of pharmacologic management of death rattle are anticholinergic agents, also known as muscarinic receptor blockers.[213,214] These drugs include scopolamine, hyoscyamine, glycopyrrolate, and atropine. The primary difference in these drugs is whether they are tertiary amines that cross the blood–brain barrier (scopolamine, atropine) or quaternary amines that do not (hyoscyamine, glycopyrrolate). Atropine, a widely available drug, is frequently used in home care for the treatment of death rattle; a common approach is 1% atropine ophthalmic solution, one to two drops sublingually every 4 hours as needed.[11] Scopolamine (hyoscyamine hydrobromide), a muscarine receptor antagonist, has been reported to more potently inhibit production of bronchial secretions and causes less tachycardia.[215] Scopolamine and atropine can cause central effects such as sedation, confusion, or paradoxical excitation, especially in elderly patients. Hyoscine butylbromide, a semisynthetic derivative of scopolamine, is effective in treating respiratory tract secretions, has peripheral effects similar to scopolamine, and has no central adverse effects.[216]

Recent research has studied the relative effectiveness and frequency of adverse effects of atropine, scopolamine, and hyoscine butylbromide for treating death rattle in terminally ill patients. In an open-label, multisite, prospective, phase III trial, 333 terminally ill patients with death rattle were randomly assigned to receive 0.5 mg atropine, 20 mg hyoscine butylbromide, or 0.25 mg scopolamine, initiated in subcutaneous bolus followed by continuous administration. In patients in all three study arms, death rattle decreased to a non-disturbing intensity or disappeared after 1 hour in 42%, 42%, and 37% of cases, respectively (p = 0.72); effectiveness improved throughout treatment without significant differences among the treatment groups.[217] Although this study is the largest randomized controlled trial of anticholinergics for death rattle to date, it has numerous limitations, including its unblinded design, failure to standardize across sites, and lack of a placebo control.[218] Indeed, although other randomized controlled trials have been few and small in sample size, they have failed to establish the superiority of one drug (including placebo) compared with another.[219] One might conclude, then, that the anticholinergics are equally ineffective in alleviating death rattle. Given the scant and inconclusive evidence, a 2008 Cochrane review updated in 2010 to include the above study advised that clinicians have an ethical obligation to closely monitor patients for lack of therapeutic benefit and adverse effects, discontinuing ineffective or detrimental treatments. More important than treatment with anticholinergics may be discussing death rattle with family members, so as to reduce their distress; these conversations should address cause, implications, and caregivers' fears and concerns.[220]

MEDICATIONS AND OTHER INTERVENTIONS

As the patient nears the EOL, the clinician should review all medications being administered to the patient and continue only those that contribute to increased comfort. Similarly, implanted defibrillators, and possibly pacemakers as well, can be deactivated. Diagnostic tests and functions (e.g., transfusions, needle sticks, intake and output, blood glucose monitoring, oxygen saturation monitoring, suctioning) can be discontinued if deemed unnecessary for symptom control and comfort.[11] In deciding which medications to discontinue, all medications should be reconsidered for their benefit to the patient, not only those that were introduced for symptom control in the palliative phase of the illness. For example, for type I diabetes, insulin may be necessary to prevent hyperglycemia to spare the patient unquenchable thirst. Essential medications should be obtained in a form that can be administered to someone who may not predictably be swallowing. Alternative formulations include sublingual, subcutaneous, intravenous, transdermal, intranasal, and rectal. Doses of medications retained for symptom management should be increased as necessary to optimize comfort.

Nutrition and Hydration

As patients are actively dying, any nutritional supplements and any parenteral hydration should be reviewed. Almost always, parenteral hydration should be stopped, with appropriate advice to the family, because overhydration will worsen respiratory symptoms and enteral fluids will potentially cause secretions in the gut that may cause vomiting.

MANAGEMENT OF AGITATION

Physical agitation can occur in the patient's final days. The clinician should first ensure that this agitation is not a result of pain, urinary retention, or constipation. Palliative sedation can be considered if these causes are ruled out, or if agitation persists despite their treatment. First, informed consent should be obtained from the patient, his or her family, or other surrogate; this process should involve discussion of goals of treatment, the patient's status, prognosis, and expected outcomes. Family members or surrogates should fully understand that palliative sedation will render the patient unconscious; they should be allowed to voice feelings and concerns related to this scenario.

Treatment of terminal agitation may include a regular dose of a long-acting benzodiazepine. Benzodiazepines can precipitate or worsen delirium, and they should be used with care. In rare circumstances, palliative sedation may be required; this should be administered in a monitored setting in consultation with a palliative medicine specialist. For palliative sedation, recommended drugs and doses are thiopental at an initial infusion rate of 20 mg/hour to 80 mg/hour (range, 160 mg/hour to 440 mg/hour), or midazolam at an initial infusion rate of 0.4 mg/hour to 0.8 mg/hour (range, 20 mg/hour to 102 mg/hour).[11]

COMMUNICATION WITH THE FAMILY AND/OR CAREGIVERS

Communication with the family or with other loved ones involved in the last stages of caregiving should be a key focus for health professionals as a patient nears death. What does the family expect? How well do they understand the patient's condition and the dying process? A trusted clinician should clearly—but compassionately—describe the process of dying. Patients should be reassured that, in most cases, the person dying gently slips into a coma and life ebbs away with no dramatic manifestations of dying.[221] The clinician should emphasize that, at this important phase, the sole focus of care is the dying person's comfort—and that current medical practice has multiple strategies for ensuring a comfortable death.

MANAGEMENT OF CARE FOR THE UNCONSCIOUS PATIENT

Even when a patient is unconscious, clinical staff should carefully assess him or her to ensure comfort. This cannot be done from the door of the patient's room. An examination is required, with special attention to the face (is it relaxed?), respiration (is it regular, not labored?) and positioning (is the patient positioned comfortably?). The clinician should continue to explain to the patient what is happening in the clinical

---

KEY POINTS

- At the very end of life, the patient's comfort should be the primary focus. Unconscious patients should be treated with the same degree of care, concern, and communication as conscious patients.
- Physical care should address mouth care and musculoskeletal positioning, with attention given to maintaining skin integrity and comfort.
- Death rattle can be addressed with the careful administration of anticholinergic agents, as well as with attentive nursing care, positioning, and suctioning.
- All medications, medical interventions, nutritional supplements, and hydration efforts should be reviewed to continue only those that directly contribute to comfort.
- If agitation occurs, clinicians should determine the source, if possible, and address appropriately.
- The wishes of family members with regard to being present at the time of death should be respected and facilitated to the greatest degree possible.

examination, as if he or she were conscious; it is important for family members to understand that people, even when unconscious, may still recognize their voices and their touch. The clinician should also reassure the family that symptom control medications would be continued to ensure the patient's comfort even though consciousness is lost. Especially if continued at the same dose, there is no concern that these medications will hasten death.

Many family members have a strong desire to be present at the time of death. This specific time point can be difficult to predict, even as the patient's body shuts down. The need to be present varies from family to family, and within families, from one individual to another. If family members have a particular wish to be present at the patient's time of death, the clinician may want to set up a vigil roster to ensure that one member of the family is always present during the patient's last days.

CARE AFTER DEATH

The clinician's role does not end immediately on the death of the patient. Follow-through with the patient's body, logistical considerations, and family members and other caregivers are crucial last steps in EOL care. The clinicians and medical staff involved in the patient's EOL care should reflect upon the quality of the patient's death, with a "good death" defined as one that minimized distress and suffering for the patient, family members, and other caregivers; honored the patient's and family's desires; and upheld standards of care clinically, ethically, and culturally.[11]

Immediately after the patient's death, the clinician should allow the family time with the body, if they so desire. Treatment of the body should be respectful and culturally sensitive. If not addressed previously, plans for eye donation (allowable in many cancers except some leukemias and eye malignancies) and autopsy are discussed, addressing any family member or caregiver concerns. The clinician files a death certificate, completes any other required forms, and conveys information to the funeral director as needed. Additionally, he or she should inform the patient's other health care providers of the death.

Attention should be directed to family members and other caregivers. The normal bereavement process should be described to them; information regarding available bereavement support should be provided, and referral can be made to appropriate services. Palliative care providers can help the oncologist identify family members who may be at risk for complicated bereavement, and they can follow through with requisite care. Some family members may want to discuss their own cancer risk based on their loved one's recent experience. Formal expressions of condolences on the patient's death, such as with a card, phone call, or brief letter, can be immensely meaningful and supportive to family members and caregivers.

SUMMARY

As a patient enters the final weeks and days of life, all involved—the patient, family members, other caregivers, and physicians—face unique challenges. With survival no longer a priority, emphasis shifts toward optimizing the comfort of the patient through effective management of physical symptoms, provision of psychosocial support, and facilitation of spiritual resolution. The ultimate goal of palliative and EOL care is to maintain physical comfort and quality of life, so that the patient and his or her loved ones can share in the life remaining, the disease experience, and the process of death in a meaningful way.

Palliative and EOL care are best delivered through a multidisciplinary team approach to ensure high quality care of the whole person. Relevant expertise includes medical oncology, primary care, nursing, psychology, psychiatry, social work, and spiritual care; at times, a cultural liaison or interpreter, geriatrician, specialist from another discipline (e.g., pulmonology), complementary/alternative medicine provider, or other practitioner may be part of the care team.

Providing relief from pain and other physical symptoms is essential; appropriate treatment plans should be based on comprehensive and ongoing assessment of symptoms. Psychiatric issues, which are prevalent among patients with advanced disease, also must be identified and addressed in a timely fashion to minimize patient and family distress, which can be considerable in these circumstances. In addition, the psychosocial and spiritual concerns of patients who are terminally ill or receiving palliative care must be considered equal in magnitude to their physical concerns. The patient's family members, too, may need guidance as they struggle to manage their own emotions and to provide meaningful support for the patient. To help ensure the best possible care for the patient, family, and caregivers, the physician must not only possess clinical expertise in palliative and EOL care, but must also be prepared to function as a calm, empathetic, and communicative presence—the role requires both *skill* to alleviate the burdens associated with advanced illness and dying and *wisdom* to be present and to make appropriate referrals.

In light of emerging data, it is expected that the principles of palliative care will be applied earlier in the cancer care trajectory. The approaches described here must be appropriately modified to fit the needs of the patient with cancer receiving concurrent anticancer treatments and palliative care.

References

1. Temel JS, Greer JA, Muzikansky A, et al. Early palliative care for patients with metastatic non-small-cell lung cancer. *N Engl J Med.* 2010;363:733-742. PMID: 20818875.

2. Abernethy AP, Currow DC, Fazekas BS, et al. Specialized palliative care services are associated with improved short- and long-term caregiver outcomes. *Support Care Cancer.* 2008;16:585-597. PMID: 17960433.

3. Christakis NA, Iwashyna TJ. The health impact of health care on families: a matched cohort study of hospice use by decedents and mortality outcomes in surviving, widowed spouses. *Soc Sci Med.* 2003;57:465-475. PMID: 12791489.

4. Smith TJ, Temin S, Alesi ER, et al. American Society of Clinical Oncology Provisional Clinical Opinion: The Integration of Palliative Care into Standard Oncology Care. *J Clin Oncol.* 2012;30:880-887. PMID: 22312101.

5. Kamal AH, Bull J, Stinson CS, et al. Conformance with supportive care quality measures is associated with better quality of life in patients with cancer receiving palliative care. *J Oncol Pract.* 2013;9:e73-76. PMID: 23942504.

6. Seow H, Sussman J, Martelli-Reid L, et al. Do high symptom scores trigger clinical actions? An audit after implementing electronic symptom screening. *J Oncol Pract.* 2012;8:e142-e148. PMID: 23598849.

7. Mercadante S, Costanzo BV, Fusco F, et al. Breakthrough pain in advanced cancer patients followed at home: a longitudinal study. *J Pain Symptom Manage.* 2009;38:554-560. PMID: 19692200.

8. Meuser T, Pietruck C, Radbruch L, et al. Symptoms during cancer pain treatment following WHO-guidelines: a longitudinal follow-up study of symptom prevalence, severity and etiology. *Pain.* 2001;93:247-257. PMID: 11514084.

9. Vainio A, Auvinen A. Prevalence of symptoms among patients with advanced cancer: an international collaborative study. Symptom Prevalence Group. *J Pain Symptom Manage.* 1996;12:3-10. PMID: 8718910.

10. Gordon DB, Dahl JL, Miaskowski C, et al. American pain society recommendations for improving the quality of acute and cancer pain management: American Pain Society Quality of Care Task Force. *Arch Intern Med.* 2005;165:1574-1580. PMID: 16043674.

11. Levy MH, Adolph MD, Back A, et al. Palliative care. *J Natl Compr Canc Netw.* 2012;10:1284-1309. PMID: 23054879.

12. Ferrell B, Levy MH, Paice J. Managing pain from advanced cancer in the palliative care setting. *Clin J Oncol Nurs.* 2008;12:575-581. PMID: 18676325.

13. Bieri D, Reeve RA, Champion GD, et al. The Faces Pain Scale for the self-assessment of the severity of pain experienced by children: development, initial validation, and preliminary investigation for ratio scale properties. *Pain.* 1990;41:139-150. PMID: 2367140.

14. Herr K, Spratt KF, Garand L, et al. Evaluation of the Iowa pain thermometer and other selected pain intensity scales in younger and older adult cohorts using controlled clinical pain: a preliminary study. *Pain Med.* 2007;8:585-600. PMID: 17883743.

15. Petzke F, Radbruch L, Zech D, et al. Temporal presentation of chronic cancer pain: transitory pains on admission to a multidisciplinary pain clinic. *J Pain Symptom Manage.* 1999;17:391-401. PMID: 10388244.

16. Portenoy RK, Hagen NA. Breakthrough pain: definition, prevalence and characteristics. *Pain.* 1990;41:273-281. PMID: 1697056.

17. Portenoy RK, Payne R, Coluzzi P, et al. Oral transmucosal fentanyl citrate (OTFC) for the treatment of breakthrough pain in cancer patients: a controlled dose titration study. *Pain.* 1999;79:303-312. PMID: 10068176.

18. Hagen NA, Fisher K, Victorino C, et al. A titration strategy is needed to manage breakthrough cancer pain effectively: observations from data pooled from three clinical trials. *J Palliat Med.* 2007;10:47-55. PMID: 17298253.

19. Babul N, Darke AC, Hagen N. Hydromorphone metabolite accumulation in renal failure. *J Pain Symptom Manage.* 1995;10:184-186. PMID: 7543126.

20. Quigley C. Hydromorphone for acute and chronic pain. *Cochrane Database Systematic Reviews* 2002;(1):CD003447. PMID: 11869661.

21. Moulin DE, Johnson NG, Murray-Parsons N, et al. Subcutaneous narcotic infusions for cancer pain: treatment outcome and guidelines for use. *CMAJ.* 1992;146:891-897. PMID: 1371946.

22. Moulin DE, Kreeft JH, Murray-Parsons N, et al. Comparison of continuous subcutaneous and intravenous hydromorphone infusions for management of cancer pain. *Lancet.* 1991;337:465-468. PMID: 1704089.

23. Leppert W. The role of methadone in cancer pain treatment–a review. *Int J Clin Pract.* 2009;63:1095-1109. PMID: 19570126.

24. Shaiova L, Berger A, Blinderman CD, et al. Consensus guideline on parenteral methadone use in pain and palliative care. *Palliat Support Care.* 2008;6:165-176. PMID: 18501052.

25. Shaiova L. The role of methadone in the treatment of moderate to severe cancer pain. *Support Cancer Ther.* 2005;2:176-180. PMID: 18628169.

26. Ripamonti C, Groff L, Brunelli C, et al. Switching from morphine to oral methadone in treating cancer pain: what is the equianalgesic dose ratio? *J Clin Oncol.* 1998;16:3216-3221. PMID: 9779694.

27. Bruera E, Pereira J, Watanabe S, et al. Opioid rotation in patients with cancer pain. A retrospective comparison of dose ratios between methadone, hydromorphone, and morphine. *Cancer.* 1996;78:852-857. PMID: 8756381.

28. Kaiko RF, Foley KM, Grabinski PY, et al. Central nervous system excitatory effects of meperidine in cancer patients. *Ann Neurol.* 1983;13:180-185. PMID: 6187275.

29. Sittl R, Likar R, Nautrup BP. Equipotent doses of transdermal fentanyl and transdermal buprenorphine in patients with cancer and noncancer pain: results of a retrospective cohort study. *Clinical Therapy.* 2005;27:225-237. PMID: 15811486.

30. Skaer TL. Transdermal opioids for cancer pain. *Health Qual Life Outcomes.* 2006;4:24. PMID: 16573839.

31. Mercadante S, Porzio G, Ferrera P, et al. Sustained-release oral morphine versus transdermal fentanyl and oral methadone in cancer pain management. *Eur J Pain.* 2008;12:1040-1046. PMID: 18353696.

32. Kornick CA, Santiago-Palma J, Schulman G, et al. A safe and effective method for converting patients from transdermal to intravenous fentanyl for the treatment of acute cancer-related pain. *Cancer.* 2003;97:3121-3124. PMID: 12784350.

33. Bennett MI. Effectiveness of antiepileptic or antidepressant drugs when added to opioids for cancer pain: systematic review. *Palliat Med.* 2011;25:553-559. PMID: 20671006.

34. Anderson KO, Cohen MZ, Mendoza TR, et al. Brief cognitive-behavioral audiotape interventions for cancer-related pain: Immediate but not long-term effectiveness. *Cancer.* 2006;107:207-214. PMID: 16708359.

35. Dyspnea. Mechanisms, assessment, and management. a consensus statement. American Thoracic Society. *Am J Respir Crit Care Med.* 1999;159:321-340. PMID: 9872857.

36. Ben-Aharon I, Gafter-Gvili A, Paul M, et al. Interventions for alleviating cancer-related dyspnea: a systematic review. *J Clin Oncol.* 2008;26:2396-2404. PMID: 18467732.

37. Eckenhoff JE, Oech SR. The effects of narcotics and antagonists upon respiration and circulation in man. A review. *Clin Pharmacol Ther.* 1960;1:483-524. PMID: 13819208.

38. Santiago TV, Pugliese AC, Edelman NH. Control of breathing during methadone addiction. *Am J Med.* 1977;62:347-354. PMID: 842554.

39. Weil JV, McCullough RE, Kline JS, et al. Diminished ventilatory response to hypoxia and hypercapnia after morphine in normal man. *N Engl J Med.* 1975;292:1103-1106. PMID: 1128555.

40. Kryger MH, Yacoub O, Dosman J, et al. Effect of meperidine on occlusion pressure responses to hypercapnia and hypoxia with and without external inspiratory resistance. *Am Rev Respir Dis.* 1976;114:333-340. PMID: 973724.

41. Santiago TV, Johnson J, Riley DJ, et al. Effects of morphine on ventilatory response to exercise. *J Appl Physiol: Resp Environ Exerc Physiol.* 1979;47:112-118. PMID: 468650.

42. Kamal AH, Maguire JM, Wheeler JL, et al. Dyspnea review for the palliative care professional: assessment, burdens, and etiologies. *J Palliat Med.* 2011;14:1167-1172. PMID: 21895451.

43. Bruera E, MacEachern T, Ripamonti C, et al. Subcutaneous morphine for dyspnea in cancer patients. *Ann Intern Med.* 1993;119:906-907. PMID: 8215003.

44. Abernethy AP, McDonald CF, Frith PA, et al. Effect of palliative oxygen versus room air in relief of breathlessness in patients with refractory dyspnoea: a double-blind, randomised controlled trial. *Lancet.* 2010;376:784-793. PMID: 20816546.

45. Asch DA, Faber-Langendoen K, Shea JA, et al. The sequence of withdrawing life-sustaining treatment from patients. *Am J Med.* 1999;107:153-156. PMID: 10460047.

46. Mercadante S, Ferrera P, Girelli D, et al. Patients' and relatives' perceptions about intravenous and subcutaneous hydration. *J Pain Symptom Manage.* 2005;30:354-358. PMID: 16256899.

47. Ersek M. Artificial nutrition and hydration. *J Hosp Palliat Nurs.* 2003;5:221-230.

48. Lundholm K, Daneryd P, Bosaeus I, et al. Palliative nutritional intervention in addition to cyclooxygenase and erythropoietin treatment for patients with malignant disease: Effects on survival, metabolism, and function. *Cancer.* 2004;100:1967-1977. PMID: 15112279.

49. McCann RM, Hall WJ, Groth-Juncker A. Comfort care for terminally ill patients. The appropriate use of nutrition and hydration. *JAMA.* 1994;272:1263-1266. PMID: 7523740.

50. Ganzini L, Nelson HD, Schmidt TA, et al. Physicians' experiences with the Oregon Death with Dignity Act. *N Engl J Med.* 2000;342:557-563. PMID: 10684915.

51. Pasman HR, Onwuteaka-Philipsen BD, Kriegsman DM, et al. Discomfort in nursing home patients with severe dementia in whom artificial nutrition and hydration is forgone. *Arch Intern Med.* 2005;165:1729-1735. PMID: 16087820.

52. Casarett D, Kapo J, Caplan A. Appropriate use of artificial nutrition and hydration–fundamental principles and recommendations. *N Engl J Med.* 2005;353:2607-2612. PMID: 16354899.

53. Duerksen DR, Ting E, Thomson P, et al. Is there a role for TPN in terminally ill patients with bowel obstruction? *Nutrition.* 2004;20:760-763. PMID: 15325683.

54. Burge FI. Dehydration symptoms of palliative care cancer patients. *J Pain Symptom Manage.* 1993;8:454-464. PMID: 7525778.

55. Ellershaw JE, Sutcliffe JM, Saunders CM. Dehydration and the dying patient. *J Pain Symptom Manage.* 1995;10:192-197. PMID: 7629413.

56. Morita T, Tei Y, Tsunoda J, et al. Determinants of the sensation of thirst in terminally ill cancer patients. *Support Care Cancer.* 2001;9:177-186. PMID: 11401102.

57. Bruera E, Sala R, Rico MA, et al. Effects of parenteral hydration in terminally ill cancer patients: a preliminary study. *J Clin Oncol.* 2005;23:2366-2371. PMID: 15800328.

58. Lawlor PG. Delirium and dehydration: some fluid for thought? *Support Care Cancer.* 2002;10:445-454. PMID: 12353122.

59. Mercadante S, Ripamonti C, Casuccio A, et al. Comparison of octreotide and hyoscine butylbromide in controlling gastrointestinal symptoms due to malignant inoperable bowel obstruction. *Support Care Cancer.* 2000;8:188-191. PMID: 10789958.

60. Morita T, Hyodo I, Yoshimi T, et al. Association between hydration volume and symptoms in terminally ill cancer patients with abdominal malignancies. *Ann Oncol.* 2005;16:640-647. PMID: 15684225.

61. Bruera E, Hui D, Dalal S, et al. Parenteral hydration in patients with advanced cancer: a multicenter, double-blind, placebo-controlled randomized trial. *J Clin Oncol.* 2013;31:111-118. PMID: 23169523.

62. Morita T, Shima Y, Miyashita M, et al. Physician- and nurse-reported effects of intravenous hydration therapy on symptoms of terminally ill patients with cancer. *J Palliat Med.* 2004;7:683-693. PMID: 15588360.

63. Lanuke K, Fainsinger RL, DeMoissac D. Hydration management at the end of life. *J Palliat Med.* 2004;7:257-263. PMID: 15130203.

64. Ferris FD, von Gunten CF, Emanuel LL. Competency in end-of-life care: last hours of life. *J Palliat Med.* 2003;6:605-613. PMID: 14516502.

65. Brard L, Weitzen S, Strubel-Lagan SL, et al. The effect of total parenteral nutrition on the survival of terminally ill ovarian cancer patients. *Gyn Oncol.* 2006;103:176-180. PMID: 16564074.

66. Chiu TY, Hu WY, Chuang RB, et al. Nutrition and hydration for terminal cancer patients in Taiwan. *Support Care Cancer.* 2002;10:630-636. PMID: 12436222.

67. Bruera E, MacDonald N. To hydrate or not to hydrate: how should it be? *J Clin Oncol.* 2000;18:1156-1158. PMID: 10694570.

68. Conill C, Verger E, Henríquez I, et al. Symptom prevalence in the last week of life. *J Pain Symptom Manage.* 1997;14:328-331. PMID: 9409097.

69. Regnard CFB, Hockley JM. *Flow Diagrams in Advanced Cancer and Other Diseases.* London: E. Arnold; 1995.

70. Roe JW, Leslie P, Drinnan MJ. Oropharyngeal dysphagia: the experience of patients with non-head and neck cancers receiving specialist palliative care. *Palliat Med.* 2007;21:567-574. PMID: 17942494.

71. Bruera E, Neumann CM. Management of specific symptom complexes in patients receiving palliative care. *CMAJ.* 1998;158:1717-1726. PMID: 9676549.

72. Bruera E, Belzile M, Neumann C, et al. A double-blind, crossover study of controlled-release metoclopramide and placebo for the chronic nausea and dyspepsia of advanced cancer. *J Pain Symptom Manage.* 2000;19:427-435. PMID: 10908823.

73. European Medicines Agency. European Medicines Agency recommends changes to the use of metoclopramide. Available at: http://www.ema.europa.eu/ema/index.jsp?curl=pages/news_and_events/news/2013/07/news_detail_001854.jsp. Accessed April 3, 2014.

74. Bruera E, Seifert L, Watanabe S, et al. Chronic nausea in advanced cancer patients: a retrospective assessment of a metoclopramide-based antiemetic regimen. *J Pain Symptom Manage.* 1996;11:147-153. PMID: 8851371.

75. Pereira J, Bruera E. Chronic nausea. In Bruera E, Higginson IJ (eds). *Cachexia-Anorexia in Cancer Patients.* Oxford: Oxford Medical Publications, Oxford University Press; 1996.

76. Loprinzi C, Jatoi A. Antiemetic properties of megestrol acetate. *J Palliat Med.* 2006;9:239-240. PMID: 16629544.

77. Jackson WC, Tavernier L. Olanzapine for intractable nausea in palliative care patients. *J Palliat Med.* 2003;6:251-255. PMID: 12854942.

78. Licup N. Olanzapine for nausea and vomiting. *Am J Hosp Palliat Care.* 2010;27:432-434. PMID: 20508243.

79. Lundberg JC, Passik S. Controlling opioid-induced nausea with olanzapine. *Primary Care and Cancer.* 2000;20:35-37.

80. Passik SD, Kirsh KL, Theobald DE, et al. A retrospective chart review of the use of olanzapine for the prevention of delayed emesis in cancer patients. *J Pain Symptom Manage.* 2003;25:485-488. PMID: 12727048.

81. Passik SD, Lundberg J, Kirsh KL, et al. A pilot exploration of the antiemetic activity of olanzapine for the relief of nausea in patients with advanced cancer and pain. *J Pain Symptom Manage.* 2002;23:526-532. PMID: 12067777.

82. Pirl WF, Roth AJ. Remission of chemotherapy-induced emesis with concurrent olanzapine treatment: a case report. *Psychooncology.* 2000;9:84-87. PMID: 10668063.

83. Srivastava M, Brito-Dellan N, Davis MP, et al. Olanzapine as an antiemetic in refractory nausea and vomiting in advanced cancer. *J Pain Symptom Manage.* 2003;25:578-582. PMID: 12782438.

84. Perkins P, Dorman S. Haloperidol for the treatment of nausea and vomiting in palliative care patients. *Cochrane Database Systematic Reviews.* 2009;(2):CD006271. PMID: 19370630.

85. Mercadante S. The role of octreotide in palliative care. *J Pain Symptom Manage.* 1994;9:406-411. PMID: 7525789.

86. Cowan JD, Palmer TW. Practical guide to palliative sedation. *Curr Oncol Rep.* 2002;4:242-249. PMID: 11937015.

87. Cowan JD, Walsh D. Terminal sedation in palliative medicine–definition and review of the literature. *Support Care Cancer.* 2001;9:403-407. PMID: 11585266.

88. Fainsinger RL, Waller A, Bercovici M, et al. A multicentre international study of sedation for uncontrolled symptoms in terminally ill patients. *Palliat Med.* 2000;14:257-265. PMID: 10974977.

89. Potter J, Hami F, Bryan T, et al. Symptoms in 400 patients referred to palliative care services: prevalence and patterns. *Palliat Med.* 2003;17:310-314. PMID: 12822846.

90. Choi YS, Billings JA. Opioid antagonists: a review of their role in palliative care, focusing on use in opioid-related constipation. *J Pain Symptom Manage.* 2002;24:71-90. PMID: 12183097.

91. Mostafa SM, Bhandari S, Ritchie G, et al. Constipation and its implications in the critically ill patient. *Br J Anaesth.* 2003;91:815-819. PMID: 14633751.

92. Smith S. Evidence-based management of constipation in the oncology patient. *Eur J Oncol Nurs.* 2001;5:18-25. PMID: 12849044.

93. Sykes NP. The relationship between opioid use and laxative use in terminally ill cancer patients. *Palliat Med.* 1998;12:375-382. PMID: 9924600.

94. Goodman M, Low J, Wilkinson S. Constipation management in palliative care: a survey of practices in the United kingdom. *J Pain Symptom Manage.* 2005;29:238-244. PMID: 15781174.

95. Kyle G. Constipation and palliative care - where are we now? *Int J Palliat Nurs.* 2007;13:6-16. PMID: 17353846.

96. Richmond J. Prevention of constipation through risk management. *Nurs Stand.* 2003;17:39-46; quiz 47-38. PMID: 12600129.

97. Wirz S, Klaschik E. Management of constipation in palliative care patients undergoing opioid therapy: is polyethylene glycol an option? *Am J Hosp Palliat Care.* 2005;22:375-381. PMID: 16225360.

98. Drossman D, Thompson W, Talley N, et al. Identification of sub-groups of functional gastrointestinal disorders. *Gastroenterol Int.* 1990;3:159-172.

99. Sykes NP. Methods for clinical research in constipation. In Max M, Lynn J (eds). *Interactive Textbook on Clinical Symptom Research.* Bethesda, MD: National Institutes of Health; 2004. http://painconsortium.nih.gov/symptomresearch/chapter_3/sec8/cnss8pg3.htm. Accessed June 16, 2014.

100. Fallon M, O'Neill B. ABC of palliative care. Constipation and diarrhoea. *BMJ.* 1997;315:1293-1296. PMID: 9390060.

101. Ross H. Constipation: cause and control in an acute hospital setting. *Br J Nurs.* 1998;7:907-913. PMID: 9849157.

102. Friedrichsen M, Erichsen E. The lived experience of constipation in cancer patients in palliative hospital-based home care. *Int J Palliat Nurs.* 2004;10:321-325. PMID: 15365483.

103. Dunlop G. A study of the relative frequency and importance of gastrointestinal symptoms and weakness in patients with far advanced cancer: Student paper. *Palliat Med.* 1989;4:37-44.

104. Holmes S. Use of a modified symptom distress scale in assessment of the cancer patient. *Int J Nurs Stud.* 1989;26:69-79. PMID: 2707983.

105. Hurdon V, Viola R, Schroder C. How useful is docusate in patients at risk for constipation? A systematic review of the evidence in the chronically ill. *J Pain Symptom Manage.* 2000;19:130-136. PMID: 10699540.

106. Glia A, Lindberg G. Quality of life in patients with different types of functional constipation. *Scand J Gastroenterol.* 1997;32:1083-1089. PMID: 9399387.

107. Brown L, Lawrie I, D'Sa VB, et al. Constipation: patient perceptions compared to diagnostic tools. *Palliat Med.* 2006;20:717-718. PMID: 17060272.

108. Asai T. Constipation: does it increase morbidity and mortality in critically ill patients? *Crit Care Med.* 2007;35:2861-2862. PMID: 18043207.

109. Dipalma JA, Cleveland MV, McGowan J, et al. A randomized, multicenter, placebo-controlled trial of polyethylene glycol laxative for chronic treatment of chronic constipation. *Am J Gastroenterol.* 2007;102:1436-1441. PMID: 17403074.

110. Lee-Robichaud H, Thomas K, Morgan J, et al. Lactulose versus Polyethylene Glycol for Chronic Constipation. *Cochrane Database Systematic Reviews.* 2010;(7):CD007570. PMID: 20614462.

111. Lembo A. Peripheral opioids for functional GI disease: a reappraisal. *Dig Dis.* 2006;24:91-98. PMID: 16699267.

112. Shaiova L, Rim F, Friedman D, et al. A review of methylnaltrexone, a peripheral opioid receptor antagonist, and its role in opioid-induced constipation. *Palliative and Supportive Care.* 2007;5:161-166. PMID: 17578067.

113. Webster L, Jansen JP, Peppin J, et al. Alvimopan, a peripherally acting mu-opioid receptor (PAM-OR) antagonist for the treatment of opioid-induced bowel dysfunction: results from a randomized, double-blind, placebo-controlled, dose-finding study in subjects taking opioids for chronic non-cancer pain. *Pain.* 2008;137:428-440. PMID: 18164818.

114. Mercadante S, Ferrera P, Casuccio A. Effectiveness and tolerability of amidotrizoate for the treatment of constipation resistant to laxatives in advanced cancer patients. *J Pain Symptom Manage.* 2011;41:421-425. PMID: 20833504.

115. Rubiales AS, Hernansanz S, Gutiérrez C, et al. Neostigmine for refractory constipation in advanced cancer patients. *J Pain Symptom Manage.* 2006;32:204-205. PMID: 16939843.

116. Liu M, Wittbrodt E. Low-dose oral naloxone reverses opioid-induced constipation and analgesia. *J Pain Symptom Manage.* 2002;23:48-53. PMID: 11779668.

117. Lai TK, Cheung MC, Lo CK, et al. Effectiveness of aroma massage on advanced cancer patients with constipation: a pilot study. *Complement Ther Clin Pract.* 2011;17:37-43. PMID: 21168113.

118. Baines M, Oliver DJ, Carter RL. Medical management of intestinal obstruction in patients with advanced malignant disease. A clinical and pathological study. *Lancet.* 1985;2:990-993. PMID: 2414614.

119. Beattie GJ, Leonard R, Smyth JF. Bowel obstruction in ovarian carcinoma: a retrospective study and review of the literature. *Palliat Med.* 1989;3:275-280.

120. Castaldo TW, Petrilli ES, Ballon SC, et al. Intestinal operations in patients with ovarian carcinoma. *Am J Obstetrics and Gynecology.* 1981;139:80-84. PMID: 7457527.

121. Krebs HB, Goplerud DR. Mechanical intestinal obstruction in patients with gynecologic disease: a review of 368 patients. *Am J Obstetrics and Gynecology.* 1987;157:577-583. PMID: 3631159.

122. Kyllönen LE. Obstruction and perforation complicating colorectal carcinoma. An epidemiologic and clinical study with special reference to incidence and survival. *Acta Chir Scand.* 1987;153:607-614. PMID: 3434101.

123. Lund B, Hansen M, Lundvall F, et al. Intestinal obstruction in patients with advanced carcinoma of the ovaries treated with combination chemotherapy. *Surg Gynecol Obstet.* 1989;169:213-218. PMID: 2475912.

124. Phillips RK, Hittinger R, Fry JS, et al. Malignant large bowel obstruction. *Br J Surg.* 1985;72:296-302. PMID: 3986481.

125. Solomon HJ, Atkinson KH, Coppleson JV, et al. Bowel complications in the management of ovarian cancer. *Aust N Z J Obstet Gynaecol.* 1983;23:65-68. PMID: 6578779.

126. Tunca JC, Buchler DA, Mack EA, et al. The management of ovarian-cancer-caused bowel obstruction. *Gyn Oncol.* 1981;12:186-192. PMID: 7297929.

127. Ventafridda V, Ripamonti C, Caraceni A, et al. The management of inoperable gastrointestinal obstruction in terminal cancer patients. *Tumori.* 1990;76:389-393. PMID: 1697993.

128. Mercadante S. Pain in inoperable bowel obstruction. *Pain Digest.* 1995;5:9-13. PMID:.

129. Feuer DJ, Broadley KE, Shepherd JH, et al. Systematic review of surgery in malignant bowel obstruction in advanced gynecological and gastrointestinal cancer. The Systematic Review Steering Committee. *Gyn Oncol.* 1999;75:313-322. PMID: 10600282.

130. Dormann A, Meisner S, Verin N, et al. Self-expanding metal stents for gastroduodenal malignancies: systematic review of their clinical effectiveness. *Endoscopy.* 2004;36:543-550. PMID: 15202052.

131. Holt AP, Patel M, Ahmed MM. Palliation of patients with malignant gastroduodenal obstruction with self-expanding metallic stents: the treatment of choice? *Gastrointest Endosc.* 2004;60:1010-1017. PMID: 15605026.

132. Ripamonti C. *Bowel Obstruction.* Philadelphia, PA: Lippincott-Raven; 1998.

133. Mangili G, Franchi M, Mariani A, et al. Octreotide in the management of bowel obstruction in terminal ovarian cancer. *Gyn Oncol.* 1996;61:345-348. PMID: 8641613.

134. Mercadante S, Maddaloni S. Octreotide in the management of inoperable gastrointestinal obstruction in terminal cancer patients. *J Pain Symptom Manage.* 1992;7:496-498. PMID: 1283750.

135. Riley J, Fallon MT. Octreotide in terminal malignant obstruction of the gastrointestinal tract. *Eur J Palliat Care.* 1994;1:23-25.

136. Currow DC, Clark K, Cartmill J, et al. A multi-site, fixed dose, parallel arm, double-blind, placebo controlled, block randomised trial of the addition of infusional octreotide or placebo to regular ranitidine and dexamethasone

137. Fainsinger RL, Spachynski K, Hanson J, et al. Symptom control in terminally ill patients with malignant bowel obstruction (MBO). *J Pain Symptom Manage.* 1994;9:12-18. PMID: 7513322.

138. Ripamonti C, Twycross R, Baines M, et al. Clinical-practice recommendations for the management of bowel obstruction in patients with end-stage cancer. *Support Care Cancer.* 2001;9:223-233. PMID: 11430417.

139. Feuer DJ, Broadley KE. Corticosteroids for the resolution of malignant bowel obstruction in advanced gynaecological and gastrointestinal cancer. *Cochrane Database Systematic Reviews.* 2000;(2):CD001219. PMID: 10796761.

140. Kaneishi K, Kawabata M, Morita T. Olanzapine for the relief of nausea in patients with advanced cancer and incomplete bowel obstruction. *J Pain Symptom Manage.* 2012;44:604-607. PMID: 22771132.

141. Davis MP, Furste A. Glycopyrrolate: a useful drug in the palliation of mechanical bowel obstruction. *J Pain Symptom Manage.* 1999;18:153-154. PMID: 10517034.

142. Twycross RG. *Palliative Care Formulary.* Oxford: Radcliffe Medical Press; 1998.

143. Abernethy AP. Pain and sleep: establishing bi-directional association in a population-based sample. *Pain.* 2008;137:1-2. PMID: 18410992.

144. Holland JC, Andersen B, Breitbart WS, et al. Distress management. *J Natl Compr Canc Netw.* 2013;11:190-209. PMID: 23411386.

145. Schroepfer TA. Critical events in the dying process: the potential for physical and psychosocial suffering. *J Palliat Med.* 2007;10:136-147. PMID: 17298262.

146. Cheng MJ, King LM, Alesi ER, et al. Doing palliative care in the oncology office. *J Oncol Pract.* 2013;9:84-88. PMID: 23814515.

147. Mack JW, Cronin A, Keating NL, et al. Associations between end-of-life discussion characteristics and care received near death: a prospective cohort study. *J Clin Oncol.* 2012;30:4387-4395. PMID: 23150700.

148. Weeks JC, Catalano PJ, Cronin A, et al. Patients' expectations about effects of chemotherapy for advanced cancer. *N Engl J Med.* 2012;367:1616-1625. PMID: 23094723.

149. Glare P, Virik K, Jones M, et al. A systematic review of physicians' survival predictions in terminally ill cancer patients. *BMJ.* 2003;327:195-198. PMID: 12881260.

150. Lamont EB, Christakis NA. Prognostic disclosure to patients with cancer near the end of life. *Ann Intern Med.* 2001;134:1096-1105. PMID: 11412049.

151. Anselm AH, Palda V, Guest CB, et al. Barriers to communication regarding end-of-life care: perspectives of care providers. *J Crit Care.* 2005;20:214-223. PMID: 16253789.

152. Clayton JM, Butow PN, Tattersall MHN. When and how to initiate discussion about prognosis and end-of-life issues with terminally ill patients. *J Pain Symptom Manage.* 2005;30:132-144. PMID: 16125028.

153. Thorne S, Hislop TG, Kuo M, et al. Hope and probability: patient perspectives of the meaning of numerical information in cancer communication. *Qual Health Res.* 2006;16:318-336. PMID: 16449684.

154. Moxey A, O'Connell D, McGettigan P, et al. Describing treatment effects to patients. *J Gen Intern Med.* 2003;18:948-959. PMID: 14687282.

155. Young JM, Davey C, Ward JE. Influence of 'framing effect' on women's support for government funding of breast cancer screening. *Aust N Z J Public Health.* 2003;27:287-290. PMID: 14705283.

156. Weeks JC, Cook EF, O'Day SJ, et al. Relationship between cancer patients' predictions of prognosis and their treatment preferences. *JAMA.* 1998;279:1709-1714. PMID: 9624023.

157. Curtis JR, Patrick DL, Caldwell ES, et al. Why don't patients and physicians talk about end-of-life care? Barriers to communication for patients with acquired immunodeficiency syndrome and their primary care clinicians. *Arch Intern Med.* 2000;160:1690-1696. PMID: 10847263.

158. Knauft E, Nielsen EL, Engelberg RA, et al. Barriers and facilitators to end-of-life care communication for patients with COPD. *Chest.* 2005;127:2188-2196. PMID: 15947336.

159. Heyland DK, Dodek P, Rocker G, et al. What matters most in end-of-life care: perceptions of seriously ill patients and their family members. *CMAJ.* 2006;174:627-633. PMID: 16505458.

160. Wenrich MD, Curtis JR, Ambrozy DA, et al. Dying patients' need for emotional support and personalized care from physicians: perspectives of patients with terminal illness, families, and health care providers. *J Pain Symptom Manage.* 2003;25:236-246. PMID: 12614958.

161. Petticrew M, Bell R, Hunter D. Influence of psychological coping on survival and recurrence in people with cancer: systematic review. *BMJ.* 2002;325:1066. PMID: 12424165.

162. Jacobsen J, Jackson VA. A communication approach for oncologists: understanding patient coping and communicating about bad news, palliative care, and hospice. *J Natl Compr Canc Netw.* 2009;7:475-480. PMID: 19406044.

163. Baile WF, Buckman R, Lenzi R, et al. SPIKES-A six-step protocol for delivering bad news: application to the patient with cancer. *Oncologist.* 2000;5:302-311. PMID: 10964998.

164. Vaidya VU, Greenberg LW, Patel KM, et al. Teaching physicians how to break bad news: a 1-day workshop using standardized parents. *Arch Pediatr Adolesc Med.* 1999;153:419-422. PMID: 10201727.

165. Chaturvedi SK, Loiselle CG, Chandra PS. Communication with relatives and collusion in palliative care: a cross-cultural perspective. *Indian J Palliat Care.* 2009;15:2-9. PMID: 20606848.

166. Xue D, Abernethy AP. Management of dyspnea in advanced lung cancer: recent data and emerging concepts. *Curr Opin Support Palliat Care.* 2010;4:85-91. PMID: 20440205.

167. Butler LD, Koopman C, Cordova MJ, et al. Psychological distress and pain significantly increase before death in metastatic breast cancer patients. *Psychosom Med.* 2003;65:416-426. PMID: 12764215.

168. Solano JP, Gomes B, Higginson IJ. A comparison of symptom prevalence in far advanced cancer, AIDS, heart disease, chronic obstructive pulmonary disease and renal disease. *J Pain Symptom Manage.* 2006;31:58-69. PMID: 16442483.

169. Wilson KG, Chochinov HM, Skirko MG, et al. Depression and anxiety disorders in palliative cancer care. *J Pain Symptom Manage.* 2007;33:118-129. PMID: 17280918.

170. Akechi T, Okuyama T, Sugawara Y, et al. Screening for depression in terminally ill cancer patients in Japan. *J Pain Symptom Manage.* 2006;31:5-12. PMID: 16442477.

171. Maguire P, Walsh S, Jeacock J, et al. Physical and psychological needs of patients dying from colo-rectal cancer. *Palliat Med.* 1999;13:45-50. PMID: 10320875.

172. Sise MJ, Sise CB, Sack DI, et al. Surgeons' attitudes about communicating with patients and their families. *Curr Surg.* 2006;63:213-218. PMID: 16757376.

173. Chibnall JT, Bennett ML, Videen SD, et al. Identifying barriers to psychosocial spiritual care at the end of life: a physician group study. *Am J Hosp Palliat Care.* 2004;21:419-426. PMID: 15612233.

174. Levinson W, Gorawara-Bhat R, Lamb J. A study of patient clues and physician responses in primary care and surgical settings. *JAMA.* 2000;284:1021-1027. PMID: 10944650.

175. Vodermaier A, Linden W, Siu C. Screening for emotional distress in cancer patients: a systematic review of assessment instruments. *J Natl Cancer Inst.* 2009;101:1464-1488. PMID: 19826136.

176. Dumont I, Dumont S, Mongeau S. End-of-life care and the grieving process: family caregivers who have experienced the loss of a terminal-phase cancer patient. *Qual Health Res.* 2008;18:1049-1061. PMID: 18650561.

177. Dumont S, Turgeon J, Allard P, et al. Caring for a loved one with advanced cancer: determinants of psychological distress in family caregivers. *J Palliat Med.* 2006;9:912-921. PMID: 16910806.

178. Rivera HR. Depression symptoms in cancer caregivers. *Clin J Oncol Nurs.* 2009;13:195-202. PMID: 19349266.

179. Rabow MW, Hauser JM, Adams J. Supporting family caregivers at the end of life: "they don't know what they don't know". *JAMA.* 2004;291:483-491. PMID: 14747506.

180. Stein MD, Crystal S, Cunningham WE, et al. Delays in seeking HIV care due to competing caregiver responsibilities. *Am J Public Health.* 2000;90:1138-1140. PMID: 10897195.

181. Wilkinson A. The carer experience in end-of-life caregiving- a discussion of the literature. *Cancer Forum.* 2010; 34.

182. Rose K. How informal carers cope with terminal cancer. *Nurs Stand.* 1997;11:39-42. PMID: 9165899.

183. Bair MJ, Robinson RL, Katon W, et al. Depression and pain comorbidity: a literature review. *Arch Intern Med.* 2003;163:2433-2445. PMID: 14609780.

184. Lin EH, Katon W, Von Korff M, et al. Effect of improving depression care on pain and functional outcomes among older adults with arthritis: a randomized controlled trial. *JAMA.* 2003;290:2428-2429. PMID: 14612479.

185. Abernethy A, Burns C, Wheeler J, et al. Defining distinct caregiver subpopulations by intensity of end-of-life care provided. *Palliat Med.* 2009;23:66-79. PMID: 18996981.

186. Bainbridge D, Krueger P, Lohfeld L, et al. Stress processes in caring for an end-of-life family member: application of a theoretical model. *Aging and Mental Health.* 2009;13:537-545. PMID: 19629778.

187. Redinbaugh EM, Baum A, Tarbell S, et al. End-of-life caregiving: what helps family caregivers cope? *J Palliat Med.* 2003;6:901-909. PMID: 14733682.

188. Aizer AA, Chen MH, McCarthy EP, et al. Marital status and survival in patients with cancer. *J Clin Oncol.* 2013;31:3869-3876. PMID: 24062405.

189. Tao H, Ellenbecker CH, Chen J, et al. The influence of social environmental factors on rehospitalization among patients receiving home health care services. *ANS Adv Nurs Sci.* 2012;35:346-358. PMID: 23107991.

190. Emanuel EJ, Fairclough DL, Slutsman J, et al. Understanding economic and other burdens of terminal illness: the experience of patients and their caregivers. *Ann Intern Med.* 2000;132:451-459. PMID: 10733444.

191. Sekelja N, Butow PN, Tattersall MH. Bereaved cancer carers' experience of and preference for palliative care. *Support Care Cancer.* 2010;18:1219-1228. PMID: 19821168.

192. Noorani NH, Montagnini M. Recognizing depression in palliative care patients. *J Palliat Med.* 2007;10:458-464. PMID: 17472517.

193. Periyakoil VS, Hallenbeck J. Identifying and managing preparatory grief and depression at the end of life. *Am Fam Physician.* 2002;65:883-890. PMID: 11898960.

194. Breitbart W, Rosenfeld B, Pessin H, et al. Depression, hopelessness, and desire for hastened death in terminally ill patients with cancer. *JAMA.* 2000;284:2907-2911. PMID: 11147988.

195. Delgado-Guay M, Parsons HA, Li Z, et al. Symptom distress in advanced cancer patients with anxiety and depression in the palliative care setting. *Support Care Cancer.* 2009;17:573-579. PMID: 19005686.

196. Hotopf M, Chidgey J, Addington-Hall J, et al. Depression in advanced disease: a systematic review Part 1. Prevalence and case finding. *Palliat Med.* 2002;16:81-97. PMID: 11969152.

197. Chochinov HM, Wilson KG, Enns M, et al. "Are you depressed?" Screening for depression in the terminally ill. *Am J Psychiatry.* 1997;154:674-676. PMID: 9137124.

198. Lloyd-Williams M, Friedman T, Rudd N. An analysis of the validity of the Hospital Anxiety and Depression scale as a screening tool in patients with advanced metastatic cancer. *J Pain Symptom Manage.* 2001;22:990-996. PMID: 11738161.

199. Lloyd-Williams M, Dennis M, Taylor F. A prospective study to compare three depression screening tools in patients who are terminally ill. *Gen Hosp Psychiatry.* 2004;26:384-389. PMID: 15474638.

200. Lloyd-Williams M, Shiels C, Dowrick C. The development of the Brief Edinburgh Depression Scale (BEDS) to screen for depression in patients with advanced cancer. *J Affect Disord.* 2007;99:259-264. PMID: 17055588.

201. Mitchell AJ. Are one or two simple questions sufficient to detect depression in cancer and palliative care? A Bayesian meta-analysis. *Br J Cancer.* 2008;98:1934-1943. PMID: 18506146.

202. Massie M, Holland J, Glass E. Delirium in terminally ill cancer patients. *Am J Psychiatry.* 1983;140:1048-1050. PMID: 6869591.

203. Minagawa H, Uchitomi Y, Yamawaki S, et al. Psychiatric morbidity in terminally ill cancer patients. A prospective study. *Cancer.* 1996;78:1131-1137. PMID: 8780554.

204. Bruera E, Miller L, McCallion J, et al. Cognitive failure in patients with terminal cancer: a prospective study. *J Pain Symptom Manage.* 1992;7:192-195. PMID: 1517640.

205. Moryl N, Carver AC, Foley KM. Management of cancer pain. In Kufe DW, Pollock RE, Weischselbaum RR, et al (eds). *Holland-Frei Cancer Medicine, 6th ed.* Hamilton, Ontario: BC Decker, Inc.; 2003;1113-1123.

206. Trzepacz PT, Baker RW, Greenhouse J. A symptom rating scale for delirium. *Psychiatry Res.* 1988;23:89-97. PMID: 3363018.

207. Inouye SK, van Dyck CH, Alessi CA, et al. Clarifying confusion: the confusion assessment method. A new method for detection of delirium. *Ann Intern Med.* 1990;113:941-948. PMID: 2240918.

208. Albert MS, Levkoff SE, Reilly C, et al. The delirium symptom interview: an interview for the detection of delirium symptoms in hospitalized patients. *J Geriatr Psychiatry Neurol.* 1992;5:14-21. PMID: 1571069.

209. Breitbart W, Rosenfeld B, Roth A, et al. The Memorial Delirium Assessment Scale. *J Pain Symptom Manage.* 1997;13:128-137. PMID: 9114631.

210. Folstein MF, Folstein SE, McHugh PR. "Mini-mental state". A practical method for grading the cognitive state of patients for the clinician. *J Psychiatr Res.* 1975;12:189-198. PMID: 1202204.

211. McNamara P, Minton P, Twycross R. The use of midazolam in palliative care. *Palliat Med.* 1991;5:244-249.

212. Truog RD, Berde CB, Mitchell C, et al. Barbiturates in the care of the terminally ill. *N Engl J Med.* 1992;327:1678-1682. PMID: 1279424.

213. Bennett M, Lucas V, Brennan M, et al. Using anti-muscarinic drugs in the management of death rattle: evidence-based guidelines for palliative care. *Palliat Med.* 2002;16:369-374. PMID: 12380654.

214. Hughes AC, Wilcock A, Corcoran R. Management of "death rattle". *J Pain Symptom Manage.* 1996;12:271-272. PMID: 8942121.

215. O'Donnell V. Symptom Management: The pharmacological management of respiratory tract secretions *Int J Palliat Nurs* 1998;4:199-203.

216. Bausewein C. Comparative cost of hyoscine injections. *Palliat Med.* 1995;9:256. PMID: 7582183.

217. Wildiers H, Dhaenekint C, Demeulenaere P, et al. Atropine, hyoscine butyl-bromide, or scopolamine are equally effective for the treatment of death rattle in terminal care. *J Pain Symptom Manage.* 2009;38:124-133. PMID: 19361952.

218. Abernethy AP, Clark K, Currow DC. How should we conduct and interpret phase III clinical trials in palliative care? *J Pain Symptom Manage.* 2010;39:e6-8. PMID: 19875269.

219. Wee B, Hillier R. Interventions for noisy breathing in patients near to death. *Cochrane Database Systematic Reviews.* 2008;23:CD005177. PMID: 18254072.

220. Wee BL, Coleman PG, Hillier R, et al. The sound of death rattle II: how do relatives interpret the sound? *Palliat Med.* 2006;20:177-181. PMID: 16764222.

221. Gazelle G. A good death: not just an abstract concept. *J Clin Oncol.* 2003;21:95s-96s. PMID: 12743208.

1 EPIDEMIOLOGY AND PREVENTION
SELF-EVALUATION

EPIDEMIOLOGY AND PREVENTION QUESTIONS

1-1 A recent study in the *Journal of Clinical Oncology* focused on patients with stage III colon cancer who were randomly assigned to two different adjuvant chemotherapy regimens and followed for disease recurrence and death. The study queried 1,038 patients in the trial regarding the use of multivitamins and found that 49.9% reported using multivitamins during adjuvant chemotherapy. The use of multivitamins, compared to nonuse, was not associated with disease-free survival or overall survival.

What kind of study is this?
- A. Case-control study
- B. Cohort study
- C. Cross-sectional study
- D. Randomized trial

1-2 A study is conducted to determine the effect of familial aggregation of cancer on the risk of testicular cancer. Interviews are conducted with 194 patients with testicular cancer and also with 194 control participants, and detailed family histories of cancer are obtained from each. Of the 194 men with testicular cancer, 21 report the occurrence of testicular cancer in one of their first-degree male relatives, while 13 of the control participants report such a history.

Of what bias may this be an example?
- A. Lead-time bias
- B. Recall bias
- C. Selection bias
- D. Healthy worker bias

1-3 We have made significant progress in reducing the incidence rates of a number of cancers. However, for which of the following cancers are the incidence rates continuing to rise in the United States?
- A. Lung cancer
- B. Colon cancer
- C. Gastric cancer
- D. Melanoma

1-4 Lung cancer remains the primary cause of cancer-related mortality in the United States. Which of the following interventions is not likely to reduce mortality for this disease?
- A. Annual chest x-ray screening for heavy smokers
- B. Annual low-dose computed tomography (CT) screening for heavy smokers
- C. Reducing or preventing teenage cigarette smoking
- D. Strict regulation of asbestos exposure among construction workers

1-5 Tobacco is responsible for close to one-third of cancers in the United States. Thus, the reduction in cigarette smoking prevalence is having a profound effect on current and future cancer rates.

Which of the following is currently considered the second most important cause of cancer in the United States?
- A. Hepatitis B virus
- B. Human papillomavirus
- C. Obesity
- D. Low intake of fruits and vegetables

1-6 Low-prevalence, high-penetrance genes for cancer—such as *BRCA1, BRCA2*, and the retinoblastoma gene—share certain characteristics, such as early age at onset of the cancers.

Which of the following characteristics do they also share?
- A. X-linked dominant
- B. X-linked recessive
- C. Autosomal dominant
- D. Autosomal recessive

1-7 A total of 100 patients are screened for cancer using a newly developed test with the following results: eight results are true-positives; one result is false-positive; one result is false-negative; and 90 results are true-negatives.

Which of the following formulas calculates the sensitivity of the test?
A. 90 divided by (1 + 90)
B. 8 divided by (1 + 90)
C. 90 divided by (90 + 8)
D. 8 divided by (8 + 1)

1-8 When a heavy smoker discontinues smoking, it can take 10 or more years before his or her risk of lung cancer begins to fall significantly.

Why is this?
A. Cigarette smoke contains tumor initiators
B. Cigarette smoke contains tumor promoters
C. Cigarette smoke contains nicotine
D. Cigarette smoke contains acetone and benzene

1-1 B

A cohort study compares two groups on the basis of exposures. In this example, the basis is whether they were exposed to multivitamins or not. The outcomes were survival. The cohort study uses patients who were included within a randomized trial.

Suggested Reading

Ng K, Meyerhardt JA, Chan JA, et al. Multivitamin use is not associated with cancer recurrence or survival in patients with stage III colon cancer: findings from CALGB 89803. *J Clin Oncol.* 2010;28:4354-4363. PMID: 20805450.

1-2 B

Studies are subject to a number of biases, some of which are important to recognize. This is an example of recall bias: the individual with the disease will recall and report information differently than a control participant. The affected sibling may, in fact, have better information about family history, but the two are reporting differently from each other, which will lead to biased results.

Suggested Reading

Chang ET, Smedby KE, Hjalgrim H, et al. Reliability of self-reported family history of cancer in a large case-control study of lymphoma. *J Natl Cancer Inst.* 2006;98:61-68. PMID: 16391372.

1-3 D

Melanoma has been increasing due to a combination of factors, including migration to southern states and increased skin screening. There has not been a concomitant increase in mortality from melanoma. Lung cancer rates are falling because of the decreased prevalence of tobacco smoking, whereas colon cancer rates are decreasing because of the increased use of colon cancer screening and the removal of adenomatous polyps. Gastric cancer has been on a steady decline for decades, presumably reflecting changes in dietary patterns and a decrease in peptic ulcer disease.

1-4 A

Several randomized trials in the past have shown no benefit for lung cancer screening with plain chest x-rays. This was recently confirmed with another randomized trial evaluating chest x-ray screening as part of the PLCO study. The NLST study did show a 20% reduction in lung cancer mortality for heavy smokers who underwent annual screening with low-dose CT scans. Use of tobacco is a major risk factor for lung cancer, so any successful efforts to reduce tobacco use, such as reducing teen smoking, will have beneficial effects on lung cancer mortality. Likewise, asbestos is a well-known occupational lung carcinogen and its regulation will also reduce lung cancer mortality rates.

Suggested Reading

Oken MM, Hocking WG, Kvale PA, et al. Screening by chest radiograph and lung cancer mortality: the Prostate, Lung, Colorectal, and Ovarian (PLCO) randomized trial. *JAMA.* 2011;306:1865-1873. PMID: 22031728.

National Lung Screening Trial Research Team, Aberle DR, Adams AM, et al. Reduced lung-cancer mortality with low-dose computed tomographic screening. *N Engl J Med.* 2011;365:395-409. PMID: 21714641.

1-5 C

Many experts consider obesity the second most important cancer risk factor, after tobacco, in the United States. It increases the risk for a variety of cancers through a number of mechanisms, including breast and endometrial cancers, adenocarcinoma of the esophagus, and prostate cancer.

Suggested Reading

Schottenfeld D, Beebe-Dimmer JL, Buffler PA, et al. Current perspective on the global and United States cancer burden attributable to lifestyle and environmental risk factors. *Annu Rev Public Health.* 2013;34:97-117. PMID: 23514316.

1-6 C

These genetic syndrome genes are typically tumor suppressor genes, which are autosomal dominant.

Suggested Reading

Lux MP, Fasching PA, Beckmann MW. Hereditary breast and ovarian cancer: review and future perspectives. *J Mol Med (Berl).* 2006; 84:16-28. PMID: 16283147.

1-7   D

When screening for a disease with a test, the following outcomes are possible:

	Disease Present	Disease Absent
Positive Result	True-positive (A)	False-positive (B)
Negative Result	False-negative (C)	True-negative (D)

The specificity is the proportion of people without the disease who have a negative test result: D divided by (B + D; answer A). Answers B and C are not really meaningful statistics. Sensitivity is the proportion of people with the disease who have a positive test result: A divided by (A + C; answer D). In this example, the sensitivity is 8 divided by 9, or 89%.

1-8   A

The long delay in the decline of risk for lung cancer stems from the fact that cigarette smoke is an initiator. Initiators are carcinogens that affect the early stages of the carcinogenic process and hence have their effect years before the malignancy actually appears. Hence, the decline in risk upon cessation of smoking follows a reverse pattern, requiring years before their initiating effect has dissipated. Cigarette smoke also contains promoters, but they are not responsible for this long delay.

2 MOLECULAR BIOLOGY
SELF-EVALUATION

MOLECULAR BIOLOGY QUESTIONS

2-1 A 72-year-old man develops progressive dyspnea on exertion. His peripheral blood exam shows pancytopenia and a bone marrow aspirate, and biopsy reveals 7% abnormal myeloblasts, as well as erythroid and megakaryocytic dysplasia. He is diagnosed with myelodysplastic syndrome and begins treatment with 5-azacytidine.

Which of the following statements best describes the epigenetic regulatory mechanism targeted by 5-azacytidine?
- A. High levels of histone acetylation are found in actively transcribed genes
- B. DNA methylation in cytosine-phosphate-guanine (CpG) islands silences the expression of tumor suppressor genes
- C. Histone phosphorylation alters chromatin structure
- D. Mismatch repair gene mutations cause genome instability

2-2 A 65-year-old woman presents with a T10 spinal compression fracture, elevated serum beta 2-microglobulin, and a bone marrow aspirate that reveals sheets of plasma cells. She is diagnosed with multiple myeloma, and you suggest therapy with a regimen containing the proteasome inhibitor bortezomib.

Which statement best explains bortezomib's mechanism of action?
- A. The proteasome repairs DNA damage in cancer cells
- B. The proteasome degrades microRNAs (miRNAs) that regulate oncogene expression
- C. Bortezomib prevents the attachment of ubiquitin to cyclin D
- D. The attachment of ubiquitin to proteins signals their degradation by the proteasome

2-3 A 32-year-old woman with asymptomatic leukocytosis is found to have Philadelphia chromosome–positive chronic myelogenous leukemia (CML).

Which of the following statements best describes chromosomal translocations found in cancers?
- A. Translocations can deregulate oncogene expression by placing them in proximity to strong regulatory regions associated with immunoglobulin genes
- B. Translocations are only found in leukemias and lymphomas
- C. Translocations often activate *p53* gene expression
- D. Translocations never lead to gene fusions

2-4 The patient in Question 2-3 is treated with imatinib and experiences a complete molecular response.

Which of the following statements about using molecular testing to assess response and minimal residual disease (MRD) is correct?
- A. Classical cytogenetics is the most sensitive testing modality for detecting minimal residual disease
- B. Whole-genome sequencing using next-generation technology is the method of choice for monitoring a continued response to imatinib
- C. Real-time reverse transcriptase-polymerase chain reaction (RT-PCR) can detect and quantify the *BCR-ABL* fusion product in rare cells within peripheral blood and bone marrow
- D. Fluorescence in situ hybridization (FISH) cannot detect gene fusions such as *BCR-ABL*

2-5 A 38-year-old woman with a history of a childhood sarcoma develops breast carcinoma. Her family history is consistent with Li-Fraumeni syndrome, and she is found to have a germ-line mutation in one allele of the *p53* gene.

Which of the following statements best describes *p53* mutations in cancers?
- A. Despite their association with poor prognosis, *p53* mutations are very rare in cancers
- B. *p53* amplification in ovarian cancers contributes to tumor progression by increasing p53 activity
- C. *p53*'s central roles in regulating cell division and DNA repair are compromised by mutations in cancers
- D. The *p53* protein is a GTPase-activating protein (GAP), and *p53* mutations increase RAS enzymatic activity by affecting p53 GAP-activity

2-6 A 53-year-old man presents with a colorectal adeno-carcinoma, and PCR-based testing of his tumor DNA revealed the presence of microsatellite instability and a mutation in a DNA mismatch repair gene.

Which of the following statements best applies to the relationship between DNA repair pathways and tumorigenesis?
- A. Mutations in tumor suppressor genes involved in DNA repair promote carcinogenesis through increased genetic instability
- B. DNA repair genes associated with mutations in familial colon cancer syndromes are never mutated in sporadic colon cancers
- C. Microsatellite instability is a hallmark of Fanconi anemia
- D. Germ-line mutations that impair each of the three major DNA repair pathways (double-strand break repair, nucleotide excision repair, mismatch repair) lead to similar cancer syndromes

2-7 A 58-year-old woman with non-small cell lung cancer undergoes next-generation–based DNA sequencing of her tumor and normal DNA.

Which of the following statements best describes the evolving roles of next-generation sequencing and precision therapy?
- A. Whole-genome sequencing is required to identify all of the coding sequence mutations in a tumor
- B. Exome sequencing reveals rare mutations in a cancer type that predict response to targeted therapies
- C. Next-generation sequencing of tumors provides limited information because it only detects point mutations
- D. Next-generation sequencing cannot be used for guiding therapy because of the long time frame required for its completion

2-8 The sequencing of the patient's tumor described in Question 2-7 is found to have an activating point mutation in the epidermal growth factor receptor (EGFR) and the patient is treated with gefinitib.

Which of the following statements best describes the molecular mechanism associated with gefinitib response?
- A. Activation of apoptosis through inhibition of the BCL-2 protein
- B. Reactivation of the p53 tumor suppressor protein
- C. Inhibition of mitogenic signaling driven by RAS
- D. Activation of the WNT pathway

2-1   B

Epigenetic modifications to chromatin play critical roles in regulating gene expression. DNA methylation with CpG islands is associated with gene repression and is an important mechanism that silences tumor suppressor gene expression in cancer cells. 5-azacytidine is a cytosine nucleotide analog that inhibits DNA methylation and re-establishes the expression of genes suppressed by methylation. Although histone acetylation is an epigenetic modification that increases gene expression and is targeted by histone deacetylase inhibitors such as vorinostat, it is not affected by 5-azacytidine. Histone phosphorylation and DNA mismatch repair are not affected by 5-azacytidine.

Suggested Reading

Yoo CB, Jones PA. Epigenetic therapy of cancer: past, present and future. *Nat Rev Drug Discov.* 2006;5:37-50. PMID: 16485345.

Kouzarides T. Chromatin modifications and their function. *Cell.* 2007; 128:693-705. PMID: 17320507.

Laird PW. Cancer epigenetics. *Hum Mol Genet.* 2005;14 Spec No 1:R65-76. PMID: 15809275.

2-2   D

The proteasome is a large proteolytic structure that degrades cellular proteins after they become conjugated to poly-ubiquitin chains. The ubiquitin-proteasome system (UPS) degrades numerous proteins involved in cell division, differentiation, and apoptosis, and tumors contain mutations in UPS components. Bortezomib was the first approved proteasome inhibitor, and second-generation proteasome inhibitors, such as carfilzomib, are now in use and in clinical trials. These agents function by inhibiting proteases that are contained within the proteasome, but they do not inhibit the attachment of ubiquitin to target proteins. The proteasome does not degrade miRNAs or repair DNA damage.

Suggested Reading

Micel LN, Tentler JJ, Smith PG, et al. Role of ubiquitin ligases and the proteasome in oncogenesis: novel targets for anticancer therapies. *J Clin Oncol.* 2013;31:1231-1238. PMID: 23358974.

Kortuem KM, Stewart AK. Carfilzomib. *Blood.* 2013;121:893-897. PMID: 23393020.

Nakayama KI, Nakayama K. Ubiquitin ligases: cell-cycle control and cancer. *Nat Rev Cancer.* 2006;6:369-381. PMID: 16633365.

2-3   A

Translocations are DNA rearrangements that join together DNA regions that are normally found on different chromosomes. Translocations activate oncogenes by two primary mechanisms. The first involves placing oncogene transcription under the control of strong regulatory elements that normally function within the translocated partner gene. Examples of this mechanism include translocations between *MYC* and *BCL2* with immunoglobulin genes in Burkitt and mantle cell lymphoma, respectively. The second mechanism involves the joining of the coding sequences of two different genes together, such that a fusion transcript is produced that encodes a novel fusion protein, such BCR-ABL in CML t(9;22) and PML-retinoic acid receptor-alpha in acute promyelocytic leukemia t(15;17). In addition to the well-known translocations found in hematologic cancers, translocations also contribute to the pathogenesis of solid tumors, such as those involving *ERG* in prostate cancer and *EWS* in Ewing sarcoma. The *p53* gene is commonly disabled by loss-of-functions mutations in cancers and is not activated by translocation.

Suggested Reading

Look T. Genes altered by chromosomal translocations in leukemia and lymphomas. In Vogelstein B, Kinzler KW (eds). *The Genetic Basis of Human Cancer.* New York: McGraw-Hill Professional, 2002;57-92.

Nambiar M, Kari V, Raghavan SC. Chromosomal translocations in cancer. *Biochim Biophys Acta.* 2008;786:139-152. PMID: 18718509.

2-4   C

The ability of molecular testing to detect fusion products in very small cell populations allows for the sensitive and quantitative monitoring of diseases such as CML. PCR detection of the BCR-ABL transcript is a key tool for monitoring both response and relapse of Philadelphia chromosome–positive acute myeloid leukemia or acute lymphocytic leukemia. RT-PCR methods can detect a single CML cell within 1 million normal cells and are the most sensitive means of detecting residual disease. FISH analyses that employ BCR-ABL–specific probes can analyze hundreds of cells in a sample and are also used to detect MRD or disease relapse in these patients. Indeed, FISH is often used to detect gene rearrangements in hematopathology labs. In contrast, the number of cells that can be practically analyzed by classical cytogenetics is at least an order of magnitude less than FISH, and its sensitivity is not adequate for detecting MRD. Although whole-genome sequencing can certainly detect translocations, it is not a suitable approach for such a focused molecular analysis.

Suggested Reading

Chung NG, Buxhofer-Ausch V, Radich JP. The detection and significance of minimal residual disease in acute and chronic leukemia. 2006. *Tissue Antigens*. 2006;68:371-385. PMID: 17092250.

Schrappe M. Minimal residual disease: optimal methods, timing, and clinical relevance for an individual patient. 2012. *Hematology Am Soc Hematol Educ Program*. 2012;2012:137-142. PMID: 23233572.

2-5   C

The p53 protein has pivotal roles in checkpoint pathways that impinge on cell division and DNA repair, and its activity instigates complex cellular responses including apoptosis, senescence, and cell cycle arrest. Mutations that disable *p53* are the most common mutations in tumors, and these include point mutations, insertions/deletions, and transversions. In contrast, the amplifications described in option B cause increased expression of dominant oncogenes, but are not associated with *p53* alterations in cancers. The p53 protein is a transcription factor and does not function as a Ras-GAP.

Suggested Reading

Lane DP. Exploiting the p53 pathway for the diagnosis and therapy of human cancer. *Cold Spring Harb Symp Quant Biol*. 2005; 70:489-497. PMID: 16869788.

Vousden KH, Prives C. Blinded by the Light: The Growing Complexity of p53. *Cell*. 2009;137:413-431. PMID: 19410540.

Muller PA, Vousden KH. p53 mutations in cancer. *Nat Cell Biol*. 2013;5:2-8. PMID: 23263379.

2-6   A

All three DNA repair pathways are mutated in various cancers and each contributes to familial cancer syndromes. Mutations affecting nucleotide excision repair lead to sunlight sensitivity and cancer-prone disorders such as xeroderma pigmentosum. Defects in double-strand break repair genes compromise homologous recombination and lead to syndromes such as Fanconi anemia. Finally, mismatch repair mutations cause microsatellite instability and are found in hereditary nonpolyposis colon cancer. Thus, mutations within each DNA repair pathway produce distinct cancer-prone syndromes. Importantly, the same DNA repair genes that are mutated in the germline in rare hereditary cancers are also targeted by somatic mutations in sporadic cancers. Each of these DNA repair systems contributes to maintaining genome integrity, and mutations that impair their functions contribute to tumorigenesis through genetic instability, which facilitates the accumulation of the many mutations needed for neoplastic progression.

Suggested Reading

Hartwell L, Weinert T, Kadyk L, et al. Cell cycle checkpoints, genomic integrity, and cancer. *Cold Spring Harb Symp Quant Biol*. 1994; 59:259-263. PMID: 7587077.

Abbas T, Keaton MA, Dutta A. Genomic instability in cancer. *Cold Spring Harb Perspect Biol*. 2013;5:a012914. PMID: 23335075.

Lukas J, Lukas C, Bartek J. Mammalian cell cycle checkpoints: signalling pathways and their organization in space and time. *DNA Repair (Amst.)*. 2004;3:997-1007. PMID: 15279786.

2-7   B

Next-generation sequencing refers to new technologies that produce enormous amounts of sequence data from complex biologic samples such as tumors. Unlike earlier methods, such as the Sanger dideoxy sequencing that was used to complete the original human genome sequence, each of these new technologies incorporates amplification of individual DNA molecules bound to chips or beads, followed by massively parallel sequencing. These approaches can be applied to whole genomes, to coding genes (exomes), to limited DNA sequences, or to all expressed genes (transcriptome). Exome sequencing allows all of the mutations in coding sequences to be identified without the need for a more extensive genome-wide analysis. Unlike previous sequencing methods, next-generation sequencing can also be used to identify changes in copy number (gains and losses) as well as structural changes in tumors, such as translocation. These advances are transforming virtually all aspects of cancer genomics. For example, the rapid turnaround time of exome sequencing or more limited sequencing approaches allows the use of targeted therapy to be guided by the precise mutations present in a patient's tumor tissue. Moreover, large collaborative efforts such as The Cancer Genome Atlas are cataloging all mutations that contribute to many common cancer types.

Suggested Reading

Schuster SC. Next-generation sequencing transforms today's biology. *Nature Methods*. 2008;5:16-18. PMID: 18165802.

Meyerson M, Gabriel S, Getz G. Advances in understanding cancer genomes through second generation sequencing. *Nat Rev Genet*. 2010;11:685-696. PMID: 20847746.

Chin L, Hahn WC, Getz G, et al. Making sense of cancer genomic data. 2011. *Genes Dev*. 2011;25:534-555.PMID: 21406553.

2-8   C

"Precision oncology" refers to the use of agents that target the molecular lesions found in specific cancers. Gefitinib is a small molecule that inhibits EGFR's kinase activity and blocks its signaling. Recent studies have shown that gefitinib has efficacy in non-small cell lung cancer that harbors *EFGR* mutations but not in tumors that do not carry this mutation. These types of studies highlight the potential of targeted agents to achieve responses and the importance of identifying patients whose tumors have the specific mutations that render them sensitive to a targeted therapy. The EGFR is a receptor tyrosine kinse that instigates mitogenic signaling pathway involving Ras and its downstream effectors. EGFR is not involved with BCL-2, WNT, or p53 activity.

Suggested Reading

Numico G, Silvestris N, Grazioso Russi E. Advances in EGFR-directed therapy in head and neck cancer. *Front Biosci (Schol Ed)*. 2011;3: 454-466. PMID: 21196389.

Sequist LV, Lynch TJ. EGFR tyrosine kinase inhibitors in lung cancer: an evolving story. *Annu Rev Med*. 2008;59:429-442.PMID: 17716025.

3 CLINICAL PHARMACOLOGY SELF-EVALUATION

CLINICAL PHARMACOLOGY QUESTIONS

3-1 A 62-year-old woman began capecitabine treatment for metastatic colon cancer. She is taking a beta blocker for hypertension and warfarin for atrial fibrillation. Ten days after the administration of capecitabine, the patient developed watery diarrhea, stomatitis, generalized weakness, altered mental status, and pancytopenia (white blood cell [WBC] count 2.0×10^3; hemoglobin 9.6 g/dL; platelets 21×10^3).

The most likely reason for the marked toxicity observed is:
- A. Leptomeningeal central nervous system metastases
- B. An inherited deficiency in the dihydropyrimidine dehydrogenase (DPD) enzyme
- C. Thromboembolic stroke
- D. An inherited polymorphism of uridine diphosphate glucuronosyl-transferase 1A1 (UGT1A1)

3-2 A 60-year-old man with a diagnosis of non-small cell lung cancer presents with progressive metastatic disease after treatment with carboplatin/paclitaxel followed by single-agent gemcitabine. His past medical history is notable for a history of large cell lymphoma and status post-allogeneic transplant at age 42. His post-transplant course was complicated by the development of mild graft-versus-host disease, chronic mild active hepatitis B, and atrial fibrillation. His current medications include prednisone, fluconazole, diltiazem, omeprazole, and megestrol. A computed tomography (CT) scan demonstrates two enhancing lesions in the left lobe of the liver as well as multiple bilateral lung nodules. Laboratory exam demonstrates normal liver enzymes; complete blood count (CBC) demonstrates a hemoglobin of 10.3 g/dL, WBC 6.5, with an absolute neutrophil count (ANC) of 4,000. Peripheral smear demonstrates no dacrocytes. Serum creatinine is 1.1.

One week after the administration of the first dose of vinorelbine, the patient presents to the emergency department with febrile neutropenia and sepsis.

Which of the following is the most likely factor causing the patient's condition?
- A. Presence of a functional polymorphism in the hepatic *CYP3A4* gene leading to absent CYP3A activity
- B. Marrow infiltration by lung cancer
- C. A drug-drug interaction limiting the clearance of vinorelbine
- D. Impaired clearance by the kidneys

3-3 A 72-year-old woman with a history of ischemic cardiomyopathy (ejection fraction 35%) presents with newly diagnosed metastatic breast cancer. Three years ago, she presented with an invasive ductal carcinoma, grade 2, forming a 3.5-cm mass. A sentinel lymph node biopsy was negative. The tumor cells were positive (10% to 25% nuclear staining) for estrogen receptor (ER), negative for progesterone receptor (PR), and negative for HER2. After mastectomy, she received adjuvant anastrozole. On examination, her liver is enlarged. A chemistry panel demonstrates elevated liver enzymes with aspartate aminotransferase (AST) of 230 U/L (normal, 8 to 48 U/L) and total bilirubin of 2.5 mg/dL (normal, < 1.0 mg/dL). A CT demonstrates multiple confluent hepatic metastases without evidence of intrahepatic biliary dilatation. A CT-guided biopsy demonstrates adenocarcinoma, consistent with breast primary. ER, PR, and HER2 are negative.

Which of the following would be the most appropriate treatment now?
A. Paclitaxel (175 mg/m^2) administered once every 3 weeks
B. Paclitaxel (80 mg/m^2) administered weekly, with careful monitoring of blood counts
C. Doxorubicin (60 mg/m^2) and cyclophosphamide (600 mg/m^2) administered once every 3 weeks
D. Fulvestrant (500 mg) intramuscularly monthly

3-4 A 50-year-old man is seen after receiving the first cycle of infusional fluorouracil/leucovorin/oxaliplatin/irinotecan (FOLFOXIRI) for metastatic pancreas cancer. During this first cycle, which was given 3 weeks ago, he developed febrile neutropenia, with an ANC nadir of 100 cells/μL. Results of a CBC today show a total WBC count of 1,200/μL with an ANC of 450 cells/μL, a platelet count of 175,000/μL, and a hematocrit of 36 g/dL. He has had no mucositis, nausea, vomiting, bloody stool, or rash. The results of baseline liver and renal function studies (obtained before the first cycle of treatment) were normal, except for a total bilirubin of 1.9 mg/dL. His only other medication is metoprolol for hypertension.

Which of the following would you recommend once the patient's neutrophil count recovers to a normal value?
A. Give no additional fluorouracil
B. Give capecitabine instead of the fluorouracil-based combination
C. Reduce subsequent doses of irinotecan
D. Discontinue leucovorin

3-5 In the clinical scenario described in Question 3-4, what is the most likely reason for the severe toxicity observed?
A. A polymorphism in the promoter of the UGT1A1*28
B. DPD deficiency
C. Metoprolol-induced inhibition of fluorouracil metabolism
D. There is no likely explanation

3-6 Which of the following best describes a pharmacodynamic endpoint?
A. The relationship between an administered dose and the maximum plasma concentration achieved
B. The pharmacokinetic interaction of two drugs administered simultaneously
C. The relationship of an administered dose of a drug and a change in a biologic target
D. The relationship between an administered dose and drug clearance

3-7 A 24-year-old man with osteogenic sarcoma of the femur is being treated with high-dose methotrexate chemotherapy. He was admitted to the hospital 3 days ago for his second cycle of treatment. On admission, his serum creatinine level was 1.0 mg/dL (normal, 0.7 mg/dL to 1.5 mg/dL). He was started on intravenous fluids with 150 mEq/L of sodium bicarbonate in 5% dextrose in water (D5W), which resulted in a urinary pH of 8.0 (normal, 4.5 to 8.0). High-dose methotrexate was given at a dose of 12 g/m2 over 4 hours.

Twenty-four hours after the start of the methotrexate infusion, leucovorin rescue was started.

Now, 48 hours after the start of the methotrexate administration, his serum creatinine level is 2.5 mg/dL, and his serum methotrexate level is in the toxic range at 12 μmol/L. Serum uric acid level is 6.4 mg/dL (normal, 3.0 mg/dL to 7.0 mg/dL). He continues to receive intravenous fluids to achieve an alkaline urinary pH.

Which of the following interventions do you recommend?
A. Increase the amount of bicarbonate to 300 mEq/L of sodium bicarbonate in 5% dextrose in water (D5W)
B. Begin glucarpidase
C. Administer methylene blue
D. Begin rasburicase

3-8   A 38-year-old woman presents to your office after recently being diagnosed with ER-positive metastatic breast cancer with metastases to bone. She is currently taking tamoxifen and goserelin as well as monthly zoledronic acid. Shortly after diagnosis, she develops symptoms of depressed mood.

Which of the following antidepressants are contraindicated for this patient?

A.   Paroxetine

B.   Citalopram

C.   Escitalopram

D.   Venlafaxine

3-1   B

Capecitabine is a prodrug that is activated through three steps leading to the generation of fluorouracil (5-FU) in target cells. The DPD enzyme is responsible for the elimination of approximately 85% of administered dose of 5-FU. Mutations in the *DPD* gene are rare but, when present, are associated with severe 5-FU toxicity. The syndrome of DPD deficiency manifests as diarrhea, stomatitis, mucositis, neurotoxicity, and, in some cases, death. This is a true pharmacogenetic syndrome, with symptoms being unrecognizable until exposure to the drug occurs.

Suggested Reading

Ezzeldin H, Diasio R. Dihydropyrimidine dehydrogenase deficiency, a pharmacogenetic syndrome associated with potentially life-threatening toxicity following 5-fluorouracil administration. *Clin Colorectal Cancer.* 2004;4:181-189. PMID: 15377401.

Van Kuilenburg AB, Vreken P, Beex LV, et al. Heterozygosity for a point mutation in an invariant splice donor site of dihydropyrimidine dehydrogenase and severe 5-fluorouracil related toxicity. *Eur J Cancer.* 1997;33:2258-2264. PMID: 9470816.

3-2   C

Vinorelbine is a vinca alkaloid that is approved for the treatment of non-small cell lung cancer. Vinorelbine is metabolized by the liver and the CYP3A4/3A5 enzyme substantially contributes to the metabolism of vinorelbine. This patient likely has some mild liver impairment, given his history of chronic hepatitis B. Most importantly, he is currently taking two drugs (fluconazole and diltiazem) that are known to either moderately or potently inhibit CYP3A, which will dramatically inhibit the clearance of vinorelbine by CYP3A. Answer A is incorrect, as no functional polymorphisms in the *CYP3A4* gene have been identified that lead to absent CYP3A4 enzyme activity. Answer B is incorrect, as the patient presented with a normal WBC count and a smear that did not demonstrate stigmata of marrow infiltration (dacrocytes negative), suggesting that the observed neutropenia is drug-related. Answer D is incorrect, as vinorelbine is not excreted by the kidneys and increased clearance would reduce exposure to the parent drug.

Suggested Reading

Kajita J, Kuwabara T, Kobayashi H, et al. CYP3A4 is mainly responsible for the metabolism of a new vinca alkaloid, vinorelbine, in human liver microsomes. *Drug Metab Dispos.* 2000;28:1121-1127. PMID: 10950859.

Beulz-Riché D, Grudé P, Puozzo C, et al. Characterization of human cytochrome P450 isoenzymes involved in the metabolism of vinorelbine. *Fundam Clin Pharmacol.* 2005;19:545-553. PMID: 16176333.

3-3   B

Paclitaxel is approved for the first-line therapy of metastatic breast cancer and a prospective study demonstrated a significant improvement in response rates and time to progression for the weekly regimen as compared to the every-3-week regimen. Additionally, the presence of multiple liver metastases and hepatic dysfunction make answer A an incorrect choice, as paclitaxel is cleared by the liver, and total bilirubin is a good predictor of paclitaxel elimination capacity and of individual susceptibility to paclitaxel-related myelosuppression in patients with cancer with moderate to severe liver impairment. Answer C is incorrect, as doxorubicin and cyclophosphamide are cleared by the liver, making full dose administration of these drugs the incorrect option. Additionally, this option is relatively contraindicated, given the presence of cardiomyopathy. Answer D is incorrect, as the repeat biopsy demonstrated that the tumor was ER-negative, and fulvestrant is not approved for ER-negative breast cancer.

Suggested Reading

Seidman AD, Berry D, Cirrincione C, et al. Randomized phase III trial of weekly compared with every-3-weeks paclitaxel for metastatic breast cancer, with trastuzumab for all HER-2 overexpressors and random assignment to trastuzumab or not in HER-2 nonoverexpressors: final results of Cancer and Leukemia Group B protocol 9840. *J Clin Oncol.* 2008;26:1642-1649. PMID: 18375893.

Joerger M, Huitema AD, Huizing MT, et al. Safety and pharmacology of paclitaxel in patients with impaired liver function: a population pharmacokinetic-pharmacodynamic study. *Br J Clin Pharmaco.* 2007;64:622-633. PMID: 17935602.

3-4   C

3-5   A

This 50-year-old patient had marked neutropenia and infection after treatment with FOLFOXIRI. The results of laboratory studies demonstrate an elevated total bilirubin, consistent with Gilbert syndrome. Patients with these laboratory parameters are frequently found to be homozygous for the *UGT1A1*28* allele, a common polymorphism that decreases UGT1A1 enzyme function and, therefore, the efficiency of bilirubin glucuronidation. In the case of irinotecan, patients with this genetic variant have impaired SN-38 glucuronidation and a higher risk of severe neutropenia. This patient is unlikely to be DPD deficient, given the lack of severe diarrhea, the quick recovery phase, and the absence of mucositis.

For Question 3-4, C is the best answer, as irinotecan dose reduction will reduce the risk of severe neutropenia.

Suggested Reading

Pizzolato JF, Saltz LB. The camptothecins. *Lancet*. 2003;361:2235-2242. PMID: 12842380.

Innocenti F, Undevia SD, Iyer L, et al. Genetic variants in the UDP-glucuronosyltransferase 1A1 gene predict the risk of severe neutropenia of irinotecan. *J Clin Oncol*. 2004;22:1382-1388. PMID: 15007088.

3-6   C

Pharmacodynamic endpoints are increasingly important in clinical research, and it is important to understand their precise meaning. The best definition is specifically the effect of a drug on a particular biologic target, making C the best option.

Suggested Reading

Colburn WA, Lee JW. Biomarkers, validation and pharmacokinetic-pharmacodynamic modelling. *Clin Pharmacokinet*. 2003;42:997-1022. PMID: 12959633.

Workman P. How much gets there and what does it do?: The need for better pharmacokinetic and pharmacodynamic endpoints in contemporary drug discovery and development. *Curr Pharm Des*. 2003;9:891-902. PMID: 12678873.

3-7   B

Glucarpidase, a recombinant form of the bacterial enzyme carboxypeptidase G2, converts methotrexate into glutamate and 2,4-diamino-N(10)-methylpteroic acid, which are inactive metabolites that can be eliminated from the body through nonrenal pathways. The drug is administered as a single intravenous injection of 50 U/kg. Clinicians need to be aware that leucovorin should not be administered within 2 hours before or after a glucarpidase dose because leucovorin is a substrate for glucarpidase. Other alternatives include hemodialysis. Methylene blue is reported to reverse or ameliorate ifosfamide-induced neurotoxicity, but is not used for the treatment of methotrexate-induced toxicity. Rasburicase is approved for use by the U.S. Food and Drug Administration for the prevention and treatment of tumor lysis syndrome.

Suggested Reading

Widemann BC, Schwartz S, Jayaprakash N, et al. Efficacy of glucarpidase (carboxypeptidase g2) in patients with acute kidney injury after high-dose methotrexate therapy. *Pharmacotherapy*. 2014;34:427-439. Epub 2013 Oct 17. PMID: 24132809.

3-8   A

Tamoxifen undergoes metabolic activation from a weak antiestrogen to a potent antiestrogen, endoxifen. This activation step is dependent upon CYP2D6, a phase I enzyme that is highly variable. Approximately 7% to 10% of white patients lack functional CYP2D6 enzyme (poor metabolizers) and have low endoxifen concentrations. Additionally, the coadministration of potent CYP2D6 inhibitors, such as paroxetine, inhibits the metabolic activation of tamoxifen to endoxifen. There are conflicting data regarding the association between CYP2D6 enzyme activity and tamoxifen antitumor activity; however, a secondary analysis of the prospective Austrian Breast and Colorectal Study Group 8 (ABCSG 8) trial demonstrated a significantly higher likelihood of recurrence or death for CYP2D6 poor metabolizers compared to extensive metabolizers in women treated with adjuvant tamoxifen for 5 years, but not in women receiving adjuvant anastrozole. The concurrent administration of paroxetine has been associated with a higher risk for recurrence or death in women treated with tamoxifen. The correct answer is A, as paroxetine is a potent CYP2D6 inhibitor. All of the other choices are drugs that are expected to have minimal or no CYP2D6 inhibition.

Suggested Reading

Mürdter TE, Schroth W, Bacchus-Gerybadze L, et al. Activity levels of tamoxifen metabolites at the estrogen receptor and the impact of genetic polymorphisms of phase I and II enzymes on their concentration levels in plasma. *Clin Pharmacol Ther*. 2011;89:708-717. PMID: 21451508.

Kelly CM, Juurlink DN, Gomes T, et al. Selective serotonin reuptake inhibitors and breast cancer mortality in women receiving tamoxifen: a population based cohort study. *BMJ*. 2010;340:c693. PMID: 20142325.

Goetz MP, Suman VJ, Hoskin TL, et al. CYP2D6 metabolism and patient outcome in the Austrian Breast and Colorectal Cancer Study Group trial (ABCSG) 8. *Clin Cancer Res*. 2013;19:500-507. PMID: 23213055.

4 PRINCIPLES OF BIOLOGIC THERAPY
SELF-EVALUATION

PRINCIPLES OF BIOLOGIC THERAPY QUESTIONS

4-1 Which of the following is true regarding the activation of antitumor T cells?
- A. The primary costimulatory signal is delivered through the cytotoxic T-lymphocyte antigen 4 (CTLA-4) receptor on the T cell after engagement of ligands on antigen-presenting cells
- B. Engagement of the CD28 receptor on the T cell by the B7-2 ligand results in inhibition of the response
- C. Engagement of the programmed death (PD)-1 receptor with its ligand, PD-L1, on antigen-presenting cells results in inhibition of the response
- D. Engagement of CD28 on the activated T cell by CTLA-4 on the tumor results in inhibition of T-cell function

4-2 You start a patient with stage III melanoma on standard high-dose adjuvant interferon-alfa (IFN-α). At follow-up 1 week later, she is pleased to report that other than a mild fever after the initial infusion, she is tolerating therapy quite well.

You remind her that the following side effects may increase during the 12 months of administration:
- A. Myalgia
- B. Fever
- C. Fatigue
- D. Chills

4-3 A 78-year-old man who has metastatic lung cancer is hospitalized for febrile neutropenia that occurred on a weekly intravenous chemotherapy program, which has achieved a disease response. The febrile neutropenia was successfully managed with antibiotics. You are considering hematopoietic growth factor support.

Which of the following therapeutic options would be most appropriate?
- A. Sargramostim administered when white count reaches less than 500 mm^3
- B. Sargramostim administered daily while on chemotherapy
- C. Filgrastim administered beginning 1 day after chemotherapy infusion and stopping 1 day prior to the next infusion
- D. Pegfilgrastim administered weekly beginning the day after infusion

4-4 Which of the following is true regarding the use of antitumor monoclonal antibodies?
- A. Most are of the human immunoglobulin (Ig) G1 subclass, the subclass that is the least effective at mediating antibody-dependent cellular cytotoxicity (ADCC)
- B. Those used initially were mouse and generated human–anti-mouse antibody response
- C. They have short serum half-lives, on the order of minutes to hours
- D. They should not be administered in combination with other monoclonal antibodies

4-5   A 38-year-old man with metastatic renal cell carcinoma (RCC) comes to you seeking a second opinion after a tyrosine kinase inhibitor currently being evaluated in a clinical trial was recommended to him. The patient finds the idea of immunotherapy more appealing and wants to know more about interleukin (IL)-2.

Which of the following are true regarding IL-2?
A.   IL-2 was approved on the basis of improved survival
B.   To improve survival, IL-2 is best combined with chemotherapy
C.   Because of ease of administration, IL-2 is preferred over other treatments
D.   IL-2 is one of few treatments that can produce durable responses in patients with metastatic RCC

4-6   A 54-year-old woman with metastatic melanoma who is receiving ipilimumab develops significant fatigue after the second of four planned infusions. Thyroid function tests are abnormal. You prescribe oral pred-nisone, and her symptoms improve within 3 days. At follow-up, thyroid function tests also normalize.

Which of the following is true?
A.   The development of endocrinopathy is associated with a durable clinical response
B.   Abnormalities in thyroid function are caused by the direct uptake of ipilimumab by the thyroid
C.   Ipilimumab should be permanently discontinued if systemic corticosteroids are necessary to manage toxicity
D.   Clinical benefit can be achieved after systemic corticosteroids are administered

4-7   A 71-year-old woman presents with adenopathy and is diagnosed with follicular lymphoma. She is started on rituximab. During her first infusion she developed dyspnea. The infusion was stopped until dyspnea resolved. Rituximab was restarted at a slower rate, and she was able to complete this and five other weekly infusions and achieved a complete clinical response. At follow-up 14 months later, recurrent adenopathy was found. Repeat biopsy confirmed follicular lymphoma.

When considering treatment options, which of the following should influence your decision regarding retreatment with rituximab?
A.   Response rates associated with retreatment are essentially equivalent to those for initial treatment
B.   The reaction to the initial infusion is a contraindication for retreatment
C.   Administering a noncross-reactive antibody, such as alemtuzumab, is preferred
D.   Retreating with rituximab is likely to cause neutropenia

4-8   A 56-year-old woman with stage IV head and neck cancer experienced disease progression after che-motherapy. She then received palliative radiotherapy to a painful vertebral metastasis. Thereafter, she began cetuximab. She is premedicated with diphen-hydramine and has received eight weekly infusions. Except for a rash, she is tolerating therapy well. Recent scans document stable disease.

Which of the following is true?
A.   The development of rash predicts resistance to cetuximab
B.   Increasing frequency of dosing from weekly to daily can increase response rate
C.   Dermatologic toxicity precludes administration of radiation in combination with cetuximab
D.   Monoclonal antibodies may be able to improve survival in the absence of tumor regression

4-1   C

During the priming phase of T-cell activation, antigens are presented to the T-cell receptor as peptide fragments within major histocompatibility complex (MHC) molecules on antigen-presenting cells. The primary costimulatory signal is delivered through the CD28 receptor on the T cell after engagement of its ligands, B7-1 or B7-2, on the antigen-presenting cells. Engagement of the CTLA-4 receptor on the T cell by the same B7-1 or B7-2 ligands results in inhibition of the response. Engagement of the PD-1 receptor with one of its two ligands, PD-L1 and PD-L2, on the antigen-presenting cell also results in inhibition of the response. PD-L1 is also expressed by tumors. During the effector phase, engagement of PD-1 on the activated T cell by PD-L1 on the tumor results in inhibition of T-cell function. These immune checkpoints have become important therapeutic targets.

Suggested Reading

Wolchok JD, Yang AS, Weber JS. Immune regulatory antibodies: are they the next advance? *Cancer J.* 2010;16:311-317. PMID: 20693841.

4-2   C

Although its effect on overall survival is not clear, IFN is routinely applied in the adjuvant setting for patients with stage III melanoma after primary surgery. Flu-like symptoms, fever, chills, and myalgia usually abate as IFN therapy is continued. Fatigue and depression usually develop later and progress with continued therapy. Frequent laboratory assessments are necessary to monitor hepatic function and granulocyte counts.

Suggested Reading

Kirkwood JM, Manola J, Ibrahim J, et al. A pooled analysis of Eastern Cooperative Oncology Group and Intergroup trials of adjuvant high-dose interferon for melanoma. *Clin Cancer Res.* 2004;10: 1670-1677. PMID: 15014018.

Hurley KE, Chapman PB. Helping melanoma patients decide whether to choose adjuvant high-dose interferon-alpha2b. *Oncologist.* 2005; 10:739-742. PMID: 16249355.

4-3   C

Because of the sensitivity of rapidly dividing myeloid cells, filgrastim and sargramostim should be administered no earlier than 24 hours after the administration of cytotoxic chemotherapy and no later than 24 hours before the administration of chemotherapy. Pegfilgrastim should not be administered in the period between 14 days before and 24 hours after administration of cytotoxic chemotherapy. Hematopoietic cytokines, including sargramostim, are best administered to patients sufficiently in advance of the nadir to allow adequate time for cell formation and maturation.

Suggested Reading

Smith TJ, Khatcheressian J, Lyman GH, et al. 2006 update of recommendations for the use of white blood cell growth factors: an evidence-based clinical practice guideline. *J Clin Oncol.* 2006;24:3187-3205. PMID: 16682719.

4-4   B

Monoclonal antibodies that were used initially were developed in mice and generated human–anti-mouse antibody response. Fully human antibodies are now in use. Most are of the human IgG1 subclass, the subclass that is the most effective at engaging Fc receptors on natural killer (NK) cells and macrophages, and mediating ADCC. Monoclonal antibodies have long serum half-lives, on the order of days to weeks. Although monoclonal antibodies are administered as monotherapy, combinations of monoclonal antibodies with chemotherapy are in common use. Pertuzumab targets the extracellular dimerization domain of HER2 and thereby blocks ligand-dependent heterodimerization of HER2 with other HER family members. It has been approved for use in combination with trastuzumab, which also binds HER2, and docetaxel for the treatment of patients with HER2-positive metastatic breast cancer.

Suggested Reading

Baselga J, Cortés J, Kim SB, et al. Pertuzumab plus trastuzumab plus docetaxel for metastatic breast cancer. *N Engl J Med.* 2012;366:109-119. PMID: 22149875.

Gianni L, Pienkowski T, Im YH, et al. Efficacy and safety of neoadjuvant pertuzumab and trastuzumab in women with locally advanced, inflammatory, or early HER2-positive breast cancer (NeoSphere): a randomised multicentre, open-label, phase 2 trial. *Lancet Oncol. 2012;* 13:25-32. PMID: 22153890.

4-5   D

High-dose IL-2 (aldesleukin) immunotherapy received approval based on its ability to produce durable responses in a small subset of patients with advanced RCC (and advanced melanoma). An overall response rate of 15% and a complete response rate of 6% were observed in initial studies. Many of these responses were durable, suggesting that some patients were cured. High-dose aldesleukin treatment produces significant adverse effects that require inpatient hospitalization and restricts its application to select patients treated at centers experienced in its administration. Although response rates of the combination of IL-2 and chemotherapy ("biochemotherapy") were higher than chemotherapy alone, survival was not improved.

Suggested Reading

Klapper JA, Downey SG, Smith FO, et al. High-dose interleukin-2 for the treatment of metastatic renal cell carcinoma: a retrospective analysis of response and survival in patients treated in the surgery branch at the National Cancer Institute between 1986 and 2006. *Cancer.* 2008;113:293-301. PMID: 18457330.

4-6   D

Immune-related adverse events (IRAEs) produced by ipilimumab, likely the result of breaking immune tolerance upon CTLA-4 blockade, have included endocrinopathy in approximately 5% of patients, as well as colitis/diarrhea, dermatitis, and hepatitis. Inflammatory myopathy, nephritis, and uveitis also have been reported occasionally. These side effects are generally reversible and manageable by following specific treatment guidelines that include symptomatic therapies or systemic corticosteroids. Therapy can usually be resumed after toxicity resolves, and corticosteroid dose can be tapered. The relationship between endocrinopathy and other IRAEs and durable clinical response has not been established. Objective response rates have been low, in the 10% to 15% range. Predictive biomarkers are being investigated. It is unknown if systemic corticosteroid therapy has an attenuating effect on ipilimumab activity. However, clinical antitumor responses have been maintained in patients treated with corticosteroids who have discontinued ipilimumab therapy.

Suggested Reading

Hodi FS, O'Day SJ, McDermott DF, et al. Improved survival with ipilimumab in patients with metastatic melanoma. *N Engl J Med.* 2010;363:711-723. PMID: 20525992.

Robert C, Thomas L, Bondarenko I, et al. Ipilimumab plus dacarbazine for previously untreated metastatic melanoma. *N Engl J Med.* 2011; 364:2517-2526. PMID: 21639810.

4-7   A

Response rates associated with retreatment have been essentially the same as with initial cycles of treatment (40% to 50%). Although neutralizing antibodies to the chimeric protein are possible, they have rarely been reported. Dyspnea, although common during initial infusion, does not presage more serious sequelae, and treatment can usually continue uninterrupted. Alemtuzumab is a monoclonal antibody directed at CD52, not CD20. It is approved for use to treat chronic lymphocytic leukemia. CD20 is not expressed by neutrophils, and neutropenia would not be predicted with rituximab monotherapy. Rituximab will cause lymphopenia.

Suggested Reading

Davis TA, Grillo-López AJ, White CA, et al. Rituximab anti-CD20 monoclonal antibody therapy in non-Hodgkin's lymphoma: safety and efficacy of re-treatment. *J Clin Oncol.* 2000;18:3135-3143. PMID: 10963642.

Hainsworth JD, Litchy S, Shaffer DW, et al. Maximizing therapeutic benefit of rituximab: maintenance therapy versus re-treatment at progression in patients with indolent non-Hodgkin's lymphoma— a randomized phase II trial of the Minnie Pearl Cancer Research Network. *J Clin Oncol.* 2005;23:1088-1095. PMID: 15657401.

4-8   D

Through effects on the growth cycle, the antitumor effects of monoclonal antibodies can be cytostatic. Antibodies against growth factor receptors also may modify other important processes in cancer progression, such as invasion and metastasis. Thus, improved survival can be achieved in the absence of tumor regression. Antibodies have elimination half-lives often on the order of days to weeks and usually are not administered daily. Although active as monotherapy, monoclonal antibodies have been effectively applied with myelosuppressive and immunosuppressive treatment modalities, and are usually applied clinically with chemotherapy and radiotherapy. Although dermatologic toxicity can be problematic, cetuximab is approved for use with radiotherapy for patients with head and neck cancer. There is evidence that the development of a skin rash for patients receiving cetuximab is predictive of treatment benefit.

Suggested Reading

Adams GP, Weiner LM. Monoclonal antibody therapy of cancer. *Nat Biotechnol.* 2005;23:1147-1157. PMID: 16151408.

5 CLINICAL TRIALS AND BIOSTATISTICS
SELF-EVALUATION

CLINICAL TRIALS AND BIOSTATISTICS QUESTIONS

5-1   Many recently published journal articles report results of studies attempting to establish genetic associations in prostate cancer; more specifically, the association of gene expression with prostate-specific antigen (PSA) levels. In one study, the correlation between *SPIFE* and PSA was based on samples from 120 men, with $r = 0.70$ and $p = 0.01$. In another study, the correlation between *PIKX* and PSA was based on samples from 500 men, with $r = 0.15$ and $p < 0.0001$. In yet another study, the correlation between *GRIZL* and PSA was based on samples from 20 men, with $r = 0.9$ and $p = 0.31$.

Assuming all of the studies were methodologically sound, which of the following best describes what one can conclude about which gene might be most promising for further study?
A. *SPIFE* has the most promising association with PSA
B. *PIKX* has the most promising association with PSA
C. *GRIZL* has the most promising association with PSA
D. All of the genes have promising associations with PSA

5-2   The Kaplan-Meier curve is the universal standard for presenting results on survival outcomes from clinical trials and other clinical studies. Which of the following statements about a Kaplan-Meier curve is NOT true?
A. It can be used to estimate the median survival time
B. It can be used to estimate the probability of survival at a particular point in time
C. Only patients that have had at least 1 year of follow-up should be used to estimate 1-year survival
D. The curve is related to the underlying hazard rate analyzed in Cox regression

5-3   The report of a clinical trial may provide some or all of the following results from a Cox regression analysis: sample size, hazard ratio, p-value, and confidence interval. For example, a trial of two agents for colon cancer might report that 300 patients were randomly assigned, with a mortality hazard ratio (HR) for the experimental versus standard arm equal to 0.65 (95% CI 0.45 to 0.94; $p = 0.02$).

Which of these pieces of information, by itself, is the most informative as to the outcome of the trial?
A. HR = 0.65
B. HR = 0.65 and sample size of 300
C. $p = 0.02$
D. 95% CI 0.45 to 0.94

5-4   A phase II trial demonstrated promising results in stage III breast cancer with iDRUG added as adjuvant therapy to a standard regimen. A partial/complete response rate of 40% was observed in a study of 40 women, compared to the 25% expected from historical experience. A randomized trial was conducted in 400 women comparing standard therapy plus iDRUG to standard therapy plus placebo. The study had 90% power to detect a 15% difference in survival at 3 years. The results were disappointing and showed virtually no differences in overall survival.

Which of the following is the most unlikely explanation for the difference between the two trials?
A. Overrepresentation of better-risk patients in the phase II trial may have resulted in a response rate that was not really comparable to prior experience
B. The good results of the phase II trial were an anomaly due to chance
C. The results of the phase III trial were worse than they should have been due to chance
D. There is not a good correlation between short-term tumor response and long-term survival

5-5 A study evaluating long-term toxicity of two therapeutic regimens was conducted among 1-year survivors of a randomized trial. The surviving patients were assessed for a variety of symptoms and several measures of quality of life (QOL), and more than 80% of surviving patients participated on both arms. The abstract reported that patients on the arm receiving standard therapy plus an experimental adjuvant therapy had a higher rate of myalgia (p = 0.05) and headache (p = 0.04) than on the arm receiving standard therapy plus placebo.

What additional information would be most helpful in interpreting this finding?

A. Whether the patients were blinded as to the treatment arm they were on
B. How many separate symptoms and QOL measures were assessed
C. What proportions of patients were alive at 1 year in each arm
D. How many patients were randomly assigned to each arm

5-6 A retrospective analysis of a large cohort of patients with lung cancer showed an association between high levels of FLOPx and poorer survival. A phase I study of a drug targeting the FLOPx receptor was conducted. Patients on this study demonstrated a decrease in FLOPx levels after treatment compared to pretreatment levels, with minimal toxicity.

What additional piece of information would be most useful in evaluating whether to conduct a larger-scale phase II study of the drug?

A. A prospective study demonstrating the same association with survival as in the retrospective study
B. The results from patients with lung cancer participating in the phase I study
C. A biologic hypothesis causally linking FLOPx levels to tumor progression
D. The results of a phase I study with a placebo arm as well as an active-drug arm

5-7 A retrospective analysis of 300 patients with lung cancer was undertaken to identify factors predicting tumor response (complete or partial) at 8 weeks. In univariate analysis, the two strongest predictors were having serum fluff in the lowest quartile with an odds ratio (OR) of 1.5 (p = 0.01) and favorable histology (OR = 2.0; p = 0.002). Multivariate analysis of these two factors yielded the same results.

If the response rate in patients with unfavorable characteristics for both of those factors is 20%, what is the estimated response rate in patients with both favorable factors present?

A. 30%
B. 43%
C. 60%
D. 80%

5-1   A

Although the correlation of *PIKX* expression with PSA is highly statistically significant, due to the large sample size, the correlation is exceedingly weak and likely has little biological significance. An *r* value of 0.15 corresponds to an r^2 of 0.02, meaning that *PIKX* expression explains only 2% of the variation in PSA level. The *r* value of 0.7 associated with *SPIFE*, however, corresponds to an r^2 of nearly 50%, which is a very strong correlation that appears to be statistically significant in a reasonably large sample. Although the *r* value of 0.9 associated with *GRIZL* is highest, it is derived from a small sample and could well be due to chance.

Suggested Reading

Guyatt G, Walter S, Shannon H, et al. Basic statistics for clinicians: 4. Correlation and regression. *CMAJ.* 1995;152:497-504. PMID: 7859197.

5-2   C

Clearly, the Kaplan-Meier curve estimates the survival probability at a particular point in time. If the survival probability drops below 50%, then it can be used to estimate the median survival time as well. One of the most important features of the Kaplan-Meier curve is that it uses information from *all* patients, including those who have not yet died. There is no minimum amount of follow-up required, and including patients with short follow-up does not bias the estimated curve, although it increases the imprecision of the survival estimates. There is a direct functional relationship between a survival and the underlying hazard of death; however, the survival curve is easier to represent graphically and to understand.

Suggested Reading

Green S, Benedetti J, Smith A, et al. *Clinical Trials in Oncology, 3rd ed*. Boca Raton, FL: Chapman & Hall/CRC Taylor & Francis Group, 2012; 23-30.

5-3   D

A hazard ratio of 0.65 certainly suggests a superior effect of the experimental arm, but without some measure of precision there is no way to know whether the result is due to chance. Conversely, the statistically significant p-value of 0.02 suggests the result is not due to chance, but without some measure of the size of the effect it is impossible to know the clinical significance of the result. The combination of hazard ratio and reasonably large sample size only suggests that the result might be significant. The confidence interval, however, indicates both the magnitude of the effect and the fact that it must be statistically significant, since the upper bound of the 95% confidence interval is less than 1.0. In fact, both the hazard ratio and the p-value could be determined from the confidence interval. The hazard ratio is the geometric mean of the upper and lower confidence limits; the p-value computation is slightly more complicated.

Suggested Reading

Guyatt G, Jaeschke R, Heddle N, et al. Basic statistics for clinicians: 1. Hypothesis testing. *CMAJ.* 1995;152:27-32. PMID: 7804919.

Guyatt G, Jaeschke R, Heddle N, et al. Basic statistics for clinicians: 2. Interpreting study results: confidence intervals. *CMAJ.* 1995; 152:169-173. PMID: 7820798.

5-4   C

When the results of a phase II and a phase III trial differ, it is almost always the case that the "fault" lies in the phase II trial. Selection factors certainly play a role in the results of a phase II trial, but even if the patients are perfectly representative of the patient population that are to be enrolled in a phase III trial, chance can produce an observed response rate higher (or lower) than the true rate associated with the regimen. The observed response rate of 40% is inconsistent with a true response rate of 25%, but could be reasonably produced by a true response rate of 30%. Finally, even if the phase II trial has a representative sample of the target patient population, and the observed response rate is close to the true response rate in this population, a favorable result with respect to short-term tumor response may or may not translate to a longer-term survival benefit. The phase III trial in this example clearly had sufficient power to detect a modest treatment benefit, and failed to do so. It would be difficult to argue that the result of the phase III trial is incorrect.

Suggested Reading

Friedman LM, Furberg CD, DeMets DL. *Fundamentals of Clinical Trials, 2nd ed*. New York, NY: Springer-Verlag; 1998.

Fleming TR, DeMets DL. Surrogate end points in clinical trials: are we being misled? *Ann Intern Med.* 1996;125:605-613. PMID: 8815760.

Piantadosi S. *Clinical Trials: A Methodologic Perspective, 2nd ed.* Hoboken, NJ: John Wiley & Sons, 2005; 211-221.

5-5   B

Although it would be interesting to know the size of the study, neither the number of patients randomly assigned nor the number of patients who were 1-year survivors is critical. QOL studies can certainly be biased by patient knowledge of the treatment arm, but this was a study of an adjuvant agent and even the patients on the placebo arm received significant active therapy. In this case, knowing the number of endpoints analyzed would be very important. The reported results are only marginally statistically significant, and could well be produced by chance by screening a large number of symptoms and QOL measures. Even if only a small number of endpoints was analyzed, it would weaken the significance of these findings. For example, a Bonferroni correction applied to the testing of five endpoints would require a significance level of 0.01 for each endpoint in order to achieve an overall significance level of 0.05. It is not necessary to actually make an explicit adjustment, but knowing the number of comparisons is critical for placing the results in context.

Suggested Reading

Waalen J, Beutler E. Beware of multiple comparisons: a study of symptoms associated with mutations of the HFE hemochromatosis gene. *Clin Chim Acta*. 2005;361:128-134. PMID: 15993396.

5-6   C

A prospective study would not add significant useful information, other than to rule out the possibility that the retrospective finding was a chance observation. It is also highly unlikely that the effect of a drug on a biomarker is due to a placebo effect. Although the results in patients with lung cancer from the phase I study would be interesting to know, the number of patients would likely be small and not necessarily informative. However, unless there is a plausible biologic hypothesis that would place FLOPx in the causal pathway to tumor progression and subsequent survival, the previous studies by themselves do not establish the drug as a good candidate for phase II study. For example, if FLOPx is only a marker of tumor progression, then reducing FLOPx will have no effect on outcome. Although it is clear that many phase II studies are undertaken without such biologic rationale, they are certainly less likely to prove successful than those that are motivated by a foundation comprised of relevant correlative studies and solid biologic hypotheses.

Suggested Reading

Fleming TR, DeMets DL. Surrogate end points in clinical trials: are we being misled? *Ann Intern Med*. 1996;125:605-613. PMID: 8815760.

Piantadosi S. *Clinical Trials: A Methodologic Perspective, 2nd ed*. Hoboken, NJ: John Wiley & Sons, 2005; 211-221.

5-7   B

The effect of combining two risk factors in a multivariate logistic regression model is the product of the two effects. In this case the OR for response with both favorable factors present would be $1.5 \times 2.0 = 3.0$, compared to neither favorable factor present. This does not mean that the probability (risk) of response is increased 3-fold, however, unless that probability is quite small. If the response rate in the reference group is 20%, this corresponds to odds of 0.25 (0.2/0.8); thus, the odds in the comparison group is 0.75 (3.0 x 0.25). Finally, an odds of 0.75 translates to a response rate of 43% (0.75/1.75), or a rate ratio of 2.15. In contrast to typical cases in epidemiology, where the odds ratio can usually be treated as a risk ratio, one should be careful to distinguish the two in most clinical research settings.

Suggested Reading

Motulsky H. *Intuitive Biostatistics: A Nonmathematical Guide to Statistical Thinking, 3rd ed*. New York, NY: Oxford University Press, 2014; 233-250.

6 BREAST CANCER
SELF-EVALUATION

BREAST CANCER QUESTIONS

6-1 A 35-year-old premenopausal woman with a known *BRCA2* mutation has never had cancer. Regarding future cancer screening for her, which of the following have been shown to detect cancer at an earlier stage?
A. Annual bilateral breast magnetic resonance imaging (MRI)
B. Biannual transvaginal ultrasound
C. Annual magnetic resonance cholangiopancreatography (MRCP)
D. Biannual serum CA-125 assessment

6-2 A 47-year-old woman was premenopausal at the time of diagnosis of a 2.8-cm, high-grade, invasive ductal cancer which was estrogen receptor (ER)–positive, progesterone receptor (PR)–positive, and HER2-negative. The single sentinel lymph node was negative. Her last menstrual period was the month prior to beginning chemotherapy. Now, 5 months later, she is discussing endocrine therapy.

What is the best therapeutic option for her?
A. Anastrozole
B. Tamoxifen
C. Anastrozole for 2 years followed by tamoxifen
D. Combination tamoxifen and anastrozole

6-3 A 45-year-old woman developed pulmonary metastasis 2 years after completing trastuzumab and chemotherapy as adjuvant treatment for stage II breast cancer.

The optimal first-line therapy for her includes:
A. Pertuzumab alone
B. Trastuzumab alone
C. Pertuzumab, trastuzumab, and a taxane
D. Trastuzumab, lapatinib, and a taxane

6-4 The Oncotype DX recurrence score is helpful in determining which of the following in early-stage breast cancer:
A. The added benefit of chemotherapy to tamoxifen in adjuvant treatment
B. The added benefit of aromatase inhibitors (AI) to tamoxifen
C. The probability of carrying a *BRCA* mutation
D. The likelihood of having axillary lymph node involvement in addition to the sentinel lymph node

6-5 A 40-year-old woman underwent an excisional breast biopsy (lumpectomy) and sentinel lymph node sampling following a core biopsy, which showed invasive breast cancer. The pathology revealed a 2.5-cm invasive ductal cancer that involved one out of four sentinel lymph nodes. The invasive carcinoma was ER-positive, PR-positive, and HER2-negative.

Which of the following will optimize local-regional control of her disease?
A. A completion axillary lymph node dissection
B. A completion mastectomy
C. Whole-breast radiation therapy (WBRT)
D. A bilateral mastectomy

6-6 A 75-year-old healthy woman was diagnosed with a 1.4-cm invasive lobular carcinoma which is ER-positive, PR-positive, and HER2-negative. Lymphovascular invasion is absent and zero out of two sentinel lymph nodes were involved with disease. She was offered 5 years of an AI as adjuvant therapy and is agreeable to this therapy.

Which of the following are appropriate options for local therapy of her breast cancer?
A. Lumpectomy alone
B. Lumpectomy and WBRT
C. Complete mastectomy
D. All of the above

6-7 A 53-year-old postmenopausal woman was diagnosed with a 2.0-cm ductal carcinoma in situ (DCIS) that was a high nuclear grade, ER-positive, PR-positive, and HER2-positive. In addition to her primary breast surgery and radiation, which of the following would you recommend?

A. Anastrozole for 5 years
B. Trastuzumab for 1 year
C. Tamoxifen for 5 years
D. Raloxifene for 5 years

6-8 A 30-year-old premenopausal woman was told that she carries a *BRCA2* mutation. You counsel her about her increased risk of developing the following malignancies except:

A. Glioblastoma
B. Breast cancer
C. Ovarian cancer
D. Melanoma

6-9 A 45-year-old woman presents to your office with a 3-week history of right breast enlargement, pain, erythema, and skin thickening. Skin and breast biopsy confirm a triple-negative inflammatory breast cancer. There is no evidence of metastatic disease.

Which of the following is true about this subtype of breast cancer?

A. A sentinel node biopsy should be done before therapy
B. Chemotherapy should be given before radiation and surgery
C. A modified radical mastectomy with full axillary dissection should be done prior to adjuvant chemotherapy
D. Combined chemotherapy and radiation should be given immediately

6-10 A healthy, asymptomatic 56-year-old woman is diagnosed with a 1.9-cm invasive ductal carcinoma with lymphovascular involvement and two negative sentinel nodes. It is ER-negative, PR-negative, and HER2-positive.

Prior to initiating adjuvant systemic therapy, you recommend the following tests:

A. An echocardiogram, bone scan, and computed tomography (CT) of the chest, abdomen, and pelvis
B. An echocardiogram and positron emission tomography (PET)/CT
C. An echocardiogram
D. An echocardiogram, PET/CT, and MRI of the brain

6-11 You have been treating a 49-year-old woman with a 4.0-cm invasive ductal carcinoma which is ER- and PR-negative, but HER2-positive. Two out of nine axillary lymph nodes were involved with disease. She has completed chemotherapy with trastuzumab and is requesting a discussion about additional HER2-directed therapy.

Which of the following treatments will you recommend for this patient?

A. Trastuzumab for 2 years
B. Combination trastuzumab and lapatinib for 1 year
C. Trastuzumab for 1 year
D. Combination pertuzumab, trastuzumab, and lapatinib for 1 year

6-12 An 80-year-old woman was seen in the office for a new diagnosis of breast cancer. She lives alone and rarely leaves the house. She has not had medical care since she delivered her son 50 years ago. She now complains of increasing erythema of the right breast associated with ulceration of the skin and retraction of the entire breast. She is unclear about how long these changes have been present. A biopsy of the breast reveals an invasive lobular carcinoma that is ER-positive, PR-positive, and HER2-negative. A fine needle aspiration (FNA) of her palpable right axillary adenopathy is positive for malignancy.

You recommend the following initial treatment:

A. Doxorubicin and cyclophosphamide
B. Letrozole
C. Modified radical mastectomy
D. Ovarian suppression and tamoxifen

6-13 You have been asked to comment on adjuvant systemic therapy for a healthy 55-year-old postmenopausal woman with a 1.5-cm invasive ductal carcinoma that is ER-positive, PR-negative, and HER2-negative. Two of three sentinel lymph nodes are involved with disease.

You recommend the following adjuvant systemic therapy:

A. Endocrine therapy alone with an AI for 5 years followed by tamoxifen for 5 years
B. Combination chemotherapy without endocrine therapy
C. Ovarian suppression and an AI for 5 years without chemotherapy
D. Combination chemotherapy followed by endocrine therapy

6-14 A 55-year-old postmenopausal woman was diagnosed with a 1.5-cm ER-positive invasive ductal cancer 9 years ago. She received treatment with tamoxifen for 5 years and now has evidence of bone metastasis. A biopsy of the bone is positive for a recurrent breast cancer which is ER-positive, PR-negative, and HER2-negative. She has no other evidence of disease and complains of back pain controlled with ibuprofen.

You recommend palliative therapy with the following:
A. Exemestane and everolimus
B. Capecitabine
C. Letrozole
D. A bone-modifying agent (i.e., denosumab or zoledronic acid) alone

6-15 Your patient, a 40-year-old premenopausal woman, has completed adjuvant chemotherapy and is starting tamoxifen. She will begin radiation therapy to her right breast because she had a lumpectomy as primary surgery. She is interested in reviewing your recommendations for follow-up imaging for her breast cancer.

You recommend the following:
A. An annual mammogram and breast MRI
B. An annual mammogram
C. An annual mammogram, bone scan, and CT scan of the chest and abdomen
D. An annual mammogram and PET/CT

6-1   A

Annual MRI screening has been shown to detect breast cancer at an earlier stage compared with mammographic screening alone. The current recommendation for screening among women with *BRCA* mutations is annual mammogram and annual breast MRI. Transvaginal ultrasound and CA-125 monitoring have not been shown to detect ovarian cancer at an earlier stage. MRCP is often used to evaluate pancreatic intraductal papillary mucinous neoplasms associated with familial cancer syndromes, but it has not been shown to be an effective screening tool for pancreas cancer that is often associated with *BRCA2* mutations.

Suggested Reading

Warner E, Hill K, Causer P, et al. Prospective study of breast cancer incidence in women with a BRCA1 or BRCA2 mutation under surveillance with and without magnetic resonance imaging. *J Clin Oncol.* 2011;29:1664-1669. PMID: 21444874.

6-2   B

Return of ovarian function following chemotherapy-induced amenorrhea can occur as long as 2 years following completion of chemotherapy. In addition, the administration of AIs can prompt an increase in gonadotropin secretion, which will interfere with the efficacy of the AI. For this reason, the initial endocrine therapy following chemotherapy is chosen based upon the initial menopausal status of the patient. Since this patient was premenopausal at the time of diagnosis, she should receive tamoxifen therapy.

Suggested Reading

Smith IE, Dowsett M, Yap YS, et al. Adjuvant aromatase inhibitors for early breast cancer after chemotherapy-induced amenorrhoea: caution and suggested guidelines. *J Clin Oncol.* 2006;24:2444-2447. PMID: 16735701.

6-3   C

The results from the CLEOPATRA trial demonstrated improvement in disease-free survival (DFS) and overall survival (OS) with combination pertuzumab, trastuzumab, and docetaxel therapy administered as first-line treatment for patients with HER2-positive metastatic breast cancer. The U.S. Food and Drug Administration and National Comprehensive Cancer Network have modified the regimen to include any taxane therapy; however, front-line treatment for HER2-positive recurrent disease now includes the dual HER2-targeting agents of pertuzumab and trastuzumab. Single-agent trastuzumab is occasionally utilized in this regimen, but with minimal efficacy and no effect on OS.

Suggested Reading

Baselga J, Cortés J, Kim SB, et al. Pertuzumab plus trastuzumab plus docetaxel for metastatic breast cancer. *N Engl J Med.* 2012;366:109-119. PMID: 22149875.

6-4   A

The Oncotype DX Recurrence Score utilizes a multistep high-throughput reverse transcriptase (RT)-polymerase chain reaction (PCR) gene expression assay evaluating 16 genes involving proliferation and hormone expression, as well as five reference genes. This test has been validated as a predictive tool in determining the added benefit of chemotherapy to tamoxifen in adjuvant treatment.

Suggested Reading

Paik S, Tang G, Shak S, et al. Gene expression and benefit of chemotherapy in women with node-negative, estrogen receptor-positive breast cancer. *J Clin Oncol.* 2006;24:3726-3734. PMID: 16720680.

Albain KS, Barlow WE, Shak S, et al. Prognostic and predictive value of the 21-gene recurrence score assay in postmenopausal women with node-positive, oestrogen-receptor-positive breast cancer on chemotherapy: a retrospective analysis of a randomised trial. *Lancet Oncol.* 2010;11:55-65. PMID: 20005174.

6-5   C

Breast-conserving surgery and WBRT is comparable to mastectomy in terms of OS. The ACOSOG Z0011 trial demonstrated adequate disease control without a need to completely dissect the axilla if one to three sentinel lymph nodes were involved and breast-conserving WBRT was performed. Removal of the uninvolved contralateral breast has not been shown to improve survival.

Suggested Reading

Giuliano AE, Hunt KK, Ballman KV, et al. Axillary dissection vs no axillary dissection in women with invasive breast cancer and sentinel node metastasis: a randomized clinical trial. *JAMA.* 2011;305:569-575. PMID: 21304082.

6-6   D

In elderly women older than age 70, radiation can be avoided following breast conservation in ER-positive disease when adjuvant endocrine therapy is given. Although local disease was higher without radiation, breast cancer–related death was not increased. Lumpectomy and radiation is comparable to mastectomy in terms of OS.

Suggested Reading

Fisher B, Anderson S, Bryant J, et al. Twenty-year follow-up of a randomized trial comparing total mastectomy, lumpectomy, and lumpectomy plus irradiation for the treatment of invasive breast cancer. *N Engl J Med.* 2002;347:1233-1241. PMID: 12393820.

Hughes KS, Schnaper LA, Bellon JR, et al. Lumpectomy plus tamoxifen with or without irradiation in women age 70 years or older with early breast cancer: long-term follow-up of CALGB 9343. *J Clin Oncol.* 2013;31:2382-2387. PMID: 23690420.

6-7　C

Tamoxifen is the only endocrine therapy that has been shown to reduce the incidence of new primary breast cancer, both ipsilateral and contralateral, in women diagnosed with DCIS and treated with lumpectomy and radiation therapy. The benefit of tamoxifen appears to be limited to ER-positive DCIS. Both anastrozole and trastuzumab are currently being evaluated in clinical trials.

Suggested Reading

Allred DC, Anderson SJ, Paik S, et al. Adjuvant tamoxifen reduces subsequent breast cancer in women with estrogen receptor-positive ductal carcinoma in situ: a study based on NSABP protocol B-24. *J Clin Oncol.* 2012;30:1268-1273. PMID: 22393101.

6-8　A

Hereditary breast cancer syndromes are associated with the autosomal-dominant inheritance of germ-line mutations in various genes, such as *BRCA1* and *BRCA2*. *BRCA2* mutations are associated with a higher risk of several malignancies including breast, ovarian, fallopian tube, pancreas, melanoma, and prostate cancers. Glioblastoma is associated with *p53* mutations in Li-Fraumeni syndrome.

Suggested Reading

Breast Cancer Linkage Consortium. Cancer risks in BRCA2 mutation carriers. *J Natl Cancer Inst.* 1999;91:1310-1316. PMID: 10433620.

6-9　B

Inflammatory breast cancer is a clinicopathologic diagnosis wherein there is a rapid onset, usually within a 3-month duration, of breast erythema, edema, and enlargement in the setting of a pathologically confirmed diagnosis of invasive breast cancer. The disease is inoperable at the time of diagnosis; therefore, the standard treatment is neoadjuvant chemotherapy followed by modified radical mastectomy and radiation.

Suggested Reading

Dawood S, Merajver SD, Viens P, et al. International expert panel on inflammatory breast cancer: consensus statement for standardized diagnosis and treatment. *Ann Oncol.* 2011;22: 515-523. PMID: 20603440.

6-10　C

The likelihood of presenting with distant metastasis when diagnosed with stage I disease (T1c, N0) is less than 1%; therefore, extensive radiographic studies for staging is not indicated in an asymptomatic patient. Given this patient's hormone receptor–negative and HER2-positive disease, a trastuzumab-containing regimen should be offered as adjuvant therapy. Trastuzumab carries a risk of congestive heart failure; therefore, baseline echocardiogram is indicated and should be repeated during adjuvant treatment.

Suggested Reading

Slamon D, Eiermann W, Robert N, et al. Adjuvant trastuzumab in HER2-positive breast cancer. *N Engl J Med.* 2011;365: 1273-1283. PMID: 21991949.

Perez EA, Romond EH, Suman VJ, et al. Four-year follow-up of trastuzumab plus adjuvant chemotherapy for operable human epidermal growth factor receptor 2-positive breast cancer: joint analysis of data from NCCTG N9831 and NSABP B-31. *J Clin Oncol.* 2011;29:3366-3373. PMID: 21768458.

6-11　C

Adjuvant HER2-directed therapy includes 1 year of trastuzumab. Longer and shorter durations of trastuzumab have not been shown to be more beneficial. Combination HER2-directed therapy remains investigational.

Suggested Reading

Goldhirsch A, Gelber RD, Piccart-Gebhart MJ, et al. 2 years versus 1 year of adjuvant trastuzumab for HER2-positive breast cancer (HERA): an open-label, randomised controlled trial. *Lancet.* 2013; 382:1021-1028. PMID: 23871490.

6-12　B

Invasive lobular cancer is often hormone receptor–positive and carries a more indolent natural history. This patient's history describes a neglected primary breast cancer which is often successfully treated with primary endocrine therapy. In a postmenopausal woman, neoadjuvant endocrine therapies with AIs are superior to tamoxifen.

Suggested Reading

Barnadas A, Gil M, Sánchez-Rovira P, et al. Neoadjuvant endocrine therapy for breast cancer: past, present and future. *Anticancer Drugs.* 2008;19:339-347. PMID: 18454044.

6-13   D

Adjuvant chemotherapy is administered as adjuvant treat-ment for lymph node–positive disease, regardless of menopausal status or hormone receptor status. It is given prior to endocrine therapy when the disease is hormone receptor–positive.

Suggested Reading

Early Breast Cancer Trialists' Collaborative Group (EBCTCG). Effects of chemotherapy and hormonal therapy for early breast cancer on recurrence and 15-year survival: an overview of the randomised trials. *Lancet.* 2005;365:1687-1717. PMID: 15894097.

6-14   C

In hormone receptor–positive metastatic disease, endocrine therapy is as effective as chemotherapy unless there is vis-ceral crisis. Therefore, in this patient with a long disease-free interval with bone-only disease that is ER-positive, endocrine therapy is the treatment of choice. Combination therapy with exemestane and everolimus has been found to be benefi-cial after disease progression following a nonsteroidal AI. Although the bone-modifying agents denosumab and zolen-dronic acid have anticancer properties, they are not used alone as therapy for metastatic disease.

Suggested Reading

Baselga J, Campone M, Piccart M, et al. Everolimus in postmenopausal hormone-receptor-positive advanced breast cancer. *N Engl J Med.* 2012;366:520-529. PMID: 22149876.

Van Poznak CH, Temin S, Yee GC, et al. American Society of Clinical Oncology executive summary of the clinical practice guideline update on the role of bone-modifying agents in metastatic breast cancer. *J Clin Oncol.* 2011;29:1221-1227. PMID: 21343561.

6-15   B

Standard surveillance for patients who have completed adju-vant therapy includes breast imaging in order to detect a new primary cancer. Annual mammograms are indicated, with MRI imaging only beneficial in high-risk individuals. Radio-graphic imaging to detect systemic metastasis has not been found to be efficacious and should be limited to evaluation of new onset symptoms.

Suggested Reading

Khatcheressian JL, Hurley P, Bantug E, et al. Breast cancer follow-up and management after primary treatment: American Society of Clinical Oncology clinical practice guideline update. *J Clin Oncol.* 2013;31:961-965. PMID: 23129741.

7 LUNG CANCER
SELF-EVALUATION

LUNG CANCER QUESTIONS

7-1 A 60-year-old man with a 70-pack per year smoking history presents with cough and weight loss. Computed tomography (CT) reveals a right upper lobe lung mass, mediastinal lymphadenopathy, and three liver lesions. Biopsy of a liver lesion shows a poorly differentiated squamous cell carcinoma. His performance status (PS) is 1. The patient is motivated for therapy.

Which of the following is the best treatment option for this patient?
A. Carboplatin/paclitaxel
B. Carboplatin/paclitaxel/bevacizumab
C. Cisplatin/pemetrexed
D. Erlotinib
E. Chemoradiation

7-2 A 32-year-old white woman who has never smoked has a chest x-ray for a chronic nonproductive cough that shows a large left lower lobe mass. Positron emission tomography (PET)-CT reveals bilateral pulmonary nodules that are 18-fluorodeoxyglucose (FDG)-avid with a dominant 5-cm FDG-avid left lower lobe mass. Fine-needle aspiration of the left lower lobe reveals lung adenocarcinoma (immunohistochemistry [IHC] markers, CK7-positive, CK20-negative, TTF1-positive). There is insufficient tissue for molecular analysis. Physical exam is negative. She presents to your clinic relatively asymptomatic with a PS of 1.

Which of the following is the best next step for this patient with stage IV lung adenocarcinoma?
A. Cisplatin/pemetrexed
B. Erlotinib
C. Core biopsy of left lower lobe mass for epidermal growth factor receptor (EGFR) activating mutation and anaplastic lymphoma kinase (ALK) fluorescence in situ hybridization (FISH) testing
D. Carboplatin/paclitaxel

7-3 A 54-year-old woman with a five-pack per year smoking history presents to the emergency department with cough and shortness of breath. CT-angiogram to rule out pulmonary embolism reveals a central right main-stem bronchus lung mass within 2 cm of the carina and mediastinal adenopathy. PET-CT shows the lung mass as well as an FDG-avid 3-cm right paratracheal node and a 2-cm subcarinal node, with no evidence of distant metastases. Bronchoscopy with endobronchial ultrasound biopsy of both the R4 and the subcarinal node confirms lung adenocarcinoma. Magnetic resonance imaging (MRI) of the brain is negative for intracranial metastases. *EGFR* mutation testing is positive for an *L858R* point mutation. Clinical stage (according to the American Joint Committee on Cancer 7th edition staging manual) is IIIA (T3N2M0). At tumor board, your thoracic surgeon determines right pneumonectomy is the only surgical option. At follow-up in clinic, the patient is clinically stable and she has a PS of 1.

Which of the following is the best treatment option for this patient with stage IIIA non-small cell lung cancer (NSCLC)?
A. Right pneumonectomy followed by adjuvant chemotherapy
B. Concurrent chemoradiation
C. Erlotinib
D. Sequential chemotherapy followed by radiation
E. Chemoradiation followed by right pneumonectomy

7-4 A 62-year-old woman with a 70-pack per year smoking history and chronic obstructive pulmonary disease presents to your clinic for routine follow-up. Physical exam shows oxygen saturation of 97% on room air and prolonged expiratory phase but is otherwise unremarkable. She requests a screening study for lung cancer.

Which of the following is the best screening test for lung cancer in this patient?
A. Chest x-ray
B. Low-dose non-contrast CT of the chest
C. PET-CT
D. Serum carcinoembryonic antigen
E. Routine screening for lung cancer should not be offered to this patient

7-5 A 66-year-old woman with a 50-pack per year smoking history presents to your clinic. She was recently diagnosed with lung adenocarcinoma metastatic to the liver and bone. Zubrod PS is a 2 based on bone pain, weight loss, and declining activity level. Molecular testing for an *EGFR*-activating mutation and *ALK* gene rearrangement was negative.

Which of the following is the best treatment option for this patient?
A. Navelbine
B. Cisplatin and etoposide
C. Carboplatin and pemetrexed
D. Pemetrexed alone
E. Docetaxel

7-6 A 42-year-old Asian woman presents to your clinic with cough and shortness of breath. A CT of the chest, abdomen, and pelvis shows bilateral pulmonary nodules. Biopsy of a pulmonary nodule shows lung adenocarcinoma (IHC: CK7-positive, CK20-negative, TTF1-positive). *EGFR* mutation testing is positive for an exon 19 deletion. MRI of the brain shows no intracranial metastatic disease, and nuclear medicine bone scan is negative. Zubrod PS is 1. Erlotinib is chosen for first-line therapy.

What benefit will erlotinib provide compared with with platinum-based chemotherapy in this first-line setting?
A. Improved response rate alone
B. Improved response rate, progression-free survival (PFS), and overall survival (OS)
C. Improved response rate and PFS
D. Improved OS alone

7-7 A 45-year-old man presents to your clinic. He recently had progression of his metastatic lung adenocarcinoma on carboplatin, paclitaxel, and bevacizumab. You order a repeat biopsy of his large peripheral lung lesion. Molecular testing is positive for an *ALK* gene rearrangement. His PS is 1.

What is the best next treatment for this patient?
A. Pemetrexed
B. Docetaxel
C. Crizotinib
D. Erlotinib
E. Gemcitabine

7-8 A patient presents to you with chronic cough. Chest x-ray shows a hilar mass. This is followed by a PET-CT that shows an FDG-avid 4-cm right hilar mass, mediastinal adenopathy, and right supraclavicular adenopathy.

What do you order for pathologic diagnosis?
A. Mediastinoscopy for biopsy and mediastinal lymph node staging
B. Biopsy of right supraclavicular node
C. Bronchoscopy with endobronchial biopsy of an accessible mediastinal lymph node
D. CT-guided core biopsy of hilar mass by interventional radiology

7-9 A patient presents to your clinic with unresectable advanced malignant pleural mesothelioma with epithelioid histology. The patient's PS is 1.

What is the best systemic treatment for this patient?
A. Cisplatin/gemcitabine
B. Cisplatin/pemetrexed
C. Navelbine
D. Cisplatin alone

7-10 What is the most common finding from rebiopsy in *EGFR*-mutated cancers at time of clinical resistance to erlotinib?

A. HER2 amplification
B. MET amplification
C. Secondary T790M *EGFR* mutation
D. *PIK3CA* mutation
E. Small cell lung cancer histologic transformation

7-11 A 63-year-old patient with a 100-pack per year smoking history presents with cough and shortness of breath. CT of the chest shows a 4-cm hilar right lung mass and mediastinal adenopathy. Mediastinoscopy shows a right paratracheal node positive for small cell lung cancer. PET-CT shows liver and bone metastases. An MRI of the brain shows no intracranial metastatic disease. The patient completes six cycles of cisplatin/etoposide chemotherapy with an excellent partial response in all areas of tumor and improvement of symptoms.

What is the best next step for this patient?
A. Maintenance cisplatin/etoposide until progression
B. Observation only
C. Initiation of topotecan
D. Referral to a radiation oncologist for prophylactic cranial irradiation

7-12 A 54-year-old man with a 60-pack per year smoking history presents with a 4-cm right lower lobe lung lesion on PET-CT. An MRI of the brain shows no evidence of intracranial metastatic disease. A right lower lobe video-assisted thoracic surgical lobectomy is performed. Pathology returns moderately differentiated squamous cell lung carcinoma. Two of three hilar nodes are positive. None of the five mediastinal lymph nodes sampled during surgery show cancer. He follows up with you in clinic 1 month later and has fully recovered from surgery. His PS is 0, and all laboratory values are within the reference range.

What do you recommend to the patient as the next step?
A. Observation
B. Adjuvant chemotherapy with cisplatin/vinorelbine
C. Adjuvant chemotherapy with carboplatin/ paclitaxel
D. Adjuvant chemotherapy with cisplatin/ pemetrexed
E. Testing for ERCC1 by IHC and treatment with adjuvant chemotherapy if ERCC1 expression is low

7-13 In addition to *ALK* translocations, which of the following molecular aberrations predict sensitivity to crizotinib?
A. *ROS1* translocation
B. *KRAS* mutation
C. *PIK3CA* mutation
D. HER2 amplification

7-14 A 58-year-old East Asian woman presents to your clinic with worsening dry cough and dyspnea on exertion. The patient has never smoked and has metastatic lung adenocarcinoma treated with erlotinib for 2 months. Her tumor has an *EGFR*-activating mutation (exon 19 deletion), and she previously had an excellent clinical and radiographic response to erlotinib with improvement in cough, shortness of breath, appetite, and energy level. Physical exam reveals bilateral crackles, normal heart exam, and no lower extremity edema. CT shows extensive bilateral interstitial infiltrates. Echocardiogram shows normal heart function.

What is the most likely diagnosis?
A. Cardiogenic pulmonary edema
B. Development of lymphangitic spread of lung cancer
C. Interstitial pneumonitis from erlotinib
D. Pulmonary embolus

7-1   A

Platinum-based doublet chemotherapy has been demonstrated to improve survival in patients with advanced-stage NSCLC, with a variety of regimens showing similar results. However, pemetrexed-based regimens have shown inferior efficacy in squamous histology NSCLC. The anti-vascular endothelial growth factor (VEGF) antibody bevacizumab is contraindicated in squamous NSCLC because of increased life-threatening and fatal hemoptysis in squamous cell lung cancer. Erlotinib is approved for first-line treatment of patients with tumors harboring EGFR-activating mutations but only approved past first-line as maintenance therapy and as treatment after progression on one or two previous lines of chemotherapy based on trials such as SATURN and BR21, which demonstrated a modest OS benefit seen in patients with NSCLC regardless of EGFR mutation status.

Suggested Reading

Belani CP, Lee JS, Socinski MA, et al. Randomized phase III trial comparing cisplatin-etoposide to carboplatin-paclitaxel in advanced or metastatic non-small cell lung cancer. Ann Oncol. 2005;16:1069-1075. PMID: 15860487.

Sandler A, Gray R, Perry MC, et al. Paclitaxel-carboplatin alone or with bevacizumab for non-small-cell lung cancer. N Engl J Med. 2006;355:2542-2550. PMID: 17167137.

Shepherd FA, Rodrigues Pereira J, Ciuleanu T, et al. Erlotinib in previously treated non-small-cell lung cancer. N Engl J Med. 2005;353:123-132. PMID: 16014882.

Cappuzzo F, Ciuleanu T, Stelmakh L, et al. Erlotinib as maintenance treatment in advanced non-small-cell lung cancer: a multicentre, randomised, placebo-controlled phase 3 study. Lancet Oncol. 2010;11:521-529. PMID: 20493771.

Scagliotti GV, Parikh P, von Pawel J, et al. Phase III study comparing cisplatin plus gemcitabine with cisplatin plus pemetrexed in chemotherapy-naive patients with advanced-stage non-small-cell lung cancer. J Clin Oncol. 2008;26:3543-3551. PMID: 18506025.

7-2   C

Rebiopsy for molecular testing for EGFR-activating mutations and ALK gene rearrangements should be performed in patients with advanced NSCLC with an adenocarcinoma component and inadequate tumor tissue for analysis, regardless of clinical characteristics. Randomized clinical trials have shown that in patients with cancers harboring an EGFR-activating mutation, first-line therapy with an EGFR tyrosine kinase inhibitor (TKI) is superior for response and PFS compared with platinum-based chemotherapy. Conversely, in patients with cancers demonstrating wild-type EGFR, results with chemotherapy are superior.

Suggested Reading

Mok TS, Wu YL, Thongprasert S, et al. Gefitinib or carboplatin-paclitaxel in pulmonary adenocarcinoma. N Engl J Med. 2009;361:947-957. PMID: 19692680.

Rosell R, Carcereny E, Gervais R, et al. Erlotinib versus standard chemotherapy as first-line treatment for European patients with advanced EGFR mutation-positive non-small-cell lung cancer (EURTAC): a multicentre, open-label, randomised phase 3 trial. Lancet Oncol. 2012;13:239-246. PMID: 22285168.

Lindeman NI, Cagle PT, Beasley MB, et al. Molecular testing guideline for selection of lung cancer patients for EGFR and ALK TKIs: guideline from the College of American Pathologists, International Association for the Study of Lung Cancer, and Association for Molecular Pathology. J Thorac Oncol. 2013;8:823-859. PMID: 23552377.

7-3   B

Concurrent administration of platinum-based chemotherapy and thoracic radiation is considered standard of care for patients with stage III multistation N2 NSCLC, although trimodality approaches (preoperative chemoradiation followed by surgery) have also been employed in this setting. In the intergroup phase III trial by Albain et al comparing trimodality therapy with chemoradiation, PFS was superior in the surgical arm, but OS was equivalent. In a retrospective analysis, OS in those patients requiring pneumonectomy favored chemoradiation, whereas the reverse was true in patients treated with lobectomy. Thus, in this patient with a central lesion requiring pneumonectomy and multistation N2 disease, chemoradiation is the most appropriate therapy.

Suggested Reading

Curran WJ, Jr., Paulus R, Langer CJ, et al. Sequential vs. concurrent chemoradiation for stage III non-small cell lung cancer: randomized phase III trial RTOG 9410. J Natl Cancer Inst. 2011;103:1452-1460. PMID: 21903745.

Albain KS, Swann RS, Rusch VW, et al. Radiotherapy plus chemotherapy with or without surgical resection for stage III non-small-cell lung cancer: a phase III randomised controlled trial. Lancet. 2009;374:379-386. PMID: 19632716.

7-4 B

The recent National Lung Screening Trial showed a 20% reduction in lung cancer–related mortality and a 6.7% reduction in rate of death from any cause with low-dose CT of the chest in patients age 55 to 74 with at least a 30-pack per year smoking history. Since a great majority of abnormalities identified on screening are nonmalignant, an organized multidisciplinary team approach to evaluation of findings from CT screening is highly recommended.

Suggested Reading

National Lung Screening Trial Research Team, Aberle DR, Adams AM, et al. Reduced lung-cancer mortality with low-dose computed tomographic screening. *N Engl J Med.* 2011;365:395-409. PMID: 21714641.

Humphrey LL, Deffebach M, Pappas M, et al. Screening for lung cancer with low-dose computed tomography: a systematic review to update the US Preventive services task force recommendation. *Ann Intern Med.* 2013;159:411-420. PMID: 23897166.

7-5 C

Patients with a PS of 2 fare poorly compared with those with a PS of 0 to 1, regardless of the therapeutic approach. Nevertheless, recent studies suggest that platinum-based combination chemotherapy is still preferable for first-line therapy. In a recent clinical trial, patients with PS of 2 were randomly assigned to receive carboplatin (area under the curve 5) and pemetrexed compared with pemetrexed alone. OS and PFS were prolonged with carboplatin and pemetrexed followed by pemetrexed maintenance therapy compared with pemetrexed alone.

Suggested Reading

Lilenbaum RC, Herndon JE, 2nd, List MA, et al. Single-agent versus combination chemotherapy in advanced non-small-cell lung cancer: the cancer and leukemia group B (study 9730). *J Clin Oncol.* 2005;23:190-196. PMID: 15625373.

Zukin M, Barrios CH, Pereira JR, et al. Randomized phase III trial of single-agent pemetrexed versus carboplatin and pemetrexed in patients with advanced non-small-cell lung cancer and Eastern Cooperative Oncology Group performance status of 2. *J Clin Oncol.* 2013;31:2849-2853. PMID: 23775961.

7-6 C

Multiple randomized phase III trials have shown improved response rate and PFS for first-line EGFR TKIs compared with chemotherapy in patients with cancers harboring *EGFR*-activating mutations. None of the trials show improved OS, perhaps reflecting crossover between trial arms. Nevertheless, the EURTAC trial demonstrates equivalent OS whether patients with *EGFR*-mutated *NSCLC* receive erlotinib as first-line or second-line treatment after crossover. Importantly, despite favorable clinical and pathologic characteristics for EGFR TKI benefit, the IPASS trial showed inferior PFS when East Asian patients with adenocarcinoma—mainly women and never-smokers, who had cancers negative for *EGFR* mutation—were treated with an EGFR TKI instead of platinum chemotherapy.

Suggested Reading

Mok TS, Wu YL, Thongprasert S, et al. Gefitinib or carboplatin-paclitaxel in pulmonary adenocarcinoma. *N Engl J Med.* 2009;361:947-957. PMID: 19692680.

Rosell R, Carcereny E, Gervais R, et al. Erlotinib versus standard chemotherapy as first-line treatment for European patients with advanced EGFR mutation-positive non-small-cell lung cancer (EURTAC): a multicentre, open-label, randomised phase 3 trial. *Lancet Oncol.* 2012;13:239-246. PMID: 22285168.

7-7 C

A patient whose disease progressed on first-line chemotherapy and whose tumor harbors an *ALK* translocation should be treated with crizotinib based on high response rates and prolongation of PFS when compared with pemetrexed or docetaxel in a recent randomized phase III trial.

Suggested Reading

Kwak EL, Bang YJ, Camidge DR, et al. Anaplastic lymphoma kinase inhibition in non-small-cell lung cancer. *N Engl J Med.* 2010;363:1693-1703. PMID: 20979469.

Shaw AT, Yeap BY, Solomon BJ, et al. Effect of crizotinib on overall survival in patients with advanced non-small-cell lung cancer harbouring ALK gene rearrangement: a retrospective analysis. *Lancet Oncol.* 2011;12:1004-1012. PMID: 21933749.

Shaw AT, Kim DW, Nakagawa K, et al. Crizotinib versus chemotherapy in advanced ALK-positive lung cancer. *N Engl J Med.* 2013;368: 2385-2394. PMID: 23724913.

7-8 B

Of the answer choices, option B is the least invasive location to biopsy and would provide the most useful pathologic staging. If the supraclavicular node is positive, the patient would have stage IIIB (N3 disease), which would exclude surgery as a treatment option.

Suggested Reading

Ettinger DS, Akerley W, Borghaei H, et al. Non-small cell lung cancer, version 2.2013. *J Natl Compr Canc Netw.* 2013;11:645–53. PMID: 23744864.

7-9 B

In a randomized phase III trial, patients with unresectable mesothelioma treated with cisplatin/pemetrexed had a longer OS with the combination than with cisplatin alone (12.1 vs. 9.3 months; p = 0.02).

Suggested Reading

Vogelzang NJ, Rusthoven JJ, Symanowski J, et al. Phase III study of pemetrexed in combination with cisplatin versus cisplatin alone in patients with malignant pleural mesothelioma. *J Clin Oncol.* 2003; 21:2636-2644. PMID: 12860938.

7-10 C

Secondary *T790M EGFR* mutations are present in more than 50% of patients with acquired resistance to erlotinib. This point mutation sterically hinders erlotinib from fastening to the ATP-binding site of *EGFR*. It is less clear how often *T790M* represents the actual mechanism of resistance, as several *T790M*-directed drugs have failed in the clinic. In addition, a recent trial of afatinib plus cetuximab based on a T790-positive preclinical model shows equivalent activity regardless of *T790M* status. All of the other answer choices can also occur as a mechanism of EGFR TKI resistance but are less frequent.

Suggested Reading

Sequist LV, Waltman BA, Dias-Santagata D, et al. Genotypic and histological evolution of lung cancers acquiring resistance to EGFR inhibitors. *Sci Transl Med.* 2011;3:75ra26. PMID: 21430269.

Kosaka T, Yatabe Y, Endoh H, et al. Mutations of the epidermal growth factor receptor gene in lung cancer: biological and clinical implications. *Cancer Res.* 2004;64:8919-8923. PMID: 15604253.

7-11 D

Prophylactic cranial irradiation for patients with extensive-stage small cell lung cancer that responds to chemotherapy reduced the incidence of brain metastases and improved median OS (5.4 vs. 6.7 months) and time to symptomatic brain metastases (hazard ratio 0.27; p < 0.001).

Suggested Reading

Aupérin A, Arriagada R, Pignon JP, et al. Prophylactic cranial irradiation for patients with small-cell lung cancer in complete remission. Prophylactic Cranial Irradiation Overview Collaborative Group. *N Engl J Med.* 1999;341:476-484. PMID: 10441603.

Slotman B, Faivre-Finn C, Kramer G, et al. Prophylactic cranial irradiation in extensive small-cell lung cancer. *N Engl J Med.* 2007;357:664-672. PMID: 17699816.

7-12 B

The patient has stage II disease based on hilar lymph node involvement. Multiple clinical trials and meta-analysis have shown the benefit of adjuvant cisplatin-based chemotherapy in this setting. The benefit of adjuvant carboplatin-based therapy is less proven. Pemetrexed is often given with cisplatin as adjuvant therapy in nonsquamous histology extrapolating from data in the metastatic setting, but this is less effective in squamous histology. Selecting therapy based on ERCC1 expression remains unproven.

Suggested Reading

Pignon JP, Tribodet H, Scagliotti GV, et al. Lung adjuvant cisplatin evaluation: a pooled analysis by the LACE Collaborative Group. *J Clin Oncol.* 2008;26:3552-3559. PMID: 18506026.

Douillard JY, Rosell R, De Lena M, et al. Adjuvant vinorelbine plus cisplatin versus observation in patients with completely resected stage IB-IIIA non-small-cell lung cancer (Adjuvant Navelbine International Trialist Association [ANITA]): a randomised controlled trial. *Lancet Oncol.* 2006;7:719-727. PMID: 16945766.

Arriagada R, Bergman B, Dunant A, et al. Cisplatin-based adjuvant chemotherapy in patients with completely resected non-small-cell lung cancer. *N Engl J Med.* 2004;350:351-360. PMID: 14736927.

7-13 A

ROS1 gene rearrangements are a recently discovered molecular aberration present in about 2% of NSCLC tumors. *ROS1* is an orphan tyrosine kinase with sequence homology to *ALK*. Gene rearrangements of *ROS1* lead to constitutive activation of this tyrosine kinase. Like many oncogene-addicted lung cancers, *ROS1*-rearranged tumors commonly arise in younger nonsmokers with lung adenocarcinoma histology. As with *ALK*, crizotinib has activity in lung cancers with *ROS1* gene rearrangements, with high response rates noted in clinical trials.

Suggested Reading

Bergethon K, Shaw AT, Ignatius Ou SH, et al. ROS1 rearrangements define a unique molecular class of lung cancers. *J Clin Oncol.* 2012;30:863-870. PMID: 22215748.

7-14 C

The patient's symptoms represent an uncommon but serious side effect from erlotinib. Pneumonitis appears to be more frequent in East Asian patients. Erlotinib should be discontinued and supportive care initiated, including consideration of corticosteroids.

Suggested Reading

Yoneda K, Shelton DK, Beckett LA, et al. Independent review of interstitial lung disease associated with death in TRIBUTE (paclitaxel and carboplatin with or without concurrent erlotinib) in advanced non-small cell lung cancer. *J Thorac Oncol.* 2007;2: 537–543. PMID: 17545850.

8 HEAD AND NECK CANCERS
SELF-EVALUATION

HEAD AND NECK CANCERS QUESTIONS

8-1 A 56-year-old man presents with a right-sided sore throat for 3 weeks. He saw his primary care physician 2 weeks ago and was prescribed a course of antibiotics, without relief. He denies any history of tobacco exposure or alcohol intake. Examination reveals an exophytic mass in the right tonsillar area and bilateral level II lymph nodes measuring between 3 and 4 cm. A fine needle aspiration of the right-sided neck lymph node shows human papillomavirus (HPV) p16 positivity and basaloid poorly differentiated squamous cell carcinoma.

Which statement regarding the prognosis of this patient is most accurate?
A. Stage IVA disease represents an incurable presentation of this malignancy
B. p16 expression portends a favorable prognosis
C. p16 expression is associated with chemo-radioresistance
D. Tobacco smoking exposure has no influence on the favorable prognosis associated with p16 expression by the tumor cells

8-2 A 68-year-old man presents with a nonhealing sore in the left lateral tongue for 2 months. He has a history of chewing betel nut for many years. Biopsy of the lesion reveals squamous cell cancer. He undergoes a wide excision of the lesion and a supraomohyoid neck dissection of the ipsilateral neck. Operative pathology reveals a 2.1-cm squamous cell carcinoma with negative margins. Lymph node dissection reveals four out of 24 nodes positive for metastatic disease. The largest involved lymph node was 0.7 cm in size and extracapsular extension was identified.

Which of the following is the most appropriate therapy for this patient?
A. No further therapy is necessary
B. Radiation therapy to the primary site
C. Radiation therapy to the primary site and both sides of the neck
D. Concurrent cisplatin with radiation therapy to the primary site and both sides of the neck

8-3 A 37-year-old Asian man presents with a lump in the left posterior neck for the past 2 months. He has noted fullness in his left ear after a recent trip overseas that involved a 10-hour flight. On examination he has a 4-cm level V palpable lymph node. Nasopharyngoscopy reveals a friable left-sided nasopharyngeal mass. Biopsy of this lesion reveals an undifferentiated cancer. Computed tomography (CT) of the neck reveals a large left-sided nasopharyngeal mass eroding the clivus and multiple bilateral cervical lymph nodes, with the largest noted in the retropharyngeal area measuring 5 cm with central necrosis. Positron emission tomography (PET)/CT scan confirms these findings and no evidence of distant metastases is noted.

Which of the following is the most appropriate therapy for this patient?
A. Radiation therapy to the primary site after bilateral neck dissection
B. Induction chemotherapy with 5-fluorouracil (5-FU) plus mitomycin followed by radiation therapy to the primary site and bilateral neck nodes
C. Concurrent chemotherapy with radiation therapy followed by three cycles of adjuvant chemotherapy
D. Radiation therapy to the primary site and regional nodes followed by adjuvant chemotherapy with cisplatin and 5-FU

8-4 A 62-year-old woman with a 70 pack-year history of smoking presents with hoarseness and difficulty swallowing for the past 3 months. She is accompanied by her daughter who reports that her mother has lost 14 lbs over the past 6 months. She is active, and is able to live independently. Laryngoscopy reveals a large hypopharyngeal mass that is biopsied and confirms the clinical suspicion of squamous cell carcinoma. A chest radiograph shows multiple bilateral nodules varying in size from 1 to 2 cm. Biopsy of a peripheral nodule reveals similar histology as the hypopharyngeal mass.

What is the best treatment strategy for this patient?
A. Close observation with insertion of percutaneous endoscopic gastrostomy tube to facilitate nutrition
B. Weekly intravenous administration of high-dose methotrexate
C. Combination chemotherapy with cetuximab, cisplatin, and 5-FU
D. Radiation therapy to the hypopharynx with concomitant cisplatin

8-5 A 58-year-old woman with a long history of metastatic papillary thyroid cancer presents with worsening cough and shortness of breath for the past 3 months. Her prior treatments have included thyroidectomy, neck node dissection, and radioactive iodine ablative treatment. She recently underwent external beam radiation therapy to the right main stem bronchus where an endobronchial lesion was causing post-obstructive pneumonia. A recent radioactive iodine (RAI) scan was negative. CT reveals progressive pulmonary metastases and a moderate-sized right pleural effusion.

What is the best systemic treatment choice for this patient?
A. Chemotherapy with doxorubicin and cisplatin
B. Sorafenib
C. Vandetanib
D. RAI

8-6 A 47-year-old man presents with bilateral otalgia and progressive soreness of the throat over the past 6 weeks. He has a 40 pack-year history of smoking and says he consumes alcohol on the weekends. On examination he is noted to have a large tumor in the right base of tongue and bilateral bulky adenopathy, with the largest node being 7 cm in size. He is seeking a second opinion to enquire about the role of induction chemotherapy in the management of his high-risk oropharyngeal squamous cell carcinoma. No evidence of metastatic disease is noted on a PET/CT scan.

What is the most appropriate statement about the role of induction therapy in this patient?
A. Induction therapy has no role in the management of his locally advanced oropharyngeal cancer
B. Induction therapy followed by radiation therapy is superior to concomitant chemotherapy and radiation therapy
C. Induction therapy with taxanes, cisplatin, and 5-FU is superior to induction therapy with cisplatin and 5-FU
D. Induction therapy is equivalent to adjuvant postradiation therapy

8-7 A 56-year-old woman with a history of metastatic medullary carcinoma of the thyroid presents for evaluation of progressive weight loss and worsening diarrhea uncontrolled with antidiarrheals. She is status post-external beam radiation therapy to symptomatic lung lesions and her most recent serum carcinoembryonic antigen and calcitonin levels are progressively rising. Germ-line mutation analysis does not show any *RET* mutations.

Which of the following is an appropriate treatment option for this patient?
A. RAI
B. Cabozantinib
C. Sorafenib
D. Imatinib

8-8 An 83-year-old woman presents with a rapidly enlarging neck mass over the past 3 weeks associated with progressive shortness of breath, hoarseness, and throat pain. Physical examination reveals a 10-cm hard mass in the left lobe of the thyroid gland. Laryngoscopy reveals direct extension of the fixed mass into the anterior trachea. Chest radiograph reveals innumerable subcentimeter bilateral nodules. She was living independently until 1 month ago. Fine needle aspiration of the thyroid mass reveals anaplastic thyroid cancer.

What is the most appropriate treatment approach for this patient?

A. Surgical en bloc resection of the thyroid, anterior tracheal wall with reconstruction followed by chemotherapy

B. External beam radiation therapy to the neck

C. Vandetanib

D. Brentuximab vedotin

8-1   B

HPV-associated oropharyngeal cancers carry an excellent prognosis. Despite being staged as stage IVA disease, this is still considered locoregional disease and treated with curative intent. p16 expression is known to be associated with improved outcome for these tumors. Patients with p16-expressing squamous cell head and neck cancer with up to 10 pack-year tobacco smoke exposure had substantially better overall survival when compared with more than 10 pack-years.

Suggested Reading

Kumar B, Cordell KG, Lee JS, et al. EGFR, p16, HPV Titer, Bcl-xL and p53, sex, and smoking as indicators of response to therapy and survival in oropharyngeal cancer. *J Clin Oncol.* 2008;26:3128-3137. PMID: 18474878.

Gillison ML, Zhang Q, Jordan R, et al. Tobacco smoking and increased risk of death and progression for patients with p16-positive and p16-negative oropharyngeal cancer. *J Clin Oncol.* 2012;30:2102-2111. PMID: 22565003.

8-2   D

Postoperative chemoradiation therapy would be considered standard of care for this scenario. The addition of chemotherapy to the radiation therapy in the postoperative setting would be recommended for positive margins and/or extracapsular extension of disease in neck nodes.

Suggested Reading

Bernier J, Cooper JS, Pajak TF, et al. Defining risk levels in locally advanced head and neck cancers: a comparative analysis of concurrent postoperative radiation plus chemotherapy trials of the EORTC (#22931) and RTOG (# 9501). *Head Neck.* 2005;27:843-850. PMID: 16161069.

8-3   C

Concurrent chemotherapy with radiation therapy is the mainstay of therapy of locally advanced nasopharyngeal cancer. Although the value of the additional adjuvant three cycles of chemotherapy after conclusion of concurrent chemotherapy is unclear, it still remains a standard treatment option.

Suggested Reading

Al-Sarraf M, LeBlanc M, Giri PG, et al. Chemoradiotherapy versus radiotherapy in patients with advanced nasopharyngeal cancer: phase III randomized Intergroup study 0099. *J Clin Oncol.* 1998;16:1310-1317. PMID: 9552031.

Chen L, Hu CS, Chen XZ, et al. Concurrent chemoradiotherapy plus adjuvant chemotherapy versus concurrent chemoradiotherapy alone in patients with locoregionally advanced nasopharyngeal carcinoma: a phase 3 multicentre randomised controlled trial. *Lancet Oncol.* 2012;13:163-171. PMID: 22154591.

8-4   C

Improved overall survival has been demonstrated by the combination of cetuximab, cisplatin, and 5-FU compared with cisplatin and 5-FU. In individuals with good performance status, combination chemotherapy with such a regimen would be one of the standard recommended first-line therapies. When methotrexate is used as a single agent, it is typically not recommended in high doses, but rather in a dose range of 40 mg/m^2 weekly.

Suggested Reading

Vermorken JB, Mesia R, Rivera F, et al. Platinum-based chemotherapy plus cetuximab in head and neck cancer. *N Engl J Med.* 2008;359:1116-1127. PMID: 18784101.

8-5   B

The U.S. Food and Drug Administration (FDA) recently approved sorafenib for the treatment of locally recurrent or progressively metastatic differentiated thyroid cancer that does not respond to RAI. Standard chemotherapy is typically ineffective. Vandetanib was recently approved by the FDA for the treatment of advanced symptomatic medullary thyroid cancer.

Suggested Reading

Brose MS, Nutting C, Jarzab B, et al. Sorafenib in locally advanced or metastatic patients with radioactive iodine-refractory differentiated thyroid cancer: The Phase III Decision Trial. *J Clin Oncol.* 2013;31(suppl; abstr 4).

8-6   C

Both concurrent systemic chemotherapy with cisplatin plus radiation therapy and induction therapy with taxanes, cisplatin, and 5-FU followed by radiation therapy with or without concomitant chemotherapy are considered standard options in this scenario. However, when induction chemotherapy is utilized, two randomized phase III trials have shown superior results with a three-drug regimen of taxanes, cisplatin, and 5-FU when compared with the two-drug regimen of cisplatin and 5-FU.

Suggested Reading

Vermorken JB, Remenar E, van Herpen C, et al. Cisplatin, fluorouracil, and docetaxel in unresectable head and neck cancer. *N Engl J Med.* 2007;357:1695-1704. PMID: 17960012.

Posner MR, Hershock DM, Blajman CR, et al. Cisplatin and fluorouracil alone or with docetaxel in head and neck cancer. *N Engl J Med.* 2007;357:1705-1715. PMID: 17960013.

8-7 B

Cabozantinib is an oral tyrosine kinase inhibitor (TKI) that has recently been approved by the FDA for the treatment of progressive metastatic medullary thyroid cancer. In the pivotal study, patients treated with cabozantinib experienced a substantial improvement in progression-free survival of 11.2 months compared with 4.0 months in the placebo arm. Vandetanib is another oral TKI that targets vascular endothelial growth factor receptor, *RET*, and EGFR and has also been recently approved for its activity and advance medullary thyroid cancer. Both of these agents have been approved for progressive disease, and indolent or asymptomatic disease states may not require immediate initiation of therapy.

Suggested Reading

Elisei R, Schlumberger MJ, Müller SP, et al. Cabozantinib in progressive medullary thyroid cancer. *J Clin Oncol*. 2013;31:3639-3646. PMID: 24002501.

Haddad R. How to incorporate new tyrosine kinase inhibitors in the treatment of patients with medullary thyroid cancer. *J Clin Oncol*. 2013;31:3618-3620. PMID: 24002516.

8-8 B

Anaplastic thyroid cancer of the thyroid with presence of metastatic disease carries a dismal prognosis. Treatment is primarily with supportive and palliative intent. External beam radiation therapy alone to the enlarging neck mass for symptom management with or without radiation-sensitizing chemotherapy are reasonable options. Vandetanib is approved for advanced medullary thyroid cancer. Brentuximab vedotin is FDA-approved for the management of anaplastic large cell lymphoma and relapsed Hodgkin lymphoma.

GASTROINTESTINAL CANCERS
SELF-EVALUATION

GASTROINTESTINAL CANCERS QUESTIONS

9-1 A 62-year-old man with a longstanding history of gastroesophageal reflux disease develops progressive dysphagia over 3 months. An upper endoscopy identifies a partially obstructing mass right above the gastroesophageal junction. Biopsies confirm the presence of a moderately differentiated adenocarcinoma, and immunohistochemistry (IHC) for HER2 classifies the cancer as HER2 3+. Subsequent endoscopic ultrasound (EUS) characterizes the tumor as a T3 lesion, with one periesophageal lymph node suspicious for tumor involvement. A positron emission tomography/computed tomography (PET/CT) scan demonstrates tracer accumulation in the area of the primary tumor and one periesophageal lymph node. No evidence for distant metastatic disease is found. The patient does not have any major comorbidities.

What is the most appropriate next step in the treatment of this patient?
A. Surgery in the form of a Ivor-Lewis esophagectomy with subsequent adjuvant chemoradiotherapy
B. Neoadjuvant chemotherapy with a fluoropyrimidine/cisplatin/trastuzumab combination followed by esophagectomy and postoperative chemotherapy
C. Neoadjuvant chemoradiotherapy with a fluoropyrimidine/cisplatin/trastuzumab combination followed by esophagectomy
D. Neoadjuvant chemoradiotherapy with carboplatin/paclitaxel followed by esophagectomy

9-2 A 57-year-old woman with a history of well-controlled diabetes and hypertension notices unintentional weight loss of 5 kg over 2 months as well as progressive upper abdominal discomfort. A CT scan shows diffuse thickening of the gastric wall as well as multiple intrahepatic lesions up to 2 cm in maximum diameter and suspicion for peritoneal tumor implants. An upper endoscopy identifies a rigid stomach wall with superficial erosions. Deep biopsies of the stomach lining confirm the presence of a diffusely infiltrating, poorly differentiated adenocarcinoma (linitis plastica), HER2 1+ by IHC, and *KRAS* wild-type.

Which of the following treatment regimens would not be appropriate as first-line therapy in this setting?
A. EOX (epirubicin, oxaliplatin, capecitabine)
B. DCF (docetaxel, cisplatin, 5-fluorouracil)
C. FOLFOX (leucovorin, 5-fluorouracil, oxaliplatin) plus cetuximab
D. Cisplatin plus 5-fluorouracil
E. ECF (epirubicin, cisplatin, 5-fluorouracil)

9-3 A 62-year-old man with a good performance status and no relevant comorbidities was diagnosed with a metastatic gastric adenocarcinoma, HER2-negative, with liver and peritoneal metastases. He was started on FOLFOX with partial response of metastatic sites after 2 months and stable disease after 4 months of therapy per CT criteria. He has been tolerating the treatment well with only mild diarrhea and transient, cold-induced sensory neuropathy as the main side effects. A CT scan after 6 months of therapy (12 cycles) demonstrates progression of disease with increased size of liver metastases. The patient is still in good performance status and is motivated to receive further therapy.

What would not be an appropriate next step in the treatment of this patient?
A. Best supportive care alone
B. Second-line chemotherapy with irinotecan
C. Second-line chemotherapy with docetaxel or paclitaxel
D. Second-line therapy with ramucirumab

9-4 A 45-year-old woman with a history of alcohol and drug abuse 10 years ago has developed upper abdominal discomfort during the last month. She now presents with obstructive jaundice and a 2-cm mass in the head of the pancreas per CT imaging without evidence for distant metastases. An EUS-guided biopsy confirms the presence of an adenocarcinoma. Since no involvement of major arterial blood vessel is found, the patient is taken to surgery for a Whipple resection. Pathology confirms the presence of a poorly differentiated adenocarcinoma, 2.5 cm in maximum diameter, with one of 13 resected peripancreatic lymph nodes involved by cancer and free resection margins.

What would an appropriate adjuvant therapy be for this patient?

A. Radiation plus continuously infused 5-fluorouracil for 6 weeks to a target radiation dose of 50.4 Gy in 28 fractions

B. Gemcitabine for a planned duration of 24 weeks (six 4-weekly cycles)

C. FOLFIRINOX (leucovorin, 5-fluorouracil, oxaliplatin, irinotecan) for a planned duration of 24 weeks (12 2-weekly cycles)

D. Gemcitabine plus nab-paclitaxel for a planned duration of 24 weeks (six 4-weekly cycles)

9-5 A 50-year-old man with a history of hypertension and new onset of diabetes on metformin is diagnosed with a metastatic, moderately differentiated adenocarcinoma of the body of the pancreas. He has multiple liver metastases and retroperitoneal lymphadenopathy. He is being referred to a medical oncologist to discuss treatment options for his advanced cancer. Upon presentation his main complaints are upper abdominal pain and a loss of appetite. He has a good performance status and is highly motivated to start therapy.

For the discussion with the patient, which of the following statements is evidence-based?

A. In metastatic pancreas cancer, systemic chemotherapy does not improve survival outcomes compared with best supportive care, but can improve tumor-related symptoms

B. Gemcitabine as a single agent has been found to be superior to FOLFOX as first-line therapy

C. The use of FOLFIRINOX as first-line therapy is associated with an improvement in median overall survival of over 4 months compared with gemcitabine alone

D. Gemcitabine plus nab-paclitaxel has been found to be associated with higher response rate, but identical overall survival, compared with FOLFIRINOX in a phase III trial

9-6 A 64-year-old patient with a 20-year history of hepatitis C and mild cirrhosis (Child-Pugh A) who is being monitored with yearly alpha-fetoprotein (AFP) levels and abdominal magnetic resonance imaging (MRI) shows an increase in AFP levels from 18 ng/dL to 200 ng/mL. The MRI identifies a new 4-cm lesion in the periphery of the right liver lobe with imaging characteristics supportive of a hepatocellular carcinoma (HCC). No other new focal abnormalities can be found in the liver.

What is the best next step in the treatment of this patient?

A. Ultrasound-guided biopsy of the suspicious intrahepatic lesion

B. PET/CT scan to rule out distant metastases

C. Transarterial chemoembolization (TACE) of the liver followed by surgical resection of the liver lesion

D. Radiofrequency ablation of the liver lesion

E. Surgical resection of the liver lesion

9-7 A 35-year-old woman who smokes with a 15-year history of inflammatory bowel disease accompanies her 45-year-old sister who has been diagnosed with an advanced intrahepatic cholangiocarcinoma to an appointment. She is very concerned that she might develop the same malignant disease as her sister and asks you for advice.

In your discussions with the patient's sister, what could be the most important factor predisposing her for the development of a cholangiocarcinoma?

A. Her young age

B. Her smoking history

C. Her family history

D. Her history of inflammatory bowel disease

E. She is not at a higher risk for the development of a cholangiocarcinoma compared with the average population

9-8 A 32-year-old patient develops bright red blood per rectum. A colonoscopy identifies two synchronous nonobstructing masses in the colon: one in the sigmoid, another in the ascending colon. No polyps are found. Biopsies confirm the presence of moderately differentiated adenocarcinomas in both locations. A CT scan shows large, 5-cm masses in the colonic tumor locations with peritumor lymphadenopathy, but no evidence for distant metastases. Since the patient is an adoptee, no details on a family history of colon cancers are available.

Which test would confirm or rule out the presence of a hereditary nonpolyposis colon cancer (HNPCC; Lynch syndrome) in this patient?
A. IHC determination of mismatch repair enzyme protein expression levels in the tumor tissue
B. Analysis of microsatellite instability in tumor tissue by polymerase chain reaction
C. *BRAF* mutation analysis and methylation status of the promoter region of genes encoding mismatch repair enzymes
D. Analysis of microsatellite instability in nontumor tissue
E. Sequencing of the adenomatous polyposis colon (*APC*) gene in nontumor tissue

9-9 A 78-year-old woman notices intermittent blood in her bowel movements, gradually increasing abdominal pain, and new constipation. A colonoscopy reveals an almost completely obstructing mass in the sigmoid, 25 cm from the anal verge. Biopsies show a poorly differentiated adenocarcinoma with mucinous features. A CT scan of abdomen and pelvis demonstrates no signs of distant metastatic disease. A chest x-ray demonstrates no intrapulmonary lesions suspicious for metastases. The patient undergoes a laparoscopic sigmoid resection without complications. Final pathology confirms an adenocarcinoma with mucinous components, poorly differentiated with invasion through the bowel wall into adipose tissue. Of 15 resected lymph nodes, three show tumor involvement. The tumor is found to be *KRAS* wild-type and *BRAF* wild-type per mutation analysis. The patient lives alone after her husband died 3 years ago and is able to run her household without external help. She has comorbidities in the form of well-controlled diabetes and hypertension as well as osteoarthritis.

What would be the appropriate considerations for potential adjuvant therapy in this patient?
A. In view of the patient's age and comorbidities, adjuvant chemotherapy should not be considered
B. FOLFOX for 6 months (12 cycles) has shown to improve survival in elderly patients with stage III colon cancer compared with 5-fluorouracil/leucovorin alone and should be strongly considered in this situation
C. In *KRAS* wild-type colon cancers, the addition of cetuximab to a chemotherapy backbone leads to improvement in disease-free, but not overall, survival in the adjuvant setting
D. Fluoropyrimidines alone (5-fluorouracil/leucovorin or capecitabine) without oxaliplatin can be considered an adequate adjuvant therapy in elderly patients with stage III colon cancers

9-10 A 57-year-old man was diagnosed with a stage III right-sided colon cancer (pT3 pN1 M0) 9 months ago. After right hemicolectomy, he underwent adjuvant therapy with modified FOLFOX6 for 12 cycles; the last two cycles, however, were administered without oxaliplatin because of persistent grade 2 sensory neurotoxicity. He now returns to a medical oncologist for his first assessment after completion of adjuvant chemotherapy. He states that the sensory symptoms have almost completely resolved. He only has some mild numbness in his toes, which does not interfere with his daily activities. Laboratory studies are within normal range with the exception of mild anemia, platelets at 115,000/mL, and a carcinoembryonic antigen (CEA) level of 8.4 mg/dL. A CT scan reveals multiple intrahepatic lesions and enlarged retroperitoneal lymph nodes; both findings are new compared with scans obtained immediately prior to his colon surgery. A biopsy of one of the liver lesions confirms the presence of a metastatic adenocarcinoma consistent with a colon primary. *KRAS* exon 2 analysis reveals a mutation in codon 12.

What is the best treatment approach for this patient?
A. Start systemic chemotherapy with FOLFOX plus bevacizumab
B. Start systemic chemotherapy with FOLFIRI plus bevacizumab
C. Start systemic chemotherapy with FOLFIRI plus cetuximab
D. Start systemic chemotherapy with FOLFOXIRI
E. Start systemic chemotherapy with FOLFIRI plus aflibercept

9-11 A 63-year-old otherwise healthy patient notices blood in her bowel movement and changes in her bowel habits with intermittent constipation followed by a period of loose stools. She has also developed the feeling of perianal pressure, in particular while sitting. During a digital rectal exam, her gynecologist felt a mass at about 3 cm from the anal verge. A colonoscopy reveals a partially obstructing mass in the mid-rectum; biopsies confirm a moderately differentiated adenocarcinoma. The rest of the colon could only be partially visualized because of a suboptimal bowel preparation. A pelvic MRI classifies the tumor as a T3 lesion with multiple enlarged lymph nodes in the perirectal region. Further imaging scans do not identify distant metastases, and the patient's serum CEA is elevated at 10.3 mg/dL. The tumor is classified as *KRAS* wild-type, *BRAF* wild-type.

What is the best next step in the management of this patient's newly diagnosed rectal cancer?
A. Low-anterior resection with protective ileostomy and subsequent adjuvant chemoradiotherapy
B. Neoadjuvant chemotherapy with FOLFOX followed by low-anterior resection and postoperative chemoradiotherapy
C. Neoadjuvant chemoradiotherapy with a fluoropyrimidine/oxaliplatin regimen followed by surgical resection and further adjuvant chemotherapy with FOLFOX
D. Neoadjuvant chemoradiotherapy with a fluoropyrimidine (continuously infused 5-fluorouracil or capecitabine) as radiation sensitizer followed by rectal resection and adjuvant oxaliplatin-based chemotherapy

9-12 A 55-year-old woman has noticed intermittent episodes of diarrhea for almost 15 years, which have been characterized as related to irritable bowel syndrome. During the last year she has noticed progressive ankle edema for which she was advised to wear compression stockings; she has also been put on a mild diuretic with transient success. Upon further questioning she reveals that she had noticed hot flashes for "quite some time," which she thought were related to menopause. Physical exam reveals a well-nourished patient without appreciable peripheral lymphadenopathy and no jaundice. She has positive hepatojugular reflux, prominent S3 upon auscultation, enlarged liver palpable 5 cm under the right costal margin, and bilateral 2+ ankle edema.

Which of the following tests is <u>not</u> indicated in the further work-up for this patient?
A. Echocardiogram
B. PET/CT scan
C. 24-hour urine on 5-hydroxyindoleacetic acid (5-HIAA)
D. CT scan of abdomen and pelvis
E. Octreoscan

9-1   D

For patients with esophageal adenocarcinomas, a trimodality approach with neoadjuvant radiation plus chemotherapy followed by surgery is superior to surgery alone. A weekly carboplatin/paclitaxel combination parallel to radiation has evolved as standard of care with better tolerability than the previously used 5-fluorouracil/cisplatin combination. Postoperative radiation after esophagectomy should be avoided since the radiation field would have to include the mediastinum with the pulled-up stomach after Ivor-Lewis resection; preoperative radiation is preferred. Although the addition of trastuzumab to chemotherapy is standard of care in the management of metastatic gastroesophageal cancer with HER2 overexpression, its role in the neoadjuvant and adjuvant setting is not established yet, but currently is being investigated in clinical trials.

Suggested Reading

Bang YJ, Van Cutsem E, Feyereislova A, et al. Trastuzumab in combination with chemotherapy versus chemotherapy alone for treatment of HER2-positive advanced gastric or gastro-oesophageal junction cancer (ToGA): a phase 3, open-label, randomised controlled trial. *Lancet.* 2010;376:687-697. PMID: 20728210.

Wolff CS, Castillo SF, Larson DR, et al. Ivor Lewis approach is superior to transhiatal approach in retrieval of lymph nodes at esophagectomy. *Dis Esophagus.* 2008;21:328-333. PMID: 18477255.

van Hagen P, Hulshof MC, van Lanschot JJ, et al. Preoperative chemoradiotherapy for esophageal or junctional cancer. *N Engl J Med.* 2012;366:2074-2084. PMID: 22646630.

Tepper J, Krasna MJ, Niedzwiecki D, et al. Phase III trial of trimodality therapy with cisplatin, fluorouracil, radiotherapy, and surgery compared with surgery alone for esophageal cancer: CALGB 9781. *J Clin Oncol.* 2008;26:1086-1092. PMID: 18309943.

9-2   C

Various combination regimens have been established as standard of care in first-line therapy of advanced gastric cancer. These combinations routinely include a fluoropyrimidine (5-fluorouracil or capecitabine) plus a platinum agent (cisplatin or oxaliplatin). Whether the addition of epirubicin enhances the activity of a fluoropyrimidine/platinum regimen is controversial, but commonly used in clinical practice based on phase III trials mainly conducted in the United Kingdom. DCF was shown to be superior to cisplatin plus 5-fluorouracil, but at the cost of higher toxicity. The addition of epidermal growth factor receptor (EGFR) antibodies (panitumumab or cetuximab) to chemotherapy in this setting has not been shown to improve outcomes, but might potentially be detrimental (presumably because increased toxicity associated with the use of EGFR antibodies requires dose reductions of the chemotherapy backbone). The *KRAS* status is not predictive of the activity of EGFR antibodies in gastric cancers. Trastuzumab is not indicated since the tumor does not demonstrate HER2 overexpression.

Suggested Reading

Wagner AD, Grothe W, Haerting J, et al. Chemotherapy in advanced gastric cancer: a systematic review and meta-analysis based on aggregate data. *J Clin Oncol.* 2006;24:2903-2909. PMID: 16782930.

Cunningham D, Starling N, Rao S, et al. Capecitabine and oxaliplatin for advanced esophagogastric cancer. *N Engl J Med.* 2008;358: 36-46. PMID: 18172173.

Van Cutsem E, Moiseyenko VM, Tjulandin S, et al. Phase III study of docetaxel and cisplatin plus fluorouracil compared with cisplatin and fluorouracil as first-line therapy for advanced gastric cancer: a report of the V325 Study Group. *J Clin Oncol.* 2006;24:4991-4997. PMID: 17075117.

Lordick F, Kang YK, Chung HC, et al. Capecitabine and cisplatin with or without cetuximab for patients with previously untreated advanced gastric cancer (EXPAND): a randomised, open-label phase 3 trial. *Lancet Oncol.* 2013;14:490-499. PMID: 23594786.

9-3   A

In patients with metastatic gastric cancer and good performance status, second-line therapy with either irinotecan or a taxane has shown to be superior in terms of overall survival and symptom control compared with best supportive care alone and should be considered standard of care, in particular in patients with a tumor response to first-line therapy. Ramucirumab, a human monoclonal antibody against vascular endothelial growth factor receptor (VEGFR) 2, has likewise shown to improve survival compare with best supportive care in a phase III trial.

Suggested Reading

Fuchs CS, Tomasek J, Yong CJ, et al. Ramucirumab monotherapy for previously treated advanced gastric or gastro-oesophageal junction adenocarcinoma (REGARD): an international, randomised, multicentre, placebo-controlled, phase 3 trial. *Lancet.* 2014;383: 31-39. PMID: 24094768.

Park SH, Lim DH, Park K, et al. A multicenter, randomized phase III trial comparing second-line chemotherapy (SLC) plus best supportive care (BSC) with BSC alone for pretreated advanced gastric cancer (AGC). *J Clin Oncol.* 2011;29:15s (suppl; abstr 4004).

Thuss-Patience PC, Kretzschmar A, Bichev D, et al. Survival advantage for irinotecan versus best supportive care as second-line chemotherapy in gastric cancer--a randomised phase III study of the Arbeitsgemeinschaft Internistische Onkologie (AIO). *Eur J Cancer.* 2011;47:2306-2314. PMID: 21742485.

Kang JH, Lee SI, Lim do H, et al. Salvage chemotherapy for pretreated gastric cancer: a randomized phase III trial comparing chemotherapy plus best supportive care with best supportive care alone. *J Clin Oncol.* 2012;30:1513-1518. PMID: 22412140.

9-4   B

Radiation plus bolus 5-fluorouracil/leucovorin (Mayo Clinic regimen) represents a historic approach based on studies with small numbers of patients that has been abandoned in favor of a gemcitabine-based adjuvant therapy. The German CONKO-1 phase III trial documented the superiority of adjuvant gemcitabine to surgery alone with long-term benefits in overall survival. The question of whether radiation therapy added to gemcitabine in the adjuvant setting is associated with improved outcome is currently being investigated in clinical trials. FOLFIRINOX and a gemcitabine/*nab*-paclitaxel combination have been shown to be superior to gemcitabine alone in the palliative setting, but their role as adjuvant therapy is not established yet.

Suggested Reading

Kalser MH, Ellenberg SS. Pancreatic cancer. Adjuvant combined radiation and chemotherapy following curative resection. *Arch Surg.* 1985;120: 899-903. PMID: 4015380.

Oettle H, Neuhaus P, Hochhaus A, et al. Adjuvant chemotherapy with gemcitabine and long-term outcomes among patients with resected pancreatic cancer: the CONKO-001 randomized trial. *JAMA.* 2013; 310:1473-1481. PMID: 24104372.

Regine WF, Winter KA, Abrams RA, et al. Fluorouracil vs gemcitabine chemotherapy before and after fluorouracil-based chemoradiation following resection of pancreatic adenocarcinoma: a randomized controlled trial. *JAMA.* 2008;299:1019-1026. PMID: 18319412.

Conroy T, Desseigne F, Ychou M, et al. FOLFIRINOX versus gemcitabine for metastatic pancreatic cancer. *N Engl J Med.* 2011;364:1817-1825. PMID: 21561347.

9-5   C

In patients considered candidates for systemic chemotherapy based on age, performance status, and comorbidities, systemic chemotherapy improves overall survival compared with best supportive care. The old standard of care, single-agent gemcitabine, has been replaced by more active combination regimens like FOLFIRINOX and gemcitabine/*nab*-paclitaxel, which both have shown improvement in overall survival in randomized phase III trials compared with gemcitabine alone. FOLFIRINOX improved median overall survival from 6.8 to 11.1 months compared with gemcitabine. To date, no direct randomized head-to-head comparison between FOLFIRINOX and gemcitabine/*nab*-paclitaxel has been conducted in metastatic pancreas cancer.

Suggested Reading

Burris HA, 3rd, Moore MJ, Andersen J, et al. Improvements in survival and clinical benefit with gemcitabine as first-line therapy for patients with advanced pancreas cancer: a randomized trial. *J Clin Oncol.* 1997;15:2403-2413. PMID: 9196156.

Conroy T, Desseigne F, Ychou M, et al. FOLFIRINOX versus gemcitabine for metastatic pancreatic cancer. *N Engl J Med.* 2011;364:1817-1825. PMID: 21561347.

Von Hoff DD, Ervin T, Arena FP, et al. Increased survival in pancreatic cancer with nab-paclitaxel plus gemcitabine. *N Engl J Med.* 2013;369: 1691-1703. PMID: 24131140.

Pelzer U, Schwaner I, Stieler J, et al. Best supportive care (BSC) versus oxaliplatin, folinic acid and 5-fluorouracil (OFF) plus BSC in patients for second-line advanced pancreatic cancer: a phase III-study from the German CONKO-study group. *Eur J Cancer.* 2011;47:1676-1681. PMID: 21565490.

9-6   E

The patient's medical background (hepatitis C), the increase in AFP level, and the radiographic criteria of sequential MRI studies confirm the presence of HCC; no biopsy is needed here. The sensitivity of PET imaging in HCCs is low and PET is not recommended in the staging of HCC. TACE is useful as palliative therapy for unresectable, liver-limited HCC with adequate liver function but is not an appropriate approach for a resectable solitary HCC lesion. The risk for local recurrence after radiofrequency ablation is high for lesions larger than 3 cm in diameter and should only be considered if surgical resection is impossible. The best approach for this patient is upfront resection of the liver lesion. The role of sorafenib as adjuvant therapy is currently being evaluated in clinical trials.

Suggested Reading

Llovet JM, Burroughs A, Bruix J. Hepatocellular carcinoma. *Lancet.* 2003;362:1907-1917. PMID: 14667750.

Llovet JM, Ricci S, Mazzaferro V, et al. Sorafenib in advanced hepatocellular carcinoma. *N Engl J Med.* 2008;359:378-390. PMID: 18650514.

Germani G, Pleguezuelo M, Gurusamy K, et al. Clinical outcomes of radiofrequency ablation, percutaneous alcohol and acetic acid injection for hepatocelullar carcinoma: a meta-analysis. *J Hepatol.* 2010;52:380-388. PMID: 20149473.

Llovet JM, Bruix J. Systematic review of randomized trials for unresectable hepatocellular carcinoma: chemoembolization improves survival. *Hepatology.* 2003;37:429-442. PMID: 12540794.

9-7   D

Patients with inflammatory bowel disease are at risk for the development of primary sclerosing cholangitis, which predisposes for cholangiocarcinomas. These cancers occur most commonly in woman older than age 50. Smoking has not been established as a risk factor for the development of cholangiocarcinomas, and familial syndromes associated with biliary cancers are rare.

Suggested Reading

Shaib Y, El-Serag HB. The epidemiology of cholangiocarcinoma. *Semin Liver Dis.* 2004;24:115-125. PMID: 15192785.

LaRusso NF, Shneider BL, Black D, et al. Primary sclerosing cholangitis: summary of a workshop. *Hepatology.* 2006;44:746-764. PMID: 16941705.

Valle J, Wasan H, Palmer DH, et al. Cisplatin plus gemcitabine versus gemcitabine for biliary tract cancer. *N Engl J Med.* 2010;362: 1273-1281. PMID: 20375404.

9-8   D

The case of a young patient with two large synchronous colon cancers without further colon polyps raises the suspicion for a hereditary syndrome, particularly HNPCC. HNPCC is characterized by a germ-line mutation of gene encoding mismatch repair enzymes, *MSH-2*, *MLH-1*, *PMS-1*, *PMS-2*, and *MSH-6*. Germ-line mutations can be found in all cells of an affected individual, whereas somatic mutations can only be found in tumor tissue. Absence of protein expression levels of mismatch repair genes and microsatellite instability can be a consequence of a mutation in the genes encoding for these proteins or a result of a methylation of the gene promoter region. Although HNPCC accounts for less than 5% of all colon cancer cases, 15% of sporadic cancers can present with an HNPCC-like phenotype due to methylation of the gene promoter region, mainly of *MLH-1*. These cancers are commonly right-sided and commonly harbor a *BRAF* mutation. The clinical setting here would not be consistent with a familial adenomatous polyposis syndrome, which is characterized by a germ-line mutation of *APC*.

Suggested Reading

Kinzler KW, Vogelstein B. Lessons from hereditary colorectal cancer. *Cell.* 1996;87:159-170. PMID: 8861899.

Goel A, Arnold CN, Niedzwiecki D, et al. Characterization of sporadic colon cancer by patterns of genomic instability. *Cancer Res.* 2003; 63:1608-1614. PMID: 12670912.

Vasen HF, Möslein G, Alonso A, et al. Guidelines for the clinical management of Lynch syndrome (hereditary non-polyposis cancer). *J Med Genet.* 2007;44:353-362. PMID: 17327285.

Lindor NM, Burgart LJ, Leontovich O, et al. Immunohistochemistry versus microsatellite instability testing in phenotyping colorectal tumors. *J Clin Oncol.* 2002;20:1043-1048. PMID: 11844828.

9-9   D

Elderly patients experience approximately the same benefit from fluoropyrimidine-based adjuvant chemotherapy as younger patients. However, the addition of oxaliplatin to 5-fluorouracil/leucovorin has not been shown to improve outcomes in patients older than age 70 and should only be reserved for very fit patients older than age 70. It is important to point out in this setting that the pivotal MOSAIC trial, which established FOLFOX as standard of care in the adjuvant therapy of stage III colon cancers, excluded patients older than age 75. The addition of cetuximab to FOLFOX did not improve disease-free or overall survival in two phase III trials even when patients were selected based on their *KRAS* status.

Suggested Reading

André T, Boni C, Mounedji-Boudiaf L, et al. Oxaliplatin, fluorouracil, and leucovorin as adjuvant treatment for colon cancer. *N Engl J Med.* 2004;350:2343-2351. PMID: 15175436.

Sargent DJ, Goldberg RM, Jacobson SD, et al. A pooled analysis of adjuvant chemotherapy for resected colon cancer in elderly patients. *N Engl J Med.* 2001;345:1091-1097. PMID: 11596588.

Tournigand C, André T, Bonnetain F, et al. Adjuvant therapy with fluorouracil and oxaliplatin in stage II and elderly patients (between ages 70 and 75 years) with colon cancer: subgroup analyses of the Multicenter International Study of Oxaliplatin, Fluorouracil, and Leucovorin in the Adjuvant Treatment of Colon Cancer trial. *J Clin Oncol.* 2012;30:3353-3360. PMID: 22915656.

Jackson McCleary NA, Meyerhardt J, Green E, et al. Impact of older age on the efficacy of newer adjuvant therapies in >12,500 patients (pts) with stage II/III colon cancer: Findings from the ACCENT Database. *J Clin Oncol.* 2009;27:15s (suppl; abstr 4010).

9-10 B

The clinical course suggests that the metastases evolved during the adjuvant therapy with FOLFOX, so an oxaliplatin-based treatment regimen as the first step in this obviously palliative setting would not be indicated. In addition, even if the sensory neurotoxicity has largely resolved, the prior cumulative exposure to oxaliplatin would limit the duration of any palliative oxaliplatin-based therapy. EGFR monoclonal antibodies like cetuximab and panitumumab are not active in *KRAS*-mutated colon cancers and should be avoided. Aflibercept in combination with FOLFIRI is indicated for the second-line therapy of patients whose disease progressed on prior oxaliplatin-based first-line therapy in the palliative setting. Although the patient's scenario does not perfectly mirror this indication, one could argue that failure of an oxaliplatin-based adjuvant therapy within 6 months would allow aflibercept to be considered in this setting. However, in view of the large body of evidence of bevacizumab in advanced colorectal cancer and the lack of data confirming a superiority of aflibercept compared with bevacizumab, FOLFIRI plus bevacizumab is the preferred option here.

Suggested Reading

Tournigand C, André T, Achille E, et al. FOLFIRI followed by FOLFOX6 or the reverse sequence in advanced colorectal cancer: a randomized GERCOR study. *J Clin Oncol.* 2004;22:229-237. PMID: 14657227.

Hurwitz H, Fehrenbacher L, Novotny W, et al. Bevacizumab plus irinotecan, fluorouracil, and leucovorin for metastatic colorectal cancer. *N Engl J Med.* 2004;350:2335-2342. PMID: 15175435.

Bennouna J, Sastre J, Arnold D, et al. Continuation of bevacizumab after first progression in metastatic colorectal cancer (ML18147): a randomised phase 3 trial. *Lancet Oncol.* 2013;14:29-37. PMID: 23168366.

Van Cutsem E, Tabernero J, Lakomy R, et al. Addition of aflibercept to fluorouracil, leucovorin, and irinotecan improves survival in a phase III randomized trial in patients with metastatic colorectal cancer previously treated with an oxaliplatin-based regimen. *J Clin Oncol.* 2012;30:3499-3506. PMID: 22949147.

9-11 D

Based on a pivotal German phase III trial, neoadjuvant chemoradiotherapy has become standard of care for low- and mid-rectal cancers because, compared with surgery followed by chemoradiotherapy, the neoadjuvant approach reduced the risk for local recurrence by about 50%, was associated with less acute and long-term toxicity, and allowed a higher rate of sphincter conservation. This last point, however, has not routinely been replicated in subsequent studies. Fluoropyrimidines represent the standard chemotherapy administered parallel to radiation therapy (commonly 50.4 Gy in 28 fractions), with capecitabine and continuously infused 5-fluorouracil being appropriate choices. The addition of oxaliplatin as a potential radiosensitizer in the neoadjuvant setting has been investigated in several trials with consistently negative results for short-term outcome parameters (pathologic complete response), but it significantly increased toxicity and should not be used in this setting. Neoadjuvant chemotherapy alone without radiation is currently being investigated in clinical trials.

Suggested Reading

Sauer R, Becker H, Hohenberger W, et al. Preoperative versus postoperative chemoradiotherapy for rectal cancer. *N Engl J Med.* 2004;351:1731-1740. PMID: 15496622.

Hofheinz RD, Wenz F, Post S, et al. Chemoradiotherapy with capecitabine versus fluorouracil for locally advanced rectal cancer: a randomised, multicentre, non-inferiority, phase 3 trial. *Lancet Oncol.* 2012;13:579-588. PMID: 22503032.

Aschele C, Cionini L, Lonardi S, et al. Primary tumor response to preoperative chemoradiation with or without oxaliplatin in locally advanced rectal cancer: pathologic results of the STAR-01 randomized phase III trial. *J Clin Oncol.* 2011;29:2773-2780. PMID: 21606427.

Gérard JP, Azria D, Gourgou-Bourgade S, et al. Comparison of two neoadjuvant chemoradiotherapy regimens for locally advanced rectal cancer: results of the phase III trial ACCORD 12/0405-Prodige 2. *J Clin Oncol.* 2010;28:1638-1644. PMID: 20194850.

9-12   B

The patient's symptoms strongly suggest a metastatic carcinoid with longstanding high levels of serotonin that likely have already led to right-heart insufficiency because of tricuspid valve fibrosis. In patients with newly diagnosed carcinoids and suspected cardiac involvement, an echocardiogram is mandatory to evaluate if the next step in the management of the patient's situation might actually require surgical valve replacement. A PET/CT scan is not indicated since carcinoids and most well-differentiated neuroendocrine cancers are not 18-fluorodeoxyglucose (FDG)-avid and appear negative on PET scans. Quantification of the 24-hour urine excretion of 5-HIAA, a serotonin metabolite, is part of the routine initial work-up of suspected carcinoids. Serum chromogranin A can also be used as a tumor marker for further follow-up if indicated. The role of octreoscans in the initial staging of carcinoids has been questioned, but it can be valuable to identify an occult intestinal primary malignancy that should be resected to prevent subsequent bowel obstruction if surgery is appropriate in the clinical setting.

Suggested Reading

Kulke MH, Siu LL, Tepper JE, et al. Future directions in the treatment of neuroendocrine tumors: consensus report of the National Cancer Institute Neuroendocrine Tumor clinical trials planning meeting. *J Clin Oncol.* 2011;29:934-943. PMID: 21263089.

Rinke A, Müller HH, Schade-Brittinger C, et al. Placebo-controlled, double-blind, prospective, randomized study on the effect of octreotide LAR in the control of tumor growth in patients with metastatic neuroendocrine midgut tumors: a report from the PROMID Study Group. *J Clin Oncol.* 2009;27:4656-4663. PMID: 19704057.

Modlin IM, Kidd M, Drozdov I, et al. Pharmacotherapy of neuroendocrine cancers. *Expert Opin Pharmacother.* 2008;9: 2617-2626. PMID: 18803449.

10 GENITOURINARY CANCERS
SELF-EVALUATION

GENITOURINARY CANCERS QUESTIONS

10-1 A 67-year-old man with hypertension and a 50-pack per year smoking history develops gross painless hematuria and is prescribed a course of antibiotics for a presumed urinary tract infection. The hematuria persists and he is referred to a urologist who performs a cystoscopy, revealing a 3-cm mass on the posterior wall of the bladder, and a transurethral biopsy of the mass, with pathology consistent with muscle-invasive urothelial carcinoma. A computed tomography (CT) scan shows a diffusely thick-walled bladder with no evidence of suspicious lymphadenopathy.

What of the following is the next best step in management?
A. Intravesical bacille Calmette-Guérin (BCG)
B. Cisplatin-based combination chemotherapy
C. Radiation therapy
D. Repeat transurethral biopsy

10-2 An 80-year-old woman with multiple comorbidities including coronary artery disease, hypertension, and diabetes mellitus is diagnosed with a muscle-invasive bladder cancer. A CT scan reveals no hydronephrosis and no adenopathy. Although she is a surgical candidate, the patient wishes to avoid surgery.

Which of the following is the most appropriate counseling strategy for the patient?
A. Trimodality bladder preservation is associated with an inferior survival compared to radical cystectomy
B. Trimodality bladder preservation should be avoided in patients with muscle-invasive bladder cancer
C. Cisplatin chemotherapy is the only radiosensitizing agent for bladder preservation demonstrated to offer a survival benefit
D. Approximately one-third of patients treated with a bladder preservation approach will require cystectomy

10-3 A 57-year-old man is diagnosed with metastatic bladder cancer involving lung, bone, and lymph nodes. He does not have any coexisting medical problems, and his Karnofsky performance status is 90%. Laboratory studies reveal a normal hemoglobin, elevated total leukocyte count, and normal albumin.

Which of the following variables may be used to predict survival?
A. Lung metastases
B. Performance status
C. Hemoglobin
D. Lymph node metastases
E. All of the above

10-4 A 58-year-old woman who is obese and currently uses tobacco reports a 15-lb unintentional weight loss over the past 3 months, right-sided back pain, and intermittent gross hematuria. A CT scan shows a large centrally necrotic mass in the lower pole of the right kidney measuring up to 15 cm, extensive peritoneal nodules, soft tissue implants, multiple pulmonary nodules, and two liver lesions. An ultrasound-guided biopsy of a liver lesion reveals metastatic renal cell carcinoma (RCC), clear cell variant. Laboratory studies are significant for a hemoglobin of 8.2 g/dL, an elevated lactate dehydrogenase (LDH), and a platelet count of 600 x 10^9/L.

Which of the following therapies is associated with an overall survival benefit?
A. Sorafenib
B. Sunitinib
C. Bevacizumab and interferon
D. Temsirolimus
E. Pazopanib

10-5 A 72-year-old man with metastatic clear cell RCC develops progression of lung metastases after 7 months on pazopanib. Everolimus is started, and a CT scan reveals stable disease after 2 months. Several weeks later, he reports dyspnea on exertion with an aggravating dry cough. A chest x-ray reveals pulmonary nodules and increased interstitial markings.

What is the next best step in disease management?
A. Discontinue everolimus and start axitinib
B. Hold everolimus and start prednisone
C. Continue everolimus at a reduced dose
D. Continue everolimus and add sunitinib

10-6 A 65-year-old man with a past medical history significant for diabetes mellitus and chronic fatigue syndrome is diagnosed with metastatic RCC involving lung and bone. He has mild bone pain and otherwise only reports baseline moderate fatigue.

Which represents the best treatment plan?
A. Pazopanib
B. Sunitinib
C. Everolimus
D. Axitinib

10-7 A 64-year-old man with no significant past medical history presents to the emergency room with 3 days of back pain and difficulty walking. On examination, he appears uncomfortable, with lumbar spine tenderness to palpation and bilateral lower extremity weakness. Magnetic resonance imaging of the spine reveals extensive diffuse multilevel osseous metastatic disease throughout the entire spine with epidural extension of tumor noted from L2 through L4, with resultant mild to moderate compression of the spinal cord and mild cord edema. His prostate-specific antigen (PSA) level is 560 ng/mL.

What is the next most appropriate step in management?
A. Administer leuprolide acetate
B. Start bicalutamide
C. Consult neurosurgery
D. Administer zoledronic acid
E. Administer denosumab

10-8 A 68-year-old man with a past medical history of hypertension and gout sees his primary care physician for a routine visit and undergoes a digital rectal examination that reveals an enlarged prostate with a left-sided nodule (clinical T3 examination). His PSA level is 19 ng/mL. He undergoes a transrectal ultrasound-guided biopsy that reveals adenocarcinoma of the prostate—Gleason score 4+5 involving five of 12 cores with perineural invasion present. A CT scan of the abdomen and pelvis and a bone scan reveal no evidence of metastatic disease.

What is the next most appropriate step in management?
A. Brachytherapy
B. External beam radiation therapy
C. External beam radiation therapy with androgen deprivation therapy for 6 months
D. External beam radiation therapy with androgen deprivation therapy for 3 years

10-9 A 70-year-old man with a past history of coronary artery disease and hypertension has castrate-resistant prostate cancer with bone-only metastases and receives six cycles of docetaxel chemotherapy. A bone scan reveals progression of disease. He reports moderate rib pain and is using a long-acting narcotic for pain control.

Which treatment is associated with a survival benefit and an improvement in quality of life?
A. Strontium-89
B. Samarium-153
C. Radium dichloride-223
D. Denosumab
E. Zoledronic acid

10-10 A 21-year-old man notices an enlarging left testis over the past 3 months and more recent development of left-sided back pain. He sees his primary physician, who orders a testicular ultrasound that reveals an enlarged heterogeneous left testis measuring 5.4 by 3.2 by 3.0 cm. He is referred to a urologist, who orders tumor markers, revealing an alpha-fetoprotein level of 850 ng/mL, human chorionic gonadotropin level of less than 5 U/L, and an LDH level of 500 U/L (less than 1.5 times the upper limit of normal). A CT scan reveals a large, predominantly cystic 8.5- by 7.2-cm para-aortic retroperitoneal mass. A left radical inguinal orchiectomy is performed, revealing a mixed germ cell tumor (30% yolk sac, 20% embryonal carcinoma, and 50% mature cystic teratoma) involving the spermatic cord (pT3). He receives three of a planned four cycles of etoposide/cisplatin (EP) with normalization of tumor markers and develops worsening back pain. A CT scan reveals enlargement of the retroperitoneal mass.

Which represents the next best step in management?
A. Administer final cycle of EP chemotherapy
B. Salvage chemotherapy with paclitaxel/ifosfamide/ cisplatin (TIP)
C. High-dose chemotherapy with stem cell rescue
D. Retroperitoneal lymph node dissection

10-11 A 26-year-old man with a past history of ulcerative colitis develops right testicular pain after a long bicycle ride. He takes ibuprofen with minimal relief, and after 2 weeks of persistent discomfort, he sees his primary care physician. His physician palpates an enlarged firm right testis and orders an ultrasound demonstrating a heterogeneous testicular mass measuring 2.8 by 1.8 by 2.4 cm. A right radical inguinal orchiectomy is performed revealing a pure seminoma limited to the testis with vascular/lymphatic invasion present. Serum tumor markers, chest x-ray, and a CT scan of the abdomen and pelvis are normal.

Which is the preferred management plan?
A. Surveillance
B. Bleomycin/etoposide/cisplatin (BEP) for two cycles
C. Radiation therapy
D. Retroperitoneal lymph node dissection

10-12 A 37-year-old man with a past history of a stage IIC nonseminomatous germ cell tumor diagnosed 7 years earlier and treated with BEP for three cycles followed by a retroperitoneal lymph node dissection with no evidence of viable germ cell tumor develops mid-back pain and is referred for a CT scan of the abdomen and pelvis that reveals a 5-cm retroperitoneal mass. Serum tumor markers are normal and a biopsy reveals metastatic germ cell tumor.

Which of the following is the next best step in management?
A. Salvage chemotherapy with vinblastine/ifosfamide/ cisplatin
B. High-dose chemotherapy followed by stem cell rescue
C. Surgical resection of the mass
D. Radiation therapy

10-1   B

The patient has been diagnosed with muscle-invasive bladder cancer, a potentially lethal phenotype. There is no role for repeat transurethral resection or for intravesical therapy, which is used to treat noninvasive bladder cancer. Radiation therapy alone is a suboptimal treatment for invasive bladder cancer, although the use of a trimodality bladder preservation strategy—which includes a complete transurethral resection followed by concurrent chemotherapy and radiation therapy—does represent an option. In two randomized clinical trials and a meta-analysis, neoadjuvant cisplatin-based chemotherapy prior to radical cystectomy has been shown to offer a survival benefit in patients with muscle-invasive bladder cancer.

Suggested Reading

Grossman HB, Natale RB, Tangen CM, et al. Neoadjuvant chemotherapy plus cystectomy compared with cystectomy alone for locally advanced bladder cancer. *N Engl J Med.* 2003;349:859-866. PMID: 12944571.

International Collaboration of Trialists, Medical Research Council Advanced Bladder Cancer Working Party (now the National Cancer Research Institute Bladder Cancer Clinical Studies Group), European Organisation for Research and Treatment of Cancer Genito-Urinary Tract Cancer Group, et al. International phase III trial assessing neoadjuvant cisplatin, methotrexate, and vinblastine chemotherapy for muscle-invasive bladder cancer: long-term results of the BA06 30894 trial. *J Clin Oncol.* 2011;29:2171-2177. Epub 2011 Apr 18. PMID: 21502557.

Advanced Bladder Cancer (ABC) Meta-analysis Collaboration. Neoadjuvant chemotherapy in invasive bladder cancer. update of a systematic review and meta-analysis of individual patient data advanced bladder cancer (ABC) meta-analysis collaboration. *Eur Urol.* 2005;48:202-205; discussion 5-6. PMID: 15939524.

10-2   D

A trimodality bladder preservation approach may be considered in select patients with T1 and muscle-invasive bladder cancer and includes a complete transurethral resection followed by concurrent chemotherapy and radiation. Although trimodality bladder preservation has not been formally compared to radical cystectomy, survival outcomes appear comparable. Alternative noncisplatin regimens have demonstrated a benefit in patients, including a recently published randomized trial including 5-fluorouracil and mitomycin plus radiotherapy versus radiotherapy alone. Approximately one-third of patients initiated on a bladder preservation approach will undergo a radical cystectomy because of an initial incomplete response or recurrent muscle-invasive disease.

Suggested Reading

Balar A, Bajorin DF, Milowsky MI. Management of invasive bladder cancer in patients who are not candidates for or decline cystectomy. *Ther Adv Oncol.* 2011;3:107-117. PMID: 21904567.

Efstathiou JA, Spiegel DY, Shipley WU, et al. Long-term outcomes of selective bladder preservation by combined-modality therapy for invasive bladder cancer: the MGH experience. *Eur Urol.* 2012;61: 705-711. PMID: 22101114.

James ND, Hussain SA, Hall E, et al. Radiotherapy with or without chemotherapy in muscle-invasive bladder cancer. *N Engl J Med.* 2012;366:1477-1488. PMID: 22512481.

10-3   E

Several prognostic models have been developed to predict survival in patients with metastatic bladder cancer. An early model incorporating two variables—Karnofsky performance status (less than 80%) and presence of visceral metastases (lung, liver, or bone)—demonstrated survival times for patients who had zero, one, or two risk factors of 33 months, 13.4 months, and 9.3 months, respectively. More recently, two nomograms for predicting survival in patients with metastatic urothelial cancer include the following pretreatment variables: the presence and number of visceral metastases, albumin, performance status, hemoglobin, site of the primary tumor, lymph node metastases, and leukocyte count.

Suggested Reading

Bajorin DF, Dodd PM, Mazumdar M, et al. Long-term survival in metastatic transitional-cell carcinoma and prognostic factors predicting outcome to chemotherapy. *J Clin Oncol.* 1999;17: 3173-3181. PMID: 10506615.

Galsky MD, Moshier E, Krege S, et al. Nomogram for predicting survival in patients with unresectable and/or metastatic urothelial cancer who are treated with cisplatin-based chemotherapy. *Cancer.* 2013;119:3012-3019. PMID: 23720216.

Apolo AB, Ostrovnaya I, Halabi S, et al. Prognostic model for predicting survival of patients with metastatic urothelial cancer treated with cisplatin-based chemotherapy. *J Natl Cancer Inst.*2013;105:499-503. PMID: 23411591.

10-4 D

The prognosis of a newly diagnosed patient with metastatic RCC may be used to guide disease management. Poor prognostic factors for survival in the cytokine era included no prior nephrectomy, low performance status, low hemoglobin level, high corrected serum calcium, and high serum LDH. For patients with zero, one to two, and three or more risk factors, the median survival times were 24 months (good risk), 12 months (intermediate risk), and 5 months (poor risk). Newer prognostic models for patients with metastatic RCC treated in the current targeted therapy era include these prognostic factors in addition to others such as platelet count, alkaline phosphatase, and number and sites of metastatic disease. Although all of the listed agents represent potential first-line treatment strategies, temsirolimus is the only agent demonstrating a survival benefit in untreated patients with three or more of six poor prognostic factors (elevated LDH, low hemoglobin, elevated corrected serum calcium, time from initial diagnosis of less than 1 year, a low performance status, and metastases in multiple organs).

Suggested Reading

Motzer RJ, Mazumdar M, Bacik J, et al. Survival and prognostic stratification of 670 patients with advanced renal cell carcinoma. *J Clin Oncol.* 1999;17:2530-2540. PMID: 10561319.

Heng DY, Xie W, Regan MM, et al. Prognostic factors for overall survival in patients with metastatic renal cell carcinoma treated with vascular endothelial growth factor-targeted agents: results from a large, multicenter study. *J Clin Oncol.* 2009;27:5794-5799. Epub 2009 Oct 13. PMID: 19826129.

Heng DY, Xie W, Regan MM, et al. External validation and comparison with other models of the International Metastatic Renal-Cell Carcinoma Database Consortium prognostic model: a population-based study. *Lancet Oncol.* 2013;14:141-148. PMID: 23312463.

Hudes G, Carducci M, Tomczak P, et al. Temsirolimus, interferon alfa, or both for advanced renal-cell carcinoma. *N Engl J Med.* 2007;356: 2271-2281. PMID: 17538086.

10-5 B

Mammalian target of rapamycin (mTOR) inhibitors including everolimus are associated with reversible noninfectious pneumonitis. In the setting of symptomatic pneumonitis, prescription of a corticosteroid and either holding or reducing the dose of everolimus are appropriate options. In a retrospective review of 310 patients with metastatic RCC treated with temsirolimus and/or everolimus, noninfectious pneumonitis occurred in 23% of patients treated with everolimus. Symptoms include cough, dyspnea, and fever. In patients with grade 1 (mild) pneumonitis defined as asymptomatic—radiographic findings only—everolimus may be continued without dose adjustment with close monitoring, including radiographic and clinical assessment.

Suggested Reading

Atkinson BJ, Cauley DH, Ng C, et al. Mammalian target of rapamycin (mTOR) inhibitor-associated non-infectious pneumonitis in patients with renal cell cancer: predictors, management, and outcomes. *BJU Int.* 2014;113:376-382. PMID: 24053120.

White DA, Camus P, Endo M, et al. Noninfectious pneumonitis after everolimus therapy for advanced renal cell carcinoma. *Am J Respir Crit Care Med.* 2010;182:396-403. PMID: 20194812.

10-6 A

Although both sunitinib and pazopanib represent potential first-line treatment options for metastatic RCC, a recently reported randomized phase III noninferiority trial comparing the efficacy and safety of pazopanib and sunitinib demonstrated similar progression-free survival. However, the safety profile favored pazopanib with less fatigue, hand-foot syndrome, and thrombocytopenia. Health-related quality-of-life measures also favored pazopanib. Everolimus and axitinib are used after progression on first-line therapy.

Suggested Reading

Motzer RJ, Hutson TE, Cella D, et al. Pazopanib versus sunitinib in metastatic renal-cell carcinoma. *N Engl J Med.* 2013;369: 722-731. PMID: 23964934.

Motzer RJ, Escudier B, Oudard S, et al. Efficacy of everolimus in advanced renal cell carcinoma: a double-blind, randomised, placebo-controlled phase III trial. *Lancet.* 2008;372:449-456. Epub 2008 Jul 22. PMID: 18653228.

Rini BI, Escudier B, Tomczak P, et al. Comparative effectiveness of axitinib versus sorafenib in advanced renal cell carcinoma (AXIS): a randomised phase 3 trial. *Lancet.* 2011;378:1931-1939. PMID: 22056247.

10-7 C

Spinal cord compression related to metastatic cancer is an oncologic emergency. The diffuse bone involvement and elevated PSA are consistent with metastatic prostate cancer. In a randomized trial of surgery followed by radiotherapy compared with radiotherapy alone in patients with spinal cord compression caused by metastatic cancer, significantly more patients in the surgery group than in the radiotherapy group were able to walk after treatment. Administration of leuprolide acetate is associated with an initial testosterone flare and is contraindicated in the setting of impending or existing cord compression, and bicalutamide monotherapy will not reliably treat cord compression. Both zoledronic acid and denosumab are used to decrease skeletal-related complications in patients with bone metastases.

Suggested Reading

Patchell RA, Tibbs PA, Regine WF, et al. Direct decompressive surgical resection in the treatment of spinal cord compression caused by metastatic cancer: a randomised trial. *Lancet.* 2005;366:643-648. PMID: 16112300.

Saad F, Gleason DM, Murray R, et al. Long-term efficacy of zoledronic acid for the prevention of skeletal complications in patients with metastatic hormone-refractory prostate cancer. *J Natl Cancer Inst.* 2004;96:879-882. PMID: 15173273.

Fizazi K, Carducci M, Smith M, et al. Denosumab versus zoledronic acid for treatment of bone metastases in men with castration-resistant prostate cancer: a randomised, double-blind study. *Lancet.* 2011;377:813-822. Epub 2011 Feb 25. PMID: 21353695.

10-8 D

The management options for localized prostate cancer include watchful waiting or active surveillance, radical prostatectomy, and radiation therapy. In the setting of high-risk prostate cancer as defined in this patient by a Gleason score of 9 and a cT3 examination, watchful waiting or active surveillance is not an appropriate option. Brachytherapy is also not appropriate as monotherapy in patients with locally advanced prostate cancer. Based on the pretreatment features including Gleason score, clinical stage, and number of involved cores, the risk of lymph node involvement is approximately 50% (www.nomograms.org). Randomized trials have demonstrated a survival benefit associated with long-term androgen deprivation therapy (2 to 3 years) with radiation therapy compared to radiation therapy alone in locally advanced disease. Additionally, long-term androgen deprivation therapy is associated with a survival benefit over short-term (4 to 6 months) therapy.

Suggested Reading

Bolla M, Collette L, Blank L, et al. Long-term results with immediate androgen suppression and external irradiation in patients with locally advanced prostate cancer (an EORTC study): a phase III randomised trial. *Lancet.* 2002;360:103-106. PMID: 12126818.

Horwitz EM, Bae K, Hanks GE, et al. Ten-year follow-up of radiation therapy oncology group protocol 92-02: a phase III trial of the duration of elective androgen deprivation in locally advanced prostate cancer. *J Clin Oncol.* 2008;26:2497-2504. Epub 2008 Apr 14. PMID: 18413638.

Bolla M, de Reijke TM, Van Tienhoven G, et al. Duration of androgen suppression in the treatment of prostate cancer. *N Engl J Med.* 2009;360:2516-2527. PMID: 19516032.

10-9 C

In a recently reported randomized trial of the alpha-emitter radium dichloride-223 compared with placebo in men with metastatic castrate-resistant prostate cancer with symptomatic bone metastases, overall survival was significantly improved with radium-223 with a median survival of 14.9 months versus 11.3 months for men treated with placebo (HR 0.70, 95% CI 0.58, 0.83; $p < 0.001$). Time to first symptomatic skeletal event and all other main secondary endpoints were improved with radium-223. A significantly greater percentage of patients treated with radium-223 compared to placebo had an improvement in quality of life as measured by the Functional Assessment Cancer Therapy—Prostate questionnaire. The bone-seeking radiopharmaceutical agents strontium-89 and samarium-153 have been shown to reduce pain without a survival benefit. Both denosumab and zoledronic acid are used for the prevention of skeletal-related events without a survival benefit.

Suggested Reading

Parker C, Nilsson S, Heinrich D, et al. Alpha emitter radium-223 and survival in metastatic prostate cancer. *N Engl J Med.* 2013;369: 213-223. PMID: 23863050.

Fizazi K, Carducci M, Smith M, et al. Denosumab versus zoledronic acid for treatment of bone metastases in men with castration-resistant prostate cancer: a randomised, double-blind study. *Lancet.* 2011;377:813-822. Epub 2011 Feb 25. PMID: 21353695.

10-10 D

The patient has a good-risk mixed nonseminomatous germ cell tumor and is appropriately treated with etoposide/cisplatin chemotherapy for a planned four cycles. The development of worsening back pain during treatment with normalization of tumor markers and an enlarging retroperitoneal mass is consistent with a growing teratoma syndrome. This requires an immediate retroperitoneal lymph node dissection.

Suggested Reading

Logothetis CJ, Samuels ML, Trindade A, et al. The growing teratoma syndrome. *Cancer.* 1982;50:1629-1635. PMID: 6288220.

Jeffery GM, Theaker JM, Lee AH, et al. The growing teratoma syndrome. *BR J Urol.* 1991;67:195-202. PMID: 2004236.

Tongaonkar HB, Deshmane VH, Dalal AV, et al. Growing teratoma syndrome. *J Surg Oncol.* 1994;55:56-60. PMID: 8289455.

10-11 A

The management of early-stage germ cell tumors is risk-stratified based on the tumor type (i.e., seminoma or nonseminoma) and the likelihood of retroperitoneal lymph node involvement. For clinical stage I seminoma, the likelihood of disease relapse is between 15% to 20%, mostly in the retroperitoneum. The patient has a stage IB (pT2N0M0S0) seminoma, and the management options include surveillance, single-agent carboplatin for one or two cycles, and radiation therapy to the retroperitoneum. The preferred management in a compliant patient is surveillance based on the potential for late risks including secondary malignancies associated with radiation and the unknown potential late risks and limited follow-up with single-agent carboplatin. Two cycles of BEP or a retroperitoneal lymph node dissection represent options for the management of early-stage nonseminoma, not seminoma. Radiation therapy is contraindicated in the setting of inflammatory bowel disease.

Suggested Reading

Motzer RJ, Agarwal N, Beard C, et al. NCCN clinical practice guidelines in oncology: testicular cancer. *J Natl Compr Canc Netw.* 2009;7: 672-693. PMID: 19555582.

Nichols CR, Roth B, Albers P, et al. Active surveillance is the preferred approach to clinical stage I testicular cancer. *J Clin Oncol.* 2013;31: 3490-3493. PMID: 24002502.

de Wit R, Bosl GJ. Optimal management of clinical stage I testis cancer: one size does not fit all. *J Clin Oncol.* 2013;31:3477-3479. PMID: 24002512.

10-12 C

The majority of relapses occur within 2 years of initial therapy; however, 2% to 3% of patients present with a late relapse, with most occurring more than 5 years after initial treatment. Late relapse is associated with a high degree of resistance to salvage chemotherapy and with an overall poor prognosis. The majority of late relapses involve lung or retroperitoneal nodes, and lack of a prior retroperitoneal lymph node dissection or an inadequate dissection are associated with an increased risk for late relapse. Improved outcomes in late relapse are associated with complete surgical excision of disease.

Suggested Reading

Sharp DS, Carver BS, Eggener SE, et al. Clinical outcome and predictors of survival in late relapse of germ cell tumor. *J Clin Oncol.* 2008;26: 5524-5529. Epub 2008 Oct 20. PMID: 18936477.

George DW, Foster RS, Hromas RA, et al. Update on late relapse of germ cell tumor: a clinical and molecular analysis. *J Clin Oncol.* 2003;21:113-122. PMID: 12506179.

11 GYNECOLOGIC CANCERS
SELF-EVALUATION

GYNECOLOGIC CANCERS QUESTIONS

11-1 A 50-year-old woman with newly diagnosed endo-metrial adenocarcinoma comes to you for consultation. The pathology report states that there is loss of *MSH2* by immunohistochemistry (IHC). In addition to discussing the management of her endometrial cancer you recommend genetic counseling.

For which of the following cancers may this patient be at increased genetic risk?
A. Lobular breast cancer
B. Clear cell renal cell carcinoma
C. Medullary thyroid carcinoma
D. Adenocarcinoma of the colon

11-2 A 60-year-old woman presents with postmenopausal bleeding. She undergoes total hysterectomy, bilateral salpingo-oophorectomy, and lymph node dissection. Pathology shows grade 3 endometrioid adenocarcinoma with 50% invasion into the myometrium, and lymphovascular invasion. None of the resected lymph nodes are involved by cancer.

What is your recommendation for treatment?
A. No additional treatment
B. Adjuvant megestrol acetate
C. Adjuvant whole-pelvis radiation or platinum-taxane chemotherapy
D. Adjuvant whole-abdomen radiation

11-3 A 62-year-old woman with stage IV, suboptimally debulked ovarian carcinoma is receiving paclitaxel/carboplatin treatment. At her office visit for the fourth cycle, she complains of worsening peripheral neuropathy. She cannot button her blouse, and the neuropathy pain in her feet wakes her several times during the night.

Which symptom management option do you recommend?
A. Continue current dose and schedule of paclitaxel/carboplatin; start gabapentin treatment for the neuropathy complaints
B. Discontinue paclitaxel, continue carboplatin
C. Discontinue paclitaxel, substitute nanoparticle albumin-bound (nab)-paclitaxel, continue carboplatin
D. Continue paclitaxel, substitute cisplatin for the carboplatin

11-4 A 48-year-old woman presents with abnormal vaginal bleeding. On exam she has a palpable right adnexal mass. Endometrial biopsy shows endometrial carcinoma. She undergoes hysterectomy, bilateral salpingo-oophorectomy, and complete surgical staging. The pathology review shows a 4-cm granulosa cell tumor of the right ovary and an International Federation of Gynecology and Obstetrics (FIGO) grade 1 endometrioid adenocarcinoma of the endometrium with no myometrial invasion. The rest of the surgical specimens are negative for tumor involvement.

What is your recommendation for further treatment?
A. Observation, no further active treatment
B. Estrogen replacement therapy for 5 years
C. Adjuvant bleomycin/etoposide/cisplatin (BEP)
D. Adjuvant paclitaxel/carboplatin

11-5 A 75-year-old woman presents with postmenopausal bleeding. Endometrial biopsy suggests carcinoma. She undergoes total hysterectomy, bilateral salpingo-oophorectomy, and staging. Final pathology shows uterine carcinosarcoma with deep myometrial invasion. All other surgical specimens are negative for tumor involvement. Post-resection imaging shows no evidence of disease.

What is your treatment recommendation?
A. No additional treatment
B. Adjuvant two-drug platinum or taxane-based chemotherapy
C. Adjuvant whole-abdomen radiation
D. Adjuvant whole-pelvis radiation

11-6 A 48-year-old woman presents for gynecologic evaluation, reporting mild, persistent pelvic pressure and bloating. On pelvic examination, the cervix appears normal. A Pap smear yields cells suspicious for adenocarcinoma with features suggestive of serous carcinoma; human papillomavirus (HPV) testing is negative for all high-risk subtypes. Sonography shows small pelvic ascites and a right adnexal mass. CA-125 is 1,536 u/mL. Her family history is negative for colon cancer and endometrial cancer; a paternal aunt had breast cancer at age 50. The patient's body mass index (BMI) is 24.

Which of the following is the most likely diagnosis?
A. HPV-negative adenocarcinoma of the cervix, with metastasis to the right ovary
B. Endometrial adenocarcinoma with endocervical and right ovarian involvement
C. Fallopian tube carcinoma
D. Vaginal adenocarcinoma

11-7 A 70-year-old woman has recurrent uterine carcinosarcoma. She initially presented with stage III disease. After complete resection, she received treatment with paclitaxel/carboplatin. One month after her sixth cycle of chemotherapy she developed bloating, ascites, and elevation of her CA-125 to 2,489 u/mL. She denied pain, had a performance status of 80%, and wanted to pursue second-line therapy. Four days ago she started treatment with ifosfamide. Her family reports that the patient is alert and appears comfortable but not quite "herself," with episodes of confusion when she seems to be talking to someone who is not in the room. She has had no hematuria. Pretreament laboratory values showed hemoglobin of 9.9 mg/dL; creatinine of 1.4; albumin of 2.9; and normal levels of sodium, potassium, calcium, aspartate aminotransferase (AST), alanine aminotransferase (ALT), bilirubin, and alkaline phosphatase.

Which of the following is the likely explanation of her symptoms?
A. Ifosfamide toxicity
B. Brain metastases
C. Hypercalcemia of malignancy
D. Narcotic overdose

11-8 A 66-year-old woman presents with cough and dyspnea on exertion. Computed tomography (CT) imaging shows multiple bilateral lung metastases, measuring up to 7 cm. Biopsy shows high-grade leiomyosarcoma. The patient reports a hysterectomy for enlarging fibroids 2 years ago. Review of the uterine pathology shows high-grade leiomyosarcoma.

Which of the following statements about treatment for high-grade uterine leiomyosarcoma has been demonstrated in the prospective clinical trial setting to be true?
A. Doxorubicin plus ifosfamide yields superior overall survival outcomes compared with single-agent doxorubicin
B. Fixed-dose rate gemcitabine plus docetaxel achieves objective response in about one-third of patients
C. Fixed-dose rate gemcitabine plus docetaxel yields higher objective response rate compared to doxorubicin
D. Adjuvant fixed-dose rate gemcitabine plus docetaxel followed by doxorubicin improves overall survival compared to observation for uterus-limited disease

11-9 A 32-year-old woman presents with a large pelvic mass. She undergoes right salpingo-oophorectomy, with preservation of the left ovary and uterus. Pathology shows ovarian dysgerminoma. The operative note states there were no other visibly suspicious areas of disease.

Which of the following will you recommend for management of her disease?

A. Treatment with platinum-based chemotherapy

B. Re-operation for completion hysterectomy, left salpingo-oophorectomy and staging; chemotherapy recommendations to be made according to final tumor staging

C. Whole-pelvis radiation

D. Oral contraceptive treatment for prevention of a second ovarian malignancy

11-1   D

Endometrial carcinoma is part of hereditary nonpolyposis colon cancer (Lynch) syndrome and is often the first diagnosed cancer among women with Lynch syndrome. Certain histologic characteristics and patient age may suggest the possibility of a Lynch syndrome endometrial cancer. Demonstrating loss of one of the mismatch repair enzyme proteins by IHC can further corroborate the possibility of Lynch syndrome. Patients should be referred for genetic counseling and testing. Patients with endometrial carcinoma who have Lynch syndrome are at increased risk for colon cancer.

A genetic increased risk for lobular breast cancer is found in patients with E-cadherin germ-line mutations. Such patients are also at risk for gastric cancer. Patients with Lynch syndrome are at increased risk for urothelial cell tumors but not renal cell carcinomas. Medullary thyroid carcinoma is part of the multiple endocrine neoplasia 2 (MEN2) familial syndrome.

Suggested Reading

Vasen HF, Stormorken A, Menko FH, et al. MSH2 mutation carriers are at higher risk of cancer than MLH1 mutation carriers: a study of hereditary nonpolyposis colorectal cancer families. *J Clin Oncol.* 2001;19:4074-4080. PMID: 11600610.

Bonadona V, Bonaïti B, Olschwang S, et al. Cancer risks associated with germline mutations in MLH1, MSH2, and MSH6 genes in Lynch syndrome. *JAMA.* 2011;305:2304-2310. PMID: 21642682.

11-2   C

Patients with endometrial cancer that does not involve lymph nodes are classified by uterine factors (grade, lymphovascular invasion, depth of myometrial invasion) and age to determine which patients are considered "high-intermediate risk" (HIR). HIR patients have a 12% to 20% risk of recurrence and it is standard to offer such patients some form of adjuvant therapy. Whole-pelvis radiation therapy has been the standard of care, although there are data suggesting that vaginal brachytherapy may be adequate, and a recent phase III study compared paclitaxel/carboplatin adjuvant chemotherapy to whole-pelvis radiation in this population. Neither megestrol acetate nor observation would be considered adequate treatment for this HIR patient.

Suggested Reading

Keys HM, Roberts JA, Brunetto VL, et al. A phase III trial of surgery with or without adjunctive external pelvic radiation therapy in intermediate risk endometrial adenocarcinoma: a Gynecologic Oncology Group study. *Gynecol Oncol.* 2004;92:744-751. PMID: 14984936.

Nout RA, Smit VT, Putter H, et al. Vaginal brachytherapy versus pelvic external beam radiotherapy for patients with endometrial cancer of high-intermediate risk (PORTEC-2): an open-label, non-inferiority, randomised trial. *Lancet.* 2010;375:816-823. PMID: 20206777.

11-3   B

This patient had at least grade 2 neuropathy, attributable to paclitaxel. The paclitaxel should be discontinued for this cycle; continuing paclitaxel at the current dose would risk further impairment of function, which may not be reversible. Substitution of nab-paclitaxel is incorrect since this agent is associated with a similar or even higher risk for neurotoxicity compared to paclitaxel. Substituting cisplatin for carboplatin is incorrect since the risk for neurotoxicity is higher with cisplatin compared with carboplatin.

Suggested Reading

Gradishar WJ, Tjulandin S, Davidson N, et al. Phase III trial of nanoparticle albumin-bound paclitaxel compared with polyethylated castor oil-based paclitaxel in women with breast cancer. *J Clin Oncol.* 2005;23:7794-7803. PMID: 16172456.

11-4   A

Granulosa cell tumors are frequently unilateral. These tumors are often estrogen-producing and may present with abnormal vaginal bleeding due to endometrial hyperplasia or due to a concurrent estrogen-stimulated endometrial carcinoma. Patients with granulosa cell tumors are at risk for recurrence, although the time to recurrence can be very long, sometimes exceeding 10 years from the original diagnosis. It would not be considered standard to give estrogen replacement therapy to women with this hormone-sensitive tumor, thus B is incorrect. While BEP, and more recently paclitaxel/carboplatin, has demonstrated activity in advanced granulosa cell tumors, adjuvant BEP or adjuvant paclitaxel/carboplatin would not generally be recommended for stage I, newly diagnosed granulosa cell tumors; thus C is incorrect. Similarly, a grade 1, stage IA endometrial carcinoma in a 42-year-old patient would not require adjuvant therapy, therefore D is incorrect.

Suggested Reading

Schumer ST, Cannistra SA. Granulosa cell tumor of the ovary. *J Clin Oncol.* 2003;21:1180-1189. PMID: 12637488.

11-5 B

Adjuvant ifosfamide/cisplatin for all stages of uterine carcinoma yielded higher overall survival compared with adjuvant whole-abdomen radiation, thus C is incorrect. Paclitaxel/carboplatin achieved high objective response rates as first-line treatment for patients with measurable disease, and is being compared to ifosfamide/paclitaxel as adjuvant therapy in a phase III trial.

Adjuvant chemotherapy with paclitaxel/carboplatin, paclitaxel/ifosfamide, or ifosfamide/cisplatin is appropriate for completely resected carcinosarcoma (stage I, II, III, or IV), thus B is correct.

Suggested Reading

Wolfson AH, Brady MF, Rocereto T, et al. A gynecologic oncology group randomized phase III trial of whole abdominal irradiation (WAI) vs. cisplatin-ifosfamide and mesna (CIM) as post-surgical therapy in stage I–IV carcinosarcoma (CS) of the uterus. *Gynecol Oncol.* 2007;107:177-185. PMID: 17822748.

Powell MA, Filiaci VL, Rose PG, et al. Phase II evaluation of paclitaxel and carboplatin in the treatment of carcinosarcoma of the uterus: a Gynecologic Oncology Group study. *J Clin Oncol.* 2010;28: 2727-2731. PMID: 20421537.

11-6 C

Fallopian tube cancer may present with adenocarcinoma cells on Pap smear due to shedding of the malignant cells from the tubal lumen. The high CA-125 level suggests an ovarian or fallopian tube cancer, although it may be elevated in other Mullerian cancers. The serous features suggest ovarian or fallopian tube primary cancer, although some endometrial carcinomas may be classified as serous. The family history supports the possibility of a fallopian tube or ovarian primary. Cervix cancer, both adenocarcinomas and squamous cell carcinomas, are nearly always associated with HPV (thus A is incorrect). Endometrial carcinoma may also present with a positive Pap smear but the patient's low BMI, young age, and lack of family history make this diagnosis less likely than a tubal or ovarian primary.

Suggested Reading

Mulvany NJ, Mitchell G, Allen DG. Adenocarcinoma cells in Pap smears. *Pathology.* 2009;41:411-418. PMID: 19900079.

11-7 A

Risk factors of ifosfamide central nervous system toxicity include older age, low albumin, and renal insufficiency—all of which are present in this patient. Brain metastases are extremely rare in carcinosarcoma; hypercalcemia of malignancy would be unlikely to develop over 4 days, and narcotic overdose is unlikely in a patient who is not taking pain medications and who is fully alert.

Suggested Reading

Kettle JK, Grauer D, Folker TL, et al. Effectiveness of exogenous albumin administration for the prevention of ifosfamide-induced encephalopathy. *Pharmacotherapy.* 2010;30:812-817. PMID: 20653357.

11-8 B

Fixed-dose rate gemcitabine plus docetaxel has demonstrated high objective response rates, ranging from 27% as second-line therapy to 35% as first-line therapy, in several prospective trials and is an accepted first-line treatment for metastatic uterine leiomyosarcoma. Doxorubicin with or without ifosfamide is also an accepted first-line treatment. These two regimens have not been directly compared in a prospective clinical trial. In soft-tissue sarcoma, doxorubicin plus ifosfamide may achieve higher objective response rates compared to single-agent doxorubicin, but this has not translated into higher overall survival rates. A prospective phase II trial of fixed-dose rate gemcitabine plus docetaxel followed by doxorubicin suggested that adjuvant therapy may improve progression-free survival but a phase III trial with an observation control arm is required in order to determine whether this regimen can improve overall survival. Currently, standard management after resection of uterus-limited disease is observation.

Suggested Reading

Hensley ML, Wathen JK, Maki RG, et al. Adjuvant therapy for high-grade, uterus-limited leiomyosarcoma: results of a phase 2 trial (SARC 005). *Cancer.* 2013;119:1555-1561. PMID: 23335221.

Hensley ML, Blessing JA, Mannel R, et al. Fixed-dose rate gemcitabine plus docetaxel as first-line therapy for metastatic uterine leiomyosarcoma: a Gynecologic Oncology Group phase II trial. *Gynecol Oncol.* 2008;109:329-334. PMID: 18534250.

Hensley ML, Blessing JA, Degeest K, et al. Fixed-dose rate gemcitabine plus docetaxel as second-line therapy for metastatic uterine leiomyosarcoma: a Gynecologic Oncology Group phase II study. *Gynecol Oncol.* 2008;109:323-328. PMID: 18394689.

11-9   A

This patient has a malignant ovarian germ cell tumor. As with male germ cell tumors, treatment of these malignancies with platinum-based chemotherapy has improved patient outcomes. Most dysgerminomas are unilateral, and in young women, fertility-sparing surgery is generally appropriate (thus B is incorrect). Indeed, fertility and pregnancy outcomes after cancer treatment are favorable for this population. C is incorrect because data show high chance for cure with chemotherapy and the pelvic radiation would be highly likely to impair future fertility. D is incorrect because the protective effect of oral contraceptives pertains to epithelial ovarian cancer rather than to germ cell tumors.

Suggested Reading

Zhang R, Sun YC, Zhang GY, et al. Treatment of malignant ovarian germ cell tumors and preservation of fertility. *Eur J Gynaecol Oncol.* 2012;33:489-492. PMID: 23185794.

Williams SD, Kauderer J, Burnett AF, et al. Adjuvant therapy of completely resected dysgerminoma with carboplatin and etoposide: a trial of the Gynecologic Oncology Group. *Gynecol Oncol.* 2004; 95:496-499. PMID: 15581952.

Weinberg LE, Lurain JR, Singh DK, et al. Survival and reproductive outcomes in women treated for malignant ovarian germ cell tumors. *Gynecol Oncol.* 2011;121:285-289. PMID: 21256579.

12 MALIGNANT MELANOMA
SELF-EVALUATION

MALIGNANT MELANOMA QUESTIONS

12-1 A 36-year-old man with stage III melanoma is receiving high-dose interferon (IFN) therapy. He has completed 4 weeks of daily intravenous therapy and is now in the second month of subcutaneous maintenance therapy with IFN-alpha-2b. Laboratory studies from yesterday revealed a normal complete blood count (CBC) and differential count but the serum bilirubin was 1.9 mg/dL, the aspartate aminotransferase was 510 units/mL, and the alanine aminotransferase (ALT) was 480 units/mL. He feels well except for fatigue. His physical examination last week was within normal limits.

Which of the following should you recommend regarding therapy?
A. Continue with current treatment plan
B. Discontinue IFN therapy permanently
C. Continue IFN therapy but reduce to 75% of the current dose
D. Hold IFN until liver function tests normalize, then restart IFN at a 50% dose reduction

12-2 A 34-year-old woman was recently diagnosed with a 0.53-mm–thick melanoma. There was no ulceration, it was a Clark level III, and the mitotic count was zero. The melanoma occurred on her right posterior calf. The patient had blood work performed that included a CBC, chemistry panel, and lactate dehydrogenase, all of which were normal.

Which of the following is appropriate for this patient?
A. No imaging studies
B. Computed tomography (CT) scan of the chest/abdomen/pelvis and magnetic resonance imaging (MRI) of the brain
C. Positron emission tomography (PET)/CT scan and MRI of the brain
D. Bone scan, CT scan of the chest/abdomen/pelvis, and brain MRI

12-3 A 64-year-old man was recently diagnosed with stage IV melanoma. Staging work-up showed multiple liver, lung, and bone metastases. Symptoms at this time include mild shortness of breath (SOB), cough, significant bone pain, and an 8-lb weight loss. Mutation testing for *BRAF* confirmed *BRAF V600K* mutation.

What treatment would you recommend now?
A. Dabrafenib
B. Trametinib
C. Imatinib
D. Sorafenib

12-4 You have been treating a 62-year-old man with stage IV melanoma with ipilimumab. He has completed four cycles of therapy, which he tolerated well except for mild skin rash. His dose of ipilimumab was 3 mg/kg. He had follow-up CT scans that showed a slight increase in the size of metastatic lung nodules and subcutaneous nodules. He has no new sites of metastases. Prior testing for *BRAF* mutation showed no mutation. The patient has no symptoms at this time.

What do you recommend?
A. Continue ipilimumab at 3 mg/kg
B. Continue ipilimumab but increase the dose to 10 mg/kg
C. Begin treatment with vemurafenib
D. Monitor and repeat CT scans in 8 weeks

12-5 You are seeing a 55-year-old woman with stage IV melanoma. You are recommending treatment with ipilimumab.

Which of the following side effects should be discussed?
A. Fever, congestive heart failure, and diarrhea
B. Diarrhea, skin rash, endocrinopathies
C. Fever, chills, depression, neutropenia, and abnormal liver function tests
D. Neutropenia, peripheral edema, and pleural effusion

12-6 You are seeing a 63-year-old woman with stage IV melanoma. You are recommending treatment with vemurafenib.

Which of the following side effects should be discussed?
A. Diarrhea, myelosuppression, thyroid dysfunction
B. Cardiac dysfunction, fever, skin rash
C. Photosensitivity, squamous cell skin cancer, skin rash, arthralgias
D. Nausea, vomiting, weight loss

12-7 A 40-year-old woman presents with a mild cough, fatigue, and some weight loss. She was treated for melanoma on her left lower leg 3 years ago. Imaging studies reveal multiple pulmonary nodules. A CT-guided biopsy confirms the diagnosis of metastatic melanoma.

Analysis of the tumor for which of the following would be most useful in determining treatment options?
A. *KIT*
B. *BRAF*
C. *NRAS*
D. *MEK*

12-8 A 48-year-old man was recently diagnosed with stage IV melanoma. Staging work-up showed multiple liver, lung, and bone metastases. Brain MRI demonstrated two central nervous system (CNS) brain metastases, a 1.5-cm right frontal lobe lesion, and a 2.0-cm right temporal lobe lesion. Symptoms at this time include mild SOB, cough, and significant bone pain. The patient has no neurologic symptoms. Mutation testing for *BRAF* confirmed *BRAF V600E* mutation.

Which of the following is the best systemic therapeutic option?
A. Temozolomide
B. Dabrafenib
C. Interleukin (IL)-2
D. Ipilimumab

12-9 A 48-year-old woman presents to your office for a second opinion regarding the management of her melanoma. Three years ago she was treated for a malignant melanoma on her right upper arm. The melanoma was 0.78 mm thick; there was no ulceration, mitotic count was 1 mitosis/mm^2, and it was a Clark level III. She was treated with wide excision that showed no residual melanoma, and was then observed. She now presents with an enlarged right axillary lymph node that measures 2.5 cm by 2 cm. A fine needle aspiration (FNA) of the lymph node is positive for melanoma. Staging work-up including CT scans of the chest, abdomen, and pelvis confirmed the enlarged axillary lymph node but no other sites of disease.

Which of following would you recommend to this patient now?
A. Axillary lymph node dissection
B. High-dose IFN
C. IL-2
D. Radiation therapy to the axillary lymph node basin
E. Sentinel lymph node sampling procedure

12-1   D

High-dose IFN therapy is associated with significant toxicity. Patients experience flu-like symptoms such as fatigue, fever, chills, myalgias, anorexia, nausea, vomiting, and headache. Significant laboratory abnormalities include elevated hepatic transaminases, neutropenia, elevated triglycerides, thyroid dysfunction, and anemia. It is critical that patients undergoing treatment with IFN be monitored closely and that the dose of IFN is modified appropriately for toxicity. Therefore, it is recommended that patients undergoing treatment with high-dose IFN have liver function tests monitored weekly during the induction phase and monthly during the maintenance phase of treatment. If the hepatic transaminases (ALT/SGOT) increase to greater than five times the upper limit of normal, then IFN treatment should be temporarily discontinued until they normalize. IFN treatment should be restarted at 50% of the previous dose. Similarly, if granulocytes decrease to less than 500/mm^3, treatment should be held until normalization and the IFN dose should be reduced by 50%.

Suggested Reading

Kaufman HL, Kirkwood JM, Hodi FS, et al. The Society for Immunotherapy of Cancer consensus statement on tumour immunotherapy for the treatment of cutaneous melanoma. *Nat Review Clin Oncol.* 2013;10:588-598. PMID: 23982524.

Ascierto PA, Gogas HJ, Grob JJ, et al. Adjuvant interferon alfa in malignant melanoma: an interdisciplinary and multinational expert review. *Crit Rev Oncolog Hematol.* 2013;85:149-161. PMID: 22874771.

12-2   A

The staging evaluation of a patient with a low-risk melanoma should include a physical examination and a skin exam. Routine blood work and imaging is not routinely recommended. The majority of patients who present with melanoma do not have distant metastatic disease at presentation; therefore, extensive evaluations with CT scans to search for distant metastases have an extremely low yield and, consequently, are not indicated in asymptomatic patients. More extensive staging evaluation with CT scans of the chest/abdomen/pelvis can be considered in patients with high-risk disease (thick primary melanoma greater than 4 mm thick or node-positive disease) in whom the risk of distant metastatic disease is higher.

Suggested Reading

Coit DG, Thompson JA, Andtbacka R, et al. Melanoma, version 4.2014. *J Natl Compr Cancer Netw.* 2014;12:621-629. PMID: 24812131.

12-3   A

In this patient with symptomatic metastatic melanoma, the most appropriate choice would be a BRAF inhibitor. Dabrafenib treatment is associated with an approximately 60% response rate, although the response rate in patients with *V600K* mutation is lower than the response rate for patients with *V600E* mutation. Clinical benefit has been seen within 72 hours of administration. Trametinib is a recently approved MEK inhibitor; however, single-agent objective response rates are lower than those reported for dabrafenib. Similarly, sorafenib, although it targets BRAF and other kinases, has little activity in melanoma. Imatinib targets cKIT so it is not an appropriate choice.

Suggested Reading

Ascierto PA, Minor D, Ribas A, et al. Phase II trial (BREAK-2) of the BRAF inhibitor dabrafenib (GSK2118436) in patients with metastatic melanoma. *J Clin Oncol.* 2013;31:3205-3211. PMID: 23918947.

12-4   D

The patterns of response to immunotherapy appear to be distinct from chemotherapy and molecularly targeted therapy. Patients receiving treatment with ipilimumab may have transient worsening of disease on radiologic studies prior to disease stabilization or regression. Immune-related response criteria have been proposed as the traditional RECIST criteria may not be appropriate for immune-based therapies. Therefore, it is important that therapy with ipilimumab not be abandoned early or new therapies started too soon, as there can be a delayed response to ipilimumab. In this patient with slight increase in disease and no new symptoms, monitoring the patient and repeating scans in about 8 weeks would be very appropriate. Although maintenance therapy with ipilimumab every 3 months has been evaluated in clinical trials, maintenance ipilimumab is not U.S Food and Drug Administration (FDA) approved. Similarly, high-dose ipilimumab is currently being studied in clinical trials but is not FDA approved. There is no role for vemurafenib, a BRAF inhibitor, as the patient's melanoma does not have a *BRAF* mutation.

Suggested Reading

Hodi FS, O'Day SJ, McDermott DF, et al. Improved survival with ipilimumab in patients with metastatic melanoma. *N Engl J Med.* 2010;363:711-723. PMID: 20525992.

Robert C, Thomas L, Bondarenko I, et al. Ipilimumab plus dacarbazine for previously untreated metastatic melanoma. *N Engl J Med.* 2011;364:2517-2526. PMID: 21639810.

Oxnard GR, Morris MJ, Hodi FS, et al. When progressive disease does not mean treatment failure: reconsidering the criteria for progression. *J Natl Cancer Inst.* 2012;104:1534-1541. PMID: 22927506.

12-5   B

Ipilimumab is associated with significant toxicities that are immune-related adverse events. These immune-mediated reactions may involve any organ system; however, the most common immune-adverse reactions are enterocolitis, hepatitis, dermatitis, neuropathy, and endocrinopathy. Treatment of immune-mediated toxicity requires interruption of ipilimumab and use of corticosteroids depending upon severity of symptoms. The FDA has created a Risk Evaluation and Mitigation Strategy to provide additional information regarding side effects and management of ipilimumab-associated adverse events. Therefore, it is recommended that patients undergoing treatment with ipilimumab be monitored closely with physical exams, review of symptoms, and blood tests including liver and thyroid function before and during treatment. Dose modification occurs through withholding a dose, not dose reduction.

Suggested Reading

Robert C, Thomas L, Bondarenko I, et al. Ipilimumab plus dacarbazine for previously untreated metastatic melanoma. *N Engl J Med.* 2011;364:2517-2526. PMID: 21639810.

12-6   C

The most frequent adverse events of vemurafenib are arthralgias, rash, nausea, photosensitivity, pruritus, and hand-foot syndrome. Cutaneous squamous cell carcinomas or keratoacanthoma can occur in approximately 25% of patients treated with vemurafenib. Based upon the frequent skin-associated adverse events, patients undergoing treatment with vemurafenib should be counseled to perform regular self-examination of their skin and report any new or changing skin lesions to their physicians. Additionally, patients starting therapy should be advised of sun protective measures. Dermatologic skin exams should be performed prior to initiation of therapy and every 2 months during therapy. Arthralgias and arthritis associated with vemurafenib at times require treatment with corticosteroids.

Suggested Reading

Chu EY, Wanat KA, Miller CJ, et al. Diverse cutaneous side effects associated with BRAF inhibitor therapy: a clinicopathologic study. *J Am Acad Dermatol.* 2012;67:1265-1272. PMID: 22609219.

12-7   B

BRAF V600 is the most common somatic mutation in melanoma, occurring in about 50% of patients. This mutation also tends to occur in younger patients with melanoma; therefore, it is the most likely mutation in this patient. Importantly, BRAF inhibitors (vemurafenib, dabrafenib) are effective therapies for patients with *BRAF*-mutant melanoma and are now FDA-approved based upon survival benefit demonstrated in randomized phase III clinical trials. *KIT* is uncommonly mutated in melanoma, occurring in fewer than 3% of melanomas. *KIT* mutations are most frequent in acral (occurring on palms and soles or subungual) melanoma, mucosal melanoma, or cutaneous melanomas associated with chronic sun exposure. In this patient, testing for *BRAF* mutation first is most appropriate. Although *NRAS* mutations occur in 20% of patients with melanoma, there are no FDA-approved treatments for this patient population at this time. *MEK* mutations are extremely rare in melanoma. Many institutions are now testing for multiple cancer-related somatic mutations using next-generation sequencing platforms, which allow for testing of multiple genes simultaneously.

12-8   B

Melanoma brain metastases are extremely common. Approximately 50% of patients will eventually develop clinical evidence of brain metastases. Recent studies have shown activity of ipilimumab, dabrafenib, and vemurafenib in patients with brain metastases. In addition, temozolomide, which crosses the blood-brain barrier, has been used to treat patients with CNS metastases but has very limited clinical activity. Treatment of patients with brain metastases requires a multidisciplinary team with radiation oncology and neurosurgery to determine optimal local and systemic therapy.

In this patient with symptomatic metastatic melanoma involving both brain and other sites, the most appropriate choice for therapy would be treatment with a BRAF inhibitor. Dabrafenib treatment is associated with an approximately 60% response rate. Although ipilimumab may be useful for this patient, given the extent of symptoms, a BRAF inhibitor is preferred. Use of high dose IL-2 for patients with CNS metastases has not been well studied and is generally avoided.

Suggested Reading

Hauschild A, Grob JJ, Demidov LV, et al. Dabrafenib in BRAF-mutated metastatic melanoma: a multicentre, open-label, phase 3 randomised controlled trial. *Lancet.* 2012;380:358-365. PMID: 22735384.

12-9   A

In patients who present with palpable regional adenopathy, an FNA should be used as the initial step to confirm the clinical suspicion of regional metastasis from melanoma. If the staging work-up is negative for stage IV disease, then the patient should proceed to a therapeutic lymph node dissection, in this case an axillary dissection. Surgery is the main treatment for this patient. In addition, surgery helps prevent local complications from the enlarged lymph nodes. Radiation therapy could be considered after a therapeutic lymph node dissection, but not in place of surgery. Postoperative radiation has been shown to reduce the risk for local recurrence in some studies, but does affect overall survival. Some consider postoperative radiation if there are many nodes involved and/or extracapsular extension of the melanoma. Regional radiation does increase the risk for lymphedema. The results of a randomized clinical trial of postoperative radiation therapy compared with observation were recently published. Risk for lymph node field relapse was significantly reduced in the adjuvant radiation therapy group compared with the observation group (20 relapses in the radiotherapy groups vs. 34 in the observation group; hazard ratio 0.56, 95% CI 0.32 to 0.98) but no difference in relapse-free survival or overall survival was observed. There is no role for sentinel lymph node procedure in a patient with a palpable lymph node. After surgery, one could consider IFN or participation in a clinical trial, but surgery should be completed prior to considering adjuvant therapy.

Suggested Reading

Wong SL, Balch CM, Hurley P, et al. Sentinel lymph node biopsy for melanoma: American Society of Clinical Oncology and Society of Surgical Oncology joint clinical practice guideline. *J Clin Oncol.* 2012;30:2912-2918. PMID: 22778321.

Burmeister BH, Henderson MA, Ainslie J, et al. Adjuvant radiotherapy versus observation alone for patients at risk of lymph-node field relapse after therapeutic lymphadenectomy for melanoma: a randomised trial. *Lancet Oncol.* 2012;13:589-597. PMID: 22575589.

13 SARCOMA
SELF-EVALUATION

SARCOMA QUESTIONS

13-1 A 34-year-old man presents with left hip pain that intensifies with activity. A radiograph of the pelvis demonstrates a lytic process adjacent to the acetabulum. He was previously healthy and has no chronic medical conditions. His family history is notable for a sister who died of acute leukemia in her 20s and a maternal grandfather who had brain cancer in his 40s.

What will a biopsy of the lytic process most likely identify?
A. Multiple myeloma
B. Ewing sarcoma
C. Osteosarcoma
D. Giant cell tumor of bone

13-2 A 58-year-old woman is receiving imatinib (400 mg daily) as treatment for metastatic gastrointestinal stromal tumor (GIST). Tumor genotyping identified mutation in exon 9 of *KIT*. After 2 years of stable disease, computed tomography (CT) demonstrates enlargement of multiple enhancing lesions in the liver and peritoneum. She acknowledges taking the medication daily as prescribed, is not using herbal or vitamin supplements, and has no significant adverse drug effects. Two months after increasing the dose to 400 mg twice daily, CT demonstrates further enlargement of multiple masses and development of new masses.

What is the most appropriate next treatment for this patient?
A. Sunitinib (50 mg daily) for 4 weeks followed by 2 weeks without drug every 6 weeks
B. Regorafenib (160 mg daily) for 3 weeks followed by 1 week without drug every 4 weeks
C. Referral to surgical oncologist
D. Increase imatinib to 600 mg twice daily

13-3 A 23-year-old woman presents with right flank pain. Routine complete blood count (CBC), chemistry panel, and urinalysis are normal and a pregnancy test is negative. A contrast-enhanced CT of the chest, abdomen, and pelvis is normal except for an enhancing 8-cm perinephric mass involving the kidney. A CT-guided core needle biopsy is obtained and shows a small blue cell tumor. The tumor cells stain for CD99 in the cytoplasmic membrane. Fluorescence in situ hybridization testing identifies a translocation involving *FLI-1* and *EWS* on chromosomes 11 and 22, respectively, confirming a diagnosis of Ewing sarcoma. A radionuclide bone scan is normal.

In addition to nephrectomy, what is the most appropriate treatment for this patient?
A. No therapy
B. Biologic therapy with interleukin-2
C. Cyclophosphamide, doxorubicin, and vincristine alternating with ifosfamide and etoposide
D. Doxorubicin and ifosfamide

13-4 A 54-year-old previously healthy man presents with severe fatigue, shortness of breath on exertion, and pallor. Routine blood testing reveals hemoglobin of 6 gm/dL and mean cell volume of 74 fL. Serum ferritin is less than 10 ng/mL. Endoscopy identifies an ulceration in the stomach but mucosal biopsy is nondiagnostic. CT of the abdomen and pelvis reveals a 12-cm enhancing, vascular mass arising from the gastric fundus but is otherwise normal. He undergoes partial gastrectomy and the mass is removed intact. The pathologist reports the presence of a GIST, 11 cm in greatest dimension, 4 mitoses per 50 high-power microscopic fields (HPF) of view, the presence of CD117 (*KIT*) and CD34, and absence of desmin on immunohistochemistry. Molecular testing detects a deletion in exon 11 of *KIT*. Surgical margins are reported as close but negative. Imatinib at a dose of 400 mg daily for 3 years is recommended as adjuvant therapy.

The effect of 3 years compared with 1 year of imatinib in patients with resected high-risk GIST in a randomized trial demonstrated:
A. Delay in time to tumor recurrence but no difference in overall survival
B. Improvement in overall survival at 5 years but no improvement in recurrence-free survival
C. Improvement in recurrence-free and overall survival at 5 years
D. No difference in recurrence-free or overall survival

13-5 A 42-year-old man is being treated for metastatic GIST. After 3 years of stable disease on imatinib (400 mg daily), CT demonstrates enlargement of multiple tumors. His treatment is changed to sunitinib. After 12 weeks of sunitinib, CT demonstrates further enlargement of multiple masses and the appearance of new masses. Treatment is changed to regorafenib.

What adverse event is most likely to occur with regorafenib treatment?
A. Oral mucositis
B. Peripheral edema
C. Diarrhea
D. Hand-foot skin reaction

13-6 A 28-year-old woman presents with 3 months of increasing numbness and paresthesia in her right forearm and hand. Complete physical exam is notable for weakness in forearm and wrist extension, multiple neurofibromas, café-au-lait skin marks, freckles in the axilla and groin, and a firm mass in the right axilla. Breast examination is normal. CT identifies a 6-cm mass in the axilla.

Upon biopsy of the axillary mass, what is the most likely diagnosis?
A. Adenocarcinoma
B. Malignant peripheral nerve sheath tumor
C. Leiomyosarcoma
D. Lymphoma

13-7 A 26-year-old man presents with worsening right knee pain and stiffness. One year earlier he underwent curettage and cementation of a lytic area in the proximal tibia. A pathologist diagnosed giant cell tumor of bone. CT of the knee identifies a 1-cm area of bone lysis adjacent to the bone cement. The opinion from the treating orthopedic oncologist is that surgical management would require resection of the proximal tibia and endoprosthestic reconstruction of the knee. He is referred for treatment with denosumab. He has had a normal dental examination and cleaning in the past 6 months.

What adverse event is most likely to occur after initiating denosumab therapy?
A. Osteonecrosis of the jaw
B. Hypocalcemia
C. Hypophosphatemia
D. Infection

13-8 A 42-year-old man presents with scattered brown macular lesions smaller than 1 cm in size involving the thighs and legs. On examination he has palpable adenopathy in the groin and mild pitting edema in the legs. The remainder of the examination is normal. CBC reveals lymphopenia, CD4 count is 50 cells/μL, a rapid HIV test is positive, and HIV viral load is 50,000 copies/mL. Biopsy of a skin lesion demonstrates an endothelial proliferation and presence of human herpesvirus-8. He is started on triple antiretroviral therapy. One month after starting therapy, he develops rapidly enlarging adenopathy in the groin, significant worsening of lower extremity edema, and enlargement of the skin lesions. HIV viral load is undetectable and CD4 count is improved.

What is the most appropriate next step for this patient's therapy?

A. Change antiretroviral therapy
B. Discontinue antiretroviral therapy and start liposomal doxorubicin
C. Continue antiretroviral therapy and start liposomal doxorubicin
D. Continue antiretroviral therapy and refer for radiation

13-9 A 68-year-old woman is being treated for metastatic leiomyosarcoma. She previously received palliative chemotherapy with first-line doxorubicin and ifosfamide, second-line gemcitabine and docetaxel, and third-line dacarbazine. Her Eastern Cooperative Oncology Group (ECOG) performance score is 1, and cardiac, renal, and hepatic functions are normal. Pazopanib (800 mg daily) is started.

What measurement is most likely to benefit from treatment compared to best supportive care?

A. Prolongation in time to tumor progression but no improvement in overall survival
B. Prolongation in time to tumor progression and improvement in overall survival
C. Improvement in overall survival but no effect on tumor progression
D. Significant reduction in the volume of sarcoma

13-1   C

The patient has a primary bone process resulting in demineralization and destruction of bone matrix. His young age and family medical history suggests a familial cancer predisposition syndrome and meets the definition for Li-Fraumeni syndrome pedigree. There is a high likelihood of germ-line mutation in *TP53*. Patients with Li-Fraumeni syndrome are at high risk of developing sarcoma, including osteosarcoma, rhabdomyosarcoma, leiomyosarcoma, and pleomorphic sarcoma. Osteosarcoma often results in disorganized bone formation but may manifest as a principally lytic process. There is no known genetic predisposition associated with Ewing sarcoma; however, Ewing sarcoma is much more common in white individuals than in other races. Multiple myeloma and giant cell tumor of bone are lytic bone lesions but are not associated with Li-Fraumeni syndrome.

Suggested Reading

Malkin D. Li-fraumeni syndrome. *Genes Cancer.* 2011;2:475-484. PMID: 21779515.

Tinat J, Bougeard G, Baert-Desurmont S, et al. 2009 version of the Chompret criteria for Li Fraumeni syndrome. *J Clin Oncol.* 2009; 27:e108-e109. PMID: 19652052.

Mitchell G, Ballinger ML, Wong S, et al. High frequency of germline *TP53* mutations in a prospective adult-onset sarcoma cohort. *PLoS ONE.* 2013;8:e69026. PMID: 23894400.

Ognjanovic S, Olivier M, Bergemann TL, et al. Sarcomas in TP53 germline mutation carriers: a review of the IARC TP53 database. *Cancer.* 2012;118:1387-1396. PMID: 21837677.

13-2   A

The patient has metastatic GIST with evidence of multifocal progression of tumor. Imatinib (400 mg daily) is the standard first-line drug therapy for treatment of locally advanced or metastatic GIST. Approximately 35% of patients with metastatic GIST harboring mutation in exon 9 of *KIT* demonstrated objective response to treatment with imatinib in one large trial. Retrospective analyses of patients with *KIT* exon 9–mutant GIST crossing over to the higher dose of 400 mg twice daily of imatinib demonstrated significant benefit in approximately 50% of the patients, and dose escalation is a reasonable first step in a patient who has no significant adverse effects on the lower dose. In a phase I trial of imatinib in patients with sarcoma, dose-limiting toxicities were encountered at daily doses of 1,000 mg. An antitumor advantage of 1,200 mg per day versus 800 mg per day has not been established. Surgical debulking has not obtained long-term control of GIST in patients with multifocal tumor progression. Sunitinib is the only drug approved for second-line use in patients with GIST resistant to imatinib or in patients who are intolerant of imatinib.

Suggested Reading

Demetri GD, van Oosterom AT, Garrett CR, et al. Efficacy and safety of sunitinib in patients with advanced gastrointestinal stromal tumour after failure of imatinib: a randomised controlled trial. *Lancet.* 2006;368:1329-1338. PMID: 17046465.

DeMatteo RP, Maki RG, Singer S, et al. Results of tyrosine kinase inhibitor therapy followed by surgical resection for metastatic gastrointestinal stromal tumor. *Ann Surg.* 2007;245:347-352. PMID: 17435539.

Patel S, Zalcberg JR. Optimizing the dose of imatinib for treatment of gastrointestinal stromal tumors: lessons from the phase 3 trials. *Eur J Cancer.* 2008;44:501-509. PMID: 18234488.

van Oosterom AT, Judson I, Verweij J, et al. Safety and efficacy of imatinib (STI571) in metastatic gastrointestinal stromal tumours: a phase I study. *Lancet.* 2001;358:1421-1423. PMID: 11705489.

13-3   C

The patient has an extraskeletal Ewing sarcoma. In adults, Ewing sarcoma frequently arises in soft tissue sites. There is no evidence of metastasis on tumor staging studies. The patient is at high risk for sarcoma recurrence without chemotherapy. Treatment with drugs that included ifosfamide and etoposide improved relapse-free and overall survival in patients with localized Ewing sarcoma and is the preferred treatment. Ifosfamide treatment carries a higher risk of renal damage, including renal failure, and is more toxic if administered in setting of reduced glomerular filtration rate or prior nephrectomy. In the scenario presented, ifosfamide should be administered prior to nephrectomy. Increasing dose density by shortening time between chemotherapy cycles demonstrated improvement in relapse-free survival rate in patients with localized Ewing sarcoma. Doxorubicin and ifosfamide is an accepted standard regimen for treatment of soft tissue sarcoma but is inadequate for treatment of extraskeletal Ewing sarcoma.

Suggested Reading

Womer RB, West DC, Krailo MD, et al. Randomized controlled trial of interval-compressed chemotherapy for the treatment of localized Ewing sarcoma: a report from the Children's Oncology Group. *J Clin Oncol.* 2012;30:4148-4154. PMID: 23091096.

Grier HE, Krailo MD, Tarbell NJ, et al. Addition of ifosfamide and etoposide to standard chemotherapy for Ewing's sarcoma and primitive neuroectodermal tumor of bone. *N Engl J Med.* 2003;348: 694-701. PMID: 12594313.

13-4   C

A randomized trial of 1 year versus 3 years of imatinib at a dose of 400 mg daily following resection of a high-risk GIST demonstrated improvement in relapse-free survival and overall survival rates. High risk is defined as tumor size larger than 10 cm or tumor mitotic count higher than 10 per 50 HPF of view, or tumor size 5 cm to 10 cm and mitotic count 5 to 10 per 50 HPF of view, or rupture of tumor. At 5 years from study entry, 66% of the patients receiving imatinib for 3 years compared with 48% of the patients receiving imatinib for 1 year were alive and recurrence-free, and 92% of the patients receiving imatinib for 3 years compared with 82% of patients assigned to 1 year of therapy were alive. Only 4% of patients developed recurrence of GIST during treatment with imatinib. However, significant side effects from adjuvant imatinib may occur, and approximately 25% of patients assigned to imatinib for 3 years discontinued treatment early for reasons other than tumor recurrence.

Suggested Reading

Joensuu H, Eriksson M, Sundby Hall K, et al. One vs three years of adjuvant imatinib for operable gastrointestinal stromal tumor: a randomized trial. *JAMA.* 2012;307:1265-1272. PMID: 22453568.

13-5   D

Hand-foot skin reaction was the most common adverse event, occurring in more than 50% of patients with GIST treated in a phase II or randomized phase III trial. Severe hand-foot skin reaction occurred in 20% of the patients treated with regorafenib and in none of the patients receiving placebo. Hypertension of any grade was the next most common adverse event, which developed in 49% of patients with GIST treated with regorafenib compared with 17% of patients treated with placebo. Diarrhea and fatigue occurred in approximately 40% of patients treated with regorafenib, but severe cases were infrequent. Oral mucositis was reported in fewer than 40% of patients and was higher than grade 1 in fewer than 10%. Peripheral edema is more likely to occur from imatinib than regorafenib. Regorafenib carries a black-box warning for severe or fatal hepatotoxicity, and liver function should be monitored before and during treatment.

Suggested Reading

Demetri GD, Reichardt P, Kang YK, et al. Efficacy and safety of regorafenib for advanced gastrointestinal stromal tumours after failure of imatinib and sunitinib (GRID): an international, multicentre, randomised, placebo-controlled, phase 3 trial. *Lancet.* 2013; 381:295-302. PMID: 23177515.

George S, Wang Q, Heinrich MC, et al. Efficacy and safety of regorafenib in patients with metastatic and/or unresectable GI stromal tumor after failure of imatinib and sunitinib: a multicenter phase II trial. *J Clin Oncol.* 2012;30:2401-2407. PMID: 22614970.

Belum VR, Wu S, Lacouture ME. Risk of hand-foot skin reaction with the novel multikinase inhibitor regorafenib: a meta-analysis. *Invest New Drugs.* 2013;31:1078-1086. PMID: 23700287.

13-6   B

This patient has stigmata of neurofibromatosis type-1 (NF-1). Neurofibromatosis type-1 is the most common autosomal dominant disorder and stems from loss-of-function mutations in the tumor-suppressor gene neurofibromin-1. Neurofibromin-1 is a negative regulator of the Ras/mitogen-activated protein kinase pathway. Patients with NF-1 may develop multiple café-au-lait macules, axillary and/or inguinal freckling, Lisch nodules in the iris, optic gliomas, and benign peripheral nerve sheath tumors including cutaneous neurofibromas, subcutaneous neurofibromas, and plexiform neurofibromas. Patients with NF-1 are also at increased risk of developing malignant tumors, including malignant peripheral nerve sheath tumors, GIST, rhabdomyosarcoma, and pheochromocytomas. GISTs arising in patients with NF-1 have a predilection for the duodenum and small intestine. There is significant phenotypic variability in affected patients, with a lifetime risk of developing malignant peripheral nerve sheath tumor of about 10% to 15%. Malignant peripheral nerve sheath tumor should be suspected in patients with NF-1 who have an enlarging, symptomatic mass associated with a nerve. Lymphoma may arise in young patients in the axilla but usually does not cause neurologic symptoms. Leiomyosarcoma may arise in the upper extremity or axilla and adenocarcinoma may involve axillary nodes, but these diseases are not associated with NF-1 and usually occur in older individuals.

Suggested Reading

Laycock-van Spyk S, Thomas N, Cooper DN, et al. Neurofibromatosis type 1-associated tumours: their somatic mutational spectrum and pathogenesis. *Hum Genomics*. 2011;5:623-690. PMID: 22155606.

Evans DG, Baser ME, McGaughran J, et al. Malignant peripheral nerve sheath tumours in neurofibromatosis 1. *J Med Genet*. 2002;39:311-314. PMID: 12011145.

13-7   B

Denosumab is a fully human monoclonal antibody that inhibits receptor activator of nuclear factor kappa-B (RANK) ligand, preventing activation of RANK, which disrupts osteoclast maturation and activation. Treatment of patients with locally advanced or metastatic giant cell tumor of bone with denosumab led to a high rate of disease stabilization and reduction in markers of bone destruction in phase II trials. The most common adverse event overall was hypocalcemia, which occurred in 5% of patients despite supplementation with vitamin D and calcium. The most common severe adverse event was hypophosphatemia, which occurred in 3% of patients. Osteonecrosis of the jaw is an infrequent but serious complication of treatment with denosumab. The RANK/RANK ligand axis is involved in lymphocyte development and activation, but infection was rarely associated with denosumab treatment in patients with giant cell tumor of bone.

Suggested Reading

Chawla S, Henshaw R, Seeger L, et al. Safety and efficacy of denosumab for adults and skeletally mature adolescents with giant cell tumour of bone: interim analysis of an open-label, parallel-group, phase 2 study. *Lancet Oncol.* 2013;14;901-908. PMID: 23867211.

Thomas D, Henshaw R, Skubitz K, et al. Denosumab in patients with giant-cell tumour of bone: an open-label, phase 2 study. *Lancet Oncol.* 2010;11:275-280. PMID: 20149736.

13-8 C

This patient has extensive Kaposi sarcoma involving the lower extremities. Kaposi sarcoma in the setting of HIV infection is an AIDS-defining condition. Kaposi sarcoma is associated with human herpesvirus-8 infection and is most prevalent in HIV-seropositive men who have sex with men but may also occur in the absence of HIV infection in elderly patients. In patients who are HIV-positive and are not receiving antiretroviral therapy, Kaposi sarcoma is associated with low CD4 counts and high copy number of HIV. The introduction of highly active antiretroviral therapy (HAART) in these patients leads to regression of Kaposi sarcoma in the majority of patients, which is often durable. In approximately 5% to 10% of patients with HIV initiating HAART, an immune reconstitution inflammatory syndrome develops, leading to a sudden flare in Kaposi sarcoma growth despite control of HIV with therapy. In this setting it is appropriate to continue HAART and begin chemotherapy. Because HIV is responding to HAART, it would not be appropriate to discontinue or change antiretroviral therapy. Radiation may be helpful in controlling skin lesions of limited distribution but is unlikely to control extensive lesions or lymphedema.

Suggested Reading

Aversa SM, Cattelan AM, Salvagno L, et al. Treatment of AIDS-related Kaposi's sarcoma. *Crit Rev Oncol Hematol.* 2005;53:253-265. PMID: 15718150.

Bower M, Nelson M, Young AM, et al. Immune reconstitution inflammatory syndrome associated with Kaposi's sarcoma. *J Clin Oncol.* 2005;23: 5224-5228. PMID: 16051964.

Northfelt DW, Dezube BJ, Thommes JA, et al. Pegylated-liposomal doxorubicin versus doxorubicin, bleomycin, and vincristine in the treatment of AIDS-related Kaposi's sarcoma: results of a randomized phase III clinical trial. *J Clin Oncol.* 1998;16:2445-2451. PMID: 9667262.

Stewart S, Jablonowski H, Goebel FD, et al. Randomized comparative trial of pegylated liposomal doxorubicin versus bleomycin and vincristine in the treatment of AIDS-related Kaposi's sarcoma. International Pegylated Liposomal Doxorubicin Study Group. *J Clin Oncol.* 1998;16:683-691. PMID: 9469358.

13-9 A

Pazopanib is a pan-tyrosine kinase inhibitor that interrupts activity of vascular endothelial growth factor and platelet-derived growth factor receptors, among others. A phase III randomized, placebo-controlled trial of pazopanib (800 mg daily) was conducted with 369 patients with advanced soft tissue sarcoma progressing despite previous standard chemotherapy. The median progression-free survival was significantly different in the group receiving pazopanib (4.6 months) versus the group receiving placebo (1.6 months); however, overall survival was not different (12.5 months for the group receiving pazopanib vs. 10.7 months for the group receiving placebo). Kaplan-Meier analysis estimated 10% of patients receiving pazopanib were free from tumor progression 1 year after starting therapy. Objective partial tumor responses occurred in only 6% of patients receiving pazopanib. Pazopanib was discontinued in 14% of patients because of adverse events. The most common adverse events in the group receiving pazopanib were fatigue, diarrhea, and nausea, which occurred in the majority of patients. Possible serious complications from pazopanib included multiorgan failure, cardiac toxicity, pneumothorax, and venous thromboembolism. Pazopanib prescribing information carries a black-box warning for severe and fatal hepatotoxicity.

Suggested Reading

van der Graaf WT, Blay JY, Chawla SP, et al. Pazopanib for metastatic soft-tissue sarcoma (PALETTE): a randomised, double-blind, placebo-controlled phase 3 trial. *Lancet.* 2012;379:1879-1886. PMID: 22595799.

Sleijfer S, Ray-Coquard I, Papai Z, et al. Pazopanib, a multikinase angiogenesis inhibitor, in patients with relapsed or refractory advanced soft tissue sarcoma: a phase II study from the European organisation for research and treatment of cancer-soft tissue and bone sarcoma group (EORTC study 62043). *J Clin Oncol.* 2009;27:3126-3132. PMID: 19451427.

14 CENTRAL NERVOUS SYSTEM TUMORS
SELF-EVALUATION

CENTRAL NERVOUS SYSTEM TUMORS QUESTIONS

14-1 A 35-year-old woman without prior health problems suddenly experienced the onset of transient headache and dizziness, followed shortly by loss of consciousness and a generalized tonic-clonic seizure. Emergency department evaluation included a computed tomography (CT) scan of her head that revealed a mass lesion in the right frontal lobe with patchy enhancement and slight mass effect. Subsequent magnetic resonance imaging (MRI) revealed similar findings. She underwent anterior right frontal lobe resection with gross total removal of tumor. Pathology revealed an anaplastic oligodendroglioma characterized by 1p and 19q deletion by fluorescent in situ hybridization (FISH) as well as an *IDH1* mutation detected by immunohistochemical stains. Postoperatively, other than fatigue, she had no neurologic deficits.

Which of the following is the most appropriate treatment now?
A. Radiation therapy plus procarbazine/CCNU (lomustine)/vincristine (PCV) chemotherapy
B. Temozolomide alone
C. Radiation therapy alone
D. PCV alone

14-2 A 59-year-old man noted word-finding difficulty. On neurologic examination he is found to have expressive aphasia. MRI revealed a ring-enhancing mass lesion in the left frontotemporal lobe. He underwent subtotal resection of a small portion of the tumor. Pathology revealed glioblastoma. Methylguanine methyltransferase (*MGMT*) promoter was methylated.

The initial treatment demonstrated to result in improved survival in similar patients is:
A. Radiation therapy alone
B. Radiation therapy with concurrent temozolomide
C. Radiation therapy with concurrent temozolomide followed by six cycles of post-radiation temozolomide
D. Radiation therapy with concurrent temozolomide and bevacizumab followed by adjuvant temozolomide and bevacizumab

14-3 A 78-year-old man noted gradually increasing weakness in his left leg over a 3-week period of time. MRI of the head revealed a 5-cm irregularly enhancing mass in the posterior right frontal lobe. Subtotal resection resulted in transient worsening of his weakness, but his strength returned to baseline during the immediate postoperative period. Pathology revealed glioblastoma. *MGMT* promoter methylation status is pending at the time of your consultation with the patient. The patient has a history of hypercholesterolemia treated with a statin, but he has had no cardiovascular events. He has no other comorbidities.

Which of the following is appropriate as initial therapy?
A. Temozolomide alone if the tumor *MGMT* promoter is unmethylated
B. Radiation therapy alone given as 40 Gy in 15 fractions if *MGMT* promoter status is unknown
C. Radiation therapy plus PCV chemotherapy
D. Radiation therapy with 60 Gy in 30 fractions with stereotactic radiation boost to the residual tumor

14-4 A 48-year-old woman was diagnosed with a right parietal lobe glioblastoma in mid-January. *MGMT* promoter was methylated. Postoperative imaging performed 24 hours after subtotal resection revealed residual tumor with minimal mass effect. She completed radiation therapy, consisting of 60 Gy in 30 fractions, with concurrent temozolomide (once-daily 75 mg/m^2 with radiation) at the end of March. She tolerated concurrent radiation plus temozolomide treatment well, experiencing only minimal fatigue, constipation, and anorexia without weight loss. She returned to the clinic in April to begin post-radiation temozolomide. At the time of her April visit, the MRI revealed increased contrast enhancement, increased T2 signal, and no change in the extent of mass effect, restricted diffusion, or cerebral blood volume compared with her postoperative MRI. The patient's symptoms have not changed since prior to initiating therapy.

Which of the following is the best treatment strategy for this patient?
A. Discontinue temozolomide and begin irinotecan and bevacizumab
B. Discontinue temozolomide and begin single-agent irinotecan
C. Biopsy the area of increased contrast enhancement and determine treatment based on the genomic profile
D. Continue post-radiation adjuvant temozolomide as planned

14-5 A 61-year-old man presents with new onset severe headaches and right-arm incoordination. MRI reveals a solitary, intensely homogeneous contrast enhancement with significant mass effect. Biopsy reveals large B-cell lymphoma. Staging evaluation reveals no evidence of systemic lymphoma.

The most appropriate initial treatment is:
A. Cyclophosphamide/doxorubicin/vincristine/prednisone plus rituximab (R-CHOP)
B. Radiation plus temozolomide
C. High-dose methotrexate-based chemotherapy
D. Radiation therapy with concurrent high-dose methotrexate

14-6 A 47-year-old woman was diagnosed with T2N1M0, HER2-positive, estrogen receptor (ER)/progesterone receptor (PR)–negative breast cancer 2 years ago. Following lumpectomy, she received adjuvant doxorubicin, cyclophosphamide, paclitaxel, and trastuzumab followed by radiation therapy to the breast and axilla with continued trastuzumab. She has remained free of recurrent disease until the present time. She now returns to your office complaining of persistent headaches, vomiting, and difficulty concentrating. She has no additional symptoms and review of systems is unremarkable. Physical examination reveals a left supraclavicular lymph node suspicious for recurrent disease. MRI of the head reveals a solitary uniformly contrast-enhancing mass in the anterior right temporal lobe with marked edema and mass effect, including early uncal herniation. CT scan of the chest, abdomen, and pelvis is negative for malignancy. Biopsy of the supraclavicular node confirms the diagnosis of recurrent HER2-positive, ER/PR-negative breast cancer.

The most appropriate recommendation for initial treatment is:
A. Resection of the right temporal lobe mass
B. Whole-brain radiation
C. Trastuzumab emtansine
D. Lapatanib

14-7 A 45-year-old man presented with a 6-month history of intermittent left-arm and hand numbness lasting 3 to 5 minutes with subsequent development of left-hand incoordination, most commonly noted when using his computer keyboard. He sought medical attention and MRI of the head revealed a right parietal mass with scattered foci of wispy contrast enhancement. Subtotal resection revealed an anaplastic astrocytoma. The postoperative course was unremarkable.

Which of the following statements is true?
A. The most appropriate course at the present time is careful observation
B. *IDH* mutational analysis will assist in discussing prognosis
C. *MGMT* promoter methylation status will determine the most appropriate treatment recommendations
D. Median life expectancy for this patient is 12 to 18 months

14-1 A

While temozolomide clearly has antitumor activity in patients with anaplastic oligodendroglioma, the only beneficial adjuvant chemotherapy treatment is PCV when added to radiation therapy. In two separate phase III trials, PCV plus radiation was associated with improved survival in patients with 1p and 19q deletions. Radiation alone for this patient population results in inferior outcomes. Neither PCV alone nor temozolomide alone has been established as equivalent to the combination of radiation and PCV for patients with 1p/19q codeletion and *IDH* mutation. Thus, radiation plus adjuvant PCV is the current standard of care for patients with anaplastic oligodendroglioma with 1p/19q deletions.

A current international phase III trial for patients with anaplastic oligodendroglioma and 1p/19q deletion is investigating other adjuvant options. In this study patients are randomly assigned to radiation therapy plus PCV (control arm), or radiation therapy plus temozolomide, or, in a small cohort of patients, temozolomide alone followed by radiation therapy upon tumor progression. Patients with oligodendrogliomas whose tumors lack 1p/19q deletions or *IDH* mutations do not appear to derive benefit from adjuvant PCV chemotherapy.

Suggested Reading

Cairncross G, Wang M, Shaw E, et al. Phase III trial of chemoradiotherapy for anaplastic oligodendroglioma: long-term results of RTOG 9402. *J Clin Oncol.* 2013;31:337-343. PMID: 23071247.

van den Bent MJ, Brandes AA, Taphoorn MJ, et al. Adjuvant procarbazine, lomustine, and vincristine chemotherapy in newly diagnosed anaplastic oligodendroglioma: long-term follow-up of EORTC brain tumor group study 26951. *J Clin Oncol.* 2013;31:344-350. PMID: 23071237.

Cairncross JG, Wang M, Jenkins RB, et al. Benefit from procarbazine, lomustine, and vincristine in oligodendroglial tumors is associated with mutation of IDH. *J Clin Oncol.* 2014;32:783-790. PMID: 24516018.

14-2 C

Temozolomide given concurrently with radiation therapy, followed by adjuvant temozolomide given daily for 5 days every 28 days for six cycles, prolongs survival compared with radiation alone. It is not known whether radiation with concurrent temozolomide without subsequent adjuvant temozolomide is effective. Final results of two recently completed phase III clinical trials demonstrated no survival benefit when bevacizumab is added to standard therapy with radiation and concurrent temozolomide followed by six cycles of post-radiation temozolomide.

Suggested Reading

Hegi ME, Diserens AC, Gorlia T, et al. MGMT gene silencing and benefit from temozolomide in glioblastoma. *N Engl J Med.* 2005;352:997-1003. PMID: 15758010.

Stupp R, Hegi ME, Mason WP, et al. Effects of radiotherapy with concomitant and adjuvant temozolomide versus radiotherapy alone on survival in glioblastoma in a randomised phase III study: 5-year analysis of the EORTC-NCIC trial. *Lancet Oncol.* 2009;10:459-466. PMID: 19269895.

Fine HA. Bevacizumab in glioblastoma–still much to learn. *N Engl J Med.* 2014;379:764-765. PMID: 24552324.

Chinot OL, Wick W, Mason W, et al. Bevacizumab plus radiotherapy-temozolomide for newly diagnosed glioblastoma. *N Engl J Med.* 2014;370:709-722. PMID: 24552318.

Gilbert MR, Dignam JJ, Armstrong TS, et al. A randomized trial of bevacizumab for newly diagnosed glioblastoma. *N Engl J Med.* 2014;370:699-708. PMID: 24552317.

14-3 B

Phase III data suggest that in elderly patients, treatment with temozolomide alone is associated with superior survival only in patients with *MGMT* promoter methylation. Methylation status was not associated with different outcomes in patients who received radiation therapy alone. Previous studies have also demonstrated that survival following an abbreviated course of radiation therapy (40 Gy in 15 fractions) is very similar to that observed after a longer course (60 Gy in 30 fractions) in elderly patients. It remains uncertain if elderly patients benefit from radiation plus temozolomide or PCV. One phase III trial demonstrated no survival benefit with the addition of stereotactic radiation therapy to standard radiation therapy.

Suggested Reading

Wick W, Platten M, Meisner C, et al. Temozolomide chemotherapy alone versus radiotherapy alone for malignant astrocytoma in the elderly: the NOA-08 randomised, phase 3 trial. *Lancet Oncol.* 2012;13:707-715. PMID: 22578793.

Roa W, Brasher PM, Bauman G, et al. Abbreviated course of radiation therapy in older patients with glioblastoma multiforme: a prospective randomized clinical trial. *J Clin Oncol.* 2004;22:1583-1588. PMID: 15051755.

Laperriere N, Weller M, Stupp R, et al. Optimal management of elderly patients with glioblastoma. *Cancer Treat Rev.* 2013; 39:350-357. PMID: 22722053.

Souhami L, Seiferheld W, Brachman D, et al. Randomized comparison of stereotactic radiosurgery followed by conventional radiotherapy with carmustine to conventional radiotherapy with carmustine for patients with glioblastoma multiforme: report of Radiation Therapy Oncology Group 93-05 protocol. *Int J Radiat Oncol Biol Phys.* 2004;60:853-860. PMID: 15465203.

14-4 D

Pseudoprogression is a relatively common imaging finding in patients receiving radiation and temozolomide for glioblastoma, and may be more common in patients with *MGMT* promoter methylation. Because the patient is asymptomatic, and there is no increased mass effect, restricted diffusion, or increased perfusion, there is not compelling evidence that she has true tumor progression, so continuing adjuvant temozolomide with the presumptive diagnosis of pseudoprogression is reasonable. Temozolomide alone is not known to cause pseudoprogression; rather, radiation (with or without temozolomide) causes pseudoprogression. Not only is biopsy unnecessary and potentially hazardous in this patient, but early biopsy cannot reliably distinguish progressive tumor from residual tumor and pseudoprogression, and genomic profiling in glioblastoma has not yet been validated as a diagnostic assay that accurately predicts response to subsequent therapy.

Suggested Reading

Brandes AA, Franceschi E, Tosoni A, et al. MGMT promoter methylation status can predict the incidence and outcome of pseudoprogression after concomitant radiochemotherapy in newly diagnosed glioblastoma patients. *J Clin Oncol.* 2008;26:2192-2197. PMID: 18445844.

Brandsma D, Stalpers L, Taal W, et al. Clinical features, mechanisms, and management of pseudoprogression in malignant gliomas. *Lancet Oncol.* 2008;9:453-461. PMID: 18452856.

14-5 C

While systemic lymphoma is most appropriately treated with R-CHOP, primary central nervous system (CNS) lymphoma does not respond as favorably. High-dose methotrexate, alone or in various combination regimens, remains the primary therapeutic agent for primary CNS lymphoma. Initial therapy with whole-brain radiation is usually not indicated in primary CNS lymphoma because of the risk of neurocognitive injury and because the response to high-dose methotrexate may be excellent. Temozolomide plus radiation is appropriate treatment for glioblastoma but not for primary CNS lymphoma. The risk of CNS injury is substantially increased with the use of both whole-brain radiation and methotrexate, so answer D is incorrect.

Suggested Reading

Batchelor T, Carson K, O'Neill A, et al. Treatment of primary CNS lymphoma with methotrexate and deferred radiotherapy: a report of NABTT 96-07. *J Clin Oncol.* 2003;21:1044-1049. PMID: 12637469.

DeAngelis LM, Seiferheld W, Schold SC, et al. Combination chemotherapy and radiotherapy for primary central nervous system lymphoma: Radiation Therapy Oncology Group Study 93-10. *J Clin Oncol.* 2002;20:4643-4648. PMID: 12488408.

Rubenstein JL, Gupta NK, Mannis GN, et al. How I treat CNS lymphomas. *Blood.* 2013;122:2318-2330. PMID: 23963042.

14-6   A

Previous studies have demonstrated that patients who undergo resection of solitary metastases have superior survival compared with those treated with radiation alone. Moreover, this patient has symptoms and imaging findings of significantly increased intracranial pressure. She needs immediate surgical consultation. While there is some evidence that stereotactic radiation may be appropriate for solitary brain metastases, the presence of significant mass effect is a contraindication to stereotactic radiation, and whole-brain radiation would not be appropriate in the absence of tumor resection. The efficacy of trastuzumab emtansine for brain metastases remains unclear, and lapatinib alone without surgery with or without radiation therapy would not be appropriate.

Suggested Reading

Patchell RA, Tibbs PA, Walsh JW, et al. A randomized trial of surgery in the treatment of single metastases to the brain. *N Engl J Med.* 1990;322:494-500. PMID: 2405271.

Patchell RA, Tibbs PA, Regine WF, et al. Postoperative radiotherapy in the treatment of single metastases to the brain: a randomized trial. *JAMA.* 1998;280:1485-1489. PMID: 9809728.

14-7   B

Recent studies have determined that patients with *IDH*-mutant anaplastic astrocytoma have markedly better outcomes than those without *IDH* mutations. However, associations between *IDH* mutations and the effect of specific therapies upon outcome have not yet been noted. For patients with anaplastic astrocytoma, standard therapy continues to be immediate radiation therapy, therefore, unlike treatment of patients with low-grade glioma, observation is not appropriate. The benefit of adding temozolomide to radiation therapy is being assessed in an ongoing phase III trial. To date, the utility of *MGMT* promoter methylation status to direct therapy has not been established. Finally, even patients with *IDH* wild-type tumors can be expected to have median life expectancy exceeding 2 years.

Suggested Reading

Yan H, Parsons DW, Jin G, et al. IDH1 and IDH2 mutations in gliomas. *N Engl J Med.* 2009;360:765-773. PMID: 19228619.

Kizilbash SH, Giannini C, Voss JS, et al. Impact of adjuvant temozolomide and IDH mutation status among patients with anaplastic astrocytoma. *J Clin Oncol.* 31;2013 (suppl; abstr 2025).

European Organisation for Research and Treatment of Cancer. NCT00626990. Radiation Therapy with or without Temozolomide in Treating Patients with Anaplastic Glioma. http://clinicaltrials.gov/show/NCT00626990. Accessed June 13, 2014.

15 LEUKEMIAS
SELF-EVALUATION

LEUKEMIAS QUESTIONS

15-1 A 58-year-old otherwise fit man presents with fatigue. On physical examination, a 2-cm nontender cervical lymph node is detected in his right neck, and the exam is otherwise normal. A complete blood count (CBC) shows a white blood cell count of 96,000/mm³, of which more than 90% are mature-appearing lymphocytes with occasional prolympho-cytes. His hematocrit is 43% and his platelet count is 372,000/mm³.

An appropriate work-up of this individual would include which of the following?

A. Studies of the peripheral blood for immunophenotype, immunoglobulin (Ig) heavy chain status, and fluorescence in situ hybridization (FISH) for 11q, 13q, and 17q

B. Bone marrow aspiration and biopsy for morphology, and studies of immunophenotype, Ig heavy chain status, and FISH for 11q, 13q, and 17q

C. Studies of peripheral blood for immunophenotype, Ig heavy chain status, and FISH for 11q, 13q, and 17q, as well as bone marrow aspiration and biopsy for morphology

D. Bone marrow aspiration and biopsy for morphology and studies of immunophenotype, Ig heavy chain status, and FISH for 11q, 13q, and 17q, as well as a lymph node biopsy

E. Studies of peripheral blood for immunophenotype, Ig heavy chain status, and FISH for 11q, 13q, and 17q, as well as bone marrow aspiration and biopsy for morphology, and a chest and abdominal computed tomography (CT) scan

15-2 A 27-year-old woman presents with bleeding gums and easy bruising. She was found to have a hemato-crit of 29%, a white blood cell count of 3,800/mm³ with 5% peripheral promyelocytes, and a platelet count of 48,000/mm³. A bone marrow exam shows morphologic and molecular evidence of promyelocytic leukemia. She was administered all-trans retinoic acid (ATRA). Infection prophylaxis includes a quinolone and sulfamethoxazole plus trimethoprim. Seven days after starting therapy, the patient presents with fever and increasing shortness of breath that has developed over several days. Her white blood cell count has risen to 15,000/mm³ with 20% promyelocytes and metamyelocytes.

A chest x-ray shows diffuse pulmonary infiltrates. What would be the most appropriate next step?

A. Add daunorubicin to therapy

B. Add arsenic trioxide to therapy

C. Perform a bronchoscopy

D. Add posaconazole for antifungal coverage

E. Temporarily discontinue ATRA and add dexamethasone

15-3 A 74-year-old woman presents with increasing fatigue and peripheral edema, and is found to have a hema-tocrit of 26%, a white blood cell count of 40,000/mm³ with circulating lymphoblasts, and a platelet count of 90,000/mm³. A bone marrow biopsy shows Philadelphia (Ph)-positive acute lymphocytic leuke-mia (ALL). She has a prior history of congestive heart failure.

What therapy would you recommend for her?

A. Supportive care only

B. Low-dose cytarabine

C. Dasatinib plus dexamethasone

D. Vincristine, prednisone, L-asparaginase, daunorubicin, and imatinib

E. Gemtuzumab ozogamicin

15-4 A 45-year-old man was found to have a hematocrit of 30%, a platelet count of 800,000/mm³, and a white blood cell count of 75,000/mm³, the majority of which were mature granulocytes, at his annual examination. A bone marrow examination showed myeloid hyperplasia and FISH confirmed the presence of a t(9;22) translocation in 90% of metaphases. The diagnosis of chronic-phase chronic myeloid leukemia (CML) was made and the patient was started on 400 mg per day of imatinib. After 6 months of therapy, the patient is being restudied. His CBC has returned to normal values, but a repeat bone marrow shows persistence of the Ph-positive chromosome in 25% of metaphases. He has tolerated therapy without any side effects.

Based on this result, what treatment strategy do you recommend?
A. Continue imatinib at 400 mg once daily
B. Increase the dose of imatinib to 600 mg once daily
C. Increase the dose of imatinib to 800 mg once daily
D. Switch to nilotinib at 400 mg twice daily
E. Switch to dasatinib at 100 mg once daily

15-5 An 83-year-old man presents with fatigue, shortness of breath, and increasing angina, and is found to have a hematocrit of 23%, a white blood cell count of 27,000/mm³, and a platelet count of 85,000/mm³. A bone marrow examination shows acute myeloid leukemia (AML) with complex cytogenetics including monosomy 7 and monosomy 11. The patient has a known past history of coronary artery disease, hypertension, and peripheral vascular disease. His Eastern Cooperative Oncology Group (ECOG) performance status is 2.

Which of the following options would you recommend?
A. Supportive care only
B. Low-dose cytarabine
C. Imatinib
D. Conventional induction with cytarabine (200 mg/m² per day for 7 days) and daunorubicin (60 mg/m² per day for 3 days)
E. Conventional induction with cytarabine, but with reduced-dose daunorubicin (45 mg/m² per day for 3 days)

15-6 A 43-year-old woman presents with a 2-month history of fatigue, bleeding gums when brushing her teeth, and easy bruising. A CBC shows a white blood cell count of 45,000/mm³, a platelet count of 24,000/mm³, and a hematocrit of 27%. Examination of the peripheral smear shows that at least 50% of the cells are myeloblasts. A bone marrow examination shows a hypercellular marrow with 65% myeloblasts consistent with a diagnosis of AML. Routine cytogenetics fail to detect any abnormalities.

Which further tests are indicated?
A. Polymerase chain reaction testing for t(9;22)
B. Genome-wide expression array analysis
C. Immunophenotyping
D. Mutational analysis of *NPM1, FLT3,* and *CEBPA*
E. Lumbar puncture

15-7 A 68-year-old woman presents with extreme fatigue. She is found to have a hematocrit of 17%, but other features of her CBC are normal. A bone marrow examination is performed and shows a mildly hyperplastic marrow with erythroid dysplasia and 3% myeloblasts. Cytogenetics show del(5)(q31-33). The serum erythropoietin level is elevated. She is transfused with 2 units of packed red blood cells.

What would be the most appropriate next step?
A. Observation
B. Treatment with erythropoietin
C. Treatment with lenalidomide
D. Treatment with azacytidine
E. Treatment with decitabine

15-8 A 67-year-old man was diagnosed with chronic-phase CML 4 years ago and was treated with 400 mg per day of imatinib. He tolerated therapy well and his peripheral counts returned to normal within 3 months, and after 1 year of therapy his bone marrow had become cytogenetically normal. Over the last 6 months, his peripheral count has risen back to 50,000/mm³ and his spleen has enlarged to the point of causing early satiety. In addition, a bone marrow analysis now shows myeloid hyperplasia with 5% myeloblasts and Ph positivity in 80% of the metaphases. A sample sent for mutational analysis indicates presence of a *G250* mutation.

What would be an appropriate next step?
A. Increase the imatinib dose to 800 mg per day
B. Switch to interferon-alpha
C. Switch to dasatinib
D. Treat with cytarabine plus daunorubicin
E. Switch to decitabine

15-9 A 53-year-old man presents with pallor, easy bruising, and bleeding gums. A CBC shows a white blood cell count of 2,100/mm^3 with 20% promyelocytes, a hematocrit of 20%, and a platelet count of 24,000/mm^3. FISH examination of the marrow is positive for t(15;17). The patient has a past history of coronary artery disease with two previous myocardial infarctions. He has congestive heart failure requiring medical therapy.

What therapy would you recommend as initial treatment?

A. Reduced-dose daunorubicin (45 mg/m^2 per day for three cycles) and standard-dose cytarabine
B. Standard-dose daunorubicin (90 mg/m^2 per day for three cycles) and standard-dose cytarabine
C. Reduced-dose daunorubicin (45 mg/m^2 per day for three cycles) with standard-dose cytarabine and ATRA
D. Standard-dose daunorubicin (90 mg/m^2 per day for three cycles) with standard-dose cytarabine and ATRA
E. ATRA and arsenic trioxide

15-10 A 27-year-old black woman presents with fever and recurrent infections. A work-up shows a white blood cell count of 36,000 mm^3 with 70% myeloblasts. A bone marrow examination shows 80% myeloblasts and cytogenetics indicate that all metaphases have the t(6;9) translocation. The patient is treated with daunorubicin (90 mg/m^2 per day) for 3 days combined with cytarabine (200 mg/m^2 per day for 7 days). Twenty-eight days later, she has recovered normal counts and a repeat bone marrow shows a complete remission with normal cytogenetics. She is an only child and an unrelated donor search is unable to identify any matched or single-antigen mismatched donors, but a two-antigen mismatched cord unit with an adequate CD34+ cell count was found.

What would be the best form of subsequent therapy?

A. Treat with four cycles of cytarabine (400 mg/m^2 per day for 5 days)
B. Treat with four cycles of cytarabine (400 mg/m^2 per day for 5 days) combined with dasatinib (100 mg/day for 14 days)
C. Treat with four cycles of cytarabine (3 g/m^2 every 12 hours) every other day for six doses
D. Treat with four cycles of cytarabine (3 g/m^2 every 12 hours) every other day for six doses, followed by 6 months of azacitidine maintenance (75 mg/m^2 per day) for 5 days
E. Proceed to an umbilical cord blood transplant

15-1 A

This patient likely has chronic lymphocytic leukemia (CLL). Immunophenotyping of the peripheral blood is required to establish the diagnosis. Typically the cells will be positive for the B-cell markers CD19, CD20, and CD23, and the T-cell marker CD5. This helps to distinguish the disease from mantle cell lymphoma, which does not express CD23, and T-cell prolymphocytic leukemia, which expresses additional T-cell markers. Since the patient is symptomatic, he will likely be offered therapy for his disease. Thus, additional tests are useful to help select therapy and provide prognostic information. Ig heavy chain status is a useful prognostic factor, with more aggressive disease associated with unmutated heavy chain status. A FISH panel for abnormalities of 11q, 13q, and 17q not only provides prognostic information, but may help in the selection of therapy. Abnormalities of 13q are associated with a more favorable prognosis, whereas abnormalities of 11q and 17q are associated with more aggressive disease. For patients with 11q and 17q abnormalities, more aggressive regimens like fludarabine/cyclophosphamide/rituximab are recommended. A bone marrow examination might provide useful information if the patient had a significant cytopenia. Neither CT scan nor lymph node biopsy is indicated.

Suggested Reading

Döhner H, Stilgenbauer S, Benner A, et al. Genomic aberrations and survival in chronic lymphocytic leukemia. *N Engl J Med.* 2000;343:1910-1916. PMID: 11136261.

15-2 E

This patient likely has the so-called retinoic acid syndrome associated with the sudden maturation of promyeloblasts. The syndrome usually responds rapidly to dexamethasone, following which ATRA can be restarted. A similar syndrome has been seen with the use of arsenic trioxide for acute promyelocytic leukemia.

Suggested Reading

Tallman MS, Andersen JW, Schiffer CA, et al. Clinical description of 44 patients with acute promyelocytic leukemia who developed the retinoic acid syndrome. *Blood.* 2000;95:90-95. PMID: 10607690.

15-3 C

The addition of the tyrosine kinase inhibitor imatinib mesylate to conventional chemotherapeutic regimens has increased complete response rates in Ph-positive ALL, equaling those seen in Ph-negative ALL, but the effect of the addition of imatinib mesylate on the duration of remission is not yet known. Dasatinib, a second-generation BCR-ABL tyrosine kinase inhibitor, has demonstrated efficacy in relapsed/refractory adult Ph-positive ALL. Therapy with dasatinib and prednisone alone without chemotherapy appears sufficient to allow the majority of older patients with Ph-positive ALL to achieve an initial hematologic remission. Given this patient's age and presence of peripheral edema, it would probably be preferable to avoid the concomitant chemotherapy.

Suggested Reading

Foà R, Vitale A, Vignetti M, et al. Dasatinib as first-line treatment for adult patients with Philadelphia chromosome-positive acute lymphoblastic leukemia. *Blood.* 2011;118:6521-6528. PMID: 21931113.

15-4 A

The patient is tolerating imatinib well and has reached an appropriate 6-month milestone with normalization of his peripheral counts with less than 35% of Ph-positive metaphases in the marrow. By 12 months, one would expect to see a complete cytogenetic response and a 2-log reduction in BCR-ABL fusion product.

Suggested Reading

Baccarani M, Deininger MW, Rosti G, et al. European LeukemiaNet recommendations for the management of chronic myeloid leukemia: 2013. *Blood.* 2013;122:872-884. PMID: 23803709.

15-5 B

Given the patient's age and performance status, and the very low response rate of AML with a monosomal karyotype, conventional chemotherapy either at normal or reduced doses is unlikely to help this patient. In a randomized trial, low-dose cytarabine was superior to supportive care alone.

15-6   D

Assuming this patient experiences a complete remission, analysis of the mutational status of *NPM1, FLT3,* and *CEBPA* will be the most important determinants of whether she should subsequently be treated with hematopoietic cell transplantation. Patients with AML with normal cytogenetics but either with mutations in *CEBPA,* or with mutations in *NPM1* without an *FLT3* mutation, are in the favorable-risk category and have equivalent prospects for long-term survival when treated with subsequent consolidation chemotherapy or with transplantation. Patients with all other combinations (*CEBPA, NPM1* wild-type, or mutated *FLT3*) appear to benefit with transplantation in first remission.

Suggested Reading

Döhner H, Estey EH, Amadori S, et al. Diagnosis and management of acute myeloid leukemia in adults: recommendations from an international expert panel, on behalf of the European LeukemiaNet. *Blood*. 2010;115:453-474. PMID: 19880497.

15-7   C

Lenalidomide, an analog of thalidomide, has been approved for the treatment of transfusion-dependent low-risk or intermediate-risk 1 myelodysplastic syndrome that is associated with del(5)(q31-33). In the pivotal study, 64% of patients became transfusion-independent and 75% experienced a cytogenetic response, one-half of which were complete responses. Erythropoietin seldom works in patients with already elevated erythropoietin levels. Response rates to azacytidine or decitabine are much lower than with lenalidomide in this setting.

Suggested Reading

Goldstone AH, Richards SM, Lazarus HM, et al. In adults with standard-risk acute lymphoblastic leukemia, the greatest benefit is achieved from a matched sibling allogeneic transplantation in first complete remission, and an autologous transplantation is less effective than conventional consolidation/maintenance chemotherapy in all patients: final results of the International ALL Trial (MRC UKALL XII/ECOG E2993). *Blood*. 2008;111: 1827-1833. PMID: 18048644.

15-8   C

Mutations in the ABL–tyrosine kinase domain cannot usually be overcome with dose escalation. Chronic-phase CML with the *G250* mutation generally maintains sensitivity to dasatinib. While the patient's disease might respond to interferon, complete responses to interferon are less frequent and the toxicities are generally much greater than those seen with dasatinib. Neither conventional AML therapy nor decitabine are indicated in this setting.

Suggested Reading

Branford S, Melo JV, Hughes TP. Selecting optimal second-line tyrosine kinase inhibitor therapy for chronic myeloid leukemia patients after imatinib failure: does the BCR-ABL mutation status really matter? *Blood*. 2009;114:5426-5435. PMID: 19880502.

15-9   E

This patient has favorable-risk acute promyelocytic leukemia. Although the disease is very sensitive to daunorubicin, recent studies have shown that outcomes similar to those achieved with standard chemotherapy–containing regimens can occur with a combination of ATRA and arsenic trioxide. Given this patient's cardiac condition, avoidance of an anthracycline is appropriate.

Suggested Reading

Lo-Coco F, Avvisati G, Vignetti M, et al. Retinoic acid and arsenic trioxide for acute promyelocytic leukemia. *N Engl J Med*. 2013;369: 111-121. PMID: 23841729.

15-10 E

AML with t(6;9) is a very high-risk category of disease with a poor cure rate when treated with conventional chemotherapy. Neither concomitant dasatinib nor azacitidine maintenance has been shown to improve outcome of chemotherapy for patients with this subtype of AML. Because of both genetic diversity and under-representation in the donor registry, matched unrelated donors can be found for only a minority of black patients. With recent advances in supportive care measures, the outcome of transplantation using umbilical cord blood approaches that observed when using matched, unrelated donors.

Suggested Reading

Scaradavou A, Brunstein CG, Eapen M, et al. Double unit grafts successfully extend the application of umbilical cord blood transplantation in adults with acute leukemia. *Blood*. 2013;121: 752-758. PMID: 23223509.

16 LYMPHOMAS
SELF-EVALUATION

LYMPHOMAS QUESTIONS

16-1 A 78-year-old man with type II diabetes mellitus and congestive heart failure presents to his physician for a routine visit. He is asymptomatic. His examination reveals a 1.5-cm right cervical node, which he first noted three months ago. An excisional biopsy of the right cervical node reveals grade 1 follicular lymphoma (FL). His complete blood count (CBC), lactate dehydrogenase (LDH) level, and beta 2 microglobulin level are all normal. Computed tomography (CT) scans of the chest, abdomen, and pelvis reveal no other adenopathy, but a bone marrow biopsy contains low-level involvement with FL (5% of marrow cellularity).

What is the most appropriate management for this patient?
A. Watchful waiting
B. Chlorambucil therapy
C. Rituximab weekly for 4 weeks followed by maintenance rituximab every 2 months for 2 years
D. Rituximab plus bendamustine every 28 days for six cycles

16-2 A 45-year-old woman presents with abdominal pain and diffuse adenopathy. Physical examination demonstrates multiple 2- to 6-cm lymph nodes in bilateral cervical, axillary, and inguinal regions and massive, tender hepatosplenomegaly. A positron emission tomography (PET)/CT scan also demonstrates a 12-cm retroperitoneal mass that encases the aorta, inferior vena cava, and left ureter. There is mild left-sided hydronephrosis. Her CBC is normal, but her LDH is elevated (450 U/L; normal range, 0 to 190 U/L), as is her beta 2 microglobulin. A left axillary lymph node biopsy reveals grade 2 FL with a Ki67 proliferation index of 40%.

Which of the following FL treatment regimens is most likely to be associated with prolonged hematologic toxicity, long-term hematopoietic stem cell damage, and secondary malignancies?
A. Rituximab, cyclophosphamide, vincristine, and prednisone (R-CVP)
B. Rituximab, cyclophosphamide, doxorubicin, vincristine, and prednisone (R-CHOP)
C. Rituximab plus bendamustine (R-bendamustine)
D. Rituximab and fludarabine with mitoxantrone

16-3 An asymptomatic 35-year-old man presents with a 4-cm right cervical mass. A biopsy reveals mixed cellularity Hodgkin lymphoma (HL). A PET/CT scan confirms right cervical lymphadenopathy as well as a 4-cm anterior mediastinal mass and right axillary adenopathy (1.5- to 3-cm nodes). A CBC is normal, but the erythrocyte sedimentation rate is elevated at 55 mm/hour (normal range, 0 to 20 mm/hour). There is no infradiaphragmatic disease, and other staging tests are normal.

Which of the following treatment options is most appropriate?
A. Subtotal nodal radiotherapy (36 Gy)
B. Doxorubicin/bleomycin/vinblastine/dacarbazine (ABVD) for two cycles followed by 20 Gy of involved nodal radiotherapy
C. ABVD for four cycles followed by 30 Gy of involved nodal radiotherapy
D. Bleomycin/etoposide/doxorubicin/cyclophosphamide/vincristine/procarbazine/prednisone (BEACOPP) for four cycles followed by 30 Gy of involved nodal radiotherapy

16-4 A 42-year-old man presents with mild shortness of breath, a sensation of chest pressure, and night sweats. A staging workup with fluorodeoxyglucose (FDG)-PET/CT imaging reveals a 7-cm anterior mediastinal mass, retroperitoneal adenopathy, and FDG-avid splenic nodules. The bone marrow is uninvolved. Lab testing reveals a normal CBC, differential, and albumin but a slightly elevated sedimentation rate (45 mm/hour). A biopsy demonstrates classical Hodgkin lymphoma with typical Hodgkin Reed-Sternberg cells. He is treated with six cycles of ABVD chemotherapy and achieves a complete remission. Two years later, his disease relapses with right cervical adenopathy and intra-abdominal adenopathy. He is treated with three cycles of ifosfamide, carboplatin, and etoposide (ICE) chemotherapy and achieves a complete remission documented by FDG-PET/CT at the end of treatment.

How would you treat this patient now?
A. No further therapy
B. Administer brentuximab vedotin every 3 weeks for six cycles
C. Consolidate with autologous stem cell transplantation (ASCT)
D. Consolidate with allogeneic stem cell transplantation (alloSCT)

16-5 A 48-year-old woman presents with a rapidly growing 5-cm left cervical lymph node that is biopsied, revealing diffuse large B-cell lymphoma (DLBCL). The Ki67 proliferation index is 60% and fluorescence in situ hybridization (FISH) studies reveal no obvious chromosomal abnormalities. Staging studies including FDG-PET/CT scans and bone marrow biopsies document stage IIIA disease with several 2- to 4-cm abdominal lymph nodes. The CBC and LDH are normal. The patient is treated with six cycles of R-CHOP and achieves a complete remission as documented by an end-of-treatment FDG-PET/CT.

How would you treat this patient now?
A. No further therapy; perform surveillance imaging with FDG-PET/CT every 6 months for 2 years
B. No further therapy; perform surveillance imaging with contrast-enhanced CT of the chest, abdomen, and pelvis no more frequently than every 6 months for 2 years
C. Administer maintenance rituximab intravenously every 2 to 3 months for 2 years
D. Consolidate the patient's complete remission with high-dose therapy and ASCT

16-6 A 48-year-old woman presents with profound fatigue, drenching night sweats, and a rapidly growing 5-cm left cervical lymph node. A biopsy shows DLBCL. The Ki67 proliferation index is 95% and FISH studies reveal rearrangements affecting both the *c-Myc* oncogene and the *BCL2* gene. Staging studies with PET/CT scans and bone marrow biopsies document several 2- to 4-cm abdominal lymph nodes, as well as marrow involvement with DLBCL. The CBC is normal, but the LDH level is elevated at 600 U/L (normal range, up to 200 U/L).

Which statement most accurately describes the expected clinical course for this patient?
A. The patient has a 60% chance of cure with R-CHOP chemotherapy
B. The patient is unlikely to be cured with R-CHOP but has a more than 60% chance of cure with aggressive chemotherapy regimens such as R-hyperCVAD or R-CODOX-M/IVAC
C. The patient has a more than 60% chance of cure with aggressive chemotherapy (R-hyperCVAD or R-CODOX-M/IVAC) followed by ASCT
D. The patient has a poor chance of long-term disease-free survival with any current treatment strategy

16-7 A 65-year-old man is noted to have an elevated white blood cell count (25,000) on a routine blood test, with a normal hematocrit and platelet count. The white cell differential shows that 90% of the cells are abnormal lymphoid cells. Physical examination reveals diffuse lymphadenopathy in the cervical, axillary, and inguinal regions with the largest node being 4 cm in diameter. CT scans confirm these enlarged nodes as well as documenting multiple 2- to 4-cm mesenteric and retroperitoneal nodes and moderate splenomegaly. A bone marrow examination reveals diffuse infiltration with neoplastic lymphocytes identical to those in the blood.

Which of the following tests would establish a diagnosis of mantle cell lymphoma?
A. Flow cytometry of the blood showing monoclonal B cells expressing low levels of surface immunoglobulin G with kappa light chain restriction, low levels of CD20, and positivity for CD5, CD19, and CD23
B. FISH testing of the blood and marrow revealing a translocation between chromosomes 8 and 22
C. A lymph node biopsy showing high levels of cyclin D1 expression
D. Immunohistochemical analysis of a lymph node biopsy revealing *p53* overexpression

16-8 A 45-year-old man presents with stage IIIA anaplastic large T-cell lymphoma. He is treated with CHOP chemotherapy for six cycles and achieves a complete remission. His disease relapses 3 years later and he is treated with three cycles of ICE chemotherapy, followed by consolidation with ASCT. He achieves a second remission but disease recurs again 2 years later.

How would you treat the patient now?
A. Denileukin diftitox
B. Romidepsin
C. Pralatrexate
D. Brentuximab vedotin

16-9 A 60-year-old woman presents complaining of abdominal distension and early satiety. A physical examination reveals splenomegaly with a spleen tip descending four fingerbreadths below the left costal margin. Blood testing reveals moderate pancytopenia (hematocrit 30, leukocyte count 2,000/μL, neutrophil count 750/μL, and platelet count 50,000/μL). Circulating atypical lymphocytes with a ruffled border and villous projections are seen on the blood smear. Blood chemistries, including LDH and beta 2 microglobulin levels, are normal. FDG-PET/CT confirms splenomegaly but reveal no adenopathy. A bone marrow aspirate and biopsy demonstrate sparse infiltration with neoplastic lymphocytes representing 10% to 20% of marrow cells. Flow cytometry of the neoplastic lymphocytes reveals normal levels of surface immunoglobulin, CD19, CD20, and CD22 without expression of CD5, CD10, CD11c, CD103, or CD123.

Of the following treatment options, which would you choose for this patient?
A. Watchful waiting
B. Laparoscopic splenectomy
C. R-CHOP chemotherapy given every 3 weeks for six cycles
D. Lenalidomide and dexamethasone for six cycles

16-10 A 35-year-old man with AIDS presents with a 3-cm right infraclavicular mass. He feels well, is working full time, and denies fever, drenching sweats, or weight loss. He has been treated with highly active combination antiretroviral therapy (HAART) for 1 year and has no recent opportunistic infections. An excisional biopsy of the infraclavicular mass demonstrates DLBCL expressing monoclonal surface immunoglobulin, CD19, and CD20 without CD10. FISH testing reveals no rearrangements of *c-Myc* or *Bcl2*. PET/CT demonstrates pathologic adenopathy in the mediastinum (4 cm), retroperitoneum (3 cm), and a 4-cm extranodal mass in the right psoas muscle. His leukocyte count is 4,500/μL, with a platelet count of 150,000/μL, neutrophil count of 2,500/μL, hematocrit of 34, CD4 count of 500/μL, and an undetectable HIV viral load by polymerase chain reaction testing. His bone marrow biopsy shows involvement with DLBCL.

How would you treat this patient's lymphoma?
A. Supportive care
B. Reduced-dose, anthracycline-based therapy with rituximab (e.g., dose-adjusted R-EPOCH or R-CHOP)
C. Full-dose anthracycline-based therapy (R-CHOP or DA-EPOCH-R) plus intrathecal prophylaxis (e.g., methotrexate)
D. Full-dose anthracycline-based therapy with intrathecal prophylaxis (e.g., methotrexate) followed by consolidation with ASCT

16-1 A

The patient has asymptomatic, low tumor burden, stage IVA grade 1 FL. He does not fulfill any of the National Comprehensive Cancer Network (NCCN) guidelines or any of the Groupe d'Etude des Lymphomes Folliculaires criteria for initiation of therapy of FL. These guidelines recommend that patients with grade 1 to 2 FL be initially observed without therapy unless they have symptoms (drenching sweats, pain, fever), high tumor bulk (largest node bigger than 7 cm or three nodes bigger than 3 cm), impairment of normal organ function (e.g., ureteral or bile duct obstruction), pleural effusions, ascites, massive splenomegaly, or cytopenias. Several randomized phase III clinical trials have investigated the utility of immediate institution of chemotherapy (including chlorambucil) or rituximab immunotherapy in patients with newly diagnosed FL. None of these studies have demonstrated an improvement in overall survival (OS) with immediate treatment. Consequently, watchful waiting remains a standard approach for patients with asymptomatic, low tumor burden FL, especially those who are elderly and have multiple comorbidities, like this patient.

Suggested Reading

Zelenetz AD, Abramson JS, Advani RH, et al. *NCCN Clinical Practice Guidelines in Oncology (NCCN Guidelines®) Non-Hodgkin's Lymphomas*, Version 2.2013. Rockledge, PA: National Comprehensive Cancer Network, 2013.

Brice P, Bastion Y, Lepage E, et al. Comparison in low-tumor-burden follicular lymphomas between an initial no-treatment policy, prednimustine, or interferon alfa: a randomized study from the Groupe d'Etude des Lymphomes Folliculaires. Groupe d'Etude des Lymphomes de l'Adulte. *J Clin Oncol.* 1997;15:1110-1117. PMID: 9060552.

Press OW. Follicular Lymphoma. In: Kaushansky K, Lichtman M, Beutler E et al (eds). *Williams' Hematology, 8th ed.* New York: McGraw-Hill, Medical Publications Division; 2010;1565-1574.

16-2 D

This patient is markedly symptomatic, has a high tumor burden, and threatened end organ damage due to ureteral obstruction with hydronephrosis. Therefore, prompt initiation of an effective regimen is indicated. Several acceptable front-line regimens for FL exist, including R-CVP, R-CHOP, and R-bendamustine. Two large phase III clinical trials have compared R-CVP, R-CHOP, and rituximab plus fludarabine-containing regimens for treatment of grade 1 to 2 FL, and both demonstrated that regimens with fludarabine and rituximab had significantly more hematologic toxicity and a higher risk of secondary malignancies than the alkylator-based regimens R-CVP or R-CHOP. R-CHOP provides superior progression-free survival (PFS) compared to R-CVP, but there is no difference in OS, so most authorities still believe that both regimens are acceptable. R-CHOP and R-bendamustine have been compared in two randomized studies, and both concluded that R-bendamustine is at least as effective as R-CHOP and may be less toxic. Although treatment of FL remains controversial, most authorities are now reluctant to use fludarabine-based regimens as front-line therapy for indolent lymphomas other than chronic lymphocytic leukemia/small lymphocytic lymphoma, where it remains the standard of care for young, fit patients.

Suggested Reading

Salles G, Seymour JF, Offner F, et al. Rituximab maintenance for 2 years in patients with high tumour burden follicular lymphoma responding to rituximab plus chemotherapy (PRIMA): a phase 3, randomised controlled trial. *Lancet.* 2011;377:42-51. PMID: 21176949.

Federico M, Luminari S, Dondi A, et al. R-CVP versus R-CHOP versus R-FM for the initial treatment of patients with advanced-stage follicular lymphoma: results of the FOLL05 trial conducted by the Fondazione Italiana Linfomi. *J Clin Oncol.* 2013;31:1506-1513. PMID: 23530110.

Press OW, Palanca-Wessels MC. Selection of first-line therapy for advanced follicular lymphoma. *J Clin Oncol.* 2013;31:1496-1498. PMID: 23530108.

Rummel MJ, Niederle N, Maschmeyer G, et al. Bendamustine plus rituximab versus CHOP plus rituximab as first-line treatment for patients with indolent and mantle-cell lymphomas: an open-label, multicentre, randomised, phase 3 non-inferiority trial. *Lancet.* 2013;381:1203-1210. PMID: 23433739.

16-3 C

This patient has stage IIA classical HL with some unfavorable features, as defined by the German Hodgkin Disease Study Group—namely an elevated sedimentation rate and more than two sites of involved disease. Eich et al randomly assigned nearly 1,400 such patients to four cycles of either ABVD or BEACOPP followed by either 20 or 30 Gy of involved field radiation. ABVD for four cycles followed by 30 Gy of irradiation was as effective and less toxic than BEACOPP$_{baseline}$ followed by involved field radiotherapy. Four cycles of ABVD plus 20 Gy of involved field radiotherapy was significantly inferior to four cycles of ABVD plus 30 Gy of involved field radiotherapy or to BEACOPP followed by either 20 or 30 Gy of radiation. Subtotal nodal radiotherapy for early-stage HL which has largely been abandoned as an approach due to its increased risk of inducing late toxicities and secondary malignancies, contributing to a worse OS than combined modality regimens. Patients with early-stage (I-IIA) HL with no risk factors (normal sedimentation rate, no more than two sites of disease, no large mediastinal masses or tumor bulk) can be satisfactorily treated with only two cycles of ABD and 20 Gy of radiotherapy, but this minimal approach is not appropriate for patients exhibiting adverse risk features, like this patient. Some physicians might prefer to treat this patient using four to six cycles of ABVD alone without any radiotherapy, as guided by interim FDG-PET. However, this approach is still somewhat controversial and is not offered as an option here. Approaches eliminating radiotherapy altogether are especially appropriate for women younger than 25 who have a markedly increased risk of developing breast cancer if treated with thoracic radiotherapy.

Suggested Reading

Eich HT, Diehl V, Görgen H, et al. Intensified chemotherapy and dose-reduced involved-field radiotherapy in patients with early unfavorable Hodgkin's lymphoma: final analysis of the German Hodgkin Study Group HD11 trial. *J Clin Oncol.* 2010;28:4199-4206. PMID: 20713848.

Meyer RM, Gospodarowicz MK, Connors JM, et al. ABVD alone versus radiation-based therapy in limited-stage Hodgkin's lymphoma. *N Engl J Med.* 2012;366:399-408. PMID: 22149921.

Engert A, Plütschow A, Eich HT, et al. Reduced treatment intensity in patients with early-stage Hodgkin's lymphoma. *N Engl J Med.* 2010; 363:640-652. PMID: 20818855.

16-4 C

This patient has had a chemotherapy-sensitive relapse of classical HL and now is in a second complete remission. Two randomized trials have demonstrated markedly superior PFS when such patients receive consolidation therapy with high-dose chemotherapy and ASCT compared with patients treated conservatively without transplantation. More recent data suggest that patients who are FDG-PET-negative after ICE or gemcitabine/vinorelbine/liposomal doxorubicin (GVD) chemotherapy and then receive consolidation therapy with ASCT have a long-term PFS as high as 75% to 80%. No study has shown improved outcomes with alloSCT compared to ASCT for HL, and alloSCT is associated with higher transplant-related morbidity and mortality, hence answer D is not a good choice. Brentuximab vedotin is a very exciting new anti-CD30 targeted antibody-drug conjugate that is approved for patients who have disease relapse following ASCT or who are not transplant candidates, but no randomized trials have yet been conducted to suggest it can displace the current standard of care (ASCT) for this population of patients.

Suggested Reading

Schmitz N, Pfistner B, Sextro M, et al. Aggressive conventional chemotherapy compared with high-dose chemotherapy with autologous haemopoietic stem-cell transplantation for relapsed chemosensitive Hodgkin's disease: a randomised trial. *Lancet.* 2002;359:2065-2071. PMID: 12086759.

Linch DC, Winfield D, Goldstone AH, et al. Dose intensification with autologous bone-marrow transplantation in relapsed and resistant Hodgkin's disease: results of a BNLI randomised trial. *Lancet.* 1993; 341:1051-1054. PMID: 8096958.

Moskowitz CH, Matasar MJ, Zelenetz AD, et al. Normalization of pre-ASCT, FDG-PET imaging with second-line, non-cross-resistant, chemotherapy programs improves event-free survival in patients with Hodgkin lymphoma. *Blood.* 2012;119:1665-1670. PMID: 22184409.

Younes A, Gopal AK, Smith SE, et al. Results of a pivotal phase II study of brentuximab vedotin for patients with relapsed or refractory Hodgkin's lymphoma. *J Clin Oncol.* 2012;30:2183-2189. PMID: 22454421.

16-5 B

The role of surveillance imaging of patients with lymphoma in complete remission is rapidly evolving. Most studies show little benefit of routine monitoring of patients in remission with either contrast-enhanced CT or PET/CT. Current NCCN guidelines for DLBCL recommend performing PET/CT imaging at baseline before initiation of induction chemotherapy and again 6 to 8 weeks after the end of treatment. If any subsequent surveillance imaging is to be performed after documentation of complete remission, NCCN guidelines suggest it should be done with contrast-enhanced CT scans, and that it be done no more frequently than every 6 months for 2 years to minimize risks of radiation exposure to patients and unnecessary health care costs. After 2 years in complete remission, further surveillance imaging is discouraged unless there are symptoms or signs worrisome for relapse. Authorities including the NCCN guideline committee and an international working group specifically discourage the common practice of surveillance imaging of patients in complete remission using FDG-PET/CT because of the high false-positive rate, due to detection of minor infectious or inflammatory conditions, which are FDG-avid, leading to unnecessary anxiety and biopsies. Randomized controlled trials have shown no benefit of maintenance rituximab in patients with good-risk DLBCL, like this patient. A recent phase III study suggests that patients with DLBCL in the highest-risk category (International Prognostic Index [IPI] of 4 to 5) may benefit from consolidation with ASCT, but this conclusion was based on a retrospective analysis of a small subset of patients, and patients with lower IPIs did not benefit. (This patient has an IPI of 1, based on stage III disease without other high-risk features such as advanced age, elevated LDH, poor performance status, or multiple extranodal sites of disease.)

Suggested Reading

Zelenetz AD, Abramson JS, Advani RH, et al. *NCCN Clinical Practice Guidelines in Oncology (NCCN Guidelines®) Non-Hodgkin's Lymphomas*, Version 2.2013. Rockledge, PA: National Comprehensive Cancer Network, 2013.

Cheson BD. Role of functional imaging in the management of lymphoma. *J Clin Oncol.* 2011;29:1844-1854. PMID: 21482982.

Cheson BD, Pfistner B, Juweid ME, et al. Revised response criteria for malignant lymphoma. *J Clin Oncol.* 2007;25:579-586. PMID: 17242396.

Habermann TM, Weller EA, Morrison VA, et al. Rituximab-CHOP versus CHOP alone or with maintenance rituximab in older patients with diffuse large B-cell lymphoma. *J Clin Oncol.* 2006;24:3121-3127. PMID: 16754935.

Stiff PJ, Unger JM, Cook JR, et al. Autologous transplantation as consolidation for aggressive non-Hodgkin's lymphoma. *N Engl J Med.* 2013;369:1681-1690. PMID: 24171516.

16-6 D

This patient has a double-hit lymphoma, which is classically defined by a chromosomal breakpoint affecting the MYC/8q24 locus in combination with another recurrent breakpoint, usually t(14;18)(q32;q21) involving *BCL2* or a rearrangement involving the *BCL6* locus. These abnormalities are best detected by FISH. Morphologically, double-hit lymphomas may either appear to be DLBCLs or have an appearance intermediate between Burkitt lymphoma and DLBCL (B-cell lymphoma unclassifiable with features intermediate between Burkitt lymphoma and DLBCL). Double-hit lymphomas typically present aggressively with rapidly growing diffuse adenopathy, B symptoms, multiple sites of extranodal disease, a high Ki67 proliferative index, and an elevated LDH. Double-hit lymphomas usually respond transiently to conventional chemotherapy regimens (R-CHOP), but remissions are typically not durable, with most studies reporting a 5-year PFS of less than 25%. Most authorities now treat these cases with aggressive chemotherapy (R-hyperCVAD, R-CODOX-M/IVAC) followed by ASCT or alloSCT, but even these approaches are usually not satisfactory. Recently, multiple publications have demonstrated that overexpression of the Myc and BCL2 proteins as detected by immunohistochemistry also defines a poor-risk group of patients with aggressive lymphoma. It is important to recognize, however, that the group of patients defined by immunohistochemistry as double-protein overexpressors is not the same group of patients defined by FISH as double-hit lymphomas. Only 5% to 10% of patients with DLBCL are double-hit lymphomas by FISH, whereas approximately 30% of patients with DLBCL overexpress both proteins by immunohistochemistry. Furthermore, immunohistochemistry for MYC is a variable assay with relatively poor reproducibility, and MYC staining and interpretation must be standardized prior to routine use for prognostication in DLBCL.

Suggested Reading

Aukema SM, Siebert R, Schuuring E, et al. Double-hit B-cell lymphomas. *Blood.* 2011;117:2319-2331. PMID: 21119107.

Johnson NA, Slack GW, Savage KJ, et al. Concurrent expression of MYC and BCL2 in diffuse large B-cell lymphoma treated with rituximab plus cyclophosphamide, doxorubicin, vincristine, and prednisone. *J Clin Oncol.* 2012;30:3452-3459. PMID: 22851565.

Green TM, Young KH, Visco C, et al. Immunohistochemical double-hit score is a strong predictor of outcome in patients with diffuse large B-cell lymphoma treated with rituximab plus cyclophosphamide, doxorubicin, vincristine, and prednisone. *J Clin Oncol.* 2012;30:3460-3467. PMID: 22665537.

16-7   C

Mantle cell lymphoma may be difficult to differentiate clinically at the time of presentation from chronic lymphocytic leukemia/small lymphocytic lymphoma, marginal zone lymphoma, or lymphoplasmacytic lymphoma. Mantle cell lymphoma is best diagnosed by either demonstration of cyclin D1 overexpression by immunohistochemistry or presence of the t(11;14) translocation by FISH. This translocation juxtaposes the immunoglobulin heavy chain region on chromosome 14 with the cyclin D1 gene (BCL1) on chromosome 11. Flow cytometry is also very helpful if the typical mantle cell lymphoma immunophenotype is expressed, namely, strong expression of monoclonal immunoglobulin on the cell surface as well as strong expression of CD5, CD19, CD20, and CD22, with absence of expression of CD10 and CD23. The immunophenotype in answer A would be typical of chronic lymphocytic leukemia (not mantle cell lymphoma), with low levels of surface immunoglobulin and CD20 expression in association with expression of both CD5 and CD23. The FISH test in answer B implies juxtaposition of the c-Myc oncogene and the lambda immunoglobulin light chain gene and would be more commonly seen in Burkitt lymphoma and virtually never seen in mantle cell lymphoma. p53 overexpression is seen in a large assortment of malignancies, including mantle cell lymphoma, where it confers a poor prognosis but is not useful in establishing a diagnosis.

Suggested Reading

Pérez-Galán P, Dreyling M, Wiestner A. Mantle cell lymphoma: biology, pathogenesis, and the molecular basis of treatment in the genomic era. Blood. 2011;117:26-38. PMID: 20940415.

Press OW, Grogan TM, Fisher RI. Evaluation and management of mantle cell lymphoma. Adv Leuk and Lymphoma. 1996;6:3-11.

16-8   D

A recent study treated 58 patients with relapsed or refractory anaplastic large-cell lymphoma (ALCL) with brentuximab vedotin, yielding an overall response rate of 86% and a complete remission rate of 57%. This data led to its U.S. Food and Drug Administration approval for this indication in 2011. No other regimen has been shown to have comparable results in relapsed or refractory ALCL. Denileukin diftitox is an interleukin 2-diphtheria toxin fusion protein that is approved for relapsed or refractory cutaneous T-cell lymphomas but not ALCL. Romidepsin and pralatrexate have significant activity in peripheral T-cell lymphomas (particularly peripheral T-cell lymphoma not otherwise specified and angioimmunoblastic T-cell lymphoma) and cutaneous T-cell lymphomas, but no large series evaluating their use in ALCL have been reported. The few data that are available with these other agents do not suggest comparable activity to brentuximab vedotin for this histology.

Suggested Reading

Pro B, Advani R, Brice P, et al. Brentuximab vedotin (SGN-35) in patients with relapsed or refractory systemic anaplastic large-cell lymphoma: results of a phase II study. J Clin Oncol. 2012;30: 2190-2196. PMID: 22614995.

Piekarz RL, Frye R, Prince HM, et al. Phase 2 trial of romidepsin in patients with peripheral T-cell lymphoma. Blood. 2011;117: 5827-5834. PMID: 21355097.

O'Connor OA, Pro B, Pinter-Brown L, et al. Pralatrexate in patients with relapsed or refractory peripheral T-cell lymphoma: results from the pivotal PROPEL study. J Clin Oncol. 2011;29:1182-1189. PMID: 21245435.

16-9 B

This is a typical case of splenic marginal zone lymphoma with villous lymphocytes. This disease is an indolent lymphoma characterized by infiltration of the spleen and marrow with neoplastic lymphocytes, which typically have a low proliferation index. Lymph nodes are usually minimally enlarged. The peripheral blood often shows circulating malignant lymphocytes, which may exhibit villous projections. The major clinical manifestations usually relate to splenomegaly with abdominal distension, splenic discomfort, early satiety, and cytopenias due to splenic sequestration. Answer A is inappropriate in this case because the patient is symptomatic. Splenectomy is recommended for front-line therapy of patients with symptomatic disease by the NCCN guidelines and usually results in relief of symptoms and reversal of cytopenias that commonly lasts for many years. Immunization for encapsulated organisms (pneumococcus, haemophilus influenzae, hepatitis B, etc.) is advisable prior to splenectomy. This case presentation has some features of hairy cell leukemia including splenomegaly and cytopenias, but hairy cell lymphoma is much more common in males than females, and the immunophenotype of this case does not demonstrate expression of classic hairy cell leukemia markers (CD11c, CD103, or CD123). If patients with splenic marginal zone lymphoma are poor surgical candidates or refuse surgery, systemic therapy is also usually effective. In such circumstances, most authorities would administer rituximab monotherapy initially (as recommended by NCCN guidelines) since this disease is very sensitive to CD20 antibody therapy and toxicity is minimal. Other systemic regimens, including R-CHOP (answer C), would also be expected to be effective, but R-CHOP is considerably more toxic than rituximab monotherapy and hence less preferred. Lenalidomide and dexamethasone are commonly used for multiple myeloma, but their roles in splenic marginal zone lymphoma are poorly defined.

Suggested Reading

Zelenetz AD, Abramson JS, Advani RH, et al. *NCCN Clinical Practice Guidelines in Oncology (NCCN Guidelines®) Non-Hodgkin's Lymphomas*, Version 2.2013. Rockledge, PA: National Comprehensive Cancer Network, 2013.

Iannitto E, Tripodo C. How I diagnose and treat splenic lymphomas. *Blood.* 2011;117:2585-2595. PMID: 21119113.

Thieblemont C, Felman P, Berger F, et al. Treatment of splenic marginal zone B-cell lymphoma: an analysis of 81 patients. *Clin Lymphoma.* 2002;3:41-47. PMID: 12141954.

16-10 C

Recent studies have demonstrated that patients with HIV who have aggressive lymphomas with CD4 counts above 200/μL have remission rates and PFS comparable to similar patients without HIV, if treated with conventional regimens. Most HIV lymphoma authorities currently prefer the DA-EPOCH-R regimen based on nonrandomized studies conducted at the National Cancer Institute and retrospective analyses performed by the AIDS Malignancy Consortium, although rigorous proof that DA-EPOCH-R is superior to R-CHOP is not yet available. Patients with AIDS-associated aggressive lymphomas have a high risk of central nervous system involvement, especially if they present with multiple extranodal sites of disease, as in this case (bone marrow, psoas muscle), so intrathecal prophylaxis is advisable. Early studies in the pre-HAART era suggested that patients with AIDS-related lymphomas should be treated with attenuated doses of chemotherapy (answer B), but this is no longer true and such an approach is now discouraged. Palliative care alone is clearly inappropriate for this patient with a good performance status and normal CD4 count, who would have a high chance of durable complete remission with standard therapy. Answer D is inappropriate since this patient has a sufficiently good prognosis with standard therapy that up-front ASCT is difficult to justify. Controversy persists about the role of rituximab in treating patients with AIDS-related lymphomas, but the current consensus is that rituximab administration is safe in patients with CD4 counts above 50/μL and that outcomes are improved if this antibody in included in treatment regimens.

Suggested Reading

Dunleavy K, Wilson WH. How I treat HIV-associated lymphoma. *Blood.* 2012;119:3245-3255. PMID: 22337719.

Barta SK, Lee JY, Kaplan LD, et al. Pooled analysis of AIDS malignancy consortium trials evaluating rituximab plus CHOP or infusional EPOCH chemotherapy in HIV-associated non-Hodgkin lymphoma. *Cancer.* 2012;118:3977-3983. PMID: 22180164.

17 MULTIPLE MYELOMA
SELF-EVALUATION

MULTIPLE MYELOMA QUESTIONS

17-1 A 40-year-old man is found to have a serum monoclonal (M) protein of 2.5 g/dL during the course of work-up for an elevated erythrocyte sedimentation rate. Immunofixation characterizes the protein as immunoglobulin (Ig) A lambda. Hemoglobin, creatinine, and calcium levels are normal. Skeletal survey shows no lytic lesions. The serum free light chain (FLC) ratio is elevated at 110 (normal range, 0.26 to 1.65). He is asymptomatic. A bone marrow biopsy reveals 70% infiltration by lambda plasma cells.

What is the best treatment option for this patient?
A. Initiate systemic therapy for multiple myeloma
B. Close observation every 3 to 4 months
C. Repeat testing in 6 months, and if unchanged repeat labs every 12 months
D. Plasmapheresis

17-2 Which of the following abnormalities attenuate the adverse prognosis associated with 17p deletion in myeloma?
A. t(11;14)
B. t(4;14)
C. Trisomies of chromosomes 5, 7, and 11
D. 1q amplification
E. 1p deletion

17-3 Which of the following strategies can decrease the risk of developing neuropathy frequently seen with bortezomib therapy, without substantially compromising efficacy?
A. Administration on a once-weekly schedule
B. Intravenous route of administration
C. Concurrent administration of 500 mL of normal saline
D. Combining bortezomib with thalidomide

17-4 Pomalidomide is indicated for the treatment of which of the following conditions?
A. Newly diagnosed myeloma
B. Relapsed Waldenström macroglobulinemia
C. Maintenance therapy following transplantation in high-risk myeloma
D. Disease refractory to both lenalidomide and bortezomib
E. Preventive therapy in smoldering myeloma

17-5 A 54-year-old man was found to have intermediate-risk myeloma with the t(4;14) translocation.

Appropriate therapeutic options for initial therapy in this patient include:
A. Lenalidomide plus dexamethasone, followed by autologous transplantation
B. Thalidomide plus dexamethasone, followed by autologous transplantation
C. Bortezomib-based therapy, followed by autologous transplantation
D. Carfilzomib, lenalidomide, and dexamethasone
E. Carfilzomib, pomalidomide, and dexamethasone

17-6 A 50-year-old man is found on laboratory testing to have an M protein of 1.5 g/dL. His physician determines a diagnosis of monoclonal gammopathy of undetermined significance (MGUS) after a full work-up, including bone marrow studies and a bone survey.

Which of the following factors is not a major prognostic factor for risk of progression in MGUS?
A. Serum (FLC) ratio
B. Size of serum M protein
C. Type of serum M protein
D. Age

17-7 A 63-year-old woman presents with an enlarged tongue, pedal edema, and shortness of breath. Serum electrophoresis shows no M protein. Urine electrophoresis shows total urine protein excretion of 3.5 g/24 hours, consisting of primarily albumin, plus a small M lambda paraprotein. A bone marrow biopsy shows 5% clonal lambda plasma cells, but is otherwise negative. Echocardiogram shows thickened ventricular walls.

The most appropriate next step in the diagnostic evaluation will consist of:
A. Fat aspirate
B. Endomyocardial biopsy
C. Renal biopsy
D. Magnetic resonance imaging (MRI) of the heart
E. Repeat bone marrow biopsy

17-1   A

Patients with 60% or higher clonal plasma cell involvement of the marrow should be treated for multiple myeloma, regardless of the presence or absence of end-organ damage, because these patients will almost inevitably develop such damage within 2 years, and have a median time to symptomatic disease of approximately 8 months. Close observation every 3 to 4 months is the standard of care for smoldering myeloma, but given this level of plasma cell involvement, the patient needs to be considered as having myeloma requiring therapy. Repeat testing in 6 months, and then observation every 12 months, is only appropriate for MGUS. A high serum FLC ratio places the patient at risk for renal failure, but plasmapheresis is not indicated without symptoms.

Suggested Reading

Rajkumar SV, Larson D, Kyle RA. Diagnosis of smoldering multiple myeloma. *N Engl J Med.* 2011;365:474-475. PMID: 21812699.

Rajkumar SV, Merlini G, San Miguel JF. Haematological cancer: Redefining myeloma. *Nat Rev Clin Oncol.* 2012;9:494-496. PMID: 22850755.

17-2   C

Trisomies ameliorate the adverse prognosis associated with high-risk cytogenetics in myeloma. t(11;14) is associated with standard-risk myeloma, but its presence does not ameliorate adverse prognosis associated with high-risk cytogenetics. All the other abnormalities are associated with an adverse prognosis.

Suggested Reading

Kumar S, Fonseca R, Ketterling RP, et al. Trisomies in multiple myeloma: impact on survival in patients with high-risk cytogenetics. *Blood.* 2012;119:2100-2105. PMID: 22234687.

17-3   A

The once-weekly schedule has been shown in randomized trials to decrease the risk of severe neuropathy that is associated with bortezomib therapy. The subcutaneous route of administration has been shown to produce a lower risk of severe neuropathy compared with intravenous administration. Intravenous administration with normal saline supplementation is often used to reduce side effects associated with carfilzomib, not bortezomib. Combining bortezomib and thalidomide can increase the risk of neuropathy, as thalidomide is also associated with a propensity for nerve damage.

Suggested Reading

Mateos MV, Oriol A, Martínez-López J, et al. Bortezomib, melphalan, and prednisone versus bortezomib, thalidomide, and prednisone as induction therapy followed by maintenance treatment with bortezomib and thalidomide versus bortezomib and prednisone in elderly patients with untreated multiple myeloma: a randomised trial. *Lancet Oncol.* 2010;11:934-941. PMID: 20739218.

Palumbo A, Bringhen S, Rossi D, et al. Bortezomib-melphalan-prednisone-thalidomide followed by maintenance with bortezomib-thalidomide compared with bortezomib-melphalan-prednisone for initial treatment of multiple myeloma: a randomized controlled trial. *J Clin Oncol.* 2010;28:5101-5109. PMID: 20940200.

Moreau P, Pylypenko H, Grosicki S, et al. Subcutaneous versus intravenous administration of bortezomib in patients with relapsed multiple myeloma: a randomised, phase 3, non-inferiority study. *Lancet Oncol.* 2011;12:431-440. PMID: 21507715.

17-4   D

Pomalidomide is approved for the treatment of multiple myeloma refractory to both lenalidomide and bortezomib. It is not indicated in newly diagnosed myeloma or in the treatment of relapsed Waldenström macroglobulinemia. Lenalidomide, not pomalidomide, is used as post-transplant maintenance therapy and as preventive therapy in smoldering myeloma.

Suggested Reading

Lacy MQ, Hayman SR, Gertz MA, et al. Pomalidomide (CC4047) plus low-dose dexamethasone as therapy for relapsed multiple myeloma. *J Clin Oncol.* 2009;27:5008-5014. PMID: 19720894.

Lacy MQ, Allred JB, Gertz MA, et al. Pomalidomide plus low-dose dexamethasone in myeloma refractory to both bortezomib and lenalidomide: comparison of 2 dosing strategies in dual-refractory disease. *Blood.* 2011;118:2970-2975. PMID: 21690557.

17-5   C

In various trials, the prognosis of t(4;14) myeloma has been shown to be improved only when patients receive early therapy with a bortezomib-based regimen followed by stem cell transplantation. Although carfilzomib is a proteasome inhibitor, data are limited on its use for initial therapy of t(4;14) myeloma, and there are no randomized data available to support the use of carfilzomib as initial therapy in myeloma.

Suggested Reading

Cavo M, Tacchetti P, Patriarca F, et al. Bortezomib with thalidomide plus dexamethasone compared with thalidomide plus dexamethasone as induction therapy before, and consolidation therapy after, double autologous stem-cell transplantation in newly diagnosed multiple myeloma: a randomised phase 3 study. *Lancet.* 2010;376:2075-2085. PMID: 21146205.

17-6   D

Age is not associated with the risk of progression in MGUS. In contrast, the size and type of the M protein and the serum FLC ratio are all important prognostic factors in MGUS. The risk of progression to myeloma or a related disorder is higher with increasing size of the M protein. IgM and IgA MGUS have a higher risk of progression than IgG MGUS. An abnormal FLC ratio is associated with a substantially higher risk of progression.

Suggested Reading

Rajkumar SV, Kyle RA, Therneau TM, et al. Serum free light chain ratio is an independent risk factor for progression in monoclonal gammopathy of undetermined significance. *Blood.* 2005;106:812-817. PMID: 15855274.

Kyle RA, Therneau TM, Rajkumar SV, et al. A long-term study of prognosis in monoclonal gammopathy of undetermined significance. *N Engl J Med.* 2002;346:564-569. PMID: 11856795.

17-7   A

The most likely diagnosis in this patient is Ig light chain (AL) amyloidosis. Although biopsy of the heart or kidney may provide the diagnosis, a fat aspirate is the most appropriate next step because of the ease of the procedure and low risk for complications. The fat aspirate has a high sensitivity for AL amyloidosis. Confirmation of the presence of amyloidosis in the fat aspirate is usually followed by a more detailed analysis to determine the nature of the deposit by mass spectroscopy. An MRI study will not provide a specific diagnosis, and a repeat bone marrow biopsy is likely to be of low yield.

Suggested Reading

Gertz MA. Immunoglobulin light chain amyloidosis: 2013 update on diagnosis, prognosis, and treatment. *Am J Hematol.* 2013;88:416-425. PMID: 23605846.

18 HEMATOPOIETIC CELL TRANSPLANTATION

SELF-EVALUATION

HEMATOPOIETIC CELL TRANSPLANTATION QUESTIONS

18-1 A 67-year-old man with myelodysplasia (International Prognostic Scoring System risk category, intermediate-2) seeks advice about whether to be treated with a hypomethylating agent or to pursue hematopoietic cell transplantation (HCT) from a human leukocyte antigen (HLA)-matched unrelated donor. He has no significant comorbidities.

Which of the following statements is most accurate?
A. Compared with hypomethylating agent therapy, transplantation offers overall and quality-adjusted survival benefit
B. Compared with hypomethylating agent therapy, transplantation offers overall survival benefit but, because of chronic graft-versus-host disease (GVHD), no quality-adjusted benefit
C. The largest overall and quality-adjusted survival benefit is seen with a strategy of initial hypomethylating agent therapy followed by transplantation upon treatment failure
D. There is no role for unrelated donor transplantation in patients older than age 65

18-2 A 33-year-old woman presents with epistaxis, gingival bleeding, and easy bruising. Fourteen months earlier, she underwent a single-antigen mismatched cord blood transplant following a myeloablative preparative regimen for acute myeloid leukemia (AML) in first remission. She was cytomegalovirus (CMV) sero-positive pretransplant. At 1 year post-transplant, she was in remission, completely engrafted, and off all medications. She now presents with severe thrombocytopenia (platelets, 8,000/mm³) but an otherwise normal peripheral smear. She has no splenomegaly. A bone marrow examination shows slightly increased numbers of megakaryocytes but is otherwise normal.

What is the most likely diagnosis?
A. Early graft rejection
B. Incipient relapse of her AML
C. CMV reactivation
D. Idiopathic thrombocytopenic purpura
E. Chronic GVHD

18-3 A 50-year-old man with very high-risk (monosomal karyotype) AML in first remission is being evaluated for a matched unrelated bone marrow donor. In the course of the evaluation, he develops a runny nose but no other symptoms. His physical examination is normal, as is a chest x-ray, but a nasopharyngeal swab reveals respiratory syncytial virus (RSV).

What is the most appropriate choice?
A. Delay the transplant until symptoms clear
B. Delay the transplant until a repeat nasopharyngeal swab is virus-free
C. Delay the transplant and begin systemic vibavirin
D. Proceed to transplant with the patient on prophylactic ribavirin

18-4 A 25-year-old man with Philadelphia chromosome–positive acute lymphocytic leukemia in first remission is being evaluated for a myeloablative transplant. A matched unrelated donor has been identified.

Which of the following statements is correct concerning the choice of bone marrow versus peripheral blood stem cells?
A. Compared with marrow, peripheral blood results in faster engraftment, less graft rejection, and improved survival
B. Compared with marrow, peripheral blood results in more chronic GVHD and poorer survival
C. Compared with marrow, peripheral blood results in faster engraftment, more chronic GVHD, and equivalent survival
D. Compared with marrow, peripheral blood results in more chronic GVHD, a lower risk of malignant relapse, and equivalent survival
E. Compared with marrow, peripheral blood results in faster engraftment, more chronic GVHD, a lower risk of malignant relapse, and equivalent survival

18-5 A 61-year-old woman received a transplant from her HLA-identical brother for mantle cell lymphoma in second remission following a reduced-intensity conditioning regimen with tacrolimus and mycophenolate mofetil as GVHD prophylaxis. She engrafted promptly and had no complications over the early post-transplant period. At 1 month the mycophenolate was discontinued, and at 3 months tapering of the tacrolimus was initiated and was completed at 6 months. Approximately 2 months after the taper was completed, she noted the onset of dry eyes and a skin rash. Physical examination revealed a skin rash with morphea-like features over 15% of her body and signs of keratoconjunctivitis. The rest of her physical exam and laboratory tests, including a complete blood count and liver function tests, were normal.

What initial therapy would you recommend?
A. Prednisone (1 mg/kg/day)
B. Tacrolimus
C. Prednisone plus tacrolimus
D. Tacrolimus and mycophenolate mofetil
E. Cyclosporine eye drops and steroid skin cream

18-1   A

In a study of 514 patients age 60 to 70 with myelodysplastic syndromes (MDS), for patients with low/intermediate-1 MDS, hypomethylating agent therapy was associated with greater life expectancy. However, for patients with intermediate-2/high-risk MDS, transplantation was associated with greater life expectancy than nontransplant therapies. Quality-adjusted life expectancy analyses also favored transplantation.

Suggested Reading

Cutler CS, Lee SJ, Greenberg P, et al. A decision analysis of allogeneic bone marrow transplantation for the myelodysplastic syndromes: delayed transplantation for low-risk myelodysplasia is associated with improved outcome. *Blood.* 2004;104:579-585. PMID: 15039286.

18-2   D

Approximately 5% of recipients of cord-blood transplants will develop an autoimmune disease at some point post-transplant. The most common forms are idiopathic thrombocytopenia purpura and autoimmune hemolytic anemia. No clinical feature distinguishes these disorders from those developing in the nontransplant setting, although they tend to respond less well to conventional therapies.

Suggested Reading

Daikeler T, Labopin M, Ruggeri A, et al. New autoimmune diseases after cord blood transplantation: a retrospective study of EUROCORD and the Autoimmune Disease Working Party of the European Group for Blood and Marrow Transplantation. *Blood.* 2013;121:1059-1064. PMID: 23247725.

18-3   B

As many as 40% of patients with upper respiratory tract RSV will progress to pneumonia in the setting of HCT, with 45% of pneumonias proving fatal. Thus, patients should not receive a transplant when they have active RSV. Elimination of symptoms does not ensure absence of virus. It is uncertain whether systemic ribavirin alters the course of disease.

18-4   C

In the only prospective randomized trial available, compared to marrow, peripheral blood was associated with faster engraftment, a lower risk of graft rejection, more chronic GVHD, and equivalent risks of relapse and mortality.

Suggested Reading

Anasetti C, Logan BR, Lee SJ, et al. Peripheral-blood stem cells versus bone marrow from unrelated donors. *N Engl J Med.* 2012;367:1487-1496. PMID: 23075175.

18-5   E

With only dry eyes and 15% body rash, this patient's global severity score of chronic GVHD would be rated as mild. Such patients are not at a high risk of mortality and can be treated with local therapy.

Suggested Reading

Socie G, Ritz J, Martin PJ. Current challenges in chronic graft-versus host disease. *Biol Blood Marrow Transplant.* 2010;16:S146-S151. PMID: 19836455.

19 CANCER IN ELDERLY PATIENTS
SELF-EVALUATION

CANCER IN ELDERLY PATIENTS QUESTIONS

19-1 A 68-year-old man presents to the emergency department with profound fatigue and epistaxis. The patient says he has had "low blood" for a few months. His medications include 5 mg of amlodipine per day, 500 mg of acetaminophen as needed for pain, and 10 mg of zolpidem as needed to sleep. On exam, the patient's blood pressure is 126/80, pulse is 70, temperature is 37.8 degrees, and respirations are 12. He has pale mucus membranes and had dried blood in his nares. His lungs are clear to auscultation. He is in sinus rhythm and has no murmurs or edema. On exam his white blood count (WBC) is 1.3 K/µL, his hemoglobin is 7.6 g/dL, and his platelet count is 8,000 K/µL. Review of a peripheral blood film shows circulating myeloblasts and a bone marrow biopsy confirms acute myeloid leukemia.

Which of the following is the most appropriate next step in the treatment of this patient?
A. Evaluation for stem cell transplantation
B. Induction chemotherapy with cytarabine and an anthracycline
C. Hydroxyurea (500 mg orally)
D. Imatinib (400 mg a day orally)

19-2 A 75-year-old woman is found on routine mammography to have a new spiculated mass in the upper outer quadrant of the right breast. After lumpectomy, the primary lesion is noted to be 2.4 cm in maximum dimension; estrogen receptor (ER), progesterone receptor (PR), and HER2 status are all negative. Sentinel lymph node biopsy shows two axillary lymph nodes with cancer. She has no comorbidities. On physical exam she has a well-healed incisions on the right breast and axilla. Her lungs are clear to auscultation. Imaging studies show no evidence of metastases. The patient has seen the radiation oncologist, who recommends radiation therapy.

What therapy would do you recommend?
A. Complete mastectomy
B. Axillary lymph node dissection followed by tamoxifen for 5 years
C. Four cycles of doxorubicin and cyclophosphamide (AC) followed by paclitaxel
D. Six cycles of capecitabine chemotherapy

19-3 A 72-year-old man with stage IV adenocarcinoma of the lung presents to your clinic for assessment. He has a history of hypertension, atrial fibrillation, and bilateral total knee replacement surgery. The patient takes hydrochlorothiazide (25 mg a day), metoprolol (25 mg once daily), warfarin (5 mg every night), and acetaminophen (325 mg as needed for pain). He walks with a cane and lives with his wife of 44 years, who is recovering from a recent stroke. He is able to care for himself without any assistance, and is able to drive to all his appointments.

What measures can help the treating oncologist decide if the patient can tolerate chemotherapy?
A. Cardiology evaluation
B. Using granulocyte colony-stimulating factor (G-CSF)
C. Comprehensive geriatric assessment
D. Neuropsychiatric testing

19-4 A 74-year-old man presents with left cervical adenopathy and drenching night sweats over a duration of 3 months. He has lost 20 lbs over the past 3 weeks. The patient undergoes an excisional left supraclavicular lymph node biopsy and this confirms a diffuse large B-cell lymphoma that is CD20+. Positron emission tomography scan reveals activity in the mediastinum and para-aortic lymph nodes. A bone marrow biopsy is negative for lymphomatous involvement. Laboratory studies indicate his WBC is 7.3 K/µL, his hemoglobin is 12.0 g/dL, and his platelet count is 175,000 K/µL. Lactate dehydrogenase is 450 µL. Creatinine is 0.8 mg/dL. The patient is very functional, independent, and has no comorbidities. He plays golf twice weekly and is very keen on preserving his quality of life.

Which of the following do you recommend?
A. Involved field radiation therapy to the left neck
B. Cyclophosphamide, doxorubicin, vincristine, and prednisone (CHOP) for six cycles
C. Dose-attenuated CHOP plus rituximab for four cycles followed by radiation to the left neck
D. CHOP plus rituximab for six cycles

19-5 A 79-year old women presents with a new diagnosis of Philadelphia chromosome–positive chronic phase chronic myeloid leukemia. Her oncologist starts her on imatinib (400 mg orally once a day). The patient has diarrhea six to seven times per day and has profound arthralgia in the bilateral knees and ankles. She is also on metoprolol (12.5 mg orally) for hypertension, and on pantoprazole (20 mg orally) for gastroesophageal reflux disease. Despite loperamide, the patient has loose stools six to seven times per day. She weighs 115 lbs and is 64 inches tall. Labs show WBC is 9.6 K/μL, hemoglobin is 11.0 g/dL, and platelet count is 240,000 K/μL. Her creatinine is 1.0 mg/dL (stable from 8 weeks ago at start of therapy when it was 1.0 mg/dL) and her liver enzymes are all normal.

Which of the following may help ameliorate the severity of the patient's side effects?
A. Recalculate the dose of imatinib based on creatinine clearance and decrease it to 200 mg once daily
B. Add atropine/diphenoxylate to loperamide and admit for intravenous fluids
C. Discontinue pantoprazole
D. Add oxycodone (5 mg every 6 hours by mouth) for arthralgias

19-1   B

This patient has acute myeloid leukemia, likely from an underlying myelodysplastic syndrome. Hydroxyurea, an antimetabolite, has been used for palliative therapy in patients with high WBC counts and in elderly patients unfit for therapy. Imatinib is not indicated in acute myeloid leukemia. One needs information about additional prognostic factors (cytogenetics and molecular mutation studies) before deciding if the patient needs a stem cell transplant evaluation. At this time, the aim is to achieve a complete remission; this may be achieved with induction chemotherapy with 7 days of cytarabine and 3 days of an anthracycline.

Suggested Reading

Appelbaum FR, Gundacker H, Head DR, et al. Age and acute myeloid leukemia. *Blood.* 2006;107:3481-3485. PMID: 16455952.

Rowe JM. Optimal induction and post-remission therapy for AML in first remission. *Hematology Am Soc Hematol Educ Program.* 2009; 396-405. PMID: 20008225.

19-2   C

The patient has a T2N1aM0 (stage IIA) breast cancer. She has high-risk disease by virtue of negative ER, PR, and HER2 status. There is no indication for a complete mastectomy or axillary lymph node dissection followed by tamoxifen since the patient is ER/PR-negative. The patient has an excellent performance status and no comorbid medical conditions, thus, a recommendation for adjuvant chemotherapy is reasonable. In older women with early-stage breast cancer, six cycles of capecitabine was found to be inferior to AC or cyclophosphamide/methotrexate/5-fluorouracil (CMF) chemotherapy. The Adjuvant! Online tool predicts that the 10-year survival probability will increase from about 35% to about 50% with this therapy.

Suggested Reading

Muss HB, Woolf S, Berry D, et al. Adjuvant chemotherapy in older and younger women with lymph node–positive breast cancer. *JAMA.* 2005; 293:1073-1081. PMID: 15741529.

Extermann M, Balducci L, Lyman GH. What threshold for adjuvant therapy in older breast cancer patients? *J Clin Oncol.* 2000;18: 1709-1717. PMID: 10764431.

Muss HB, Berry DA, Cirrincione CT, et al. Adjuvant chemotherapy in older women with early-stage breast cancer. *N Engl J Med.* 2009; 360:2055-2065. PMID: 19439741.

19-3   C

The patient has a few comorbidities and an elderly caregiver who is recovering from a recent stroke. He walks with a cane but is able to drive. There is evidence that elderly patients with stage IV lung cancer do benefit from chemotherapy, demonstrated in the ELVIS and MILES clinical trials. Comprehensive geriatric assessment (CGA) includes assessment tools to predict the functional age of patients with cancer based on functional status, comorbidities that may interfere with cancer therapy, nutritional status, polypharmacy, psychological and cognitive status, socioeconomic issues, and geriatric syndromes. Health care professionals can incorporate the CGA parameters along with laboratory tests and tumor and patient variables to predict for chemotherapy toxicity.

Suggested Reading

Hurria A, Cirrincione CT, Muss HB, et al. Implementing a geriatric assessment in cooperative group clinical cancer trials: CALGB 360401. *J Clin Oncol.* 2011;29:1290-1296. PMID: 21357782.

Hurria A, Togawa K, Mohile SG, et al. Predicting chemotherapy toxicity in older adults with cancer: a prospective multicenter study. *J Clin Oncol.* 2011;29:3457-3465. PMID: 21810685.

Extermann M, Boler I, Reich RR, et al. Predicting the risk of chemotherapy toxicity in older patients: the Chemotherapy Risk Assessment Scale for High-Age Patients (CRASH) score. *Cancer.* 2012;118:3377-3386. PMID: 22072065.

19-4   D

The patient has at least stage III diffuse large B-cell lymphoma and thus has no indication for local field radiation. The practice-changing GELA study in patients with diffuse B-cell lymphoma has been conducted in patients age 60 to 80 and compared CHOP with CHOP plus rituximab (R-CHOP). The patients who received R-CHOP had a higher complete response rate (76% vs. 63%), 2-year event-free survival, and overall survival, thus making R-CHOP the standard of care for this group of patients.

Suggested Reading

Coiffier B, Lepage E, Briere J, et al. CHOP chemotherapy plus rituximab compared with CHOP alone in elderly patients with diffuse large-B-Cell lymphoma. *N Engl J Med.* 2002;346:235-242. PMID: 11807147.

19-5   A

The patient's creatinine clearance based on the Cockcroft-Gault equation is 37.6 mL/minute. Thus, the full dose of imatinib at 400 mg daily may be too toxic for the patient, causing her to have significant diarrhea and arthralgias. Decreasing the dose by 50% to 200 mg per day may be able to achieve the effect required (a major molecular remission). In addition, this may decrease the side effects and preserve her quality of life.

Suggested Reading

Lichtman SM, Wildiers H, Launay-Vacher V, et al. International Society of Geriatric Oncology (SIOG) recommendations for the adjustment of dosing in elderly cancer patients with renal insufficiency. *Eur J Cancer.* 2007;43:14-34. PMID: 17222747.

Russo D, Malagola M, Skert C, et al. Treatment of chronic myeloid leukemia elderly patients in the tyrosine kinase inhibitor era. *Curr Cancer Drug Targets.* 2013;13:755-767. PMID: 23941515.

20 SYMPTOM MANAGEMENT
SELF-EVALUATION

SYMPTOM MANAGEMENT QUESTIONS

20-1 A patient with a history of hormone receptor–positive breast cancer has substantial hot flashes and requests a nonhormone treatment option.

Which of the following can be shared with the patient?
A. No antidepressant drug has been approved by the U.S. Food and Drug Administration (FDA) for the treatment of hot flashes
B. Venlafaxine decreases hot flashes more than gabapentin
C. In a randomized cross-over clinical trial, women with a history of breast cancer chose venlafaxine over gabapentin, by a 2:1 margin
D. Paroxetine decreases hot flashes and can be safely given with tamoxifen

20-2 Mrs. Smith, a patient with advanced pancreas cancer, has an Eastern Cooperative Oncology Group performance status of 2 and malignant ascites, which is minimally symptomatic.

Which of the following is true?
A. Furosemide should be started
B. Spironolactone should be started
C. A detailed discussion of prognosis and treatment options, if not already performed, is in order
D. A permanent paracentesis catheter should be inserted to keep ascites to a minimum

20-3 Mrs. Jones is scheduled to receive adjuvant therapy with doxorubicin and cyclophosphamide. She plans to receive therapy through a peripheral venous line. There are plans to give her a neurokinin (NK)-1 receptor antagonist, in addition to granisetron and dexamethasone.

Which of the following is true?
A. She should be given intravenous fosaprepitant, as a one-time dose of this agent is more effective than 3 days of oral aprepitant, more convenient, and may be better covered by her insurance
B. Neither intravenous fosaprepitant nor oral aprepitant causes venous irritation to any substantial degree
C. Oral aprepitant is preferred, given the substantial amount of venous toxicity that has recently been ascribed to intravenous fosaprepitant
D. Venous toxicity with intravenous fosaprepitant seems to be similar in patients receiving doxorubicin-based chemotherapy and patients receiving cisplatin-based chemotherapy

20-4 Which of the following is true regarding the treatment of anorexia/cachexia?
A. Megestrol acetate stimulates appetite much better than dexamethasone
B. Megestrol acetate increases the incidence of nausea and vomiting
C. Megestrol acetate can cause adrenal suppression
D. Megestrol acetate increases survival in patients with cancer anorexia/cachexia

20-5 Mr. Black has stage III colon cancer and is about to start leucovorin/5-fluorouracil/oxaliplatin (FOLFOX) chemotherapy. He asks whether there are any agents that have been proven to be helpful for decreasing neuropathy from this treatment.

Which of the following can be shared with the patient?
A. Intravenous calcium/magnesium infusions have been proven to decrease neuropathy in this situation
B. Glutathione has been proven to decrease neuropathy in this situation
C. Acetyl-L-carnitine has been proven to decrease neuropathy in this situation
D. There are no proven therapies to decrease the incidence of FOLFOX neuropathy

20-6 Mrs. Johnson has multiple lytic bone breast cancer metastases and a decision has been made to start her on a bone-modifying agent.

Which of the following can be shared with the patient?
A. Zoledronate causes more hypocalcemia than does denosumab
B. Zoledronate appears to decrease the time to the first skeletal-related event compared with denosumab
C. Denosumab appears to be particularly beneficial in patients with multiple myeloma
D. The 2011 ASCO guidelines dictate that there is not enough evidence to recommend either a bisphosphonate or denosumab compared with the other

20-7 It is well accepted that 5-hydroxytryptamine (5-HT) receptor antagonists are helpful agents to decrease the incidence of chemotherapy-induced nausea and vomiting.

Which of the following is true regarding palonosetron, a newer-generation agent?
A. ASCO 2011 antiemetic guidelines have now established that palonosetron is more effective than other 5-HT3 receptor antagonists for patients who are receiving moderately emetogenic chemotherapy but not receiving an NK1 receptor antagonist
B. Antiemetic guidelines have now established that palonosetron is more effective than other 5-HT3 receptor antagonists for patients that are receiving moderately emetogenic chemotherapy whether or not they are receiving an NK1 receptor antagonist
C. Palonosetron does not have a longer half-life than do other available 5-HT3 receptor antagonists
D. Palonosetron does not have a higher binding affinity than do other available 5-HT3 receptor antagonists

20-8 Cryotherapy consists of using ice to cool tissues to decrease local exposure to chemotherapy drug concentrations and, thus, decrease local toxicity.

Which of the following are true regarding cryotherapy?
A. Oral cryotherapy does not decrease bolus 5-fluorouracil (5-FU)-induced oral mucositis
B. Finger cryotherapy does decrease docetaxel-induced nail toxicity
C. Scalp cryotherapy is clearly contraindicated in patients with breast cancer and has been shown to be associated with an increased incidence of subsequent scalp metastases
D. There is no evidence that ocular cryotherapy might decrease 5-FU-associated ocular toxicity

20-9 Mrs. Pham is receiving adjuvant chemotherapy for breast cancer and notes that she is fatigued to the point that it is interfering with her quality of life. She wants to know if she can do anything for this.

What advice can you provide for her?
A. She should conserve her energy and avoid regular exercise
B. A trial of methylphenidate is reasonable to try
C. A trial of either modafinil or armodafinil is reasonable to try
D. Randomized placebo-controlled clinical trials support that a ginseng preparation can decrease fatigue in this clinical scenario

20-10 Patients receiving paclitaxel can experience pain on the few days that follow each dose, which usually resolves after a few days.

What can a patient be told about this pain?
A. It is clearly related to muscle and/or joint pathology associated with the paclitaxel and, thus, is called paclitaxel-associated arthralgia/myalgia
B. Considerable data support that this phenomena is a form of acute neuropathy, similar to oxaliplatin being associated with an acute, largely reversible neuropathy
C. Opioid medications are contraindicated for the treatment of this problem
D. There are no available data to support that the degree of pain in an individual patient is positively associated with the amount of eventual chronic peripheral neuropathy that patients develop

20-1   C

A clinical trial looked at the efficacy of gabapentin compared with venlafaxine, utilizing patient preference as its primary endpoint. Patients were randomly assigned to receive venlafaxine or gabapentin in relatively standard doses recommended by previous placebo-controlled clinical hot flash trials. Patients were treated for 4 weeks and then had a 2-week washout period, before being crossed over to the alternative treatment. Although both agents appeared to reduce hot flashes to similar extents (approximately a 65% reduction) and had similar amounts of toxicities, 68% of patients preferred venlafaxine compared with 32% who preferred gabapentin (p = 0.01). The authors concluded that venlafaxine should be recommended as an initial treatment but that some patients did better with gabapentin, supporting a trial of this medication if venlafaxine was not efficacious enough.

In 2013, paroxetine was FDA-approved for the treatment of hot flashes. However, this drug should not be used with tamoxifen as it inhibits CYP2D6, the enzyme that converts tamoxifen to its more active form, endoxifen.

Suggested Reading

Bordeleau L, Pritchard KI, Loprinzi CL, et al. Multicenter, randomized, cross-over clinical trial of venlafaxine versus gabapentin for the management of hot flashes in breast cancer survivors. *J Clin Oncol.* 2010;28:5147-5152. PMID: 21060031.

20-2   C

Malignant ascites is usually seen in patients with advanced cancer. Diuretics can be useful in selected patients. Spironolactone is the initial diuretic to consider, with furosemide added afterwards. However, the goal of diuretic therapy is to decrease the symptoms of ascites, as opposed to getting rid of all asymptomatic ascites. Although diuretic therapy can be helpful in some patients, in many patients with advanced disease, diuretic therapy is more burdensome than beneficial. Thus, prior to starting diuretic therapy in such a patient, a detailed discussion of prognosis and treatment options is the first order of business. If the patient is symptomatic, then paracentesis can be performed. If repeat paracentesis is necessary, then a more permanent paracentesis catheter can be considered. This is only needed in a minority of patients.

20-3   C

NK-1 receptor antagonists can be helpful for patients receiving doxorubicin and cyclophosphamide. Oral aprepitant and intravenous fosaprepitant are relatively equivalent in terms of their ability to provide antiemetic efficacy.

New information has supported that there is a substantial amount of venous toxicity associated with the use of intravenous fosaprepitant if the drug and chemotherapy are given through peripheral intravenous lines as opposed to central intravenous lines. For this reason, oral aprepitant is recommended. Available data suggest that venous toxicity with intravenous fosaprepitant is much milder in patients receiving cisplatin-based regimens, as opposed to doxorubicin-based regimens.

Suggested Reading

Fujii T, Nishimura N, Kanai H, et al. Impact of fosaprepitant use on dermal and vascular adverse events in anthracycline-based regimens administered through peripheral lines. *J Clin Oncol.* 2013;31 (suppl; abstr 9629).

Leal AD, Kadakia KC, Looker S, et al. Fosaprepitant-induced phlebitis: a focus on patients receiving doxorubicin/cyclophosphamide therapy. *Support Care Cancer.* 2014;22:1313-1317. PMID: 24402411.

20-4   C

Although it is not well appreciated, numerous publications have demonstrated that megestrol acetate causes adrenal suppression. Thus, covering stress situations with steroids is recommended. At this time, it is common to stop megestrol acetate abruptly, as opposed to weaning it.

Data support that megestrol acetate has antiemetic properties, as opposed to causing nausea/vomiting. Megestrol acetate stimulates appetite to a relatively similar degree as dexamethasone but has less steroidal-associated toxicity. There are no good data to support that megestrol acetate increases survival in patients with cancer anorexia/cachexia.

Suggested Reading

Subramanian S, Goker H, Kanji A, et al. Clinical adrenal insufficiency in patients receiving megestrol therapy. *Arch Intern Med.* 1997; 157:1008-1011. PMID: 9140272.

Loprinzi CL, Jensen MD, Jiang NS, et al. Effect of megestrol acetate on the human pituitary-adrenal axis. *Mayo Clin Proc.* 1992;67: 1160-1162. PMID: 1469926.

Loprinzi CL, Jatoi A. Antiemetic properties of megestrol acetate. *J Palliat Med.* 2006;9:239-240. PMID: 16629544.

Loprinzi CL, Kugler JW, Sloan JA, et al. Randomized comparison of megestrol acetate versus dexamethasone versus fluoxymesterone for the treatment of cancer anorexia/cachexia. *J Clin Oncol.* 1999;17:3299-3306. PMID: 10506633.

20-5   D

There are no proven therapies known to decrease the instance of FOLFOX neuropathy, aside from dose reduction. There had been considerable excitement regarding intravenous calcium and magnesium, but a recently published placebo-controlled, double-blinded clinical trial provides convincing data that there was no substantial benefit for calcium and magnesium in this situation. Although there is preliminary information suggesting that glutathione might be helpful for decreasing oxaliplatin-induced neuropathy, no definitive studies have been completed. There is no good information that acetyl-L-carnitine can decrease oxaliplatin-induced neuropathy.

Suggested Reading

Loprinzi CL, Qin R, Dakhil SR, et al. Phase III randomized, placebo-controlled, double-blind study of intravenous calcium and magnesium to prevent oxaliplatin-induced sensory neurotoxicity (N08CB/Alliance). *J Clin Oncol.* 2014;32:997-1005. PMID: 24297951.

20-6   D

The 2011 updated ASCO guideline did not feel that there was enough evidence to recommend either a bisphosphonate or denosumab compared with the alternate one. Although there is evidence that denosumab is a bit better at preserving bone, there is no evidence, to date, that denosumab can decrease the incidence of bone fractures, and it is quite a bit more expensive than bisphosphonates. Zoledronate causes less hypocalcemia than does denosumab. Zoledronate appears to be better in patients with multiple myeloma, with a hazard ratio of 2.26 (95% CI 1.13, 4.50), related to overall survival data.

Suggested Reading

Van Poznak CH, Temin S, Yee GC, et al. American Society of Clinical Oncology executive summary of the clinical practice guideline update on the role of bone-modifying agents in metastatic breast cancer. *J Clin Oncol.* 2011;29:1221-1227. PMID: 21343561.

West H. Denosumab for prevention of skeletal-related events in patients with bone metastases from solid tumors: incremental benefit, debatable value. *J Clin Oncol.* 2011;29:1095-1098. PMID: 21343550.

20-7   A

Palonosetron has a longer half-life than do older 5-HT3 receptor antagonists and has a higher binding affinity. ASCO 2011 antiemetics guidelines now recommend it over older 5-HT3 receptor antagonists for patients with moderately emetogenic chemotherapy, if they are not receiving an NK1 receptor antagonist. If they are receiving an NK1 receptor antagonist, then a less expensive, older 5-HT3 receptor antagonist is thought to be adequately effective.

Suggested Reading

Basch, E, Hesketh PJ, Kris MG, et al. Antiemetics: American Society of Clinical Oncology clinical practice guideline update. *J Oncol Pract.* 2011;7:395-398. PMID: 22379425.

20-8   B

Cryotherapy has been helpful for decreasing toxicity in a number of situations. This includes decreasing mucositis in patients receiving bolus-dose 5-FU. It can also decrease docetaxel-induced nail toxicity, demonstrated by randomized trials whereby one upper extremity received cryotherapy and the other did not, then comparing the fingernails by photographs. It has been demonstrated to decrease alopecia in multiple trials. The incidence of scalp metastases in patients with solid tumors is very low, and available data suggest that the incidence is not any different in patients receiving scalp cryotherapy compared with patients who are not. There is a single published trial that provided data supporting that ocular cryotherapy can decrease 5-FU-induced ocular toxicity.

Suggested Reading

Kadakia KC, Rozell SA, Butala AA, et al. Supportive cryotherapy: a review from head to toe. *J Pain Symptom Manage.* 2014;47: 1100-1115. Epub 2013 Nov 7. PMID: 24210702.

Grevelman EG, Breed WP. Prevention of chemotherapy-induced hair loss by scalp cooling. *Ann Oncol.* 2005;16:352-358. PMID: 15642703.

Loprinzi CL, Wender DB, Veeder MG, et al. Inhibition of 5-fluorouracil-induced ocular irritation by ocular ice packs. *Cancer.* 1994;74: 945-948. PMID: 8039123.

Scotté F, Tourani JM, Banu E, et al. Multicenter study of a frozen glove to prevent docetaxel-induced onycholysis and cutaneous toxicity of the hand. *J Clin Oncol.* 2005;23:4424-4429. PMID: 15994152.

Scotté F, Banu E, Medioni J, et al. Matched case-control phase 2 study to evaluate the use of a frozen sock to prevent docetaxel-induced onycholysis and cutaneous toxicity of the foot. *Cancer.* 2008; 112:1625-1631. PMID: 18286527.

20-9 D

Cancer fatigue is a major clinical problem for many patients with cancer, both in the adjuvant setting and in patients with advanced disease. The available evidence suggests that regular exercise is beneficial in patients with fatigue, understanding that patients should not overdo things. Psychostimulants such as methylphenidate, modafinil, and armodafinil have been studied to a relatively marked degree. The bulk of data available support that these drugs are not helpful for attenuating cancer-related fatigue. Alternatively, two placebo-controlled, double-blinded clinical trials have supported that ginseng can decrease fatigue in patients with cancer. Noting this, not all ginseng preparations are the same. Being an herbal product, ginseng preparations are not regulated. The ginseng used in the two positive clinical trials was supplied by the Ginseng Board of Wisconsin; similar ginseng preparations can be obtained from their website. The study dose was 2,000 mg/day, divided into two doses of 1,000 mg each, at breakfast and at lunch.

Suggested Reading

Barton DL, Soori GS, Bauer BA, et al. Pilot study of Panax quinquefolius (American ginseng) to improve cancer-related fatigue: a randomized, double-blind, dose-finding evaluation: NCCTG trial N03CA. *Support Care Cancer*. 2010;18:179-187. PMID: 19415341.

Barton DL, Liu H, Dakhil, SR, et al. Wisconsin Ginseng (Panax quinquefolius) to improve cancer-related fatigue: a randomized, double-blind trial, N07C2. *J Natl Cancer Inst*. 2013;105:1230-1238. Epub 2013 July 13. PMID: 23853057.

20-10 B

Paclitaxel produces a disabling syndrome of subacute aches and pains in a majority of patients, which had been commonly referred to as arthralgias and myalgias. These symptoms generally begin 1 to 3 days after administration and are self-limited, usually resolving within a week. Symptoms have been described in large axial muscular and joint regions and generally are not accompanied by objective musculoskeletal or neurologic examination changes. The symptom location, temporal relationship, and self-limited nature of the syndrome make paclitaxel-induced acute pain syndrome (APS) distinct from paclitaxel-associated peripheral neuropathy.

In the more distant past, the exact characterization of paclitaxel-induced APS had not been well defined. There had been very little known about how exactly patients characterize these symptoms or how these symptoms compare or contrast to symptoms of neuropathy. Given that paclitaxel, administered to rats, causes dorsal root ganglion injury by 24 hours, it was hypothesized that the APS may well be related to nerve pathology, as opposed to muscle and/or joint pathology. To address this topic, 18 patients who noted the presence of subacute aches and pains following paclitaxel participated in structured interviews to characterize their symptoms. Eighty-three percent of the patients (15/18) specifically denied joint or muscle pain. The pain commonly started 1 to 2 days after the paclitaxel infusion, with the median duration of pain being 4 to 5 days. Patients commonly described the discomfort as "aching" or "deep pain" that was "radiating," "stabbing," or "shooting." The pain was usually generalized and located in the back, hips, shoulders, thighs, legs, and feet and, at times, radiated down the legs, arms, or back. It was concluded that the subacute paclitaxel-induced pain appeared to be related to a pathologic process in nerve tissue (e.g., sensitization of nociceptors or nociceptive fibers) as opposed to a musculoskeletal injury. Although this hypothesis has not yet been confirmed by neurologic testing in humans, new supporting data has revealed that the degree of APS pain after the first dose of paclitaxel, in individual patients, positively correlates with the degree of more classic peripheral neuropathy 12 to 18 weeks later. Opioid medications are helpful for the treatment of this problem.

Suggested Reading

Loprinzi CL, Maddocks-Christianson K, Wolf SL, et al. The Paclitaxel acute pain syndrome: sensitization of nociceptors as the putative mechanism. *Cancer J*. 2007;13:399-403. PMID: 18032978.

Loprinzi CL, Reeves BN, Dakhil SR, et al. Natural history of paclitaxel-associated acute pain syndrome: prospective cohort study NCCTG N08C1. *J Clin Oncol*. 2011;29:1472-1478. PMID: 21383290.

Reeves BN, Dakhil SH, Sloan JA, et al. Further data supporting that the paclitaxel-associated acute pain syndrome is associated with the development of peripheral neuropathy: NCCTG Trial N08C1. *Cancer*. 2012;118:5171-5178. PMID: 22415454.

21 PALLIATIVE AND END-OF-LIFE CARE
SELF-EVALUATION

PALLIATIVE AND END-OF-LIFE CARE QUESTIONS

22-1 A 62-year-old man is being treated with gemcitabine for metastatic pancreatic adenocarcinoma. He receives close support from several family members, including his wife and three adult children. At least two caregivers accompany the patient to every office appointment, chemotherapy infusion, and lab draw. The family members always keep a list of questions to ask during each visit, routinely report updates between office visits to your clinical team, and keep a daily log of his body temperature and drug side effects to review with you.

Which one of the following statements is most correct?
A. Patients with higher levels of depression often have family members with lower levels of depression, signaling that caregivers tend to be immune to the emotional state of their loved ones
B. Only a small percentage of adults are caregivers for family members with serious illness
C. Depressive symptoms of caregivers can be reduced by clinicians demonstrating that their input has value and that their feelings and concerns are being heard
D. Close caregiver involvement often results in more frequent readmissions to the hospital

22-2 A 72-year-old man with metastatic adenocarcinoma of the lung is currently being treated with single-agent docetaxel in the second-line setting. His distant sites of disease include a 3-cm right hepatic lobe lesion and several areas of bone metastases in his axial spine. His Eastern Cooperative Oncology Group (ECOG) performance status is 2. On a routine visit between chemotherapy cycles, his family notes that the patient continues to lose weight, most recently 15 lbs during the last month. He denies any nausea or changes in bowel frequency. Examination demonstrates normal bowel sounds. The patient's family asks you about supplementing his nutrition to address the unintentional weight loss.

Which one of the following statements is most correct?
A. Artificial nutrition and hydration generally improves patient quality of life
B. Patients near the end of life often experience hunger or thirst
C. Feeding is an emotionally charged issue for loved ones and caregivers, which requires close support and education by oncology professionals
D. As patients progress towards death, less interest in food requires some form of medical intervention

22-3 A 76-year-old man recently experienced disease progression on single-agent docetaxel plus prednisone for hormone-refractory prostate cancer. He is a nonsmoker with no personal or family history of cardiac disease. He complains of sharp pain in his lower back related to known bone metastases. He has lost 15 lbs during the last 3 weeks. He has no appetite, only taking a few small bites a few times per day. He also complains of dyspnea, noting that this has gotten worse as his overall energy level has dropped. He spends more than 75% of his day in bed. In the office, his resting oxygen saturation is 95%. With exertion it reduces to 93%.

Which one of the following statements is true about the treatment of dyspnea?
- A. Benzodiazepines are the pharmacologic mainstay of dyspnea treatment
- B. Evidence suggests that supplemental oxygen through nasal cannula should be given to all patients with dyspnea in the end-of-life setting
- C. Respiratory depression and resultant worsening of hypoxemia are not a major concern when using opioids for dyspnea treatment
- D. Dyspnea is a subjective symptom that requires documentation of tachypnea or hypoxemia before opioids are prescribed

22-4 A 22-year-old woman with metastatic HER2 non-overexpressed, hormone receptor–negative breast cancer is beginning second-line chemotherapy. She experienced progression after only 3 months of stable disease after completing first-line therapy. Now her functional status has remarkably changed, from an ECOG 0 to an ECOG 2. She spends most of your office visits discussing logistics and side effects of chemotherapy, occasionally mentioning that she is "fighting so I can watch my 5-year-old graduate high school."

Which of the following statements is true regarding patient-centered communication?
- A. Difficult conversations about limitations of therapy and poor prognosis are a must in this clinical situation, even if the patient does not want to discuss it
- B. Patients can often clearly articulate the intentions of cancer-directed therapy, obviating the need to check in with the patient occasionally about her understanding
- C. Discussing your assessment of her prognosis, in the terms she would like, will take away her hope
- D. Assessing the patient's and caregiver's understanding of the illness, the meaning of its severity, and perceptions of potential outcomes are important steps in conducting a difficult conversation

22-5 A 47-year-old woman with platinum-resistant recurrent ovarian cancer has significant abdominal pain. She is having regular bowel movements. She is on a regimen of long-acting opioids only, taken twice daily without any complementary breakthrough medications. You notice this, and decide to add a short-acting breakthrough opioid for incident pain that occurs a few times per day. She is currently on a fentanyl transdermal patch at 37 μg per hour, tolerating it well.

Which of the following is the most appropriate breakthrough pain regimen?
- A. Oxycodone/acetaminophen (5 mg/500 mg), one tablet every 1 to 2 hours as needed
- B. Transmucosal fentanyl (400 μg) every 1 to 2 hours as needed
- C. Hydromorphone (2 mg) every 1 to 2 hours as needed
- D. Immediate-release morphine sulfate (15 mg) every 1 to 2 hours as needed

22-6 A 66-year-old woman receives a new diagnosis of metastatic squamous cell lung cancer. She establishes oncology care with a large multispecialty physician practice, which includes palliative care specialists. Her treatment plan includes carboplatin and paclitaxel, which is scheduled to begin next week.

Which of the following statements is true about palliative care?
- A. Palliative care, either provided by the oncologist or through a specialty consult, should be reserved for the end-of-life setting when a patient is no longer receiving antineoplastic therapy
- B. One randomized controlled trial demonstrated a survival advantage of more than 2 months with the incorporation of palliative care to usual oncology care
- C. Adding a palliative care physician to the patient's care team should only occur after the oncologist has signed off, since the opposing goals of each discipline can seem confusing to a patient
- D. The focus of palliative care is on the patient only; referrals are always made to other team members such as social workers or counselors to address the needs of caregivers

22-1   C

Increasing attention is being given to the role of caregivers in supporting positive outcomes for patients with cancer. Caregivers often are the "front-line" members of the oncology team, reporting back to clinical professionals on issues of symptoms, performance status, and goals of care. Significant evidence demonstrates that caregivers suffer from the effects of poor emotional states of their loved ones. This is observed as higher levels of depression among caregivers of patients who also exhibit depressive symptoms.

Oncology teams will need to further incorporate the needs and distress of caregivers into the comprehensive cancer care plan as the number of caregivers grows and their influence on patient outcomes becomes better understood. For example, higher intensity and frequency of caregiving practices are associated with lower hospital readmissions. Because of this, oncology teams are increasingly realizing that support of caregivers is an effective way to reduce unnecessary health care utilization while supporting patient-centered cancer care. This support of caregivers at its most basic level involves listening to caregivers, soliciting input and suggestions, and frequently reminding caregivers that their efforts are appreciated and valued.

Suggested Reading

Rabow MW, Hauser JM, Adams J. Supporting family caregivers at the end of life: "they don't know what they don't know". *JAMA*. 2004;291:483-491. PMID: 14747506.

Dumont S, Turgeon J, Allard P, et al. Caring for a loved one with advanced cancer: determinants of psychological distress in family caregivers. *J Palliat Med*. 2006;9:912-921. PMID: 16910806.

Rivera HR. Depression symptoms in cancer caregivers. *Clin J Oncol Nurs*. 2009;13:195-202. PMID: 19349266.

22-2   C

Artificial nutrition and hydration is an issue often brought up by concerned patients and family members when loss of weight, energy, and functional status occur in the advanced cancer setting. These concerns are not unfounded, since feeding is often considered an important caregiving duty by loved ones and patients often are disturbed by weight loss associated with progressive disease. Further, the act of sharing a meal is considered a ubiquitous activity in many cultures; loved ones eat together in times of joy (e.g., weddings, holiday parties) and in times of sadness (e.g., funerals). This makes any discussions of not pursuing artificial means to supplement a patient's own drive and desire for eating potentially distressful.

Patients and families often need open and direct education regarding the potential risks and outcomes related to artificial nutrition and hydration. Clinicians should reassure patients and families that loss of appetite, generally without an increase in a sense of hunger, is a normal part of the disease process. As no study has conclusively demonstrated that any intervention can improve quality of life or survival, caregivers should be counseled on the gap between the lack of efficacy from such interventions and the common side effects from gastric tubes and other feeding devices. Further, although most patients do not experience an escalation of hunger or thirst near the end of life, dry mouth is common, necessitating good oral care.

Just as patients and caregivers are transitioning thinking from quantity of life to quality of life, this analogy can often be translated to eating, where the quality of foods eaten (i.e., "What do I want to eat?") should outweigh the quantity (i.e., "How much did I eat?").

Suggested Reading

Mercadante S, Ferrera P, Girelli D, et al. Patients' and relatives' perceptions about intravenous and subcutaneous hydration. *J Pain Symptom Manage*. 2005;30:354-358. PMID: 16256899.

Ersek M. Artificial nutrition and hydration: clinical issues. *J Hosp Palliat Nurs*. 2003;5:221-230.

Casarett D, Kapo J, Caplan A. Appropriate use of artificial nutrition and hydration–fundamental principles and recommendations. *N Engl J Med*. 2005;353:2607-2612. PMID: 16354899.

22-3   C

Dyspnea is a highly subjective symptom that does not require corroboration of anatomic or physiologic abnormalities, such as low oxygen saturations or abnormal chest imaging. It is a common symptom in patients with advanced cancer, independent of whether progressive disease has affected the lung parenchyma, resulted in a pleural effusion, or affected the cardiorespiratory circuit.

In the end-of-life setting, opioids (either oral or parenteral) are the most frequently used interventions for dyspnea. Morphine remains the mainstay, and is generally well tolerated when used for this purpose. Morphine has been found neither to depress the respiratory rate nor to result in severe sedation or obtundation. It is a well-accepted intervention for treating patient-reported dyspnea near the end of life and a common component of the hospice toolbox for symptom control.

Palliative oxygen is also often prescribed to relieve refractory dyspnea in patients with cancer. Although it is indicated for severely hypoxemic patients, it does not confer greater benefit than does air for mildly hypoxemic or nonhypoxemic patients. Additionally, the burden of oxygen therapy, which includes cost, tubing, confinement to a concentrator, and exaggeration of the "sick role," may outweigh its advantages.

Suggested Reading

Ben-Aharon I, Gafter-Gvili A, Paul M, et al. Interventions for alleviating cancer-related dyspnea: a systematic review. *J Clin Oncol.* 2008;26:2396-2404. PMID: 18467732.

Currow DC, Abernethy AP, Frith PA. Morphine for management of refractory dyspnoea: authors' reply. *BMJ.* 2003;327: 1288-1289. PMID: 14644985.

Abernethy AP, McDonald CF, Frith PA, et al. Effect of palliative oxygen versus room air in relief of breathlessness in patients with refractory dyspnoea: a double-blind, randomised controlled trial. *Lancet.* 2010;376:784-793. PMID: 20816546.

22-4   D

Effective, clear communication between clinicians and patients starts with first asking permission to have the conversation. Then, it involves clearly assessing and addressing any issues in the patient's perceptions of their illness and ensuring that their understanding aligns with that of the medical team. This requires frequently checking in regarding their knowledge of the facts ("I have stage IV cancer"), the meaning of those facts ("Stage IV means this is not a curable cancer"), and the plan for their care ("I am receiving chemotherapy to help me live a bit longer").

A common misconception is that direct and open conversations with patients about bad news may take away their "hope" or "fight." In fact, these conversations, performed in a timely way and prior to a medical crisis, can reduce unwanted, unnecessary, and overly aggressive end-of-life care that often impedes meeting the patient's goals of care. These goals may include dying at home or spending the last chapters of life next to family and friends instead of in the hospital. Recent studies also demonstrate that patients may be overly optimistic in their estimations of life expectancy and achievable outcomes from chemotherapy in metastatic disease settings. Checking in frequently with patients to both clarify misperceptions and build rapport by demonstrating a concerted interest in how care is aligning with their goals is important in these settings.

Suggested Reading

Glare P, Virik K, Jones M, et al. A systematic review of physicians' survival predictions in terminally ill cancer patients. *BMJ.* 2003;327:195-198. PMID: 12881260.

Lamont EB, Christakis NA. Prognostic disclosure to patients with cancer near the end of life. *Ann Intern Med.* 2001;134: 1096-1105. PMID: 11412049.

Anselm AH, Palda V, Guest CB, et al. Barriers to communication regarding end-of-life care: perspectives of care providers. *J Crit Care.* 2005;20:214-223. PMID: 16253789.

22-5 D

It is the standard of care to provide all patients with short-acting breakthrough opioids to complement long-acting sustained-release products (e.g., sustained-release morphine). When opioids are prescribed, the breakthrough dose is usually 10% to 20% of the total daily around-the-clock sustained-release dose; the exceptions to this calculation are short-acting fentanyl products, for which the short-acting dose is typically the lowest dose in which the product is available (e.g., 200 µg of transmucosal fentanyl). For the patient described, the current 37-µg transdermal fentanyl dose is equivalent to approximately 100 mg of oral morphine per day. A standard breakthrough dose, being at 10% to 20% of this total opioid dose per day, would best be achieved through 15 mg of immediate-release morphine. Data support that oral "as needed" short-acting analgesics can be given at hourly intervals, if pain is not relieved and the patient is not drowsy. This is because the maximal effect should be apparent by 1 hour.

Oxycodone/acetaminophen at a 5-mg/500-mg dose, one tablet every 4 hours as needed, is only equivalent to approximately 7.5 mg of oral morphine, which is insufficient to provide adequate analgesia for breakthrough pain. A 400-µg dose of transmucosal fentanyl available every 4 hours as needed is too high a starting dose; this medication should be titrated upward from a starting dose of 200 µg. Hydromorphone at 2 mg is also an insufficient dose, since it is equivalent to only approximately 7.5 mg of oral morphine.

Suggested Reading

Zeppetella G. Opioids for the management of breakthrough cancer pain in adults: a systematic review undertaken as part of an EPCRC opioid guidelines project. *Palliat Med.* 2011;25:516-524. PMID: 21708858.

Davies AN. The management of breakthrough cancer pain. *Br J Nurs.* 2011;20:803-804, 806-807.

Dickman A. Integrated strategies for the successful management of breakthrough cancer pain. *Curr Opin Support Palliat Care.* 2011;5:8-14. PMID: 21325998.

Ryan M, Moynihan TJ, Loprinzi CL. As-needed morphine: yes, but at what dose and at what interval? *J Clin Oncol.* 2005;23:3849-3852. PMID: 15923580.

22-6 B

Palliative care is an approach that emphasizes quality of life across several domains, including symptom management and psychosocial distress, considering both the patient and their caregivers as the unit of care. Oncologists, who support the palliative care needs of patients through frequent assessment and timely management of symptoms, provide support to caregivers and family members, and assist with advanced care planning, most often deliver this type of care. Sometimes specialty palliative care services are needed to address highly complex or unique issues, such as pain refractory to usual oral opioids or complex family dynamics (frequent conflict, etc.).

Since the landmark clinical trial demonstrating a survival advantage with palliative care added to usual oncology care, there has been an increased emphasis on incorporating palliative care concurrent with treatment-focused care. For most patients, this involves attention to both aspects of care, either concurrently with the oncology team and palliative care team, or with both services provided by oncology professionals. Palliative care is considered an essential component of comprehensive cancer care, which should begin from the moment of diagnosis and extend all the way through either survivorship care or support of the bereaved after a patient's death.

Suggested Reading

Smith TJ, Temin S, Alesi ER, et al. American Society of Clinical Oncology provisional clinical opinion: the integration of palliative care into standard oncology care. *J Clin Oncol.* 2012;30:880-887. PMID: 22312101.

Temel JS, Greer JA, Muzikansky A, et al. Early palliative care for patients with metastatic non-small-cell lung cancer. *N Engl J Med.* 2010;363:733-742. PMID: 20818875.

INDEX

Note: Page numbers followed by f and t indicate figures and tables, respectively.

COMMONLY USED ABBREVIATIONS

The following abbreviations are commonly used throughout *ASCO-SEP®*. See specific chapters for expansions of abbreviated drug names, trial names, and infrequently used acronyms.

ACRIN: American College of Radiology Imaging Network
ACS: American Cancer Society
AIDS: acquired immune deficiency syndrome
AJCC: American Joint Committee on Cancer
ASCO: American Society of Clinical Oncology
ASTRO: American Society for Radiation Oncology
AUC: area under the curve
BMI: body mass index
CALGB: Cancer and Leukemia Group B
CDC: U.S. Centers for Disease Control and Prevention
CI: confidence interval
COG: Children's Oncology Group
CT: computed tomography
DFS: disease-free survival
ECOG: Eastern Cooperative Oncology Group
EORTC: European Organisation for Research and Treatment of Cancer
FDA: U.S. Food and Drug Administration
FDG: fluorodeoxyglucose
HIV: human immunodeficiency virus
HPV: human papillomavirus
HR: hazard ratio
MCQ: multiple-choice question
MRI: magnetic resonance imaging
NCCN: National Comprehensive Cancer Network
NCCTG: North Central Cancer Treatment Group
NCI: U.S. National Cancer Institute
NCIC: National Cancer Institute of Canada
NSABP: National Surgical Adjuvant Breast and Bowel Project
OR: odds ratio
OS: overall survival
PCR: polymerase chain reaction
PET: positron emission tomography
PFS: progression-free survival
RFS: recurrence-free survival
RTOG: Radiation Therapy Oncology Group
SWOG: Southwest Oncology Group
TNM: tumor/node/metastasis
UICC: Union for International Cancer Control
USPSTF: U.S. Preventive Services Task Force